Psychological Assessment and Testing

Expanding upon and updating the first edition, this comprehensive guide instructs readers on how to effectively conduct psychological assessment and testing in their practice, efficiently advancing a case from the initial referral and clinical interview, through the testing process, and leading to informed diagnosis and treatment recommendations. This second edition incorporates updated editions of all major tests, pertinent revisions from the DSM–5, more in-depth analysis of testing topics, and coverage of new constructs that are the targets of psychological testing relevant to outpatient mental health practice. Readers will learn about the fundamentals of assessment, testing, and psychological measurement, the complete process of psychological testing using a broad range of major tests, supplemented by interpretive flowcharts and case examples. Downloadable practice and report forms, along with data tables with pre-drafted interpretive excerpts for all tests are also available for immediate use in clinical practice.

Psychologists in both practice and training will come away with the tools and knowledge needed to successfully conduct psychological assessment and testing within the contemporary mental health field.

John M. Spores, Ph.D., J.D., is a professor of psychology at Purdue University Northwest, USA. He is also a licensed psychologist and attorney-at-law in the state of Indiana.

Psychological Assessment and Testing
A Clinician's Guide

Second Edition

John M. Spores

Routledge
Taylor & Francis Group

NEW YORK AND LONDON

Second edition published 2022
by Routledge
605 Third Avenue, New York, NY 10158

and by Routledge
2 Park Square, Milton Park, Abingdon, Oxon, OX14 4RN

Routledge is an imprint of the Taylor & Francis Group, an informa business

© 2022 Taylor & Francis

First edition published by Springer Publishing Company 2013

Library of Congress Cataloging-in-Publication Data
Names: Spores, John M., author.
Title: Psychological assessment and testing : a clinician's guide / John M. Spores.
Description: Second edition. | New York, NY : Routledge, 2022. | Includes bibliographical references and index.
Identifiers: LCCN 2021058214 (print) | LCCN 2021058215 (ebook) | ISBN 9780367346041 (hardback) |
    ISBN 9780367346058 (paperback) | ISBN 9780429326820 (ebook)
Subjects: LCSH: Psychological tests. | Mental illness—Diagnosis. | Psychiatric rating scales.
Classification: LCC RC473.P79 S66 2022 (print) | LCC RC473.P79 (ebook) | DDC 616.8/0475—dc23/eng/20211228
LC record available at https://lccn.loc.gov/2021058214
LC ebook record available at https://lccn.loc.gov/2021058215

ISBN: 978-0-367-34604-1 (hbk)
ISBN: 978-0-367-34605-8 (pbk)
ISBN: 978-0-429-32682-0 (ebk)

DOI: 10.4324/9780429326820

Typeset in Bembo
by Apex CoVantage, LLC

Access the Support Material: www.routledge.com/9780367346058

To Billie.

Contents

Preface

The objective of this book is to teach both the theory and practice of psychological assessment and testing in mental health. To facilitate the latter component, this book provides a generous quantity of modifiable electronic word processing files of all the practice forms, report forms, and test data tables presented throughout Parts I and II. The intended audience includes those who wish to learn and practice psychological assessment and testing in the mental health field, most especially those majoring in psychology at the advanced undergraduate and graduate levels of training, along with those who are already fully credentialed. It is also intended for mental health therapists who do not engage in testing themselves, but who desire such knowledge in order to be well informed when referring their clients for assessment and testing services. Specifically, the materials in this book instruct readers how to conduct assessments such that a proper targeted test battery is ordered, how to ask for and obtain insurance preauthorization for the appropriate quantity of testing units (i.e., time), how to schedule appointments, and finally, how to effectively score, report, interpret, integrate, and summarize the test results in addressing the diagnostic questions and issues raised. Useful prior courses include basic statistics and research methods, and perhaps an additional course in psychological measurement.

The book begins with an introduction chapter that provides an overview of the organization and structure of the ensuing material. Thereafter, the book is apportioned into two large parts. Part I consists of Chapters 2 through 4, which together cover the psychological assessment and testing process from start to finish, including a visual flowchart outlining five specific steps that constitute the entire sequence, along with practice and report forms needed to move the case along to termination. New to this edition are four initial assessment forms designed for early childhood, middle and late childhood, adolescence, and adulthood, rather than the dichotomous childhood and adulthood forms presented in the first edition. These four initial assessment report forms are reviewed in detail throughout Part I, along with several supplemental report forms that assist in transforming the original into a final psychological assessment report with incorporated test data forms presented throughout Part II.

Part II contains the core subject matter, which is comprised of Chapters 5 through 13. Together, these chapters present all of the tests that comprise this book's inventory, including clear definitions of the constructs measured, historical background (where applicable), reasons for inclusion within a test battery, development of the instrument, test organization and structure, norm reference samples, administration, scoring, reporting of the data, and interpretation of the data yield. Each instrument comes with detailed test data tables designed to be incorporated into the final psychological assessment report, including pre-drafted interpretive excerpts following each of the data tables to facilitate and guide the effective integration and summary of the results. In addition, interpretive flowcharts for either single tests, or a series of similar tests, are available for download on Routledge's e-resources website. They are each reviewed in the book so that test reporting, interpretation, integration, and summarization can proceed efficiently and precisely, and ultimately contribute to accurate psychodiagnostic conclusions and treatment recommendations.

Also new to this edition in Part II are chapters covering screening tests, developmental (i.e., infant) tests, projective tests that are empirically scored, and malingering tests. The latest editions of each test and/or their scoring systems are also included, at least as of the date this book manuscript was submitted for publication on or about November 1, 2021. This includes the MMPI–3 for ages 18 years through adulthood, which published in the fall of 2020. The reader will note that occasionally when a particular test has very recently been published into its newest edition, both it and the immediate predecessor is also included in this book. This is based upon the assumption that the majority of clinicians may continue to use, or be trained upon, the prior test, this being due to such factors as greater familiarity with the previous test, the current relatively sparse independent supporting data for the newest edition, and/or because a financial investment has been made in the prior edition and the user would prefer to obtain more use of the test before moving to the next edition. For example, the MMPI–2–RF is also included in the book as a companion to the newest MMPI–3. It is also instructive to observe how tests are modified into updated editions.

Finally, a number of enhancements are available on Routledge's e-resources website to supplement the book. They consist of (a) test interpretive flowcharts, (b) case examples, and (c) electronic forms for actual testing practice. The interpretive flowcharts provide a visual guide that presents a clear, logical, and efficient strategy for reporting test scores and evincing meaning from the data yield for each major test or test series. Regarding case studies, there are four in total, one selected for each major developmental period. For each case, a complete initial and final psychological assessment report is provided such that readers have concrete examples of how the system presented in this book is intended to work. Finally, the electronic forms are apportioned into three classes as follows: (a) practice forms ($n = 10$), (b) report forms ($n = 9$), and (c) test data tables ($n = 91$). The practice forms assist in moving a case from its initial referral to termination (e.g., Referral for Psychological Testing; Consent for Psychological Testing Services). The report forms provide an initial report outline for each major developmental period, along with supplemental forms that help transform the initial into a final report (e.g., Initial Psychological Assessment-Report Adulthood Form; Assessment and Test Battery List-Adolescence). Lastly, the test data tables are modifiable electronic versions of the forms presented throughout Part II, which are designed to efficiently report test scores within a final psychological assessment report, including excerpts that guide interpretation of the data (e.g., NEPSY–II Full Battery for Ages 5–16; MCMI–IV for Ages 18–85). Referral sources very much appreciate psychological testing reports that efficiently incorporate the actual empirical data that contributed to the psychologist's conclusions. These test data tables accomplish this objective. The author is confident that this book, along with its generous quantity of forms, will contribute to the effective learning and practice of psychological assessment and testing in the mental health field.

About the Author

John M. Spores is a professor of psychology at Purdue University Northwest (PNW) located in northwest Indiana. He is also a practicing clinical psychologist (Indiana Psychologist License #20040638A) and a licensed attorney (Indiana Bar #21404–64, Inactive Status, In Good Standing). In 1990, he received a Ph.D. in clinical psychology, including a minor in developmental psychology, from Purdue University at West Lafayette, Indiana. He subsequently earned a J.D. degree from Valparaiso University School of Law, also in Indiana, which was conferred in 1998. He teaches a wide range of courses, including introductory and advanced statistics for psychology, research methods in psychology, personality psychology, forensic psychology, abnormal psychology, and psychotherapy. In practice, he specializes in psychological assessment and testing. Professor Spores lives with his loving family, including his wife, Billie Ladas Spores, M.A., V.R.C., his son, Andrew John Spores, who is matriculating at Butler University in Indianapolis, majoring in computer science, his daughter, Demetra Spores, who is matriculating at Loyola University in Chicago, majoring in forensic science, and his dogs, Max (who passed), Moe, and Macy Spores. He and his family members are active in the Greek Eastern Orthodox Christian religion.

Acknowledgments

First, I wish to recognize my son Andrew J. Spores, who assisted in the computerized design of several flowcharts and figures incorporated into this title. Second, I wish to acknowledge my daughter Demetra Spores, whose consultation regarding the organization and structure of this book was invaluable, including the case studies that are available on Routledge's e-resources website. Third, I wish to thank my wife Billie Spores for her assistance in proofreading for grammar and sentence structure, and making needed modifications in the Glossary, Name Index, and Subject Index parts of the book. I was blessed with a very caring, supportive, and patient family, who exhibited continuing forbearance throughout the writing of this book.

Finally, I wish to acknowledge both Sarah Gore, Editor, and Priya Sharma, Editorial Assistant, of Routledge Taylor & Francis Group, for their invaluable support and guidance in the final draft and organization of this book, including both the print and e-resources parts. The original manuscript was extremely lengthy and complex, and the final published work benefitted immensely from their advisement and ongoing feedback.

1 Introduction

Overview

This chapter has two goals. First, it introduces the principal objective of this book and its related tasks. Second, it provides an overview of the book's general organization, which is specifically designed to meet the aforementioned objective.

Principal Objective

At its most fundamental level, this book is written to instruct readers how to effectively practice *psychological assessment* and *psychological testing* in the contemporary field of mental health. In order to accomplish this goal, a number of tasks are explicated throughout the book such that they are learned and eventually mastered. These tasks are as follows. First, a preliminary listing of the diagnostic questions and issues of a case that has been referred for testing must be obtained. Second, an initial clinical interview must be conducted in order to further refine the diagnostic questions, identify whether further testing is needed or required, and if the answer is in the affirmative, to select a targeted test battery that will efficiently, yet completely, address the enumerated issues. This may require the utilization of screening tests in order to address some or all of the presenting assessment issues, or alternatively, to bolster the request for follow-up testing. In instances where the initial clinical assessment is sufficient, a report needs to be proximately generated with diagnoses and recommendations so that intervention can be initiated in an efficient and timely manner.

On the other hand, if further assessment is deemed necessary, a targeted test battery must be judiciously selected, along with the proper psychological services billing codes and number of units needed (i.e., time). Third, *preauthorization (PA)* for the requested services and units must be obtained from insurance carriers, with a preparedness and strategy for appeal should some or all testing units be denied. Fourth, test administration appointments must be scheduled and completed within a coherent order and a reasonable time frame. Fifth, the garnered test scores must be incorporated into a formal report such that the results are presented within an organized, clear, and logical sequence of data integration, and use of an interpretive strategy in search of converging evidence, which culminates in a final diagnostic summary that serves as an impetus for treatment planning. Finally, effective communication of the results must be accomplished, with the ability to realize when supplementary testing is needed in order to address any enduring unresolved issues.

There are several major themes that run through the entire book as does a motif within an artistic or literary composition. First, the concept of efficiency is emphasized at each stage of the assessment and testing process. Second, clarity is another idea that is applied to all of the aforesaid tasks. This is especially applicable to the many psychological constructs that are measured by the tests incorporated into this book's inventory. Briefly, a *construct* is an abstract idea used to organize, interpret, and explain observed facts (e.g., intelligence, personality). Third, although psychological assessment and testing are both thoroughly defined and described, this is foremost a pragmatic and practice-oriented book. Therefore, the subject matter is teeming with practice forms that inform precisely how to negotiate each step in the assessment process, along with data tables designed for each test that can be inserted into formal psychological reports. The latter are designed to present each test's data yield within a readily comprehensible and organized framework, with diligently defined constructs, and narrative excerpts that assist in guiding the interpretation and report generation process.

After readers have scrutinized and mastered this book's subject matter and supporting materials, and assuming proper supervised training, they will be fully capable and confident in practicing psychological assessment and testing in the mental health field. Furthermore, a wealth of supplementary materials is available on the Routledge e-resource website (see subsequently). Of note, this book incorporates a prudently selected inventory of tests that together have

DOI: 10.4324/9780429326820-1

proven capable of resolving innumerable assessment dilemmas most frequently encountered in contemporary mental health. However, the knowledge gained by reading this book and utilizing it in practice will readily generalize to other psychological tests and assessment cases. Next, the general organization of the book is presented, which is intended to inform readers as to how the prior stated objective and its related tasks shall be accomplished.

Organization of the Book

The book begins with this introduction, followed by two broad parts and their more narrowly defined conceptually related topics in the form of chapters (see Figure 1.1).

The latter represent the core subject matter of the book. The final grouping of items is comprised of supplementary materials that have been uploaded to the e-resource portion located on the Routledge website, which are designed to facilitate actual clinical practice, hence being consistent with the book's pragmatic emphasis. Each is described in more detail subsequently.

Part I: The Psychological Assessment and Testing Process: Practice Forms and Report Forms

Part I delineates a five-stage sequence of psychological assessment and testing, which begins at the point of accepting a testing referral and proceeding through to case termination. To help explain the sequence, an analogy is made to the process of scientific investigation, which begins with an important question that is in need of an answer, and ends with publication of the results. In Figure 1.1, Chapter 2 begins the part with a succinct overview of the process, which consists of five interrelated stages. Here, the objective is to provide a scheme or mental map of how these stages are integrated into a coherent whole. Two complementary flowcharts afford a visual framework of the sequence. The first highlights the specific tasks to be accomplished, while the second enumerates the associated practice forms to be employed at each stage. These forms have been diligently designed and continually modified over the course of several thousand cases, hence helping to ensure that they indeed facilitate actual clinical practice. Of course, they may be readily modified to suit a practitioner's varying needs and types of cases. Lastly, Chapter 2 serves as a prelude to Chapters 3 and 4, which together comprise Part I and describe this five-stage sequence in significantly greater detail.

Chapter 3 proceeds from the initial referral through drafting an "Initial Psychological Assessment Report" by means of a *semi-structured clinical interview*, along with selecting a targeted test battery, the proper type of testing services and units of time, submitting any rating forms to examinees and collaterals, and scheduling the psychological test administration appointments; that is, proceeding through the first three stages (see Figure 1.1). At this juncture, there is a natural pause in the assessment and testing process. Therefore, it is logical to conclude Chapter 3 at this point and subsequently transition quite readily into Chapter 4, which continues the sequence with test administration and scoring services, along with the efficient and efficacious strategy of simultaneous test interpretation and report generation (i.e., test evaluation services).

The discussion then focuses on how the initial report evolves into a "Final Psychological Assessment Report." Although this concerns the manner in which some of the previous initial report sections are modified, the major

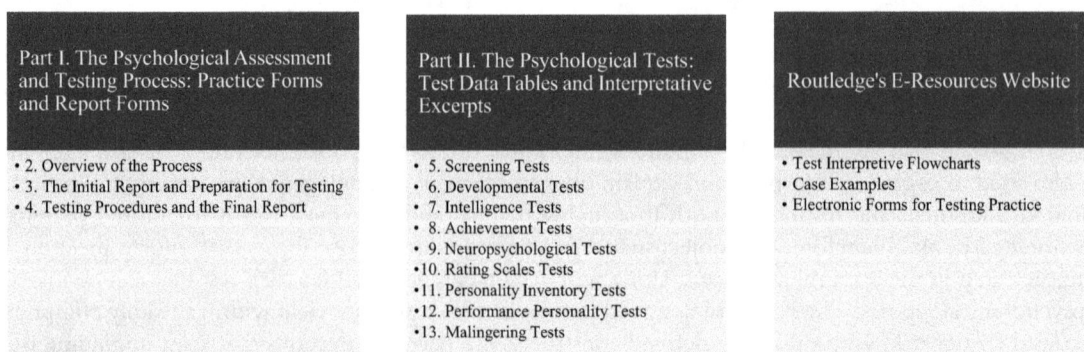

Part I. The Psychological Assessment and Testing Process: Practice Forms and Report Forms

• 2. Overview of the Process
• 3. The Initial Report and Preparation for Testing
• 4. Testing Procedures and the Final Report

Part II. The Psychological Tests: Test Data Tables and Interpretative Excerpts

• 5. Screening Tests
• 6. Developmental Tests
• 7. Intelligence Tests
• 8. Achievement Tests
• 9. Neuropsychological Tests
• 10. Rating Scales Tests
• 11. Personality Inventory Tests
• 12. Performance Personality Tests
• 13. Malingering Tests

Routledge's E-Resources Website

• Test Interpretive Flowcharts
• Case Examples
• Electronic Forms for Testing Practice

Figure 1.1 Visual Organization of Parts I and II of the Print Version of the Book, Along with the Supplementary E-Resources

Note. Chapter 1 is an introductory chapter that summarizes the objective and organization of the book. Arabic numbers represent a continuous sequence of chapters within their respective major sections. E-resources consist of supplemental materials uploaded onto the Routledge website, which include all practice forms, report forms, and test data tables presented throughout the book, here in modifiable Microsoft Word format, hence, rendering them ideal for continued use in actual clinical practice.

focus is on the incorporation of several new sections and information therein, including test data tables, interpretive excerpts, an integrative summary of results, a final diagnostic summary, addressing any leftover unresolved referral questions, and inserting logically related treatment recommendations. This chapter ends with a discussion regarding communication of the results, which focuses most especially on the final written report and further supplemented by optional oral feedback. After completing Part I, readers will have assimilated a clear and coherent understanding of the manner in which psychological assessment and testing proceeds within the mental health field, both characteristically and with occasional modifications encountered due to special case circumstances and referral requests.

Part II: The Psychological Tests: Test Data Tables and Interpretation

Part II provides a meticulous presentation of each test selected for inclusion within this book. Table 1.1 succinctly lists these tests, which are categorized according to a combination of format and/or measured construct. This scheme also serves as a conceptual organization for the whole of Part II. Because Table 1.1 serves as convenient outline for this core part, the information contained therein shall be introduced next.

The following information is enumerated in Table 1.1 in said order: (a) chapter numbers; (b) chapter titles that reveal the genre of tests contained therein according to format and/or construct measured; (c) titles of each test that comprise

Table 1.1 Part II: List of Tests

Chapter Number and Category of Tests	Title	Age Range*
9. Screening Tests	Conners Early Childhood, Behavior, Short Version, Parent Form	2:0–6:11
	Conners 3rd Edition, ADHD Index Version, Parent Form	6:0–18:11
	Conners' Adult ADHD Rating Scales, Screening Version, Self-Report Form	18:0–80:11
	Wechsler Memory Scale, Fourth Edition, Brief Cognitive Status Exam	16:0–90:11
	Mini-Mental State Examination, Second Edition	18:0+
	Clinical Assessment of Behavior, Parent Form	2:0–18:11
	Personality Assessment Screener	18:0+
	Sentence Completion Test–Child	7:0–12:11
	Sentence Completion Test–Adolescent	13:0–18:11
	Kinetic Drawing System for Family and School	5:0–20:11
10. Developmental Tests	Bayley Scales of Infant and Toddler Development, Third Edition and Fourth Edition	0:1–3:6
	Adaptive Behavior Assessment System, Third Edition	0:1–89:0
	Vineland Adaptive Behavior Scales, Third Edition	0:1–90:11+
	Autism Diagnostic Observation Schedule, Second Edition	1:0+–40:11+
11. Intelligence Tests	Stanford–Binet Intelligence Scales, Fifth Edition	2:0–85:11
	Wechsler Preschool and Primary Scale of Intelligence, Fourth Edition	2:6–7:7
	Wechsler Intelligence Scale for Children, Fifth Edition	6:0–16:11
	Wechsler Adult Intelligence Scale, Fourth Edition	16:0–90:11
12. Achievement Tests	Wechsler Individual Achievement Test, Third Edition and Fourth Edition	4:0–50:11
	Woodcock–Johnson IV Tests of Achievement	2:0–90:11+
13. Neuropsychological Tests	NEPSY–II	3:0–16:11
	Neuropsychological Assessment Battery	18:0–97:11
	Wechsler Memory Scale, Fourth Edition	16:0–90:11
	Conners Kiddie Continuous Performance Test, Second Edition	4:0–7:11
	Conners Continuous Performance Test, Third Edition	8:0–89:11+
	Conners Continuous Auditory Test of Attention	8:0–83:11+
14. Rating Scales Type Tests	Conners Early Childhood	2:0–6:11
	Conners Comprehensive Behavior Rating Scales	6:0–18:11
	Conners' Adult ADHD Rating Scales, Long Version	18:0–50:0+
	Gilliam Autism Rating Scale, Third Edition	3:0–22:11
	Gilliam Asperger's Disorder Scale	3:0–22:11
	Sensory Processing Measure–Preschool	2:0–5:11
	Sensory Processing Measure	5:0–12:11
	Trauma Symptom Checklist for Young Children	3:0–12:11
	Trauma Symptom Checklist for Children	8:0–16:11
	Trauma Symptom Inventory, Second Edition	18:0–90:11

(Continued)

Table 1.1 (Continued)

Chapter Number and Category of Tests	Title	Age Range*
15. Personality Inventory Tests	Millon Pre-Adolescent Clinical Inventory	9:0–12:11
	Millon Adolescent Clinical Inventory, Second Edition	13:0–18:11
	Millon Clinical Multiaxial Inventory, Fourth Edition	18:0–85:11
	Millon Behavioral Medicine Diagnostic, Bariatric Norms	18:0–85:11
	Minnesota Multiphasic Personality Inventory, Adolescent Edition, Restructured Form	14:0–18:11
	Minnesota Multiphasic Personality Inventory, Second Edition, Restructured Form	18:0–89:11
	Minnesota Multiphasic Personality Inventory, Third Edition	18:0–80+
	NEO Personality Inventory, Third Edition	12:0–85:11
16. Performance Personality Tests	Children's Apperception Test, Ninth and Revised Edition, Color Edition	3:0–10:11
	Roberts, Second Edition	6:0–18:11
	Rorschach Performance Assessment System	6:0–86:11
17. Malingering Tests	Structured Interview of Reported Symptoms, Second Edition	18:0–84:11
	Test of Memory Malingering	16:0–84:11

Note. * number to the left of colon = years; number to the right of colon = months (e.g., 18:0–89:11 means that the test's age range is from 18 years 0 months through 89 years 11 months, inclusive).

each chapter; and (4) test age ranges. The age ranges are reported in conventional fashion, with yearly units listed on the left of the colon and monthly units listed on the right side. For instance, 18:0 translates into 18 years 0 months. Taken together, this listing represents all of the psychological measures selected for the book's test inventory, all of which have demonstrated relevance, precision, accuracy, and utility. *Utility* is a vital concept in clinical testing practice as it emphasizes pragmatism; that is, utility addresses the issue of whether or not a test can be administered, scored, and interpreted in a timely and efficient manner. Irrespective of test *reliability* (i.e., consistency and precision) and *validity* (i.e., measuring the construct it claims to measure or accuracy), if a test is excessively cumbersome and consumes a significant amount of time to use, it is not likely to be used in contemporary mental health practice where a premium is placed upon time.

Consistent with the need for efficiency, each test listed in Table 1.1 is described in Part II in terms of the following: (a) what data is most relevant to report; (b) how such data can be efficiently, precisely, and comprehensively presented and interpreted within a formal report by inserting previously prepared data tables with pre-drafted interpretive excerpts; (c) how the results can be progressively integrated into an accurate diagnostic summary; and (d) how such information can ultimately lead to effective and meaningful treatment recommendations. For each test, forms that contain data tables have been prepared wherein an examiner can facilely input the most critical quantitative yield into a formal report, which is supplemented by (a) pre-drafted narrative excerpts that summarize common score patterns and profiles within and across the data tables, and (b) an overall interpretive strategy (frequently supplemented by visual flowcharts that may be accessed from e-resources available on Routledge's website). These data tables and interpretive excerpts have been drafted and continually modified by means of actual practice such that they present the data in a clear and coherent manner.

In essence, and consistent with the book's prime objective, the intention is to instruct how the data yield from each of these tests can be reported and interpreted so as to maximize diagnostic precision, accuracy, and especially utility. A psychological testing report, irrespective of how well composed, represents a fruitless venture if not done in a reasonable and timely manner. Therefore, these qualities are emphasized throughout the book, especially notable within Part II.

As can be seen in Table 1.1, the chapters that comprise Part II are organized according to (a) *test format* (e.g., rating scale type tests), (b) type of major construct measured (e.g., neuropsychological tests), or (c) a combination of both test format and major construct measured (e.g., performance personality tests). Next, a pithy review of the tests in Table 1.1 will be presented. The intent here is to provide the reader with a mental scheme of all the tests to be encountered in Part II, including their format and measured constructs. Of note, the tests that are contained in this listing are those that have proven to be most efficacious in actual mental health testing practice.

Screening Tests

Chapter 5 covers *screening tests*, which are primarily employed at the examiner's discretion in order to supplement assessment information gathered by means of an initial clinical interview, mental status examination, and behavioral observations. Their principal objective is to help determine if further testing for one or more suspected disorders is warranted. The felicitous use of screening data can help establish *medical necessity*[1] for subsequent formal testing, which is a standard used by insurance carriers in determining PA for all mental healthcare services, including psychological testing. Screening tests also show examinees what psychological testing entails, at least in part, and thus (a) effectively acclimates them to the process, and (b) simultaneously helps to establish the *rapport* needed for gathering reliable and valid data. Considering that these instruments tend to be utilized so early in the process of assessment, it is logical to begin Part II with this class of tests.

Developmental Tests

Chapter 6 consists of *developmental tests* that measure skills and abilities that are expected to first appear and become increasingly sophisticated according to various age ranges, especially during the early formative years. These skills and expected age ranges are commonly referred to as *developmental milestones*; that is, phylogenetic checkpoints in human development that determine what the average person is able to do at a particular age or age range. Such tests are principally used to (a) identify individuals in early childhood who are at risk for the later onset of various types of *neurodevelopmental disorder*, and (b) diagnose individuals who are manifesting deficits or delays in various lines of development.

Therefore, Table 1.1 includes two tests of infant development capable of measuring cognitive, language, motor, social-emotional development, along with adaptive behavior from the ages of 1 month through 3 years 6 months. There are also two *adaptive behavior* measures in this class of tests designed to identify delays in the execution of daily activities that are required for self-sufficiency or autonomous functioning (see Table 1.1).

Intelligence Tests

Intelligence is defined as the ability to learn from experience, acquire knowledge, and use resources effectively in order to adapt and solve problems (see Wechsler, 1975; Sternberg & Kaufman, 1998). This is consistent with the manner in which the *intelligence tests* in the book's inventory define this construct. The need to measure people's intelligence was responsible for launching the psychological testing movement in the early 1900s, and continues to represent a vital contribution to contemporary mental health practice in the quest for resolving many issues concerning *differential diagnosis*, especially those concerning more complex aspects of cognitive functioning; for example, *intellectual disability (ID)* or *specific learning disorder (SLD)*. The intelligence tests listed in Table 1.1 have a long and impressive history. Furthermore, as a class they cover the vast majority of the entire lifespan; specifically, from the age of 2 years 0 months through late adulthood (see Table 1.1).

Achievement Tests

As opposed to mental ability or mental competence, which is measured by intelligence tests, *achievement tests* measure an individual's degree of acquired knowledge and proficiency in basic academic subjects. Academic training in our complex technological information age has become increasingly vital and relevant to overall adaptation, functioning, and adjustment. Hence, referrals for the detection of *communication disorders*, *language disorders*, and SLDs in the mental health field have increased substantially. In part, this is due to school systems being inundated by referrals for learning disability testing. This is also consistent with fairly recent estimates in the United States, which indicate that nearly 6.5 million students between 2009 and 2010 were diagnosed with a SLD (U.S. Department of Education, National Center for Education Statistics, 2012).

Although the *Diagnostic and Statistical Manual of Mental Disorders, Fourth Edition, Text Revision (DSM–IV–TR*; American Psychiatric Association, 2000) emphasized an *ability-achievement discrepancy analysis* as an essential criterion for diagnosing learning disorders, DSM–5 has simplified process; namely, assuming that the presence of intellectual disability, educational deprivation, and sensory impairment has been ruled out, a *standard score* equal to or less than 78 (i.e., with a *mean* of 100, *standard deviation* of 15), indicates the presence of a learning disorder "with the greatest degree of diagnostic certainty" (American Psychiatric Association, 2013, p. 69). Therefore, this book includes two major achievement tests, both of which provide standard scores consistent with new DSM–5 guidelines (see Table 1.1).

Neuropsychological Tests

Neurodevelopmental and *neurocognitive disorders* share the involvement of brain dysfunction, disease, damage, or delay as an inherent component of the symptom profile. Although these two classes of neuropsychological impairment are more prevalent during the two extremes of the life span, respectively, they can manifest at virtually any age. The implication is that all test inventories should have available comprehensive *neuropsychological tests* that measure key brain-behavior relationships across the majority of the lifespan; especially ages 3 years 0 months through late adulthood. Prior to age three years, a well-designed test of infant development (see prior) suffices in measuring such delays or impairments, principally because so much maturation has yet to be manifested. Therefore, at such a young age range, the major focus is on measuring failures to obtain expected developmental gains, and not so much on loss of obtained function.

To meet this need, two comprehensive neuropsychological tests are included as part of this book's inventory, each of which provide measures of key neurocognitive abilities, including (a) attention, (b) language, (c) memory, (d) visuospatial abilities, and (e) executive functioning (see Table 1.1). All of these are implicated in such types of *psychopathology* as *major neurocognitive disorder, minor neurocognitive disorder, attention-deficit/hyperactivity disorder (ADHD)*, and *language disorder*. Among these neurocognitive abilities, *memory* (i.e., the process of retaining and retrieving information) is perhaps the most essential as it (a) has a pervasive deleterious effect on functioning when impaired, and (b) is considered an essential symptom among the neurocognitive disorders (American Psychiatric Association, 2013). Therefore, a test that focuses on measuring this fundamental construct, along with its underlying hierarchical structure (see Chapter 9), is included in this class of specialized tests.

Lastly, *continuous performance tests* (CPTs) are extremely useful measures of attention, sustained attention (i.e., vigilance), impulse control, and sustained impulse control, which primarily contribute to the accurate diagnosis of ADHD. Their distinctive features include the following: (a) performance-based and fully automated in terms of administration and scoring; (b) uninterrupted presentation of visual or auditory stimuli that are repetitive and without breaks; and (c) production of a prodigious data yield. Such tasks are ideal for detecting symptoms consistent with a diagnosis of ADHD. Included in the book's test inventory are three CPT instruments, which together cover ages 4 years 0 months through adulthood.

Rating Scales Tests

Rating scales are convenient standardized tests that can facilitate differential diagnosis, especially concerning cases during the formative years; specifically, ages 2 years 0 months through 18 years 11 months. This is principally due to wide variations in abilities and skill sets observed across these developmental years, particularly during early childhood, including widespread individual differences in impulse control, emotion regulation, and attention span. The rating scales included in the book's test inventory have all been normed using pertinent standardization samples, and on characteristics that can significantly affect the behaviors and symptoms measured. Most typically, such norm reference samples are stratified according to proportions of age, gender, race/ethnicity, socioeconomic status (SES), parental years of education, and region of the country, which are reported by the U.S. Census Bureau statistics in proximity to that instrument's publication date. Rating scales are also efficient in terms of time and the capability of using multiple observers as sources for data collection in order to improve reliability or precision (i.e., interrater reliability checks).

Comparable to many of the screening tests discussed prior, a number of these rating scales are multidimensional in that they simultaneously measure an array of syndromes and problems, including inattention, depression, anxiety, autism, learning problems, and, for older children and adolescents, all of the major DSM–5 clinical disorders with the exception of *psychosis*. The remaining rating scales are unidimensional in that they concentrate on one key complex construct or disorder that is frequently encountered in mental health practice, although in a comprehensive and detailed fashion that augments diagnosis and facilitates treatment planning; for example, *sensory processing (integration) disorders*, trauma-related disorders.

Personality Inventory Tests

Personality traits are average tendencies in thinking, feeling, and behavior, which are relatively consistent over time and across situations, and which describe individual differences among people (e.g., see Larsen & Buss, 2021). *Personality inventory tests* are principally designed to measure maladaptive traits by having respondents indicate the degree to which they agree or endorse a set of standardized statements, typically *True–False* or more of a range from *Strongly Disagree* to *Strongly Agree*. Because these instruments primarily target problematic traits, by extension they provide data pertinent to the diagnosis of *personality disorders*, which consist of continuing patterns of aberrant thinking, feeling, and behavior, manifest both cross-situational and temporal consistency, and cause dysfunction (American Psychiatric Association, 2000, p. 686).

Second, these tests are also capable of measuring the presence of a variety of *clinical disorders* or *clinical syndromes*, defined as interrelated clusters of essential and nonessential signs and symptoms, that cause dysfunction, with an identifiable onset, and a tendency to be responsive to treatment (American Psychiatric Association, 2000, 2013). The theory behind many of these inventories, especially explicit in the Millon series (see, e.g., Millon, Grossman, & Millon, 2015), is that personality psychopathology increases the risk for various clinical disorders. In mental health practice, these personality inventories can be employed to diagnose both types of psychopathology; namely, personality disorders and clinical disorders.

Third, several inventories are capable of measuring maladaptive traits consistent with the *Five-Factor Model* (*FFM*), a taxonomy of personality traits that has received the most attention, empirical support, and acceptance from personality researchers (Costa & McCrae, 1995; Goldberg, 1981; McCrae & John, 1992; Saucier & Goldberg, 1996), and which has been espoused by the DSM–5 as an alternative dimensional model for personality disorder diagnosis (American Psychiatric Association, 2013, Section III, Emerging Measures and Models, Alternative DSM–5 Model for Personality Disorders, pp. 761–781). Inclusion of these measures shows how this book focuses on contemporary practice and incorporates new developments in the field of psychological testing.

Performance Personality Tests

Performance personality tests require examinees to respond to a set of standardized instructions to either (a) interpret, (b) complete, and/or (c) create stimuli, which ultimately provides information regarding their personality traits, signs, symptoms, and/or psychological adjustment. In essence, rather than asking examinees to describe themselves in terms of the extent to which they agree or disagree with a set of pre-drafted statements, or whether such statements are true or false as applied to themselves, as is done when using the personality inventories described prior, they elicit a sample of behavior under controlled standardized conditions, which then produces quantitative data and/or qualitative information about their psychological functioning. For example, rather than answering "true" to the statement, "I feel sad most of the time," an examinee may repeatedly perceive damaged, torn, injured, or dead objects, coded as a *morbid special score* (viz., *MOR*), among a series of ten standardized inkblots when asked, "What might this be?" Both are components of a depressive disorder, although are obtained in quite different ways. This genre of measures obtain data according to the latter format and are frequently referred to as *implicit personality tests* because examinees may not be consciously aware of what they are revealing. For instance, an examinee who provides numerous morbid responses to inkblots may not be aware that they are pessimistic and perhaps even depressed.

Performance tests are vital to include within an inventory of tests because they rely much less on the degree of cooperation, honesty, and introspective ability on the part of examinees. Therefore, as long as the individual responds in some meaningful manner, the results are much more likely to be interpretively useable. Of note, this is consistent with the concept of *psychological determinism*, in which it is assumed that all responses to stimuli indicate something meaningful about personality structure and/or functioning. However, this distinct advantage is weighed against the significantly greater time and effort that must be expended for proper training, administration, scoring, and interpretation that these instruments require and even demand. As will become apparent, these tests measure diagnostic clinical syndromes and personality disorders much more indirectly than do the personality inventories and rating scale type tests. In consequence, they require significantly greater degrees of diagnostic inference, thus accounting for the greater time and interpretive effort they consume when used in actual clinical practice.

There are three performance personality tests in this book's listing, which together cover ages 3 years 0 months through adulthood (see Table 1.1). They all utilize empirical scoring systems from which interpretation and diagnostic inferences can be produced. Hence, data tables with interpretive excerpts are also available for each of these measures.

Malingering Tests

As defined, *malingering* consists of the following two elements: (a) the feigning of symptoms or disability; and (b) for identifiable personal gain. The first element, *feigning* is defined as, "the deliberate fabrication or gross exaggeration of psychological or physical symptoms without any assumptions about its goals" (Rogers, 2008, p. 6). There are two tests in the book's inventory that are specifically and uniquely designed to determine the likelihood that feigning is present in a particular case, which is the first element of malingering. In the event feigning is determined to be present, information from the clinical interview and other assessment methods (e.g., neuroimaging, medical records) must ultimately determine whether the second element of malingering is met; that is, is there probative evidence of personal gain.

Although the majority of cases referred for psychological testing involve individuals who genuinely desire an accurate psychological diagnosis, primarily because symptoms are *ego dystonic* and people desire effective treatment, there are some who feign both signs and symptoms to accomplish the ulterior motive of personal gain. This is especially the case when one or more of the following issues are present, although pending and as yet unresolved: (a) disability claims; (b) forensic personal injury litigation; (c) forensic criminal competency or insanity litigation; or (d) *secondary gain*. The latter is defined as any form of positive or negative reinforcement an individual would receive contingent upon the presence of severe psychopathological signs or symptoms (e.g., attention, sympathy, avoiding responsibility). Therefore, a consummate psychological test inventory for mental health practice should include empirical measures that specifically target feigning, the first element of malingering.

There are two malingering tests in the book's inventory (see Table 1.1). One is based upon a *structured interview* format and is designed to measure the likelihood that the examinee is feigning psychiatric symptoms. The other is a performance-based test of memory that appears difficult on its face, although can be passed by those with severe neurocognitive dysfunction. Together, both tests cover the two major kinds of feigning that clinicians may encounter in mental health practice; that is, clinical disorders via self-reported *symptoms*, and neurocognitive disorders via *signs* of memory impairment.

E-Resources on Routledge Website

The third and final portion of the book is devoted to the provision of supplementary materials, all of which are accessible on Routledge's online electronic resources website (see Figure 1.1). These include visual flowcharts that illustrate the interpretive process for most tests listed in Table 1.1, case examples, and electronic files of all practice forms, report forms, and data tables presented throughout the book. These are summarized next.

Interpretive Flowcharts

Many of the tests included in this book are rather complex in terms of structure. This should not be surprising when one considers that many tests measure multifaceted psychological constructs with hierarchical organizations (e.g., intelligence, neurocognition). To facilitate the interpretive process, visual flowcharts have been created to assist readers in systematically navigating through the many variables measured by these tests. That is, the chapters in Part II verbally describe how each test or series of tests should be most efficiently interpreted. This narrative description is further supplemented by the test data tables (see below) that also have interpretive excerpts, which provide guidance as to the manner in which test scores should be reported and interpreted. The flowcharts represent a third resource uniquely designed to visually map the interpretive process for readers, which may be downloaded for added assistance during practice.

Case Examples

This portion of e-resources provides one complete case demonstration for each of the following four developmental periods: (a) early childhood; (b) middle and late childhood; (c) adolescence; and (d) adulthood. In addition to the four complete cases, there is a second adolescent case that shows how the judicious use of a screening measure can resolve the test referral issues. Here, the prime objective is to demonstrate how actual testing cases proceed through the five stages that comprise the psychological assessment and testing process as delineated in this book. The more particular focus is showing readers how the initial report is transformed into a final report that incorporates test data, final diagnoses, and treatment recommendations.

Electronic Forms

There are a total of three major types of forms presented throughout this book, all of which are designed to facilitate psychological assessment and testing practice. Two of these are presented throughout Part I as follows: (a) moving a case along from the initial referral to termination (e.g., Form 3.1. Referral for Psychological Testing); and (b) completing an initial assessment report for each of the aforementioned developmental periods (e.g., Form 3.5. Initial Psychological Assessment Report: Adolescence Form) and transitioning it into a final report. Third, test data tables are presented throughout Part II and consist of the following two components: (a) tables designed to present test scores effectively within a formal report; and (b) interpretive excerpts inserted after each data table. The latter helps to guide test interpretation, integration, and a summary of the results. Hence, all of these forms are available in electronic, and thus modifiable, Microsoft Word 2016 documents, and may be downloaded to effectuate clinical testing practice.

Recapitulation

Chapter 1 began with the principal objective of this book, which is essentially to teach the effective and efficient practice of psychological assessment and testing within the contemporary mental health field. This includes: (a) testing individuals across the entire lifespan, from infancy through older adulthood; and (b) providing a wide array of tests and testing services, including psychological, neuropsychological, and developmental (see Table 1.1). The remainder of the chapter elaborated upon the book's organization, which delineated its two major parts and e-resources on Routledge's website (see Figure 1.1).

Key Terms

- ability–achievement discrepancy analysis
- achievement test/s
- attention–deficit/hyperactivity disorder (ADHD)
- clinical disorder/s
- clinical syndrome/s
- communication disorder/s
- construct/s
- continuous performance test/s (CPTs)
- developmental milestone/s
- developmental test/s
- differential diagnosis
- ego dystonic
- feigning
- Five-Factor Model (FFM)
- implicit personality test/s
- intellectual disability (ID)
- intelligence
- intelligence test/s
- language disorder
- major neurocognitive disorder/s
- malingering
- mean
- medical necessity
- memory
- minor neurocognitive disorder/s
- morbid special score (*MOR*)
- neurocognitive disorder/s
- neurodevelopmental disorder/s
- neuropsychological test/s
- performance personality test/s
- personality disorder/s
- personality inventory test/s
- personality trait/s
- preauthorization (PA)
- psychological assessment
- psychological determinism
- psychological testing
- psychopathology
- psychosis
- rapport
- rating scale/s
- reliability
- score/s
- screening test/s
- secondary gain

- semi-structured clinical interview
- sensory processing (integration) disorder/s
- sign/s
- specific learning disorder/s (SPD)
- standard deviation
- standard score/s
- symptom/s
- syndrome/s
- test format
- utility
- validity

Note

1. Medical necessity will be discussed in earnest in Chapter 3, which focuses on selecting a relevant and efficient test battery, determining the types of testing services and time required, and meeting the requirements for PA.

See Routledge's e-resources website for forms. (www.routledge.com/9780367346058)
References

American Psychiatric Association. (2000). *Diagnostic and statistical manual of mental disorders* (4th ed., text rev., DSM–IV–TR). Washington, DC: Author.

American Psychiatric Association. (2013). *Diagnostic and statistical manual of mental disorders* (5th ed., DSM–5). Arlington, VA: Author.

Costa, P. T., Jr., & McCrae, R. R. (1995). Solid ground in the wetlands of personality: A reply to Block. *Psychological Bulletin, 117*, 216–220.

Goldberg, L. R. (1981). Language and individual differences: The search for universals in personality lexicons. In L. Wheeler (Ed.), *Review of personality and social psychology* (vol. 2, pp. 141–165). Beverly Hills, CA: Sage.

Larsen, R. J., & Buss, D. M. (2021). *Personality psychology: Domains of knowledge about human nature* (7th ed.). New York, NY: McGraw-Hill.

McCrae, R. R., & John, O. P. (1992). An introduction to the Five-Factor Model and its applications. *Journal of Personality, 60*, 175–215.

Millon, T., Grossman, S. D., & Millon, C. (2015). *Millon clinical multiaxial inventory manual* (4th ed., MCMI–IV). Minneapolis, MN: Pearson.

Rogers, R. (2008). An introduction to response styles. In R. Rogers & S. D. Bender (Eds.), *Clinical assessment of malingering and deception* (4th ed., p. 6). New York, NY: The Guilford Press.

Saucier, G., & Goldberg, L. R. (1996). The language of personality: Lexical perspectives on the five-factor model. In J.S. Wiggins (Ed.), *The five-factor model of personality: Theoretical perspectives* (pp. 21–50). New York: The Guilford Press.

Sternberg, R. J., & Kaufman, J. C. (1998). Human abilities. *Annual Review of Psychology, 49*, 479–502.

U.S. Department of Education, National Center for Education Statistics (NCES). (2012). *Digest of education statistics, 2011*. Washington, DC: Author.

Wechsler, D. (1975). *The collected papers of David Wechsler*. New York, NY: Academic Press.

Part I

The Psychological Assessment and Testing Process

Practice Forms and Report Forms

Part I covers the process of psychological assessment and testing in the mental health field in its entirety; that is, tracking the sequence of steps from the initial point of referral to test feedback and case termination. In particular, Chapter 2 provides an overview of the process, which is supplemented by a visual flowchart. This is intended to serve as an initial mental map or scheme, which is elaborated upon in detail by the succeeding two chapters that partition the sequence into two approximately equivalent parts. First, Chapter 3 delineates the steps taken from the initial referral through obtaining preauthorization (PA) for the requested testing services. Second, Chapter 4 describes the process from the point of test administration through test feedback and the proper termination of a case. The principal objective of Part II and its trilogy of chapters is to inform the reader as to how psychological assessment and testing is practiced in the contemporary mental health field. It is specifically designed to set the stage for Part II, which describes all of the tests appearing in Table 1.1, including data tables, interpretation strategies, and narrative excerpts that are to be integrated into final psychological assessment and testing reports.

DOI: 10.4324/9780429326820-2

2 Overview of the Process

Overview

This chapter begins Part I of this book, which delineates the psychological assessment and testing[1] process from the point of the initial referral to the communication of the final results. The objective of this particular chapter is to provide a general overview or road map of this sequence, including (a) steps that are required, and (b) alternative routes through the process contingent upon the particular case facts. Figure 2.1 illustrates this process within a visual flowchart, which also integrates practice forms and report forms at strategic points that have been diligently prepared according to (a) actual clinical testing practice, (b) current criteria and procedures for coding and billing psychological assessment and testing services, and (c) pertinent statutory guidelines. This overview prepares the reader for the ensuing two chapters in Part I, which describe these steps and forms in much more detail such that they may be used in clinical testing practice.

In particular, Chapter 3 takes the reader from the point of the initial referral through obtaining the permission to proceed with testing (i.e., either by insurance *preauthorization* (*PA*) or an agreed upon self-pay or pro-bono arrangement). Next, Chapter 4 takes the reader from test administration through communication of the results, also in sufficient detail for practice purposes. Finally, both Chapters 3 and 4 review the practice forms in greater of detail such that the language contained therein and their objectives are fully comprehensible for proper clinical use. Of note, these forms may be modified to meet that particular agency or practice procedures and/or case circumstances.

Flowchart of the Psychological Assessment and Testing Process

This section outlines each step in the psychological assessment and testing sequence. That is, the tasks involved and objectives for each of the steps are summarized. In addition, any forms that are needed to facilitate the completion of a particular step are introduced.

Receiving the Initial Referral for Psychological Testing

The initial referral for testing officially begins the psychological assessment and testing process (Stage 1). Such referrals can be classified as either external or internal. First, an *external referral* originates from a source that is not formally affiliated with the psychologist's private practice, group practice, or community agency. Examples include referrals from an examinee's[2] *pediatrician*, *primary care physician* (*PCP*), *neurologist*, school personnel, court of law, family member, or even a self-referral. In Figure 2.1, such referral is depicted in the upper left portion of the flowchart in which the solid-lined box titled, "External Referral for Psychological Testing," is proceeded by a down arrow leading to a solid-lined box titled, "Admissions." Here, the case becomes active and is thereafter sent on to the solid-lined box titled, "Initial Clinical Interview for Testing." That is, the request for such services is determined from the point of admissions and ensued by an initial clinical interview for psychological testing.

In contrast, an *internal referral* occurs in instances where a psychologist's colleague within the same group practice or community agency is asking for testing services. This sequence is portrayed in the upper right portion of Figure 2.1. In such circumstance, individuals are first referred by themselves or *collaterals*[3] for some type of mental health services, as depicted by the solid-lined box titled, "Person Requesting Mental Health Services," and have proceeded through a similar admissions process that activates their case (see left-pointing connecting arrow to "Admissions"). The principal difference is that the admissions staff do not yet refer for psychological testing, but rather for an initial clinical interview and beginning treatment intervention (e.g., psychiatric, psychotherapeutic, couples counseling, substance abuse counseling).

Regarding the specific identity of the referral source, external types are much more wide ranging and may include self-referrals, family members, close friends, employers, vocational rehabilitation counselors (VRCs), medically

DOI: 10.4324/9780429326820-3

```
┌─────────────────┐                                      ┌──────────────┐      ┌────────────────┐
│ External Referral│                                     │  Admissions  │◄─────│     Person      │
│ for Psychological│                                     │              │      │ Requesting Mental│
│     Testing     │                                      └──────────────┘      │ Health Services │
└─────────────────┘                                                            └────────────────┘
        │                    Stage 1
        ▼                            ┌──────────────────┐
┌─────────────────┐                  │ Internal Referral│       ┌──────────────────┐
│                 │                  │ for Psychological│◄──────│ Mental Health     │
│   Admissions    │──────────────────│     Testing      │       │ Clinician         │
│                 │                  │  (Forms 3.1, 3.2)│       │ Assessment (and   │
└─────────────────┘                  └──────────────────┘       │ Treatment)        │
                                                                 └──────────────────┘
                                                                   Transfer   │
                         ┌──────────────────┐   ┌──────────────────┐          │
                         │ Initial Clinical │   │ Communicate Findings │      │      ┌──────────┐
   Stage 2               │ Interview for    │──►└──────────────────┘──────────────► │Discharge │
                         │    Testing       │                                        └──────────┘
                         │(Form 3.3, 3.4, 3.5, or│   ┌──────────────────┐
                         │  3.6;  Form 3.7) │- - ► │  Initial-Final   │
                         └──────────────────┘      │  Psychological   │
                                 │                 │ Assessment Report│
                                 ▼                 └──────────────────┘
                         ┌──────────────────┐                                  Transfer
                         │ Preparation for  │
   Stage 3               │ Testing and      │
                         │ Scheduling Appointments│
                         │ (Forms 3.8, 3.9, 3.10, 3.11)│          ┌──────────────────┐      Key:
                         └──────────────────┘                     │ Initial Psychological│
        Form 7.12          - - - - - - - - - - - - - ►            │ Assessment Report │   ──► Required Step
                                 │                                └──────────────────┘
                                 ▼                                                        ····► Potential Step
                         ┌──────────────────┐   ┌──────────────────┐
                         │ Request for      │   │ Testing Denied or Units│            ─·─► Report
                         │ Testing          │····►│ Requested Reduced │
                         │ Preauthorization │   └──────────────────┘
                         │      (PA)        │            │
                         └──────────────────┘            ▼
                                 │             ┌──────────────────┐
                                 ▼             │ Peer-to-Peer     │
                         ┌──────────────────┐  │ Consultation;    │
                         │ Testing PA Obtained or│◄│ Letter of Appeal │
                         │ Otherwise Negotiated with│ └──────────────────┘
                         │    Examinee      │
                         └──────────────────┘
                                 │    ┌──────────────────────────────────┐
                                 ◄────│ Scheduling Appointments          │  Stage 5
                                      │ (if not done after initial clinical interview)│
                                      └──────────────────────────────────┘
                                 ▼
                         ┌──────────────────┐   ┌──────────────────┐      ┌──────────────────┐
                         │ Test Administration, Scoring,│──►│ Final Psychological│──►│ Billing All Test Hours│
   Stage 4               │ Interpretation, and Final│   │ Assessment Report │   └──────────────────┘
                         │ Report  Generation│      └──────────────────┘
                         │(Form 3.3, 3.4, 3.5, or 3.6  in Final│  ┌──────────────────┐   ┌──────────┐
                         │      Format)     │─────►│ Communicate Findings │─►│Discharge │
                         └──────────────────┘      └──────────────────┘      └──────────┘
```

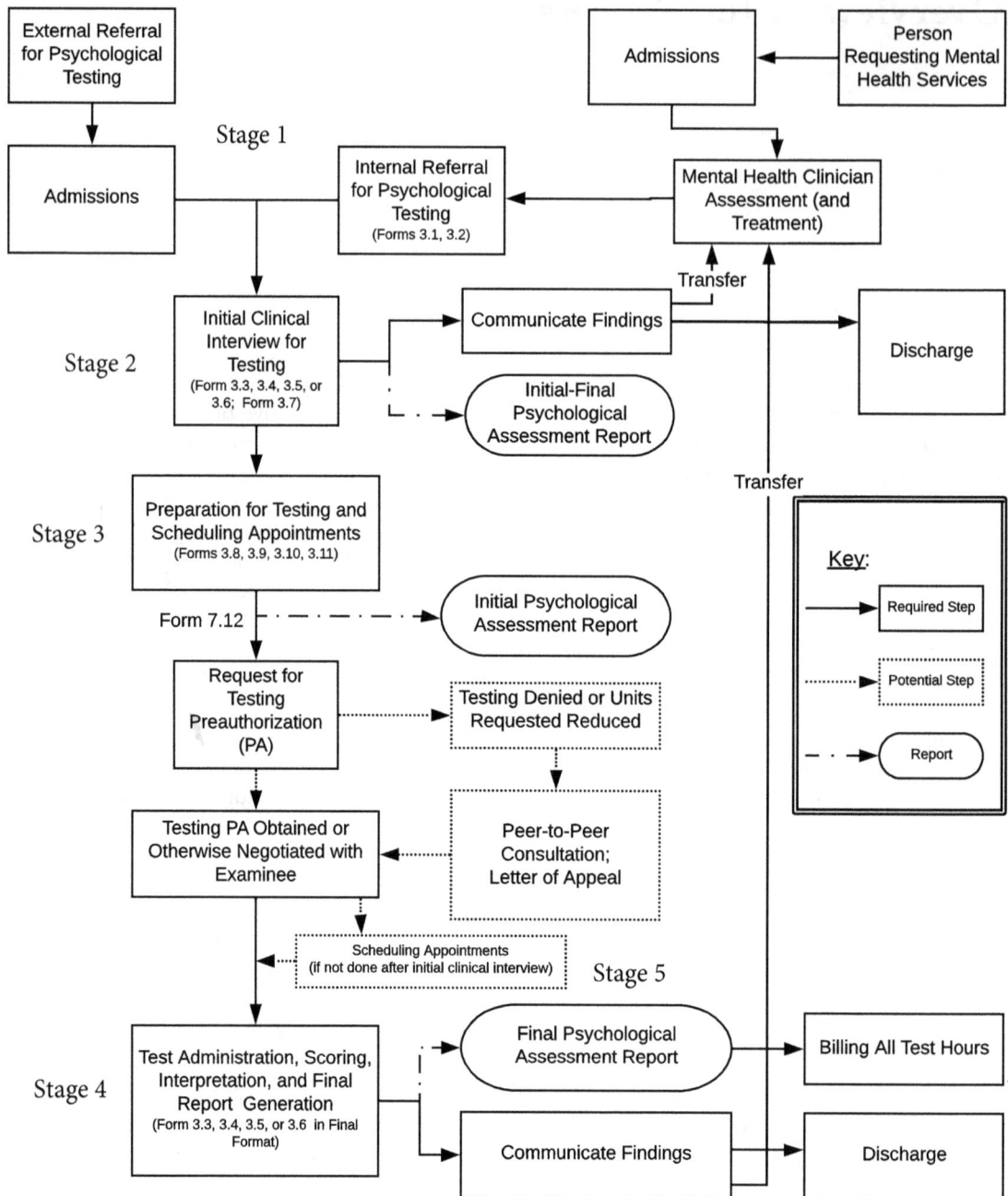

Figure 2.1 Flowchart of the Psychological Assessment and Testing Process

Note. Form 3.1 = Referral for Psychological Testing; Form 3.2 = Authorization for Disclosure of Protected Health Information; Form 3.3 = Initial Assessment-Early Childhood (Ages 2–5; 24–71 Months); Form 3.4 = Initial Assessment- Middle-to-Late Childhood (Ages 6–12 Years); Form 3.5 = Initial Assessment-Adolescence (Ages 13–18 Years); Form 3.6 Initial Assessment-Adult (19 Years–Older); Form 3.7 = List of Available Psychological Tests; Form 3.8 = Consent for Psychological Testing Services; Form 3.9 = Scheduling Appointments for Psychological Test Administration; Form 3.10a = Psychological Testing Instructions to Examinee (& Collaterals)- Scheduling Appointments before Preauthorization; Form 3.10b = Psychological Testing Instructions to Examinee (& Collaterals)-Scheduling Appointments after Preauthorization; Form 3.11 = Proof of Appointment Note-School or Work.

training health care providers, mental health care clinicians, educational staff, court referrals, and so on. Internal referral sources are most likely mental health clinicians who are not trained to provide psychological testing services, including a *psychiatrist, nurse practitioner, clinical social worker, case manager,* or *admissions specialist.* Although less frequently, such referrals may also originate from psychologists who choose not to engage in testing practice even though they possess the requisite training, or psychologists who prefer to avoid testing their own psychotherapy clients (i.e., avoiding a dual-role per ethical guidelines).

Finally, irrespective of whether the referral is external or internal, the following information is essential to obtain in this inaugural step: (a) examinee test-related demographic information; (b) the diagnostic and related issues and questions that need to be addressed; and (c) the rationale as to why formal psychological testing is being requested. For such information, Form 3.1 has been prepared and is aptly titled, "Referral for Psychological Testing," which is a succinct one-page referral sheet reviewed in detail later in Chapter 3. For an external referral, admissions staff would either complete this form or otherwise document such information in some alternate format. For an internal referral, the treating clinician would complete this form or otherwise provide this information.

Lastly, a *release of information (ROI)* form should be completed at this juncture for (a) the examinee, and (b) each other entity who is to receive a formal written copy of the final report that is not part of the same practice (i.e., external referral sources only). The single page Form 3.2 titled, "Authorization for Disclosure of Mental Health Information," is designed for such purpose and consists of language that is consistent with applicable federal law (e.g., see Confidentiality of Substance Use Disorder, 2020; The Health Insurance Portability and Accountability Act of 1996, 2000, 2020; Missouri Bar, 2006). Next, an initial clinical interview for testing needs to be done by the psychologist who accepts the referral.

Initial Clinical Interview for Testing: Use of the Clinical Method

Subsequent to documenting the referral for testing information, the primary objective of the ensuing step (Stage 2) is to complete an initial psychological assessment report by means of a clinical interview, including (a) mental status examination and behavioral observations, and (b) discretionary screening tests (see also Chapters 3 & 5). In Figure 2.1, this is depicted in the following two ways: (a) by the solid-lined arrow connecting the "Admissions" step to the "Initial Clinical Interview for Testing" step (viz., external referral); and (b) by the solid-lined arrow connecting the "Mental Health Clinician Assessment (and Treatment)" step, to the "Internal Referral for Testing" step, and finally to the "Initial Clinical Interview for Testing" step (viz., internal referral). Here, the *clinical method* (i.e., mental health professionals utilizing their expert training and experience) is employed to determine one of the following: (a) if a case's diagnostic issues are adequately addressed in order to proceed directly to treatment; or, more likely; (b) if a case is in need of follow-up psychological testing to properly address as yet unresolved diagnostic concerns. To proceed with the clinical method, four versions of a semi-structured initial clinical interview have been prepared, each of which differ somewhat according to the particular developmental period. In increasing order of age, they are as follows: (a) Form 3.3 titled, "Initial Psychological Assessment Report, Early Childhood (Ages 2–5 Years; 24–71 Months)"; (b) Form 3.4 titled, "Initial Psychological Assessment Report, Middle and Late Childhood (Ages 6–12 Years)"; (c) Form 3.5 titled, "Initial Psychological Assessment Report, Adolescence (Ages 13–18 Years)"; and (d) Form 3.6 titled, "Initial Psychological Assessment Report, (19 Years–Older)."

These forms are specifically designed to answer the following questions: (a) is psychological testing needed to address the diagnostic issues and questions; and, if yes, (b) what kind of testing services and how much time is required. To facilitate the process, the outlines include (a) pre-drafted narrative statements that are most frequently given by examinees and collaterals, (b) are worded in the normative direction, and (c) contain multiple selection (e.g., gender, handedness) and fill-in-the-blank (e.g., date of birth, age, grade level, birth weight) sentences for efficiency of use. The purpose of the latter is to guide the selection and insertion of key data. In this manner, these particular interview forms provide an effective guide for semi-structured interviewing, ensuring that vital information is investigated and documented, while facilitating efficient report writing as the pre-drafted statements usually need only minor degrees of modification to be consistent with interviewees' actual responses. The particulars of these forms are reviewed in Chapter 3, including a comparison and contrast across the different age ranges.

Initial–Final Psychological Assessment Report

In the event that the testing psychologist is satisfied with the evidence garnered by means of the clinical interview alone, the results can be immediately reviewed orally with the examinee and any collaterals, and the results reduced to writing in a report felicitously titled, "Initial–Final Psychological Assessment Report." This phrasing denotes that the initial interview was sufficient and doubles as the final report. However, this oral and written feedback must also include treatment recommendations for it to legitimately be considered a complete and final report. Thereafter, the examinee is either discharged for follow-up with the external referral source (see solid-lined arrow proceeding from "Initial Clinical Interview for Testing" to "Communication," and finally, to "Discharge") or referred back to the mental health clinician who requested testing within the same practice (see solid-lined arrow proceeding from "Initial Clinical Interview for Testing" to "Communication," and finally, to "Mental Health Clinician Assessment [and Treatment]").

Decision to Pursue Formal Psychological Testing

In contrast, the more likely decision is to request follow-up psychological testing. This is not surprising since in most cases a clinical interview will have already been done and deemed insufficient for developing comprehensive diagnostic conclusions. In those instances where a clinical interview has not yet been done, the referral for testing will have probably been precipitated by (a) a complex differential diagnostic issue, and/or (b) questions that require, or are significantly bolstered by the use of standardized testing (e.g., specific learning disability, neurocognitive disorder, need for a rapid personality disorder diagnosis, assessing risk of re-offense). In such instances, the objective is to narrow the scope of testing as much as possible such that all remaining diagnostic issues can be adequately addressed with the fewest number of measures, types of testing services, and number of units (i.e., testing time). This principle is analogous to the use of the least restrictive (or invasive) alternative treatment to achieve the desired therapeutic effects.

Here, the testing psychologist is fundamentally presented with a balancing test; that is, to select the type and number of testing units that most effectively balances precision and accuracy with *efficiency* (i.e., cost effectiveness). *Precision* reflects reliability or test consistency while *accuracy* refers to validity or truthfulness of the results (Price, 2017). Hence, the balancing test is as follows: As the type and number of testing units increase, precision and accuracy increase while efficiency declines. Another way to frame this dilemma is by the question, "How much precision and accuracy is needed to sufficiently address the identified diagnostic issues and questions?" Of course, this will depend upon many variables, including the relative importance of the pertinent constructs (e.g., assessing risk of re-offending, violence, or suicide), the complexity of the diagnostic issues (e.g., how many psychological constructs are involved), and the quality of tests designed to measure such constructs.

In order to resolve the aforementioned balancing test or related question, each interview form (viz., Forms 3.3–3.6) concludes with the following information: (a) a listing of the most common diagnoses to select from as being either provisional or to represent the targets of follow-up testing; (b) a listing of tests normed for that age cohort by name, along with the types of testing services and number of units (i.e., time) required to administer, score, and interpret each test; and (c) a method for aggregating the types of testing services and units needed for the test battery as a whole. In addition, Form 3.7 titled, "List of Available Psychological Tests," provides an enumeration of all tests available to a psychologist who is preparing to provide such professional service. In this instance, such listing comprises all of the tests that are covered in detail in Part II, and which were previously introduced in Table 1.1. In Form 3.7, the tests are similarly catalogued by (a) the general type of psychological construct measured (e.g., intelligence), (b) the type of test format (e.g., rating scales tests), or (c) a combination of both construct measured and test format (e.g., performance personality tests), whichever identifies them most readily. In addition to providing a complete catalogue of all available tests, the age range for each test is reported. Such information is not included in the interview forms for purposes of brevity and because over time, this information becomes encoded into the long-term memory of the examiner through the process of over-learning. However, Form 3.7 is designed as a quick reference guide if needed to help make fine discriminations among the tests in terms of (a) the constructs measured, and (b) the ages for which they are designed.

Preparation for Testing and Scheduling Appointments

At this juncture, the psychologist has done the following: (a) determined that psychological testing is needed; (b) what disorders are to be the focus of testing; (c) selected the tests and subtests to be included in the targeted test battery; and (d) identified the type of testing services and number of units needed for answering the remaining diagnostic questions and issues. To move forward, a number of tasks must be done to prepare adequately for the planned testing. This is illustrated in Figure 2.1 by the solid-lined arrow connecting the "Initial Interview for Testing" step with the "Preparation for Testing and Scheduling Appointments" step (Stage 3). In particular, this current step focuses on (a) obtaining informed consent for the testing plan, and if granted, (b) submitting any needed measures for completion outside of sessions, and (c) scheduling the needed follow-up testing appointments.

Informed consent requires that clients be apprised of all the pertinent facts, roles, and expectations of all involved parties to a new procedure, such that they can render a reasonably prudent decision of whether or not to participate. In this circumstance, sharing with clients what has thus far been determined would generally satisfy the tenets of informed consent. Therefore, the psychologist should first review the provisional diagnosis. A *provisional diagnosis* is one that is (a) imprecise to some degree and in need of refinement, (b) usually based upon insufficient or conflicting information, (c) intended to be temporary or time-limited, and (d) anticipated to change pending the addition of diagnostically pertinent data. The most commonly used provisional diagnoses are those that are more general, although provide some direction in that they identify a general class of disorder (e.g., *other specified neurodevelopmental disorder*). However, a more specific historical diagnosis that is now in question due to increasingly contradictory information (e.g., *attention-deficit/hyperactivity disorder* or *ADHD*) can also be amended as being provisional. Briefly, an *historical diagnosis* is one that a client has been given at some time prior to a subsequent psychological assessment.

Thereafter, an oral review of the suspected disorders that are in need of testing with the examinee and any collaterals is a logical next step, including some of the conflicting facts that impede a more definitive diagnosis. Next, the tests and subtests being requested should be reviewed orally, including their format, required respondents, estimated time investment, and most importantly, what data the measures will generally contribute to clarify the diagnostic picture. Although this sounds involved, it can be done rather efficiently within a few minutes, including adequately addressing any questions the examinee and collaterals may have. Once such information is provided, the following two objectives have been accomplished: (a) the criteria for the "informed" portion of informed consent has been met; and (b) the examinee and any collaterals are more likely to agree and be cooperative with the testing procedures. The latter is vital for purposes of test reliability and validity.

Before proceeding any further, it makes most sense now to obtain the "consent" portion of informed consent. For this, Form 3.8 has been prepared titled, "Consent for Psychological Testing Services," which enumerates all of the specific types of information needed to be conveyed for such agreement. Form 3.8 also serves as a convenient checklist for the psychologist, including a review of the planned recipients of the final report. After the examinee or collateral (e.g., parent or guardian) signs this form, the psychologist or *support staff*[4] may co-sign as witness. It is important for the psychologist to highlight the clause that permits the examinee to withdraw consent at any time thereafter by written notice for documentation purposes.

Once informed consent is granted, rating scales tests that can or must be completed outside of session should be submitted to the examinee and any collaterals, reviewing with them the instructions for both completing them and then submitting them. Next is the scheduling issue. Technically, scheduling can be done at this juncture or after PA by the insurance carrier(s) has been obtained. Both methods are viable, although the former may be preferable for various reasons, especially the following: (a) convenience; (b) providing continuity and greater client engagement in the process versus the perception of delay; (c) being more consistent with submitting rating scales tests for completion immediately upon conclusion of the initial clinical interview; and (d) the simplicity of canceling and rescheduling test administration appointments if there are unanticipated delays in obtaining PA. Therefore, this discussion shall proceed with the understanding that scheduling will be done at this point, with a brief note on the alternative scheduling method when this juncture is reached later in the flowchart.

Here, the scheduling process is facilitated by Form 3.9 titled, "Scheduling Appointments for Psychological Test Administration." This is to be completed by the testing psychologist subsequent to selecting the test battery and obtaining informed consent for this newly planned mental health service. Form 3.9 is in both fill-in-the blank and checklist format to expedite its completion. Essentially, this form provides sufficient information to enable support staff to schedule the number, duration, and type of testing appointments needed in a particular case.

Thereafter, Form 3.10a titled, "Psychological Testing Instructions to Examinee (& Collaterals): Scheduling Appointments before Preauthorization," provides detailed written instructions for examinees and any collaterals that inform them how testing proceeds from this point, including a reiteration of the total number of testing units and time that is being requested, the PA procedure, and the submission of any rating scales tests. Alternatively, if scheduling is to follow insurance preauthorization, Form 3.10b titled, "Psychological Testing Instructions to Examinee (& Collaterals): Scheduling Appointments after Preauthorization," is to be completed and provided as it reverses the sequence: that is, (a) PA first, then (b) scheduling appointments. In such instance, the scheduling form (viz., Form 3.9) should be retained in the examinee's *medical record*[5] for use by support staff after PA or alternative financial arrangements have been reconciled. Lastly, prior to sending the examinee and any collaterals to support staff for scheduling, they may need a note that establishes their attendance at the initial assessment and absence from school or work responsibilities. Form 3.11 titled, "Proof of Appointment Note: School or Work," is designed for this purpose and for any subsequent appointments they attend.

Once the examinee and any collaterals exit the interview room for scheduling, the "Initial Psychological Assessment Report" should be completed immediately thereafter and prior to the next case on that psychologist's schedule. The principal reason for this practice is that there will be no other point in time in which the psychologist's memory traces for the interview information will be stronger. Therefore, the initial report will be composed more rapidly and the information will be more accurate (see the discussion on completing the final report later in this chapter). The final form needed prior to the preauthorization step is one that effectively records the ongoing progress of the testing case.

In particular, Form 3.12 titled, "Psychological Assessment and Testing Services Record Form," is fundamentally designed to track the provision of services from the initial clinical interview to termination (i.e., an historical summary of all testing services provided). This one-page document consists of key information to facilitate case tracking, including examinee name, medical record number (MRN), insurance carrier, and number and type of units requested and approved. The latter will be covered in detail in Chapter 3, including how to select and aggregate the various testing service units and time. Here, it will suffice simply to mention that having such information readily available as a face sheet, or in an otherwise prominent location within the case file (be it electronic or in hard copy format), will assist immensely in keeping apprised of case progress.

Request for Testing Preauthorization

The Figure 2.1 box titled, "Request for Testing Preauthorization (PA)," is enclosed with solid lines to emphasize that it is both a required an integral step in the flowchart. Unfortunately, the PA process tends to be remarkably variable and contingent upon the provisions contained within examinee's health insurance policy. The best-case scenario is that psychological testing services are (a) covered, and that (b) PA is not required (see Figure 2.1, "Request for Testing Preauthorization (PA)," broken dotted-line down arrow to, "Testing PA Obtained or Otherwise Negotiated with Examinee"). Of course, the most unfavorable outcome is that such services are not covered, thus resulting in an automatic denial. In between these two extremes, the testing request can be either denied outright, or the units requested reduced due to a determination by the insurance carrier that the criteria used in defining what is *medically necessary* have either not been met, or only partially met (see Figure 6.1, broken dotted-line arrow connected to, "Testing Denied or Units Requested Reduced"). In such instance, insurance companies typically offer two types of appeal in the following order: (a) a peer-to-peer consultation, most frequently scheduled and done by phone; and (b) a formal letter of appeal (see Figure 2.1, broken dotted-line arrow connected to, "Peer-to-Peer Consultation; Letter of Appeal").

Peer-to-peer consultation is done with a psychologist who has read the initial report and will discuss the reasons the requested testing was denied or number of units reduced. If additional diagnostic information can be offered that rectifies the noted deficiencies, in whole or part (e.g., additional developmental delay information), the decision may be immediately reversed or modified with added units being approved. If the needed diagnostic information is immediately unavailable but can be obtained at a later date (e.g., collecting screening data that empirically shows the likelihood of a disorder), it can be integrated into a follow-up letter of appeal with added units potentially being later approved. In any case, proceeding with the planned test battery as scheduled according to the units approved is the most frequent outcome (see Figure 2.1, "Testing PA Obtained or Otherwise Negotiated with Examinee"). However, if an adverse decision of complete denial is upheld, whether testing is not covered by the policy or is deemed not medically necessary, the examinee can proceed on a self-pay, reduced-fee basis; possibly supplemented by the psychologist reducing the number of requested units. This issue will be discussed further in Chapter 4.

Before moving on to the next intricate step, a final note on scheduling appointments after PA is needed. In the event scheduling was deferred pending PA or negotiating alternative arrangements, the examinee or any collaterals should be contacted by support staff using the scheduling form (viz., Form 3.9) that was filed as part of the medical record. This is depicted in Figure 2.1 by the broken dotted-line box titled, "Scheduling Appointments (if not done after initial clinical interview), along with the subsequent broken dotted-line arrow."

Test Administration, Scoring, Interpretation, and Final Report Generation

Once PA or the negotiation of alternative financial arrangements has been resolved, the next step consolidates four essential sub-steps that should be undertaken in close succession, including (a) test administration, (b) scoring, (c) interpretation, and (d) generation of the final report. This is depicted in Figure 2.1 by the solid dark-lined box titled, "Test Administration, Scoring, Interpretation, and Final Report Generation," which explicitly encloses all four sub-steps together as one grouping (Stage 4). With few exceptions (e.g., attending to emergency cases), the cardinal objective here is to have the "Final Psychological Assessment Report" done, signed, and filed as a formal document within the examinee's medical record in proximity (i.e., ideally later on the same day) as the final test administration appointment.

This can be accomplished by following the tasks outlined in Table 2.1, which can be converted, in whole or in modified part, as a "to-do" checklist for the testing psychologist. Task 1 is actually a scheduling strategy that works in practice, and which facilitates the completion of the remaining tasks. Essentially, the work day is first partitioned into halves; hence, a traditional eight-hour work day would be apportioned into first and second four-hour intervals. The first four-hour time block would then be filled with either (a) one- or two-hour test administration appointments (see Chapter 3 regarding advised duration of test administration appointments), or (b) initial clinical interviews to begin new testing cases. The second four-hour time block would be cleared for test scoring, interpretation, and

Table 2.1 Psychological Test Scoring, Interpretation, and Final Report Generation Tasks

Task #	Task Label	Task Description
1	**Organization of Schedule**	(a) 1st half of day test administration appointments one to two hours duration; (b) 2nd half of day cleared for scoring, interpretation, and report generation.
2[a]	**Examinee Arrival**	Examiner notified of examinee arrival for final administration session.
3[a]	**Cursory Review of Case File**	(a) Initial report—test battery, suspected disorders and diagnostic questions/issues; (b) check for any previously given rating scales.
4[a]	**Greet Examinee/Collaterals**	(a) Ask for any previously given rating scales; (b) ensure any rating scales are properly completed; (c) ask if attendance note is needed.
5[a]	**Test Administration**	Test administration session (typical one to two hours).
6[a]	**Conclude Appointment**	(a) Estimate time final report will be done (e.g., later the same day); (b) review the intended recipients of final report and communication plans.
7[b]	**Modify Initial Report**	(a) Proof and scrutinize the case facts; (b) make modifications to read as the final report (e.g., add test battery listing).
8[b]	**Test Scoring**	Score all tests (use computer test scoring software when available).
9[b]	**Review Test Data**	(a) List the test data from most-to-least pertinent in addressing the diagnostic issues; (b) modify the initial listing of tests as indicated by their data quality.
10[b]	**Incorporate Body of Final Report**	Final report section, "Test Data and Interpretation," enter data tables and their scores for each test available in electronic form in Section III of this book.
11[b]	**Test Interpretation**	(a) Interpret scores immediately after each table; (b) highlight patterns within the table (from general-to-specific); (c) then highlight patterns across tables.
12[b]	**Recapitulation**	Final report section, "Summary of Results": (a) highlight essential findings; (b) connect findings to final diagnoses and treatment recommendations.
13[b]	**Final Diagnostic Summary**	Final report section, "Final DSM–5 Diagnostic Summary": (a) List final diagnoses (principal, secondary, etc.); (b) list prognosis and reasons therefore.
14[b]	**Treatment Recommendations**	Final report section, "Treatment Recommendations": (a) Insert appropriate recommendation (see Chapter 5); (b) ensure added disorders are addressed.

Note: [a] denotes that the task should be completed during the 1st half of the daily schedule; [b] denotes that the task should be done during the cleared 2nd half of the work day.

final report generation services as delineated below and in further detail in Chapter 4. In this manner, testing services can be typically completed on the final date of test administration services while simultaneously initiating new testing cases. In addition to such pragmatism, this practice exploits the workings of human *memory*. Specifically, the psychologist has done the following within the previous one to four hours: (a) reviewed the tested-for diagnoses and test battery to prepare for test administration; (b) administered the final tests (including observations of diagnostically relevant behaviors); and (c) proofread the entire initial report with the incorporation of modifications that begin its transformation into a final formal report. According to two prominent theories of memory and forgetting, there is no other point in time in which recall for the case information will be more easily accessible and accurate.

First, decay theory and the idea of memory traces. *Memory traces* refer to physical changes in the brain, likely due to communication within and between neurons, which form upon exposure to pertinent information (Brown, 1958; Peterson & Peterson, 1959). According to *decay theory*, these memory traces will begin to rapidly weaken and fade when the following two events are permitted to occur: (a) time from exposure to the information elapses; and (b) there is no opportunity for further exposure or use. Hence, another term for decay theory is *disuse*; that is, memories that are not afforded the opportunity to be used will eventually fade, weaken, and disappear.

Second, *interference theory* posits that long-term memory (LTM) traces become increasingly inaccessible as competing information accumulates (Anderson & Neely, 1996). *Proactive interference* occurs when previously learned information competes with current information; in this instance, previously similar cases. More on point, *retroactive interference* occurs when newer information hinders previously learned information; here, any current or new cases seen after a final test administration. Both decay and *interference* theories of memory, in addition to logical and practical experience, make a cogent argument for scoring, interpretation, and report generation to occur in proximity to the final testing appointment. The proposed system in Figure 2.1 accomplishes this and makes the process so much more feasible, efficient (i.e., faster), precise (i.e., reliable), accurate (i.e., valid), and perhaps most of all, enjoyable. It also provides examinees, any collaterals, and referral sources with a remarkably efficient and responsive service.

Continuing with Table 2.1, Tasks 2 through 4 properly prepare the psychologist and the examinee (and/or collaterals) for the test administration session(s). These are essential because psychologists are asked to provide professional services to multiple cases within and across days and weeks, with caseloads of 40 to 50 patients at any one time.

Whatever the specifics, having some system of rapidly reacquainting oneself with a case is essential. The circumscribed one- to two-hour test administration duration in Task 6 (Table 2.1) is intended to reduce *error variance* in the test scores due to examinee fatigue and/or waning motivation. Testing experience shows that if a test battery exceeds two hours, typically a neuropsychological case, it is best to schedule two appointments on separate days, even if they are one day apart.

Accurate test scores supersede the need for rapid but less than reliable and valid results. Besides, the efficiency incorporated into other aspects of this targeted assessment and testing process (see Figure 2.1) sufficiently compensates for any delay of one or several days. Even if afforded short breaks during longer testing sessions, examinees become both mentally and emotionally fatigued, especially older and younger cases. Taking standardized tests, especially those that are performance-based (e.g., intelligence, memory) are notably stressful and emotionally invasive. For example, formerly active and independent adults have broken down and cried during neuropsychological test administration when they could not immediately recall more than one or two words of a short story. In addition, clients are repeatedly thankful for not scheduling sessions that exceed two hours when planning testing appointments. Lastly, scheduling in excess of two hours will not be a frequent occurrence using the system portrayed in Figure 2.1.

Task 7 in Table 2.1 serves multiple purposes as follows: (a) correcting any clerical or factual errors in the initial report; (b) modifying and incorporating headings, subheadings, and information into the initial report such that it begins and continues its transformation into the final version; and (c) refreshing one's memory of the case details such that the data to be scored immediately subsequent can be interpreted within a meaningful cognitive framework or context. This is demonstrated in Chapter 4 and throughout the case examples available on Routledge's e-resources website.

Task 8 in Table 2.1 states explicitly that *computer test scoring software* is to be used when available. In most or all cases it proves to be cost effective. In contrast, using *computer test interpretive software* is to be avoided for two reasons. First, the fee for this service is usually cost prohibitive, typically three times the rate of simple scoring software. Second, the interpretative statements are simply triggered by the presence of certain scores, score ranges, and score patterns, and do not consider context. Therefore, they are often both contradictory, stereotyped, ambiguous, and consist of *Barnum statements* (see Larsen & Buss, 2021) that generally apply to all people and are not discriminatory. This is partly due to the computer's failure to integrate and resolve inconsistencies or seemingly paradoxical results; a unique ability reserved by the human mind. Additionally, if they also become part of the client's medical record, they can be difficult to explain ethically speaking.

Once all of the tests are scored, Task 9 in Table 2.1 indicates that their data should be visually scanned for patterns, especially those that (a) most closely address the principal diagnostic issues and questions, and (b) are most reliable and valid. Chapter 4 provides specific guidelines for how to prioritize the order of tests in the body of the final report. Once the initial order is selected, Task 10 in Table 2.1 states that they should be incorporated into the main section of the final report titled, "Test Data and Interpretation." This is the point in which the practice of simultaneous test score reporting and interpretation is done. In particular, data tables for each test are incorporated into the report. Immediately after each data table, an interpretive summary should be composed (i.e., Task 11 in Table 2.1), first describing score patterns within the table and proceeding from making general inferences to those that are more specific (e.g., "these observer-based results are consistent with a depressive disorder, which is of moderate degree, and with secondary anxious distress"), ensued by making connections between the tables (e.g., "these results are also consistent with previous performance-based test results showing evidence of depression"). In this manner, the reader is able to closely follow the relevant data, along with the underlying thought process and rationale of the examiner. Inconsistencies within and between the data tables can also be effectively addressed immediately after they become apparent and highlighted.[6] Here, the testing psychologist integrates the *statistical method* (also known as the *actuarial assessment*) in rendering diagnoses, which is defined as using empirical or quantitative data in determining the presence of psychopathology, integrated with that of the prior clinical method. That is, test data should rarely (if ever) be interpreted in the absence of (a) contextual developmental history information, (b) mental status examination, and (c) use of some degree of clinical judgment.

Task 12 in Table 2.1 is a recapitulation of the essential findings reported within a section titled, "Summary of Results," which is inserted immediately after the report body and prior to the final diagnoses. It may be in either a narrative or bullet-point format. The latter tends to be more effective in complex diagnostic cases with multiple issues or questions. This part of the final report is analogous to the abstract section of a journal article written in American Psychological Association (APA) style (American Psychological Association, 2019). It should thus remain succinct. Task 13 in Table 2.1 indicates that the supported diagnoses should be enumerated in order from most to least prominent. This is done in a separate section titled, "Final DSM–5 Diagnostic Summary." Therefore, the first most prominent disorder is designated as the *principal diagnosis*, followed by disorders in declining degree of significance. Greater detail of what to include in the diagnostic summary and how it can be effectively organized is provided in Chapter 4.

Finally, Task 14 in Table 2.1 regards proposals for intervention, which should be enumerated in a concluding section of the final report felicitously titled, "Treatment Recommendations." Both traditional and evidence-based treatment approaches can be employed in the form of specific recommendations. At this juncture, what remains is reviewing the new sections of the final report for accuracy, signing it, and making the titled "Final Psychological Assessment Report" a formal part of the client's medical record.

Billing for Psychological Testing Services

If test scoring, interpretation, and final report generation indeed occur on the last date of test administration services, then billing can proceed immediately after such document is made an official part of the medical record. This is depicted in Figure 2.1 by the solid arrows connecting the solid boxes as follows: "Test Administration, Scoring, Interpretation, and Final Report Generation" ◊ "Final Psychological Assessment Report" ◊ "Billing All Test Hours." This is vital because billing should occur on a date of *face-to-face service*. Face-to-face service means that the client (a) is physically present, (b) is provided preauthorized professional services (here, test administration), and (c) is participating in a formally scheduled appointment. Alternatively, if billing is done on a date after which scoring, interpretation, and report generation is done, there is a significant risk that payment for services will be denied. Therefore, billing all test hours in the manner delineated above is most efficacious, ethical, accepted by third party payers, and averts the need for back-dating billing for testing services to the last date of face-to-face contact, which is permitted but can increase the risk of billing errors.

Communication of the Results

All of the prior work in completing a testing case is rather fruitless unless the results can be communicated (a) effectively, and (b) in a timely manner. The psychological assessment and testing process delineated in Figure 2.1 is designed, especially to accomplish both of these facets of communication; that is, the rapid transmission of valuable information (Stage 5). In particular, the examinee and any collaterals may either pick up the final report physically (including later that same day if feasible), or be mailed a copy. Also, copies of the final report can be immediately mailed, faxed, or sent in PDF format by email attachment to the referring clinician(s), along with all other third parties designated by virtue of the completed ROI documents (see Form 3.2).

The format and tenor of the final report, being largely factual and interpreted in objective terms, can in the vast majority of cases be properly released in timely fashion and without modifications, editing, or major deletions. This will be emphasized in more detail and with examples in Chapter 4 and throughout the case examples that are available on Routledge's e-resources website. Irrespective of the case being an external or internal referral, it is typically left to the discretion of examinees and any collaterals as to whether or not they desire a face-to-face oral feedback session.

For internal referrals, examinees most frequently review the results with their mental health clinicians who referred them in the first place, and who will be providing the ongoing treatment. In effect, the internal referral source is in the dual role of (a) treating clinician, and (b) case manager; that is, the clinician who is responsible for (a) making all needed referrals for *adjunctive services*, and (b) tracking the client's overall ongoing progress. This is portrayed in Figure 2.1 by (a) the broken dotted-line box titled "Communicate Findings," denoting that this is an optional step, ensued by the long, solid dark-lined, initially horizontal, then turning upward in a long vertical direction that connects "Communicate Findings" back to "Mental Health Clinician Assessment (and Treatment)." In that context, the client (previously the examinee) and clinician (who is also the case manager) can discuss the results and negotiate any needed changes in the overall treatment plan.

Regarding external referrals, communication works in similar fashion, with the exception that some cases may need assistance in scheduling follow-up mental health and/or adjunctive services. In such instances, examinees should be asked if any collaterals who read through the report would want either (a) a face-to-face oral feedback session, and/or (b) an appointment with one or more mental health clinicians within the agency or practice who can provide any services listed in the final report's treatment recommendations. This practice is not ideal in the sense that all testing cases are not routinely provided with both written and oral feedback. However, in the practical world, some clients do very much appreciate the cost savings realized by forgoing a feedback session and proceeding immediately to treatment. Also, clients have become increasingly savvy regarding mental health disorders and psychological testing in this information age, and can sufficiently comprehend much of this information on their own (or at least the essence of the results). Clients that neither want nor need further mental health services within the agency should be discharged immediately, as denoted by the solid arrow proceeding from "Communicate Findings" to "Discharge."

Finally, cases in which face-to-face feedback sessions are indicated include those with (a) a significant and complex amount of standardized test scores (e.g., testing for *specific learning disorders* or *SLDs*), or (b) results having profound implications for ongoing assessment and treatment (e.g., neuropsychological test results that are positive for Alzheimer's dementia). Chapter 4 will provide more details regarding communication issues and how they may be managed.

Analogizing the Practice of Scientific Research with Psychological Assessment and Testing

A concluding analogy is useful here for pedagogical reasons; that is, to view psychological assessment and testing comparable to that of scientific investigation. Science has developed over thousands of years and is based on the assumption of *orderliness*; namely, that the world operates in an orderly and lawful manner. Science works by means of a combination of rationalism and empiricism, which seeks to discover these laws of nature (Gravetter & Foranzo, 2019; Graziano & Raulin, 2013; Shaughnessy, Zechmeister, & Zechmeister, 2015). *Rationalism* is the use of logic and reason to derive new from old knowledge, and is vital for building theories. In complementary fashion, *empiricism* relies on the collection of facts and evidence for knowledge and is used in science to test its theories. Together, these two means of acquiring knowledge have defined the scientific process. Next, the process of scientific investigation is analyzed further and compared with that of psychological assessment and testing as outlined in this chapter. The objective is to show their close resemblance.

Table 2.2 juxtaposes the steps of scientific research and psychological assessment and testing. Each assessment and testing case can be viewed as a single-case experimental design.

Instead of a conducting a literature review and developing hypotheses, the testing psychologist conducts an initial clinical interview and develops predictions as to which diagnoses can be initially ruled out, and which are predicted to be present by use of the clinical method (i.e., use of rationalism, logic, and reasoning). In both cases, these predictions are then *operationally defined* by the selection of psychological tests that measure the relevant constructs in a reliable and valid (usually quantitative) manner. Rather than have the study approved by an *institutional review board* (*IRB*), consisting of a group of faculty and citizenry who ensure that the proposed study is ethical and can provide useful scientific knowledge, the requested psychological tests are reviewed by a third party insurance company who ensures that such testing meets the criteria for *medical necessity* (i.e., that its findings will it have a positive impact on treatment). In both cases, empirical data are collected under controlled, standardized conditions, and thereafter statistically analyzed to determine if the predictions are supported. In scientific research, this is followed by discussing the implication of the results, along with proposals to resolve additional questions raised by the current research. Similarly, the final psychological assessment report discusses implications of the results in the form of treatment recommendations. Lastly, in both cases, the results are communicated in written and oral fashion.

The point is that the process of psychological assessment and testing, as depicted in Figure 2.1, works in close correspondence with the scientific method. This includes the benefits that come from maximizing scientific objectivity with increases in precision and accuracy that are derived from standardized psychological testing. Next, Chapters 3 and 4 review the steps in Figure 2.1 in more detail, including a closer examination of the introduced practice forms.

Table 2.2 Comparison Between Scientific Research and Psychological Assessment and Testing

Step	Scientific Research	Psychological Assessment and Testing
1	Literature review to identify conceptual definitions variables and hypotheses	Clinical interview to identify provisional and hypothesized diagnoses
2	Developing operational definitions of variables to be manipulated/measured	Developing operational definitions of constructs to be measured
3	Obtaining approval to run the study from an institutional review board (IRB)	Obtaining approval for testing from an insurance carrier
4	Data collection	Test administration
5	Statistical analysis of data	Test scoring and interpretation
6	Manuscript write-up with results, discussion, and recommendations for further study	Final report generation with diagnoses and treatment recommendations

Recapitulation

Chapter 2 provided an overview of the psychological assessment and testing process, which included five stages as follows: (a) referral for testing; (b) completing the initial clinical interview and psychological assessment report; (c) scheduling the test administration appointments; (d) completing the final psychological assessment report; and (e) communication of the results. The major steps in the sequence were illustrated in Figure 2.1 in the form of a flow-chart, including both required and potential steps depending upon the case facts. Also introduced were the practice and report forms that facilitate the completion of particular steps. The objective was to provide a cognitive roadmap of the entire process and prepare the way for the succeeding chapters in Part I of this book. Finally, the psychological assessment and testing process was compared with that of scientific inquiry in psychology. The purpose here was to demonstrate the objectivity, precision, and accuracy such practice brings to psychological assessment, diagnosis, and treatment planning within the mental health services. Subsequently, Chapter 3 discusses the steps from the initial referral through scheduling appointments (including obtaining PA) for the requested psychological test battery. The discussion is sufficiently detailed in order to prepare the reader for actual practice, including the content, organization, and purpose of each practice and report form introduced in this chapter. Thereafter, Chapter 4 explicates the remaining steps, in particular, focusing on the transformation of the initial report into the final version and communicating the results.

Key Terms

- accuracy
- actuarial assessment
- adjunctive service/s
- admissions specialist
- attention-deficit/hyperactivity disorder (ADHD)
- Barnum statements
- case manager
- clinical method
- clinical social worker
- collaterals
- computer test interpretive software
- computer test scoring software
- decay theory
- disuse
- efficiency
- empiricism
- external referral
- face-to-face service
- historical diagnosis
- informed consent
- institutional review board (IRB)
- interference
- interference theory
- internal referral
- medical necessity
- medical record
- medically necessary
- memory
- memory trace/s
- neurologist
- nurse practitioner
- operationally defined
- orderliness
- other specified neurodevelopmental disorder
- pediatrician
- preauthorization (PA)

- precision
- primary care physician (PCP)
- principal diagnosis
- proactive interference
- provisional
- provisional diagnosis
- psychiatrist (M.D. or D.O.)
- release of information (ROI)
- retroactive interference
- specific learning disorder/s (SLD)
- statistical method
- support staff

Notes

1. In this context, assessment refers to an assortment of techniques, methods, or tests, which together assist in understanding a person's psychological, biological, and sociological functioning, who may be manifesting a mental health or developmental disorder. Defined in this way, assessment is the broader classification within which testing represents a more specific component. Therefore, in contrast to other authors (e.g., see Cohen & Swerdlik, 2018), the phrase psychological assessment and testing is used because it proceeds in the same logical direction as does test interpretation; that is, from general to specific.
2. When referring to individuals who are the focus of psychological assessment and testing services, the felicitous term examinee (and occasionally testee) is used. It is both more accurate and more consistent, as opposed to alternating between the terms patient and client. The latter two terms are used when referring to individuals who are receiving more general mental health services.
3. I use the term collateral for any individual who (a) accompanies an examinee during an initial clinical interview and provides relevant assessment information, and/or (b) provides data on one or more psychological measures that contributes to diagnosis (i.e., observer-based data). Most often, this includes a close family member, such as a parent, caregiver, teacher, spouse, partner, or adult child. However, it is a convenient summary term for any individual that fills such a role (e.g., a case manager or caseworker).
4. Support staff refers to those principally responsible for scheduling appointments, or at least it is a frequent part of their job responsibilities. Most often this includes front desk staff, who also answer phones, take messages, and compose letters for communication purposes, although may also refer to admissions staff that schedule cases to be newly activated.
5. Because this author practices psychological assessment and testing within a community mental health center, which includes medically trained mental health clinicians (i.e., psychiatrist, psychiatric nurses, and nurse practitioners), he identifies a client's case file as a medical record. Mental health record may be preferred if, for example, a group or private practice consists of only non-medical mental health clinical staff.
6. I am cognizant of the arguments against presenting results in a test-by-test format, including a lack of test integration, potential inconsistencies among test scores, and a greater emphasis on numbers as opposed to the individual (Mendoza, 2001; Groth-Marnat, 2003; Groth-Marnat & Wright, 2016; Sattler, 2001, 2008, 2014; Tallent, 1992, 1993; Wright, 2010). However, the approach here (a) integrates the data gradually as the data are presented, (b) identifies and resolves score inconsistencies immediately as they are presented, and (c) refers repeatedly to the examinee as well as the data sources within the narrative interpretations following each data table. Furthermore, this approach presents the reader with vital supplementary information, including confidence intervals, percentile ranks, and clear definitions of the constructs that the data are purportedly measuring, in addition to the summary of results appearing just prior to the diagnostic summary, hence affording full context to the meaning of the standard scores. Consequently, the reader is maximally aware of both *how* and *why* the examiner arrived at the conclusions stated in the report. These points are further expounded upon throughout the book.

References

American Psychological Association. (2019). *Publication manual of the American Psychological Association* (7th ed.). Washington, DC: Author.

Anderson, M. C., & Neely, J. H. (1996). Interference and inhibition in memory retrieval. In E. L. Bjork & R. A. Bjork (Eds.). *Handbook of perception and cognition. Memory* (2nd ed., pp. 237–313). San Diego, CA: Academic Press. https://doi.org/10.1016/B978-012102570-0/50010-0

Brown, J. (1958). Some tests of the decay theory of immediate memory. *Quarterly Journal of Experimental Psychology, 10*, 12–21.

Cohen, R. J., & Swerdlik, M. E. (2018). *Psychological testing and assessment: An introduction to tests and measurement* (9th ed.). New York, NY: McGraw-Hill Education.

Confidentiality of Substance Use Disorder, 42 Code of Federal Regulations (C.F.R.) Part 2 (§§ 2.1–2.4). Retrieved February 23, 2020, from www.law.cornell.edu/cfr/text/42/part-2

Gravetter, F. J., & Foranzo, L. B. (2019). *Research methods for the behavioral sciences* (6th ed.). Boston, MA: Cengage Learning, Inc.

Graziano, A. M., & Raulin, M. L. (2013). *Research methods: A process of inquiry* (8th ed.). Upper Saddle River, NJ: Pearson Education.

Groth-Marnat, G. (2003). The psychological report. In R. Fernandez-Ballesteros (Ed.), *Encyclopedia of psychological assessment* (pp. 812–817). Thousand Oaks, CA: Sage Publications.

Groth-Marnat, G., & Wright, A. J. (2016). *Handbook of psychological assessment* (6th ed.) Hoboken, NJ: John Wiley & Sons.

Larsen, R. J., & Buss, D. M. (2021). *Personality psychology: Domains of knowledge about human nature* (7th ed.). New York, NY: McGraw-Hill.

Mendoza, J. (2001). Reporting the results of the neuropsychological evaluation. In C. G. Armengol, E. Kaplan, & E. J. Moes (Eds.), *The consumer-oriented neuropsychological report* (pp. 95–122). Lutz, FL: Psychological Assessment Resources.

Missouri Bar. (2006). *HIPAA privacy authorization form.* Jefferson City, MO: Author. Retrieved from http://members.mobar.org/pdfs/publications/public/hipaa.pdf

Peterson, L. R., & Peterson, M. J. (1959). Short-term retention of individual items. *Journal of Experimental Psychology, 58,* 193–198.

Price, L. R. (2017). *Psychometric methods: Theory into practice.* New York, NY: The Guilford Press.

Sattler, J. M. (2001). *Assessment of children: Cognitive functions* (4th ed.) San Diego, CA: Author.

Sattler, J. M. (2008). *Assessment of children: Cognitive functions* (5th ed.) San Diego, CA: Author.

Sattler, J. M. (2014). *Fundamentals of behavioral, social, and clinical assessment of children* (6th ed.). San Diego, CA: Author.

Shaughnessy, J. J., Zechmeister, E. B., & Zechmeister, J. S. (2015). *Research methods in psychology* (10th ed.). New York, NY: McGraw Hill Education.

Tallent, N. (1992). *The practice of psychological assessment.* Englewood Cliffs, NJ: Prentice-Hall.

Tallent, N. (1993). *Psychological report writing.* (4th ed.). Englewood Cliffs, NJ: Prentice-Hall.

The Health Insurance Portability and Accountability Act of 1996 (HIPPA), Pub. L. 104–191., Stat. 1936. Web. February 15, 2020.

The Health Insurance Portability and Accountability Act of 1996 (HIPAA), 45 C.F.R. Parts 160 & 164 (2000). Retrieved from http://ecfr.gpoaccess.gov/cgi/t/text/text-idx?c=ecfr&rgn= div5&view=text&node=45:1.0.1.3.72&idno=45

Wright, A. J. (2010). *Conducting psychological assessment: A guide for practitioners.* Hoboken, NJ: John Wiley & Sons.

See Routledge's e-resources website for forms. (www.routledge.com/9780367346058)

3 The Initial Report and Preparation for Testing

Overview

This chapter covers in detail the first several steps of the psychological assessment and testing process outlined in Figure 2.1. Therefore, it begins with the point of initial referral (Stage 1) through either of the following: (a) obtaining preauthorization (PA) for some or all of the requested testing services and units; or (b) negotiating a reduced-fee and remuneration schedule through a self-payment arrangement. Following the initial assessment, the preferred next step is that testing appointments will be scheduled immediately after the *clinical interview* has been completed, although some commentary will be devoted to discussing the option of scheduling them after PA or other self-pay arrangements has been resolved (Stage 3). Furthermore, much more attention will be devoted to the content and objectives of the practice forms that were previously introduced in Chapter 2.

The Referral for Psychological Testing (Stage 1)

As stated in Chapter 2, testing referrals can be dichotomized into those that are external or internal. By definition, external referral sources are significantly more variable, ranging from lay people (e.g., self, family member, supervisor), non-health care professionals (e.g., educational staff, courts, attorneys), general health care professionals (e.g., primary care physicians, neurologists), and both medical (e.g., psychiatrists) and non-medical (e.g., psychologists, clinical social workers) mental health professionals. Internal referral sources are usually limited to medical and non-medical mental health counselors and clinicians. Another differential between external and internal referrals is that the latter has more likely initiated some type of mental health treatment, at least to some degree. Irrespective of the type of referral, however, the essential objective at this incipient stage of the assessment process is to clearly define the referral source's diagnostic issues and any related referral questions. This information serves to focus and guide the clinical interview, its consequential line of questioning, and the substance of the initial psychological assessment report. Furthermore, the diagnostic issues and any related questions must be stated in a form that can be viably addressed by psychological test data.

Form 3.1 titled, "Referral for Psychological Testing," was designed to guide a referral source in providing such information using both fill-in and checklist items. In the event of an external referral that specifically requests psychological or neuropsychological testing services, admissions staff may use this form as a guide in activating the case. Likewise, this form may be completed by admissions staff when it becomes clear that psychological testing is needed either prior to, or simultaneous with, other mental health services (e.g., psychiatric services for severe depressive symptoms with associated memory problems, along with neuropsychological testing to rule out a possible co-occurring neurocognitive disorder). Once external referral sources become more cognizant of the availability of psychological testing services, and assuming subsequent reports are both helpful and timely, more such referrals will undoubtedly follow. In such occurrences, meeting with referral sources to share this form and how it may be completed can facilitate the request for further testing cases. Regarding internal referrals, this form may be presented to mental health colleagues during an in-service training session in order to educate them how to properly complete this document and present diagnostic issues and questions in a form most conducive to psychological testing practice.

In addition to obtaining information concerning the diagnostic issues and questions, it is also important to identify to whom the final results will be released. If such information is not obtained at some time prior to completion of the final report, there is a risk of an unnecessary delay in its release and subverting the objective of providing both valid and timely results. Therefore, although early in the process, this is likely to be the most felicitous opportunity to obtain the necessary release of information (ROI) forms. Next, the testing referral form and its content is examined in detail.

DOI: 10.4324/9780429326820-4

Referral for Psychological Testing (Form 3.1)

Form 3.1 titled, "Referral for Psychological Testing," is designed to be a succinct guide for referral sources to organize their differential diagnostic issues and questions regarding a case, and to avert improper referrals. It is assumed that all health practitioners have limited time such that a protracted form would either discourage referrals or, more likely, result in it being submitted in incomplete fashion. Therefore, its design represents an attempt at a reasonable balance between obtaining essential referral information and minimizing time to complete the form.

The first portion of the form is devoted to obtaining necessary examinee identifying information. Date of birth (DOB) is essential for classifying the case into one of the four available initial clinical interview forms that are differentiated according to as many developmental periods (discussed at length subsequently). DOB and other identifying information, such as gender, is also relevant to matching the examinee to proper psychological tests and their associated norms. Knowing the referral date is useful when tracking case progress and is noted in the initial and final reports (see below). A realistic goal is to complete an entire testing case within a four- to six-week duration, from the initial referral (Stage 1) to completion and release of the final report (Stage 5). If successful, this would represent convincing evidence to referral sources and the public of reliable and timely psychological service.

The enclosed dark-lined boxed section of the document is intended to emphasize the importance of providing insurance information. As will become apparent when discussing the specific criteria for medical necessity, being cognizant of an examinee's insurance carrier is vital because they vary considerably in terms of (a) what services are covered, and if so, (b) the particular criteria employed in determining whether testing is medically necessary (i.e., varying from liberal to extremely stringent). Other information here is (a) identity of the referring clinician (with instructions to print this information as many clinician signatures are illegible), and (b) the reason(s) for the testing referral. The latter are presented within a structured checklist format, which permits referring clinicians to quickly indicate one or more of the most frequently recognized reasons for testing that contribute to medical necessity. That is, the enumerated reasons for testing contain language that many third-party payers generally consider as acceptable and justifiable for purposes of preauthorizing test hours. As will become apparent, this same language is incorporated into the initial clinical report forms such that the ones marked by the referral source can be retained as part of the medical record for all testing cases. An "other" option is added for any reason that is not covered by the former three standard alternatives.

Following the dark-lined box is a series of fill-in items. These are meant to guide referring clinicians in presenting diagnostic issues that are conducive to psychological testing. Thus, *working diagnoses* are those currently listed for the client by the referring clinician (if any). As will be clarified among the remaining fill-in items, some, all, or none of these diagnoses may be in question. Next, *diagnoses to be ruled out* are intended for those that are suspected but not yet corroborated by supporting evidence. In contrast, *diagnoses to be ruled in/confirmed* are intended for those that are already listed as part of the working diagnoses, although are now in question and in need of corroborating evidence in order to remain a genuine part of the treatment plan. Thereafter, *diagnoses to be screened for* are intended for those that are suspected, although usually to a lesser extent than those to be ruled out because only a brief examination is being requested. For such request, a clinical interview and optional rapid screening measure administered during or sometime after this first meeting will suffice (see Chapter 5 for a detail presentation of screening measures). If results are positive, two courses of action are available. First, this positive screening result can be noted in (a) the summary of results, (b) the final DSM–5 diagnostic summary, and (c) the treatment recommendations in the form of more comprehensive follow-up testing services. Second, this disorder can automatically become a rule out diagnosis and therefore be pursued as part of the psychological test battery. Although more efficient, this alternative should best be undertaken only if prearranged between the testing psychologist and the referral source. To do otherwise risks being presumptuous as the referral source may have good reason for not requesting a more complete testing approach (e.g., a client's lack of insurance coverage and limited finances, simply wanting to determine if such disorder could be quickly ruled out).

Near the bottom of the Form 3.1, the referring clinician's signature renders the document official and includes a date line in the event the aforementioned date of referral is not entered (i.e., referring clinicians have a proclivity for not entering in all requested information thus justifying very occasional redundancy). Finally, there is a final small section for support staff use only, which includes a fill-in line for recording the scheduled date of the *initial clinical interview*. Support staff should record their initials here in the event errors in scheduling are in need of being corrected efficiently. Regarding external referrals, admission staff would complete this form and either schedule the initial appointment themselves, or forward it to front desk staff for scheduling with the testing psychologist. If this is an internal referral, the clinician would complete Form 3.1 and forward it to front desk staff for subsequent scheduling. The final destination for Form 3.1 is the testing psychologist, who now is apprised of such referral and the information contained therein, including the date and time of the initial clinical interview. At this juncture, the process is approaching the "Initial Clinical Interview for Testing," labeled box in Figure 2.1, which represents the beginning of Stage 2. But before reaching this stage, the requisite ROIs should be completed, along with obtaining PA for the initial clinical interview.

This broaches the vital topic of Current Procedural Terminology codes for psychological assessment and testing services. Briefly, *Current Procedural Terminology* (*CPT*) are numerical codes and service descriptions published and maintained by the American Medical Association (see Citardi, 2009). CPT represents a uniform coding system that enables health providers report an array of assessment and treatment procedures to various entities, especially insurance companies for billing purposes. Accredited organizations such as the American Psychological Association adopt these codes as central to their provision of specified health-related services, which by law they are permitted to provide the public. In measurement terms, these codes represent data on a *nominal scale* that identify categorically defined procedures (e.g., initial clinical interviews, psychological testing services). Later, the discussion delves more deeply into CPT codes when focusing on obtaining PA for the initial clinical interview, and thereafter, for various psychological testing services. But first, the ROIs.

Authorization for Disclosure of Mental Health Information (Form 3.2)

Form 3.2 titled, "Authorization for Disclosure of Mental Health Information," is designed to be accordant with applicable laws governing the release of health information (Confidentiality of Substance Use Disorder, 42 C.F.R. Part 2, 2020; *Health Insurance Portability and Accountability Act of 1996 [HIPPA]*, 2000, 2020). For instance, 42 C.F.R. Part 2 represents added protection from prosecution for individuals who have disclosed that they have a substance use disorder, especially involving illicit drugs. This is cited in the second dark-lined box in Form 3.2.

This document similarly begins with the examinee's identifying information, including name, DOB, address, and phone. This is ensued by language indicating whether information is to be either (a) released to the agency or practice identified subsequently, or (b) released from the agency or practice identified subsequently. In this case, the former is always marked and, at minimum, the examinee or pertinent collateral (e.g., parent or guardian of a minor child) will be entered on the "Name of Agency/Person," blank line of the document. A separate Form 3.2 is to be completed and signed for each entity that (a) is to receive a final written copy of the final report, and (b) is not an employee or independent contractor of the testing psychologist's practice or agency. If an agency is cited (e.g., a school), it is prudent to identify an individual recipient who will be responsible for securing the released confidentially sensitive information. Examinees or their legal representatives should sign one to themselves to establish a record of all parties that have been authorized to receive a copy.

The first dark-lined box is designed in a checklist-type format. It first asks for whether authorization is for (a) all years for which the client has received mental health services (the usual selection) or (b) only one or more specified years. Next comes the checklist of various portions of the medical record to be released. For psychological testing cases, the following are usually the most pertinent selections: (a) Psychological/Psychiatric Assessment (i.e., the initial clinical interview, mental status examination and behavioral observations, and any screening data); (b) Psychological Test Results (i.e., the final report); and (c) Medications. The latter is included because medications are typically enumerated in both the initial and final reports. The purpose of the release is usually, "Continuity of Care." *Continuity of care* refers to the degree to which a team of professionals communicate and cooperate with each other in order to maximize the quality of an individual's treatment over time. Because Form 3.2 permits the sharing of vital psychological information concerning examinees (e.g., adaptive behavioral functioning, intellectual functioning), it makes it more probable that their quality of care will be remarkably enhanced. This is why the utility of a psychological assessment report is contingent upon both (a) the precision of its results, and (b) its timeliness. That is, "Does the report address all identified diagnostic issues in a valid and timely manner?"

Instructions as to the manner in which the selected information is to be delivered appears between the two dark-lined boxes, including the date needed (e.g., court date, school meeting, date of follow-up appointment with the external referral source), along with a preference for either (a) picking the report up physically on site, or (b) by mail. The second dark-lined box delineates the general rules governing the disclosure of health information, including any limitations and date in which the examinee or collateral would like the ROI to expire. This contains a useful provision that, in the event a date of expiration is not selected, Form 3.2 expires automatically 60 days from the date services have been terminated (i.e., the examinee has been officially discharged from the agency or practice). This latter provision can be modified to suit the particular facility's needs or desires (e.g., after all financial obligations have been satisfied).

Finally, the individuals who by law possess the authority to afford such consent are required to sign and date Form 3.2, including their relationship to the examinee (e.g., self, mother, father). This is ensued by a witness signature, which is typically provided by the individual who assists the examinee or collateral in completing the ROI. The examinee's medical record should at this juncture consist of (a) a completed referral form with a scheduled date and time certain for the initial clinical interview, and (b) a separate ROI for each external entity who is to receive the final psychological assessment report.

Preauthorization of the Initial Clinical Interview for Testing

Mental health parity laws have been passed by most states, which require health insurance carriers to cover mental health disorders as equivalent to physical illnesses, diseases, or injuries. Therefore, if an individual manifests a mental health disorder such a major depression, it is covered no differently than that of a fractured leg. Furthermore, the *Paul Wellstone-Pete Domenici Mental Health Parity and Addiction Equity Act of 2008* became federal law, which precluded insurance companies from charging more for mental health services versus medical services. However, insurance companies responded by instituting the same criteria for preauthorizing mental health treatment as is done for physical disorders; namely, *medical necessity*.

Fortunately, PA of an initial clinical interview is either not required, or if it is, the criterion is simply that signs of a mental health disorder may be present. This is because an initial assessment is considered to be a routine outpatient procedure. In particular, there are two types of initial mental health assessments: nonmedical and medical. The *CPT* code for the former is *90791, psychiatric diagnostic evaluation without medical services*, while the latter is *90792, psychiatric diagnostic evaluation with medical services*. The 90791 CPT code is billed when done by a non-medical mental health clinician, including a psychologist, clinical social worker, and mental health counselor. The 90792 code must be done by a psychiatrist or other medically trained clinician. There are no time ranges for these codes. That is, they are event-based and not time-based. Both require the same face-to-face services as follows: (a) complete medical and psychiatric history; (b) *mental status examination (MSE)*; (c) establishment of a psychodiagnosis; (d) evaluation of the individual's ability to respond to treatment (i.e., *prognosis*); (e) initial treatment plan; and (f) done once when first detecting a disorder. As will become apparent, the initial psychological assessment report forms (i.e., Forms 3.3–3.6) cover all of this information, in addition to that for meeting the much more stringent medical necessity criteria for psychological testing services.

Concerning an initial clinical interview for testing, all subsequent testing-related CPT codes require a comprehensive diagnostic evaluation done by the testing psychologist prior to test administration, scoring, and evaluation services. This is consistent with testing practice in which test data are routinely interpreted within the context of information garnered from an initial clinical interview. The frequency of initial assessments permitted by most insurance companies is once per calendar year per provider. Of concern for internal referrals, however, some insurance companies consider two mental health clinicians within the same agency or practice to derive from the same "provider," which is defined as the agency. Thus, if a psychiatrist provides a CPT code 90792 initial assessment medical service, then refers to a testing psychologist within the same practice who performs a CPT code 90791 service to initiate psychological testing one month later, the latter may be denied reimbursement because they were done in the same calendar year. This seems to vary somewhat depending upon the particular policy terms.

External referrals do not have this concern as the referring clinician is by definition a different provider than that of the testing psychologist. An example billing code and descriptive phrase for such an initial clinical interview for psychological testing is as follows: "CPT Code 90791, Psychological Testing Eval." This is a required service to be done prior to pursuing psychological test administration, scoring, and evaluation services (see subsequently). In Figure 2.1, Stage 2 has been reached as the "Initial Clinical Interview for Testing." Next, the discussion focuses on how to complete this specially designed initial clinical interview. Forms 3.3, 3.4, 3.5, and 3.6 shall serve as guides. First, however, an overall stratagem is provided that shows how to complete this interview, including the manner in which to begin the written report in preparation for meeting the examinee and any collaterals.

The Initial Clinical Interview for Testing (Stage 2)

Generating the Initial Psychological Assessment Report (Forms 3.3, 3.4, 3.5, and 3.6)

In this section, how to complete the initial clinical interview for testing will be discussed in detail by making repeated references to Forms 3.3, 3.4, 3.5, and 3.6. Although these forms are very similar in outline, there are some differences in content coverage associated with varying developmental tasks. For example, collecting detailed information regarding early developmental milestones are emphasized when assessing a 3-year-old for suspected *autism-spectrum disorder (ASD)*, whereas occupational history and functioning are relevant when assessing a 45-year-old for potential *neurocognitive disorder*. Therefore, general comments are made for shared content areas while differences among the forms are explicitly identified and explicated.

In addition, although this type of interview is comparable to that of a more general initial clinical interview done by any mental health clinician, it differs significantly in focus and objective. Most apparently, the ultimate objective of a psychological assessment and testing case is for the psychologist to address all of the presented diagnostic issues and questions as sufficiently as possible. In such instance, the psychologist's job is done once this goal is met and such information is communicated to pertinent individuals; that is, this psychologist will not be providing any actual treatment intervention other than possibly giving feedback according to the tenets of therapeutic assessment (see Finn, 2007; Finn, Fischer, & Handler, 2012). In consequence, differences in outline between a clinical interview for testing versus a more standard clinical interview can become increasingly apparent.

Finally, Forms 3.3 through 3.6 contain pre-drafted statements, fill-in-the-blanks, and multiple-choice options. Fill-ins are typically denoted by a sequence of periods as ". . .," pound signs as "#," and empty slashes as "//"; the latter usually for dates in the format of MM/DD/YYYY as month/day/year. Multiple choice alternatives are denoted by words or phrases separated by slashes as follows: "Gender: male/female." The pre-drafted statements are those most frequently provided by respondents to interview questions. The gist of interview questions themselves can be deduced by the pre-drafted statements. The majority of these tend to be in the normal or asymptomatic direction, although some of the more common symptomatic statements are provided as a multiple-choice option. Presenting the interview forms in this style accomplishes the following two objectives: (a) it guides a semi-structured interview for needed content; and (b) it speeds the written documentation of pertinent facts.

More specifically, the interview process should unfold as follows: (a) adhere as closely as possible to the organization of the interview form (i.e., according to the order of the sections); and (b) allow for some flexibility in shifting among the report sections when following the respondents' provision of facts in order to develop rapport. For instance, the examinee's parent may provide vital developmental information (e.g., preterm birth) when discussing the presenting symptoms. Here, the interviewer may choose to either of the following: (a) inform the parent that such information is vital and that it will be discussed soon (and thus continue with the presenting symptoms); or (b) shift to the developmental section temporarily and document such facts. The former strategy should be employed as much as possible in order to remain on task as this will prevent the inadvertent omission of vital information. However, occasionally following the respondent in order that rapport develops properly should also be used judiciously. Using this approach, psychologists should typically be able to complete the "Initial Psychological Assessment Report" within a 50-minute hour.

Next, the discussion delves more deeply into a stratagem for completing an initial clinical interview for testing. It is in the form of a sequence of questions that should be addressed as the psychologist progresses through the interview process. It is designed principally for psychologists who are less experienced and/or who otherwise desire more guidance in the area of assessment and testing practice. Although it is detailed, with time and practice this step-by-step approach will become overlearned, more automatic, nonconscious, and rapidly done,

Stratagem for Conducting the Initial Clinical Interview for Testing

Table 3.1 presents the questions that should be answered by the psychologists who conduct an initial clinical interview for testing. Questions 1, 2, and 3 help determine if the clinical interview facts, along with any screening test data, sufficiently address the diagnostic issues of a case. Although the examinee is being referred for "psychological testing," occasionally a properly done clinical interview suffices. For instance, there may be referrals to rule out *attention-deficit/hyperactivity disorder* (*ADHD*) in adults, where upon interview the symptoms of inattention, difficulties focusing, mind-wandering, and the like did not begin until well after the age of 12 years (e.g., 32 years). In such case, ADHD is immediately ruled out as the onset criterion is clearly not met. Unless there are other disorders in question, the answer to Question 1 is affirmative, and the case is essentially done.

Similarly, passing scores on the *Mini-Mental State Examination, Second Edition* (*MMSE–2*; Folstein, Folstein, White, & Messer, 2010) screening test during an initial clinical interview for testing can be used to rule out a neurocognitive disorder. Think about the savings provided to such clients, both in terms of finances, time, and the emotional invasiveness of a neuropsychological test battery. Furthermore, reviewers hired by insurance companies look favorably upon clinicians who practice in a manner consistent with the tenets of managed care. That is, they are more likely to provide PA to such providers in future cases because they demonstrate such ethical practice and do not request unnecessary testing. In either case, an "Initial–Final Psychological Assessment Report" should now be completed and the results communicated to the examinee and any collaterals (see Figure 2.1, left-to-right horizontal arrow from "Initial Clinical Interview for Testing" to both "Communicate Findings" and "Initial–Final Psychological Assessment Report").

Table 3.1 Initial Clinical Interview for Testing: Questions, Answers, and Directives

#	Content
1	Do the collected clinical interview facts address all of the diagnostic issues in this case? *If no, proceed to #2; if yes, generate the initial–final report.*★
2	Will any available screening tests, when integrated with the clinical interview facts, potentially address all of the diagnostic issues in this case? *If no, proceed to #4; if yes, use the most pertinent screening test(s).*
3	Do the screening test data, when integrated with the clinical interview facts, now address all diagnostic issues in this case? *If no, proceed to #4; if yes, generate the initial–final report.*★
4	Are there disorders that can either be ruled out, or cast in serious doubt, by the clinical interview facts (and any screening data)? *If yes, state them with a notation that either (a) no testing for them is needed, or (b) they will only be (further) screened for by the requested tests; proceed to #5.*
5	Are there disorders that can be ruled in or confirmed by the clinical interview facts (and any screening data)? *If yes, state them with optional notation that the requested tests will examine their continuing degree and pattern in order to add any useful specifiers; proceed to #6.*
6	Are there any specific referral questions being asked that are not adequately addressed by the clinical interview facts? *If yes, state them in a manner conducive to testing; proceed to #7.*
7	Which disorders are predicted to be potentially present and will consequently be the targets of psychological testing? *List them; proceed to #8.*
8	Which disorder will represent the most fitting principal diagnosis based upon the clinical interview facts (and any screening data)? *List it; proceed to #9.*
9	Which tests are needed to detect the presence of the predicted disorders? *List the minimum number and type of tests that are best able, considering the examinee and case facts, to detect the predicted disorder(s) if indeed they are present; proceed to #10.*
10	What psychological testing services and units (i.e., time) are needed to complete the tests identified in question #9? *State them (a) independently for each test, and (b) in the aggregate (i.e., # of units, cumulative time in minutes/hours); generate the initial report.*†

Note. ★ initial–final = Initial–Final Psychological Assessment Report. † initial report = Initial Psychological Assessment Report. Answers to each question and consequential directions are in italics.

However, in practice the answers to Questions 1, 2, and 3 are typically negative and some degree of testing is more frequently necessitated. This is understandable, especially for internal referrals, because a comprehensive assessment has already been done without the capability of addressing all diagnostic issues and questions, not to mention some additional but failed attempts at treatment intervention. If such technique was not sufficient for diagnostic clarification, it is unlikely that a comparable clinical interview will suffice. Still, maximum efficiency should continue to be an underlying objective. To this end, Questions 4 and 5 attempt to narrow the focus of testing by (a) ruling out or casting serious doubt upon one or more suspected disorders, and (b) ruling in or confirming one or more suspected disorders. If a disorder is in serious doubt (e.g., ASD), it can either be deferred pending the testing for other, more likely disorders (e.g., *social anxiety disorder*), or it can be merely screened for in the requested test battery. In either case, the goal is to narrow as much as possible the diagnoses that are to be the target of testing, which in turn effectively reduces the type of testing services and number of units (i.e., time) needed.

Question 6 ensures that any related diagnostic questions are not overlooked when deciding which tests are needed. Question 7 asks the psychologist to list the remaining suspected disorders, which are to be the targets of testing and will directly influence selection of the test battery. Because the initial clinical interview represents a billable psychological service (viz., CPT code 90701 Diagnostic Evaluation), it must be attached to a principal diagnosis that the insurance company considers to be legitimately reimbursable. Although these vary among the various insurance companies, the vaguely defined "unspecified" diagnoses should be avoided because they are frequently rejected as billable disorders for want of detail. If the examinee already carries a more narrowly defined specific diagnosis, this can be listed as being the *principal diagnosis* pending psychological testing, in which case an additional *provisional diagnosis* designation can be added if so desired. This term can be inserted within the diagnostic section title to denote that the listed disorders in the initial assessment report are together considered *working diagnoses* that are subject to change pending the test results (see below).

Finally, Questions 9 and 10 guide psychologists' critical decision-making concerning a test battery, along with the needed testing services and units (i.e., time). This topic is covered subsequently when this portion of the forms are reviewed in the next section. In particular, the tests for each of the four developmental periods are enumerated near the end of the respective forms, along with the recommended type of services and units (i.e., time) needed for each test separately. Lastly, these forms provide a table that is used to aggregate the requested testing services and units. With this information, the "Initial Psychological Assessment Report" can now be reduced to writing, hence completing Stage 2. Next, the content of Forms 3.3 through 3.6 are reviewed, concluding with a vital section that discusses how to (a) select an efficient although effective test battery, and (b) request the appropriate type and number of test services and units (i.e., time).

Preparing the Initial Psychological Assessment Report (Stage 2)

Prior to greeting the examinee and any collaterals, the relevant information on Form 3.1, "Referral for Psychological Testing," should first be perused and entered into one of the initial clinical interviews for testing forms. This section examines the first entries that the testing psychologist incorporates into the initial report before even meeting the examinee and any collaterals in a face-to-face encounter.

Selecting the Correct Initial Psychological Assessment Report Form

The first consideration is the prospective examinee's *chronological age (CA)*, which is defined as a person's time on earth since date of birth. In chronological order (denoted years:months), the forms partition the lifespan into four developmental periods as follows: (a) Form 3.3, early childhood[1] (i.e., 2:0–5:11); (b) Form 3.4, middle and late childhood (i.e., 6:0–12:11); (c) Form 3.5, adolescence (13:0–18:11); and (d) Form 3.6, adulthood (19:0 and older). These developmental periods have been routinely recognized by developmental psychologists (see, e.g., Sigelman & Rider, 2018, Table 1.1, p. 6), and in practical experience comports felicitously with standardization samples employed by various psychological tests (see Form 3.7, "List of Available Psychological Tests").

However, it can be noticed that the adult form begins at age 19 years as opposed to 18 years. This is because as shown by experience, the majority of examinees who are 18 years continue to be largely dependent upon their parents who typically play an active role in the assessment process (e.g., attending the initial clinical interview and providing observer-report test data). In fact, many developmentalists define the end of adolescence as either 18 years or when an individual becomes relatively autonomous. Additionally, some major personality test developers use age 18 years as part of both the adolescent and adult versions of their personality tests (see, e.g., *Minnesota Multiphasic Personality Inventory–Adolescent–Restructured Form* [*MMPI–A–RF*]; Archer, Handel, Ben-Porath, & Tellegen, 2016; and the *Minnesota Multiphasic Personality Inventory, Second Edition, Restructured Form* [*MMPI–2–RF*]; Ben-Porath & Tellegen, 2008, 2011), hence further recognizing age 18 years as potentially part of either the adolescent or adult period. Lastly, due to the fact that standardized tests apportion their norm-reference samples based upon narrowly defined age groupings, all of these initial clinical interview forms require the computation of both years and months.

Computation of an examinee's CA proceeds from the current year-month-day minus the examinee's birth year-month-day. If such subtraction requires borrowing, a month is equivalent to 30 days, while a year is equivalent to 12 months. Thus, if the date of the interview is July 19, 2020, and the examinee's DOB is December 28, 1999, the computation would proceed as follows: 2020/07/19–1999/12/28 = 2019/19/19–1999/12/28 = 2019/18/49–1999/12/28 = 20/06/21 = 20 years 6 months. In the final result, the number of months is never rounded up. As such, from the beginning of a case the examiner is cognizant of which interview form to employ, along with the proximity of an individual to a possible older year and developmental period. This can be vital information to know in advance in cases where the prospective examinee is on the threshold of both a new form and perhaps an older set of norms. For example, if a child is 7 years 11 months at the time of the initial examination, then requesting the *Conners Kiddie Continuous Performance Test, Second Edition (K–CPT 2*; Conners, 2015) for subsequent ADHD testing is likely to be ill-advised as the norms for this test do not extend to 8 years 0 months. Although this does not occur often, not planning for such adjustments can lead to unnecessary complications, including being required to resubmit for PA of different and properly normed tests, and the potential need for rescheduling due to having insufficient time for test administration (i.e., tests for older age groups often require additional administration time). Once CA is determined, the proper form can be opened and prepared for the actual interview.

Entering the Examinee Demographic Information

After selecting the proper developmental period and form, and prior to creating and saving the document, the examinee's basic demographic information pertinent to testing should be entered. First, the examinee name, medical record number (MRN), and date should be entered. Second, the computed CA in years and months and DOB should be entered. Third, gender should be selected by deleting the on that does not match what is on the referral form. It is at this point that the electronic word processing document should be titled and saved to guard against losing significant amounts of information.

Organizing and Storing Psychological Assessment and Testing Electronic Files and Word Processing Documents

All client medical record documents should be stored onto an external portable drive, alternately termed a *thumb drive, USB drive, flash drive, memory stick,* or *USB stick* (hereafter, thumb drive), which is connected to a lap top computer through a USB port available on most personal computers. In addition to a laptop being portable and thus mobile, it is also battery powered and will remain on in the event of a power outage. Furthermore, a thumb drive that is password protected is highly recommended. Using such a device affords maximum protection for such highly sensitive medical record information because it can be removed from the hard drive after use, including added password protection, and thereafter stored in a locked file cabinet. Finally, client files should never remain on a computer hard drive and, if possible, all computers upon which client files are worked upon and stored, even temporarily (as in scoring software), should be encrypted. Briefly, *encryption* is a process that encodes data so that only select people who possess the correct password or secret key can read it. Encryption software is readily available on the internet.

In terms of organizing the thumb-drive files, three subfolders can be used as follows: (a) "Initial Assessments"; (b) "Final Assessments"; and (c) "Supplementary Assessments." The first two report types are self-explanatory, although demonstrate that both initial and final report versions of a case should be retained in order to create a case history that matches the entries made on Form 3.12, "Psychologist Assessment and Testing Services Record." Both versions can also be scanned into an electronic medical records software program used by a mental health agency or group practice, which of course should also be encrypted. Supplementary assessments are done when the final report data indicate that further testing is needed. One of the risks of targeted testing is that occasionally there may be an additional issue that either first presents itself after the first test battery is done (e.g., testing for ADHD is negative, although test data now suggest a possible specific learning disorder that escaped prior detection), or does not fully resolve an original diagnostic question (e.g., there are conflicting data among the tests concerning the presence of a particular disorder). For any additional testing that continues a particular active case, the following title, "Supplementary Psychological Assessment Report," can be used and saved within a "Supplementary Assessments" subfolder.

Within each of the three aforementioned subfolders, additional subfolders can be created for all letters of the alphabet A through Z. Examinees' reports are then placed in the subfolder letter that matches the first letter of their last names. For instance, let us assume that George H. Pappas completed an initial clinical interview, psychological testing, and then supplementary testing. His three files would be respectively saved within the letter "P" subfolders as follows: I_Pappas, George H. 2003768; F_ Pappas, George H. 2003768; and S_ Pappas, George H. 2003768. The first letter prior to the underscore denotes the type of report, I for Initial, F for Final, and S for Supplementary, ensued by this examinee's last name, first name, middle initial (if available), and medical record number (MRN).

Entering the Key Referral Information

Although the aforementioned demographics were important in starting and saving the document, the ensuing key referral information from Form 3.1 should next be incorporated into the initial report: "Examiner"; "Referral Source"; "Referral Date"; "Reasons for Psychological Testing Referral"; "Stated Diagnostic Objectives for Psychological Testing"; "Referral Questions"; "Referral Comments"; and finally, "Pertinent/Presenting Symptoms." Note that the examiner's identity is logically inserted between the examinee's identifying information and that of the referral source. In this manner, the three principal parties to the assessment are listed in proximity at the beginning of the report where such information is salient. The most common referral sources' professional degrees are listed after blank dotted-lines reserved for their names. The names of frequent referral sources can be inserted here to avoid having to repeatedly type them in full. The referral date should be entered as it appears on the referral form. It represents the date that officially begins the assessment and testing process. The objective would be to complete such services within six weeks of this date for evidence of timely service. Next, of vital importance are the reasons for the testing referral.

REASONS FOR PSYCHOLOGICAL TESTING REFERRAL

This section is vital because such information directly pertains to establishing whether or not psychological testing, if ultimately requested, will meet the standards of medical necessity. As stated previously, insurance policies and companies vary significantly in terms of the standards they apply for determining PA for psychological testing. In general, commercial insurance criteria are less stringent compared to government assistance policies (e.g., Medicaid). Therefore, the most stringent criteria for determining medical necessity across the various insurance policies was investigated, which influenced the design of the initial clinical interview report forms so that they addressed each of them. Table 3.2 enumerates the medical necessity criteria for standard psychological testing, while Table 3.3 does the same for more specialized neuropsychological testing.

Note that the language used in the "Reasons for Psychological Testing Referral" section is consistent with those listed in Table 3.3 in determining the medical necessity for testing PA. Also note that these reasons are entered verbatim in the initial assessment forms (i.e., Forms 3.3–3.6) as they first appear in Form 3.1, "Referral for Psychological

Table 3.2 General Criteria for Determining Whether Psychological Testing is Medically Necessary

#	Criterion
1	Testing to help establish *diagnosis* and *treatment planning* for a *mental disorder* when such information is not available from either (a) a comprehensive psychiatric evaluation, (b) a comprehensive medical or behavioral health (i.e., psychological) evaluation, or (c) administration of at least one norm-referenced rating scale involving the examinee and ancillary sources (e.g., family, school, health care providers).
2	*Standardized testing* with *published norm-referenced* data that matches the demographic characteristics of the examinee (e.g., chronological age, gender).
3	Evidence that test results will have a *timely* and *direct impact* on the treatment plan for the examinee who is actively engaged in treatment.
4	Testing is not for the primary purpose of educational planning, testing for learning disorders, vocational testing, disability evaluations, and court referrals (e.g., custody, competency to stand trial).

Note. In general, all four of the above criteria must be met for psychological testing to be determined to be medically necessary.

Table 3.3 General Criteria for Determining Whether Neuropsychological Testing is Medically Necessary

#	Criterion
1	When there is evidence of mild deficits on *standard mental status testing*, and more precise testing is needed to establish the presence of abnormalities or distinguish any deficits from the normal aging process.
2	If there exists evidence from either a *medical or neurological evaluation* within the previous six months that neuropsychological testing will have a *timely* and *direct impact* on the treatment plan for the examinee.
3	When neuropsychological test data can help with other assessment techniques (e.g., neuroimaging) in determining diagnosis.
4	When any acute causes of brain dysfunction have been ruled out (e.g., drug intoxication).
5	When the examinee is a candidate for neurosurgery.
6	When the examinee has been diagnosed with a medical condition that is either a recognized etiological factor for, or is associated with, a neurocognitive disorder (e.g., TBI, dementia, cerebrovascular disease, Parkinson's disease, HIV infection, MS).

Note. In general, criterion 1 is required plus at least one of the other listed criteria. TBI = traumatic brain injury; HIV = human immunodeficiency virus; MS = multiple sclerosis.

Testing." Therefore, the testing psychologist can simply retain those marked by the referral source and enter anything added into the "Other" option. They essentially include (a) helping to establish diagnosis and treatment planning for a mental disorder not available by previous clinical assessments, (b) noting that there has been a poor response to treatment intervention, and (c) proposing that testing will have a timely and direct impact upon treatment planning. The poor treatment response notation in particular implies that the diagnosis needs clarification. Together, these criteria also explain why Form 3.1, "Referral for Psychological Testing," focuses upon questions regarding diagnosis. Most often, referral sources mark the reasons for testing that they believe are most relevant and add nothing further, which suggests that they are both useful and accurate. However, simply listing these criteria in an initial report is not sufficient when attempting to obtaining PA for testing; that is, they represent arguments that must be supported by relevant factual information, especially if the examiner is testing for a complex disorder such as autism. Their main function here, then, is to help focus the testing psychologist on what information and facts need to be obtained.

Table 3.3 lists some special criteria for neuropsychological testing (i.e., testing for brain-behavior relationships). Of special note, Criterion 2 indicates that a prior medical or neurological examination done recently (i.e., within six months of the interview), which indicates the presence of brain dysfunction, is extremely useful. Therefore, referral for such testing directly from a nonmedical professional or person presents a weaker case for neuropsychological testing. However, if consultation is done with a medical professional who concurs with the need for neuropsychological testing, and this is documented within the referral, a much stronger case can be made for PA. Once this is done, any one or more of the other criteria will together increase the odds that PA will be obtained even when applying the most stringent criteria enumerated in Table 3.3. For example, there was once a patient who was diagnosed with hydrocephalous (i.e., water on the brain) who was readily approved for neuropsychological testing, the purpose being to measure baseline functioning prior to neurosurgery to remove the excess fluid by means of shunt implantation (see Table 3.3, Criterion 5). As progress is made through subsequent sections of the initial interview, the reader will note the collection of information that supports the criteria listed in both Tables 3.2 and 3.3. Next examined is how the diagnostic issues and questions recorded by referral sources using the referral for testing form (i.e., Form 3.1) should be entered into the initial report.

STATED DIAGNOSTIC OBJECTIVES FOR PSYCHOLOGICAL TESTING

Form 3.1, "Referral for Psychological Testing," includes the disorders the referring clinician wishes to (a) rule out (i.e., suspects but desires supporting data), (b) rule in/confirm (i.e., has been previously or provisionally diagnosed, but is now in question and desires corroboration), and (c) obtain screening evidence (i.e., a rapid assessment of a diagnostic possibility). Here, the testing psychologist simply inserts the various disorders listed by the referral source in each item on the referral form, along with any working diagnoses. If any categories are left blank, simply insert "None" or "None noted." Note that disorders have been inserted into each category, which are either (a) most frequently listed by referral sources for a particular developmental period, and/or (b) are long and cumbersome to type. Hence, the psychologist may simply delete those that are not selected or enter those of their own preference.

Referral questions are most frequently asked by government administrative agencies, some of which include court referrals, referrals from juvenile or adult probation, and especially a state sponsored child welfare or protective services department.[2] In fact, agencies such as the latter present multiple questions consistent with their legal charge of protecting children. In Form 3.13, listed are some of the special reasons for referral and objectives (including questions) presented by a state child welfare department regarding a requested psychological testing for a parent with confirmed child neglect or abuse. The purpose is to share such an example and to recommend that this or a similar form be composed if such referrals are received on a continuing basis. It can be a significant time saver. This form will be discussed later in more detail. In contrast, "Referral Comments" are much more frequent and, although usually succinct, share or highlight case facts that help explain the underlying rationale for the testing referral, such as "Family psychiatric history of bipolar disorder" (i.e., I wonder if the client is showing signs of bipolar psychopathology) or "Client previously diagnosed with autism without testing" (i.e., I wonder if this is a misdiagnosis).

As stated prior, the Form 3.1, "Current Working Diagnosis," item is frequently left blank, especially for external referrals who are not mental health clinicians. However, some of these clinicians tend to put in information that resemble comments, such as "disruptive behavior," or "anger outbursts." In such case, this information can be placed in the comments section. Also, if a disorder is placed in working diagnosis that also appears in rule out, that disorder can be moved from rule out to rule in/confirm since logically that is what the clinician actually intends.

Final Preparations to the Initial Report

The "Individuals Providing Assessment Information" section was most recently added to the initial report. This was in reaction to the many initial interviews that have been done with both the examinee and collaterals. When evaluating minors, the inclusion of at minimum one primary caretaker (typically a parent) is advised. With adults, collaterals can be permitted to attend the initial interview per request of the examinee, including spouses, committed couples, adult children, and the like. Based upon experience, collaterals provide valuable information from a third person perspective, along with interpersonal dynamics that are diagnostically useful. As such, it is valuable to have a written record of who was present and providing facts during the initial interview. Hence, the examinee's name can automatically be entered (as it is rare to conduct an assessment without the examinee), along with the "Contact name for scheduling" listed on the referral form when assessing a minor (typically the primary caretaker). Of note, the more formal Mr. and Ms. is used followed by surname (i.e., last name) for adults (i.e., Form 3.6), and the less formal first (i.e., given name) for minors (i.e., Forms 3.3–3.5).

Lastly, in the "Pertinent/Presenting Symptoms" section, several clusters of symptoms have been drafted for various disorders that are most prominent for each developmental period. They are in an order of decreasing frequency, with abbreviated names, acronyms, or initials in capital letters for each disorder preceding the symptom cluster for easy reference (which should be deleted in the final version of the report). Here, the testing psychologist can move the relevant clusters to the top and delete all clusters that are not listed on the referral form as being considered. In this manner, once the semi-structured interview begins, it can proceed quickly into questioning whether or not the relevant symptoms are present, and adding to or modifying to them as needed.

Also, the "pertinent" portion of the section title can be deleted if all symptoms considered are new to the case or are in question. It should be retained and the slash deleted if there are working disorders listed that are not in question. For example, if ADHD is a working diagnosis and is not being questioned by the referral source, then there is no need to ask about them and to focus only on those disorders that are suspected. In such case, the section should be titled, "Pertinent Presenting Symptoms," in order to inform the reader that the interview questions were focused only upon those disorders being targeted for potential testing. Again, this is another strategy that promotes efficiency.

At this point, all of the needed information has been incorporated into the beginnings of the initial report, even before greeting the examinee and collaterals. In addition, such information is now salient for the testing psychologist who is now well prepared to conduct an efficient semi-structured interview.

One final note, in instances where Form 3.1, "Referral for Psychological Testing," has not been completed, such information can be garnered by semi-structured clinical interviewing and/or from information collected by admissions or intake staff. Sections that do not apply, for example, a self-referral for ADHD testing, can be deleted or modified. Now, we are now ready to move through the body of the report by means of semi-structured clinical interviewing.

Semi-Structured Clinical Interviewing: Completing the Initial Psychological Assessment Report (Stage 2)

As stated above, Forms 3.3 through 3.6 are designed to be completed as a semi-structured interview. The sections that form the body of the report are in the order in which they should be covered. If examinees and any collaterals spontaneously provide information pertinent to a section other than the one presently being discussed, the psychologist may either (a) acknowledge that information's importance and reassure that such information will be asked for subsequently, or (b) move to that section of the report format and enter that information immediately. The potential problem with the latter is that the interviewer may inadvertently forget to go back to the previous point prior to the move, hence miss vital information; therefore, the latter choice is more favorable. With practice, these sections may be rearranged and/or modified in order to more felicitously match the case facts and objectives.

Filling in the Preliminary Information

After greeting the examinee and any collaterals, preliminary information not available on the referral form is first entered beginning with the section, "Examinee Demographics." Here, such data as grade in school, years of education, relationship status, occupation, and handedness is entered; the latter especially if the opportunity to watch the examinee write or draw will not be observed. Asking for handedness occasionally elicits a question regarding its relevance, to which it can be stated, "If we do testing, I need to know on which side to present the stimulus materials." Next, ask for any collaterals' names and relationships to the examinee. If other than a primary caretaker (e.g., parent, guardian), obtaining the average number of hours they spend with the examinee per week can provide a gauge as to the reliability of their observations.

Pertinent/Presenting Symptoms

Presenting symptoms are feelings, thoughts, and behaviors that are indicative of a mental health disorder, and which are based upon the subjective report of the examinee and any collaterals. As stated prior, the word "pertinent" is used when the examinee comes into the assessment with one or more well-established diagnoses that are not currently in question. In such case, this section should only cover disorders that are in question (i.e., rule out, rule in/confirm, or screen for) for purposes of efficiency. Therefore, this term should be deleted if there are no well-established diagnoses (usually from an external, non-mental health clinician).

To focus the interviewing from its initiation, two strategies can be employed; one of which was done in the preparation phase, and one which is done at this juncture. First, recall that during preparation of the initial report (see prior), the clusters of symptoms in question were retained in this section and placed in their approximate order of importance, with the most important listed first and moving down to the least important. For example, if a referral of a 16-year-old male asks for ruling out *bipolar disorder* and *conduct disorder* (*CD*), with a well-established diagnosis of ADHD, the testing psychologist would do the following: (a) utilize Form 3.5; (b) title this section, "Pertinent Presenting Symptoms"; (c) move the bipolar cluster of symptoms to the top of this section (viz., BIPOLAR); (d) followed by the conduct disorder cluster (viz., CD); and (e) deleting the remaining clusters. Again, the capitalized designations for each diagnostic cluster should be deleted in the written report as they exist merely as visual guideposts or reference points.

Second, begin interviewing for information in this section with an open-ended question concerning the most important symptom cluster. For example, if working from the referral form, succinct feedback as to the disorders in question can be provided, such as, "Your therapist states here (pointing to the referral form) that she wonders if you have ADHD. Can you tell me why she thinks so?" If working from admission notes indicating that this is a self-referral for bipolar disorder testing, the examinee may be prompted as follows, "Describe your mood for me." Soon after their response to such open-ended question or statement, which is done to begin evaluating the examinee's degree of insight, the interviewer can begin asking *leading questions* and moving down the list of symptoms in each pertinent cluster.

Leading questions are those which contain the potential answer; for example, "Do you feel distractible?" or "Does your son frequently act without thinking of the consequences of his behavior?" Although such questioning injects the confounding effects of suggestibility into respondents' answers (see Yapko, 2019), and hinders the examination of thought process because they elicit succinct, dichotomous, affirmative–negative type responses, they do significantly increase the pace of the interview, which is of prime importance. Recall that the cardinal objective at this early juncture is information gathering, whereas reliability and validity concerns can be addressed most effectively during the process of standardized testing.

Note that the particular wording of the symptom clusters is in succinct, listing-type format, with commas that permit more detailed descriptions of each major symptom. For example, consider the wording, "sadness, in the form of feeling gloomy; irritability, in the form of frequent and abrupt anger outbursts, and destroying inanimate objects." In this case, the key symptoms are sadness and irritability, which are separated by means of semi-colon, with specific descriptive elaborations of these symptoms interspersed by commas. The key symptoms mirror that of the *Diagnostic and Statistical Manual of Mental Disorders, Fifth Edition* (*DSM–5*; American Psychiatric Association, 2013), while descriptive elaborations enrich the symptom picture with more detailed evidence. The listing of key symptoms is intentional because insurance companies search for the correct wording of suspected disorders. Also note that principal clusters within a disorder are identified in italics (e.g., "social" in autism, "inattentive" in ADHD) to facilitate the diagnostic process. Like the capital letter designations that serve as guideposts, these cluster designations should be deleted after their use has expired. After all of the key symptoms have been noted, along with their descriptive elaborations, it can be asked, "Do you have any other concerns that we have not covered?" If not, they can be afforded the opportunity to add such information later as the interview process continues. The two remaining symptom-related issues here are (a) onset and course, and (b) degree of insight.

Symptom Onset and Course

First, *onset* is the time in which at least some of the pertinent symptoms first became noticeable. This is a difficult question for examinees and collaterals to answer because they must rely on *long-term memory (LTM)* without the benefit of cues or hints (i.e., a *recall task*). How does such memory work? There is strong evidence for the *constructive processing theory* of LTM retrieval (Hyman, 1993; Hyman & Loftus, 1998, 2002). According to this theory, LTMs are built and recreated each time they are encoded, retrieved, and then encoded once again to incorporate new information and/or exclude previous details. Because LTMs are ever-changing reconstructions, they can become increasingly distorted over time. Therefore, examinees need encouragement, reassurance, and prompts that assist them in providing their best or educated guess. The following, or something akin to such query, can be effective: "When was the time you first thought to yourself that there may be a problem that needs professional intervention?" As encouragement, it can be stated that even a best guess is more useful than no information. This usually prompts examinees and collaterals to search for salient events in their LTM as clues for symptom onset, analogous to identifying landmarks when giving directions, such as beginning to receive calls from preschool teachers about their 4-year-old's acting out behavior, or failing a college course for the first time. It can also be emphasized that not all of the symptoms must be present in order to be considered a bona fide time of onset; one or two prominent symptoms will suffice. Finally, although only one symptom onset subsection appears in italics, the psychologist should establish separate onsets for each major symptom cluster, especially if they are fundamentally different disorders. This is most typically the case when a *neurodevelopmental disorder*, most typically ADHD, is being queried, along with a potential comorbid mood disorder. Stated differently, the interviewer should not automatically assume that all principal symptom clusters have the same or similar onset. Psychological disorders that have varying ages of onset as part of their diagnostic criteria should invariably be investigated as to when they first evolved.

After onset for each major cluster has been estimated, their subsequent course should be investigated. For convenience, some of the more common patterns have been inserted, including chronic, symptoms becoming more apparent with age, and other variations. These can be selected in whole, part, or modified form. They are especially important to note for diagnoses that consider course as an inherent part of the diagnostic criteria (e.g., *major depressive disorder*, single versus recurrent; *generalized anxiety disorder*, which is chronic by definition).

Level of Insight

Lastly, "Level of Insight" appears on Forms 3.4, 3.5, and 3.6. Although this aspect of the assessment can be done in the "Mental Status Examination and Behavioral Observations" section, it can be better dealt with here while discussing examinees' subjective perception of their symptoms. Because evidence shows that children 8 years of age and older can provide reliable and valid ratings of their symptoms (see, e.g., *Conners Comprehensive Behavior Rating Scales* (*Conners CBRS*; Conners, 2008), assessing insight can begin at approximately this age.

The term *insight* is used here to refer to an individuals' ability to recognize their own mental health disorder. It is important to evaluate this aspect of an examinee because it is strongly associated with (a) degree of psychopathology, (b) motivation to work to reduce symptoms, and (c) prognosis, all of which are interrelated. Insight is best assessed in terms of a continuum as follows (proceeding from healthy to unhealthy): excellent; good; fair; poor; absent (viz., *anosognosia* or complete absence of self-awareness); and distorted. The latter two are indicative of a psychotic disorder, or at a minimum, a disorder with psychotic features, including *schizophrenia, obsessive-compulsive disorder* (*OCD*) with poor insight or with absent insight/delusional beliefs, and *mood disorders with psychotic features* (American Psychiatric Association, 2013).

Psychodynamic theory uses the related terms *ego syntonic*, meaning the symptoms are acceptable to the self, and *ego dystonic* (or *ego alien*), meaning that the symptoms are considered to be distressing, unacceptable, and even repugnant to the self (PDM–2 text). The former is considered more pathological because there is a lack of insight that symptoms are problematic, whereas in the latter case, individuals recognize their abnormality and are motivated to work to change them. Therefore, the more favorable prognosis is afforded the one who possesses insight as to their symptoms' problematic nature and the need to eradicate them.

Finally, insight can paradoxically be "too good." In this sense, this means *feigning* psychological disorder. This is a risk most typically in adult cases in which a reinforcement (e.g., disability benefits) is contingent upon the presence of severe psychopathology. A common clue that feigning is occurring is when an examinee's description of symptoms is much too facile; that is, reporting symptoms as if reading directly from the DSM–5 by means of a teleprompter. Because of the strong association between level of insight and diagnosis, it is advantageous to assess and report this aspect of examinee's functioning at this point in the initial report. Next, we move into what many clinicians refer to as the developmental history of the client, which here represents the mid-section of the clinical interview.

Health-Related

This section generally refers to the examinee's health care history, which covers psychiatric, medical, sensory, and psychological assessments and treatments. Subcategories consist of (a) psychiatric–medical (including visual and auditory functioning), and (b) psychological, and for all examinees under 19 years, (c) early intervention. This section is a fairly complicated one, although very important as it reviews any past relevant diagnoses, treatments and their degree of effectiveness, along with any evidence of genetic diatheses or vulnerabilities. However, the order of particular information varies across the developmental periods. For instance, the form having to do with early childhood (i.e., Form 3.3) leads off with a negative history of psychiatric treatment considering its very young age-range, whereas this statement appears further into the subsection for the adulthood period. The subsections are also separated into paragraphs to make the differing content more salient, although they are intended to be presented in one paragraph in the final draft of the report.

PSYCHIATRIC–MEDICAL

This subsection refers to any past outpatient and inpatient psychiatric treatment, respectively. Any current or previously prescribed psychiatric medications should be enumerated, including dosages if available, along with a subjective rating of their judged effectiveness on each of the major symptom clusters documented in the "Pertinent/Presenting Symptoms" section (see prior). The descriptors include ineffectual, poor, minimal, variable, and mixed, all separated by "/" to denote multiple choice, although a more detailed phrase can be used such as "causing symptom exacerbation." This is vital as it provides evidence that previous diagnoses have been either (a) incorrect, and/or (b) incomplete, which in turn supports the medical necessity for testing. To facilitate documentation of a previous list of medicines, which can be quite cumbersome as quite often names are multisyllabic (especially the generic versions), the most common one's prescribed are listed in Table 3.4. Note that they are alphabetized within targeted major symptom clusters (e.g., Anti-Psychotic) for (a) easier reference, and (b) suggesting the type of psychopathology for which examinees were previously treated.

A few more remarks concerning Table 3.4 are in order. First, the typical dose ranges are listed for each drug, which informs the degree to which past interventions were more or less aggressive. This fact is important because the degree to which a previous treatment was aggressive is usually commensurate with the level of symptom severity. Second, the internal horizontal and vertical borders are retained within the table, which although contravenes APA manuscript style (American Psychological Association, 2020), provides a more effective visual guide for the reader due to its greater detail. Third, some of the anti-depressant medications that double as anti-obsessional are associated with greater dosage ranges. In such cases, the smaller are incorporated into the larger ranges and reported only the

Table 3.4 Quick Reference to Psychiatric Medications

Anti-Depressants/Anti-Obsessional†

Brand Name	Generic Name	Dosage
Anafranil†	clomipramine	150–300 mg
Brintellix	vortioxetine	10–20 mg
Celexa†	citalopram	10–40 mg
Cymbalta	duloxetine	20–80 mg
Effexor	venlafaxine	75–350 mg
Elavil	amitriptyline	150–300 mg
Lexapro†	escitalopram	5–30 mg
Luvox†	fluvoxamine	50–300 mg
Paxil†	paroxetine	20–60 mg
Pristiq	desvenlafaxine	50–400 mg
Prozac†	fluoxetine	20–80 mg
Remeron	mirtazapine	15–45 mg
Wellbutrin	bupropion	150–400 mg
Zoloft†	sertraline	50–200 mg

Anti-Psychotic

Brand Name	Generic Name	Dosage
Abilify	aripiprazole	15–30 mg
Clozaril	clozapine	300–900 mg
Geodon	ziprasidone	60–160 mg
Haldol	haloperidol	2–40 mg
Invega	paliperidone	3–12 mg
Latuda	lurasidone	40–80 mg
Loxitane	loxapine	50–250 mg
Mellaril	thioridazine	150–800 mg
Navane	thiothixene	10–60 mg
Prolixin	fluphenazine	3–45 mg
Risperdal	risperidone	4–16 mg
Saphris	asenapine	10–20 mg
Seroquel	quetiapine	150–600 mg
Stelazine	trifluoperazine	2–40 mg
Thorazine	chlorpromazine	50–800 mg
Zyprexa	Olanzapine	5–20 mg

Anti-Manic/Anti-Mood Cycling

Brand Name	Generic Name	Dosage
Depakote	divalproex	750–1500 mg
Eskalith	lithium	600–2400 mg
Lamictal	lamotrigine	50–500 mg
Tegretol	carbamazepine	600–1600 mg
Trileptal	oxcarbazepine	1200–2400 mg
Symbyax	fluoxetine	6/25–12/50 mg

Attention-Deficit/Hyperactivity Disorder (ADHD)

Brand Name	Generic Name	Dosage
Adderall	d-l-amphetamine	5–40 mg
Concerta	methylphenidate	18–54 mg
Daytrana	methylphenidate	15–30 mg
Dexedrine	dextroamphetamine	5–40 mg
Focalin	dextroamphetamine	5–40 mg
Metadate	methylphenidate	5–40 mg
Quillivant XR	methylphenidate	10–60 mg
Ritalin	methylphenidate	5–50 mg
Vyvanse	lisdexamphetamine	30–70 mg

Anti-Anxiety

Ativan	lorazepam	0.5–2.0 mg
BuSpar	buspirone	5–20 mg
Inderal	propranolol	10–80 mg
Intuniv; Tenex	guanfacine	0.5–3 mg
Kapvay	clonidine	0.1–0.3 mg
Klonopin	clonazepam	0.5–2.0 mg
Librium	chlordiazepoxide	10–50 mg
Lyrica	pregabalin	25–450 mg
Minipress	prazosin	5–20 mg
Neurontin	gabapentin	200–600 mg
Tenormin	atenolo	25–100 mg
Valium	diazepam	2–10 mg
Xanax XR	alprazolam	0.25–2.0 mg

Source: Adapted from Preston, J. (Updated 2019). *Quick Reference to Psychiatric Medications.* Downloaded July 20, 2020, from http://psyd-fx.com/quick-reference-chart/quick-reference-direct/

Note. † denotes that the medication is used as both an antidepressant and anti-obsessional purposes; when dosage ranges differ for each purpose, the larger range is reported.

latter rather than listing them as an entirely separate class. This helped to keep the table smaller and more consistent with it representing a quick reference.

As an aside regarding treatment history, if the examinee has been psychiatrically hospitalized, any reported diagnoses given during such inpatient treatments should be somewhat suspect as occasionally they are given to ensure reimbursement of services provided. Take for example a patient who actually manifests borderline personality disorder and was hospitalized for severely unstable mood and a suicide attempt. In this case, a *bipolar I disorder* diagnosis may be listed as the principal disorder because many insurance policies do not cover intensive inpatient treatments for personality disorders. Therefore, the validity of such diagnoses should always be confirmed rather than automatically accepting them.

After listing both current and previous biomedical psychiatric medications and their perceived effectiveness, obtaining facts regarding an examinee's current and past medical functioning is the next logical area of focus. It is incontrovertible that physiological variables, genetics, medical disorders, diseases, and injuries can all have a formidable impact upon most, if not all, mental health disorders, either working to maintain, exacerbate, or even precipitate their occurrence. In fact, the previous distinction made between *organic mental disorders* and *nonorganic mental disorders* (also known as functional mental disorders) was dropped in the *Diagnostic and Statistical Manual of Mental Disorders, Fourth Edition* (*DSM–IV*; American Psychiatric Association, 1994), because of accumulating evidence that such distinction was meaningless. Furthermore, the current DSM–5 contains numerous disorders that are associated with medically based disorders, diseases, and injuries (e.g., *major neurocognitive disorder due to traumatic brain injury*; *major neurocognitive disorder due to Parkinson's disease*; *psychotic disorder due to another medical condition*). Of additional significance, the *vulnerability-stress model* (also known as the *diathesis-stress model*) of psychopathology, argues that genetic weaknesses can predispose individuals to later mental disorders (Barlow & Durand, 2018; Mash & Wolfe, 2019; see also Caspi et al., 2003 for empirical evidence of such model).

Genetic influence is measured by a construct called *heritability*, which is defined as the proportion of individual differences in an observed or measured trait that is due to genetic variance. The proportion ranges from 0.0, which means an absence of genetic influence or heritability on a trait (i.e., the trait is completely due to environment), to 1.0, which means that a trait is completely genetic (i.e., environment has no effect). So what are some of the pertinent facts? Succinctly, the estimated heritability of bipolar disorder, schizophrenia, and ASD is an impressive 0.80 (or 80%), which is higher than that of both Parkinson's disease and breast cancer (Burmeister, McInnis, & Zöllner, 2008). Other disorders showing a strong genetic link include *alcohol use disorder*, ADHD, *anxiety disorders*, and *MDD* (Lotan et al., 2014). Such robust evidence indicates that obtaining the examinee's individual medical history, along with family psychiatric and medical histories is both important and can be extremely informative, not only for current diagnosis, but also to help identify either the potential incipience of a major disorder, or at minimum a risk for later development of a particular disorder or class of disorders.

Therefore, irrespective of developmental period, references to the examinee's current and past medical functioning will be observed, including an enumeration of conditions and disorders more common to that cohort (e.g., tympanostomy tube placement due to repeated ear infections for childhood, neurological diseases for adults), with specific queries for *traumatic brain injury* (*TBI*) and seizure disorder. There are also additional prompts for non-psychiatric medications as they can cause negative side effects that mimic psychological symptoms (e.g., antihistamines can cause drowsiness).

Here, there are some differences among the forms that need to be highlighted. First, note that on the middle-to-late childhood and adolescence forms, there is a statement referring to when an examinee began or reached puberty, along with the evidence therefore, such as the growth spurt (Geithner, Satake, Woynarowska, & Malina, 1999), *menarche* (Thomas, Renaud, Benefice, de Meeus, & Guegan, 2001), and *semenarche* or *spermarche* (Herman-Giddens et al., 2012). This is a significant landmark in that at this juncture, the base rate of mood disorders in the population, especially depression, increases to that of adulthood according to several epidemiological studies (Brent et al., 2003, 2015; Garber et al., 2009; Kessler, Petukhova, Sampson, Zaslavsky, & Wittchen, 2012; Rhode, Lewinsohm, Klein, Seeley, & Gau, 2013; Rudolph, 2009).

Second, inserted into the adulthood format (viz., Form 3.6) is a brief reference to possible early developmental problems, such as preterm birth and low birth weight. This is because a full developmental section does not appear on this form for purposes of brevity. In addition, these early events may still be very pertinent to young adults, especially those in their late teens and early 20s considered by some developmental psychologists as being part of a cohort named, "emerging adulthood" (see Arnett, 2004, 2015). If there are considerable diagnostically relevant facts regarding an emerging adult's early development, the entire "Developmental" section that already routinely appears in all of the younger age groupings should be inserted and investigated.

Also related to general health care is sensory functioning, most especially vision and audition. It should be consistently checked whether there are potential concerns with eyesight and hearing. For instance, an inattentive child may not be able to effectively see the board in class, or children with speech delays may have chronic ear infections such that they cannot discriminate sounds. It should also be investigated whether there are any other unusual sensory impairments (e.g., olfaction or smell), or atypically high or low sensory thresholds that may be suggestive of a sensory (integration) processing disorder, which in turn can precipitate or aggravate behavioral problems. So much can be learned in little time assuming the correct questions are asked.

PSYCHOLOGICAL

The ensuing subsection under "Health-Related" regards a potential history of psychological testing, psychotherapy, professional counseling, and behavior therapy. The former should also have been previously explored during the admissions or intake process, with the advice to bring any generated written report that may have been composed. Especially relevant are any available standardized test scores, including IQ or achievement scores, and personality test data. Obtaining the actual data are extremely useful because they can serve as a baseline measure if the upcoming test battery includes the same or newer versions of the same or similar tests. For children in special education, obtaining the test report that first led to their placement is most important. Updated reports will only include data regarding progress toward the identified objectives and therefore will not be as useful. Finally, identifying the essential results or diagnoses should be done, which can be difficult as many reports tend to be verbose and without effective integration and summary.

EARLY INTERVENTION

For all developmental periods save for adulthood, questions regarding the provision of any early intervention services should be done. Here, speech therapy (ST), occupational Therapy (OT), physical therapy (PT), and development therapy (DT) are covered, along with any early educational intervention such as *Head Start*. In the author's region, there is an early education program with the name, "First Steps," which assesses young children for developmental delays and intervenes until age 3 years, at which time they "age out." Obtaining any assessment, intervention, and treatment progress information here is useful as it helps track how and what delays were manifested, and most relevantly for prognosis, the examinee's response to treatment intervention. If some of these services have or are being given in the adulthood period, (e.g., OT or PT following a stroke), they can be added within the "Health-Related," section of the adulthood form (i.e., Form 3.6) under the rubric, "Special Adjunctive Services."

In general, response to treatment concerns an examinee's *resiliency*, which is defined as an individual's ability to recover from adversity. Although assessment and testing are focused largely on pathology, the trait of resiliency must be considered as it impacts the anticipated response to treatment. The section immediately following continues the concept of development, although the focus there is on diagnostically pertinent events that may have occurred from the point of conception through the preschool years (generally from conception through age 5 years, inclusive). As such, this section is not routinely included in the adulthood form to reserve more time for exploring events later in life that may have a more proximate impact on functioning.

Developmental

The "Developmental" section appears in Forms 3.3, 3.4, and 3.5, and covers the period from *conception* (i.e., the fertilization of the ovum, which transforms it into a *zygote* or fertilized egg), the entire period of gestation or *prenatal* development, perinatal events (i.e., the time proximate to the birthing process), postnatal events, and the major developmental milestones from infancy through early childhood; hence, from conception through age 5 years. Of key concern here is any exposure of the embryo and *fetus* to *teratogens* (i.e., agents or events that can cross the placental barrier and cause birth defects), especially the former since *organogenesis* (i.e., forming of the major internal organs) occurs at this time. Other prenatal concerns include maternal malnutrition, lack of access to, or utilization of, healthcare, and maternal stress. Birth complications are also covered here, especially *anoxia* (or *asphyxia*) as loss of oxygen is the most rapid means of brain cell death. All of the vital facts surrounding birth are covered in fill-in format, including birth weight and length, length of term, and *Apgar test* scores if available.

Inserted next is a table of *developmental milestones*. The advantage of presenting these facts within a tabular format is that it makes the data more salient to the reader, especially denoting the presence of delays by means of asterisks. The milestones cover motor skills, language development, social interaction and communication, and behavioral tasks (i.e., bladder and bowel control). These facts are vital to collect when making a case for the subsequent testing of neurodevelopmental disorders, especially ASD. In the event caretakers hesitate to estimate these milestones, they can be reassured that a "best guess" is more than sufficient because the case is simply being made for testing approval, which will be much more precise and settle matters. As a final attempt, they can be provided with the normal ranges for these milestones so as to cue their LTMs, although this can increase error variance due to the suggestive nature of this approach to questioning. Still, in this case something is better than nothing. In recognition that some readers of the report may not comprehend these milestones (e.g., joint attention), specific notes provide succinct definitions immediately below the table. Of course, it is the responsibility of the testing psychologist to interpret the meaning of any delays and their support for follow-up testing.

To make interpretation easier, there are phrases separated by "/" that indicate multiple choice selections, one stating an absence of delays, some partial delays, and general delays. The latter two require some degree of elaboration, especially the partial delays alternative, because the variability in meeting the various milestones is frequently diagnostic. For example, delays in language, and social interaction and communication, with normal development among the remainder of milestones, is strongly indicative of autism, hence bolstering medical necessity for such testing. Following is a fundamental section for all developmental periods; namely, the family system.

Family

As a rule, the information in the family section should be focused upon the following: (a) objective facts regarding the examinee's current living situation, including with whom the person lives (e.g., spouse, parents, examinee's birth order, number of siblings); (b) quality of the primary family relationships; and (c) diagnostically pertinent, although potentially sensitive information, concerning historical and chronic and/or recent acute stressors occurring within, or impinging upon from the external environment, the examinee and/or family system. Initiating this section by asking for objective facts, such as who is living in the household in which the examinee resides, is a non-threatening segue into a general topic that can raise potentially sensitive issues. For example, if a testing referral is to determine a diagnosis of autism in a 5-year-old male, and the child's parents divorced one year prior, discussing family relationships has the potential of broaching unresolved conflicts within the parental dyad. Thus, being as factual as possible when beginning to gather information in this content area is a prudent strategy. Next, examining the quality of relationships within the family is a logical and natural transition.

QUALITY OF FAMILY RELATIONSHIPS

The quality of family relationships essentially addresses attachment patterns, whether this involves parent-child or adult-adult dyads. *Attachment* is the emotional bond between an individual and an intimate partner. It also represents a vital interpersonal behavioral system through which people of all ages regulate their emotions. They do this by obtaining security through what is referred to as *proximity-seeking*. Put simply, people seek comfort from their intimate partner when under stress. For children, such partner is the primary caretaker. For adults, it is their chosen emotionally intimate adult partner(s).

Although the attachment patterns found through experimental research and naturalistic observation do not map cleanly onto the two trauma-related attachment disorders listed in the DSM–5, namely, *reactive attachment disorder* (*RAD*) and *disinhibited social engagement disorder*, they do assist in conceptualizing the attachment style of the individual. For children, the four attachment styles are secure, resistant, avoidant, and disorganized-disoriented. The first three were initially discovered by Ainsworth, Blehar, Waters, and Wall (1978) using a laboratory procedure called the *Strange Situation*. Here, quality of attachment was measured by observing 1-year-old children's reactions to a series of increasingly stressful separations and reunions involving their primary caregivers and strangers. Approximately 60% of children are classified as *secure attachment* (Colin, 1996; Howe, 2011), which has the following components: (a) *proximity maintenance* (i.e., exploring but monitoring the location of the caregiver; (b) *safe haven* (i.e., retreating to the caregiver when stressed); (c) *separation distress* (i.e., showing dysphoria when involuntarily separated from the caregiver); and (d) *secure base* (i.e., not being afraid to explore the room; Hazan, Campa, & Gur-Yaish, 2006).

About 10% show *ambivalent attachment* in which children show mixed feelings toward their caregivers, not daring to leave them to explore the room, seeking but not being comforted upon their caregiver's return, and showing anger and resentment when their caregivers separate and return to them, hence resisting any attempts by their caregivers to show affection for calming purposes (Ainsworth et al., 1978). As much as 15% of children show *avoidant attachment* in which affective expression is suppressed and there is emotional distance between them and their caregivers (i.e., showing an attitude of indifference; Ainsworth et al., 1978). Lastly, about 15% of children show *disorganized-disoriented attachment*. This is considered the most disturbed type of bonding pattern as children appear dazed, confused, and may freeze and become immobilized with fear in reaction to their caregivers, hence manifesting a true approach-avoidance conflictual pattern with their primary caregiver (Hesse & Main, 2006; Main & Solomon, 1990; van IJzendoorn, Schuengel, & Bakermans-Kranenburg, 1999). Although these patterns were observed with very young children, it is not difficult to generalize them to older children when gathering information about the quality of the child-parent emotional bond, especially if the presenting problems include difficulty regulating emotions.

Comparable patterns can be applied when conceptualizing the attachment styles of examinees in both adolescence and adulthood. The impetus for such theorizing was a particular study in which it was shown how early attachment patterns appeared remarkably similar to those that manifest later in the lifespan (Hazan & Shaver, 1987). Somewhat later, a number of studies focused upon the increasingly apparent continuity between the different child attachment patterns and that of later adolescent and adult emotionally intimate relationships (see Bartholomew & Horowitz, 1991; Crowell, Fraley, & Shaver, 1999). In particular, these investigators accounted for the tendency for different attachment patterns to remain relatively consistent through the lifespan by proposing the presence of various covert mental perceptions of the self in relation to others, which were ultimately termed *internal working models*. That is, underlying each adult attachment style is a mental scheme or belief about the self in relation to others that first developed in childhood, which is used to explain its continuation into adulthood.

These mental schemes or attitudes about the self and others will become apparent subsequently when delineating the adult versions of the earlier child attachment styles. First, however, it should be pointed out that this kind of research has continued to have an important impact. For example, it was more recently employed by a group of scientists who investigated and conceptualized adult romantic relationships in terms of attachment theorizing (Fraley & Shaver, 2008; Mikulincer & Shaver, 2007). In any case, these internal working models have been proposed to explain the type of attachment style manifested in one's adult intimate interpersonal relationships, and are useful conceptual tools when used during an initial interview for testing for the two older developmental periods, namely adolescence and adulthood. The four different types of adult attachment styles are presented next.

First, the *adult secure attachment style* includes individuals who are able to trust others, and can easily form satisfying relationships. This includes maintaining a healthy balance between being attached to one's selected partners while also permitting them the freedom to be independent and explore (so to speak). The internal working model of secure adults includes a positive view of themselves and of others. Hence, they neither fear intimacy or closeness nor do they fear being rejected or abandoned. Second, the *adult avoidant attachment style* (also known as *dismissing*; Bowlby, 1973) consists of individuals who lack trust in others, are continually suspicious of others' motives, fear making commitments, and anticipate that they will be eventually disappointed, rejected, and abandoned. Therefore, they constrict or repress emotions, defend against potential rejection by avoiding emotional closeness, and are compulsive about being self-reliant and not needing others (also known as being *counter-dependent*). Their underlying internal working model consists of a positive self-image coexisting with a negative perception of others.

Third, the *adult ambivalent attachment style* (also known as *preoccupied*) is characterized by becoming excessively dependent and demanding of significant others, along with needing constant attention and reassurance. These tendencies may be attributed to an underlying sense of vulnerability and uncertainty in relationships. Because such people rely upon the affection of others to feel worthy as an individual, they are incessantly apprehensive about being rejected or abandoned, and therefore may manifest anger outbursts and anxiety attacks at the thought of losing an important relationship (Roisman, 2009). Their internal working model is comprised of a negative self-view coexisting with a positive view of others. Finally, the *adult disorganized-disoriented attachment style* (also known as *fearful*) is defined by an unpredictable amalgamation of both neediness and fear of intimacy, along with an absence of a coherent plan for developing genuine emotional attachments with others. Their internal working model consists of dual negative perceptions of the self and others (Bartholomew & Horowitz, 1991).

The point of providing this brief review on attachment patterns through the lifespan is to integrate these diagnostically useful theoretical constructs and research evidence into the clinical interview for testing content, here gathering vital and pertinent data to facilitate diagnosis and bolster the medical necessity for testing. Asking about the quality of current and previous primary family relationships can address potential attachment disorders in children, help account for symptoms of emotional dysregulation, identify the seeds of emerging personality disorders in older children and adolescents, and assist in detecting personality psychopathology in adults. Therefore, the questioning begins with the quality of current family relationships, including all significant dyads (e.g., parent-child, child-child, parent-parent, adult romantic partners, adult child-parent), including an elaboration of family system dynamics.

FAMILY STRESSORS

Finally, there needs to be a determination as to whether stressors are impacting the family that may either cause or aggravate symptoms of a psychological disorder. That is, ruling out the presence of acute and/or chronic stressors impinging upon the family is vital because they may explain the presence of symptoms masquerading as a genuine mental disorder. More specifically, *acute stressors* have an abrupt onset and are severe (e.g., martial dissolution) while *chronic stressors* are more moderate in degree but longer-lasting (e.g., poverty). For example, a child who is inattentive and cannot focus may be preoccupied with repeated conflicts occurring between parents within the home rather than having ADHD. As a more complex example, image a 40-year-old male examinee who undergoes marital dissolution five years prior with continuous interpersonal conflicts with his ex-spouse regarding custody. Then suddenly, he experiences the unexpected loss of a parent through death and exhibits symptoms of both anxiety and depression. Here, we have an acute situational stressor that is exacerbating the deleterious effects of a preexisting chronic stress overload. Rather than a specific mental disorder, such as GAD or MDD, these facts would suggest the presence of a stress-related *adjustment disorder with mixed anxiety and depressed mood*.

One difference among the clinical interview for testing forms alluded to prior is an added reference to family of origin in the adulthood version (i.e., Form 3.6), principally because the adult usually presents with two family units; the current system as an autonomous adult and the past system as a dependent minor child. Because many disorders have their roots in maladaptive family dynamics during childhood (Jones et al., 2016; Masten et al., 2010; Sroufe, 2005), this topic must be explored in some depth during the clinical interview. The relevant prompt in the form is open-ended because such dynamics vary so widely and are difficult to summarize using standardized statements. If such information is germane when assessing an adolescent, especially an older one, this information can be easily added. Also note that the prompt for assessing attachment style is located immediately after the reference to family of origin, consistent to the time in which the attachment style is first formed between infant and primary caregiver (Ainsworth, 1973; Bowlby, 1969).

A caveat here is in order if such questioning reveals diagnostically relevant dynamics of child maltreatment that here-to-fore has not been legally substantiated (e.g., physical abuse). In such a circumstance, such stressors should be phrased prudently using nonspecific terms such as, "There is a reported history of child neglect," or "There is reported sexual molestation allegedly done by a trusted adult." These qualifying words communicate to readers that the assessment is being based upon interviewees' statements for the purpose of facilitating diagnosis, not as an offer of proof or of objective fact. Regarding the perpetrator, the language should focus on the victim-perpetrator relationship and other variables that are most diagnostic (e.g., age of the victim, duration of abuse, degree of trust in the relationship, the presence of coercion, and whether the victim was supported by non-abusing family members). This rule applies irrespective of which section of the report such information is documented, for example, whether in this "Family" section, and/or within the "Presenting Symptoms" section. Following this rule will reduce the odds that the report will be used to inflame family and legal disputes, while retaining this information's diagnostic value. Following is the personality–social section of the report, which extends the attachment style analysis to non-family members.

Personality–Social

This section focuses on both personality and social relationships external to the family. Because the structure of personality and interpersonal activities change across the developmental periods, they are next partitioned into separate subsections proceeding in chronological order.

EARLY CHILDHOOD PERSONALITY AND SOCIAL FUNCTIONING

Regarding early childhood personality (i.e., Form 3.3), the construct of temperament is the focus of analysis. *Temperament* refers to early and predictable individual differences in basic response tendencies to the environment, which can be observed in infancy and form the basis of later personality (Chen & Schmidt, 2015; Rothbart, 2011; Shiner et al., 2012). Although there are a number of temperament systems, the dimensional model proposed by Mary Rothbart and colleagues (Putnam, Gartstein, & Rothbart, 2006; Rothbart, 2007, 2011; Rothbart, Ahadi, & Evans, 2000; Rothbart & Derryberry, 2002) is the one selected in assessing children's personality in early childhood because (a) it has been the subject of a considerable amount of scientific research, and (b) it is most consistent with the *Five-Factor Model* (*FFM*; McCrae & Costa, 2008) of personality used to measure personality traits in adolescence and adulthood. Therefore, this temperament model would seem most felicitous in accounting for continuities between temperament and later personality.

Specifically, Rothbart (2007, 2011) identified three temperament dimensions, the first two of which are apparent in infancy, while the third emerges in toddlerhood and continues thereafter. They are as follows. First, *surgency/extraversion* (hereafter extraversion) involves being active and confident, approaching novel situations with positive emotions, and easily and frequently interacting with people. *Negative affectivity* includes a tendency to manifest sadness, fearfulness, and irritability, along with exhibiting with low frustration tolerance, and being difficult to soothe and calm. Finally, *effortful-control* consists of the ability to focus, shift attention, inhibit responses, and appreciate activities that are low in stimulus intensity. The latter is vital in terms of being able to inhibit one's impulses and exhibiting self-control, and should be apparent between the ages of 3 and 4 years (Rothbart, 2011), followed by more complete development in adolescence (Eisenberg, Duckworth, Spinrad, & Valiente, 2014).

Therefore, these aspects of temperament should be evaluated in this section of the early childhood version. Considering that they are dimensions, each of these has an implied bipolar opposite, including extraversion–introversion, negative affectivity–positive affectivity, and effortful control–impulsivity. To be efficient, parents or primary caregivers can be simply asked to rate the child-examinee on these dimensions as low, moderate, or high, first providing them with a summary description of each, including the bipolar opposite. Low ratings imply the presence of the opposing pole. In this manner, the psychologist can develop a profile of the young examinee's early childhood personality.

Following an examination of temperament, the young child's social interaction with peers is also diagnostic. From ages 2 to 5 years, play becomes a pivotal activity for all modes of development, including sensorimotor, cognitive, and social domains (Pellegrini, 2009); to such an extent that these years have been dubbed, *the play years*. Therefore, the young child's social skills can be examined by estimating the sophistication of their play behavior.

Mildred Parten (1932) proposed a classification of play behavior among preschool children that can be employed when evaluating a young child's social abilities. From least to most sophisticated, they are as follows. First, *unoccupied play* is comprised of random or stereotyped movements, which have no meaning or purpose outside of simple stimulation. Second, *solitary play* consists of a child playing alone and involved, usually with toys or objects. Third, *onlooker play* involves a child closely attending to a peer's activity, along with making meaningful comments about what is observed. Fourth, *parallel play* concerns children playing in proximity, mirroring each other in terms of engaging in the same activity, although with little if any interaction. Fifth, *associative play* is fundamentally parallel play, although with more interaction (e.g., sharing items, such as paper to draw on), although in the absence of a mutual objective. Sixth, *cooperative play* consists of children interacting in order to achieve a common goal or objective.

In general, more recent empirical research indicates that play becomes both more social and complex from ages 2 to 5 years (Barnes, 1971; Coplan & Abreau, 2009; Rubin, Coplan, Chen, Bowker, & McDonald, 2011). In particular, at age 2 years, parallel and solitary play are more prevalent (in this order), followed by associative and very little cooperative play. At ages 3 years, parallel, associative, and cooperative play are essentially equivalent in terms of proportion, while solitary play is clearly less frequent. Finally, at age 4 to 5 years, parallel, associative, and cooperative play continue to increase in proportion, while solitary play falls behind further. Therefore, a 5-year-old child who continues to show high levels of unoccupied and solitary play is clearly delayed in social interaction and communication.

Finally, analysis of the presence of pretend play is of diagnostic usefulness because it signals the emergence of a capacity to construct internal mental representations of objects and events, and to act in accordance with those representations (Harris & Kavanaugh, 1993). *Pretend play* is one in which an object, action, or actor can represent a symbol for something else. For example, a stick can become a light saber, or a child can represent a superhero. Pretend play first emerges at 12 months, although flourishes between the ages of 2 and 5 years (Howes & Matheson, 1992; Rubin, Bukowski, & Parker, 2006). Thus, a 5-year-old child who has not yet developed this capacity is delayed both socially and cognitively.

MIDDLE AND LATE CHILDHOOD PERSONALITY AND SOCIAL FUNCTIONING

Scientific evidence shows that the early response tendencies termed temperament (see prior) develop into more complex and predictable personality traits during middle and late childhood, which in turn predicts personality and psychological adjustment in adolescence and adulthood (see, e.g., Shiner & Caspi, 2012). Thus, for example, the temperament dimension of effortful-control is related to the FFM trait dimension of conscientiousness (Hagekull & Bohlin, 1998; Rothbart, 2011; Shiner & Caspi, 2012), which predicts good psychological adjustment later in development (Eisenberg et al., 2014; Rueda, 2012). So, what aspect of personality should be focused upon during a clinical interview for testing? Erikson's psychosocial stage of ego development during ages 6 to 12 years, namely, *industry versus inferiority* (1963, 1968, 1982), is a useful theoretical guide in assessing children's ongoing personality adjustment. Here, children are focused upon mastering both cognitive and social skills, largely by means of social comparison. The degree to which they are successful in this developmental task determines their ongoing adjustment. Because examination of their academic success is focused upon in the ensuing section of "Education," this section can be used to examine their social competence.

As can be seen in Form 3.3, the "Personality–Interpersonal" section addresses fundamental social skills, including reciprocity, turn-taking, empathic ability, understanding the emotions of others, communicating needs, and, most especially, emotion regulation. Difficulties in this ability can manifest in a variety of psychopathologies, which is why it is includes here. Specifically, *emotion regulation* is defined as the processes involved in initiating, maintaining, and modifying affective responses according to situational demands (see Calkins & Mackler, 2011; Gross, 2014; Schulz & Lazarus, 2011). Developmentally speaking, infants attempt to regulate their emotions soon after birth. However, their strategies are simplistic, including turning away from unpleasant stimuli and sucking intensely upon a pacifier. Thus, they largely seek comfort from external sources, most especially their primary caregivers (Gross, 2014; Schulz & Lazarus, 2011); for example, by being stroked or rocked gently (Calkins & Hill, 2007; Cole, Michel, & Teti, 1994).

By middle-to-late childhood, emotion regulation skills should have become largely internalized by means of individuals developing their *emotional competence*, which includes creating effective patterns of affective expression, increased comprehension of emotions (both self and others), and more efficacious emotion regulation skills (Denham, Bassett, & Wyatt, 2007; Denham et al., 2003; Goodvin, Thompson, & Winer, 2015). It has been found that children who (a) express emotions appropriate to context, (b) manifest a good balance between positive and negative emotions, (c) understand their own and others feelings, and (d) manage their emotions effectively tend to be well accepted by both peers and adults (Denham et al., 2003). Therefore, these particular social skills are examined in examinees who are children because these are related, both theoretically and empirically, to psychological adjustment. That is, problems in these skills are predictive of maladjustment and psychopathology (e.g., feelings of inferiority versus industry), and documenting their presence supports the medical necessity for testing emerging personality-related skills and trends.

ADOLESCENT PERSONALITY AND SOCIAL FUNCTIONING

Identity formation and self-esteem are two aspects of adolescent personality that are most salient in the investigation of the "Personality–Interpersonal" section. Once again, Erikson's psychosocial stages of ego development (1968) can be relied upon, here *identity versus role confusion*. *Identity* refers to the manner in which people define who they are, the direction in which they are going (e.g., relationships, career), and the manner in which they fit into society at large (i.e., the various roles they play). As such, it is virtually a synonym for *self-concept* (i.e., people's descriptions of who they are). According to Erikson, adolescents should be in a process of experimentation to help form their identities because failure to do so results in confusion as to one's self-concept and thus maladjustment.

James Marcia (1966) elaborated upon Erikson's theorizing by proposing four identity statuses based upon two dimensions: commitment (yes or no) and crisis (yes or no). *Commitment* refers to when individuals have resolved all major questions and settled upon an identity, typically, around the age of 18 years. *Crisis* is when individuals have actively dealt with identity questions and investigated alternatives, once again done by age 18 years. Four identity statuses are derived from whether or not these two dimensions have been completed. *Identity achievement* refers to an individual who has gone through both crisis and commitment, which represents the healthiest outcome. *Moratorium* regards an individual who is in the midst of crisis, although has not yet reached a genuine commitment. Moratorium is considered second healthiest because it is assumed that the individual will eventually reach an achieved status; that is, assuming that the individual perseveres until an identity is achieved. *Foreclosure* concerns and individual who has made a commitment in the absence of a crisis. This implies that the commitment was premature and will likely result in a later identity crisis in the future. In this sense, it is considered to be an unhealthy resolution to the identity issue. Lastly, *diffusion* is devoid of both crisis and commitment and is the most maladaptive status.

Research indicates that identity formation proceeds slowly and over a long period of time, with most individuals not reaching identity status until the late teens or early 20s. More specifically, one study found that only 4% of 15-year-olds and 20% of 18-year-olds had achieved identity status (Meilman, 1979). However, identity formation does matter and adolescents who are especially struggling to develop a clear sense of who they are during the moratorium period of middle school and high school can manifest a variety of psychopathologies of a clinical nature. Therefore, a variety of questions can be asked that address identity formation, including how examinees describe their personality to someone who does not know them, the type of relationships they prefer, their interests, and their future goals (e.g., career, family). Such questioning also gives an indication to as to examinees' ability to introspect and their emotional competence.

While identity or self-concept refers to how people define who they are, *self-esteem* refers to their evaluation of that definition; that is, ranging from low to high. The evidence shows that, while a minority of adolescents experience a decline in self-esteem, the majority either (a) maintain moderate-to-high levels during the teenage years from 13 to 18 years, or (b) complete this developmental period with higher self-esteem than they had at the beginning (Erol & Orth, 2011; Morin, Maiano, Marsh, Nagengast, & Janosz, 2013). Evidence also indicates that moderate-to-high self-esteem during and completing adolescence (versus low self-esteem) is vital for achieving better physical and mental health, more favorable career and financial prospects, and less involvement in crime (Trzesniewski et al., 2006). Because this aspect of personality is such an important predictor of psychological adjustment and maladjustment during this developmental period, examinees can be asked to rate their overall self-esteem and to provide some reasons why they feel this way.

ADULTHOOD PERSONALITY AND SOCIAL FUNCTIONING

As stated prior, research shows that identity formation takes a considerable amount of time, at least until the late teens or early 20s. Furthermore, some people continue in a moratorium status for years into adulthood, while others reopen the question and recycle through the aforementioned identity statuses throughout young and middle adulthood (i.e., 20s through 60s; Anthis & LaVoie, 2006; Kroger, 2007). Even during late adulthood, some adults may be either reworking or strengthening their identities depending upon the circumstances (Zucker, Ostrove, & Stewart, 2002).

For these reasons, some of the same identity questions can be asked for adolescent examinees (see Form 3.5), including self-perception. However, also investigated are examinees' past experience in relationships with people and how that has contributed to their perceptions of others; including any maladaptive patterns that appear to reoccur (e.g., violations of trust, psychological abuse, becoming involved in controlling relationships, counter-dependence). Such information addresses adult examinees' identity status, attachment style (i.e., internal working model), and clues as to FFM traits (e.g., neuroticism, conscientiousness) and maladaptive personality traits suggestive of a personality disorder. For example, an adult examinee reported that if others provide her with support and care, she actively does things to subvert these efforts. When I asked why she does this, she stated, "I don't feel I deserve it." This dynamic suggests the presence of a *masochistic personality syndrome*, which should be corroborated by standardized personality testing using an appropriate norm-reference group.

Because for adults information regarding (a) identity status, (b) attachment style, and (c) maladaptive and adaptive personality traits are being simultaneously examined, this section is left in a more open-ended manner. Here, the testing psychologist should fill in what is most pertinent to the case. That is, this section should be examined and elaborated upon as needed if one or more personality disorders or personality-related issues represent a principal component of the testing referral. In contrast, this section should be deemphasized if the testing referral is more circumscribed to investigating the presence of one or more clinical syndromes (e.g., a psychotic disorder). In the latter case, noting the effects of the symptoms on social functioning would be sufficient (e.g., documenting the presence of social withdrawal as a consequence of severe anhedonia). Immediately following is the examinee's educational functioning, which addresses not only cognitive functioning but also sheds more light on social and personality functioning (e.g., achievement motivation, choice of major).

Educational

Here, the particular organization of the "Education" section for testing will be discussed. In essence, the following should be covered in this section: (a) current grade level (or highest grade completed); (b) current and typical grades earned in previous grade levels (especially noteworthy are abrupt changes in grade performance); (c) grade retentions and reasons therefore (i.e., social immaturity and/or cognitive delay); (d) special education placement, and if affirmative, type of primary and secondary classification (if any); (e) behavior-related grades or behavioral feedback by the teacher(s) (lower grade levels only); and (f) any evidence of severe behavioral misconduct, such as being asked to leave daycare or preschool, suspensions (i.e., in-school or out-of-school, the latter are more severe), or expulsions and reasons therefore. Note that achievement-related information is prioritized in the first paragraph of this section, ensued by behavioral information in the second and remaining paragraphs (if any).

ACADEMIC-RELATED INFORMATION

Distinctive patterns of grade changes suggest differing psychological disorders. First, abrupt declines subsequent to above average to superior performance suggests the presence of a stress/trauma-related, mood, anxiety, and/or substance related disorder. Second, declines beginning in third or fourth grade in only certain courses suggest a *specific learning disorder* (SLD). It is the transition to one of these two grade levels (contingent upon the particular school district curriculum) that the workload increases are significantly more than simply linear. Therefore, whatever compensatory strategies a child with an undiagnosed SLD is utilizing up to that point will likely begin to falter, resulting in declining achievement in courses that depend upon those particular skills. Third, poor grades from the initiation of formal education, especially from the point of first grade and thereafter, is suggestive of a more pervasive neurodevelopmental disorder, including *intellectual disability* (ID), ADHD, and/or ASD. Of note, the early childhood form (viz., Form 3.3) contains a statement concerning the quality of the examinee's play behavior. This is because as stated prior, these are the play years where both cognitive and social development are manifest (Pellegrini, 2009). Hence, documenting the presence of pretend play (Howes & Matheson, 1992; Rubin et al., 2006), which illustrates the acquisition of symbolic thought, is important as it supports the presence of expected cognitive advancement (i.e., preoperational thinking; see Piaget, 1926, 1952). Additional descriptors are more behavioral in quality, including "aggressive" and "isolative."

In the event the examinee is or was in special education, and was given an *Individualized Education Program* (IEP) within the United States (*Individualized Education Plan* outside the United States), then in most cases there has been some type of standardized psychoeducational testing done by the school system. Therefore, asking for a copy of the testing report that resulted in the examinee's special education placement (and not simply a progress report), is very useful because it would typically include standardized achievement and/or intelligence test (IQ) scores. If this report is not available, then asking for as much information regarding (a) the tests administered, and (b) the essential results of should be pursued.

In the early childhood form (viz., Form 3.3), there is a statement that the examinee may not yet be enrolled. If there were one or more grade retentions, it is important to determine which grade levels, and for what reasons. Grade repeats in the lowest levels (i.e., kindergarten, first grade) are usually due to either social immaturity and/or performing below grade level expectations (i.e., cognitive delays), although occasionally are they due to absenteeism associated with childhood illness. These distinctions are obviously of diagnostic import as the social immaturity suggests the presence of psychological disorders that hinder behavioral and emotional self-regulation (e.g., ADHD, *oppositional defiant disorder* (ODD), *disruptive mood dysregulation disorder* (DMDD)), while being below grade level is more indicative of ID or SPD). Of course these facts are only suggestive and must be integrated with other clinical interview data to support or reject these hypotheses.

BEHAVIOR-RELATED INFORMATION

Finally, garnering information regarding the examinee's behavior within the academic environment is also extremely diagnostic. For examinees in early childhood who are enrolled in the lowest grades (i.e., daycare and preschool through kindergarten), the primary objectives lie in obtaining (a) behavior-related grades recorded on report cards (e.g., satisfactory, in need of improvement), and (b) teachers' written comments concerning the examinee's behavior. This is because severe forms of discipline, such as school suspensions and especially expulsions, seem to be rare at these lower grade levels. Therefore, a reference to any behavior-related grades or feedback from the teacher regarding the examinee is made at this juncture. Concerning daycare and preschool environments, children who are profoundly disruptive and aggressive are typically asked to leave as they lack the resources to manage such severe psychopathology. If such has occurred, it should be documented here and/or among the presenting symptoms. A statement to that effect appears at the end of the "Educational" section in the early childhood form (viz., Form 3.3).

Beginning in middle and late childhood, there are references to (a) behavior-related grades, (b) behavioral feedback from the teacher (as with younger children), and (c) references to the need for (or lack of the need for) more severe forms of discipline, including suspensions and expulsions and the reasons therefore. The latter is important to document because school systems vary in terms of their tolerance for rule-breaking behavior. Therefore, a suspension due to possession of drug paraphernalia, suggestive of both a *substance-related disorder* and potentially *conduct disorder (CD)*, depending upon any additional major rule-breaking behaviors such as vandalism, is significantly different from a suspension that is due to being repeatedly disrespectful towards authority, which of itself is suggestive of ODD. Lastly, there is an optional statement regarding a history of being asked to leave.

The adolescence form (viz., Form 3.5) focuses investigation only upon (a) any available feedback from teacher(s), and (b) the presence or absence of the more severe forms of discipline, including suspensions and expulsions. This is due to the fact that for higher grade levels, schools no longer include behavioral grades in their academic report cards or progress reports. Because there is much more educational information, references back to preschool and daycare are not usually needed, although can be inserted if deemed relevant.

The adulthood form (viz., Form 3.6) is more typically a history of educational attainment, beginning with the year and type of high school graduation; namely high school diploma or certificate of completion. The *high school diploma* signifies that the student has met all of the curriculum and examination requirements for graduation, while the *high school certificate of completion* means that the student has passed an alternate plan of study that does not include all of the requirements for graduation. More specifically, certificates show that the student has mastered a particular vocational skill, typically associated with a job requirement (e.g., coding a type of computer language). Thereafter, any additional higher education should be documented as follows: (a) an estimated number of years of completed college coursework; (b) at which institution(s) the examinee matriculated; (c) any earned formal degrees; and (d) in what fields of study. Such documentation reveals information concerning an examinee's cognitive abilities, motives to achieve, and traits associated with a chosen major area of study.

Thereafter, pre-drafted statements regarding alternate educational paths are provided in this section of the report. These include the following: (a) discontinuing school and at what grade level; (b) achieving a high school diploma via alternative adult education or a general equivalency diploma (GED), the latter which is considered a genuine high school diploma; and, finally, (c) completing any certificate program(s), such as a Certified Nursing Assistant (CNA), Emergency Medical Technician (EMT), and Phlebotomy Certification. Lastly, it is important to document what kind of grades examinees earned through their formal academic learning, especially noting any significant changes in grades from elementary, middle, and high school through college, and exploring reasons therefore. This includes noting whether special education was provided, along with their primary classifications, especially Learning Disability and Mild Mental Handicap. In the event an examinee was classified with a learning disability within the school system, in mathematics for example, it should be listed in the DSM summary of the report with a parenthetical note so indicating the proper source; for example, F81.2 *Specific Learning Disorder, With impairment in mathematics* (per school classification).

Occupational

The "Occupational" section appears only in the adolescence and adulthood developmental periods (i.e., Forms 3.5 and 3.6). In adulthood, occupational functioning represents a fundamental area of productivity in society and is associated with both income and status. As such, it is placed prior to extracurricular activities and includes more pre-drafted prompts. In adolescence, the order is reversed and there is only one brief pre-drafted prompt due to its lesser relevance. If the examinee is younger than employment age, this section can be deleted or the "No history" phrase can be selected.

Regarding the adulthood occupational section, note that there are prompts for documenting the examinee's current employment status, employment history, and pattern of an erratic work history and reasons therefore. In addition, documenting an adult examinee's longest employment, and in what capacity, are useful diagnostic facts as they suggest a best case scenario for this individual in this area of functioning. Similarly, this information generally contributes to an estimate of *premorbid level of functioning*, which is defined as a person's most favorable degree of overall adjustment prior to the onset of abnormality. The higher such functioning, the more favorable the *prognosis* or predicted response to treatment.

Extracurricular

By definition, *extracurricular* refers to activities that are outside of the normal or expected course or career. Thus, they include such things as sports (e.g., basketball, bowling, softball), clubs (e.g., debate or chess club at school, school board member), organizations (e.g., Boy Scouts or Girl Scouts, volunteer positions), and hobbies (e.g., arts and crafts, painting, reading). Diagnostically, they signify that the individual is attempting to go beyond the normal and expected, such as school or work responsibilities. Such information sheds light upon an examinee's developing identity or self-concept (i.e., self-definition), self-esteem (i.e., low, moderate, or high) and self-confidence, and *adaptive behavioral functioning* (especially social and practical skills). Withdrawal from such involvement due to loss of interest and *anhedonia* (Solin, 1995), may represent early signs of mood disturbance such as depression (Rudolph, Hammen, & Daley, 2006).

Statements within the "Extracurricular" section regard both current and past involvement. If affirmative, those activities should be documented by listing them by name and in reverse chronological order (i.e., from most to least recent as typically done in a vita). This information should be supplemented by statements describing the quality of the examinee's participation (e.g., how good or successful), along with the degree of satisfaction or enjoyment. The focus should be on the extent to which the presenting symptoms deleteriously affected performance and/or satisfaction, which provides a convenient barometer as to their severity. If relatively unaffected vis-à-vis the presenting symptoms, such evidence signifies resilience on the part of the examinee. *Resilience* represents the ability to withstand greater degrees of stress before succumbing to various types of psychopathology. As such, it contributes to more favorable prognoses and should be documented when signs of it are revealed.

Substance Abuse

Substance use regards an examinee's pattern of consumption of any psychoactive chemical compounds that may cause or exacerbate various forms of psychopathology. *Psychoactive substances* are ingested by people for the purpose of altering mood, cognition, and/or behavior. In the majority of testing referrals from other mental health clinicians, investigation of whether or not a substance-related disorder exists has likely already been completed, and therefore is not typically part of the diagnostic issues presented. Similarly, substance abuse questions also do not arise very frequently in other types of referrals, including self-referrals. Finally, substance use issues rarely present in the youngest two developmental periods; that is early childhood and middle-to-late childhood. For the latter reason, this content area does not even appear in the two childhood forms (viz., Forms 3.3 and 3.4).

Yet, there is always a statistical risk that a *substance-related disorder* is present yet undetected. Research shows that substance use problems co-occur quite frequently with other disorders for multiple reasons. For example, someone may use drugs in an attempt to reduce symptoms of depression or anxiety, also known as *self-medicating*. In addition, psychological disorders, such as anxiety and depression, are so common that they co-exist with substance-related disorders by chance alone. Another possibility is that drug intoxication or withdrawal can cause symptoms of anxiety and depression. Therefore, substance use should be a routine and integral area of investigation in all clinical interviews done for psychological testing, beginning with adolescence cases and throughout adulthood. If there are any suggestions of substance use issues in older childhood, this section can be added to Form 3.4 and investigated.

Therefore, a "Substance Use" section appears in both the adolescent and adult clinical interviews for testing (i.e., Forms 3.5 and 3.6). If it is absolutely clear from the referral source and/or recent mental health or substance abuse evaluation reports that there is no such problem, then "Unremarkable" can be selected. However, in the vast majority of the cases, substance abuse problems are asked irrespective of the referral source's stated differential diagnostic issues and questions. In particular, it should be asked pointedly, "Have you ever had a drug or alcohol problem?" If the referral source has made absolutely no mention of substance-related problems, the aforementioned question can be prefaced by first indicating that the next questions, "are strictly routine," and are asked simply to document in the report that the issue was broached and "Denied," which is the correct selection if any such problems are disavowed. The purpose is to avoid taking the examinee by surprise and implying that there is reason to suspect that they have such a problem. If this qualification is not provided, this may have deleterious effects on the rapport needed for further information gathering and cooperation with testing.

If the examinee and/or collaterals answer in the affirmative, the following needs to be documented: (a) each substance by name individually; (b) date or age of onset; (c) estimate of severity; (d) course over time; (e) date of abstinence (if any); (f) current and past types of treatments (if any); and (g) the rated effectiveness of each attempted treatment. Of special focus should be identifying an examinee's drug of choice (e.g., cocaine) if one is indicated. This information may indicate an attempt at self-medicating (e.g., alcohol as a depressant for anxiety and tension) or providing something lacking in one's personality (e.g., a stimulant to bolster low-self-esteem and confidence). In the alternative, drug use may have been indiscriminate, in which instance this section will be more detailed and reflect the presence of impulsivity and extremely poor decision-making and judgment. In addition, the examinee's degree of insight, acknowledgment of a problem, and extent of denial, should all be assessed and documented as indicated by the final prompt in this section. Lastly, and to reiterate, although this section is not available in the two younger childhood forms, it can be inserted as needed.

Legal

In contrast to substance use, legal matters should always be investigated. However, the specific issues do vary across the developmental periods. Therefore, this section has been subdivided into (a) childhood and adolescence, and (b) adulthood.

CHILDHOOD AND ADOLESCENCE

Beginning with childhood through adolescence (i.e., Forms 3.3–3.5), the shared legally related issues are (a) minors who are declared a ward of the state for purposes of child protection and welfare (most typically under juvenile court jurisdiction), and (b) custody and guardianship determinations (usually under family court jurisdiction for minor children or adolescents). Adolescence adds a potential third issue of juvenile delinquency, which suggests the presence of CD and/or substance abuse issues.

Child Protection and Welfare   A government agency charged with protecting minors regards children who are typically in foster care, with the initial primary goal of unification with the biological parent(s). Technically, the foster parent(s) is acting as a surrogate under the authority and supervision of the state pursuant to its *parens patriae* power (i.e., "state as country as the parent"); thereafter being labeled a "Child in Need of Services" (CHINS). Hence, these facts should be documented in this section.

Custody and Guardianship   *Custody* regards the assignment of parental responsibility for the protection and care of a child. Legally speaking, custody matters concern one of two issues, including (a) who can legally provide consent for treatment (i.e., legal custody), and (b) with whom the minor child resides (i.e., physical custody). *Legal custody* is most frequently shared equally between the parents, which means that they both must provide consent for a minor's mental health services unless it constitutes emergency care (e.g., suicide prevention). However, this requires some degree of cooperation between the parents who share legal custody. If the Court deems the parental relationship to manifest immutable animosity, however, sole legal custody may then be granted to one of the parties. In either case, obtaining a copy of the most recent court order that determined how legal custody was granted is vital and should be documented in this section of the initial psychological assessment report for testing.

On the other hand, *physical custody* is typically granted to only one party according to the *best interests of the child* test, which means that the child is to be placed with the parent that is deemed ablest to meet the child's emotional and physical needs. In such case, the child resides with the "custodial parent" and has visitation with the noncustodial parent who usually also provides child support. Visitation is usually structured according to guidelines, for example (a) one night during the week to be mutually agreed by the parents, (b) every other weekend, (c) alternating holidays, and (d) half of the summer recess from school (see, e.g., Indiana Parenting Time Guidelines, 2006). Less frequently, the Court may grant the parents shared physical custody, in which case the child spends approximately 50% of the time at both parents' residences. In either case, physical custody is more relevant to the "Family" section when documenting with whom the child resides, along with associated family dynamics and any impact they may have on the presenting symptoms; whether beneficial or deleterious. Especially noteworthy is (a) whether the biological parents are cooperating or subverting each other's efforts in raising their child, and (b) whether the child is maintaining consistent visitation and contact with the noncustodial parent.

Another legal matter that may be an issue here concerns guardianship. A *guardianship* exists when the court authorizes a legal relationship between an adult and a minor child wherein the former has decision-making power and a corresponding duty of care for the latter; this includes providing consent for mental health services. Typically, the *guardian* is an extended family member, such as a grandparent, who has been intimately involved in the child's life and is knowledgeable about developmental history information. Because children and adolescents may have issues concerning child protective services intervention, custody, and guardianship, statements addressing them are provided in this section subsequent to the more common alternatives, "Unremarkable" and "Denied." Here, the unremarkable selection can be employed if the minor resides within an intact family system and there is clearly no evidence of these legal issues. The denied alternative should be used if any questioning regarding these issues was done and yielded negative responses.

Juvenile Delinquency   *Juvenile delinquency* regards a minor child or adolescent, typically between the ages of 10 and 18 years, who has committed an act that has violated the law in some way. Hence, juveniles commit *delinquent acts* and not crimes per se. There are generally two kinds of delinquent acts. The first concerns an offense that would be considered a crime if done by an adult (e.g., theft). The second is an act that would be considered perfectly legal if done by an adult, referred to as *status offenses* (e.g., alcohol possession or consumption, truancy, curfew violations). If the criminal-type offense is sufficiently egregious (e.g., murder), a motion to try the juvenile as an adult can be made, in which case the alleged act and indictment would be considered a bona-fide crime.

As such, pre-drafted phrases regarding evidence of juvenile delinquency are added to the legal section of both the middle and late childhood form and adolescence form (i.e., Forms 3.4 and 3.5). The first prompt concerns a history of being detained within a juvenile detention center (JDC) and reasons therefore. If affirmative, dates of internment and duration should be added, along with documentation of any additional behavioral problems while detained. If the examinee does not have a history of JDC detainment, a second prompt is presented for a listing of delinquent acts for which dates should be inserted, along with information regarding possible probation. Any violations of probation should not be overlooked as they inform responsiveness to treatment intervention and prognosis.

ADULTHOOD

Lastly, the adulthood form (i.e., Form 3.6) legal section focuses on criminal violations, and includes a listing of relatively common *misdemeanors* and *felonies* that should be documented if present because they show a pattern of not being able or willing to comport one's behavior in accordance with societal expectations. At minimum this may suggest impulsivity (i.e., acting without due consideration of the consequences of one's behavior), substance misuse, and/or or characterological psychopathology such as *antisocial personality* or *psychopathy* (i.e., acting antagonistically towards society). The latter is especially likely if the pattern of illicit conduct can be traced back to the age of minority. If some of these are present, it is important to distinguish between those that were only alleged versus those that represented actual convictions. The latter are likely to be less severe offenses (e.g., voluntary manslaughter) than actually occurred (e.g., second degree murder) due to plea bargaining.

Briefly, *plea bargaining* is a process that provides a way for prosecutors to (a) reduce their caseloads while (b) producing higher conviction rates that reflects positively on their work productivity. In turn, defendants are able to reduce the risk of a much harsher penalty. Assuming that defendants actually committed the more serious offenses as reflected in their original indictments, the ultimate plea agreements will tend to underestimate the true severity of their actions. Therefore, it is wise to make this correction when assessing an examinee's criminal record.

Furthermore, the age and duration of any incarcerations should also be investigated, especially noting the examinee's quality of behavior during time in prison as reflecting upon their predicted response to treatment intervention (as was pointed out when discussing a juvenile's response to detainment in JDC. Also similar to investigating JDC internments, the typical negative selection should typically be "denied" versus "unremarkable" because, as stated prior, potential legal intervention should routinely be queried supported by evidence of a relationship between mental disorder and illegal behavior (Monahan, 1992), especially substance abuse, antisocial personality, and psychotic symptoms (Link & Stueve, 1994; Modestin & Ammann, 1996; Planansky & Johnston, 1977; Wallace et al., 1998).

Mental Status Examination and Behavioral Observations

At this juncture of the clinical interview for testing, the "Mental Status Examination (MSE) and Behavioral Observations" section focuses upon data provided directly by the examinee and any collaterals. In that sense, these data represent *signs* (i.e., objectively observed manifestations) rather than symptoms (i.e., subjectively reported experiences) of psychopathology. The advantage of this information is that it does not rely upon respondents' long-term memory (LTM), which as has been previously discussed, is faulty to the extent it is based upon a reconstruction of past events versus a precise replication (Hyman, 1993; Hyman & Loftus, 1998, 2002)). However, its potential weakness and inaccuracy lies in the inferences that the clinician must make when interpreting such information. For example, when an examinee becomes "teary-eyed," is that an indication of happiness or a more negative emotion? If the latter, is it a sign of sadness, a result of frustration, or perhaps a sense of hopelessness? In such circumstances, context, clinical experience, and expertise must be relied upon and utilized. In part, context regards the consistency of signs noted in this section with those reported in the presenting symptoms section. To the extent they are consistent (i.e., reliable), this bolsters their accuracy, along with the diagnostic inference derived therefrom. In contrast, to the extent they are discordant, such divergence must be accounted for in some manner during the psychological assessment process.

While we are on the subject of process, this written section of the initial assessment report is invariably completed after the interview is finished, and the examinee and any collaterals have exited the room for either rescheduling or leaving the facility if only the initial clinical interview was needed. This provides examiners the time to reflect on their observations as they proceed through the remaining subsections that are partitioned as follows.

NOTED INFLUENCE OF PSYCHOTROPIC MEDICATIONS

This first subsection is actually an optional note, which is intended to remind examiners to qualify their inferences according to the potential effects of any psychiatric (or other) medications they may be on during the course of the interview. That is, many medically trained referral sources, whether psychiatric or non-psychiatric, may have already started biologically based treatment with a variety of psychotropic medications and for a variety of reasons. First, their patients expect some attempt to relieve their symptoms after being seen. Second, many medical practitioners use a patient's response to a particular medication to further inform diagnosis. For example, if an individual's anxiety and panic attacks are reduced after being prescribed Zoloft, this fact bolsters the diagnosis of panic disorder. So, during a clinical interview for psychological testing, we now have a diagnostic conundrum as follows.

By definition, *psychotropic medications* are capable of affecting people's minds, emotions, thoughts, and behavior. Of these, some must be prescribed and taken continuously, manifesting their therapeutic effects only after several weeks of use, and after building appropriate blood levels and restoring the balance of certain natural substances in the brain. For example, a therapeutic Lithium blood level in the treatment of bipolar psychopathology is 0.6 and 1.2 milliequivalents per liter (mEq/L; Cafasso, 2018). Another example is *Zoloft* (or *Sertraline*), which increases the level of serotonin by blocking its reuptake during interneuron communication. Others are taken *PRN*, which is a Latin term *pro re nata* that translates as, "as the thing is needed," or as-needed. Examples include *Xanax* (or *Alprazolam*), which is to be taken immediately when an individual experiences the incipience of a panic attack. This is because Xanax works by immediately binding to *GABA* receptors and stimulates its production, which is an inhibitory neurotransmitter that slows all activity; sometimes referred to as our body's natural tranquilizer (Recovery Village, 2020). Perhaps a more frequent example is *Vyvanse* (or *Lisdexamfetamine Dimesylate*), which is typically prescribed for ADHD. Specifically, Vyvanse begins to work after only 90 minutes by increasing *norepinephrine* (i.e., a stimulant) and *dopamine* (i.e., a natural substance that enhances pleasure and reward), and lasts about 14 hours due to a longer-action, steady-release chemical feature. The psychotropic effects are to improve concentration and focus, while reducing both hyperactive and impulsive behavior.

Taken together, the major implication for the assessing psychologist is that this ongoing biomedical treatment now presents what researchers commonly refer to as a *confounding variable*, which is an unintended, co-occurring factor that may also account for the observed outcome. Specifically, if an examinee is under the influence of one or more of these medications and is not showing any signs of the suspected disorder(s), the examiner can no longer be certain whether or not this is due to (a) the fact that the examinee truly does not have the disorder(s), or (b) the examinee does truly have the disorder(s) but the medication(s) are having their intended therapeutic effects. Occasionally, savvy referring medically trained clinicians occasionally do advise their patients to temporarily suspend taking a faster-acting PRN-type medication for the initial clinical interview that begins the psychological assessment process. This occurs most frequently when the clinician is a colleague who refers cases on a continuing basis. However, even in these situations, examinees will likely (and should) be under the influence of aforementioned medications that are slower-acting and must be taken continuously for maximum therapeutic effects. In fact, abrupt discontinuation of some of these slower-acting medications can be deleterious to patients' mental and physical health. For instance, an *antidepressant discontinuation syndrome* can develop if an individual abruptly stops taking a drug such as Zoloft, which consists of anxiety, insomnia, fatigue, irritability nausea, and return of depression (Hall-Falvin, 2019).

Therefore, this note is strategically positioned at the beginning of the mental status examination and behavioral observations. In particular, it informs the ultimate reader of the report of the potential influence of the medications on the examinee's behavior. However, it also makes this issue salient as psychologists are reducing their observations and associated inferences to writing. Thus, for example, consider an examinee who was interviewed and assessed in part for suspected ADHD, and was under the influence of Vyvanse that was taken three hours prior. Should the examinee appear attentive and of an average activity level, these observations can be made and then qualified by additionally stating, "such observations were done while Sally was under the influence of her prescribed medication Vyvanse." Of course, this qualifying statement would be preceded by the medication notation that begins this section of the report, in addition to the fact of Sally being prescribed Vyvanse appearing in the "Health-Related" section of the report; a cross-reference to the latter section should also be added to assist the reader.

APPEARANCE AND BEHAVIOR

Psychological disorders can directly influence examinees' overt (i.e., outward) actions and reactions, along with their physical presentations. As such, they can be clues as to the presence and type of psychopathology that are manifest in any particular case. Information here can vary along a bipolar continuum of objectivity–subjectivity, with more *objective descriptors* falling closer to observable facts upon which most people agree, while more *subjective descriptors* are based upon personal opinion upon which people can disagree. Hence, the goal here is to use observations that are as close to the objective pole as possible, including making estimates in terms of degree, such as "poor/average/good/ exceptional." When an examiner must use more subjective descriptors, it is prudent practice to follow that observation with, "as evidenced by" which provides the reader with more objective facts that support such inferences.

To begin with height and weight, both a more objective estimate in inches and pounds, respectively, and a somewhat more subjective "above/below average" designation can be seen. The latter also avoids descriptors with negative connotations, such as "overweight." For adults who are being referred to determine whether they qualify as candidates for bariatric weight-loss surgery, using these objective measures of height and weight permit the computation of body mass index (BMI). This datum determines whether the examinee meets the criteria for obesity, which in turn produces evidence for the medical necessity of psychological testing for these kinds of referral. These data should also be documented for children who may be obese, which would support a recommendation for behavioral intervention for weight loss. As such, included here is a brief discussion of body mass index, and how it can be easily incorporated into a clinical interview for psychological testing.

Documenting Body Mass Index and Obesity   For psychological testing referrals that include an obesity issue, including candidates for bariatric weight loss surgery, computing *body mass index* (*BMI*) in the "Appearance and Behavior" subsection is extremely useful. So, what is BMI and how is it computed? Furthermore, once BMI is computed, how is it used in documenting the presence of obesity?

BMI represents people's weight in kilograms divided by the square of their height in meters. BMI does not measure body fat directly, but research has shown that BMI is moderately correlated with more direct measures of body fat obtained from skinfold thickness measurements, bioelectrical impedance, densitometry (i.e., underwater weighing), dual energy x-ray absorptiometry (DXA) and other methods (Freedman, Horlick, & Berenson, 2013; Garrow & Webster, 1985; Wohlfahrt-Veje, C. et al., 2014). Furthermore, BMI appears to be as strongly correlated with various metabolic and disease outcomes as are these more direct measures of body fatness (Flegal & Graubard, 2009; Freedman, Katzmarzyk, Dietz, Srinivasan, & Berenson, 2009; Lawlor et al., 2010; Steinberger et al., 2005; Sun et al., 2010; Willett, Jiang, Lenart, Spiegelman, & Willett, 2006). In general, BMI is an inexpensive and easy-to-perform method of screening for weight category, for example underweight, normal or healthy weight, overweight, obesity, and severe (or morbid) obesity.

In terms of computing BMI, it may be done with the *U.S. standard system* (or *imperial system*) and the *metric system*. Concerning the former, BMI is calculated by dividing weight in pounds (i.e., lbs.) by height in inches (in.) squared and multiplying by a conversion factor of 703 as follows:

$$\frac{Weight\left(lbs.\right)}{Height\left(ins.\right)^{2}} \times 703 \qquad\qquad (\text{Equation 3.1})$$

For example, imagine an examinee's estimated weight is 150 pounds and height is 5 feet 5 inches (or 65 inches). The calculation would be as follows:

$$\frac{150}{65^{2}} \times 703 = 24.96$$

Regarding the metric system, BMI is calculated by dividing weight in kilograms (i.e., kg) by the height in meters (or centimeters [cm]) squared as follows:

$$\frac{Weight\,(kg.)}{Height\,(m)^2}$$

(Equation 3.2)

For example, an examinee's estimated weight is 68 kg and height is 165 m (or 1.65 m). The calculation would be as follows:

$$\frac{68}{1.65^2} = 24.98$$

The next step would be to diagnostically determine the examinee's BMI in terms of a weight class. Table 3.5 provides four BMI ranges and their associated qualitative descriptions.

In order to increase both the speed and accuracy of computing an examinee's BMI, there are a variety of websites that provide such a calculator. For example, a search term such as, "Calculation of BMI" can be entered into the Google search bar, which has in the past resulted in "Calculate Your BMI–Standard BMI Calculator–NHLBI–NIH" as one of the top search results. The website is www.nhlbi.nih.gov/health/educational/lose_wt/BMI/bmicalc.htm, which provides a calculator in both the standard and metric systems to be used for adults. Merely input the examinee's height and weight, click on "Compute BMI," and it immediately produces the associated BMI. Also on the webpage, adjacent to the BMI calculator, are the same four BMI classifications.

Another useful website for BMI calculation throughout the lifespan, beginning at age 2 years through 19 years (look for "Child & Teen BMI Calculator"), then again for adults (look for "Adult BMI Calculator"), the following website is useful: www.cdc.gov/healthyweight/bmi/calculator.html (Centers for Disease Control and Prevention, 2019). The only difference is that sex (boy or girl) and age (years and months or months only) are additional information entries, and the output includes a BMI percentile score. The adult information only requires height and weight. Interestingly, the BMI calculator results are exactly the same regardless of age. Therefore, if for some reason these websites cannot be accessed, the examinee's BMI can be computed as illustrated above and derive the same results (within rounding error). Additionally, many computer applications include electronic calculators that will make these conversions instantly, which can then be interpreted using Table 3.5. Of note, Table 3.5 uses percentile ranks to make it consistent with many of the data tables used for the psychological tests presented in Part II.

When should these objective data be computed and presented in an initial report? If the referral source references a weight issue as a component of the reason for requesting testing, then the above-referenced webpages should be bookmarked in order for the examiner to quickly compute an examinee's BMI in this subsection of the report, followed later by noting the associated weight classification in the DSM–5 diagnostic summary (see below). This information may also be included if it is believed that weight is a key issue, even if the referral source does not reference such problem.[3] More will be discussed regarding testing referrals for bariatric weight loss surgery and what many refer to as the obesity epidemic in this country (see Chapter 11).

Other Aspects of Appearance   The examinee's general appearance relative to their chronological age is also diagnostic. For example, a 40-year-old man who has struggled with years of polysubstance dependence may appear as an 80-year-old with a similar functioning central nervous system (CNS). However, this information is also applicable

Table 3.5 Body Mass Index (BMI) Interpretive Chart

BMI Score Range	Percentile Rank*	Weight Qualitative Description
40.0 and Higher	98–99**	Severely Obese (Morbid)
30.0–39.9	95–97	Obese
25.0–29.9	85–94	Overweight
18.5–24.9	5–84	Normal (Healthy)
00.0–18.5	0–4	Underweight

Source: Centers for Disease Control and Prevention (CDC). (2019, July 14). Healthy weight [Web log post]. Retrieved July 20, 2020, from www.cdc.gov/healthyweight/assessing/bmi/adult_bmi/index.html

Note. * not reported for adult cases. ** computed by interpolation.

with children and adolescents. For example, early maturing girls tend to become more self-conscious about their appearance and are apprehensive about others' reactions to them (Oldehinkel, Verhulst, & Ormel, 2011). They are also more susceptible to poor body images and mood changes (McCabe & Ricciardelli, 2004). Furthermore, late maturing boys exhibit more anxiousness and low self-worth associated with their slower growth and shorter stature (Oldehinkel et al., 2011). Younger children with ADHD may also appear younger and more immature than their chronological age (CA). Therefore, statements can be seen comparing the examinee's overall appearance with their CA.

Other facets of appearance refer to hygiene, grooming and attire, with dotted extensions that represent prompts for more specific descriptions of examinees that may provide a visual image for the reader, such as, "with shoulder length multicolored hair, multiple piercings around her lips, and wearing a multicolored t-shirt with faded blue-jeans." Poor hygiene and grooming may suggest a severe depressive disorder or *negative psychotic symptoms*.

Diagnostic Facets of Behavior   The most diagnostic facets of behavior include *gross motor skills* (i.e., large muscle movements), *fine motor skills* (i.e., small muscle movements), gait, posture, and speech. For adults, two phenomena of particular diagnostic consequence are *psychomotor* agitation and retardation, both of which are movements that arise from internal mental activity. *Psychomotor agitation* is shown by restless physical activity and caused by mental tension. It is evidenced by hand-wringing, and pulling or rubbing clothing or other objects, and is indicative of a severe mood disturbance such as a major depressive episode or manic episode (American Psychological Association, 2015, p. 860). In contrast, *psychomotor retardation* refers to a slowing down or inhibition of physical activity caused by a concomitant slowing of internal mental activity. Behaviorally, psychomotor retardation is evidenced by slow speech that includes intermittent latencies or pauses prior to giving answers, sluggishness, and slowed thinking and body movements, and is most indicative of a major depressive episode (American Psychological Association, 2015, p. 861). In consequence, reference to both phenomena have been entered, along with the tone, pacing, and volume of speech.

For childhood through adolescence, a reference has been inserted as to immature speech suggestive of a *speech sound disorder* (previously *phonological disorder*). This tendency can be easily observed during an interview by listening closely to the examinee's ability to articulate or pronounce words. Specifically, misarticulation of sounds such as [l], [r], [s], [z], [ch], [sh], or [th], or sound substitutions (e.g., [t] for [k]), and sound omissions (e.g., omitting final consonants); (American Psychological Association, 2015, pp. 792–793) are strongly suggestive of speech sound disorder. Therefore, such a prompt has been included in the three younger forms (i.e., Forms 3.3–3.5).

Additional behavior-related phenomena addressed in the younger forms include references to the adaptability of the examinee to the novel clinical interview environment (both negative and positive versions), temperament description followed by an "as evidenced by" open-ended phrase in order to prompt the examiner for supporting facts (although not in the adolescence Form 3.5 as personality is more developed at this time), noting the presence or absence of any ADHD-like signs (also on the adult form), and noting the presence or absence of joint attention as relating to potential autism (appearing only in the two youngest forms). Observations regarding temperament in the youngest two forms continues developing personality assessment as done in previous sections of the report, which serves as a reliability check. The related issue of attachment is referenced in the "Emotion–Thought–Perception" subsection as it has a strong affective component, and limited to the early childhood developmental period because the partial structure built into the clinical interview process hinders the opportunity to observe attachment-relevant evidence in action.

Finally, while the older form completes this subsection by noting the examinee's *demeanor* (i.e., conduct or behavior), including overall degree of cooperativeness (or defensiveness), the three younger forms covering childhood through adolescence reference one of two projective activities; namely, a *Kinetic Family Drawing* (KFD; Knoff & Prout, 1985) or *Sentence Completion Test* (SCT). There is convincing evidence that projective activities such as these provide diagnostically relevant information while simultaneously actively involving the child or adolescent in the assessment process (Oster, 2016). Process-type information such as attention span, frustration tolerance, anxiety level, motor coordination, problem-solving approach, degree of distractibility, and reflectivity can all be discerned by such activities (Kaufman & Lichtenberger, 2005), not to mention analysis of drawing or sentence theme content (Sattler, 2008, 2014). The latter may be addressed at the end of this entire section denoted by the prompt to the examiner, contingent upon the importance and clarity of the content analysis, along with time constraints. These two projective activities are covered in more detail in Chapter 5 as they are considered to be screening measures that may be administered during the initial clinical interview for testing.

EMOTION–THOUGHT–PERCEPTION

This subsection refers to the expressed emotion of the examinee along with thought process and content. These are next covered in said order.

Emotion   Emotion concerns two aspects of feeling, including affect and mood. First, *affect* is an expressed feeling of the moment and in reaction to external stimuli. In the clinical interview for testing, the two aspects of affect directly addressed are range (i.e., broad versus restricted) and congruence; the former addressing anxiety and mood disorders and the latter addressing the presence of psychotic elements. Second, *mood* refers to the overall emotional presentation of an examinee; metaphorically the frame surrounding the more detailed picture that represents affect. Mood can be described in terms of the following four dimensions: quality, intensity, reactivity, and stability. Here, quality is usually emphasized due to its association with the all-too-common mood disorders, including depressed (i.e., sad), normal, euphoric (i.e., elated and energized), irritable (i.e., quick to anger), and anxious (i.e., apprehensive and tense). *Melancholy* should be inserted if present, referring to a notable absence of reactivity, lost pleasure, profound despondency, excessive guilt, and *vegetative symptoms* (i.e., pertaining to fundamental physiological functions controlled by the *autonomic nervous system*, such as sleeping and appetite). This set of signs is indicative of a severe and chronic major depressive disorder, which is also known as *major depressive disorder, with melancholic features.* Euphoria is suggestive of a hypomanic episode or manic episode, depending upon its assessed intensity, while irritability can be associated with either a depressive episode (especially concerning children and adolescents; see, e.g., Rudolph & Lambert, 2007), hypomanic or manic episode, or even chronic anxiety; hence must be interpreted within the context of other signs and symptoms.

As stated prior, attachment is referenced here for examinees in early childhood as signs may become evident in the child's attempt to adapt to the novelty of the clinical interview room and clinician. For instance, if the child initially seeks security but later begins to explore the interview room using the parent as a base to explore, this may be documented as evidence of secure attachment. Other insecure styles of attachment should also be noted if apparent, and especially if consistent with other data (e.g., presenting symptoms, description of child's behavior with family members).

Thought   An examinee's *thought* or ability to think is also of diagnostic importance and similarly regards two basic facets; that is, process and content. *Thought process* is the "how" of thinking, while *thought content* is the "what" of thinking. Thought process is best dealt with first because if this aspect is severely impaired (i.e., fragmented), so will be a person's thought content. In the vast majority of testing cases, thinking is unimpaired. This is because the *prevalence* of schizophrenia and psychotic disorders is low. For example, worldwide estimates for schizophrenia range from 0.2 to 1.5% (Erlich, Smith, Horwath, & Cournos, 2014). Therefore, statements referring to thought are phrased in the negative (meaning absence of symptoms) or normal direction.

However, should anomalies in thought process become apparent, inserting aspects of abnormal language that the examinee is manifesting in oral (i.e., responses to open-ended interview questions) or written (e.g., responses to SCT open-ended items) speech is needed. The different kinds of language disturbances that mostly implicate psychotic signs of varying degrees of severity should be documented as they are manifested in an examinee's speech in real time. For example, *circumstantiality* is less severe than *loosening of associations*, because albeit dilatory, the point is eventually made without prompting or redirection, whereas in the latter case, the principal point is hopelessly lost in a seemingly infinite sequence of increasingly divergent ideas. However, some language abnormalities suggest alternate diagnoses. For instance, *flight of ideas* is frequently observed in manic episodes, *echolalia* suggests the presence of ASD, and *thought blocking* may indicate a neurocognitive disorder.

Although it is not likely that thought content will consist of ideation that would rise to the level of being *delusional* (i.e., generally defined as ideas that are in contravention of reality), it is useful to have a schematic framework of such signs when they do occur during an interview such that they are not overlooked. Their identification and discrimination (a) identifies the presence of psychotic signs, and (b) grades their degree of severity. The examiner should be alert to delusions that are non-bizarre versus bizarre and mood-congruent versus mood-incongruent. Because non-bizarre delusions can technically be true, it very much helps to have a collateral present should a psychotic disorder or psychotic features represent a component of the referral for testing. Such a resource can corroborate or dispute such beliefs professed by the examinee. Although bizarre delusions are easier to detect, they do indicate a greater degree of severity and likely poorer prognosis as it implicates not merely an absence of insight, but a grossly distorted level that would be more impervious to therapeutic intervention.

Similarly, the mood-congruent and mood-incongruent aspects of delusions are important to consider as the latter shows a significantly greater degree of psychopathology. Considering this issue more carefully, the split between emotion and thought as illustrated by mood-incongruent thinking occurs contemporaneously with a gross discrepancy between reality and fantasy: a type of psychosis with added disturbance analogous to double depression. Hence, it would be logical to assume that mood-incongruent symptoms would demonstrate a diagnostically greater degree of psychopathology. Furthermore, identifying the delusional content further facilitates efforts to narrow the diagnostic focus and the medical necessity for testing.

Before moving on to sensory-perceptual disturbances, there is a need to mention diagnostically meaningful thought content that is not delusional or psychotic. These include beliefs that may predispose towards mood and/ or anxiety disorders. Most especially, thoughts indicating pessimism, hopelessness (Barlow, 1988, 2002), helplessness (Abramson, Metalsky, & Alloy, 1989; Abramson, Seligman, & Teasdale, 1978; Miller & Norman, 1979), negative self-evaluation (Alloy et al., 2012; Beck, Epstein, & Harrison, 1983; Gotlib & Krasnoperova, 1998; Young, Rygh, Weinberger, & Beck, 2014), and negative view of others (Gotlib & Abramson, 1999; Gotlib, Joormann, & Foland-Ross, 2014) are all suggestive of depressive psychopathology. Therefore, there are statements that refer to these types of thought content, including an "as evidenced by" prompt so as to insert supporting indications if the examiner so chooses.

The general ability to *introspect* is referenced here, which can be used in lieu of, or in addition to, the degree of insight manifested by the examinee immediately subsequent to the presenting symptoms. *Introspection* is defined as the process of attempting to access one's internal thoughts, processes, perceptions, and feelings (American Psychological Association, 2015, p. 560). It represents an indispensable ability for accurately responding to many clinical interview questions, and for completing self-report personality inventory tests (see Chapter 11). Therefore, it would be important to document this fact here (or somewhere in the initial assessment report) if such test may be a part of the battery.

Perception   *Perception* occurs when cortical areas of the brain integrate and interpret incoming raw sensations. Sensory-perceptual symptoms are internal experiences that are subjectively reported by the examinee. Therefore, their presence can only be inferred indirectly from behavioral observations. These include observing that the examinee is appearing to be distracted by internal stimulation, for example, responding in a low voice or whisper as if responding in conversational mode. In such case, the reason for referral notes and presenting symptoms can alert the clinician as to the presence of sensory-perceptual disturbances, and observations of such indirect signs can result in a cogent inference that such internal disturbances are or were present.

Finally, the risk of harm to self and others must invariably be investigated and documented. Again, if there were absolutely no indications of such symptoms or signs (e.g., scratch marks on the wrists), abrupt inquiries into these staid matters can be disconcerting to examinees who have never contemplated such actions. Therefore, prefacing such questions as just being "routine" can assist and prepare the examinee in covering such material without damaging rapport. Additionally, broaching the topic as being routine (a) normalizes such symptoms, and (b) give examinees the message that they may freely discuss such issues without fear of being judged in a negative way. Of course, any affirmative responses should be followed-up to determine their (a) severity, and (b) immediacy.

Suicidal and Homicidal Ideation   Assessing risk of danger to self and others is an integral and necessary part of virtually all psychological assessments (except perhaps early childhood), whether done in general or to determine testing in particular. However, the examiner should be especially cognizant of suicidal symptoms if a mood disorder, substance use disorder, or psychopathology involving serious impulse control issues is a component of the psychological testing referral. This is because in excess of 80% of people who commit suicide manifest one or more of the aforementioned disorders and issues (Berman, 2009; Brent & Kolko, 1990; Conwell et al., 1996; Joe, Baser, Breeden, Neighbors, & Jackson, 2006; Nock, Hwang, Sampson, & Kessler, 2010). Hence, let us first examine the concepts pertinent to danger to self. *Suicidal ideation* refers to thinking about killing oneself, *suicidal plans* regard the formulation of methods designed to kill oneself, and *suicidal attempts* involve actions taken to kill oneself wherein the person survives (Kessler, Berglund, Borges, Nock, & Wang, 2005; Nock, Borges, Bromet, Alonso et al., 2008; Nock, Borges, Bromet, Cha et al., 2008; Nock, Cha, & Dour, 2011). There is also a useful distinction between those who attempt and those who gesture. Those who attempt suicide have an unequivocal desire or intent to die, whereas those who make a *suicidal gesture* do not intend to die, but wish to communicate their dire situation as a *cry for help*.

The investigation of suicidal symptoms should be systematic yet include some flexibility in terms of informative follow-up questions. First, the inquiry that broaches this topic may be along the lines of, "Have you ever had any thoughts about killing yourself?" and/or "Have you ever wished you were dead?" Asking in a direct manner effectively broaches such discussion and affords the unequivocal message that such topic is "okay" to discuss openly. Since all examinees should have previously been briefed on the limits of confidentiality during the admissions procedure, this need not be repeated at this point as being unnecessarily redundant. Second, if the response is affirmative, then investigating whether or not they have a plan ensues. This is vital because the presence of a plan implies some degree of intent. Third, if affirmative, the general rule is as follows: the more detailed the plan, the higher the risk as it indicates a more intense degree of consideration, forethought, and thus, intent. Fourth, do they have the means for carrying out the plan? If affirmative, the risk increases further. Hence, it is important here, or at least prior to completing this ongoing suicide assessment to ask, "Do you intend to act on your plan?" Of course, an affirmative response would activate an immediate referral for inpatient assessment and treatment.

Fifth, obtaining the frequency with which such thoughts occur additionally informs the degree of severity; logically, the more often people consider a course of action, the more probable they are to act upon those thoughts. Sixth, do they have a history of any prior attempts? This is based upon evidence that past attempts are strong predictors of future attempts (Berman, 2009), including one study that found a 60% increased risk in completed suicides for individuals being treated in emergency rooms for treatment of intentional self-harm (Cooper et al., 2005). If affirmative, how many attempts, when, by what means, and ensued by what intervention (if any)? Seventh, are there any completed suicides in one's family? If such information has not been covered when taking a family psychiatric history, then asking for such information here is vital because the evidence shows that the risk increases if such answer is affirmative (Brent et al., 2015; Mann et al., 2005; Nock et al., 2011). In fact, individuals with parents who attempted suicide had themselves six times the risk of an attempt compared to those without such parents (Hantouche, Akiskal, Azorin, Chatenet-Duchene, & Lancrenon, 2010). In cases where both a parent and sibling attempted suicide, the risk increases further (Brent et al., 2003). Eighth, has there been recent news of a friend, fellow student, or other peer who has committed suicide? If yes, the risk is increases, especially for adolescents as there is evidence that suicide is contagious. For example, Gould (1990) discovered an increase in completed suicides during a two-week period after there occurred a good deal of publicity concerning a suicide. Further, about 5% of all adolescent suicides are the result of imitation (Gould, 1990; Gould, Greenberg, Velting, & Shaffer, 2003).

Additional risk factors for suicide appear in various previous sections of the initial clinical interview form. First, as stated previously, if the current working or suspected diagnoses involve mood disorders (i.e., depressive or manic episodes), substance abuse, and/or disorders with a strong impulsive element, the risk increases. Second, more specific symptomatic risk factors include (a) a sense of hopelessness (Beck, 1986; Cheung, Law, Chan, Liu, & Yip, 2006; David Klonsky, Kotov, Bakst, Rabinowitz, & Bromet, 2012; Goldston, Reboussin, & Daniel, 2006; Simpson, Tate, Whiting, & Cotter, 2011), (b) a sense of not belonging or being a burden to others (van Orden et al., 2010), (c) severe personality psychopathology involving anger (Perugi et al., 2013; Soloff, Lynch, Kelly, Malone, & Mann, 2000), and some logical, although anecdotal, evidence of (d) command auditory hallucinations that instruct self-harm (Posner et al., 2008). Third, the following environmental stressors occurring in proximity to the clinical interview have also been found to increase suicide risk: (a) a poignantly shameful or humiliating event (e.g., significant failure at school or work, rejection in an attachment relationship, and unexpected arrest (Blumenthal, 1990; Conwell, Duberstein, & Caine, 2002; Joiner & Rudd, 2000); (b) physical abuse and sexual molestation (Wagner, 1997); (c) natural catastrophes (Krug et al., 1998; Matsubayashi, Sawada, & Ueda, 2012; Stratta et al., 2012); and (d) lack of social support (Posner et al., 2008).

Moving to the topic of danger to others, investigation of homicidal thoughts is also a requisite part of a mental status examination. This is supported by evidence of a moderately increased risk of violence among individuals diagnosed with a mental disorder Elbogen & Johnson, 2009; Elbogen, Dennis, & Johnson, 2016). Some specific factors that increase the risk of dangerousness to others include (a) higher anger disposition, and (b) disinhibition (especially due to alcohol and substance abuse; see Elbogen et al., 2016), (c) psychopathology involving impulsiveness (e.g., ADHD), (d) deficits in empathy (including neurocognitive impairment in the prefrontal cortex that controls empathy associated with making moral decisions; see Damasio, 2007; Decety & Skelly, 2013), (e) a history of violent behavior (Centers for Disease Control and Prevention [CDC], 2020), and (f) schizophrenia involving delusions of persecution (i.e., the previously known paranoid subtype) associated with suspiciousness and hostility (Pompili & Fiorillo, 2015). The more of these risk factors that are present in any particular case, the more important this topic be investigated and the results documented. Succinctly, if the answer is "yes," to "Have you ever had thoughts of harming someone else," then the ensuing line of questioning mirrors that for danger to self.

For both danger to self or others, if the aforementioned lines of inquiry reveal an *imminent* threat, meaning that the intended result will occur but for professional intervention, then voluntary inpatient psychiatric hospitalization should be pursued and the clinical interview for testing deferred until the acute crisis has been resolved and the individual stabilized. If the examinee resists voluntary hospitalization, then involuntary *civil commitment* is the alternative viable option; that is, when an individual can be legally declared to have a mental illness and be placed against their will in a hospital for treatment (Nunley, Nunley, Cutleh, Dentingeh, & McFahland, 2013).

The final note in this subsection regards *non-suicidal self-injury* (*NSSI*) or *self-injurious behavior* (*SIB*), which is defined as the act of deliberately inflicting harm on one's body as a means of coping with emotional pain, intense anger, and/or frustration, although without the intention of dying. Typical types of NSSI including cutting, burning, scratching, head-banging, piercing, carving, and inserting objects. This is followed by a sequence of emotional calm and catharsis, although ultimately leading to feelings of guilt and shame. Hence, the process is ultimately self-defeating, similar to psychopathology in general. Signs that an examinee is engaging in this symptom includes the appearance of patterned scars, fresh wounds, and wearing long sleeves and pants in extremely warm weather in an effort to conceal the behavior. If NSSI is not apparent among the presenting symptoms, this should be explored if borderline personality is a component of the testing referral, along with a trauma-related disorder or history, excessive guilt, intropunitiveness, expression of hopelessness or helplessness, a sense of worthlessness, behavioral or emotional instability, impulsiveness, unpredictability, frequent reports of accidental injury, and significant problems in interpersonal relationships (see, e.g., Mayo Clinic Staff, 2018).

COGNITION

While the *cognition* subsection of the mental status examination also refers to an examinee's thought process and content, the emphasis here is on mental ability or competence. This includes the following: (a) ability to orient oneself; (b) ability to recall facts and events (i.e., memory); and (c) ability to reason, acquire knowledge, learn from experience, solve problems, and adapt (i.e., intelligence). What follows is a summary of what to cover in a clinical interview for testing.

Orientation refers to examinees' basic awareness of themselves and external reality. This comprises an awareness of who they are (i.e., person), where they are (i.e., place or location), and when they are (i.e., time; American Psychological Association, 2015, p. 745). Orientation is typically normal because impairment suggests an acute psychotic state or delirium not frequently seen on an outpatient basis. Hence, statements that refer to orientation are worded exclusively in the normal direction. For the two youngest developmental periods, a qualifying phrase comparing the normal results to the examinee's age is made simply because their responses would not be expected to be as detailed, sophisticated, or accurate. For instance, most examinees in early childhood are extremely cognizant of the month and day of their birthday but not the year, most likely because the former two are more strongly associated with gifts and attention. However, this can be interpreted as a sign of what information is most salient to a child and not that of disorientation.

The *information processing* model of memory (Atkinson & Shiffrin, 1968, 2016) is a useful conceptual scheme in investigating examinees' ability to remember facts and events along three different durations of elapsed time as follows: (a) immediate (or sensory memory); (b) short-term memory (or working memory); and (c) long-term memory (or permanent/remote memory; see Figure 3.1). With the exception of referrals that request testing specifically for "memory issues," or neurocognitive disorder, it is advised that all three facets of memory be first evaluated informally. Then, if any hint of problems arise, more structured examination should be pursued. This approach provides the efficiency needed to complete the interview in a timely manner while ensuring that a memory issue is not missed.

First, concerning immediate memory (i.e., a duration of seconds), interview questions are most frequently spoken orally. Hence, such information should still be in an examinee's *auditory* (or *echoic*) *sensory memory* for a duration of 2 to 4 seconds (Schweickert, 1993). Briefly, *sensory memory* is the first stage of the process wherein an immense amount of raw information from each of our senses is encoded. If examinees are able to respond promptly and accurately to multiple questions over the course of the interview, this indicates that they are able to retain what someone said to them long enough to recognize the phrase's meaning and respond accordingly. That is, immediate memory is normal and intact. The next consideration concerns the transfer of sensory memory into short-term memory (STM) by means of attention. Because problems in this ability does hinder memory, it will be briefly discussed here so that it is accurately interpreted.

Notice in Figure 3.1, attention is required in order to transfer information from the sensory store to the STM store. *Attention* is defined as "a state in which cognitive resources are focused on certain aspects of the environment rather than on others and the central nervous system is in a state of readiness to respond to stimuli" (American Psychological Association, 2015, p. 87). Therefore, an integral component of attention is being able to focus upon only the most important information from among all of the competing sensory inputs (i.e., *selective attention*; Broadbent, 1958), because if one is deficit in this ability, critical information will be lost in a matter of seconds. It is here where the clinician should be most vigilant if the testing referral contains suspicions of disorders involving inattention. Mind-wandering, having to repeat interview questions, and losing one's train of thought are all indications of problems in attention and not of memory per se. Thus, a statement indicating no difficulties in attentional abilities is inserted between immediate and STM considerations. If there are difficulties, this statement can be easily modified to indicate the presence of inattention.

STM can be easily and quickly assessed by asking for specific information given about five minutes prior to the test question. This can include three words or colors (especially for children), something as natural as the examiner's name that is usually provided when greeting the examinee and any collaterals, or other brief new information provided within the context and scope of the interview content. Whichever is used can be either retained or inserted in

Multi Store Model - Atkinson & Shiffrin

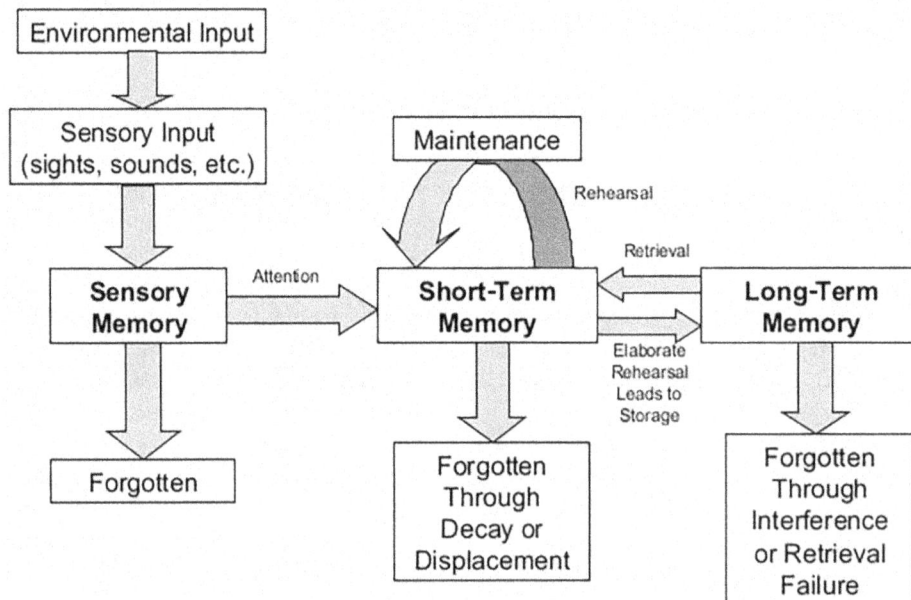

Figure 3.1 Information Processing Model of Memory

Note. The *information processing* model of memory, proposed by Atkinson and Shiffrin (1968). *Sensory memory* is the point at which information first enters the nervous system through one of the sensory systems. Sensory memory is transferred to *short-term memory* (*STM*) or *working memory* by means of attention, which retains the information for about 30 seconds or indefinitely if rehearsed continuously. If information in STM is sufficiently rehearsed or otherwise deeply processed, it will be transferred to long-term memory (LTM), where it can be retrieved later, re-worked, and stored again in modified form. This model can be applied when conducting mental status examinations and evaluating memory functioning.

Source. Downloaded March 25, 2020, by Dkahng, CC BY-SA 4.0 <https://creativecommons.org/licenses/by-sa/4.0>, via Wikimedia Commons, no changes made, *https://commons.wikimedia.org/wiki/File:Information_Processing_Model_-_Atkinson_%26_Shiffrin.jpg*

the parentheticals, or deleted entirely if the specific information used in testing is deemed unnecessary. The phrase "with interference of rehearsal" is significant because it highlights the fact that the individual's opportunity to utilize the memory strategy of *maintenance rehearsal* (i.e., repeating information in one's mind to retain it indefinitely in STM; Atkinson & Shiffrin, 1968; Rundus, 1971) was hindered, hence rendering this item a substantive test of STM (see Figure 3.1).

Finally, long-term memory (LTM) stores factual (i.e., *semantic LTM*) and eventful (i.e., *episodic LTM*) information more or less permanently; that is, there is an underlying relatively permanent change in the brain when such a memory is created. Generally speaking, memories that are a significant part of a person's life, referred to as *autobiographical memory* (e.g., year of high school or college graduation; LePort et al., 2012), and information that is learned at deeper and more meaningful levels through a process termed *elaborative rehearsal* (i.e., connecting new information to older well-learned information; Craik & Lockhart, 1972; Postman, 1975), should still be in LTM and be easily retrieved and transferred back to STM when so requested (also termed *working memory* because it represents information for which a person is currently aware and can modify before once again transferring back to LTM). Thus, LTM is technically being appraised throughout most of the clinical interview, especially within the body of the report when garnering historical information. As can be seen in each of the four initial clinical interview forms, a statement is made that LTM is normal and intact as evidenced by the examinee's ability to report a developmental history that makes chronological sense (e.g., the date of high school graduation is approximately around the time that the examinee would have been 18 years of age, and is about four years prior to their college graduation) and is coherent (e.g., stated occupation is consistent with college major).

The principal modification across the four clinical interviews for testing forms is the degree to which the examinee assumed the primary role in providing such information. In particular, an adult examinee would be expected to provide the majority of the historical information with any present collateral assuming a secondary role. In contrast, a 4-year-old child would be expected to play more of a secondary role yet still be able to contribute some LTM information, including the identification of family members, along with major events in their lives (e.g., graduations, vacations), while parents take more of a leadership role.

Lastly, the mental status examination should provide a gross estimate of an examinee's overall intellectual functioning, previously defined as the ability to acquire knowledge, learn from experience, and adapt by effective reasoning and problem-solving. Prior to the mental status examination, there are a number of facts that help estimate an examinee's intelligence, including academic achievement, occupational success and status, demonstrated perseverance and success at resolving problems one has faced in various life circumstances, and age-appropriate autonomy and independence. Here, the clinician is searching for signs of this complex psychological construct that supplement these previous facts.

As with memory, unless the testing referral includes questions regarding an examinee's level of intellectual functioning, a broad estimate is sufficient; specially to rule out or at minimum cast serious doubt about the possibility of either borderline intellectual functioning or some degree of intellectual disability. This is why the language now used as the default is "intelligence is estimated to be within normal limits," followed by the "as evidenced by" elaborative prompt. In most cases, this statement will be the most applicable. This is true even from a statistical perspective in which approximately 2% of the population falls lower than an IQ score of 70 and 14% lower than an IQ score of approximately 85 (mean = 100, standard deviation = 15).

The principal signs to be considered are the examinee's ability to reason, judgment, amount of knowledge accumulated relative to age and completed grade level, and especially their vocabulary, mostly expressive because that is more readily observable although also receptive language ability. Some of the historical indicators can be added so as to integrate some of the facts, with priority given to formal educational achievement, and supplemented by the variety and quality of their interests and extracurricular activities. The latter demonstrates multiple talents and thus types of intelligences other than those usually associated with formal abilities (e.g., verbal, visual-spatial, and logical-mathematical), including musical (e.g., band, instrument), movement (e.g., sports), interpersonal (e.g., empathy), intrapersonal (e.g., ability to introspect), natural (e.g., recognizing patterns in nature), and existential (i.e., asking questions about life and death; see Gardner, 1993, 1998, 1999a, 1999b).

PROJECTIVE EVIDENCE

Whether or not a KFD or SCT is administered, this subsection is optional, contingent upon (a) time constraints, and (b) diagnostic usefulness of the information. The early childhood form (i.e., Form 3.3) references only the KFD because a nonverbal drawing projective is more conducive to this youngest cohort. Also, the adulthood form does not contain a projective because (a) adults typically provide sufficient information via their responding to interview questions, and (b) this leaves more time for applicable screening measures that are more relevant to making the case for the medical necessity of testing. In the interests of preserving space, administering and interpreting these projectives will be discussed in Chapter 5 on screening measures.

FINAL COMMENTS

Throughout the mental status examination and behavior observations, the approach advocated is to cover each of the aforementioned subsections more informally, then delving deeper into areas that demonstrate symptoms and signs of psychopathology. Hence, for instance, ask for the presence of any suicidal ideation and, if negative, note it rapidly by retaining the standard negative previously drafted statements and phrases (i.e., absence of symptoms), including "normal and intact," "unremarkable," or "denied." In contrast, any affirmative responses should trigger follow-up questions that delve deeper into those areas (e.g., thought process or self-harm) to ensure that they are properly investigated. Using this stratagem, the psychologist can focus on the essential information and facts that form the basis of the testing referral, then render an informed decision regarding the need for screening data and subsequent psychological testing.

Initial Screening Psychological Test Data

At this section and crucial juncture of the report, the psychologist must now make some key decisions. These include the following: (a) Are screening data needed? (b) Is follow-up psychological testing needed? (c) If follow-up testing is needed, which tests are to be selected that will best address all referral diagnostic issues and questions? (d) What testing services are needed and how many units of each are needed to be requested in terms of PA? These will be addressed in such order.

CONSIDERING THE NEED FOR SCREENING TESTS

The first question facing the assessing psychologist is, "Do I need standardized screening data to supplement the clinical interview information and facts?" The various *screening tests* selected were first introduced in Chapter 1 (see Table 1.1), and are discussed in detail in Chapter 5 wherein their targeted psychological constructs, symptoms, disorders, and problem areas are delineated; some *unidimensional* (or *homogeneous*) *tests* some *multidimensional* (or *heterogeneous*) *tests* in design and structure. As stated in Chapter 1, the essential objective of a screening measure is to determine whether there exists a need for more in-depth testing for targeted disorders. Stated another way, screening data serve to accomplish one of two outcomes: (a) in the case of negative results, to essentially rule out one or more disorders; or (b) in the case of positive results, bolstering the case for the medical necessity of further testing. Therefore, there are two types of needs for screening data from the standpoint of the testing psychologist as follows: (a) to ultimately rule out one or more seemly dubious diagnoses; or (b) to help establish the medical necessity needed to obtain PA for more in-depth testing of one or more strongly suspected disorders. If the answer is "No, screening tests would not help rule out or provide further support for establishing medical necessity and PA for follow-up testing," then the psychologist would proceed directly to the next question concerning the need for formal psychological testing (see subsequently).

This section is organized as follows. First, a general balancing test is proposed for deciding whether or not to employ a screening measure during an initial assessment. Second, the more specific instances where the use of a screening measure has been advantageous is discussed. Third, the manner in which a screening measure can be used to help meet the criteria for medical necessity of subsequent testing is expanded upon. Finally, some additional considerations regarding the use of these instruments are discussed.

Use of a Balancing Test Because there are countless permutations that influence such decision, it is most pragmatic to provide a balancing test frequently utilized in determining ethical research design and in determining whether or not to pursue a treatment intervention. Such test can be stated as follows: "Does the value of the knowledge to be gained by psychological test screening data outweigh the added time, effort, expense of materials, and invasiveness to the examinee that would be required?" As will become apparent in Chapter 5, the majority of the screening tests can be administered, scored, entered into the initial report using the prepared data tables, and interpreted within an estimated range of five to ten minutes. The multidimensional tests understandably take somewhat longer, although possess computer scoring capabilities that increase the speed and accuracy of scoring. Next, a few examples of the aforementioned balancing test are offered.

Specific Instances of Using Screening Tests The most frequent set of facts that tips the balance in favor of using a screening measure consist of examinees who manifest some of the following: (a) significant difficulty describing their presenting symptoms; (b) poor historical sense (e.g., problems with LTM, difficulties establishing even approximate dates); (c) dispositional reticence; (d) extreme shyness or introversion; and (e) laconic response style (i.e., answering even open-ended questions using very few words). The case for a screening measure is further increased if examinees' insurer applies very stringent standards for meeting the medical necessity of testing. Therefore, a screening measure is typically selected if (a) more specificity is needed from the examinee, (b) further testing is deemed to be in the examinee's best interests (e.g., such data would be therapeutic), and (c) there is likely to be insufficient evidence for medical necessity considering the insurer's criteria. Next, the latter point is elaborated.

Using Screening Tests for Demonstrating the Medical Necessity of Testing One of the most vital uses of a screening measure is to make a case for the medical necessity of subsequent testing. A psychologist may be convinced that in-depth testing is needed to detect the presence of particular disorder (e.g., schizophrenia, ASD), but may not have sufficient evidence to meet the medical necessity for further testing. In such instances, a psychologist must have knowledge of the examinee's insurer and the criteria that are being applied. If such information is not known, it behooves the psychologist to assume that the most rigorous criteria for medical necessity are being applied.

Tables 3.2 and 3.3 consist of a compilation of some of the most stringent criteria among insurers. The former regards criteria for standard psychological testing (i.e., personality; psychological disorders that exclude brain injury, disease, or dysfunction), whereas the latter are applied to neuropsychological testing (i.e., specialized testing for neurocognitive disorders focused on measuring brain-behavior relationships). Let us examine these in such order.

In the case of psychological testing, the language used in Criterion 1 (Table 3.2) imply that an initial clinical interview that is focused upon detecting a "mental disorder" is assumed to be sufficient for purposes of formulating a diagnosis and treatment plan. This is consistent in peer consultations with psychologists hired by insurers who employ this standard. Specifically, psychological testing is seen as unnecessary unless (a) the data are ambiguous or mixed (e.g., school personnel are reporting symptoms of ADHD in contrast to parent screening data that are negative for this disorder), (b) there has been an ongoing treatment plan of reasonable duration that has shown insufficient positive results (i.e., thus indicating a faulty diagnosis based upon clinical interviewing), or (c) there is a suspected psychological disorder that by definition requires standardized testing (e.g., ASD, ID). Also, note in Criterion 1 (Table 3.2), the reference to the use of at minimum one standardized rating scale. In response, standardized screening tests that result in contradictory data can be successfully used, which can only be clarified by more in-depth follow-up testing.

Briefly, it would be instructive to share an argument that, although incontrovertibly true, will most certainly fail to obtain PA for psychological testing during a peer review. It refers to attacking the assumption inherent in Criterion 1 that clinical interviewing of itself is a sufficient assessment technique by pointing out the presence of *response sets* (or *noncontent responding*), or the tendency of people to answer questions in a manner that is unrelated to their content. For example, consider *acquiescence* (or *yea saying*) in which clients simply agree irrespective of question content (e.g., Question: "Are you distractible?" Answer: "Yes."). Think about how frequently clients might simply agree with the expert "doctor?" Or *social desirability*, in which clients will deny symptoms they actually have because they (consciously or unconsciously) want to appear likeable or accepted. Finally, consider a client or collateral who is motivated by *secondary gain*; that is, or reinforcement for the presence of symptoms not actually occurring. Although all of these response tendencies are well known among trained psychologists who conduct these peer reviews for insurance companies, arguing that their presence requires the use of standardized tests will do no good.

What is most effective in prevailing on a peer review call is to examine the reasons given for either an outright denial or a punitive reduction in requested testing units (i.e., time). Typically, the insurer will provide a written letter of denial or notice of a reduction of units. If it is indicated that added facts are needed for PA, then collecting and providing them during the peer review is effective (e.g., evidence multiple developmental delays for autism testing). This is why critical prompts have been included and a developmental table for the younger three developmental periods in order that such information is not inadvertently missed, which can occur during the course of a busy day that consists multiple initial assessments. Also, contacting the client and/or collateral and having them complete a screening measure, the results of which can be provided during the peer review process, is also effective. This is the reason screening tests have been added to this edition of the book.

As a general rule, if PA is given for 50% or more of the units requested, that result can be accepted and the planned battery can be pursued. Based on experience, it is not worth the time and can result in a reversal of the units previously authorized. That is, when insurance companies have their reviewers reconsider a prior decision, they can and do apply it to the entire number of units initially requested. Also, as may have already become apparent, there is a good deal of discretion built into these criteria. Hence, developing and maintaining good rapport with those who conduct peer reviews is a good practice strategy.

Once Criterion 1 has been met, the remaining three (viz., criteria 2, 3, 4) are more reasonable and viable. Criterion 2 requires standardized testing that is properly normed for the examinee that is to be tested. For this principle, note that (a) all tests in this book are standardized (see Table 1.1), (b) all tests together cover virtually the entire lifespan (hence ensuring the availability of measures for all ages), and (c) there is language at the end of each initial assessment report form documenting that the selected tests are properly normed for the examinee in question. In actuality, there are two versions of the latter, one referencing a plurality of tests, the other simply referring to one test battery. Moving to Criterion 3, another cogent argument for PA of testing is to make salient a pattern of ongoing ineffectual or failed treatment. In particular, listing all of the dates and types of treatments afforded the examinee, including the continuation or exacerbation of symptoms, successfully demonstrates that targeted testing possesses a reasonable chance of modifying, updating, and improving (i.e., directly impacting) treatment efficacy.

Lastly, Criterion 4 states that testing chiefly for academic, career, or legal planning will be summarily denied. Hence, if a testing referral pertains to any of these areas, they must address, first and foremost, mental health issues to have any chance of being afforded PA. For example, if an examinee is referred for testing to rule out a specific learning disability and the insurer in question applies Criterion 4, such testing request will surely be denied unless it can be shown that it principally serves a mental health issue. In this case, the best chance would be to document the continued exacerbation of anxiety and depression (i.e., a primary mental health issue causing dysfunction), associated with a likely undiagnosed and untreated learning disorder (i.e., a secondary academic issue), within the context of a school district which has refused to provide any psychoeducational testing (i.e., such services are not otherwise available).

Neuropsychological testing criteria (see Table 3.3) are somewhat different. These principles emphasize a mental status examination (Criterion 1) and a medical referral source (Criterion 2). First, according to Criterion 1, when planning to test for a neurocognitive disorder, memory dysfunction, or brain trauma sequelae, for example, it is imperative to administer a more formal mental status examination that includes a screening measure for neurocognitive impairment (e.g., *Wechsler Memory Scale, Fourth Edition, Brief Cognitive Status Exam, WMS–IV, BCSE*; Wechsler,

2009a, 2009b; or Mini-Mental State Examination, Second Edition, MMSE–2; Folstein et al., 2010). Positive results would show the likely presence of deficits, which would require more in-depth testing and, hence, provide the medical necessity for a full neuropsychological test battery.

Criterion 2 indicates that a referral from a physician, especially a neurologist or psychiatrist, would greatly increase the chances that medical necessity would be met because neuropsychological testing would reveal a pattern of strengths and deficits that would directly impact (i.e., guide) treatment rehabilitation services. Of course, this would also apply to Criterion 3 as neuroimaging is frequently done in medical referrals for neuropsychological testing. Criterion 4 is built into virtually all DSM–5 differential diagnostic practice; that is, ruling out the physiological effects of substances or other medical condition.

Referrals in instances where the examinee is a candidate for neurosurgery (viz., Criterion 5) does not occur often in practice. However, it is a virtual guarantee for purposes of meeting the neuropsychological criteria for medical necessity. For example, one such referral requested testing for a baseline measure in order to be able to compare pre- and post-operative neurocognitive functioning, which was afforded PA without incidence. Finally, Criterion 6 is a more specific instance of Criterion 2, here with a preexisting medical diagnosis that is known to cause a dementing process. Numerous such referrals have been sent from psychiatrists and other medical specialties, including those with HIV infection, TBI, vascular disease, and Parkinson's disease. Again, such referrals typically receive PA, especially when the initial assessment provides a thorough mental status examination with a standardized neurocognitive screening measure. As an added benefit of using such a screening measure, examinees are able to become acquainted with the test administration process, which frequently lessens their anxiety regarding the more comprehensive battery.

Additional Considerations for Using Screening Tests   Another fact pattern that tips the balance toward using a screening test is to rule out one or more diagnoses that have little if any evidence of being present. Negative screening data can reassure both the examinee and/or the referral source that a suspected disorder is indeed absent. Two examples come to mind. First, a third-grade teacher was convinced that an examinee had ADHD whereas the parent was dubious. Although the clinical interview by itself ruled out ADHD, negative standardized screening data would more effectively clarify the issue for both the parent and teacher. Second, a 7-year-old male had been diagnosed at the age of about 3 years with autism, and was referred for testing to rule it out. During the interview, this child was extremely engaging and extroverted. As it turned out, he had ADHD, which likely made him appear socially immature. In this instance a multiscale screening measure was administered, which ultimately showed via standardized scores that he had ADHD and not autism.

As an added benefit, insurance companies become cognizant of a provider's use of standardized rating scales to avoid ordering unnecessary and costly testing. In consequence, they are more likely to approve borderline cases for testing because they perceive the provider as practicing within the confines of managed care. Stated differently, as a provider, relationships are being built with both clients and those responsible for PA of clients' health care services. Developing and maintaining excellent rapport with both parties leads to a productive and rewarding practice.

One final note is in order on the use of screening tests and PA for subsequent testing. The criteria set out in the prior section are the most stringent seen in testing practice. Therefore, if all initial clinical interviews are conducted with these criteria in mind, they will most likely lead to the greatest amount of testing services and units obtaining PA. As indicated above, another strategy is to know the specified criteria in advance so as to adjust the interview to be more efficient. The former is preferred because it results in more consistency (and thus reliability) in initial clinical interviews, which usually to increases validity of the ultimate diagnostic conclusions and treatment recommendations.

To conclude the issue of whether or not screening data is needed, if the answer is negative, then the "Initial Screening Psychological Test Data" section should be deleted from the report. If used, however, the selected screening score table should be electronically inserted into that section, followed by entering the pertinent data into the table and accompanied by their interpretation immediately below.

CONSIDERING THE NEED FOR FOLLOW-UP PSYCHOLOGICAL TESTING

Once the screening question has been resolved, the next question is, "Do I need formal psychological testing?" Another way to contemplate this question is as follows: "Considering the interview information, mental status examination and behavioral observations, and any screening data that may have been added, do I have sufficient information to address all of the diagnostic issues and questions raised in this referral for testing?" The same logical balancing test applies here as it did with the use of screening measures. In words, "Does the value of the knowledge to be gained by formal psychological testing outweigh the added time, effort, expense of materials, and invasiveness to the examinee that would be required?" In cases where the referral sources are mental health clinicians or health care professionals, some degree of testing is usually justified since they have already completed their own comprehensive clinical interviews and perhaps treatment interventions with remaining unresolved diagnostic issues and questions.

In contrast to screening measures, which are by design brief and use fewer resources, more in-depth testing requires more of everything previously considered. This is one of many reasons to keep the test battery as streamlined as possible without serious detriment to the reliability and validity of the results. In general, the more targeted and efficient the requested test battery, the more likely it passes the aforementioned balancing test. However, let us first examine the process if the answer to this balancing test is as follows: "No, I do not need formal testing. The information and facts gleaned from the clinical interview in this case provided a sufficient degree of confidence in the diagnostic conclusions and treatment recommendations such that the resources required for testing are neither needed nor justified." In such case, the section titled, "Initial Psychological Assessment Summary," becomes the focal part of the report. It is to this section of the report we turn to next.

Initial Psychological Assessment Summary

This section of the report is to be used only when the initial clinical interview information, along with any screening data (although this is not a requirement), is deemed to be sufficient in addressing all of the referral diagnostic issues and questions. Such an instructional prompt appears in italics font just prior to this section within the report, which should be deleted in the final version (i.e., it merely represents an instruction to the psychologist). In contrast, if more in-depth follow-up testing is desired, which is the more common route, then this entire section is irrelevant and should be deleted, and an "Initial–Final Psychological Assessment Report" prepared (see Figure 2.1). What follows are the steps to be followed in completing this report.

ORAL FEEDBACK

First, oral feedback concerning the diagnostic conclusions and answers to referral questions should be afforded the examinee and any collaterals at a level of sophistication that they understand (see Figure 2.1, "Communicate Findings" box). Assisting them in applying the findings to the examinee's functioning in the real world has therapeutic merit (Finn, 2007; Finn et al., 2012). For example, if the interview information and screening data effectively confirm the presence of ADHD in a 9-year-old girl, a discussion can ensue as to how she can study more effectively within a distraction-minimized environment. In addition, collaterals can be assisted in not misinterpreting the examinee's behavior as being "lazy," or unmotivated.

THE INITIAL–FINAL PSYCHOLOGICAL ASSESSMENT REPORT

Oral communication of the findings should be ensued by completion of a final written report after the examinee and any collaterals exit the office (and ideally prior to working with a new case; see Figure 2.1, "Initial–Final Psychological Assessment Report" oval). The pre-drafted wording in this section begins by stating that the initial assessment evidence is sufficient and further formal psychological testing is deemed to be medically unnecessary. This should be ensued by a recapitulation of the findings, including the resolution of diagnostic issues and answers to any questions, ensued by the supporting evidence. The wording should be akin to a summary of the results section of a complete testing report or abstract section of a journal publication. Being succinct yet thorough is the objective.

In such case, the subsequent section, "Initial Psychological Assessment Summary and Follow-Up Testing Plan," should deleted as being irrelevant; that is, in this instance there is no need for such testing. Next, the "Provisional DSM–5 Diagnostic Summary" should be modified to read, "Final DSM–5 Diagnostic Summary," and "Treatment Recommendations" should supplant the, "Requested Tests, Testing Services, and Units (Time)" section. Here, a listing of appropriate treatment recommendations should be inserted. As indicated prior, the overall report should then be titled, "Initial–Final Psychological Assessment Report." This title will most effectively indicate that an initial clinical interview was done with mental status examination and behavioral observations (and any screening data), and such was sufficient to finalize the diagnostic issues and questions raised. In such a fortunate (albeit infrequent) circumstance, no further action is needed except to release this report as instructed by the previously signed ROIs.

As discussed above, the more common decision of the assessing clinician is that, "Yes, I need formal psychological testing." In this case, the "Initial Psychological Assessment Summary," section should be completely deleted. The ensuing section, "Initial Psychological Assessment Summary and Follow-Up Testing Plan," now becomes the focus of analysis. Succinctly, this section sets out the reasoning that argues in support of the need for testing, followed by a listing of the types of tests designed to address the diagnostic issues and questions. It is to this vital section that we now turn.

Initial Psychological Assessment Summary and Follow-Up Testing Plan

At this point, the psychologist has decided the formal psychological testing is warranted. To assist in establishing the medical necessity for testing and in selecting the specific measures, respectively, this section is bifurcated into two subsections as follows: (a) "Rationale for Testing"; and (b) "Requested Types of Tests." These will next be examined in such order.

RATIONALE FOR TESTING

Listed here are reasons used to justify the medical necessity for testing. This section is designed for the benefit of both the testing psychologist and reviewers who will be rendering decisions regarding the PA of testing services. For the psychologist, each listed rationale should be considered to determine if it applies to the present case. They are listed in the approximate order of use frequency, ranging from most to least selected. Their wording and order are consistent across the four initial clinical interview forms (i.e., 3.3–3.6). This is for easier reference and because their use frequency is also relatively consistent. Intended as guidelines, they can and should be modified as needed to fit the particular case facts. Each enumerated reason should be considered and used if appropriate for purposes of facilitating (a) test selection, and (b) establishing the medical necessity for each independent test in the final battery (i.e., insurance may deny certain tests in the battery for want of medical necessity). Those that do not fit the case facts should simply be deleted. Finally, any reasons not covered in the listing should be added. Next, each reason is briefly examined.

Hypothesized Disorders that are the Target of Testing First, psychological testing is principally for *differential diagnosis*, defined as the process of determining which of two or more psychological disorders are present in particular case, especially those with shared symptoms (American Psychological Association, 2015, p. 312). This is consistent with several fundamental criteria in defining medical necessity for both psychological and neuropsychological testing, all of which require targeting the detection of DSM–5 diagnoses (see Table 3.2, Criterion 1; Table 3.3, Criteria 1, 2, and 6).

Ruled Out/Casted Serious Doubt by Means of Initial Assessment A major objective of virtually all initial clinical interviews, including those for psychological testing, is in attempting to address all differential diagnostic issues and questions. Of course, this being an ideal objective, the more practical and reasonable goal is to rule out as many suspected disorders as possible. For example, somewhat frequently ADHD can be ruled out in such testing referrals due to symptoms simply not meeting the onset criteria of prior to 12 years (American Psychiatric Association, 2013, p. 60). In such cases, this usually has the beneficial effect of reducing the number of needed tests, test services, and units of time.

Ruled In/Confirmed by Means of Initial Assessment Yet another means of effectively narrowing the scope of subsequent testing is to establish the presence of one or more disorders, either fully or in part. The differential between complete or partial establishment is based upon the degree of supporting evidence using clinical expertise, experience, and judgment. For example, imagine that the referral source lists ADHD (unspecified and without a severity estimate) as a working diagnosis, and also as a diagnosis that is needed to be ruled in/confirmed. During the initial assessment, the psychologist finds the following: (a) ADHD coincides with the parent's description of the presenting symptoms; (b) both the parent and child report that Vyvanse has been effective in treating the symptoms; (c) feedback from the school to the parent has been consistently positive since the child has been on the medication; and (d) behavioral observations made by the psychologist and screening data are positive for ADHD. This set of facts leads to a reasonable conclusion that ADHD is fully established and noted as such in this portion of the report. Also, in the psychologist's judgment, knowing the presentation type and degree of symptoms is not worth pursuing, especially considering that the current treatment is sufficiently efficacious.

In contrast, assume the same fact pattern, except that a series of ADHD medications have not shown any effectiveness. In such case, it is likely that the examinee does have ADHD, although some added data would be of use. Therefore, including some quick measures of ADHD in the follow-up test battery that are (a) more in-depth than done during the initial interview, although (b) are less intensive than usually tested for without such corroborating data would be indicated (e.g., using some comprehensive rating scales for parent and teacher). Such data would help designate the type of ADHD presentation and also estimate its degree, both of which would assist in finding the proper medication and perhaps supplemental behavioral intervention. For instance, symptoms may be ADHD, combined presentation, and severe in degree, hence indicating a more aggressive approach to treatment.

In this portion of the report, note that the language used in this line of reasoning contains a fill-in for one or more diagnoses that have been ruled in/confirmed by the initial assessment. If establishment is deemed to be full, then one may delete everything after "is not medically necessary." However, if only partial corroboration has been concluded, then retaining the final sentence is necessary because it declares that subsequent test data will be examined to further clarify the diagnosis's presentation.

Masking Effects of Premorbid Psychopathology   Compared to previous DSM versions, the DSM–5 has only achieved fair levels of interrater reliability for its listed psychological disorders, which is only moderately greater than chance (Cicchetti, 1994; Fleiss, 2003; Regier et al., 2013). *Interrater reliability* is defined as the degree to which two or more independent judges arrive at the same conclusions or measurements; here, psychiatric diagnosis. One of the principal reasons that has been proposed for this low amount of agreement among clinicians refers to the high degree of symptom overlap and resulting *comorbidity* among the various disorders (Oltmanns & Emery, 2004; Krueger & Markon, 2006). For example, it has been found that between 25% and 50% of individuals with one personality disorder will have at least one other diagnosis (Oltmanns & Emery, 2004). Recognizing that this aspect of the DSM–5's nosology renders the practice of differential diagnosis significantly more challenging, especially when done without the assistance of standardized psychological testing, this particular rationale has been created.

Essentially, this line of reasoning argues that an examinee's previously diagnosed psychopathology was likely masking or obfuscating the detection of the now suspected disorder(s) due to a sharing or likeness in symptoms and signs. Therefore, this further substantiates the need for formal test instruments, which are designed to make finer discriminations using standard scores and proper standardization samples. Of course, the facts must fit this rationale in order for it be to be proposed. It works to further support the medical necessity for testing and guides the selection of needed tests.

Previous Comprehensive Assessments Unable to Provide Sufficient Differential Diagnosis   Although this argument may be inferred by three previous ones (viz., Rationale 1, 4, and 5), making the limitations of previous comprehensive evaluations more explicit bolsters the case for the medical necessity of testing. This includes the initial assessment just completed by the testing psychologist, who is here arguing that more accuracy (i.e., reliability) and precision (i.e., validity) is needed to adequately measure the presence and degree of psychopathology currently present in this case. This fact is especially important to highlight in referrals that do not offer a history of previously failed treatments. For example, many testing referrals for autism involve examinees in early or middle childhood who are showing multiple developmental delays. Because they are so young, they typically have no history of treatments, whether successful or failed. In such cases, medical necessity for testing relies upon (a) documenting symptoms and signs of a disorder that by definition require standardized testing (e.g., autism, intellectual disability, neurocognitive disorder) and/or (b) documenting ambiguity or inconsistency relating to a diagnosis (e.g., ADHD). Therefore, using this rationale when possible as a supplement to some of the other arguments.

Continued Symptoms Despite Effective Treatment of Premorbid Psychopathology   This line of reasoning is similar to that in which underlying psychopathology is masked by more salient yet similar abnormality, except that there has been an unexpected continuation of symptoms despite successful treatment for previously diagnosed disorder(s). For instance, imagine a client who is being treated for severe depressive disorder. Subsequent to a documented and incontrovertible remission of mood symptoms, the client complains of continued difficulties with concentration, difficulty focusing, mind wandering, and distractibility. Upon inquiry, it is established that these symptoms date back to childhood, although were overlooked because the individual consistently performed well in academia due to exceptional intellectual functioning. In such a case, ADHD may now be legitimately suspected. Standardized testing would provide the precision necessary to detect ADHD in the absence of residual depressive symptoms that may otherwise explain this set of circumstances. Hence, this rationale is put in to cover such testing referrals.

Other Diagnostic Questions   As may have been noticed, the phrase, "to address all diagnostic issues and any related questions," is used when referring to the objectives of psychological assessment and testing. The diagnostic issues refer to the differential diagnostic dilemmas presented in virtually all psychological testing referrals. However, the referral for testing form (Form 3.1) also includes a fill-in item that asks for any additional "questions or comments."

It is here where referral sources may add questions they want addressed that invariably are pertinent to treatment planning. For instance, "What is this client's risk for suicide?" or "Is this child capable of withstanding the stress of being examined in court as an eyewitness in a sexual abuse case?" Such questions are first entered into the "Referral Questions," section near the beginning of the report, in lower case letters and in horizontal sentence format to save space. Next, they are entered again into this argument verbatim (i.e., if asked in a manner conducive to standardized testing), or in modified form (i.e., so as to render it conducive to psychological testing).

Here, routine list of both diagnostic issues and questions employed by the Department of Child Services (DCS) in the state of Indiana is being presented in order to (a) illustrate a rather extreme example, (b) show what one can expect if one does work with such populations, and (c) illustrate how this initial assessment form can be easily modified to fit varying referral sources' idiosyncratic needs and fact patterns. In particular, Form 3.13 is dichotomized into reasons for referral titled, "Reasons for Psychological Testing Referral," and "Stated Diagnostic Objectives for Psychological Testing." These issues and questions are taken from their referral information, although are entered into the sections used in the forms titled, "Reasons for Psychological Testing Referral," and "Stated Diagnostic Objectives for Psychological Testing," respectively. The classes and statements are copied and presented in Form 3.13 and entered electronically into the proper sections of the initial assessment forms (i.e., 3.3–3.6).

Note that the reasons for testing in this particular DCS referral were partially idiosyncratic to the case, although all of the objectives are fairly standard for adult referrals. Notice also that although the majority of objectives are statements, they are actually veiled questions. For example, "Assess whether the client presents any safety risks to self or others including intentional and unintentional acts," can be rephrased as, "Is the client a danger to self or others?" If one works routinely with such agencies and cases, one should do the same as done in Form 3.13.

Also note that numbers and letters are used in enumerating such questions rather than bullet points for easier reference when addressing them both in the initial and final report. In Rationale 7, fill-in period sequences are presented where such questions can be listed either horizontally in sentence format, or vertically in list format. The latter is typically used if there are more than two questions for easier reading.

Previous Testing   Rationales 8, 9, 10, and 11 all regard the use of previous developmental or psychological testing. This comprises any testing done by early educational intervention programs, special education preschools, school psychological testing, and, most especially, prior psychological or neuropsychological testing. The various permutations are as follows.

First, if no previous psychological testing was done, this should be made salient as it further buttresses the current need for such services. In such case, select the "previous testing not done" argument and delete both 9, 10, and 11 as it is mutually exclusive to them. Second, as previously discussed, if testing was done at any time prior to the current assessment, this should be documented in as much detail as is (a) available, and (b) diagnostically useful. The more pertinent ones tend to be (a) more proximate to the current assessment, and (b) more diagnostically similar. Therefore, for instance, if a 12-year-old was assessed at the age of 3 years by a special education preschool and detected a speech delay, and subsequently was assessed and tested by the school and diagnosed with a *specific learning disorder, with impairment in reading*, the latter would be more useful in a testing referral for ADHD because it is closer in time, has a substantial 45% *comorbidity* (DuPaul, Gormley, & Laracy, 2013; see also Weyandt & Gudmundsdottir, 2015), and deleteriously affects similar areas of functioning (i.e., academic achievement; Jepsen, Fagerlund, & Mortensen, 2009; Sayal, Washbrook, & Propper, 2015). In such case, immediately delete Rationale 8.

Now, paradoxically, if such testing was done, the stronger the temporal and diagnostic-related content relationship between the previous and current assessment, the more potentially detrimental to medical necessity. In other words, if neuropsychological testing was done to rule out a dementing process with the past year, and the current referral is asking for the same diagnostic issue, it is probable that the current testing would be denied as such was recently resolved. In fact, some insurance companies will not permit a second round of testing services if it occurs within the past 6 or 12 months, depending upon the language of the policy. Here, the best hope is either to make the case for (a) a second opinion due to contradictory evidence, and/or (b) to somehow distinguish the current objective from those of the previous one. Rationales 9 and 10 both work to accomplish this objective and are not mutually exclusive.

More specifically, Rationale 9 takes the position that, although such testing was done, irrespective of how diagnostically similar (e.g., perhaps targeting the same disorders), the results are now outdated. It is a fact that even when employing the same test, a long duration or time interval between test and retest represents a confounding variable and reduces the magnitude of the *stability coefficient*. This effect is even stronger when testing younger and older examinees due to greater age-related changes in certain psychological characteristics at the extreme ends of the lifecycle (Sigelman & Rider, 2018). Another way to state this effect is that people and their symptoms change over time, sometimes significantly, along with the tests that are normed for different ages. Therefore, the greater the hiatus between the previous and current testing (i.e., especially exceeding 1 to 2 years), the more reason to select Rationale 10. Finally, Rationale 11 argues that the results of prior testing were ambiguous and hence not useful. This argument can be added to Rationale 9 and 10 to further support medical necessity for the current test battery.

Other   Here is a miscellaneous or catch-all option to be used if a rationale becomes apparent that further supports the medical necessity for testing. Following is a list of test descriptions that correspond to the specific measures enumerated in the final section of the initial report to which we rapidly approach.

REQUESTED TYPES OF TESTS

Subsequent to making the decision to pursue psychological testing, the examiner must be considering which tests are needed. With experience, these kinds of decisions will gradually become easier and more automatic, not to mention with a commensurate increase in confidence. In reality, these considerations are occurring throughout the course of the interview. In fact, in some cases, a tentative decision will be made from the original referral information and further corroborated by the clinical interview. For example, a referral asking for an assessment of a client's intelligence essentially determines the type of test needed. The only remaining question may be which particular IQ test to employ. Other cases are more complex and depend on variables such as the client's ability to introspect and be honest, and how many psychological constructs need to be measured.

This subsection once again has the dual purpose of (a) assisting the examiner in making judicious selections of the kinds of tests needed, and (b) informing the insurance carrier that each independent test selected has sufficient justification. As will become apparent, the new codes guiding the choice of test services requires a minimum of two tests within a battery (see, e.g., American Psychological Association, 2018). This dubious requirement is enforced only by the most stringent insurance carriers. As with certain psychiatric diagnoses, insurance companies reserve the right to select which of these testing codes and rules to they will enforce or honor. There are also unanswered questions as to whether a prepacked fixed test battery constitutes one test or multiple tests. The latter is why two versions of pre-drafted statements are used at the end of the initial report, which confirms that the test battery is properly normed for the examinee. This language essentially argues that fixed batteries, including a series of selected subtests from a battery constitutes more than one measure and is accordant with the new "two test" rule. This guideline is mentioned here because it needs consideration depending upon who is determining the medical necessity for PA of testing services. Again, if the examiner is not sure of this information at the time of the interview, it should be assumed that the most stringent criteria are being employed.

In making these selections, the psychologist is engaging in *deductive reasoning*, which is logic that proceeds from general principles or hypotheses to specific conclusions or facts. The general principles here are focused upon hypothesizing what (a) diagnoses are in need of testing (e.g., borderline personality versus bipolar disorder), and (b) questions to be answered (e.g., what is the examinee's risk of suicide), which represent general concepts, whereas the specific conclusions or facts focus upon which tests are needed to empirically accept or reject, or otherwise answer with data, the aforementioned predictions. This is the same process a psychological scientist engages in when forming hypotheses (e.g., *psychopaths* versus non-psychopaths do not learn from experience), then deciding how these concepts will be measured by transforming each of them into an *operational definition* (i.e., defining a variable in terms of how it will be measured or manipulated). An example would be (a) psychopathic and non-psychopathic groups formed by their scores on the psychopathic deviate scale (i.e., Scale 4) of the *Minnesota Multiphasic Personality Inventory–2* (*MMPI–2;* Butcher, Dahlstrom, Graham, Tellegen, & Kaemmer, 1989), and (b) how quickly the groups master a task involving punishment via electric shock. The former would represent the *independent variable (IV)*, while the latter would represent the *dependent variable (DV)*. In effect, the tests selected in the psychological assessment process represent operational definitions of the identified variables noted in the examiner's predicted diagnoses and conceptual questions.

One note before reviewing the various types of tests. In contrast to the prior rationale for testing section, the types of tests and their frequency usage differ across the four developmental periods and thus the four clinical interview forms (i.e., 3.3–3.6). As a result, the order listed in the adulthood form (viz., Form 3.6) is principally followed and test types interjected from the other developmental periods are done when they are most conceptually similar.

Personality Inventory Testing (Self-Report)   By design, personality inventories are explicit tests, which means that they measure symptoms and traits by means of directly asking the respondent for their degree of presence. They are also multidimensional (or heterogeneous) tests, which means that they simultaneously measure a variety of psychological constructs, including *clinical syndromes* and maladaptive (and adaptive) *personality traits*. Therefore, their advantage is efficiency, while their disadvantage is that they require certain characteristics of the respondent. Some of the more important ones include (a) the ability in introspect so as to be accurate, (b) the motivation to be honest so as to be truthful, and (c) the ability to read and comprehend the items. These are covered in detail in Chapter 11.

Personality Inventory Testing (Observer-Report)   In actuality, there is only one such test in this book, namely the *NEO Personality Inventory, Third Edition* (*NEO–PI–3*; McCrae & Costa, 2010). The design mirrors that of the self-report personality inventories. However, the one added required characteristic is that the respondent be sufficiently familiar with the examinee in order to provide accurate ratings. This can be assessed during the clinical interview. In addition, the NEO–PI–3 is focused more exclusively on both normal and abnormal personality and only risks for clinical syndromes can be inferred. That is, this test was not designed to measure the presence of clinical syndromes. This test is also covered in detail in Chapter 11.

Performance Personality Testing (Rorschach Inkblot)   It is preferred here to define the Rorschach and similar tests principally by the means in which they are administered, scored, and interpreted (see Chapter 12 for more detail). The manner in which people organize and interpret stimuli that possess varying degrees of ambiguity represents the raw data; which is thereafter converted to codes or standard scores; hence the term performance-based. Such tests require more intensive work on the part of both the examiner and examinee; that is, at minimum double the testing time. They also yield data which suggest, and thus do not measure directly, the presence of various clinical syndromes and personality disorders. Therefore, these two features represent such tests' major disadvantages. However, they excel when there is reason to believe that the examinee will not (e.g., feigning or being defensive) and/or cannot (e.g., suffers from *alexithymia*) cooperate, or when signs of impaired reality testing need to be measured as they manifest in real time versus by self-report. In that sense, they are also effective in assessing the *convergent validity* of explicit tests. See Chapter 12 for more details on the Rorschach Inkblot Test, including two scoring systems.

Trauma-Related Disorders Testing   Testing for psychopathology caused by trauma, including clinical disorders that by definition result from catastrophic experiences, along with sequelae, such as mood and personality disorders, can be most completely diagnosed by instruments designed specifically for such purpose. The test inventory presented in Table 1.1 (see Chapter 1) includes both observer-report and self-report tests designed specifically for detecting trauma and associated symptoms and disorders. Together, they cover from age 3 years through adulthood and should be included for the most accurate psychodiagnosis in cases involving trauma as part of the referral issues and/or developmental history.

Storytelling Performance Personality Testing   For cases in early through late childhood, there is a story-telling performance test that measures personality functioning and development. It comes with an empirical scoring system and is capable of measuring various dimensions of the developing personality as early as age 3 years through 10 years, inclusive. This test is presented in detail in Chapter 12 and is founded upon psychodynamic theoretical principles.

Structured Interviewing to Detect Feigning of Psychiatric Symptoms   To *feign* is to pretend, put on an appearance of, or represent fictitiously; here, concerning psychiatric symptoms. *Malingering* includes feigning as one component, although also requires the identification of a particular desired outcome. If malingering is part of the differential diagnosis as stated by the referral source, or if this becomes a likelihood during the course of an initial clinical interview for testing by identifying the desired outcome component, then a standardized measure for feigning is justified. See Chapter 13 for more details.

Rating Scales Tests   Rating scales are efficient in that an examinee's symptoms can be measured using standard scores properly normed for age and sex, and from multiple raters across different environments. Although many are multidimensional as are the personality inventories, some focus on measuring one complex disorder or construct in detail, including all of its sub-clusters (e.g., trauma-related disorders, depressive disorders, autism spectrum disorders). Therefore, they are ideal when testing children for the following two reasons: (a) their behavior is notorious for varying widely across different contexts; and (b) the younger their age, the more problems they have being both accurate and objective in rating themselves. Although they are equally efficient for adults, the two major disadvantages are that they (a) tend to result in higher *false positive* and *false negative* rates than other types of measures due to contrast effects (especially the former), and (b) some insurance companies do not consider rating scales to be bona fide psychological tests and will summarily deny their PA.

Quickly, *contrast effects* are defined as current ratings being potentially influenced by previous ratings or experiences; that is, previous positive ratings inflating current negative ratings, and previous negative ratings inflating current positive ratings (Ivancevich, 1983; Maurer, Palmer, & Ashe, 1993; Schuh, 1978; Smither, Reilly, & Buda, 1988; Wexley, Yukl, Kovacs, & Sanders, 1972). Therefore, if teachers interact with mostly "normal" children without severe behavioral problems, which statistically is most likely in general classrooms, then rating a child with such anomalous symptoms will tend to inflate their ratings of pathology simply because they become salient within the context of such normality. It is these two major disadvantages that must be considered when deliberating the inclusion of these measures. See Chapter 10 for more details regarding these measures.

Continuous Performance Testing   A *continuous performance test* (*CPT*) is fully computer automated in terms of administration and scoring, and typically presents the individual with a tedious and repetitive task, and without the opportunity for respite or rest periods. Such tests are designed principally for measuring abilities (or detecting impairments) in attention and impulse control, which are an inherent part of ADHD. Hence, CPT tests are a felicitous choice in detecting ADHD. They also possess the advantage of being objective in their performance-based automated design, and a suitable complement to ADHD rating scales that are more subjective in nature. They may also supplement a neuropsychological test battery, although for this purpose they may be unnecessarily redundant. See Chapter 9 for more regarding CPT tests.

Intelligence Testing   Individually administered tests of intelligence are useful when higher-order cognitive abilities are relevant to the differential diagnosis and/or treatment plan. This especially includes suspicion of ID as such condition will require adjustments in treatment planning, including the use of more action-oriented behavioral interventions versus those that are contingent upon insight and abstract thinking. They are also needed when testing other disorders, especially neurodevelopmental disorders that have a high comorbidity rate with ID (e.g., ASD), and neurocognitive disorders when testing individuals at the extremes of intelligence, which permits an ability-memory discrepancy analysis. See Chapter 7 for more details regarding these tests.

Adaptive Behavior Testing   The standardized measurement of adaptive behavior is an integral component of testing for ID because it is literally an element of the diagnosis, which currently also determines the degree of impairment. Adaptive behavior essentially measures to degree to which an individual can function autonomously in the real world. Therefore, if such is included in the differential diagnosis and/or is being questioned, then including such a measure should be seriously considered. As will become more apparent in Chapter 6, the adaptive behavior tests offer both a rating scales format and structured face-to-face interview format. If the examinee has insurance that does not consider rating scales to be genuine psychological tests, then the structured interview format is advised for PA. See Chapter 6 for more details.

Autism Performance Testing   Because the design of such testing is unidimensional (or homogeneous), which directly targets one albeit complex construct, the decision to utilize such a unique and valuable measure is relatively easy. Perhaps the more challenging decisions refer to what other tests are necessitated to address all differential diagnostic issues. Specifically, the comorbidity of autism with other largely neurodevelopmental disorders is impressive, and includes ID (70% rate; CDC, 2014; Charman et al., 2011; Matson & Shoemaker, 2009) and perhaps ADHD with similar deficits in *executive functioning* (Corbett, Constantine, Hendren, Rocke, & Ozonoff, 2009), which is an ability consisting of higher order planning and regulating of behavior (Russell, 1997). Therefore, intelligence testing, adaptive behavior testing, and the use of rating scales may also be considered here. More details are provided in Chapter 6.

Broad-Based Neuropsychological Testing   When a testing referral comprises differential diagnostic issues pertaining to general brain functioning, neuropsychological testing immediately becomes the prime consideration, including an array of fundamental abilities such as attention, language, learning and memory, executive functioning, visual-spatial analysis, sensory-motor ability, and social-perception. This may be directly inferred from perusing the criteria for establishing the medical necessity of this specialized testing (see Table 3.3, Criteria 2, 3, 5, and 6). If there are associated observable changes in what are considered psychiatric symptoms (e.g., hallucinations, depression, or anxiety) or in personality (e.g., increased anger outbursts and impulsivity) that are cotemporaneous with the onset of the observed neurocognitive deficits, an explicit or implicit personality test should be considered as an add-on measure so as to determine whether or not (a) a *with behavioral disturbance* specifier should be appended to a neurocognitive disorder diagnosis, and/or (b) a *personality change due to another medical condition* diagnosis is warranted. See Chapter 9 for more details regarding neuropsychological tests.

Specified Neuropsychological Testing   Regarding the younger three developmental periods, carefully selected neuropsychological subtests may assist in the diagnosis of disorders that are not formally classified within the neurocognitive general class. For example, social perception subtests that measure *theory of mind* (*ToM*) or *affect recognition* may aid in the detection of ASD. Additionally, a number of *attention* and *executive functioning* subtests can facilitate a diagnosis of ADHD. The latter are useful supplements to CPT data in testing for ADHD. Finally, language subtests can shed light upon the presence of *dyslexia* in determining a specific reading disorder. See Chapter 9 for more detail regarding these neuropsychological subtests.

Memory Testing   In the spirit of targeted testing, when the examinee and/or referral source circumscribes the diagnostic issue to complaints about memory, then tests designed to measure this single although complex construct is on order. That is, if there are no other neurocognitive complaints (e.g., of language, balance, or executive functioning), then the testing psychologist can effectively reduce the number of required units by nearly 50%. There are some excellently designed, individually administered tests of memory analogous to intelligence testing, which can provide very insightful data regarding all stages of information processing, including encoding, storage, and retrieval. If an examinee may fall at either extreme end of the normal curve concerning intellectual functioning, adding an IQ test may be a judicious selection because it permits an ability–memory discrepancy analysis. For example, an examinee with superior intelligence may perform in the average range in terms of memory ability. However, this may be significantly lower than expected for an individual with superior intelligence, hence masking the incipience of a genuine neurocognitive disorder. See Chapter 9 for more details concerning memory testing.

Performance Testing for Feigning Neurocognitive Dysfunction   Feigning psychopathology can also be manifested by intentionally showing poor performance on a neurocognitive ability task, sometimes referred to as faking bad. This can most commonly occur within the context of neuropsychological testing wherein showing disability may lead to greater rewards (e.g., more lucrative personal injury settlements, disability financial support, averting unwanted work duties or responsibilities). Therefore, in such instances, considering the inclusion of a performance-based test that is specifically designed to detect the intentional faking of memory function (i.e., neurocognitive dysfunction) would be of great assistance. This is especially the case if test administration blends naturally with other genuine neuropsychological subtests in the battery. Although some may argue that this contravenes the ethical principal of informed consent, it is ethical in the sense that its objective remains that of accurate differential diagnosis. See Chapter 13 for more detail.

Achievement Testing   Achievement tests are particularly designed to measure fundamental skills and knowledge that are taught and learned in the classroom, broadly including reading, mathematics, and written expression. In terms of differential diagnosis, they are designed to especially rule out one or more specific learning disorders (SLDs), along with discriminating these types of psychopathology from other disorders that may hinder academic performance. Recall that some of the more stringent insurance companies will summarily deny PA for anything that appears "educational" involving a minor who is enrolled in school, under the rationale that such testing remains the purview of the academic system and is not a mental health issue. As stated prior, in such cases, the best chance of obtaining PA is to document that (a) the pertinent school system has been repeatedly consulted and has refused to provide such services, and (b) the examinee's mental health continues to deteriorate to the point of becoming the primary issue (with detailed documentation of such symptoms).

Although it is uncommon to use achievement tests in this fashion, they have been incorporated as part of a comprehensive neuropsychological test battery for purposes of planning rehabilitation. In addition, testing for SLDs is more likely to receive PA for adults matriculating through higher education as it is no longer the responsibility of the academic institution and concerns overall adjustment. See Chapter 8 for more detail concerning achievement tests.

Behavioral Medicine Personality Inventory Testing (Self-Report)   *Behavioral medicine* concerns the application of psychological science to the diagnosis, treatment, and prevention of medical problems. Two medical problems, *obesity* and *chronic pain*, are increasingly common, undertreated, and costly (see, e.g., Flegal, Carroll, Kit, & Ogden, 2012; Dzau & Pizzo, 2014, respectively). This accounts for the increase in testing referrals for adults who are being considered for bariatric weight loss surgery, spinal cord stimulator surgery, spinal surgery, and treatment for chronic pain. Hence, it is prudent to have personality inventories that are either specially designed to evaluate the appropriateness of such individuals for such invasive procedures, including their particular psychological assets and needs, and/or offer appropriate standardization samples such that their scores are interpreted in a valid manner. Because these are very specialized instruments that apply only to adult cases (i.e., ages 18 years and older; Forms 3.5 and 3.6), it is rather clear when they are to be selected. The principal decision then is to select which of several competing tests, published by different authors and companies, to utilize in a particular case. See Chapter 11 for more detail.

Developmental Testing   Early detection and intervention have been laudable objectives, especially if one espouses a *developmental psychopathology* perspective. And although children's psychological disorders vary considerably in terms of symptom clusters, they all represent a type of *adaptational failure*; that is, an inability to master one or more areas of development (Rutter & Sroufe, 2000). Therefore, standardized developmental tests that specialize in measuring and detecting delays in mastering critical milestones are indispensable for examinees who are 3 years and younger. For this reason, this selection will be observed only within the early childhood period (viz., Form 3.3). See Chapter 6 for more detail regarding developmental testing.

Remaining Sections of the Initial Report for Testing

The following three aspects of the initial report for testing remain: (a) summarizing the evolving diagnostic picture (figuratively, a snapshot in time that will be modified pending the planned psychological testing); (b) identifying each test by name, type of testing services, and number of units (i.e., time) needed; and (c) aggregating the requested testing service types and units. The former is the focus of the ensuing section of the report, which is discussed immediately subsequent.

Provisional DSM–5 Diagnostic Summary

Note that the section title here varies across the four developmental periods according to the supplemental nosologies that are integrated with the DSM–5 system. Of course, the DSM–5 diagnostic codes and labels predominate for billing purposes, while the supplemental systems effectively fill in some of the remaining conceptual gaps or weaknesses (e.g., early childhood and personality disorders). Also note that the section title includes the term *provisional*, which denotes that the entire diagnostic workup is subject to some type of change, whether this be modifying the order of prominence, deleting or adding diagnoses, or simply adding or modifying the level of symptoms or specifiers, all of which are treatment related. A general provisional designation is preferable as compared to listing specific disorders for maximum flexibility.

In sequence, the general diagnostic scheme incorporated here is as follows: (a) mental health and developmental disorders (i.e., clinical syndromes, personality disorders, and IDs); (b) related medical variables and conditions; and (c) associated environmental stressors. This is consistent with the DSM–5 except that the three dimensions are labeled to make them more explicit. Each of these elements are explicated next.

MENTAL HEALTH AND DEVELOPMENTAL DISORDERS

The first dimension, *mental health and developmental disorders* is illustrative of the developmental psychopathology perspective. Its inclusion of clinical syndromes, personality disorders, and IDs essentially collapses into one dimension what were previously known in the multiaxial system as axes I and II (see, e.g., American Psychiatric Association, 2000). However, their definition has not changed. In particular, *clinical syndromes* possess several of the following characteristics: (a) identifiable and (fairly) acute onset; (b) traceable course; (c) identifiable precipitant(s); (d) responsiveness to treatment; and (e) identifiable symptom remission. Although there are exceptions, for example clinical syndromes that manifest an insidious onset and chronic course, these components capture a sufficient number of disorders so as to render the dimension conceptually useful and pragmatic.

Next, *personality disorders* concern psychopathology that begins developing in childhood, continues to escalate though adolescence, and becomes fully developed as relatively permanent problems in lifestyle with their most deleterious effects on interpersonal relationships. Finally, IDs are impairments or delays in higher-order cognitive abilities that manifest in early childhood and thereafter continue in a chronic course.

At the completion of an initial clinical interview in which testing is being requested, one of the following is typically selected: (a) an incoming working DSM–5 diagnosis assigned by the referral source for which there is convincing evidence of validity (e.g., the examinee is being specifically treated for such disorder with positive results); (b) an *other specified disorder* that best fits the presenting symptoms (e.g., *other specified anxiety disorder*, or (c) an adjustment disorder that best fits the presenting symptoms (e.g., *adjustment disorder with anxiety*). In order to facilitate selection of these diagnoses, they can be listed in the initial report form so that the desired diagnosis can be retained while the rest are deleted. The suspected disorders that were ruled out and/or ruled in/confirmed by the initial assessment are also noted for easy reference by the referral source. Examples are as follows:

Note: ADHD ruled out by initial assessment (did not meet onset criteria).

— or—

Note: ADHD confirmed by initial assessment (positive response to medication and positive screening data).

Next, any disorders can be listed that are denoted as *rule in/confirm, screen for,* and finally, *rule out,* the latter which tends to include the largest number of disorders and the focus of the requested test battery. To facilitate the selection of these, the specific disorders are listed under a general class label in italics font, which should be deleted from the final version of the initial report as they are for easy reference only.

Note that the entire range of DSM–5 disorders is not listed in the initial report as this would be cumbersome and subvert the objective of being efficient. Rather, included disorders are those that are most regularly used for that developmental period, and in the approximate order from most to least frequent. In the event a case concerns a disorder that is not included in the initial report form, then the psychologist can refer to the actual DSM–5 manual.

RELATED MEDICAL VARIABLES AND CONDITIONS

The *related medical variables and conditions* dimension is analogous to axis III in previous versions of DSM (e.g., American Psychiatric Association, 2000). However, it is bifurcated it into *current medical disorders* and *medical history variables*. The former includes physical diseases, injuries, and disorders that are current conditions being treated, and that can have an effect or relationship with the mental disorders under consideration (e.g., seizure disorder, obesity, hypothyroidism). In contrast, the latter are historical medical variables that again may have had an impact on the mental health disorders being considered (e.g., low birth weight, genetic vulnerability of bipolar disorder). Disorders that have a strong genetic component (e.g., ADHD, bipolar disorder) are included in this subclass when found in the family psychiatric history. Similarly, early abusive and/or neglectful environments that are known to have a *pathogenic* effect and increase the risk for later abnormality are included. Both of these are consistent with the vulnerability–stress (or diathesis–stress) model of psychopathology.

Lastly, the specific criteria for selected medical disorders and variables are included in italics font (e.g., $N < 37$ *wk.* adjacent to pre-term birth) to assist the testing psychologist in determining whether or not they are met, along with an antecedent parenthetical fill-in item where the garnered facts may be inserted. This italicized criterion is for guidance only and should be deleted from the final written version of the report. These guidelines assist the psychologist in rapidly determining if a particular variable or condition is present without having to memorize or research the defining criteria.

ASSOCIATED ENVIRONMENTAL STRESSORS

Associated environmental stressors are situational or external factors that either trigger the onset, or affect the progression, of psychological disorders (Schreier & Chen, 2013; Williams & Steinberg, 2011). By definition, *stressors* are interpreted by people as threatening or challenging and thus require some sort of adaptive response. In DSM–IV–TR, they were listed by category on axis IV and were routinely referred to by clinicians as "*V codes.*" Although DSM–5 has retained a categorical listing, they have increased significantly in number and are now denoted as *Z codes*, and to a lesser extent *T codes* (not to mention one atypical *E code*). A somewhat varying type and number of such codes are included for each of the four developmental periods, which should cover the majority of those needed. A pithy label in italics font appears before each general class for easy reference and should be deleted in the final version of the initial report. Of note, *borderline intellectual functioning* (code R41.83) is listed in proximity to the ID codes because its DSM–5 listing under, "Nonadherence to Medical Treatment," made little sense.

PROGNOSIS

Within the context of psychological assessment and testing, *prognosis* is the predicted course, duration, severity, and outcome of a case. This aspect of a diagnostic workup is contingent upon many variables, including the type and quantity of disorders present (e.g., single diagnosis versus comorbidity), their independent and combined severity (e.g., neurotic versus psychotic),[4] age at onset (e.g., early or late), and the relative presence or absence of risk (e.g., genetic diatheses) and resilience (e.g., superior intelligence) factors. As such, this be deferred until after the psychological testing has been completed and the diagnostic picture has been more completely clarified. A deferral regarding prognosis is the default language used in the initial report. Next concerns the choice of tests, along with the needed test services and units.

Requested Tests, Testing Services, and Units

This concluding of the initial report section informs the following critical information: (a) which tests, by name and individually, are being selected; (b) what type of testing services are requested for each test independently; (c) how many units, for each test, and for each testing service, are being requested; and finally, (d) an accrual of units and time (the latter measured in both minutes, and in hours by the half hour). Although the American Medical Association has made billing more complex and differentiated (see American Psychological Association, 2018), there are two principal advantages to the new scheme: (a) the possibility of requesting both psychological and neuropsychological testing services within the same battery (versus choosing one or the other); and (b) occasionally being able to be reimbursed for more of the actual activities involved in providing testing services. Next, an attempt is made to demonstrate these features by first briefly reviewing the previous less differentiated billing scheme used prior to 2019.

PSYCHOLOGICAL TESTING SERVICES BILLING SCHEME PRIOR TO JANUARY 1, 2019

Previous to January, 1, 2019, relevant psychological assessment and testing services and *Current Procedural Terminology* (*CPT*) billing codes were as follows: (a) *CPT Code 90801* referred to a "behavioral health evaluation" or comprehensive initial clinical interview, which was required prior to requesting any follow-up psychological testing; (b) CPT Code 96101 for psychological test services (by hourly units; e.g., four hours); and (c) CPT Code 96118 for neuropsychological test services (by hourly units; e.g., six hours). More specifically, *CPT Code 96101* was for psychological test services including the psychodiagnostic assessment of emotionality, intelligence, personality, and psychopathology, per hour, including administration (face-to-face), interpretation, and report writing (additional time other than face-to-face). In contrast, *CPT Code 96118* was for neuropsychological test services including the psychodiagnostic assessment of neurocognitive abilities, including attention, memory, language, and visual spatial, along with executive functioning and other types of cognitive functioning related to the diagnosis of brain damage or dysfunction, and secondarily, the assessment of personality and adaptive behavior functioning considered to be related to neurocognitive impairment.

There are two facets to note about these definitions. First, the dichotomy between psychological and neuropsychological testing made is occasionally awkward to accurately request the proper testing services in cases where both neurocognitive and non-neurocognitive disorders were being considered (e.g., memory impairment and personality disorder). Second, scrutiny of these definitions reveals a number of testing-related services not being acknowledged as reimbursable. For instance, technically there is no mention of scoring, treatment planning, and feedback. In fact, the major impetus for developing the new scheme was for psychologists to legitimately bill for more of their actual services conducted as part of the psychological assessment and testing process. Now, on to the new testing services billing scheme.

PSYCHOLOGICAL TESTING SERVICES BILLING SCHEME BEGINNING JANUARY 1, 2019

The aforementioned dichotomous testing codes were deemed to be too vague and antiquated (American Psychological Association, 2018), and did not accurately describe, recognize, and credit the work required when multiple hours of an array of more specific testing services were indeed provided. Hence, the following more differentiated codes were developed to correct for these deficiencies. This includes an explicit recognition for test scoring, which the previous CPT codes did not stipulate to explicitly (although was typically included by many practicing psychologists when estimating the amount of time needed, whether correctly or incorrectly), and a recognition of face-to-face test feedback as a legitimately reimbursable test-related service. However, a consequence of making the testing codes more differentiated, the previous CPT Code 96101 and CPT Code 96118 do not have a one-to-one correspondence to new code, but are differentiated into at minimum six more specific 2019 CPT codes. Furthermore, new developmental testing codes have been published, hence adding a minimum of two more codes relevant to testing covered in this book.[5]

Figure 3.2 delineates the psychological assessment and testing process, including the break-down of services, units of time, and billing CPT codes. To initiate the process, it is vital to emphasize that *all* psychological and neuropsychological testing-related billing CPT codes require a comprehensive diagnostic evaluation (i.e., an initial clinical interview as operationally defined in this chapter, Forms 3.3–3.6) by the testing psychologist prior to test administration, scoring, and evaluation services. The 2019 CPT code and descriptor is as follows: *CPT Code 90791* is a psychiatric diagnostic evaluation that must be done *prior* to pursuing psychological or neuropsychological test administration, scoring, and evaluation services (i.e., data interpretation, integration, report writing, and feedback).

Concerning the developmental test services CPT codes that will be discussed subsequently, their request may be preceded by a number of different initial assessment techniques. Some of these include assessments with developmental screening instruments (CPT Code 96110), such as a developmental milestone survey similar to the developmental milestones table included in the initial assessment forms for childhood through adolescence (i.e. Forms 3.3–3.5), along with a 15-minute routine medical examination done by a pediatrician. Therefore, although these test services do not appear to technically require a psychiatric diagnostic evaluation, they would invariably follow such assessment technique simply because it initiates virtually all ongoing mental health services. A comprehensive initial assessment would also be most efficacious in determining which kind of test service to pursue; that is, psychological/neuropsychological or developmental.

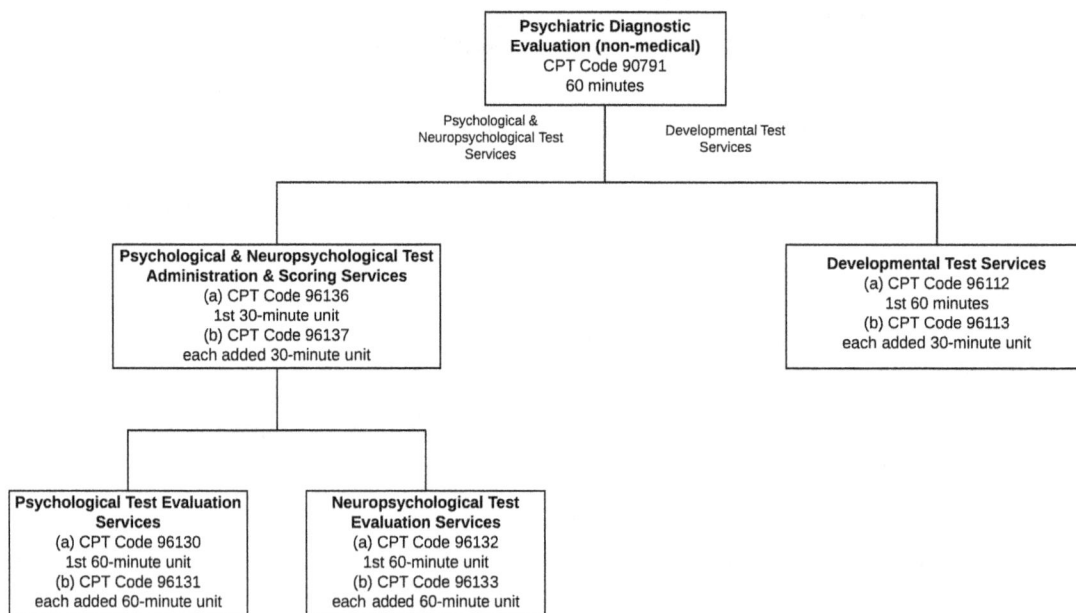

Figure 3.2 Flowchart of Current Procedural Terminology (CPT) Codes for Billing Psychological and Neuropsychological Test Services

Note. The psychiatric diagnostic evaluation is required prior to psychological/neuropsychological test services being requested, and is the technique of choice in mental health practice for developmental test services. Although it is billed as an event, the recommended time is 60 minutes for easier scheduling. After the diagnostic evaluation, a choice must be made between either psychological/neuropsychological or developmental test services (i.e., the two services do not cross-over). Each 30-minute unit requires a minimum of 16 minutes. Each 60-minute unit requires a minimum of 31 minutes. The 1st unit code must be the lead code for each date of face-to-face test services being billed, ensued by the add-on codes.

Therefore, this CPT Code 90791 is to be used for any initial clinical interview done by a qualified mental health professional (i.e., psychiatrist, nurse practitioner, psychologist, clinical social worker, or licensed professional counselor), especially here done for purposes of probably requesting psychological, neuropsychological, or developmental test services. In one mental health facility, this code is titled as, "Psychological Test Evaluation," which emphasizes its primary purpose. Although the top box in Figure 3.2 includes 60 minutes, this code technically does not have an associated time unit as a component of the code (i.e., it is billed as an event and can be of any time unit as long as the described services have been completed by the provider). Therefore, the 60 minutes is simply a recommended guidepost and may be 90 minutes in some facilities. The 60-minute unit is preferred because it comports much better with a daily work schedule that is consistently on the hour or half-hour rather than alternating between the two increments.[6]

At the next level, services bifurcate into either (a) psychological and neuropsychological test services, or (b) developmental test services. Notice that psychological and neuropsychological testing has been consolidated at the level of administration and scoring, which are typically the first two kinds of tasks provided in the sequence of test services. Additionally, developmental testing is differentiated from the former to be provided as a separate and distinct kind of test service; that is, they do not cross over or mix. Therefore, these are discussed separately in such order.

Psychological and Neuropsychological Test Services   Following Figure 3.2 regarding psychological and neuropsychological test services (left side), there exist two billing codes that cover only *test administration and scoring services*; that is, giving the test by following directions in the manual and converting the examinee's responses and behaviors into quantitative scores or codes. First, *CPT Code 96136* is defined as psychological test or neuropsychological test administration and scoring by a physician or qualified health care professional (e.g., licensed psychologist), consisting of "two or more tests," any method, first 30 minutes (i.e., a minimum of 16 to 30 minutes). It should be clarified here that this means the first 30-minutes of such services on the date provided *and* billed to the client. This is critical to understand when requesting billing units and their associated CPT codes, especially if there are multiple test administration sessions on scheduled on different dates of service. It is for this reason that all test services on a particular case are billed out (a) "on the final date of face-to-face service," and (b) after all services have been concluded. In this manner, it is known beforehand that only one CPT Code 96136 unit need be requested. Next, the definition of psychological test and neuropsychological test needs to be parsed.

The phrase *psychological test* means a psychodiagnostic assessment of emotionality, intelligence, personality, and psychopathology (excluding testing for neurocognitive disorders involving brain damage, dysfunction, or disease). Because it only applies to the first 30-minute unit, it is a partial crosswalk from the previous CPT Code 96101, which applied to all testing services then defined and all measures of time in hourly units. The phrase *neuropsychological test* means a psychodiagnostic assessment of neurocognitive abilities, including attention, memory, visual spatial, and language, along with executive functioning and other types of cognitive abilities related to a diagnosis of brain damage, dysfunction, and disease, and secondarily, the assessment of personality and adaptive behavior functioning considered to be related to the possible presence of neurocognitive impairment. In that sense, it is a similar partial crosswalk from the previous CPT Code 96118. Note here that test scoring is now explicitly recognized as a bona fide billable service.

Second, *CPT Code 96137* is defined as each additional 30 minutes of psychological or neuropsychological test administration and scoring (i.e., as previously defined), two or more tests, and any method, needed to complete such services. Therefore, any added 30-minute units needed to complete test administration and scoring would be assigned this billing code. Again, of concern is the criterion of, "two or more tests." Taken literally, this implies that single test batteries represent an illegitimate practice with which it can be disagreed. The rationale likely regards an attempt to bolster the precision of diagnostic results with a greater degree of *convergent validity*, defined as two tests that measure similar constructs deriving the same or similar results (e.g., two personality tests, of the same or different format, showing the presence of borderline personality disorder). Based upon experience, only the more stringent of the insurance companies (again which are not mandated to follow these guidelines) enforce this criterion. However, even among those who do enforce this rule, what constitutes a second test instrument is currently ambiguous and not consistently applied. This issue will be discussed further when dealing with the issue of peer-to-peer consultation for PA of testing services. For now, we will remain focused on the billing services and codes.

Before moving ahead, notice that at the test administration and scoring level, both psychological and neuropsychological services are combined into two billing codes (viz., CPT Codes 96130 and CPT Code 96131). In many facilities, CPT Code 96130 is the lead billing code because it represents the first type of testing services and unit of time provided to the examinee, again on the date in which the services are billed to the client. The CPT Code 96131 and all subsequent 30-minute units (e.g., 3 units = 90 minutes) are what are referred to as *add-on codes*. Depending upon the filing system used at the mental health facility (e.g., hard copy or electronic files), these billing codes must be added to the initial 30-minute CPT Code 96130 service in some manner (unless no such added service is needed).

The ensuing codes refer to *test evaluation services*, which consist of data interpretation, integration, decision-making, treatment planning, report generation, and interactive feedback. However, it is at this point that psychological and neuropsychological testing (i.e., as previously defined) become differentiated into their own codes, as can be seen in the bottom two left boxes in Figure 3.2. First, *CPT Code 96130* refers to psychological test evaluation services (i.e., as defined prior) by a physician or qualified health care professional (e.g., licensed psychologist), first hour (i.e., first 60-minute unit as shown in Figure 3.2). Again, there is a billing issue here as first 60-minute unit means, the first 60 minutes of such services on the date the client was billed. As stated prior, billing all test hours on the final date of face-to-face service ensures that only one of these units need to be requested when asking for types of services and units to be preauthorized by insurance. It also makes billing easier, hence reducing the odds of billing mistakes attributed to human error and either delayed or denial of remuneration for services.

Note that test *interactive feedback* to examinees and pertinent collaterals regarding test results is now recognized as a billable service under testing evaluation services, although whether this results in added units being afforded PA is another matter. That is, although test feedback is now officially recognized, insurance carriers may still provide PA for the same number of units as given prior to the billing scheme change (e.g., 2.0 hours for a Rorschach Inkblot Test irrespective of the billing scheme used). Continuing with psychological tests, *CPT Code 96131* is applied to all added 60-minute units needed to complete psychological test evaluation services as defined immediately prior. Together, these codes are partial crosswalks from the prior CPT Code 96101, which applied to all psychological testing services in hourly units.

Second, *CPT Code 96132* refers to neuropsychological test evaluation services (again as previously defined) by a physician or qualified health care professional (e.g., licensed psychologist), first 60 minutes. Finally, *CPT Code 96133* refers to all added 60-minute units needed to complete neuropsychological test evaluation services as defined previously. And again, these billing codes are partial crosswalks from the prior used CPT Code 96118 neuropsychological testing code.

Before moving on, three special notes are needed to clarify (a) what constitutes data in the aforementioned definitions of testing services, and (b) how to properly accrue and document the requested units of time. First, *data* comprise both quantitative raw and transformed standard scores, whether linear or area transformations, and qualitative classifications or descriptions (e.g., high average, borderline), along with diagnostically relevant clinical interview facts and information. Hence, data consist of all measurement scales promulgated by Stevens (1946). Second, whether they are first or added services, units of time can be legitimately billed only when the serviced time exceeds the halfway mark of the designated unit. Therefore, 30-minute units can be billed only when the actual service provided to the examinee passes the 15-minute (i.e., halfway) mark. More specifically, a 30-minute unit can be billed anywhere from 16 to 30 minutes of actual service. This means that if only 14 minutes of such service is provided, no billing for that 30-minute unit is legitimate. Similarly, a 60-minute unit can be billed only when 31 to 60 minutes of such service has been provided (i.e., passed the halfway mark).

Third, two-related notes are in order regarding the strategy of billing all test services on the final date of face-to-face service. One, it may require the psychologist to bill at an alternate time of actual service in order to bill out all units consecutively, which is the easiest to do once again to avert errors. Accuracy in billing the codes is first and foremost. Two, billing should be done of the last date of face-to-face direct service, which at times will require backdating when scoring, interpretation, and report writing are done by necessity on the following day (e.g., when crises or similar events occur). Some insurers are fastidious in the sense of providing payment only on dates of direct service, as in typical mental health assessment and treatment (e.g., psychotherapy sessions). To be both diligent and cautious in such manner will serve to avoid hindrances in receiving payment in a timely fashion for services rendered.

Developmental Test Services   Following Figure 3.2 regarding developmental test services (right side), there exist two billing codes that in this instance combine all types of tasks that comprise this sequence of test services. More specifically, a *developmental test* is defined as a standardized age-related instrument that assesses fine and/or gross motor, language, cognitive level, social, memory, and/or executive functions. This incontrovertibly includes any infant developmental test, although would arguably also apply to preschool intelligence tests (some of which are normed as low as two years) and adaptive behavior measures that are usually normed as low as one month (see Table 1.1). However, by means of many peer-to-peer consultations, it became clear that such does not include autism testing, which would fall under the rubric of psychological testing. Therefore, developmental tests are focused upon non-autism developmental issues; that is detecting early delays in developmental milestones not associated with autism.

In this case, however, there are only two testing codes. First, *CPT Code 96112* applies to the first hour (i.e., 60-minute unit) of administration, scoring, data interpretation, and report generation of developmental tests as defined prior. Interestingly, the words "interactive feedback" are not included in available descriptions. However, the issue may be moot when insurers provide only so much time per individual test irrespective of whether interactive feedback is being requested as part of the battery. Finally, *CPT Code 96113* is for all added 30-minute units needed to complete developmental test services as defined prior.

Understandably it is difficult to follow these various CPT codes and their narrative descriptions when first learning them. However, it is vital that a testing psychologist has reference to these codes and timing rules to avoid improper billing. Therefore, it is advised that one read through this narrative a second time while closely tracking the flow chart provided in Figure 3.2 to ensure more in-depth learning. Through practice, this will become increasingly overlearned and automatic.

SELECTING THE INDIVIDUAL TESTS, SERVICES, AND UNITS (FORM 3.7)

The final subsection in the initial clinical interview for testing forms contains a key so that the psychologist can interpret the testing services and units assigned to them in the subsequent listing. The four testing service types are enumerated in the form's key as follows: (a) *TAS* = Test Administration and Scoring (psychological and neuropsychological test administration and scoring); (b) *TEV* = Test Evaluation (i.e., psychological data interpretation, integration, decision-making, treatment planning, report generation, and interactive feedback); (c) *NTEV* = Neuropsychological Test Evaluation (i.e., neuropsychological data interpretation, integration, decision-making, treatment planning, report generation, and interactive feedback); (d) *DTS* = Developmental Test Services (i.e., developmental test administration, scoring, data interpretation, and report generation); and DTSA = Developmental Test Services Additional (i.e., added developmental test administration, scoring, data interpretation, and report generation). Additionally, the 2 units of time are listed in the form's key as follows: (a) each 30-minute unit is the equivalent of 16 to 30 minutes; and (b) each 60-minute unit is the equivalent of 31 to 60 minutes.

Therefore, this key is intended to be a handy reference for the psychologist to be cognizant of the most typical types of services and units needed to administer, score, interpret, report generate, and communicate the results for each test independently (then later aggregated). The units assigned to each test are located immediately under the test name and acronym. The types of services, including TAS, TEV, NTEV, DTS, and DTSA are assigned according to their principal uses. However, it is vital to ultimately code these tests according to *the principal purpose of the testing case*, not the individual test type. Therefore, although standard psychological tests (e.g., personality tests) may be initially coded as TEV (i.e., test evaluation services) in the listing, because this this their most frequent use and class, they should be recoded NTEV (i.e., neuropsychological test evaluation services) if being used to help diagnose a neurocognitive disorder with behavioral symptoms). Again, it is the principal objective of the testing case that ultimately dictates what class of evaluation services to request (i.e., either TEV, NTEV, or DTS and DTSA). Therefore, although the majority of tests have been classified according to their most typical use, with some doubling as both a psychological and developmental test, these may change depending upon the primary diagnostic objective of the testing case. In the event of case referrals that are mixed (e.g., both neurocognitive and psychological or psychological and developmental), the principal diagnostic purpose of the testing case controls; most typically this will be the more specialized objective (i.e., neuropsychological or developmental). If the referral questions are equally neuropsychological and psychological in nature, then it is best to test them independently of each other in two separate test batteries, essentially apportioning the referral into two testing cases involving the same examinee. A succinct means of stating this is that *test evaluation codes should never be mixed*; that is, they are to be all TEV, NTEV, or DTS/DTSA. The recommended time, however, should remain the same irrespective of their use and class of test evaluation service. These coding rules are illustrated in the case examples, which are available on Routledge's e-resources website.

In cases where the original use of the test is mixed, the secondary usage is listed last in the test listing. For example, two IQ tests that are normed in the two- to six-year range are primarily psychological tests, although practically it can be used to measure cognitive developmental delays. Further, the quantity of units listed are intended as estimates based upon (a) clinical experience in using each test, and (b) the number of units typically afforded PA by the most stringent insurance carriers. Again, the types of services and number of units listed are only meant as guidelines. They may be modified or adjusted depending upon the needs of the case, the context of the test battery, and the criteria employed in determining medical necessity for testing by the particular insurance carrier.

Each of the four clinical interview forms contains a list of tests properly normed for that particular cohort and in alphabetical order by test name for easy reference. Indents have been made so as to avoid hyphenating test acronyms to facilitate their identification. The dual purpose of circumscribing the list of tests to those properly normed is to (a) avoid making the list extremely long and cumbersome, and (b) assist the psychologist in choosing only those tests properly normed for that age group. However, some tests possess norms that pertain to only a limited subset of the developmental period, which is not apparent when looking at the test name and acronym. For instance, consider a case involving a 17-year, 1-month-old female being tested for *posttraumatic stress disorder* (*PTSD*). The initial clinical interview form for adolescence (viz., Form 3.5) shows two potential tests as follows: (a) *Trauma Symptom Checklist for Children* (*TSCC*; Briere, 1996); or (b) *Trauma Symptom Inventory, Second Edition* (*TSI–2*; Briere, 2011). However, the age ranges are not apparent from the test names and acronyms as they are on some tests. Hence, in such cases where the age-range information is not readily apparent from the provided listing, the psychologist can refer to Form 3.7, titled, "List of Available Psychological Tests," which provides a comprehensive listing of all tests available in the inventory from which to choose, classified by (a) the psychological construct measured (e.g., intelligence), and/or (b) the test format (e.g., rating scales tests). Further, the class labels are listed in alphabetical order whereas the tests within each class are listed by chronological age (younger to older) for easier reference. In actuality, Chapter 1, Table 1.1 serves the same function except that the tests are listed according to this book's chapter order in Part II.

Current Procedural Terminology (CPT) Testing Service Codes Totals

This section completes the initial clinical interview for testing report. After the individual tests are selected, along with their testing services and associated units, the latter must be aggregated, along with the total duration they represent in both minutes (rounded to the nearest 30-minute unit; e.g., 270 minutes) and hours (rounded to the nearest half-hour; e.g., 4.5 hours). The accrued number of units and minutes assists in comparing the amount requested and the amount obtaining PA. The total number in hours assists in scheduling and analyzing productivity (e.g., this week the author billed out 10.5 hours of testing).

Each of the four initial clinical interview forms (viz., Forms 3.3–3.6) contains a table titled, "CPT Testing Service Codes Summary: Requested Number of Units and Time," which is designed to facilitate determination of the quantity of units of each testing service that is being requested. Developmental test (DTS/DTSA) codes are listed only for the two youngest developmental periods (i.e., Forms 3.3 and 3.4). The psychologist simply enters the number of units of each test service, then sums them for a grand total in the bottom row, which includes summation of the time in both minutes and hours. A separate grand total row is provided for aggregating the DTS and DTSA units because of the fact that they do not cross over with the other codes. Therefore, entries should be made for either the psychological/neuropsychological rows or the DTS/DTSA rows, never both.

Note that "1" unit has been already inputted for the first 30-minute TAS unit and the first 60-minute TEV unit because these are most often types of services required, and thus most common. For less frequent neuropsychological test evaluation services and developmental test services, "--" symbols are inserted. Examples of how this table is to be used are given in later chapters. Here, it needs to be pointed out that this information is to be recorded into Form 3.12, titled, "*Psychological Assessment and Testing Services Record*," in the lower large section, titled, "*Psychological Assessment and Testing Service Log*." It is here where the requested services and those that ultimately obtain PA are recorded to ensure accurate billing. More will be discussed about this form in a subsequent section. Immediately beneath the table are notes that once again define the abbreviated terms (viz., TAS; TEV; NTEV; DTS; DTSA) and how to properly measure the units of time (i.e., 30 and 60). This saves time rather than being required to scroll back to the key at the beginning of this section to recall their meaning.

The last pre-drafted narratives document that the selected tests or test battery are properly normed and in their most recently developed versions. This is consistent with the criteria delineating the criteria for medical necessity (see, e.g., Table 3.2, Criterion 2). If there is only one test in the battery, or if the test selected is a fixed-battery measure as defined prior, the second selection should be chosen because it uses the phrase, "test battery." In effect, this language circumvents the unresolved issues regarding the requirement of two tests in a battery and what constitutes a single test.

At this important juncture, essentially all of the information needed to complete the "Initial Psychological Assessment Report" has been compiled, either in writing, within the interviewer's recent memory, and potentially in the form of screening test scoring results (if used). Referring to the flowchart in Figure 2.1, this means that the "Initial Clinical Interview for Testing" Stage 2 is in effect accomplished and the process it is now transitioning to the "Preparation for Testing and Scheduling Appointments" Stage 3 (including Forms 3.8–3.12), to which we now turn.

Preparation for Testing and Scheduling Appointments

Consent for Psychological Testing Services (Form 3.8)

As just indicated, the testing psychologist now has all the information needed to generate and sign the "Initial Psychological Assessment Report," whichever form was used (i.e., Forms 3.3, 3.4, 3.5, or 3.6). If a screening test was administered prior to deciding upon whether or not to pursue testing and for which disorders, then the standard score results are also available. Lastly, preliminary diagnoses should be in mind, along with the tests needed to address the diagnostic issues and any related questions not yet determined by the aforementioned assessment techniques. In order to provide feedback regarding the units (i.e., time) that will be needed, those tests can be retained in the listing and the rest deleted, along with entering the units needed into the table, "CPT Testing Service Codes Summary: Requested Number of Units and Time." This permits a quick method of adding the needed units and time for the immediate purpose of accurate oral feedback.

Therefore, although the initial assessment report is not yet fully generated in written form, everything is needed to provide the examinee and any collaterals (e.g., parents) with oral feedback necessary for obtaining informed consent to pursue follow-up testing as a new service. The attempt is to remain as succinct as possible, focusing on (a) which disorders have been ruled in and out thus far, (b) which disorders will be the focus of subsequent standardized testing (including type of presentation and severity level, (c) what types of tests are needed, (d) what these tests entail in terms of procedure and time investment (including any special instructions), and (e) how scheduling will proceed. Examples of special instructions include the following: (a) advising examinees to wear corrective eye-lenses, hearing aids, or similar devices designed to accommodate for any sensory limitations or similar handicaps during their test administration sessions; and (b) to be on or off certain medications for a defined period of time prior to and during testing (e.g., ADHD stimulant medication). Although this appears as if it would consume significant time, with practice such information can be shared well within five minutes, including addressing any questions they might have.

When oral consent is obtained, Form 3.8 titled, "Consent for Psychological Testing Services," is presented and their names entered at the top. The form can be summarized as providing written agreement to proceed with testing as just discussed. The various types of information to which they have been advised orally are presented in a numbered (and lettered) sequence for easy reference. A perusal of the types of information enumerated on the form shows that as a set, they reduce to writing all the information reviewed above, including disorders that are being targeted, types of tests being requested, time requirements, individuals involved, release of the final report highlighting the major types on information contained therein, and their ethical right to withdraw such consent at any time thereafter. The form should then be properly signed and witnessed (usually by the psychologist), and made a formal element of the testing file (whether hard copy and/or scanned as an electronic document). Of course, the examinee may request and retain a copy of this consent.

Scheduling Appointments for Psychological Test Administration (Stage 3; Form 3.9)

Once the consent process has been consummated, any rating scales that are part of the planned test battery can be distributed, including instructions as to the proper respondents (e.g., parent, teacher), estimated time for completion, and how and when to submit them. If the respondents are immediately available, (e.g., parent, self-report), then they can be asked to complete these forms prior to leaving the facility. This accomplishes two objectives as follows: (a) the forms are completed immediately to avert unnecessary delays due to the forms being forgotten or lost; and (b) the respondents become actively involved in the testing process.

Next arrives a decision point: Do I schedule the testing appointments today prior to obtaining PA for testing, or do I wait until PA has been obtained? The answer is the former because it effectively (a) maintains commitment of the examinee and any collaterals to the testing process, and (b) facilitates the scheduling process because most insurance companies maintain their PA for 90 days. A PA duration of three months is typically sufficient to cover testing appointments if scheduled immediately after the initial appointment, including perhaps one episode of cancelling and rescheduling (e.g., if the examinee or the examiner thereafter has a scheduling conflict or becomes ill). On the other hand, calling and scheduling test appointments after PA increases the chances that such appointments will be scheduled further out and closer to the PA authorization deadline. If there are any additional delays, a request to extend the PA duration may be needed, which is risky because this request may be denied as no longer meeting medical necessity standards. Therefore, as a general rule, accomplishing as much as possible at each juncture in the testing process is usually the most effective and efficient practice.

Assuming appointments will be immediately scheduled, the document to be completed is titled, "Scheduling Appointments for Psychological Test Administration," (Form 3.9). This form is designed for support staff responsible for scheduling the follow-up testing appointments. Therefore, they should be briefed as to how to read and interpret the form and its information. The needed information is demarcated into sub-categories, including fill-in and multiple-choice items, all of which increases the speed and efficiency of entering the requisite information (see Form 3.9). First, "Examinee Information" includes name, date of birth, and internal file number, along with who and how to contact for scheduling issues. This is ensued by the name and supervisor (if any) of the testing psychologist. The "Test Administration Instructions" sub-category contains the most vital information; that is, scheduling. To begin with Line 1, the "Testing appointments with psychologist," options are presented in checklist format, the first four representing the most frequent selections. Here, the most applicable alternatives should be checked, the most common being "One 1-hour" or "One 2-hour." If no such appointments are needed, the "None" option should be checked, thus proceeding to the second line.

If two separate appointments are needed for two different respondents, then the two appropriate appointments should be checked, and Line 4, "Special testing instructions" should be checked as "Yes," with the names of each respondent being associated with which appointment.

For example, perhaps one 2-hour appointment is needed to administer an IQ test to an examinee, in addition to a one 1-hour appointment to administer an adaptive behavior structured interview to a parent. In such case, the proper two appointments with the psychologist should be marked in Line 1, followed by indicating who should attend which appointment in Line 4.

Here, a practice suggestion is shared regarding test administration policy. Unless there are extenuating circumstances, test administration should not exceed two hours (or 120 minutes) in a single sitting. If a test battery selected by the psychologist happens to exceed this duration (e.g., three hours), administration should be partitioned into as many one- or two-hour appointments that would cover what is needed (e.g., one 2-hour and one 1-hour appointment). Exceeding two hours' administration time in one session risks confounding the test results with increasing fatigue and declining motivation, which reduces test reliability (or accuracy) and validity (or precision). Therefore, a series of testing appointments can be scheduled on back-to-back days or in similar proximity in order to retain efficiency while averting the aforementioned confounding effects.

Line 2, "Computer tests" refer to personality inventories that are self-administered currently by means of computer hardware and software. Some of these computer administering and scoring systems are internet-based and some are managed by means of computer software loaded onto the computer's hard drive. In previous years, such multiple-choice (i.e., True–False; degree of agreement) tests were largely administered by means of a hard copy booklet with test items and scantron answer sheet. The use of computerized versions is strongly advised in order to further reduce error variance in the resulting data. This issue is especially revisited throughout Part II when reviewing the various tests and their formats. Therefore, that is all that needs to be said about this issue here. If a previous non-computer assisted means of administration is employed for these tests, Line 2 should be modified to read as something akin to, "Self-report tests."

Note that on Line 2 in parentheses, immediately after the Phrase, "Computer tests," there appears an instruction that these measures should be completed before any testing appointments (if any) scheduled with the psychologist on Line 1. The reason is that the computer administered self-report personality inventories at the author's facility are administered by a properly trained technician during a separate scheduled appointment. This explains the final boxed sub-category allocated at the bottom of Form 3.9, titled, "Scheduled Appointments." Here, support staff enter the scheduled appointment(s), then subsequently mark whether such represents a testing appointment with the psychologist (see Line 1) or a computer test with the technician. In the event more than one personality inventory is marked, the respondent can complete both tests in one sitting because they typically can be done in under 60-minutes each; hence, less than the aforementioned 2-hour in one session principle. In the event the self-report inventory is the only test in the battery, it may be administered immediately after PA is established, hence rendering it even more efficient. In the event testing psychologists wish to personally administer these self-report inventories in order to make test-taking observations and/or answer examinee questions, the computer test entries on the form may be deleted and the administration time added to Line 1.

Some final comments about the scheduling Form 3.9 are in order before continuing with the assessment process. Line 3, "Rating scales" should also be marked as needed so that support staff are cognizant that these measures are (a) part of the requested battery, and (b) in need of being submitted at some point prior to the scheduled testing appointment(s). As stated prior, the intention of Line 4 is to document any required special testing instructions not otherwise available on the form. Examples include the need for one parent to be present and attend the testing session, and whether examinee is to be off (or on) the prescribed ADHD medication during the test administration appointment. As indicated previously, a "None" option is available after each of the test scheduling options (i.e., Lines 1, 2, and 3) and should be selected of any one or more of these do not apply.

If scheduling is to be done prior to PA, the completed Form 3.9 should be given to the examinee and any collaterals with instructions to in turn give it to the front desk staff before leaving in order to schedule the needed testing appointments. If testing is to be deferred until PA is obtained, Form 3.9 should be filed as an official part of the medical record (whether hard copy of electronically). Next, a final document that delineates test instructions in written form is reviewed.

Psychological Testing Instructions to Examinee (& Collaterals): Scheduling Appointments Before or After Preauthorization (Forms 3.10a and 3.10b)

The last form that may be given to examinees and any collaterals is a document that reduces to formal writing the test instructions just provided orally. In particular, Forms 3.10, titled, "Psychological Testing Instructions to Examinee (& Collaterals): Scheduling Appointments Before Preauthorization" (Form 3.10a) and "Psychological Testing Instructions to Examinee (& Collaterals): Scheduling Appointments After Preauthorization" (Form 3.10b) are substantively identical. The only variance is in items 1 and 2 referring to information concerning

PA and scheduling. By design, these forms are intended to educate and document the ensuing plan of action. First, they require very little information to be added. This includes only the examinee name and medical record number (MRN), date, and total number of testing units and time that the test battery will require. The latter was calculated using the clinical interview form and table titled, "CPT Testing Service Codes Summary: Requested Number of Units and Time." Second, the specific sections are enumerated by number for easy reference.

More specifically, following Form 3.10a, Item 1 on "Scheduling Information" instructs the examinee and collaterals to submit the scheduling form (i.e., Form 3.9), although also informs of an optional cancellation list wherein examinees can be contacted for appointments of a sooner date if and when they become available. This strategy is handy in facilities with a continuously high demand for services and affords hope that appointments far in the future have the potential of being moved closer in time. Item 2, "Insurance Preauthorization (PA)" informs regarding the PA process and the need for alternate plans if the requested units are denied or severely reduced or restricted. In the event of severe reductions of requested units, occasionally the most viable option is to test for some, but not all, of the suspected disorders. An example is a denial of 6 units to rule out a specific learning disability due to such testing being deemed primarily educational in nature. If 2 units of testing for a personality disorder in the same case are approved, then the examinee and any collaterals must be contacted to inform them that only the personality testing will be pursued, along with the reasons therefore.

Item 3, "Number of Testing Hours Being Requested for PA" essentially educates the examinee and any collaterals regarding the kinds of testing tasks and skills that constitute billable services, especially for those who have experience being billed for psychotherapy services. What is unique about psychological testing services and their billing is that, although fundamentally based upon units or time, a good portion of such services are not face-to-face. Thus, for example, when people are billed for a 50-minute psychotherapy session, the *CPT Code 90834, 38–52 minutes* is used (American Psychological Association, 2017). This is in accord with what is referred to as the CPT *time-rule*, which is defined as the provider choosing the billing code that is in greatest proximity to the actual clock time of the session (as opposed to *CPT Code 90832, 16–37 minutes* or *CPT Code 90837, 53 or more minutes*). In consequence, when those who have received psychological testing services are billed for units of time, which are added on and that are not face-to-face (see especially TES or testing evaluation services), misunderstandings in the form of perceived excessive billing can easily result. Therefore, the dual objectives of this section are to (a) educate regarding psychological testing services and what constitutes legitimate billable activities, and (b) inform as to the legitimate number of units and time beforehand that will be needed to complete the selected test battery. In this manner, there is a written record as to what was deemed required and ultimately billed that can be referred to in the event of any resulting questions or misunderstandings. Additionally, there is also written documentation of the obtained informed consent that works in conjunction with the test instruction form, showing evidence that the examinee and any collaterals were properly informed of the panned testing and what it entailed. Essentially, these documents work together to protect both the consumer and provider of psychological testing services.

Lastly, Item 4 titled, "Standardized Rating Scales," reminds the examinee and any collaterals of how important the standardized rating scales (if used) are to the test battery as a whole. In particular, such data are critical when the examiner is searching for both interrater reliability and convergent validity of the results. Although many of the tests provide validity scales, which are designed to detect aberrant response tendencies that may question the accuracy of the respondent's data, there remains the question of whether the ratings are consistent or accurate. Having a second and independent rater, who observes the examinee in a different context, is a vital source to analyze reliability. In any case, reminding the examinee and collaterals to complete and submit these measures as instructed, can avoid unnecessary delays and wasted materials in an attempt to complete the test battery as planned.

Lastly, a practical form that may be applied to any kind of psychological service is a proof of appointment form. Such form is intended for child clients and adults who ask for proof that they attended a healthcare related appointment. For this purpose, Form 3.11 titled,

"Proof of Appointment Note: School or Work," was created. Note that some of the blank spaces can be filled in with accurate repeating information, including the name and location of the office, time zone, psychologist's name and credentials, and the facility logo to replace the generic one that is inserted. Time zone information is useful is the practice is in proximity to a geographically defined boundary between Central Standard Time (CST) and Eastern Standard Time (EST), which is a one-hour difference. Of course, this may be deleted if not an issue. The more parsimonious the forms the more pragmatically useful they tend to be. Stage 3 is now officially done.

Completing the Initial Psychological Assessment Report

Once the test battery has been selected, the examinee and any collaterals briefed, the consent obtained (i.e., oral and written), the scheduling form completed, and any written instructions provided, the interview per se is done. The next task is to fill in portions of the initial report that were left undone, proofing and signing it, and entering it into the testing file as an official document and matter of record. This is denoted in the flowchart in Figure 2.1 by the broken dashed–dotted line in the horizontal direction (left-to-right), which emerges from the vertical down arrow that itself begins after the "Preparation for Testing and Scheduling Appointments" phase. This horizontal arrow has its distinct destination at the oval titled, "Initial Psychological Assessment Report," which represents the first of two formal reports that are essential to the testing case. This is basically a formality in reducing Stage 2 to writing.

Pragmatically speaking, if working within a 60-minute time limit, one should be done with the interview in approximately 45-minutes. This leaves 15 minutes for completing the "Initial Psychological Assessment Report" inputting any narrative notes as part of a hard copy or electronic mental health filing system, and recording billing information on a hard copy or electronic mental health services log. As will be apparent subsequently, a special record form has been designed for logging testing services (see below).

Increasingly, mental health centers and practices are utilizing an electronically based software system that combines creating narrative notes with CPT codes for billing purposes. In one facility, the completed clinical interview form is created electronically using Microsoft Word, and scanned into the electronic software system. Thus, a separate note is created for billing using the "Diagnostic Evaluation CPT Code 90791" (see Figure 3.2). Again, although this code in Figure 3.2 shows, "60 minutes," this is only author's personal recommendation and not a requirement of this code as it is event-based. That is, it either occurred in its entirety or did not occur at all. However, is mandated that a genuine comprehensive behavioral health evaluation has been done. It is difficult to image that a competently done initial evaluation is possible to do in less time.

Documenting the Provision of Psychological Assessment and Testing Services

Subsequent to the initial report and any associated billing being done, some type of summary record, log, or journal of the psychological assessment and testing services is extremely desirable. The document titled, "Psychological

Assessment and Testing Services Record" (Form 3.12; see Figure 2.1), which is inserted after the preparation for testing and appointment scheduling and prior to requesting PA, is designed to show a succinct one-page record of the following information: (a) examinee name and MRN; (b) psychologist (and supervisor if any) providing the services; (c) insurance carriers; (d) dates and types of service (including cancels and no-shows); (e) test services and units requested; (f) test services and units approved; (g) whether PA is required; and if so, (h) dates that any PA applies. As on the scheduling form, major areas of subclasses of information have been demarcated by dark-lined boxes.

The first three boxed sections are self-explanatory and such information can be entered in a matter of seconds. The fourth and final box with the subheading, "Psychological Assessment and Testing Service Log," is the most important and is itself bifurcated into a listing of dates and types of services, followed by test services requested and approved by insurance. Dates of service is self-explanatory as month/day/year (e.g., 03/12/2021 representing March 12th, 2021). Psychological services type entries are too numerous to capture based upon one standardized key, hence is left open-ended. The following can be used: (a) Initial (i.e., clinical interview); (b) Test. (i.e., testing appointment with acronyms or abbreviations for tests that were done); (c) Comp. Test (e.g., computer test, MMPI–A–RF); (d) NS (no-show); (e) CX (or cancellation); (f) FB (i.e., interactive feedback); (g) Trans. (i.e., transfer case back to internal referral source); and (h) Dis. (i.e., discharge case). The tracking of NS and CX is important to avoid rescheduling a case that continues to find reasons not to attend testing appointments, hence consuming time better spent with clients who intend to follow through with planned testing.

Perhaps the most critical information on this form is the type and number of testing services that have been requested and approved, along with the applicable dates. First, the information on the bottom far left provides a pragmatic summary of the (a) five categories of testing services (viz., TAS and TEV or NTEV; or DTS and DTSA), by (b) two durational units (viz., 30-minute and 60-minute), by 2-unit orders (viz., first and added).[7],[8]

Second, there are blank fill-in lines for the correct numbers of each CPT code requested by the testing psychologist. Note that this information should mirror the numbers inserted into the CPT computational table of the initial report. Although redundancy is seemingly antithetical to efficiency, feature can be used as an effective double-check on one's math; that is, entering and totaling the type of units and time. This is vital because the units that are being aggregated or summed are not uniform, varying from 30- to 60-minute durations. As a consequence, the same quantity of units can reflect different time totals. For example, imagine a test battery that requires 4 units of TAS and 2 units of TEV. The total number of units would equal 6 (i.e., $4 + 2 = 6$) with a total duration of 240 minutes or 4.0 hours (i.e., $[30 \times 4] + [2 \times 60] = 240$). Compare this with another test battery that requires 3 units of TAS and 3 units of TEV. Again, a total of 6 units are being requested. However, in this scenario the total duration of time would be 270 minutes or 4.5 hours (i.e., $[3 \times 30 = 90] + [3 \times 60 = 180] = 270$). Other permutations can lead to even larger discrepancies. Therefore, it is advantageous to have a rapid means of ensuring the accuracy of these calculations. As one can easily imagine, it is much easier to make corrections prior to submitting a report for PA than afterwards.

Lastly, when PA has been determined, it is prudent that these numbers be entered accurately and are easily accessible within the testing file. The principal rationale for being so diligent here is to prevent clients from being billed for requested hours that did not receive PA. Why? Two reasons are offered, one of which is lawful and the other ethical. First, recall the concept of *balance billing*, which is defined as providers charging their clients for the difference between what they deem proper for a type of service (e.g., $300.00 for an initial assessment) and what the insurer deems proper (e.g., $200.00 for an initial assessment). In this parenthetical example, the client would be charged by the provider for the difference of $100.00 (i.e., $300.00–$200.00 = $100.00). In the event the provider was contracted with the insurer to charge only what the latter deems proper, such charge would be illegal. Analogously, if the testing psychologist is working under contract with that insurer, charging the client for psychological services and units not receiving PA would be similarly illegal. Second, even if the testing psychologist is not contracted with the insurer, charging for non-preauthorized units can arguably be a violation of informed consent. That is, when clients are informed regarding the number of requested units, the implication is that such services will be covered by their insurance company. If such is not that case, and providers' intentions are to bill for all units requested (i.e., those obtaining PA and those not obtaining PA), clients should be forewarned about such discrepancy, including how much additional cost they will be responsible for due to the non-covered units. In such instances, clients can make informed decisions as to whether or not to pursue testing, in whole or in part, including signing a revised consent form with language addressing the new terms.

In these circumstances, the initially requested battery can be pursued and billing only for units that received PA. Why? First, with this psychological assessment and testing system, cases tend to balance out over the long run resulting in a reasonable financial return. Second, when one considers all the time that is consumed with informing clients of these PA circumstances, revising and resigning informed consent documents, and completing any necessary rescheduling, it is simply more pragmatic to simply provide what was planned and agreed to in the first place, and to continue being maximally productive with other cases. Third, the testing psychologist frequently has multiple clients in a single case, including the examinee and possibly one or more referral sources, not to mention the quality of one's own work. Finally, if psychologists find that their requested testing units are being continually denied at an atypically high rate, they should scrutinize the reasons given by the insurance carriers, then revise their clinical interviews accordingly. More regarding PA is discussed in the succeeding section.

Request for Testing Preauthorization

With the completion of the initial assessment report, we have reached the next stage in the assessment and test process; namely, the box titled, "Request for Test Preauthorization" (see Figure 2.1). If test administration appointments have already been scheduled, which is the advised approach, filing the request for preauthorization (PA) should be expedited in order to avoid having to reschedule appointments due to delays in the process. A number of outcomes are possible as follows (in order from most to least desirable): (a) PA for psychological testing is not required; (b) PA for psychological testing is required an all requested units are authorized (including the dates for which PA has been approved); (c) PA for psychological testing is required and most i.e., 50% to 75%) of requested units are approved (including which units approved, which not approved, and reasons therefore); (d) PA for psychological testing is required and most (i.e., 25% to 49%) of requested units are denied (including which units approved, which not approved, and reasons therefore); (e) PA for psychological testing is required and all requested units are denied; and (f) client is not insured.

Let us take these independently. In the first case, Medicaid insurance in the state of Indiana, typically applying the most stringent standards for medical necessity concerning testing, does not require PA for developmental test services. This must be an effort to support early detection and intervention. In any event, the point here is to alert one to the fact that such testing may obtain PA with many fewer obstacles than other kinds of testing, especially if other states handle PA for such testing in similar fashion. Below, some important issues are discussed associated with all requested test units being preauthorized. In such favorable instance, the assessment process immediately moves forward to the next stage; in Figure 2.1, box titled, "Testing PA Obtained or Otherwise Negotiated with Examinee."

After dealing with the most favorable circumstance, issues and strategies are discussed to use when some portion of the requested units have been denied PA. In such instance, the assessment process moves to the potential stage in Figure 2.1, broken-dotted box titled, "Testing Denied or Units Requested Reduced."

All Requested Testing Units Preauthorized: Peer-to-Peer Consultation Unnecessary

First, in the ideal case where PA is not required, the principal consideration is to resist the temptation (i.e., conscious or unconscious) to add unnecessary tests to the battery. When psychologists must repeatedly contend with insurance denials of PA for requested testing, the experience can be extremely disconcerting. Therefore, when at last there is a virtual guarantee that the requested testing will be approved, it is human nature to be more liberal in choosing the quantity of tests needed to adequately address all diagnostic issues and questions. For example, imagine a testing referral that presented a differential diagnosis between bipolar disorder and borderline personality disorder (not an infrequent request by the way). Also assume that the examinee, a 33-year-old male, is quite intelligent, verbal, possesses the ability to introspect, has no reason to be defensive or exaggerate his degree of psychopathology, and best of all, has an insurance policy in which psychological testing does not require PA.

In such case, it is the author's opinion that a *Millon Clinical Multiaxial Inventory, Fourth Edition* (MCMI–IV; Millon, Grossman, & Millon, 2015) would be sufficient and would require the following units; TAS = 1 unit, CPT Code 96136, 1st 30-minute unit; TEV = 1 unit, CPT Code 96130, 1st 60-minute unit (total minutes = 90; see Form 3.6, § Requested Tests, Testing Services, and Units (Time). However, one could rationalize the addition of the *Rorschach Performance Assessment System* (R–PAS; Mihura & Meyer, 2018; Meyer, Viglione, Mihura, Erard, & Erdberg, 2011, 2012) in order to (a) examine intrapsychic personality functioning to a greater extent, and (b) attempt to gather *convergent validity* for the diagnosis; that is, two tests of different format (i.e., an explicit and implicit personality test) that yield data supporting the same psychopathology. Although this could be justified using logic and general assessment principles, it would add the following: TAS = 4 units, CPT Code 96137, added 30-minute units; TEV = 2 units, CPT Code 96131, added 60-minute units (total added minutes 180 minutes or three hours; see Form 3.6, § Requested Tests, Testing Services, and Units (Time).

Are the added three hours it would take to employ both tests worth the attempt to bolster diagnosis? Another way to view this is in terms of cost. If testing were $200.00 per hour, then we are considering here a difference between $300.00 for the MCMI–IV alone (i.e., 200 x 1.5 = 300) versus $900.00 (200 x 4.5 = 900) for the MCMI–IV and R–PAS together; that is, three times the cost. In the real world, where testing practice must be balanced with *test utility* (i.e., the degree to which an assessment measure is useful for a specified purpose, usually balancing its costs and benefits), this makes quite a bit of difference. During training, psychology students typically administer large batteries of tests to examinees, understandably because the focus is on learning and integrating data; hence, cost is not a consideration, except perhaps in terms of time. However, in the arena of managed care and people's financial resources, both of which set pragmatic limits, cost in terms of both money and time must be considered. Here, the MCMI–IV alone can be selected. Then, if for some unanticipated reason the results are invalid or inconclusive, a second test can be requested with justification.

Second, when PA is required and all requested testing units are indeed authorized, this is an identical outcome but in reality for a more favorable reason. In particular, this means that the clinician's initial psychological assessment report provided the correct information needed to meet the medical necessity for testing. In such circumstances, it behooves the clinician to examine the report and the information contained therein and to match it with the particular insurer. Essentially, it behooves the psychologist who does a fair amount of testing to learn what particular insurers are looking for in a report, including the ones that obtain PA. Next, different scenarios in which some portion of the requested units are denied are discussed. An order from a smaller to greater proportion of units denied is followed. The amounts selected are arbitrary and intended as approximate guidelines.

Requested Units of Testing Somewhat Reduced: Peer-to-Peer Consultation Waived

First, when approximately 50% to 75% of the requested testing hours are preauthorized (i.e., 25% to 50% denied), the following two actions can be taken: (a) examine the insurer's response as to which units were denied and for what reason(s); and (b) waive the opportunity for a peer-to-peer review of the units denied (unless there remains some significant confusion as to reasons for the denial). Examining the reasons for denial further contributes to learning what particular insurers are accepting and not accepting for purposes of establishing the medical necessity for testing. For example, consider a test battery that consists of an autism rating scale, an intelligence test, an autism performance test, and an adaptive behavior structured interview in order to test for ASD and ID. Perhaps a 60-minute unit was denied because it was associated with the rating scale, which this insurer deemed as not constituting a psychological test. In such case, it should be noted that this insurer will similarly deny units associated with rating scales. Also, it is not worth the time or effort to schedule a peer-to-peer phone consultation in an attempt to gain the denied unit.

Requested Units of Testing Significantly Reduced or All Are Denied: Peer-to-Peer Consultation Pursued

In instances where about 25% to 50% of the units are preauthorized (i.e., 50% to 75% denied), scheduling a peer-to-peer phone consultation is a sensible idea, unless upon review it is clear why the denial occurred. Again, the dual purpose of such consultations is to learn what particular insurers are looking for and to attempt to add information so that more units are authorized. Even if such units are not afforded PA, the psychologist should follow through and complete the testing as planned. As alluded to in the prior section, the testing psychologist should aim principally for developing a solid reputation for being reliable and productive, in essence frequently servicing at least two clients; the examinee and the referral source.

Finally, in cases where all units are denied, peer-to-peer should be attempted, again unless it is absolutely clear why the units were denied and consultation would clearly be fruitless. In such cases, negotiating with the client for a reduced fee is a feasible approach. When engaging in such discussions, all attempts should be made to successfully complete the testing. Clients and referral sources will appreciate such efforts, the latter especially in the form of increased referrals.

Testing Denied After Peer-to-Peer Consultation: Letter of Appeal

As a final note in this section, if peer-to-peer consultation is unsuccessful, an optional letter of appeal should not be pursued for two reasons. First, the units that were preauthorized can potentially be reversed, hence taking an unnecessary risk. That is, appealing an adverse decision result in a review of all requested units, not simply the units that were denied. Second, appeals usually fail and are therefore not worth the time or effort.

Testing Preauthorization Obtained or Otherwise Negotiated with Examinee

Once the PA issue is resolved, and any needed self-pay options have been offered and accepted, the path is now cleared for actual psychological testing. However, if scheduling was deferred until after PA issues are resolved, examinees must now be contacted for establishing their appointment date(s) and time(s) according to the form, "Scheduling Appointments for Psychological Test Administration" (viz., Form 3.9). This is denoted in Figure 2.1 by the broken-dotted box titled, "Scheduling Appointments (if not done after initial clinical interview)." Recall that this form should be made a part of the examinee's testing file subsequent to the initial clinical interview and typically are contacted by support staff. Hopefully, there has not been a significant diminution in examinees' motivation to pursue the planned testing, which is always a risk when there is a hiatus between the initial and subsequent scheduled appointments.

Recapitulation

This chapter delineated the initial phases of the psychological assessment and testing process, from the point of the initial referral through the preauthorization procedure. The discussion began with a strategy for conducting the specialized clinical interview for testing, which was ensued by what information and facts were needed to complete the major sections of the initial assessment report. A significant focus was placed upon making key decisions, including whether follow-up testing was needed and, if so, how to select the proper tests with justification, the needed test services, units, and CPT billing codes, and how to aggregate the latter in preparation for obtaining PA from third party payers. Here, a discussion regarding the new CPT testing services and billing codes promulgated by the American Medical Association was provided. The chapter concluded with a discussion regarding the PA procedure and alternative courses of action contingent upon the number of requested units being preauthorized. Throughout the chapter, pertinent forms were presented, and their content and use detailed, in order to facilitate both comprehension and actual assessment and testing practice. Additionally, repeated references to the flowchart of the assessment and testing process in Figure 2.1, which was introduced in Chapter 2, was done in order to maximize comprehension.

Chapter 4 is essentially a continuation of this discussion, beginning where this Chapter 3 ended. Hence, it details the process from the point of test administration to communication of the findings and billing for test services rendered, again utilizing references to Figure 2.1 and focusing on the manner in which the initial assessment report transforms into its final format. The major new section of the final report regards that which comprises the test data and their interpretation. Chapter 4 shows the framework of this vital new section wherein the data tables for each test presented in Part II of this book are to be inserted. As such, although Chapter 4 is much briefer in length compared to Chapter 3, it sets the stage for the entire Part II of the book, along with the online e-resources, which integrate the prior two sections of the book with (a) interpretive flowcharts for the major tests, (b) case examples for each of the aforesaid four developmental periods, and (c) electronic modifiable practice and report forms, along with test data tables with interpretive excerpts.

Key Terms

- acquiescence (or yea saying)
- acute stressors
- adaptational failure/s
- adaptive behavioral functioning
- adjustment disorder with anxiety
- adjustment disorder with mixed anxiety and depressed mood
- adult ambivalent attachment style
- adult avoidant attachment style
- adult disorganized-disoriented attachment style
- adult secure attachment style
- affect
- affect recognition
- alcohol use disorder
- alexithymia
- ambivalent attachment
- anhedonia
- anosognosia
- anoxia (or asphyxia)
- antidepressant discontinuation syndrome
- antisocial personality
- anxiety disorders
- Apgar test
- associated environmental stressors

- associative play
- attachment
- attention
- attention-deficit/hyperactivity disorder (ADHD)
- auditory (or echoic) sensory memory
- autism-spectrum disorder (ASD)
- autobiographical memory
- autonomic nervous system
- avoidant attachment
- Behavioral Health Evaluation (CPT Code 90801)
- behavioral medicine
- best interests of the child
- bipolar disorder
- bipolar I disorder
- body mass index (BMI)
- borderline intellectual functioning
- chronic stressors
- chronological age (CA)
- circumstantiality
- civil commitment
- clinical interview
- clinical syndromes
- cognition
- commitment
- conception
- conduct disorder (CD)
- Confidentiality of Substance Use Disorder, 42 C.F.R Part 2
- confounding variable
- Conners Comprehensive Behavior Rating Scales (Conners CBRS)
- Conners Kiddie Continuous Performance Test, Second Edition (K–CPT 2)
- constructive processing theory
- continuity of care
- continuous performance test/s (CPT)
- contrast effects
- convergent validity
- cooperative play
- CPT Code 90791
- CPT Code 90792
- CPT Code 90801
- CPT Code 90832, 16–37 minutes
- CPT Code 90834, 38–52 minutes
- CPT Code 90837, 53 or more minutes
- CPT Code 96101
- CPT Code 96112
- CPT Code 96113
- CPT Code 96118
- CPT Code 96130
- CPT Code 96131
- CPT Code 96132
- CPT Code 96133
- CPT Code 96136
- CPT Code 96137
- crisis
- cry for help
- Current Procedural Terminology (CPT)
- data

- deductive reasoning
- delinquent acts
- delusional
- dependent variable
- developmental milestone/s
- developmental psychopathology
- developmental test/s
- diagnoses to be ruled in/confirmed
- diagnoses to be ruled out
- diagnoses to be screened for
- Diagnostic and Statistical Manual of Mental Disorders, Fifth Edition (DSM–5)
- Diagnostic and Statistical Manual of Mental Disorders, Fourth Edition (DSM–IV)
- differential diagnosis
- diffusion
- disinhibited social engagement disorder
- disorganized-disoriented attachment
- disruptive mood dysregulation disorder (DMDD)
- dopamine
- DTS
- DTSA
- dyslexia
- echolalia
- effortful-control
- ego dystonic (or ego alien)
- ego syntonic
- elaborative rehearsal
- emotion
- emotion regulation
- emotional competence
- encryption
- episodic LTM
- executive functioning
- extracurricular
- extraversion (or surgency)
- false negative
- false positive
- feign
- felonies
- fetus
- fine motor skills
- Five-Factor Model (FFM)
- flash drive
- flight of ideas
- foreclosure
- GABA (or gamma-Aminobutyric acid, or γ-aminobutyric acid)
- generalized anxiety disorder (GAD)
- gross motor skills
- guardian
- guardianship
- Head Start
- Health Insurance Portability and Accountability Act of 1996 (HIPPA)
- heritability
- high school certificate of completion
- high school diploma
- identity achievement.
- identity versus role confusion

- independent variable
- Individualized Education Plan (IEP)
- Individualized Education Program (IEP)
- industry versus inferiority
- information processing
- initial clinical interview
- intelligence
- interactive feedback
- internal working models
- interrater reliability
- introspection
- Journal of Social and Personal Relationships
- juvenile delinquency
- Kinetic Family Drawing (KFD)
- legal custody
- long-term memory (LTM)
- loosening of associations
- major depressive disorder (MDD)
- major depressive disorder, with melancholic features
- major neurocognitive disorder due to Parkinson's disease
- major neurocognitive disorder due to traumatic brain injury
- malingering
- masochistic personality syndrome (self-defeating personality syndrome)
- medical necessity
- melancholy
- memory stick
- menarche
- mental health and developmental disorders
- mental health parity laws
- mental status examination (MSE)
- metric system
- Mini-Mental State Examination, Second Edition (MMSE–2)
- Minnesota Multiphasic Personality Inventory, Adolescent Edition, Restructured Form (MMPI–A–RF)
- Minnesota Multiphasic Personality Inventory, Second Edition, Restructured Form (MMPI–2–RF)
- misdemeanors
- mood
- mood disorders with psychotic features
- moratorium
- multidimensional tests
- negative affectivity
- negative psychotic symptoms
- neurocognitive disorder
- neurodevelopmental disorder/s
- nominal scale
- nonorganic mental disorders
- non-suicidal self-injury (NSSI)
- norepinephrine (or noradrenaline)
- NTEV
- objective descriptors
- obsessive-compulsive disorder (OCD)
- onlooker play
- operational definition
- oppositional defiant disorder (ODD)
- organic mental disorders
- organogenesis
- orientation

- other specified anxiety disorder
- other specified disorder
- parallel play
- parens patriae
- pathogenic
- Paul Wellstone-Pete Domenici Mental Health Parity and Addiction Equity Act of 2008
- perception
- personality change due to another medical condition
- personality disorder/s
- physical custody
- plea bargaining
- posttraumatic stress disorder (PTSD)
- preauthorization (PA)
- premorbid level of functioning
- prenatal
- presenting symptoms
- pretend play
- prevalence
- principal diagnoses
- prognosis
- provisional
- provisional diagnosis/es
- psychoactive substances
- psychological test
- psychomotor
- psychomotor agitation
- psychomotor retardation
- psychopath
- psychopathy
- psychotic disorder due to another medical condition
- psychotropic medications
- reactive attachment disorder (RAD)
- recall task
- related medical variables and conditions
- resilience
- response sets (noncontent responding)
- rule/d out
- ruled in/confirmed
- schizophrenia
- screen for
- screening tests
- secondary gain
- secure attachment
- selective attention
- self-concept
- self-esteem
- self-medicating
- semantic LTM
- semenarche (or spermarche)
- sensory memory
- social anxiety disorder
- social desirability
- solitary play
- specific learning disorder, with impairment in mathematics
- specific learning disorder, with impairment in reading
- specific learning disorder/s (SLD)

- speech sound disorder (previously, phonological disorder)
- stability coefficient
- status offenses
- Strange Situation
- stressors
- subjective descriptors
- substance-related disorder
- suicidal attempts
- suicidal gesture
- suicidal ideation
- suicidal plans
- TAS
- temperament
- teratogens
- test administration and scoring services
- test evaluation services
- TEV
- the play years
- theory of mind (ToM)
- thought
- thought blocking
- thought content
- thought process
- thumb drive
- time-rule
- Trauma Symptom Checklist for Children (TSCC)
- Trauma Symptom Inventory, Second Edition (TSI–2)
- traumatic brain injury (TBI)
- U.S. standard system (or imperial system)
- unidimensional tests
- unoccupied play
- USB drive
- USB stick
- V codes
- vegetative symptoms
- vulnerability-stress model (diathesis–stress model)
- Vyvanse (or Lisdexamfetamine Dimesylate)
- Wechsler Memory Scale, Fourth Edition, Brief Cognitive Status Exam, WMS–IV, BCSE
- with behavioral disturbance
- working diagnosis/es
- Xanax (or Alprazolam)
- Z codes
- Zoloft (or Sertraline)
- zygote

Notes

1. This form can be modified downwards if a psychologist receives a testing referral for a young child less than 2 years of age, which is referred to as infancy by many developmental psychologists (Sigelman & Rider, 2018, Table 1.1, p. 6). In such instance, the title of the report should be modified to read, "Infancy and Early Childhood Form (Birth–5 Years; 0–71 Months)." The reason a fifth form covering these earliest years is not created is that referrals younger than two years are rare in outpatient mental health. This is likely due to the fact that there has not yet been sufficient development that would suggest the need for testing.
2. The names of state administrative agencies who are legally charged with protecting our children vary from state to state. In Indiana, the agency is called the Department of Child Services (DCS), which itself has changed frequently over the years. In the neighboring state of Illinois, the agency is called the Department of Child and Family Services (DCFS). Thus, when referring to DCS in the main narrative, it is meant any state agency with the legal charge of protecting children.
3. Previously, as evident in the first edition (Spores, 2012), this section was placed much earlier in the report, immediately subsequent to the presenting symptoms to be precise. The logic was that the mental status examination reflected information *directly* provided

by the examinee, which was in proximity to information *directly* reported by the examinee. However, over the past ten years of testing practice, it became increasingly apparent that screening data would need to be used in some cases in order to meet the criteria for the medical necessity of testing. Such screening data was most logically placed near the end of the initial assessment, where the medical necessity for testing argument is made. Therefore, it seemed to make more sense to move the mental status examination and behavioral observation data in proximately to the screening data as both representing signs of psychopathology.

4. This author had occasion to do some assessment consulting for a pediatrics clinic, which provided some medical knowledge that may be applied for testing referrals. Although it was very useful information, the data on height and weight was invariably in metric units. As being more comfortable with standard units, this author frequently converted from metric to standard units whether or not BMI was needed. Therefore, if the reader is in the same situation, 1 kg = 2.2046 lbs. and 1 cm = 0.39370079 inches. Hence, if an individual is 19.4 kg, then 19.4 x 2.2046 = 42.8 lbs. Further, if an individual is 104.4 cm, then 104.4 x 0.39370079 = 41.10 inches. There are also websites that offer calculators that perform these conversions. One is as follows: www.metric-conversions.org/weight/kilograms-to-pounds.htm.

5. I continue to find the distinction a useful one as follows: (a) *neurotic* refers to an individual suffering from distressing emotional symptoms although is reality based; whereas (b) an individual who is *psychotic* has lost touch with reality and thus is significantly more disturbed.

6. There are several other assessment and testing codes available, although they are not employed because they are too specialized (e.g., testing only for *aphasia*) or have an excessively poor reimbursement rate that hinders their utility. For example, CPT Code 96146 is used for automated testing via an electronic platform. Within the area of medical testing, this would apply to such tests as an x-ray. In psychology, it may be applied to both a psychological or neuropsychological instrument that is fully automated and rapidly done, such as a quick continuous performance test or computer-administered and scored standardized rating scale. The distinct advantage here is that typically no PA is required for such test. The disadvantage is the diminutive reimbursement rate (i.e., somewhere in the range of $5.00). Therefore, although it does exist, the author has never used this service,

7. Some clinicians and group practices schedule 90-minute initial clinical interviews due to the relatively large amount of information that needs to be garnered. Although, there is some virtue in such a practice, there are significant problems. The greatest difficulty is that it tends to effectively waste a 30-minute interval unless appointments are scheduled on alternating on-the-hour and on-the-half-hour increments, which can be extremely confusing to all involved. The greatest advantage is that it provides the extra time required for the more complicated cases, which can occasionally take in excess of 60 minutes and will cause the remaining appointments to be delayed. In the last analysis, it is really a matter of preference, and 60 minutes is most preferable.

8. Almost reminds one of a 3 x 2 x 2 ANOVA factorial design.

References

Abramson, L. Y., Metalsky, G. I., & Alloy, L. B. (1989). Hopelessness depression: A theory- based subtype of depression. *Psychological Review, 96*, 358–372.

Abramson, L. Y., Seligman, M. E. P., & Teasdale, J. D. (1978). Learned helplessness in humans: Critique and reformulation. *Journal of Abnormal Psychology, 87*, 49–74.

Ainsworth, M. D. S. (1973). The development of infant–mother attachment. In B. M. Caldwell & H. N. Ricciuti (Eds.), *Review of child development research* (Vol. 3). Chicago, IL: University of Chicago Press.

Ainsworth, M. D. S., Blehar, M., Waters, E., & Wall, S. (1978). *Patterns of attachment*. Hillsdale, NJ: Erlbaum.

Alloy, L. B., Bender, R. E., Whitehouse, W. G., Wagner, C. A., Liu, R. T., Grant, D. A., & Abramson, L. Y. (2012). High behavioral approach system (BAS) sensitivity, reward responsiveness, and goal-striving predict first onset of bipolar spectrum disorders: A prospective behavioral high-risk design. *Journal of Abnormal Psychology, 121*, 339–351.

American Psychiatric Association. (1994). *Diagnostic and statistical manual of mental disorders* (4th ed., DSM–IV). Washington, DC: Author.

American Psychiatric Association. (2000). *Diagnostic and statistical manual of mental disorders* (4th ed., text Rev.). Washington, DC: Author.

American Psychiatric Association. (2013). *Diagnostic and statistical manual of mental disorders* (5th ed., DSM–5). Arlington, VA: Author.

American Psychological Association. (2015). *American Psychological Association (APA) dictionary of psychology* (2nd ed.). Washington, DC: Author.

American Psychological Association. (2017). *Psychotherapy codes for psychologists*. Retrieved from www.apaservices.org/practice/reimbursement/health-codes/testing/codes-descriptions.pdf

American Psychological Association. (2018). *2019 psychological and neuropsychological testing CPT codes & descriptions: Effective January 1, 2019*. Retrieved from www.apaservices.org/practice/reimbursement/health-codes/testing/codes-descriptions.pdf

American Psychological Association. (2020). *Publication manual of the American psychological association* (7th ed.). Washington, DC: Author.

Atkinson, R. C., & Shiffrin, R. M. (2016). Human memory: A proposed system and its control processes. In R. J. Sternberg, S. T. Fiske, & D. J. Foss (Eds.), *Scientists making a difference: One hundred eminent behavioral and brain scientists talk about their most important contributions* (pp. 115–118). New York, NY: Cambridge University Press.

Anthis, K., & LaVoie, J. C. (2006). Readiness to change: A longitudinal study of changes in adult identity. *Journal of Research in Personality, 40*, 209–219.

Archer, R. A., Handel, R. W., Ben-Porath, Y. S., & Tellegen, A. (2016). *Minnesota multiphasic personality inventory, adolescent, restructured form (MMPI–A–RF): Administration, scoring, interpretation, and technical manual*. Minneapolis, MN: University of Minnesota Press.

Arnett, J. J. (2004). *Emerging adulthood: The winding road from the late teens through the twenties*. New York, NY: Oxford University Press.

Arnett, J. J. (2015). The cultural psychology of emerging adulthood. In L. A. Jensen (Ed.), *The Oxford handbook of human development and culture: An interdisciplinary perspective* (pp. 487–501). New York, NY: Oxford University Press.

Atkinson, R. C., & Shiffrin, R. M. (1968). Human memory: A proposed system and its control processes. In K. W. Spence & J. T. Spence (Eds.). *The psychology of learning and motivation* (Vol. 2, pp. 89–105). New York, NY: Academic Press.

Barlow, D. H. (1988). *Anxiety and its disorders: The nature and treatment of anxiety and panic.* New York, NY: The Guilford Press.

Barlow, D. H. (2002). *Anxiety and its disorders: The nature and treatment of anxiety and panic* (2nd ed.). New York, NY: The Guilford Press.

Barlow, D. H., & Durand, M. V. (2018). *Abnormal psychology: An integrative approach* (8th ed.). Stamford, CT: Cengage Learning.

Barnes, K. E. (1971). Preschool play norms: A replication. *Developmental Psychology, 5,* 99–103.

Bartholomew, K., & Horowitz, L. M. (1991). Attachment styles among young adults: A test of a four-category model. *Journal of Personality and Social Psychology, 61,* 226–244.

Beck, A. T. (1986). Hopelessness as a predictor of eventual suicide. *Annals of the New York Academy of Science, 487,* 90–96.

Beck, A. T., Epstein, N., & Harrison, R. (1983). Cognitions, attitudes and personality dimensions in depression. *British Journal of Cognitive Psychotherapy, 1,* 1–16.

Ben-Porath, Y. S., & Tellegen, A. (2008, 2011). *Minnesota multiphasic personality inventory–2–RF (MMPI–2–RF): Manual for administration, scoring, and interpretation.* Minneapolis: MN: University of Minnesota Press.

Berman, A. L. (2009). Depression and suicide. In I. H. Gotlib & C. L. Hammen (Eds.), *Handbook of depression* (2nd ed., pp. 510–530). New York, NY: The Guilford Press.

Blumenthal, S. J. (1990). An overview and synopsis of risk factors, assessment, and treatment of suicidal patients over the life cycle. In S. J. Blumenthal & D. J. Kupfer (Eds.), *Suicide over the life cycle: Risk factors, assessment and treatment of suicidal patients* (pp. 685–734). Washington, DC: American Psychiatric Press.

Bowlby, J. (1969). *Attachment and loss: Vol. 1. Attachment.* New York, NY: Basic Books.

Bowlby, J. (1973). *Attachment and loss: Vol. 2. Separation.* New York, NY: Basic Books.

Brent, D. A., & Kolko, D. J. (1990). The assessment and treatment of children and adolescents at risk for suicide. In S. J. Blumenthal & D. J. Kupfer (Eds.), *Suicide over the life cycle: Risk factors, assessment and treatment of suicidal patients.* Washington, DC: American Psychiatric Press.

Brent, D. A., Melhem, N. M., Oquendo, M., Burke, A., Birmaher, B., Stanley, B., . . . Mann, J. J. (2015). Familial pathways to early-onset suicide attempt: A 5.6-year prospective study. *Psychiatry, 72,* 160–168.

Brent, D. A., Oquendo, M., Birmaher, B., Greenhill, L., Kolko, D., Stanley, B., & Mann, J. J. (2003). Peripubertal suicide attempts in offspring of suicide attempters with siblings concordant for suicidal behavior. *American Journal of Psychiatry, 160,* 1486–1493.

Briere, J. (1996). *Trauma symptom checklist for children (TSCC): Professional manual.* Lutz, FL: Psychological Assessment Resources (PAR).

Briere, J. (2011). *Trauma symptom inventory, second edition (TSI–2): Professional manual.* Lutz, FL: Psychological Assessment Resources (PAR).

Broadbent, D. (1958). *Perception and communication.* Elmsford, NY: Pergamon Press.

Burmeister, M., McInnis, M. G., & Zöllner, S. (2008). Psychiatric genetics: Progress amid controversy. *Nature Reviews Genetics, 9,* 527–540.

Butcher, J. N., Dahlstrom, W. G., Graham, J. R., Tellegen, A., & Kaemmer, B. (1989). *Minnesota multiphasic personality inventory, second edition (MMPI–2): Manual for administration, and scoring.* Minneapolis, MN: NCS University of Minnesota Press.

Cafasso, J. (2018). The facts about lithium toxicity. *Healthline.* Retrieved from www.healthline.com/health/lithium-toxicity

Calkins, S. D., & Hill, A. (2007). Caregiver influences on emerging emotion regulation: Biological and environmental transactions in early development. In J. J. Gross (Ed.), *Handbook of emotion regulation.* New York, NY: The Guilford Press.

Calkins, S. D., & Mackler, J. S. (2011). Temperament, emotion regulation, and social development. In M. K. Underwood & L. H. Rosen (Eds.), *Social development. Relationships in infancy, childhood, and adolescence.* New York, NY: The Guilford Press.

Caspi, A., Harrington, H., Milne, B., Amell, J. W., Theodore, R. E., & Moffitt, T. E. (2003). Children's behavioral styles at age 3 are linked to their adult personality traits at age 26. *Journal of Personality, 71,* 495–513.

Centers for Disease Control and Prevention (CDC). (2014, March 28). Prevalence of autism spectrum disorder among children aged 8 years–autism and develop-mental disability monitoring network, 11 sites, United States, 2010. *MMWR: Morbidity and Mortality Weekly Report, 63,* 1–21.

Centers for Disease Control and Prevention (CDC). (2019, July 14). *Healthy weight [Web log post].* Retrieved from www.cdc.gov/healthyweight/assessing/bmi/adult_bmi/index.html

Centers for Disease Control and Prevention (CDC). (2020, March 2). Violence prevention: Risk and protective factors. *Author.* Retrieved from www.cdc.gov/violenceprevention/youthviolence/riskprotectivefactors.html

Charman, T., Pickles, A., Simonoff, E., Chandler, S., Loucas, T., & Baird, G. (2011). IQ in children with autism spectrum disorders: Data from the special needs and autism project (SNAP). *Psychological Medicine, 41,* 619–627.

Chen, X., & Schmidt, L. A. (2015). Temperament and personality. In M. E. Lamb (Vol. Ed.) & R. M. Lerner (Ed.), *Handbook of child psychology and developmental science, Vol. 3: Socioemotional processes* (pp. 152–200). Hoboken, NJ: John Wiley & Sons.

Cheung, Y., Law, C., Chan, B., Liu, K., & Yip, P. (2006). Suicidal ideation and suicidal attempts in a population based study of Chinese people: Risk attributable to hopelessness, depression, and social factors. *Journal of Affective Disorders, 90,* 193–199.

Cicchetti, D. V. (1994). Guidelines, criteria, and rules of thumb for evaluating normed and standardized assessment instruments in psychology. *Psychological Assessment, 6,* 284–290.

Citardi, M. (2009, December 11). *Current procedural technology: History, structure, process & controversies.* University of Texas, McGovern Medical School. Retrieved from https://med.uth.edu/orl/2009/12/11/current-procedural-technology-history-structure-process-controversies/

Cole, P. M., Michel, M. K., & Teti, L. O. (1994). The development of emotion regulation and dysregulation: A clinical perspective. In N. Fox (Ed.), The development of emotion regulation: Biological and behavioral considerations. *Monographs of the Society for Research in Child Development, 59* (Nos. 2–3, Serial No. 240).

Colin, V. (1996). *Human attachment*. New York, NY: McGraw-Hill.

Confidentiality of Substance Use Disorder, 42 C.F.R. Part 2 (2020). Retrieved from www.govinfo.gov/content/pkg/FR-2017-01-18/pdf/2017-00719.pdf

Conners, C. K. (2008). *Conners comprehensive behavior rating scales (Conners CBRS): Manual and interpretive update*. North Tonawanda, NY: Multi-Health Systems (MHS).

Conners, C. K. (2015). *Conners kiddie continuous performance test, second edition K–CPT 2): Technical manual*. North Towanda, NY: Multi-Health Systems (MHS).

Conwell, Y., Duberstein, P. R., & Caine, E. D. (2002). Risk factors for suicide in later life. *Biological Psychiatry, 52*, 193–204.

Conwell, Y., Duberstein, P. R., Cox, C., Hermmann, J. H., Forbes, N. T., & Caine, E. D. (1996). Relationships of age and axis I diagnoses in victims of completed suicide: A psychological autopsy study. *American Journal of Psychiatry, 153*, 1001–1008.

Cooper, J., Kapur, N., Webb, R., Lawlor, M., Guthrie, E., Mackway-Jones, K., & Appleby, L. (2005). Suicide after deliberate self-harm: A 4-year cohort study. *American Journal of Psychiatry, 162*, 297–303.

Coplan, R. J., & Abreau, K. A. (2009). Peer interactions and play in early childhood. In K. H. Rubin, W. M. Bukowski, & B. Laursen (Eds.), *Handbook of peer interactions, relationships, and groups*. New York, NY: The Guilford Press.

Corbett, B. A., Constantine, L. J., Hendren, R., Rocke, D., & Ozonoff, S. (2009). Examining executive functioning in children with autism spectrum disorder, attention deficit hyperactivity disorder and typical development. *Psychiatry Research, 166*, 210–222.

Craik, F. I. M., & Lockhart, R. S. (1972). Levels of processing. A framework for memory research. *Journal of Verbal Learning and Verbal Behaviour, 11*, 671–684.

Crowell, J. A., Fraley, R. C., & Shaver, P. R. (1999). Measurement of individual differences in adolescent and adult attachment. In J. Cassidy & P. R. Shaver (Eds.), *Handbook of attachment: Theory, research, and clinical applications*. New York: The Guilford Press.

Damasio, A. (2007). Neuroscience and ethics: Intersections. *American Journal of Bioethics, 7*, 3–7.

David Klonsky, E., Kotov, R., Bakst, S., Rabinowitz, J., & Bromet, E. J. (2012). Hopelessness as a predictor of attempted suicide among first admission patients with psychosis: A 10-year cohort study. *Suicide and Life-Threatening Behavior, 42*, 1–10.

Decety, J., & Skelly, L. R. (2013). The neural underpinnings of the experience of empathy: Lessons for psychopathy. In K. N. Ochsner & S. M. Kosslyn (Eds), *The Oxford handbook of cognitive neuroscience, volume 2: The cutting edges* (pp. 228–243). New York, NY: Oxford University Press.

Denham, S. A., Bassett, H. H., & Wyatt, T. (2007). The socialization of emotional competence. In J. E. Grusec, & P. D. Hastings (Eds.), *Handbook of socialization: Theory and research*. New York, NY: The Guilford Press.

Denham, S. A., Blair, K. A., DeMulder, E., Levitas, J., Sawyer, K., Auerbach-Major, S., & Queenan, P. (2003). Preschool emotional competence: Pathway to social competence? *Child Development, 74*, 238–256.

DuPaul, G. J., Gormley, M. J., & Laracy, S. D. (2013). Comorbidity of LD and ADHD: Implications of DSM–5 for assessment and treatment. *Journal of Learning Disabilities, 46*, 43–51.

Dzau, V. J., & Pizzo, P. A. (2014). Relieving Pain in America: Insights from an Institute of Medicine committee. *Journal of the American Medical Association, 312*, 1507–1508.

Eisenberg, N., Duckworth, A. L., Spinrad, T. L., & Valiente, C. (2014). Conscientiousness: Origins in childhood? *Developmental Psychology, 50*, 1331–1349.

Elbogen, E. B., Dennis, P. A., & Johnson, S. C. (2016). Beyond mental illness targeting stronger and more direct pathways to violence. *Clinical Psychological Science, 4*, 747–759.

Elbogen, E., & Johnson, S. (2009). The intricate link between violence and mental disorder: Results from the national epidemiologic survey on alcohol and related conditions. *Archives of General Psychiatry, 66*, 152.

Erikson, E. H. (1963). *Childhood and society* (2nd ed.). New York, NY: Norton.

Erikson, E. H. (1968). *Identity: Youth and crisis*. New York, NY: Norton.

Erikson, E. H. (1982). *The life cycle completed: A review*. New York, NY: Norton.

Erlich, M. D., Smith, T. E., Horwath, E., & Cournos, F. (2014). Schizophrenia and other psychotic disorders. In J. L. Cutler (Ed), *Psychiatry* (pp. 97–128). New York, NY: Oxford University Press.

Erol, R. Y., & Orth, U. (2011). Self-esteem development from age 14 to 30 years: A longitudinal study. *Journal of Personality and Social Psychology, 101*, 607–619.

Finn, S. E. (2007). *In our clients' shoes: Theory and techniques of therapeutic assessment*. New York, NY: Taylor & Francis Group.

Finn, S. E., Fischer, C. T., & Handler, L. (Eds.). (2012). *Collaborative/therapeutic assessment: A casebook and guide*. Hoboken, NJ: John Wiley & Sons.

Flegal, K. M., & Graubard, B. I. (2009). Estimates of excess deaths associated with body mass index and other anthropometric variables. *The American Journal of Clinical Nutrition, 89*, (1213–1219).

Flegal, K. M., Carroll, M. D., Kit, B. K., & Ogden, C. L. (2012). Prevalence of obesity and trends in the distribution of body mass index among US adults, 1999–2010. *Journal of the American Medical Association, 307*, 491–497.

Fleiss, J. L. (2003). *Statistical methods for rates and proportions* (3rd ed.). Hoboken, NJ: John Wiley & Sons.

Folstein, M. F., Folstein, S. E., White, T., & Messer, M. A. (2010). *Mini–mental state examination, second edition: User's manual*. Lutz, FL: Psychological Assessment Resources (PAR).

Fraley, R. C., & Shaver, P. R. (2008). Attachment theory and its place in contemporary personality theory. In O. P. John, R. W. Robins, & L. A. Pervin (Eds.), *Handbook of personality theory and research* (3rd ed.). New York, NY: The Guilford Press.

Freedman, D. S., Horlick, M., & Berenson, G. S. (2013). A comparison of the Slaughter skinfold-thickness equations and BMI in predicting body fatness and cardiovascular disease risk factor levels in children. *The American Journal of Clinical Nutrition, 98*, 1417–1424.

Freedman, D. S., Katzmarzyk, P. T., Dietz, W. H., Srinivasan, S. R., Berenson, G. S. (2009). Relation of body mass index and skinfold thicknesses to cardiovascular disease risk factors in children: The Bogalusa heart study. *The American Journal of Clinical Nutrition*, 90, (210–216).

Garber, J., Clarke, G. N., Weersing, V. R., Beardslee, W. R., Brent, D. A., Gladstone, T. R., & Iyengar, S. (2009). Prevention of depression in at-risk adolescents: A randomized con- trolled trial. *JAMA: Journal of the American Medical Association*, 301, 2215–2224.

Gardner, H. (1993). *Multiple intelligences: The theory in practice*. New York, NY: Basic Books.

Gardner, H. (1998). Are there additional intelligences? The case for naturalist, spiritual, and existential intelligences. In J. Kane (Ed.), *Education, information, and transformation* (pp. 111–131). Upper Saddle River, NJ: Merrill-Prentice Hall.

Gardner, H. (1999a). *Intelligence reframed: Multiple intelligences for the 21st century*. New York: Basic Books.

Gardner, H. (1999b, February). Who owns intelligence? *Atlantic Monthly*, 67–76.

Garrow, J. S., & Webster, J. (1985). Quetelet's index (W/H2) as a measure of fatness. *International Journal of Obesity*, *9*, 147–153.

Geithner, C. A., Satake, T., Woynarowska, B., & Malina, R. M. (1999). Adolescent spurts in body dimensions: Average and modal sequences. *American Journal of Human Biology*, *11*, 287–295.

Goldston, D., Reboussin, B., & Daniel, S. (2006). Predictors of suicide attempts: State and trait components. *Journal of Abnormal Psychology*, *115*, 842–849.

Goodvin, R., Thompson, R. A., & Winer, A. C. (2015). The individual child: Temperament, emotion, self, and personality. In M. H. Bornstein & M. E. Lamb (Eds.), *Developmental science: An advanced textbook* (7th ed., pp. 491–533). New York, NY: Psychology Press.

Gotlib, I. H., & Abramson, L. Y. (1999). Attributional theories of emotion. In T. Dagleish & M. J. Power (Eds.), *Handbook of cognition and emotion* (pp. 613–636). Chichester, U.K: John Wiley & Sons.

Gotlib, I. H., & Krasnoperova, E. (1998). Biased information processing as a vulnerability factor for depression. *Behavior Therapy*, *29*, 603–617.

Gotlib, I. H., Joormann, J., & Foland-Ross, L. C. (2014). Understanding familial risk for depression: A 25-year perspective. *Perspectives on Psychological Science*, *9*, 94–108.

Gould, M. (1990). Suicide clusters and media exposure. In S. J. Blumenthal & D. J. Kupfer (Eds.), *Suicide over the life cycle: Risk factors, assessment and treatment of suicidal patients* (pp. 517–532). Washington, DC: American Psychiatric Press.

Gould, M. S., Greenberg, T., Velting, D. M., & Shaffer, D. (2003). Youth suicide risk and preventive interventions: A review of the past 10 years. *Journal of the American Academy of Child and Adolescent Psychiatry*, *42*, 386–405.

Gross, J. J. (2014). Emotion regulation: Conceptual and empirical foundations. In J. J. Gross (Ed.), *Handbook of emotion regulation* (2nd ed., pp. 3–20). New York, NY: The Guilford Press.

Hagekull, B., & Bohlin, G. (1998). Preschool temperament and environmental factors related to the five-factor model of personality in middle childhood. *Merrill-Palmer Quarterly*, *44*, 194–215.

Hall-Flavin, D. (2019, January 29). Antidepressant withdrawal: Is there such a thing? *Mayo Foundation for Medical Education and Research (MFMER)*. Retrieved from www.mayoclinic.org/diseases-conditions/depression/expert-answers/antidepressant-withdrawal/faq-20058133

Hantouche, E., Akiskal, H., Azorin, J., Chatenet-Duchene, L., & Lancrenon, S. (2006). Clinical and psychometric characterization of depression in mixed mania: A report from the French National Cohort of 1090 manic patients. *Journal of Affective Disorders*, *96*, 225–232.

Harris, P. L., & Kavanaugh, R. D. (1993). Young children's understanding of pretense. *Monographs of the Society for Research in Child Development*, *58* (1, Serial No. 181).

Hazan, C., & Shaver, P. (1987). Romantic love conceptualized as an attachment process. *Journal of Personality and Social Psychology*, *52*, 511–524.

Hazan, C., Campa, M., & Gur-Yaish, N. (2006). Attachment across the lifespan. In P. Noller & J. A. Feeney (Eds.), *Close relationships: Functions, forms, and processes*. New York, NY: Psychology Press.

Health Insurance Portability and Accountability Act of 1996 [HIPPA], Pub.L. 104–191 (2000, 2020). Retrieved from www.hhs.gov/hipaa/for-professionals/privacy/index.html

Herman-Giddens, M. E., Steffes, J., Harris, D., Slora, E., Hussey, M., Dowshen, S. A., & Reiter, E. O. (2012). Secondary sexual characteristics in boys: Data from the Pediatric Research in Office Settings Network. *Pediatrics*, *130*, 1058–1068.

Hesse, E., & Main, M. (2006). Frightened, threatening, and dissociative parental behavior in low-risk samples: Description, discussion, and interpretations. *Development and Psychopathology*, *18*, 309–343.

Howe, D. (2011). *Attachment across the lifecourse. A brief introduction*. New York, NY: Palgrave Macmillan.

Howes, C., & Matheson, C. C. (1992). Sequences in the development of competent play with peers: Social and social pretend play. *Developmental Psychology*, *28*, 961–974.

Hyman, I. E., Jr. (1993). Imagery, reconstructive memory, and discovery. In B. Roskos-Ewoldsen, M. J. Intons-Peterson, & R. E. Anderson (Eds.), *Imagery, creativity, and discovery: A cognitive perspective* (pp. 99–121). The Netherlands: Elsevier Science.

Hyman, I. E., Jr., & Loftus, E. F. (1998). Errors in autobiographical memories. *Clinical Psychology Review*, *18*, 933–947.

Hyman, I. E., Jr., & Loftus, E. F. (2002). False childhood memories and eyewitness memory errors. In M. L. Eisen, J. A. Quas, & G. S. Goodman (Eds.), *Memory and suggestibility in the forensic interview* (pp. 63–84). Mahwah, NJ: Erlbaum.

Indiana Parenting Time Guidelines. (2006). *Indiana Rules of the Court*. Retrieved February 24, 2022, from https://www.in.gov/courts/files/rules-proposed-2021-mar-parenting.pdf.

Ivancevich, J. M. (1983). Contrast effects in performance evaluation and reward practices. *Academy of Management Journal*, *26*, 465–476.

Jepsen, J. R. M., Fagerlund, B., & Mortensen, E. L. (2009). Do attention deficits influence IQ assessment in children and adolescents with ADHD? *Journal of Attention Disorders, 12,* 551–562.

Joe, S., Baser, R., Breeden, G., Neighbors, H., & Jackson, J. (2006). Prevalence of and risk factors for lifetime suicide attempts among blacks in the United States. *Journal of the American Medical Association, 296,* 2112–2123

Joiner, T. E., Jr., & Rudd, M. D. (2000). Intensity and duration of suicidal crises vary as a function of previous suicide attempts and negative life events. *Journal of Consulting and Clinical Psychology, 68,* 909–916.

Jones, T. M., Hill, K. G., Epstein, M., Lee, J. O., Hawkins, J. D., & Catalano, R. F. (2016). Understanding the interplay of individual and social–developmental factors in the progression of substance use and mental health from childhood to adulthood. *Development and Psychopathology, 28,* 721–741.

Kaufman, A. S., & Lichtenberger, E. O. (2005). *Assessing adolescent and adult intelligence* (3rd ed.). Hoboken, NJ: John Wiley & Sons.

Kessler, R. C., Berglund, P., Borges, G., Nock, M., & Wang, P. S. (2005). Trends in suicide ideation, plans, gestures, and attempts in the United States, 1990–1992 to 2001–2003. *Journal of the American Medical Association, 293,* 2487–2495.

Kessler, R. C., Petukhova, M., Sampson, N. A., Zaslavsky, A. M., & Wittchen, H. U. (2012). Twelve-month and lifetime prevalence and lifetime morbid risk of anxiety and mood disorders in the United States. *International Journal of Methods in Psychiatric Research, 21,* 169.

Knoff, H. M., & Prout, H. T. (1985). *Kinetic drawing system for family and school: A handbook.* Los Angeles, CA: Western Psychological Services (WPS).

Kroger, J. (2007). *Identity development. Adolescence through adulthood* (2nd ed.). Thousand Oaks, CA: Sage Publications.

Krueger, R. F., & Markon, K. E. (2006). Reinterpreting comorbidity: A model-based approach to understanding and classifying psychopathology. *Annual Review of Clinical Psychology, 2,* 111–133.

Krug, E. G., Kresnow, M.-J., Peddicord, J. P., Dahlberg, L. L., Powell, K. E., Crosby, A. E., & Annest, J. L. (1998). Suicide after natural disasters. *New England Journal of Medicine, 338,* 373–378.

Lawlor, D. A., Benfield, L., Logue, J., Tilling, K., Howe, L. D., Fraser, A., . . . Sattar, N. (2010). Association between general and central adiposity in childhood, and change in these, with cardiovascular risk factors in adolescence: Prospective cohort study. *British Medical Journal, 341,* 6224.

LePort, A. K., Mattfeld, A. T., Dickinson-Anson, H., Fallon, J. H., Stark, C. E., Kruggel, F., Cahill, L., & McGaugh, J. L. (2012). Behavioral and neuroanatomical investigation of highly superior autobiographical memory (HSAM). *Neurobiology of Learning and Memory, 98,* 78.

Link, B. G., & Stueve, A. (1994). Psychotic symptoms and the violent/illegal behavior of mental patients compared to community controls. In J. Monahan & H.J. Steadman (Eds.), *Violence and mental disorder: Developments in risk assessment* (pp. 137–159). Chicago, IL: University of Chicago Press.

Lotan, A., Fenckova, M., Bralten, J., Alttoa, A., Dixson, L., Williams, R. W., van der Voet, M. (2014). Neuroinformatic analyses of common and distinct genetic components associated with major neuropsychiatric disorders. *Frontiers in Neuroscience, 8,* 331.

Main, M., & Solomon, J. (1990). Procedures for identifying infants as disorganized/disoriented during the Ainsworth Strange Situation. In M. T. Greenberg, D. Cicchetti, & E. M. Cummings (Eds.), *Attachment in the preschool years: Theory, research, and intervention.* Chicago, IL: University of Chicago Press.

Mann, J., Apter, A., Bertolote, J., Beautrais, A., Currier, D., Haas, A., & Hendin, H. (2005). Suicide prevention strategies: A systematic review. *Journal of the American Medical Association, 294,* 2064–2074.

Marcia, J. E. (1966). Development and validation of ego identity status. *Journal of Personality and Social Psychology, 3,* 551–558.

Mash, E. J., & Wolfe, D. A. (2019). *Abnormal child psychology* (7th ed.). Boston, MA: Cengage Learning.

Masten, A. S., Roisman, G. I., Long, J. D., Burt, K. B., Obradovic, J., Riley, J. R., Boelcke-Stennes, K., & Tellegen, A. (2005). Developmental cascades: Linking academic achievement and externalizing and internalizing symptoms over 20 years. *Developmental Psychology, 41,* 733–746.

Matson, J. L., & Shoemaker, M. (2009). Intellectual disability and its relationship to autism spectrum disorders. *Research in Developmental Disabilities, 30,* 1107–1114.

Matsubayashi, T., Sawada, Y., & Ueda, M. (2012). Natural disasters and suicide: Evidence from Japan. *Social Science & Medicine, 82,* 126–133.

Maurer, T. J., Palmer, J. K., & Ashe, D. K. (1993). Diaries, checklists, evaluations, and contrast effects in measurement of behavior. *Journal of Applied Psychology, 78,* 226–231.

Mayo Clinic Staff. (2018). *Self-injury/cutting.* Mayo Clinic. Retrieved from www.mayoclinic.org/diseases-conditions/self-injury/symptoms-causes/syc-20350950

McCabe, M. P., & Ricciardelli, L. A. (2004). A longitudinal study of pubertal timing and extreme body change behaviors among adolescent boys and girls. *Adolescence, 39,* 145–166.

McCrae, R. R., & Costa, P. T., Jr. (2008). The five factor theory of personality. In O. P. John, R. W. Robins, & L. A. Pervin (Eds.), *Handbook of personality* (pp. 159–181). New York: The Guilford Press.

McCrae, R. R., & Costa, P. T., Jr. (2010). *NEO inventories for the NEO personality inventory, third edition (NEO–PI–3), NEO five factor inventory, third edition (NEO–FFI–3), NEO personality inventory, revised (NEO PI–R): Professional manual.* Lutz, FL: Psychological Assessment Services (PAR).

Meilman, P. W. (1979). Cross-sectional age changes in ego identity status during adolescence. *Developmental Psychology, 15,* 230–231.

Meyer, G. J., Viglione, D. J., Mihura, J. L., Erard, R. E., & Erdberg, P. (2011). *Rorschach performance assessment system (R–PAS): Administrative, coding, interpretation, and technical manual.* Toledo, OH: Rorschach Performance Assessment System, L.L.C.

Meyer, G. J., Viglione, D. J., Mihura, J. L., Erard, R. E., & Erdberg, P. (2012). *Rorschach performance assessment system (R–PAS): Portable form quality tables and coding guide*. Toledo, OH: Rorschach Performance Assessment System, L.L.C.

Mihura, J. L., & Meyer, G. J. (Eds.). (2018). *Using the Rorschach performance assessment system (R–PAS)*. New York, NY: The Guilford Press.

Mikulincer, M., & Shaver, P. R. (2007). *Attachment in adulthood. Structure, dynamics, and change*. New York, NY: The Guilford Press.

Miller, I. W., & Norman, W. H. (1979). Learned helplessness in humans: A review and attribution-theory model. *Psychological Bulletin, 86*, 93–118.

Millon, T., Grossman, S., & Millon, C. (2015). *Millon clinical multiaxial inventory manual* (4th ed., MCMI–IV). Minneapolis, MN: Pearson.

Modestin, J., & Ammann, R. (1996). Mental disorder and criminality: Male schizophrenia. *Schizophrenia Bulletin, 22*, 69–82.

Monahan, J. (1992). Mental disorder and violent behavior: Perceptions and evidence. *American Psychologist, 47*, 511–521.

Morin, A. J. S., Maiano, C., Marsh, H. W., Nagengast, B., & Janosz, M. (2013). School life and adolescents' self- esteem trajectories. *Child Development, 84*, 1967–1988.

Nock, M. K., Borges, G., Bromet, E. J., Alonso, J., Angermeyer, M., Beautrais, A., & Williams, D. (2008). Cross-national prevalence and risk factors for suicidal ideation, plans and attempts. *British Journal of Psychiatry, 192*, 98–105.

Nock, M. K., Borges, G., Bromet, E. J., Cha, C. B., Kessler, R. C., & Lee, S. (2008). Suicide and suicidal behavior. *Epidemiologic Reviews, 30*, 133–154.

Nock, M. K., Cha, C. B., & Dour, H. J. (2011). Disorders of impulse-control and self-harm. In D. H. Barlow (Ed.), *Oxford handbook of clinical psychology* (pp. 504–529). New York, NY: Oxford University.

Nock, M. K., Hwang, I., Sampson, N. A., & Kessler, R. C. (2010). Mental disorders, comorbidity and suicidal behavior: Results from the National Comorbidity Survey Replication. *Molecular Psychiatry, 15*, 868–876.

Nunley, W., Nunley, B., Cutleh, D. L., Dentingeh, J., & McFahland, B. (2013). Involuntary civil commitment. In K. Yeager, D. Cutler, D. Svendsen, & G. M. Sills (Eds.), *Modern com- munity mental health: An interdisciplinary approach* (pp. 49–61). New York, NY: Oxford University Press.

Oldehinkel, A. J., Verhulst, F. C., & Ormel, J. (2011). Mental health problems during puberty: Tanner stage- related differences in specific symptoms: The TRAILS study. *Journal of Adolescence, 34*, 73–85.

Oltmanns, T. F., & Emery, R. E. (2004). *Abnormal psychology* (4th ed.). Upper Saddle River, NJ: Prentice Hall.

Oster, G. D. (2016). *Using drawings in clinical practice*. New York, NY: Routledge.

Parten, M. B. (1932). Social participation among preschool children. *Journal of Abnormal and Social Psychology, 27*, 243–269.

Paul Wellstone and Pete Domenici Mental Health Parity and Addiction Equity Act of 2008, H.R. 6983, 110th Congress (2007–2008). Retrieved from www.congress.gov/bill/110th-congress/house-bill/6983

Pellegrini, A. D. (2009). Research and policy on children's play. *Child Development Perspectives, 3*, 131–136.

Perugi, G., Angst, J., Azorin, J. M., Bowden, C., Vieta, E., & Young, A. H. (2013). Is comorbid borderline personality disorder in patients with major depressive episode and bipolarity a developmental subtype? Findings from the international BRIDGE study. *Journal of Affective Disorders, 144*, 72–78.

Piaget, J. (1926). *The child's conception of the world*. New York, NY: Harcourt, Brace & World.

Piaget, J. (1952). *The origins of intelligence in children*. New York, NY: International Universities Press.

Planansky, K., & Johnston, R. (1977). Homicidal aggression in schizophrenic men. *Acta Psychiatrica Scandinavica, 55*, 65–73.

Pompili, M., & Fiorillo, A. (2015, July 23). Aggression and impulsivity in schizophrenia. *Psychiatric Times, 32*, Retrieved from www. psychiatrictimes.com/schizophrenia/aggression-and-impulsivity-schizophrenia

Posner, K., Brent, D., Lucas, C., Gould, M., Stanley, B., Brown, G., Fisher, P., Zelazny, J., Burke, A., Oquendo, M., & Mann, J. (2008). *The Columbia suicide severity rating scale (C–SSRS)*. New York, NY: The Research Foundation for Mental Hygiene.

Postman, L. (1975). Tests of the generality of the principle of encoding specificity. *Memory & Cognition, 3*, 663–672.

Preston, J. (Updated 2019). *Quick reference to psychiatric medications*. Retrieved from http://psyd-fx.com/quick-reference-chart/quick-reference-direct/

Putnam, S. P., Gartstein, M. A., & Rothbart, M. K. (2006). Measurement of fine-grained aspects of toddler temperament: The early childhood behavior questionnaire. *Infant Behavior and Development, 29*, 386–401.

Recovery Village. (2020, February 7). *How Xanax works and other benzodiazepines*. Author. Retrieved from www.therecoveryvillage. com/xanax-addiction/how-xanax-works/#gref

Regier, D. A., Narrow, W. E., Clarke, D. E., Kraemer, H. C., Kuramoto, S. J., Kuhl, E. A., & Kupfer, D. J. (2013). DSM–5 field trials in the United States and Canada, part II: Test-retest reliability of selected categorical diagnoses. *American Journal of Psychiatry, 150*, 59–70.

Rhode, P., Lewinsohm, P. M., Klein, D. N., Seeley, J. R., & Gau, J. M. (2013). Key characteristics of major depressive disorder occurring in childhood, adolescence, emerging adulthood, and adulthood. *Clinical Psychological Science, 1*, 41–53.

Roisman, G. I. (2009). Adult attachment. Toward a rapprochement of methodological cultures. *Current Directions in Psychological Science, 18*, 122–126.

Rothbart, M. K. (2007). Temperament, development, and personality. *Current Directions in Psychological Science, 16*, 207–212.

Rothbart, M. K. (2011). *Becoming who we are: Temperament and personality development*. New York, NY: The Guilford Press.

Rothbart, M. K., & Derryberry, D. (2002). Temperament in children. In C. von Hofsten & L. Backman (Eds.), *Psychology at the turn of the millennium: Vol. 2. Social, developmental, and clinical perspectives*. New York, NY: Taylor & Francis.

Rothbart, M. K., Ahadi, S. A., & Evans, D. E. (2000). Temperament and personality: Origins and outcomes. *Journal of Personality and Social Psychology, 78,* 122–135.

Rubin, K. H., Bukowski, W. M., & Parker, J. G. (2006). Peer interactions, relationships, and groups. In N. Eisenberg (Vol. Ed.), & W. Damon & R. M. Lerner (Eds. in Chief), *Handbook of child psychology: Vol. 3. Social, emotional, and personality development* (6th ed.). Hoboken, NJ: John Wiley & Sons.

Rubin, K. H., Coplan, R., Chen, X., Bowker, J., & McDonald, K. L. (2011). Peer relationships in childhood. In M. E. Lamb & M. H. Bornstein (Eds.), *Social and personality development. An advanced textbook* (6th ed.). New York, NY: Psychology Press.

Rudolph, K. D. (2009). Adolescent depression. In I. H. Gotlib & C. L. Hammen (Eds.), *Handbook of depression* (2nd ed., pp. 444–466). New York, NY: The Guilford Press.

Rudolph, K. D., & Lambert, S. F. (2007). Child and adolescent depression. In E. J. Mash & R. A. Barkley (Eds.), *Assessment of childhood disorders* (4th ed., pp. 213–252). New York: The Guilford Press.

Rudolph, K. D., Hammen, C., & Daley, S. E. (2006). Adolescent mood disorders. In D. A. Wolfe & E. J. Mash (Eds.), *Behavioral and emotional disorders in adolescents: Nature, assessment, and treatment* (pp. 300–342). New York: The Guilford Press.

Rueda, M. R. (2012). Effortful control. In M. Z. Zentner & R. L. Shiner (Eds.), *Handbook of temperament.* New York, NY: The Guilford Press.

Rundus, D. (1971). An analysis of rehearsal processes in free recall. *Journal of Experimental Psychology, 89,* 63–77.

Russell, J. (Ed.). (1997). *Autism as an executive disorder.* New York, NY: Oxford University Press.

Rutter, M., & Sroufe, L. A. (2000). Developmental psychopathology: Concepts and challenges. *Development and Psychopathology, 12,* 265–296.

Sattler, J. M. (2008). *Assessment of children: Cognitive foundations* (5th ed.). San Diego, CA: J. M. Sattler.

Sattler, J. M. (2014). *Foundations of behavioral, social, and clinical assessment of children* (6th ed.). San Diego, CA: J. M. Sattler.

Sayal, K., Washbrook, E., & Propper, C. (2015). Childhood behavior problems and academic outcomes in adolescence: Longitudinal population-based study. *Journal of the American Academy of Child & Adolescent Psychiatry, 54,* 360–368.

Schreier, H. M. C., & Chen, E. (2013). Socio-economic status and the health of youth: A multilevel, multidomain approach to conceptualizing pathways. *Psychological Bulletin, 139,* 606–654.

Schuh, A. J. (1978). Contrast effect in the interview. *Bulletin of the Psychonomic Society, 11,* 195–196.

Schulz, M. S., & Lazarus, R. S. (2011). Regulating emotion in adolescence: A cognitive-mediational conceptualization. In P. K. Kerig, M. S. Schulz, & S. T. Hauser (Eds.), *Adolescence and beyond. Family processes and development.* New York, NY: Oxford University Press.

Schweickert, R. (1993). A multinomial processing tree model for degradation and reintegration in immediate recall. *Memory and Cognition, 21,* 168–175.

Shiner, R. L., & Caspi, A. (2012). Temperament and the development of personality traits, adaptation, and narratives. In M. Z. Zentner & R. L. Shiner (Eds.), *Handbook of temperament.* New York, NY: The Guilford Press.

Shiner, R. L., Buss, K. A., McClowry, S. G., Putnam, S. P., Saudino, K. J., & Zentner, M. (2012). What is temperament now? Assessing progress in temperament research on the twenty-fifth anniversary of Goldsmith et al. (1987). *Child Development, 6,* 436–444.

Sigelman, C. K., & Rider, E. A. (2018). *Life-span human development* (9th ed.). Boston, MA: Cengage Learning.

Simpson, G. K., Tate, R. L., Whiting, D. L., & Cotter, R. E. (2011). Suicide prevention after traumatic brain injury: A randomized con- trolled trial of a program for the psychological treatment of hopelessness. *The Journal of Head Trauma Rehabilitation, 26,* 290–300.

Smither, J. W., Reilly, R. R., & Buda, R. (1988). Effect of prior performance information on ratings of present performance: Contrast versus assimilation revisited. *Journal of Applied Psychology, 73,* 487–496.

Solin, W. S. (1995, April 1). I did not want to live. *Seventeen,* 154–156, 176.

Soloff, P. H., Lynch, K. G., Kelley, T. M., Malone, K. M., & Mann, J. J. (2000). Characteristics of suicide attempts of patients with major depressive episode and border- line personality disorder: A comparative study. *American Journal of Psychiatry, 157,* 601–608.

Spores, J. M. (2012). *Clinician's guide to psychological assessment and testing: With forms and templates for effective practice.* New York, NY: Springer Publishing.

Sroufe, L. A. (2005). Attachment and development: A prospective, longitudinal study from birth to adulthood. *Attachment & Human Development, 7,* 349–367.

Steinberger, J., Jacobs, D. R., Raatz, S., Moran, A., Hong, C. P., & Sinaiko, A. R. (2005). Comparison of body fatness measurements by BMI and skinfolds vs dual energy X-ray absorptiometry and their relation to cardiovascular risk factors in adolescents. *International Journal of Obesity, 29,* 1346–1352.

Stevens, S. S. (1946). On the theory of scales of measurement, *Science, 1103,* 677–680.

Stratta, P., Capanna, C., Riccardi, I., Carmassi, C., Piccinni, A., Dell'Osso, L., & Rossi, A. (2012). Suicidal intention and negative spiritual coping one year after the earthquake of L'Aquila (Italy). *Journal of Affective Disorders, 136,* 1227–1231.

Sun, Q., van Dam, R. M., Spiegelman, D., Heymsfield, S. B., Willett, W. C., & Hu, F. B. (2010). Comparison of dual-energy x-ray absorptiometric and anthropometric measures of adiposity in relation to adiposity-related biologic factors. *American Journal of Epidemiology, 172,* 1442–1454.

Thomas, F., Renaud, F., Benefice, E., de Meeus, T., & Guegan, J. (2001). International variability of ages at menarche and menopause: Patterns and main determinants. *Human Biology, 73,* 271.

Trzesniewski, K. H., Donnellan, M. B., Moffitt, T. E., Robins, R. W., Poulton, R., & Caspi, A. (2006). Low self- esteem during adolescence predicts poor health, criminal behavior, and limited economic prospects during adulthood. *Developmental Psychology, 42,* 381–390.

van IJzendoorn, M. H., Schuengel, C., & Bakermans-Kranenburg, M. J. (1999). Disorganized attachment in early childhood: Meta-analysis of precursors, concomitants, and sequelae. *Development and Psychopathology, 11*, 225–249.

Van Orden, K. A., Witte, T. K., Cukrowicz, K. C., Braithwaite, S. R., Selby, E. A., & Joiner, T. E., Jr. (2010). The interpersonal theory of suicide. *Psychological Review, 117*, 575–600.

Wagner, B. M. (1997). Family risk factors for child and adolescent suicidal behavior. *Psychological Bulletin, 121*, 246–298.

Wallace, C., Mullen, P., Burgess, P., Palmer, S., Ruschena, D., & Browne, C. (1998). Serious criminal offending and mental disorder. *British Journal of Psychiatry, 172*, 477–484.

Wechsler, D. (2009a). *Wechsler memory scale, fourth edition (WMS–IV): Administration and scoring manual.* San Antonio, TX: The Psychological Corporation (PsychCorp)-Pearson.

Wechsler, D. (2009b). *Wechsler memory scale, fourth edition (WMS–IV): Technical and interpretative manual.* San Antonio, TX: The Psychological Corporation (PsychCorp)-Pearson.

Wexley, K. N., Yukl, G. A., Kovacs, S. Z., & Sanders, R. E. (1972). Importance of contrast effects in employment interviews. *Journal of Applied Psychology, 56*, 45–48.

Weyandt, L. L., & Gudmundsdottir, B. G. (2015). Developmental and neuropsychological deficits in children with ADHD. In R. A. Barkley (Ed.), *Attention-deficit hyperactivity disorder: A handbook for diagnosis and treatment* (4th ed., pp. 116–139). New York: The Guilford Press.

Willett, K., Jiang, R., Lenart, E., Spiegelman, D., & Willett, W. (2006). Comparison of bioelectrical impedance and BMI in predicting obesity-related medical conditions. *Obesity (Silver Spring), 14*, 480–490.

Williams, L. R., & Steinberg, L. (2011). Reciprocal relations between parenting and adjustment in a sample of juvenile offenders. *Child Development, 82*, 633–645.

Wohlfahrt-Veje, C., Tinggaard, J., Winther, K. Mouritsen, A., Hagen, C., Mieritz, M. G., de Renzy-Martin, K. T., Boas, M., Petersen, J. H., & Main, K. M. (2014). Body fat throughout childhood in 2647 healthy Danish children: Agreement of BMI, waist circumference, skinfolds with dual X-ray absorptiometry. *European Journal of Clinical Nutrition, 68*, 664–670.

Yapko, M. D. (2019). *Trancework: An introduction to the practice of clinical hypnosis* (5th ed.). New York, NY: Routledge.

Young, J. E., Rygh, J. L., Weinberger, A. D., & Beck, A. T. (2014). Cognitive therapy for depression. In D. H. Barlow (Ed.), *Clinical handbook of psychological disorders: A step-by-step treatment manual* (5th ed.). New York, NY: The Guilford Press.

Zucker, A. N., Ostrove, J. M., & Stewart, A. J. (2002). College-educated women's personality development in adulthood: Perceptions and age differences. *Psychology and Aging, 17*, 236–244.

See Routledge's e-resources website for forms. (www.routledge.com/9780367346058)

4 Testing Procedures and the Final Report

Overview

This chapter covers in detail the final two stages in the psychological assessment and testing process delineated in Figure 2.1. Therefore, it resumes the process as follows: (a) Stage 4 (i.e., test administration, scoring, data reporting, data interpretation and integration, summary of results, and final report generation; and (b) Stage 5 (i.e., communication of the results). To facilitate the discussion, a sample case is provided that shows how an initial report is gradually transformed into a final written product, which is typically titled, "Final Psychological Assessment Report," or alternatively supplanting the term "Psychological" with either, "Neuropsychological," or "Developmental," depending upon the principal focus of the assessment (to be discussed subsequently).

This chapter continues detailing both the process and content of the ensuing and final steps in the assessment and testing sequence. Although it is comparatively brief in comparison to Chapter 3, it is perhaps even more vital in that it provides the framework for Part II of this book. As will become apparent, the body of the final assessment report is titled, "Test Data and Interpretation," and represents the section in which all of test scores are to be strategically inserted in the form of test data tables, and thereafter interpreted and integrated. Throughout Part II, data tables have been created for all tests presented in this book (see Table 1.1) by means of years of clinical practice. There, instructions are provided as to how they are intended to be used, reported, interpreted, integrated, and summarized in order to efficiently and effectively address an illimitable variety of diagnostic issues and questions. However, before this can be effectively done, the manner in which the initial report is transformed into a final version must first be delineated. This then is the cardinal objective of Chapter 4.

Test Administration (Stage 4)

Three important issues regarding test administration include (a) the number and duration of appointments, (b) the order of test administration, and (c) the employment of computerized test administration. The former was previously addressed in Chapter 3 when discussing the scheduling of follow-up testing appointments using Form 3.9 near the conclusion of the initial interview. It bears some elaboration here because (a) test administration appointments invariably occur after the initial assessment, and (b) some psychologists may opt for scheduling them ensuing PA of the requested hours. Next, the order of test administration appointments becomes an issue when (a) total duration exceeds two hours and/or (b) more than one respondent is required. They will be addressed subsequently in this sequence.

Number and Duration of Appointments

The majority of testing cases can be completed in one 1-hour or one 2-hour test administration session. This is consistent with the the practice of targeted testing (versus comprehensive testing) espoused in this book and consistent with the tenets of managed care. Another way of stating this is that the majority of cases should require between 3 to 6 hours of total testing services (i.e., from administration through the final report) in order to adequately address the majority of diagnostic issues and questions. In part, this is the result of significant improvements in test development, including tests with impressive degrees of *reliability* (i.e., accuracy) and *validity* (i.e., precision) compared to those in years past. Improvements in test design and structure have been effectuated by more powerful statistical procedures, software programs, and sampling methods such that fewer tests are needed to achieve acceptable degrees of test reliability and validity when measuring desired constructs (see, e.g., Furr, 2018; Irwing, Booth, & Hughes, 2018; Price, 2017).

DOI: 10.4324/9780429326820-5

Therefore, appearing in Form 3.7, Item 1, "Testing appointments with psychologist," the first two checklist options are "[] One 1-hour," and "[] One 2-hour," in recognition that these are (or should be) the most frequently chosen. The two major exceptions to this guideline include the following: (a) the need to administer a complete neuropsychological test battery, which characteristically exceeds two hours' administration time; and (b) testing for *intellectual disability* (*ID*), which requires administration of both an individually administered intelligence test and a standardized measure of adaptive behavior.

Regarding the former, most neuropsychological test batteries require about 4 hours to administer, including the *NEPSY–II, Form Ages 5 to 16, Full Battery* (Korkman, Kirk, & Kemp, 2007a, 2007b) for children and adolescents, and the *Neuropsychological Assessment Battery* (*NAB*; Stern & White, 2003a, 2003b) for adults. Note that these estimated durations are shown in the "Requested Tests, Testing Services, and Units (Time)," section of the initial assessment forms (viz., Forms 3.3–3.6) presented in Chapter 3. In such instances, selection of the,

"[] Two 2-hour," option in Form 3.9, Item 1, "Testing appointments with psychologist," is indicated, hence providing the needed total 4 hours' duration without overtaxing the examinee. Neuropsychological testing is both mentally and emotionally challenging, especially for examinees who have previously excelled in many facets of their lives and who are now experiencing for the first time deficits in memory, executive functioning, and other essential neurocognitive abilities. In fact, many examinees openly express their appreciation for the two-hour limitation. So that testing is not unnecessarily delayed, the two appointments can be scheduled on two different days that are either consecutive or in proximity to each other. This practice avoids confounding the test results with extraneous variables such as fatigue, boredom, loss of interest, and flagging motivation, while maintaining their active involvement in the test administration process.

A *diagnosis* of ID requires an IQ score of about 70 and below (mean = 100; standard deviation = 15), commensurate deficits in adaptive behavior as measured by a properly standardized instrument, and onset prior to age 18 years. The initial interview establishes the onset criterion while, in most instances, two different respondents are required for measuring the other two criteria. In cases where the examinee's insurer will not cover rating scales as part of a battery, the *Vineland Adaptive Behavior Scales, Third Edition* (*Vineland–3*; Sparrow, Cicchetti, & Saulnier, 2016) structured interview as a measure the examinee's adaptive behavior skills should be selected. Because examinees' intellectual functioning typically precludes their ability to provide reliable data concerning their adaptive behavior skills, such cases require a collateral, usually a parent or primary caretaker, to represent the respondent. Even if the examinee is able to provide such data, in the opinion of the examiner and/or if circumstances permit no other viable option, a second session with the examinee would be required if the IQ test administration exceeded 60 minutes (as on average it does) to avoid exceeding a two-hour administration. Therefore, in Form 3.9, Item 1, the, "[] One 2-hour" and "[] One 1-hour," options should be selected in testing for ID; the first to administer the IQ test to the examinee, and the second to interview the collateral concerning adaptive behavior. Furthermore, in Form 3.9, for Item 4, "Special testing instructions," the "[] Yes (specify)," option should be checked and on the fill-in line add something to the effect, "The 2-hour appointment is for the examinee and the 1-hour appointment if for the examinee's parent, to be done in any order."

One final note is needed here. Occasionally, this type of ID testing can be done in one two-hour session under the following conditions: (a) the examinee's estimated intelligence is extremely low to the degree that administration time is most likely to be curtailed to one hour or less; (b) the collateral is able to accompany the examinee to the same appointment; and (c) the examinee is able to be supervised or remain independently in a waiting room or front desk area while the collateral is providing adaptive behavior responses to interview items. Contemporary individually administered intelligence tests have been streamlined to about 75 minutes by shorter discontinue rules and fewer subtests contributing to index and full scale standard scores (see, e.g., Wechsler, 2014a, 2014b; see also Chapter 7). Therefore, an individual with sufficiently low intelligence will reach those discontinue points more rapidly, hence reducing administration time even further. Of course, the fastest way to test for ID is one hour for IQ test administration to an examinee with sufficiently low intelligence and a standardized measure of adaptive behavior in rating scale format (assuming insurance PA for this type the test format). The general rule espoused throughout this book is to employ the fewest measures in the least amount of time while not hindering test reliability and validity, and also ensuring fair and reasonable remuneration for services provided.

Order of Test Administration

Determining the most efficacious order in which to administer the particular tests is also a key issue. Following are some guidelines which are meant to maximize test reliability, validity, and *utility* as defined in prior chapters. First, highest priority should typically be given to tests that are (a) measures of ability and (b) based upon performance. These tests require maximum performance and the examinee's best effort for valid results. This includes a good deal of mental effort and perseverance on the part of the examinee. Therefore, this first guideline pertains to measures of various cognitive constructs, including intelligence, achievement, and the major neurocognitive abilities (e.g., memory, learning, attention, language, executive functioning, visual-spatial, sensorimotor, and social perception). Referring back to Form 3.7, these would apply to all tests enumerated under the following categories: (a) "Achievement Tests"; (b) "Continuous Performance Tests (CPT)"; (c) "Developmental Tests (DQ)"; (d) "Intelligence Tests (IQ)"; and (e) "Neuropsychological Tests." The latter includes the *Test of Memory Malingering* (*TOMM*; Tombaugh, 1996) because fatigue or lost motivation can lead to a *false positive* result (i.e., concluding that feigning has occurred when in fact it has not).

Second priority should be afforded to any performance personality tests in the battery. Even though personality is more stylistic in nature (e.g., narcissism, self-esteem) as compared to the aforementioned cognitive constructs, many measured traits do contain facets of ability (e.g., reality testing, social skills, social perception). Furthermore, the performance-based administration format can also be deleteriously affected by such variables as flagging motivation and alertness (see, e.g., Exner, 2001, 2003). Therefore, such tests should commonly be afforded a moderate or intermediate degree of priority superseded only by the aforementioned cognitive ability tests. In Form 3.7 then, second priority goes to the class of tests listed under, "Personality Tests–Performance."

Third priority should be given to self-report and observer-report instruments that are symptom or behaviorally focused. This is because they are relatively less reliant on performance and ability as compared to the previously mentioned cognitive and personality tests. Therefore, such measures include all tests listed under, "Personality Tests–Self-Report Inventories," in Form 3.7, along with tests that are administered via a structured interview format. Specifically, the latter include the (a) *Structured Interview of Reported Symptoms, Second Edition* (*SIRS–2*; Rogers, Sewell, & Gillard, 2010) and (b) Vineland–3 (Sparrow et al., 2016). Furthermore, the self-report personality inventories may be completed on an alternate day prior to any scheduled test administration sessions and without scheduling an appointment with the testing psychologist (i.e., administered by a properly trained technician). Structured interviews are usually completed within a 1-hour appointment. Thus, fatigue here is not typically an issue.

Taken together, the comments here regarding order of test administration are meant as guidelines based upon logic and years of testing experience. Take for example, a case in which an IQ test and performance personality test are required. If a one 2-hour appointment is scheduled, the guidelines here would indicate that the IQ test be administered first, ensued by the personality measure. On the other hand, these guidelines are meant to be flexible, and modified as the particular case facts dictate. For example, a testing psychologist may reverse the aforementioned order and administer the performance personality test first to assuage significant test anxiety that the examinee is expected to manifest when asked to provide correct answers to timed items. It is best to prepare for test administration using logically consistent guidelines, although be permitted to modify them as the unfolding case facts so indicate. In this manner, testing psychologists can adequately prepare for typical test administration but be capable of readily adjusting as needed for purposes of reliable and valid results.

Computerized Test Administration

As alluded to above, all of the tests listed under, "Personality Tests–Self-Report Inventories," can be administered by computer software. Although this will be discussed in much more detail in Chapter 11, it bears mentioning here because this technology significantly reduces error variance by rendering test administration significantly more objective and convenient for both the examinee and examiner alike. In contrast to the older booklet and scantron answer sheet format, test items are presented one-at-a-time on the screen and responses recorded by simple computer-mouse click. Written instructions are presented in a consistent, unbiased, dispassionate, and organized format prior to beginning the inventory, which can be supplemented by oral instructions provided by the examiner. Further, some self-report inventories offer audio-recorded playback of items, which can accommodate examinees with *dyslexia, specific learning disorder, with impairment in reading,* or visual impairment. Use of such computer assisted technology results in shorter administrative times and reductions in errors of responding to item content (see, e.g., Ben-Porath & Tellegen, 2008, 2011; Pearson, 2020). As will also become apparent, such administration is cost effective because it is paired with computer scoring that is done in seconds and with reduced error; a topic to which the discussion now turns.

Test Scoring (Stage 4)

Computerized software scoring programs are readily available for most standardized psychological tests. For example, approximately 80% to 90% of the tests listed in Table 1.1 have computer scoring capability. Judicious use of such technology maximizes both efficiency and accuracy in test scoring, the latter by significantly reducing the probability of human error. Irrespective of price, it is prudent for all psychologists who are (or will be) engaged in testing practice to purchase a standardized test's computer-scoring software when available as it is remarkably cost effective. Immediately subsequent to entering the data into such programs (i.e., usually raw scores), score computations and transformations are accomplished in a matter of seconds and can be either saved as electronic files or printed out in hard copy format.

Many scoring programs can be loaded on a personal computer hard drive and provide unlimited scoring. Increasingly, however, computer scoring is done on the publisher's website. Here, the psychologist opens an account and purchases a desired number of computer scores for a test. Many such services provide both computer test administration and scoring when self-administered. These services will be discussed in more detail in Part II when each of the tests in Table 1.1 are presented with their data tables.

In contrast to computer administration and scoring (when available), psychologists should be advised against purchasing test interpretation and report writing software. The skill of effectively interpreting test data consists of an interactive logical process, which requires contextual information obtained during the initial clinical interview in order to resolve conflicts and ambiguities among the garnered test data. The data tables prepared for each standardized test in the proposed inventory (see Table 1.1), and which are presented throughout Part II, will facilitate the testing psychologist's thought process in this regard. Furthermore, computer interpretive statements are merely associated with specified data patterns. As test data patterns can be notoriously conflicting, so then are the resulting interpretative statements. If these are printed in written form and become part of an examinee's mental health record without qualification or resolution, they can lead to significant problems, especially if they are subpoenaed and consequently become part of a legal proceeding. Finally, test interpretation and report writing services are extremely expensive, lack cost-effectiveness, and encourage psychologists to simply enter into a final report computer-generated interpretative statements without the benefit of critical thinking or consideration if vital contextual variables.

The Final Psychological Assessment Report (Stage 4)

The "Initial Psychological Assessment Report," (see Forms 3.3–3.6) is intended to serve as the beginning framework for the "Final Psychological Assessment Report." Exhibit 4.1 is taken from Form 3.6 that was first titled, "Initial Psychological Assessment Report: Adulthood Form (19 Years–Older)," and modified into its final version, in this particular case titled, "Final Neuropsychological Assessment Report: Adulthood Form (19 Years–Older)." This is because the diagnostic issue in this sample case suggested the presence of a *neurocognitive disorder*, which required specialized *neuropsychological testing* (i.e., in contrast to psychological and developmental testing). In the more usual case of standard psychological testing, the final report would read, "Final Psychological Assessment Report," whereas if the focus was on the other form of specialized testing labeled *non-autism developmental testing*, the final report would read, "Final Developmental Assessment Report." All of these types of testing were defined in more detail in Chapter 3 when discussing the various kinds of psychological testing services promulgated and maintained by the American Medical Association CPT billing codes (see Citardi, 2009). The sample case in Exhibit 4.1 illustrates the manner in which the specialized type of testing affects the final report title.

Exhibit 4.1

Final Psychological Assessment Report Sample: Smith, John J. (Adult)

Mental Health Services
Outpatient Department
Final Neuropsychological Assessment Report[1]
Adulthood Form (19 Years–Older)

Examinee Name: Smith, John J.
Medical Record Number: 1234567
Date: May 11, 2020[2]
Examinee Demographics: Chronological age: 31 years 1 month.[3] DOB: 03/13/1989. Gender: male. Years of formal education: 12. Relationship status: divorced. Occupation: Manual Laborer. Hand dominance: right.
Examiner: John M. Spores, Ph.D., J.D., H.S.P.P.; Psychologist, Indiana #20040638A; Attorney at Law-Indiana #21404–64

Referral Source: Demetra Jones, M.D.
Referral Date: 12/12/2020.
Reasons for Psychological Testing Referral:

- There is evidence that psychological testing, based upon published normative data, will produce a timely and direct impact upon the client's existing treatment plan and how it will change.

Stated Diagnostic Objectives for Psychological Testing:
Rule Out: Mild neurocognitive disorder.
Rule In/Confirm: None.
Screen for: None.
Referral Questions: None.
Referral Comments: Memory issues.
Referral Working Diagnosis: Generalized anxiety disorder (GAD).
Individuals Providing Assessment Information: Examinee–Mr. Smith.
Pertinent Presenting Symptoms: Poor memory for recent events or information (i.e., short-term memory).
Onset and Course: Onset of these symptoms was estimated to be approximately two years ago. Subsequent course was described as gradually increasing in severity
Level of Insight: Mr. Smith demonstrated good insight regarding the problematic nature of the aforementioned symptoms (i.e., symptoms are ego dystonic). Therefore, he indicated a desire to work on change and symptom remission.
Assessment and Test Battery:[4]

1. Initial Clinical Interview (04/08/2020);
2. Mental Status Examination and Behavioral Observations (04/08/2020);[5]
3. Mini–Mental State Examination, Second Edition, Expanded Version, Blue

   Form (MMSE–2–EV–BF) (04/08/2020);[6]

4. Wechsler Memory Scale, Fourth Edition, Form Ages 16 to 69

   (WMS–IV, Ages 16–69) (05/11/2020).[7]

Health-Related:

Psychiatric–Medical: Mr. Smith is currently receiving outpatient psychiatric treatment by the referring clinician Dr. Jones, who is prescribing BuSpar (buspirone) for his chronic anxiety. The effect of these medications on the relevant presenting symptoms that precipitated this testing referral (see § Pertinent Presenting Symptoms) was described as minimal. In contrast, the medication was reported to be effective in reducing his degree of anxiety. Inpatient psychiatric intervention is negative. Mr. Smith's current medical functioning is atrial fibrillation. There were no remarkable early developmental complications. There is a negative history of severe head injuries resulting in a prolonged state of unconsciousness. There is no history of and seizure disorder. Mr. Smith is taking Apixaban (Eliquis) as a blood thinner for his heart condition. Family psychiatric-medical history is positive for the following: depressive disorder; anxiety disorder; and coronary heart disease (CHD). Vision is corrected for astigmatism and distance. Auditory functioning is normal. There is no other evidence of sensory limitations or impairments in vision, audition, proprioception, and tactile and vestibular functioning that would require testing accommodations to ensure the validity of results.
Psychological: Previous psychological testing has not been done. Professional counseling history is negative.
Family: Mr. Smith lives alone in an apartment complex. He was married for about 20 years. He has two children, a son age 8 years and a daughter age 6 years who are in the physical custody of his ex-wife. He visits his children on a regular basis according to court orders. The divorce was amicable and the two parents coordinate effectively in terms of raising their children. There was no evidence of recent or current psychosocial stressors within the family system which would account for or significantly impact the pertinent presenting symptoms.

Family of origin consists of Mr. Smith's two parents who are living, along with an older sister. He has always had caring and supportive relationships with his parents and sister.

Personality: Mr. Smith described his personality as extraverted and enjoying the company of others, although he believes that he tends to be perfectionistic with high self-standards. Because of this, he believes that he also tends to be overly self-critical. He believes this accounts for at least some of his anxiety. Relationships with people were characterized in positive terms, although he has become somewhat more withdrawn since the onset of his memory difficulties.

Educational: Mr. Smith graduated from high school with a high school diploma in 2007. Academic performance was typically average. During primary and secondary education, Mr. Smith. received general education instruction.

Occupational: Mr. Smith is employed as a steel worker doing largely manual labor. Mr. Smith is concerned that his short-term memory issues may begin to deleteriously affect the quality of his work, although his supervisor has not voiced any problems in his work productivity.

Extracurricular: Mr. Smith remains active on a men's softball team and bowling league. While in high school, he was active in several sports, including basketball and football.

Substance Use: Denied.

Legal: Denied.

Mental Status Examination and Behavioral Observations:

Appearance and Behavior: Mr. Smith's height is approximately 5 feet 8 inches, and weight is about 147 pounds. This indicates a body mass index (BMI) of 22.3, with an associated weight category of normal. General appearance was consistent with his chronological age. He was neat and clean and casually dressed, with a short sleeve blue button shirt and black pants, short dark brown hair, and black glasses. Hygiene and grooming were good. There were no indications of gross or fine motor dysfunction. Gait and posture were unremarkable. Speech was normal in tone, pacing, and volume. There was no evidence of psychomotor retardation or agitation. There was no also overt evidence of restlessness or fidgeting. His demeanor was generally cooperative and all questions were responded to in appropriate fashion.

Emotion–Thought–Perception: Affect was restricted although congruent. This was evidenced by his expressed apprehension regarding his perceived memory problems. Overall mood was dysphoric and anxious. Thought process was logical, sequential, relevant, and coherent. Thought content was reality-based and normal. Mr. Smith demonstrated the ability to introspect and examine his feelings and beliefs. Sensory-perceptual psychotic disturbances were not evident. There was no evidence of suicidal or homicidal thoughts, intentions, or plans. There was no evidence of non-suicidal self-injury (NNSI).

Cognition: Mr. Smith was oriented to person, place, and time. Immediate memory (i.e., registration) was normal and intact as he was able to continuously, promptly, and accurately respond to interview questions. No problems in selective attention were noted as Mr. Smith remained focused and responsive, providing relevant facts that adequately addressed primary and follow-up inquiries. Short-term memory (i.e., recent memory) showed some mild impairment as evidenced by his difficulty recalling specifically provided information (i.e., three words) after passage of several minutes with interference of rehearsal. Long-term memory (i.e., remote memory) was normal and intact as he was able to provide a logical and coherent personal history, including approximate dates of major events in his life, along with the identity and description of intimate relationships. Mr. Smith's intelligence is estimated to be within normal limits based upon his effective reasoning abilities, demonstrated abstract multidimensional thinking, judgment, adequate fund of knowledge, receptive and expressive vocabulary, level of academic achievement and formal education, interests, participation in extracurricular activities, and the ability to maintain gainful employment.

Initial Screening Psychological Test Data:[9]

Note. Brief standardized psychological test data were obtained during the initial assessment and presented here for screening purposes only.

MMSE–2–EV–BF:[10]

Table 1 MMSE–2–EV–BF/RF Results

Neurocognitive Function	Patient's Raw Score	Maximum Possible Raw Score
Registration	3	3
Orientation to Time	5	5
Orientation to Place	5	5
Recall	1	3
Attention and Calculation	5	5
Naming	2	2
Repetition	1	1
Comprehension	3	3
Reading	1	1
Writing	1	1
Drawing	1	1
Story Memory	4	25
Processing Speed	10	35
Total Raw Score[a]	**42**	**90**

Note. Lower raw scores indicate greater neurocognitive dysfunction. Overall neurocognitive function data are in boldface.
[a]Raw scores of 50 or less indicate the need for more comprehensive neuropsychological testing. Using this cut-off, there is 97% confidence that a true case of neurocognitive disorder is recommended for further testing.

Screening Result: Positive for Neurocognitive Disorder
Level of Consciousness: Alert/Responsive

Screening results are positive for possible neurocognitive disorder. Follow-up neuropsychological testing is indicated.[11]
Initial Psychological Assessment Summary and Follow-Up Testing Plan:[12]

Rationale for Testing

1. *Hypothesized disorders that were the target of testing.* Based upon the initial psychological assessment, it was predicted that one or more of the following disorders were present: neurocognitive disorder, including degree.
2. *Previous comprehensive assessments unable to provide sufficient differential diagnosis.* Previous comprehensive psychiatric and behavioral health evaluations had not been capable of adequately detecting the suspected neurocognitive disorder.
3. *Continued Symptoms Despite Effective Treatment of Premorbid Psychopathology.* There had been a continuation of symptoms that precipitated this request for testing despite efficacious treatment of premorbid psychopathology GAD. This indicated the presence of additional and unanticipated abnormality, which needed to be more precisely detected or clarified by formal neuropsychological testing.
4. *Previous testing not done.* Previous standardized neuropsychological testing had not been provided in order to render such differential diagnosis.

Requested Types of Tests

1. *Memory Testing.* Performance-based, standardized, neuropsychological test data, obtained directly from the examinee, which are designed to formally measure the nature and quality of one's ability to encode, store, and retrieve information.

Test Data and Interpretation:[13]

Test Administration Note. Mr. Smith wore his prescription eyeglasses throughout test administration in order to prevent sensory limitations from confounding accurate diagnostic interpretation of the resulting data.[15]

WMS–IV, Form Ages 16 to 69:[17]

Memory involves (a) receiving information from the senses, (b) organizing and storing information, and (c) retrieving information from storage. The WMS–IV measures the ability to consciously learn and remember novel information that is bound by the testing situation (i.e., declarative episodic memory). *Immediate memory* refers to short-term or temporary storage (i.e., seconds), while *delayed memory* refers to long-term or more stable storage and retrieval (i.e., 20 to 30 minutes).

Throughout administration of the performance-based test battery, Mr. Smith was observed to be sufficiently attentive, motivated, and engaged such that test results can be considered both a reliable and valid estimate of his/her psychological functioning.[16]

Table 1 Index Score Summary

Index	Index Score	90% CI	PR	Qualitative Description	Measured Abilities
Auditory Memory Index (AMI)	100	[95, 105]	50	Average	Ability to remember orally-presented information.
Visual Memory Index (VMI)	112	[107, 116]	79	High average	Ability to remember visually-presented information.
Visual Working Memory Index (VWMI)	117	[110, 122]	87	High average	Ability to remember and manipulate visually-presented information in short-term memory storage.
Immediate Memory Index (IMI)	105	[100, 110]	63	Average	Ability to remember both visually- and orally-presented information immediately after it is presented.
Delayed Memory Index (DMI)	108	[102, 113]	70	Average	Ability to remember both visually- and orally-presented information after a 20 to 30 minute delay.

Note. Index score mean = 100, standard deviation = 15. Lower scores indicate greater memory impairment. CI = confidence interval; PR = percentile rank.

Test data show consistent average to high average memory functioning. These data are adjusted for gender, age, and years of education. Further, there are notable strengths in visual types of memory. Therefore, at this juncture, there is no evidence of neurocognitive dysfunction.

Summary of Results:[17]

Taken together, the data show that Mr. Smith's overall memory functioning is measured to be well-within normal limits. In fact, profile analysis revealed a relative strength in visual working memory. Therefore, the presenting symptoms of memory difficulties are psychogenic in nature and most likely due to his history of chronic anxiety. A combined psychiatric and psychotherapeutic treatment approach is indicated by the fact that complete symptom remission has not been obtained by a single modality intervention.

Final DSM–5 *(PDM–2/Millon) Diagnostic Summary:[14]

*Diagnostic Note. When a PDM–2/Millon personality syndrome more accurately represents the examinee's diagnosis, the DSM–5 diagnostic code and label to which the PDM–2/Millon personality syndrome is linked appears first in normal font, ensued by the PDM–2/Millon personality syndrome label in italics font.

Mental Health, Developmental, and Personality Disorders (Order of Prominence: Most-to-Least):[20]

F41.1 Generalized Anxiety Disorder (*Principal Diagnosis*) (*Historical Diagnosis*)
   Note. Test data are negative for neurocognitive disorder; normal memory functioning.

Related Medical Variables and Conditions

Atrial Fibrillation
Genetic Vulnerability for: Anxiety, Depressive Disorder
Associated Environmental Stressors:
None
Prognosis:[21]
Good due to negative results for neurocognitive disorder.
Treatment Recommendations:[22]

1. *Stress Management*. Reduce stress level as follows:

   a. *Stress-Reduction Skills*. Teach the following skills:

      i. *calming*–relaxation teach various calming strategies, including progressive muscle relaxation (e.g., the ability to discriminate between tension and relaxation), deep abdominal breathing, mindful breathing, and guided imagery, and generalizing these skills to real world situations;

   ii. *problem-focused coping*–use of problem-solving techniques to resolve stressors (clearly identify the problem(s), brainstorm alternative strategies for problem resolution, prioritize strategies, apply strategies systematically until problem is sufficiently resolved);

   iii. *emotion-focused coping*–for stressors and associated stress not resolved by calming and problem-focused coping, reframe the manner in which the problem is perceived to reduce stress reaction;

   iv. *effective communication*–teach effective ways of communicating thoughts and feelings to others if stressors are interpersonal in nature;

   v. *conflict resolution*–accurately read others' verbal and nonverbal communication, hear what others are saying, be aware of your own needs, communicate your needs clearly and in a non-defensive manner, and negotiate a compromise with others' needs.

  b. *Exercise Program.* Implement a regular exercise regimen as a stress release technique.

2. *Psychiatric Follow-Up Referral–Outpatient.* Refer for follow-up biomedical psychiatric assessment to determine the need for any medication adjustments or modifications and ongoing management.

  a. If medication modifications are made, compliance should be continually monitored, including the degree of effectiveness and any negative side effects.

  b. Follow-up with the prescribing clinician according to advised intervals.

    John M. Spores, Ph.D., J.D., H.S.P.P.
    Psychologist-Indiana #20040638A
    Attorney at Law-Indiana #21404–64

Revised 05/06/2020

   Box 4.1 illustrates what test services would have been requested subsequent to the initial assessment for this sample case, including the relevant information appearing near the end of the initial assessment Forms 3.3., 3.4, 3.5, and 3.6 (i.e., without the test services key). A few aspects of this request are notable. First, test selection focuses upon memory functioning, once again consistent with a targeted approach. Had there been more extensive symptoms and signs, such as impairments in language and executive functioning, a more comprehensive neuropsychological battery would have been chosen. Second, immediately underneath the selected test name and acronym appears the type of services and units needed in order to utilize that measure. Third, the CPT table provided at the end of each initial assessment form (i.e., Forms 3.3–3.6) guides the aggregation of total units and time needed for PA and for scheduling the follow-up test administration appointment. In this case, 2 hours are needed for test administration and scoring, hence indicating the need for scheduling a one 2-hour appointment (see Form 3.9), along with 2 more hours for test interpretation and report generation. Fourth, the latter require the request for special, "neuropsychological test evaluation services" codes (i.e., NTEV codes), which also guide the correct selection of the report's name as, "Final Neuropsychological Assessment Report." Again, if this were standard psychological testing (e.g., intelligence testing), the more typical test evaluation services codes (i.e., TEV codes) would have been chosen. (See Figure 3.2 for a review of the CPT codes.) Of note, the developmental test services codes do not appear because this is an adulthood form (viz., Form 7.3) for an adult case (i.e., the examinee's chronological age is calculated at 31 years 1 month).

Box 4.1 Sample Request for Test Services

Requested Tests, Testing Services, and Units (Time):

5. Wechsler Memory Scale, Fourth Edition, Form Ages 16 to 69

   (WMS–IV, Ages 16–69)

  • TAS–4 units; NTEV–2 units

Current Procedural Terminology (CPT) Testing Service Codes Totals:

Table 1 CPT Testing Service Codes Summary: Requested Number of Units and Time

CPT Code	Service Description	Units	Cumulative Time in Minutes[a]
96136	TAS–1st 30-minute unit[b]	1	30
96137	TAS–added 30-minute units[b]	3	90
96130	TEV–1st 60-minute unit[c]	--	--
96131	TEV–added 60-minute units[c]	--	--
96132	NTEV–1st 60-minute unit[c]	1	60
96133	NTEV–added 60-minute units[c]	1	60
Grand total (TAS + TEV + NTEV)		6	240 (4.0 hours)

Note. CPT = Current Procedural Terminology; TAS = test administration and scoring services (includes both psychological and neuropsychological tests); TEV = psychological test evaluation services (i.e., *data* interpretation, integration, and report generation); NTEV = neuropsychological test evaluation services (i.e., *data* interpretation, integration, and report generation);–denotes that the service is not selected or needed, and/or is not applicable.

[a]Total amount of time requested for that service code. [b]Each 30-minute unit must include an estimated 16 to 30 minutes of the described service. [c]Each 60-minute unit must include an estimated 31 to 60 minutes of the described service.

Final reports vary depending upon the case facts. Therefore, there is no single final report form can be shown as were the initial assessment forms. Instead, the sample shown in Exhibit 4.1 represents a prototype version of a final report. Exhibit 4.1 will be referenced hereafter in order to highlight the principal modifications in content needed to transform an initial version into a final report, along with the process by which test score reporting, interpretation, integration, summarization, final diagnoses, and treatment planning is to be done using this system. In general, the changes from its initial form consist of modifications, substitutions, entirely new sections, and some deletions, and are identified by means of footnotes appearing in strategic locations in the sample report. Included within the footnotes are commentary as to the substance of the particular change.

In order to minimize the report's length while simultaneously maintaining its realism, Exhibit 4.1 concerns a hypothetical case of an adult male, John J. Smith, who was referred for an uncomplicated case of memory issues. Because the focus here is on the report and not the case per se, only basic information is provided. Although Exhibit 4.1 refers only to standard psychological testing as applied to the adulthood developmental period, it should be noted that these same principles generalize to all developmental periods and types of testing (viz., psychological and developmental). Examples of these other types of testing cases appear in Routledge's e-resources website.

Using the Initial Report as a Beginning Framework for the Final Version

As stated prior, the initial report is intended to be the starting point for final version, which will upon completion incorporate all of the relevant test data, what they mean, final diagnoses, answers to any referral questions, and treatment recommendations. Prior to test score reporting and interpretation, the examiner should first read through the initial report in order to meet the following objectives: (a) make the needed amendments as delineated subsequently; (b) proofread for any errors in the initial report and/or adding or correcting any needed information discovered subsequent to the initial assessment (e.g., submission of school psychological test reports, disability evaluations, developmental milestones); and especially; (c) refreshing one's memory for the specific facts of the case. The latter is vital when a psychologist is working with a full and dynamic caseload of perhaps 30 to 50 cases and needs to become reacquainted with the specific case details.

Modifications to the Initial Report Prior to Entering Test Data

This section delineates all of the beginning changes to the initial report prior to entering any new information, such as test data to be garnered afterward by administration. These first modifications are further apportioned into (a) initial amendments, (b) assessment and test battery lists, (c) developmental history amendments, (d) mental status examination and behavioral observations modifications, (e) screening test results amendments, and (f) initial psychological assessment summary adjustments.

Initial Amendments

First, the title of the report appearing in both the header and center top are amended to read, "Final Neuropsychological Assessment Report."[1] The particular title is contingent upon the principal objective of testing, which can also be suggested by the type of testing services that dominated the request and received *preauthorization* (*PA*) (see Chapter 3, CPT codes). The two alternate types of final testing titles are, "Final Psychological Assessment Report," if principally testing for personality and/or clinical syndromes and related diagnostic questions, and "Final Developmental Assessment Report," if primarily testing for particular non-autism neurodevelopmental delays most frequently in early childhood.

Second, the date should be changed to correspond with the date the report was completed in written form and formally signed in order to render it a legal document and officially part of the examinee's medical record.[2] Ideally, this should be the same date as the final face-to-face test administration session (see Footnotes 2 and 4). This guideline contributes to more rapid and accurate test results, as the data and case information are more readily available in the psychologist's short-term or working memory. If only self-report inventories and/or self-report and observer report symptom rating scales were included in the test battery, and the former were administered by a technician without having any further contact with the principal examiner, the date should coincide with the time the report was composed by the latter. Related to the change of date, updating the examinee's computed chronological age (CA) is most likely to be necessary as scheduled testing appointments may add one or several months to this datum.[3]

For example, assume Mr. Smith's initial appointment was done on April 8, 2020. His age would then be computed as 30 years 0 months. Because the final report was composed on May 11, 2020, his age at the conclusion of his psychological assessment is 31 years 1 month. Occasionally, such age changes are sufficient to propel an examinee into an older developmental period (e.g., early childhood to middle and late childhood), including potential changes in older versions of psychological tests (e.g., *Conners Early Childhood* [*Conners EC*; Conners, 2009] to *Conners Comprehensive Behavior Rating Scales* [*Conners CBRS*; Conners, 2008]). In such cases, it behooves the examiner to anticipate and prepare for such age changes by estimating when follow-up testing will occur and selecting the older versions as deemed necessary.

Other demographic information should be checked for any changes (e.g., relationship status) and proofread. Finally, the referral information and presenting symptoms summary should also be reviewed for any additions and corrections, and to reinforce this information in the examiner's memory. Notice that the antecedent word, "Pertinent," in the presenting symptoms section title, which is an option in all of the initial assessment forms (viz., Forms 3.3–3.6), has been retained because only those symptoms precipitating the testing referral are needed in this case. This means that the incoming working diagnosis, *generalized anxiety disorder* (*GAD*), is being assumed as valid and will be later listed as an historical diagnosis as well as the principal diagnosis pending further assessment and testing. When an examiner lists a diagnosis as historical (also denoted as, *historical diagnosis*), it represents a diagnosis that was made by a previous clinician and for which treatment is likely still being provided. Listing only the relevant new symptoms is consistent with a targeted testing approach. On the other hand, when a referring clinician does not put forth a working diagnosis, gathering all pertinent presenting symptoms is likely more appropriate, in which case the word, "Pertinent," would be deleted from the section title and simply read, "Presenting Symptoms."

This information is ensued by an entirely new section titled, "Assessment and Test Battery," which enumerates all of the assessment techniques and tests, along with their corresponding date(s) of administration. Because such a listing carries a good deal of weight in such a report, it requires the design and incorporation of additional practice forms, along with a separate subsection devoted to its delineation to which the discussion now turns.

Assessment and Test Battery Section and Forms 4.1, 4.2, 4.3, and 4.4.

A new section of the report titled, "Assessment and Test Battery,"[4] should be inserted immediately following the presenting symptoms summary. It is vital to report such information both succinctly and early in the report so that readers can discern rapidly and effortlessly what techniques were employed. After all, it is a report that is based upon test data. Hence, most readers want to know quickly what types of tests were selected, especially those who are savvy regarding psychological testing. Therefore, four assessment and test battery forms have been designed that enumerate the techniques and tests specific to each developmental period as follows: (a) early childhood (Form 4.1); (b) middle and late childhood (Form 4.2); (c) adolescence (Form 4.3), and (d) adulthood (Form 4.4).

Essentially, this form provides a list of all the techniques and tests that were utilized in garnering the information and data presented throughout the report. In addition, they are to be reported in the order they appear in the report, along with the dates they were either completed or submitted (i.e., if the date of completion is not provided or available) in parentheticals. This permits readers to track the case progress at a glance and discern if there were any remarkable hiatuses in gathering the test data. Generally speaking, the test information also includes its acronym such that the abbreviated labels can be utilized throughout the remainder of the report, along with the type of forms, versions, or editions if pertinent. The design and layout of these forms are presented subsequently and apply to all developmental periods unless otherwise specified.

In all testing cases, the list leads off with the initial clinical interview and date, followed by a separate listing for the mental status examination and behavioral observations.[5] The reasons for separating out these two techniques despite them being typically part of a routine initial assessment is as follows: (a) it emphasizes the discernment between symptoms, which are based upon the subjective report of examinees and any collaterals, and signs, which are based upon the direct clinical observation of the examiner; (b) it follows logically from listing separately any screening tests employed during the initial assessment; and (c) it permits the addition of diagnostic information to this portion of the report that is later gleaned from behavioral observations made during test administration sessions (e.g., loosening of associations, delusional thinking). The latter practice then allows the interpretation of test data to narrow its focus on the meaning of the test scores without having to broaden the analysis to behavioral observations. If this is done, the examiner should add dates to the mental status examination and behavioral observations listing to alert the reader that this was done. Of course, most examiners in their discretion choose to report test observations later when reporting the test results. This is the author's preference because test observations usually have a direct impact on the meaning of the test data.

Additional features of these forms are as follows. First, immediately following the initial clinical interview and mental status listing are all screening tests for that cohort in alphabetical order.[6] Second, all relevant tests for that age range are listed in alphabetical order. These latter listings include (a) independent tests (e.g., *Minnesota Multiphasic Personality Inventory, Second Edition, Restructured Form* (*MMPI–2–RF*; Ben-Porath & Tellegen, 2008, 2011; Tellegen & Ben-Porath, 2011), (b) different test battery types (e.g., *NEPSY–II, Full Battery* versus *NEPSY–II, General Battery*; Korkman et al., 2007a, 2007b), and (c) subtest combinations that have most frequently been used for resolving specific diagnostic issues (e.g., *NEPSY–II, Form Ages 3 to 4, Social Perception Subtests* [Korkman et al., 2007a, 2007b] for autism testing during early childhood).[7] Third, it should be emphasized that the test listings in each form are circumscribed to those appropriately normed for that developmental period. The objectives here are to (a) reduce the length of the list to more manageable proportions, and (b) reduce the likelihood of human error in inadvertently selecting inappropriately normed tests for that case.

Fourth, the techniques and tests are listed by Arabic numbers for easy reference and to help maintain the correct order of test reporting and interpretation. Fifth, the margins are indented such that they are aligned evenly and uniformly, and so that the test labels and acronyms are maintained without hyphenation for easier identification. The sixth and final feature applies to most of the forms and refers to the font theme; namely *Times New Roman* typeface at *12-point font size*. Without the need for excessive detail, this font consists of a higher degree of contrast and consists of especially useful sharp *serifs* that facilitate reading.[7]

To see how this is applied, refer back now to Exhibit 4.1. In order to insert the appropriate assessment and test battery information, Form 4.4 was chosen because it lists the techniques and tests for the adulthood period (i.e., age 19 years and older; see also Footnote 4). Specifically, the initial assessment in this hypothetical case consisted of the initial clinical interview, mental status examination and behavioral observations, and the *Mini–Mental State Examination, Second Edition, Brief Version, Blue Form* (*MMSE–2–BV–BF*; Folstein, Folstein, White, & Messer, 2010). Note that all were completed on the same initial assessment date and the MMSE–2–BV–BF was reported in sufficient detail with acronym such that the reader is able to be cognizant of which version and form was used. Also note that the "Mental Status Examination and Behavioral Observations" listing contains only the date of the initial clinical interview. This means that no additional diagnostic information was added to this section of the report based upon later observations during test administration. Again, note that the specific form of the standardized memory test was provided as there exists a version for older ages. Specifically, the *Wechsler Memory Scale, Fourth Edition, Form Ages 16 to 69* (*WMS–IV, Ages 16–69*; Wechsler, 2009a, 2009b)[8] was used here rather than the version for ages 65 to 90 years (see Chapter 9). Finally, it is apparent from this listing that the report was done on the final date of testing service, which communicates to the reader that the results were obtained in a timely fashion and likely to be more reliable and valid (compare Footnotes 2 and 7).

Developmental History Amendments

The developmental history aspects of the final report refer to all the sections beginning with, "Health-Related," through "Legal," inclusive. Upon review by the testing psychologist, most of this material here is either (a) proofread for accuracy, (b) used to insert any additional pertinent information garnered since the conclusion of the initial assessment, and (c) perused to reacquaint oneself as to the specific case facts in preparation for reporting and interpreting the data that are soon to be collected. Therefore, some comments are next offered regarding what information to emphasize and why.

First, occasional cross-references appear in the report and assist the reader in making important connections between different sections (e.g., the reference from, "Health-Related," back to the "Pertinent Presenting Symptoms," highlighting that the prescribed medication has had no positive effect on the examinee's reported anxiety problems). Second, it is important to emphasize that there has been no, or an insufficient, effect of treatment on the presenting symptoms that precipitated the referral, hence bolstering the medical necessity for testing. Third, in the "Health-Related" section, it is noted that the examinee wears corrective lens for visual difficulties. This alerts the examiner to ensure that the examinee wears these glasses (or equivalent contact lens) during test administration (although this should also have been addressed during the latter portions of the clinical interview when describing the planned test battery and scheduling). The objective is to rule out any confounding effects of peripheral nervous system (here sensory) limitations on the neuropsychological test results. As will become apparent below, an administrative narrative note documenting this fact should be made when introducing the test data (see Footnote 15 subsequently).

Fourth, the family information focuses upon eliminating stressors in this area of functioning as a partial or complete explanation for the examinee's continued memory problems (i.e., severe family stressors can escalate stress to the point of exacerbating problems in concentration and thus short-term memory). Fifth, there are no noted changes in personality that could indicate neurocognitive dysfunction. Sixth, educational history is unremarkable for historical cognitive problems, such as intellectual disability or specific learning disorders, which may account for memory difficulties (although the recent onset also argues against a long-standing cognitive problem). The general point here is that the information reported all relates in some way to the presenting symptoms and strategically eliminating variables other than neurocognitive dysfunction that may account for the continued memory complaints. Added facts that are not pertinent to this diagnostic issue are not added so as to streamline the final report as much as is warranted.

Mental Status Examination and Behavioral Observations Modifications

The mental status examination and behavioral observations section typically is proofread for accuracy and to refresh the examiner's memory of how the examinee Mr. Smith presented himself more objectively. As stated prior, any changes in mental status and behavior observed between the date of the initial assessment and the follow-up testing sessions can either be added here or, more typically, as part of test interpretation. If inserted in this section, additional dates should be added to the parenthetical associated with this section. Because the data here are established from more objective observations of the examinee's behavioral presentation (i.e., *signs* versus *symptoms* of psychopathology), the report flows naturally into the ensuing preliminary standardized screening data; whether it be performance-based as here or derived from observer or self-report test formats (see also Chapter 9).

Initial Screening Psychological Test Data

The section titled, "Initial Screening Psychological Test Data," is retained from the initial assessment form (viz., Form 3.6)[9] and the data table for the MMSE–2–BV–BF[10] (Folstein et al., 2010) is inserted here (see also Chapter 5). The full title of the screening measure, including its specified version and form, "Mini-Mental State Examination, Second Edition, Expanded Version, Blue Form (MMSE–2–EV–BF)," would appear in the initial report. However, in this final report (i.e., Exhibit 4.1) only the acronym is needed here (see Footnote 10) because the full title now appears in the earlier assessment and test battery listing (refer back to Footnote 4). The data table in the report (i.e., Table 1) efficiently lists the examinee's performance juxtaposed with the total possible points for each item and in the aggregate, along with the screening test result. This makes the results readily apparent and requires only a summary interpretation that more testing is needed.[11] Therefore, the next optional section appearing in the initial assessment form (viz., "Initial Psychological Assessment Summary" in Form 3.6), which would be retained and added to if no further testing was needed (see Chapter 3), would in this case be deleted because follow-up neuropsychological testing was required to address the diagnostic issue. The succeeding sections provide the information as to what the follow-up testing plan was, hence leading into the new sections that insert the test data and its meaning.

Initial Psychological Assessment Summary and Follow-Up Testing Plan

Recall that this section of the initial report outlined the rationale and types of tests needed to answer the relevant diagnostic issues. Although this section may now be deleted since the testing was done and PA can simply be implied, retaining such information helps explain why certain tests were selected over others (e.g., why a malingering test was added to the battery or why a more labor-intensive implicit test was chosen in favor of a more efficient explicit test). It also provides a more comprehensive picture of the entire process without requiring the reader to obtain two separate reports with overlapping information. Therefore, it is best practice to preserve this section and simply make the necessary modifications to past tense in order to clarify for the reader that it pertains to the ensuing body of the report,[12] which contains all of the new data tables and their interpretation.

In the initial report version, the "Rationale for Testing" subsection consisted of four principal reasons for testing. These included a need to detect the suspected presence of a neurocognitive disorder, which called for the precision afforded by a formal standardized measure of memory functioning that was unequivocally beyond the scope of a clinical interview. Further, it was pointed out that such procedure had not previously been provided. Thereafter, the "Requested Types of Tests" subsection followed with the logical selection of, "Memory Testing," which was defined as standardized with an attendant definition of the construct of memory; namely, "the nature and quality of one's ability to encode, store, and retrieve information." It can be argued that this section should be retained in the final report, although modified into past tense as done prior, because it provides the reader with a vital explanation for why such formal testing was needed and why such test was selected over other more comprehensive neuropsychological test batteries. It may also be supplemented with a clear definition of the construct to be measured that matches the referral's stated diagnostic issue. Briefly then, preserving this section in past tense form affords the reader a cognitive framework within which the garnered test data can be afforded greater contextual meaning.

Prior to moving on to final modifications, there is an issue that needs to be addressed. Specifically, this involves how to manage instances where the examinee's insurance has denied a majority of the requested tests and test services, but has afforded PA to a single measure for a more narrowly defined yet vital differential diagnosis (e.g., personality disorder). If the examiner believes it is important to proceed with the case without the denied tests, although also wants to communicate to the reader that a more comprehensive battery was desired, then the original list in the "Requested Types of Tests" should be retained, ensued by the statement, "Insurance did not preauthorize a sufficient number of units to use this test as originally planned and requested." This effectively instructs the reader that the examiner believed the denied tests were essential but that their use was precluded by insurance issues. The denied tests, however, should not be included in the assessment and test battery section of the final report as this gives the false impression that it was indeed administered.

Final Modifications

The final steps in modifying the initial report are as follows. First, immediately following the listed memory test, "Next, a provisional diagnostic summary is delineated that elucidates the focus of testing, along with the following," and the ensuing three bullet points appearing in all initial assessment forms (i.e., Forms 3.3–3.6) are now obsolete and should be deleted. Next, a new section titled, "Test Data and Interpretation,"[13] should be entered. This will represent the body of the report wherein the test data in tabular format (see Part II for all tests and their data tables), and their interpretation will be inserted. Finally, the title, "Provisional DSM–5 ★(PDM–2/Millon) Diagnostic Summary," should now read, "Final DSM–5 ★(PDM–2/Millon) Diagnostic Summary."[14] The only modification here is the word, "provisional" being supplanted by the word, "final" (see Footnote 14).

The file should then be saved by changing its initial file name, here, "I_Smith, John J. 1234567," to "F_Smith, John J. 1234567," with the leading letter "F" denoting a final (versus "I" for initial) report, and then saved within a subfolder labeled, "Final Psychological Assessment Reports." The document is now ready for the examiner to begin filling in the body of the final report, "Test Data and Interpretation," with the pertinent tests, their scores, and what they mean.

New Additions to the Final Report

This section covers the new portions of the final report. They include (a) the test data and interpretation body of the report, (b) the summary of results, (c) the final diagnostic summary (including any questions proposed by the referral source), and finally, (d) treatment recommendations. These are set out in more detail subsequently.

Test Data and Interpretation

Entering the test data and interpreting their meaning is perhaps the most important new section of the report from which all diagnostic conclusions and treatment recommendations are derived (see Footnote 13). As such, it can be referred to as the core or body of the report. The followed subsections focus on how this section should be organized. They include the following: (a) entering test administration narrative notes or comments that qualify the meaning of the test results; (b) general strategies for reporting the test data; (c) guidelines for how to initially order the reporting of the test data (i.e., which tests are reported from first to last); (d) additional guidelines for modifying the initial order; and (d) how to simultaneously report, interpret, and gradually integrate the findings in leading up to the summary of results.

TEST ADMINISTRATION NARRATIVE NOTES OR QUALIFYING COMMENTS

Prior to moving into the presentation of actual data, a series of narrative notes are presented that can effectively bolster the validity of the garnered test data. Form 4.5 enumerates various narrative comments concerning test administration that examiners may want or need to incorporate at strategic points in this section of the final report. In particular, Narrative Note 1 (Form 4.5) states that examinees used their sensory aids in order to ensure that any deficits could be attributed to *central nervous system* (*CNS*) dysfunction. In the sample case, a comment documenting the Mr. Smith wore his corrective lens throughout test administration effectively rules out visual limitations as a confounding variable when interpreting his memory scores.[15] Later, just prior to test interpretation, an administrative note was inserted verifying that there was nothing about the examinee's performance during testing that would question the validity of the results.[16] Other narrative notes refer to the presence or absence of medication that may have affected the examinee's performance (e.g., being off ADHD medication when taking a CPT test). Of note, clear instructions concerning examinees' proper preparation for test administration should always be given when first proposing the planned follow-up testing during the latter portion of the clinical interview. Next, the body or core of this vital section is discussed.

GENERAL STRATEGIES FOR REPORTING THE TEST DATA

This first new major section of the final report is analogous to the "Results" section of an APA formatted journal article (see American Psychological Association, 2020) wherein the primary and secondary statistical analyses are presented, typically including descriptive and inferential statistics in such order. Analogously, the "Test Data and Interpretation" section of the final report emphasizes the presentation of empirical data with carefully designed tables for each test (see Footnote 13), most frequently consisting of a set of relevant scales or subscales, standard scores (i.e., linear transformations), confidence intervals that consider error and provide estimates of significant differences when conducting profile analyses, percentile ranks (i.e., area transformations) that most lay people better understand, and qualitative descriptions.

Tabular notes follow most tables to assist the reader in interpreting the presented data for each test, which are gradually integrated with subsequently presented tabular data and their interpretation. In providing a sequence of data tables for each major test, with an increasing degree of integration in each table's ensuing interpretation, then summarizing the results and leading toward a final diagnostic presentation, readers are well informed as to precisely how the examiner arrived at these conclusions and treatment recommendations, including the ongoing thought process.

In the sample case, the WMS–IV table first presents the major indexes and their norm-based standard scores, hence comparing the examinee to peers of comparable age, education, and gender who do not manifest abnormality in memory functioning.[17] As can be seen by the qualitative descriptions, all fall within the normal range or somewhat higher. This represents the primary analysis. The secondary analysis searches for any significant differences among the examinee's index scores, sometimes referred to as an *ipsative* examination. The purpose here is to investigate any internal strengths or weaknesses the examinee might manifest, which would be of diagnostic or treatment significance. Here, the 90 % confidence interval for Visual Working Memory Index (VWMI) has no overlap with the Immediate Memory Index (IMI), hence suggesting a statistically significant difference between these two memory abilities. In this case, the primary analysis is diagnostically most imperative or on point. Notice also that the percentile ranks are all 50 or above (i.e., with 50 being the median or average score), which is another way of stating that the examinee's overall performance is well within normal limits.

In illustrating the transformation of the initial report into its final version, this sample case was kept as diagnostically straightforward and pure as possible. However, when reporting test results within a sequence of data tables, as is done here in this system,[18],[19] the issue of order becomes paramount because most batteries include more than one measure. Succinctly, the examiner must ask, "In what order do I present and interpret the test data?"

In the next subsections guidelines for ordering the test data and interpretation section are presented. They are proposed to facilitate the simultaneous reporting and interpreting of scores, along with enhancing the clarity and readability of the report. This process is apportioned into (a) the initial ordering, and (b) the subsequent modification of test

Table 4.1 Guidelines for Ordering the "Test Data and Interpretation" Section of the Final Report

#	Guideline Description

Initial Ordering

1. Performance-based neurodevelopmental and neurocognitive ability tests provided by the examinee. (viz., intelligence tests, neuropsychological tests, achievement tests, developmental tests, and continuous performance tests).

   a. Within this grouping, prioritize those tests that are most relevant to resolving the diagnostic issues presented in the case.
2. Personality inventory tests.

   a. Prioritize those tests that are most relevant to resolving the diagnostic issues presented in the case.
   b. Observer-report versions of personality inventory tests.
3. Performance personality tests.

   a. Within this grouping, prioritize those tests that are most relevant to resolving the diagnostic issues presented in the case.
4. Rating scales tests.

   a. Tests that are most relevant to resolving the diagnostic issues presented in the case (including the data needed to corroborate a vital diagnosis).
   b. Tests that are administered by closely supervised administration or via structured interview.
   c. Tests that provide validity scales showing the respondent's likely test-taking response tendency on subsequent tests.

Subsequent Ordering (after reviewing test scores)

5. Move to lower priority tests that are (a) invalid, (b) of very questionable validity due to false negative or false positive results (i.e., outlier results with explanation), or (c) of very questionable validity due to unknown or undetermined reasons (i.e., outlier results without explanation).
6. Move to a higher priority position tests that (a) confirm a key diagnosis, (b) provide credibility to a key result, (c) answer a vital referral question, or (d) provide multi- versus unidimensional data.

Note. The guideline number denotes degree of priority to be afforded the identified tests (e.g., 1 = 1st priority, 2 = 2nd priority, . . . last number = lowest priority). The guideline letter denotes degree of priority to be afforded the tests within the more general group (a = 1st priority within the more general group, . . . last letter = lowest priority within the more general group). See Form 3.7 for listing of tests.

order if needed (see Table 4.1). The first phase is based upon test characteristics that are invariant or static (i.e., factors that are an inherent part of a class of tests; see Table 1.1). Their advantage lies in their consistency or predictability of application. As such, they can be relied upon in determining their order in the assessment and test battery listing near the beginning of the report. Their disadvantage derives from the same source that produced their reliability, which can now be reframed as inflexibility. That is, there are occasions when this initial ordering becomes less than ideal.

Hence, a second set of guidelines provides the flexibility needed to occasionally adjust the initial test ordering to best meet the facts of a particular case. In the event one of these secondary guidelines does not apply (e.g., a test of cognitive ability is not included in the test battery), it should be disregarded by simply advancing to the next guideline that fits the case facts.

INITIAL GUIDELINES FOR ORDERING THE REPORT OF TEST DATA

As shown in Table 4.1, Guideline 1 states that first priority is afforded the performance-based neurodevelopmental and neurocognitive ability tests, which typically measure complex constructs that directly impact functioning in several major areas of life. In reference to Form 3.7, these would refer to the *intelligence tests*, *neuropsychological tests*, *achievement tests*, *developmental tests*, and *continuous performance tests* (*CPT*), including all subtests whether used selectively (e.g., attention and executive functioning subtests to rule out ADHD) or as part of a general or full battery (e.g., to rule out a major neurocognitive disorder). If a battery is comprised of several such tests, then the ones most central to resolving the principal diagnostic issues in the case should be prioritized (see Table 4.1, Guideline 1a). This typically means that tests targeting the most serious or pervasive potential diagnoses should go first (e.g., an IQ test to rule out *intellectual disability* [*ID*]) versus those that target the less serious diagnoses or those narrower in scope (e.g., a *Continuous Performance Test* [*CPT*] to rule out *attention-deficit/hyperactivity disorder* [*ADHD*]).

Next, Guideline 2 (Table 4.1) states that second priority goes to any self-report personality inventory tests in the battery. As will become evident in Part II, these tests carry an impressive history of test development and empirical support, including reliability, validity, and utility. Again, if a battery consists of more than one of these tests, those that resolve the most central diagnostic issues or questions in a case should be prioritized (see Table 2.2, Guideline 2a). Again, this usually (although not invariably) means the most serious types of psychopathology being questioned. However, if the referral source's major concern is clearly with a less pervasive or severe type of diagnosis or question, this should be prioritized under the assumptions that (a) the referring clinician must have a legitimate reason for emphasizing such disorder, and (b) the testing psychologist actually has two clients to which services are being provided (i.e., the examinee and the referral source). Some personality inventory tests have an observer-based version. In this book, this refers to the *NEO Personality Inventory, Third Edition* (NEO–PI–3; McCrae & Costa, 2010). Because initial preference should be afforded data that has been provided by the individual being assessed, observer-based inventories are last within this grouping (see Table 4.1, Guideline 2c). As will become apparent subsequently, validity considerations can modify this preference.

Guideline 3 in Table 4.1 gives third priority to performance personality tests (refer also to Form 3.7). This is not meant to indicate that such tests have less reliability and validity (e.g., Bornstein, 1998, 1999; Ganellen, 1996, 2007; Hughes, Gacono, & Owen, 2007; Meyer & Archer, 2001; Meyer & Handler, 1997; Viglione, 1999). The reason such tests are afforded somewhat less priority as compared to the aforementioned personality inventories has to do with a lesser degree of test utility. While the required test services for personality inventories averages 60 to 90 minutes, those needed for performance personality tests averages 120 to 180 minutes (see Forms 3.3–3.6, § Requested Tests, Testing Services, and Units [Time]). At least part of the increased test services time and effort needed for these measures can be attributed to their providing only indirect corroborating evidence regarding DSM–5 diagnostic categories (Huprich, 2006).

However, their importance to assessment and testing here should not be minimized or derogated in any way. In general, their implicit nature and low face validity renders these tests remarkably resistant to intentional efforts on the part of examinees to distort or manipulate the results (see Chapter 12). In this sense they can be an invaluable part of a particular test battery. Furthermore, the data from these tests provide important evidence regarding etiology and potential targets for treatment intervention; for example, morbid responses (MOR) on the Rorschach–CS empirically demonstrate the presence of pessimism (Exner, 2003), thus indicating the need to modify a negative cognitive style as a viable treatment objective. Once again, in the less likely event a targeted test battery consists of more than one of these tests, they should be prioritized according to the degree to which they resolve central diagnostic issues or questions in the particular case (e.g., suicide potential; see Table 4.1 Guideline 3a).

Finally, Guideline 4 (Table 4.1) affords last priority to rating scales tests, many of which are completed by observers with varying degrees of familiarity with the examinee. As indicated previously, such measures tend to be more susceptible to test-taking responses tendencies on the part of the respondent, including such phenomena as contrast effects (see Ivancevich, 1983; Maurer, Palmer, & Ashe, 1993; Schuh, 1978; Smither, Reilly, & Buda, 1988; Wexley, Yukl, Kovacs, & Sanders, 1972). Their validity scales are also more circumscribed and less reliable when compared to those of the well-researched personality tests. It is for these reasons that they are usually used as supplements to the other three test groupings, although there are exceptions as indicated subsequently.

Within this last grouping, there are three considerations for modifying their priority. First, as is typical of the other tests, those most central to resolving key diagnostic issues should go first (see Table 4.1, Guideline 4a). Second, a number of these tests are comparable to (and may even be classified the same as) the personality inventories in that they are to be administered to the examinee as respondent and under close supervision (the *Trauma Symptom Inventory, Second Edition* (TSI–2; Briere, 2011). These include measures that can be administered in either rating scale format or as structured interviews, as does the Vineland Adaptive Behavior Scales, Third Edition (Vineland–3; Sparrow, Cicchetti, & Saulnier, 2016). These features permit the examiner to guide the respondent's ratings using strategic prompts such that they may be more accurate in measuring the desired construct. Thus, they should be given greater weight over more typical rating scales tests without such components (see Table 4.1, Guideline 4b). Third, some rating scales tests provide validity data for detecting response tendencies such as exaggeration or minimization of symptoms. These rating scales tests should be given priority over those without such data because such tendencies can be effectively generalized to the latter (see Table 4.1, Guideline 4c). Hence, if the same respondent was found to over-estimate symptoms on a prior rating scale, by analogy, this tendency can be assumed to affect later ratings yielded by the same respondent.

Next to be discussed are rules for changing the initial test order contingent upon particular patterns of test results and their associated interpretations. It is not intended as an exhaustive list although can be effective guidelines due to their added flexibility. In this sense, they may be considered dynamic factors or considerations (i.e., ones that are capable of change depending upon various fact patterns).

SUBSEQUENT GUIDELINES FOR MODIFYING THE INITIAL ORDER OF TEST DATA

The principles for modifying the initial test order regard data that do one of the following: (a) provide invalid results; (b) provide questionably valid results; (c) contradict the vast majority of evidence (i.e., outlier results); (d) confirm a key diagnosis; (e) provide credibility to a key result; and (f) answer a vital referral question.

The first Guideline 5 (Table 4.1) concerns a series of related outcomes that work to move a table to a lesser priority position; that is, at or near the end of the "Test Data and Interpretation" section. The first concerns a distinct test-taking response pattern by the respondent which voids test validity. As such, the test data per se are not reported as this would be misleading. However, the validity results should be reported because that specific test was requested and administered as part of the battery. Therefore, it should appear somewhere in the final report. The second outcome refers to a data pattern that clearly contradicts the bulk of the evidence. In statistics, these are commonly referred to as *outliers*. These data are usually the result of some anomaly that usually has little or nothing to do with measuring the variable or construct of interest. Examples include a data entry error, a research participant who failed to comprehend or follow instructions, or an individual who was not typical of the population for which the sample was to represent. In the realm of psychological assessment and testing, the obtained data unexpectedly and for some analogous reason do not measure the construct of interest.

For example, the CPT tests are designed to be tedious and repetitive computer tasks without respite, as in clicking a computer mouse for all letters flashing one-by-one on a screen except for the "X." It is in such tasks that individuals with ADHD are expected to show a greater deterioration in performance as compared to those without ADHD. However, there have been children with severe ADHD, which was confirmed by interrater reliability on standardized rating scales tests and other neuropsychological subtests that measure attention and executive functioning, perform to unusual perfection on such CPT tests. Upon debriefing, it became clear that many of these children adjust to the typical tedium of this task by mentally transforming it into a video game in which the letters represent "spaceships" and the mouse clicks "firing lasers" in order to destroy the imagined invaders. Although remarkably imaginative and resilient, the test did not perform as designed, thus effectuating what is called a *false negative* result; namely, the individual's test results indicate as absence of a disorder, whereas it is in reality present. On the other hand, an individual may in effect fail a CPT test due test anxiety or feeling ill and not due to ADHD; again, referred to as a false positive result. In either case, these results do not contribute to the veracity of the final diagnostic summary and should therefore be demoted in rank order to last or near last.

Finally, occasionally outlier results occur without explanation. In such cases, these data can also be moved to a lower or lowest rank position. This will give priority to the empirical evidence that converges on what the majority of results indicate, followed by the minority of contradictory results. This is analogous to a literature review that reports the majority evidence first, followed by a minority of contradictory findings on a particular issue. Such organization will provide a more logical flow to both the examiner and reader, and be more likely to expose the reason(s) for such contradictory data (e.g., is it possibly related to test format or type of respondent).

Guideline 6 (Table 4.1) consists of a series of related reasons for moving a test's data table(s) to a higher priority position. They include (a) confirming a key diagnosis, (b) adding to the credibility of a result, (c) directly answering a referral question, and (d) providing multidimensional data that measure a variety of constructs versus one that measures one construct in detail. The latter is consistent with the general to specific stratagem to test interpretation. Examples of each are next provided.

First, let us assume that to test for ID and a personality disorder, a psychologist uses a battery that consists of (a) an IQ test, (b) a self-report personality inventory test, and (c) an adaptive behavior measure in rating scale format. In accord with Guidelines 1, 2, and 4 (Table 4.1), this would represent the initial test reporting order. However, upon scoring, the examiner finds a full-scale IQ score of 65 and adaptive behavior of 60 on the same metric, with onset prior to age 18 years already established by means of clinical interview. In addition, there is no evidence of a personality disorder. According to Guideline 6 (Table 4.1), the adaptive behavior measure would move to the second position behind the IQ test and prior to the personality inventory because it would confirm a key diagnosis of mild ID, whereas there is negative evidence for a personality disorder. Even if there were evidence of personality psychopathology, such modified order would still be viable considering that (a) ID is a more pervasive and chronic diagnosis, and (b) provides a more logical flow to the discussion (i.e., confirming one diagnosis before moving on to a second diagnostic issue).

Providing added credibility to a key result works in similar fashion although is more generalized. For instance, assume a comparable test battery to the one described prior, except that instead of an adaptive behavior measure, a performance personality test was done. Hence the initial ordering would be (a) IQ test, (b) personality inventory, and (c) performance personality test. Upon scoring, however, the IQ test shows borderline intellectual functioning, which is also shown in some of the data of the performance personality test (e.g., a simple information processing approach to interpreting Rorschach Inkblots). If borderline intelligence is a key diagnosis in the case, the performance personality test results can be justifiably moved into the second position behind the IQ test data in order to increase the credibility of the borderline intellectual functioning diagnosis. Third, in one particular case rating scale data was moved to first position in order to highlight a violence potential indicator scale (viz., Conners CBRS). Specifically, the referral source wanted the testing to address an examinee's potential for future violence. Because the rating scale data showed interrater agreement that the examinee was a high risk for violence, and such data was directly on point, these results were reported first and subsequently supported with data from a performance personality test.

Fourth and finally, a referral asked for a differential diagnosis principally involving posttraumatic stress disorder (PTSD) and secondarily a possible personality disorder. In this adult case, the examinee showed unequivocal evidence of psychological mindedness and the ability to introspect. Therefore, the *Millon Clinical Multiaxial Inventory, Third Edition* (*MCMI–III*; Millon, Millon, Davis, & Grossman, 2006a, 2006b) was selected as a multidimensional self-report personality inventory test, which covered both personality psychopathology and clinical syndromes such as PTSD, along with the TSI–2, which focuses exclusively upon the psychopathological sequelae of trauma. In this case, even though the TSI–2 addressed the referral question most adequately, the MCMI–III was reported first because its wider scope was able to initially show the presence of both *borderline personality disorder* co-occurring with PTSD. Next, the TSI–2 corroborated the PTSD diagnosis while adding valuable treatment relevant detail, including a comprehensive symptom pattern that identified specifiers (e.g., specific types of dissociative symptoms) and the severity of the disorder.

Taken together, the testing psychologist may employ guidelines 1 through 4 in Table 4.1 when forming the initial test order using Forms 4.1 through 4.4 near the beginning of the final report. In most cases, these guidelines will apply without additional modification. However, after scoring all of the tests, the examiner should scrutinize the essential results of each to determine if any subsequent modifications are needed in the original test order. Such considerations are done irrespective of the test administration order as these are separate and distinct considerations. If there are changes to the initial order, modifications are needed in the "Assessment and Test Battery," listing near the beginning of the final report. Lastly, these guidelines are not meant to be exhaustive or fixed. Exceptions and additional guidelines will undoubtedly be discovered by various testing psychologists as they practice the trade. When they occur, it is wise to record them for future reference as demonstrated in Table 4.1.

THE PRACTICE OF SIMULTANEOUS TEST DATA REPORTING, INTERPRETATION, AND INTEGRATION

Before moving on to the next section in which the essential results are summarized, the practice of what may be called simultaneous test reporting, interpretation, and integration should be carefully delineated. It is both efficient and efficacious in mental health practice where timeliness, precision, accuracy, and clarity are essential. The process begins immediately after the ordering of tests as delineated prior. It can be divided into several distinct steps.

First, the examiner should once again review the diagnostic issues and any questions presented in the case. This is to ensure that only the most relevant data are reported and interpreted so as to address the testing objectives. In the sample case (Exhibit 4.1), the fundamental issue is to determine whether a *comorbid* neurocognitive disorder had developed alongside a chronic anxiety disorder in the form of memory impairment. If positive, the derivative issues would be as follows: (a) clarify the pattern of memory dysfunction; (b) provide a measure of its degree (i.e., severity); (c) identify which DSM–5 diagnosis or diagnoses would best fit the overall data pattern; (d) note if all diagnostic issues have been addressed or is supplementary testing warranted; and (e) identify the treatment objectives.

Second, the scored data patterns of each test should be securitized to generally determine (a) what data need to be reported for each independent test, and (b) what such data indicate with regard to the diagnostic and assessment issues. In the sample case, the norm-based index scores and percentile ranks are all average or above, hence showing that overall memory functioning is normal and intact. Therefore, there is no practical need to obfuscate the results by reporting the more narrowly defined subtest scores, which also possess much less reliability and validity due to their reliance on fewer test items. A secondary analysis that might be useful would be to scrutinize any relative differences among the index scores. This is referred to as an *ipsative analysis* with the objective of investigating any relative strengths and weaknesses an examinee may possess. Here, there is one significant difference as indicated by the lack of overlap between the Visual Working Memory Index (VWMI) and Immediate Memory Index (IMI) confidence intervals, here favoring the former. The VWMI is also the highest of all the other indexes. Therefore, in the sample case the norm-referenced data are interpreted first because they directly address the principal diagnostic issue in the case, followed by the ipsative comparison.

Third, each subsequent test and its data table(s) should be interpreted both independently and in comparison to previously reported results. For example, consider a CPT test and its data for a 10-year-old male, which clearly indicate the presence of ADHD. Next, assume that rating scales completed by the examinee's parent and teacher also show the presence of ADHD. The interpretation for the latter would first indicate as follows:

"The observer-based data show the presence of ADHD, hence providing interrater agreement or reliability for such diagnosis. Furthermore, these results are consistent with those of the performance-based CPT test, which also showed clear evidence of ADHD. This included evidence of moderate impairments in inattention, sustained inattention, impulsivity, and sustained impulsivity." In this example, the rating scale test data were first interpreted independently from all other tests. Secondly, the rating scale results were integrated with the prior-mentioned CPT test, which essentially provides *convergent validity* for the ADHD diagnosis according to the *multitrait-multimethod* (*MTMM*) approach of examining *construct validity* (*MTMM*; Campbell & Fiske, 1959). That is, two tests that use different methods of data collection (i.e., performance and observer ratings) but measure the same construct (i.e., ADHD) should produce similar results (i.e., both being positive for combined ADHD, moderate degree). As applied to psychological testing, this should be interpreted as strong evidence that this child indeed has the measured construct (viz., ADHD). Not only is such analysis empirical and objective, it employs a scientifically well-established method of analyzing interrater reliability and construct validity. Furthermore, the report should be written to reflect the psychologist's thought process and reasoning as the data reporting and interpretation process continues from the first to the last test and data table. Using this method then, the analysis is heavily reliant upon reporting only the most relevant empirical data, and increasingly integrating the results with each subsequent data table in the body of the report. The ensuing section designed to bring the essential results together within one or two pithy paragraphs, and tie them to the overall treatment approach that is detailed in the final section of the report.

Summary of Results

The "Summary of Results" section represents a pithy recapitulation of the fundamental findings. More specifically, it should consist of the following components: (a) positive findings (i.e., what diagnoses were found and supported by the data); (b) negative findings (i.e., what diagnoses were ruled out or negated by a lack of evidence); (c) unresolved issues and reasons therefore (including any needed supplementary testing); (d) direct answers to referral questions; and (e) implications for the general treatment approach (see Footnote 19). Although some of the latter elements may not apply in all cases, they should be routinely considered.

This section is analogous to an abstract in an APA journal article. Rather than immediately following the title page, however, it should be composed proximately to the end of the "Test Data and Interpretation" section. For more complex cases, notes of the key findings can be recorded on a pad as the examiner progresses through the data tables with ongoing interpretation and integration of results. This helps to avoid inadvertently neglecting to include some key results (e.g., "CPT positive for ADHD, combined, moderate degree" Rorschach shows positive depression and suicide indexes; and "MMPI negative for bipolar disorder, positive for moderate depression as Rorschach"). Diagnostic specifiers that are revealed by the data should always be appended for purposes of maximum precision (e.g., type, degree, qualifiers), primarily because standardized testing possesses such capability and thus should be exploited. For example, a mood disorder *with anxious distress* alerts the treating clinician as to its presence and a consequential more guarded prognosis (American Psychiatric Association, 2013).

Occasionally, a previously unexpected disorder is suggested by the results. For example, a case may be unequivocally negative for a bipolar diagnosis in an 8-year-old female. However, rating scales tests by parent and teacher are suggestive of an *autism spectrum disorder* (*ASD*). As such, this screening result should be noted in the summary of results, along with a supplementary testing recommendation for ASD. Finally, the fundamental conclusions should be related to an advised treatment approach stated in broad terms. For example, imagine a 29-year-old male whose test results are positive for persistent depression co-occurring with inattentive ADHD of moderate severity. In such a case, the summary of results can state as follows: "Considering these results, a combined biomedical and psychotherapeutic treatment approach is indicated." This single statement would be ensued by a formal diagnosis listing both these disorders, and more specific treatment recommendations consisting of coexisting referrals to both outpatient psychiatry and psychotherapy.

Some final notes on summarizing the findings are as follows. First, the examiner should make earnest attempts not to equivocate. Readers become disconcerted when there are seemingly incessant qualifiers in such a report such as, "it appears," "it may be," and "it is possible that." Many colleagues have commented on such reports as being unclear, evasive, and lacking any substance or direction. In fact, after reading such a report, one disconcerted colleague in particular wondered in exasperation, "How is testing even useful if all they do is offer these general statements that I already knew." The point here is that one can be clear and direct in writing test results without being improperly overconfident or overly interpreting the data. Therefore, stating that the results "show the presence of bipolar II disorder, including evidence of hypomanic symptoms coexisting with severe depressive symptoms," can be direct, and based upon scientific empirical evidence. This does not mean ignoring conflicting data. Rather, make valid inferences when the data so indicate.

In the sample case (Exhibit 4.1), the "Summary of Results" section first reports the negative results, addressing the major issue of whether there is a comorbid neurocognitive disorder. Positive results are omitted because there are none here to report. The relative strength in visual working memory was next reported for purposes of reemphasizing the negative results with more detail. The inference that the presenting symptoms were *psychogenic* (versus *organic*) in nature (i.e., due to his anxiety) follows directly from the empirical evidence and leads directly to the proposed treatment approach. In particular, the facts show that a biomedical approach by itself is not sufficient for complete symptom remission. Rather, it was advised that psychotherapy be added to the treatment plan for more complete recovery and improved functioning. Notice that all of these elements are addressed within one succinct paragraph, and without a hint of equivocation or overzealousness.

Final DSM–5 Diagnostic Summary

Although the DSM–5 diagnostic summaries vary somewhat across the four developmental periods in terms of the listed secondary nosological systems (e.g., *PDM–2/Millon, DC:0–5*; see Footnote 14), they are all organized in similar fashion as follows: (a) mental health disorders (i.e., clinical syndromes), developmental disorder (i.e., neurodevelopmental disorders), and personality disorders (i.e., with the exception of the early childhood form; viz., Form 3.3); (b) related medical variables and conditions; (c) associated environmental stressors; (d) prognosis; and (e) treatment recommendations (supplants "Requested Tests, Testing Services, and Units [Time]" section of the initial report). This requires an *inductive reasoning* process, which is logic that proceeds from specific facts or instances to general principles. Here, the examiner applies the facts derived from the empirically based psychological tests to determine which categorically defined diagnoses or conceptual questions are best supported or answered.

At this juncture, it is important to point out that the examiner has proceeded through a complete cycle of scientific reasoning involving (a) the use of deductive reasoning when first developing hypotheses of which disorders are present and how they may be operationally defined by the careful selection of empirical tests, and (b) the use of inductive reasoning when applying the collected facts to those general hypotheses to determine whether or not they are supported. This emulates the same process by which psychological scientists first develop conceptual hypotheses about relationships among key variables, then use deduction to operationally define how these variables are to be measured or manipulated within the context of an experiment, and finally induction to determine if the facts support the general hypotheses.

Now, back to the process of psychodiagnosis. The mental health, developmental, and personality disorders are to be listed from most to least significant as determined by the test data. The first disorder is listed as the *principal diagnosis*, thus designating it as the one that is the most salient in one or more respects, including (a) the primary focus of testing and/or (b) the greatest in degree of severity or pervasiveness. The remaining disorders are listed in order of decreasing significance as defined prior. Notes can be made here to emphasize other vital test results, including especially (a) reminders as to which disorders were negated by the test data, and (b) which disorders need to be ruled out by supplemental testing.

In the sample case, the listed working diagnosis remains the principal disorder.[20] Additionally, an *historical diagnosis* is appended in a second parenthetical. This designation means that such disorder was not the target of the current testing battery; that is, it was diagnosed previously by another clinician (usually the referral source) and is being listed as part of the examinee's mental health services history without attesting to its validity or invalidity. Also accompanying the principal diagnosis in the sample case is a reminder note stating that the suspected neurocognitive disorder was negated by current test data. In other words, the working diagnosis is being made by default (see Footnote 20).

The related medical variables and conditions and associated environmental stressors are usually either proofread for accuracy or modified by any newly collected data. Prognosis is definitely modified from its deferred status and according to the test results. Some personality tests yield data that pertain directly to estimating and examinee's predicted response to treatment (i.e., prognosis) and should be referenced if applicable. One or more reasons justifying the prognosis should always accompany its stated status. In the sample case (Exhibit 4.1), the prognosis is favorable due to the negative results for memory dysfunction.[21] Next is the final section; namely, "Treatment Recommendations."

Treatment Recommendations

The concluding section of the final report replaces the entire section titled, "Requested Tests, Testing Services, and Units (Time)," which was used to request the types and units of testing services. Such information is now a matter of record within the examinee's medical record and without a logical place within the final report. These recommendations should follow directly from the composed summary and final diagnostic workup.

The listed treatment recommendations should follow an order from most to least significant, which usually parallels that for the enumerated diagnoses. In the sample case, Mr. Smith's memory complaints are attributed to an incomplete treatment of his anxiety disorder considering that organicity has been ruled out as an alternative explanation. Therefore, stress management is listed first because it is the added psychotherapeutic component that will hopefully assist Mr. Smith in obtaining a more complete and enduring symptom recovery.[22] Referral back to the treating clinician is secondary because it represents a continuation of biomedical intervention with a potential and more minor modification in the medication regimen. (see Footnote 22).

Final Report Generation

The prior discussion delineated the manner in which an initial psychological assessment report is transformed into its final version, including score reporting, interpreting, integrating, summarizing, diagnosing, and treatment recommending. The principal question now becomes, "When should these tasks be accomplished?" Answer: "On the same and final date of test administration services." If this is not possible, then the next day. The proximity of composing the final report to that of test administration is depicted in Figure 2.1 by the large solid-lined box with the comprehensive title, "Test Administration, Scoring, Interpretation, and Final Report Generation." As stated in a prior chapter, if a clinician fills the morning work schedule with test administration appointments, then the afternoon can be devoted to test scoring, interpretation, integration, and report generation. In consequence, the examiner will be both more efficient and accurate, and will produce timely reports on a reliable basis. Typically, the process can begin during the time remaining in the final administration appointment and subsequently finalized later that same day.

Once all of the sections have been completed, the report should be proofread for accuracy. This especially regards key data presented within the pre-designed tables for each test. Thereafter, the report should be signed by the examiner and made an official document within the examinee's medical record. All test services activity should also be documented on the "Psychological Assessment and Testing Services Record" form (i.e., Form 3.12), including the signing and entering of the final report. Stage 4 is now completed. In order to move onto the final Stage 5, the intermediate next step is to bill the requested and used testing services and units. This is the succeeding topic.

Billing All Testing Hours

The most efficient method of billing is, "all preauthorized and used test services units on the final date of face-to-face administration." As also indicated prior, billing on a date that is not associated with a provided and documented face-to-face service risks problems with insurance reimbursement. This is another reason why the final report should be generated on the concluding date of face-to-face test administration. Of further consideration, in order to avoid overlapping billing times with other clients on the same date, the time of service should be adjusted and all test units billed consecutively with a comment on the note as follows: "Time of service was modified in order to bill all test services consecutively on this final date of face-to-face test service."

In cases where more than one test administration appointment was necessitated on separate days (e.g., 03/11/2020 and 03/17/2020), the final billing narrative note should contain all dates of contact and the particular test or subtests completed. Also, in instances where the report is completed on a date after face-to-face test administration was done (e.g., 03/19/2020), the billing note can be back-dated to that last date of face-to-face administration (continuing with the previous example, this would be 3/17/2020). Using these strategies minimizes any problems with reimbursement. Final steps include communicating the findings and proper termination of the testing case.

Communicate Findings (Stage 5)

The goal the initiates Stage 5 in the assessment and testing process is to effectively communicate the results, which is depicted in Figure 2.1 by the box titled, "Communicate Findings." This is analogous to scientific investigation in which key relationships are discovered among variables (e.g., being a psychopath is associated with a tendency to fail to learn from punishment). That is, unless the information is communicated effectively (e.g., via oral presentation at a regional conference and/or written publication in a journal), it is of little use. The same is true of psychological assessment and test results. Analogously, then, the findings are also of little value unless they are communicated effectively. However, with regard to the latter, efficacious communication adds a timeliness component. The fact that such communication is both an inherent and mandatory part of psychological assessment and testing is portrayed by the solid lines of the "Communicate Findings," box in Figure 2.1. The timeliness facet, which is depicted in Figure 2.1 by the juxtaposition of the "Communicate Findings," box with the, "Final Psychological Assessment Report," oval, is especially vital in the domain of psychological assessment and testing. That is, a final report of this kind can be of the highest quality in terms of both accuracy and precision, yet it will have absolutely no impact if it is not available when needed.

Here, communication potentially concerns any one or more of the following entities: (a) the examinees and any pertinent collaterals (e.g., parents); (b) referral sources (e.g., psychotherapists, psychiatrists, neurologists, school personnel, courts, attorneys); and (c) other third parties deemed significant and/or relevant to the ongoing care of the examinee (e.g., primary care physicians, pediatricians, occupational therapists, teachers). In this sense, testing psychologists may find themselves providing services to multiple clients in any one case. This is one reason why the term examinee is used in order to best distinguish the individual being tested from all other entities who may also be relying on the same assessment and test results. Subsequently, some key issues regarding test feedback are outlined, including a general approach, followed by more specific issues concerning the aforementioned parties.

Traditional Information Giving Model of Psychological Assessment

The assessment and testing approach delineated in this book advocates a *traditional information gathering model* (see Finn & Tonsager, 1997) in which an initial clinical interview is done and followed by a narrowly devised and targeted test battery for the purposes of (a) resolving the identified diagnostic issues, (b) answering properly formulated and diagnostically related questions, and (c) designing effective treatment recommendations. As the examiner, the psychologist functions as a vehicle for an enhanced understanding of the client's problems and how they may be resolved. This should be distinguished from *collaborative therapeutic assessment* in which the examiner and examinee continually use test data therapeutically for greater self-discovery and new understandings (Finello, 2011; Finn, 2003, 2007; Finn, Fischer, & Handler, 2012; Finn & Martin, 1997; Finn & Tonsager, 2002; Fischer, 1978).

Therefore, the procedure delineated in this book makes a clear distinction between assessment and *psychotherapy*, while collaborative assessment merges the two types of services. Both are acceptable practices with alternative objectives. In the traditional information-giving system, use of the results therapeutically is left to either the referral source, where it most logically belongs, or to a clinician who initiates treatment using the assessment and test results as described here. Next, more about specific feedback issues are discussed as they may arise between the examiner and the various entities identified prior.

Examinee and Any Collaterals

In the case of self or family referrals (e.g., parents), all interested parties should receive the complete (i.e., non-redacted) written report. Here, the cardinal rule of practice is that examinees are titled to "everything" that has been written about them in a formal and legal document, and explained to them in a manner that they can comprehend. This is what a signed and filed psychological assessment and test report represents, with the addition of oral feedback to clarify content that is not readily understood by the typical layperson. That is, full and complete disclosure of the entire report should be the prevailing rule. This is based on the premise that the final report be limited to that information and data deemed immediately relevant to resolving the presented diagnostic issues and sufficiently addressing any associated referral questions. This is also assuming that care has been taken to (a) eliminate specific and unnecessary names, (b) avoid unnecessary and unsubstantiated accusations, and (c) qualify all potentially controversial but diagnostically relevant statements with (or something akin to) the phrase, "as reported by the examinee." In addition, oral feedback should invariably be both offered and encouraged. This is especially for the more complex cases that involve multiple measures, and comprise a significant number of scores and data integration. The principal reason is that self and family referral cases typically involve laypeople without training in psychometrics.

As an example of a complex case that involves a significant amount of test scores and statistics, in years past *specific learning disorders* (SLDs) were most frequently diagnosed by an *ability-achievement discrepancy analysis*. This required the use of (a) an individually administered *intelligence test*, (b) an individually administered *achievement test*, and (c) comparison between examinees' full scale IQ score (or achievement scores predicted from their full scale IQ score) and their obtained achievement scores. Any obtained achievement scores that were determined to be statistically lower than their full scale IQ score was evidence of a SLD. As one can imagine by this summary alone, such an analysis involved a multitude of by norm-based comparisons, ipsative analyses, and both *descriptive statistics* (i.e., means and standard deviations) and *inferential statistics* using *conditional probability* logic (i.e., if the difference between the full scale IQ score and the obtained achievement score would occur less than five times in 100 by chance alone, then this chance explanation is to be rejected and the difference considered meaningful or significant). It is these kinds of test batteries that necessitate communicating the results both in writing and orally using a follow-up question and answer format.

In and of itself, *feedback* is considered to be a form of *information-giving*, which works to confirm, modify, or broadens another's perspective (Evans, Hearn, Uhlemann, & Ivey, 2017). It is an interviewing therapeutic *microskill* in which evidence about specified problems or issues are provided by the interviewer or clinician. Here, it is the examiner's objective to provide such evidence in as clear and cogent manner as possible. This includes summarizing the diagnostic issues and questions presented in the case, the tests selected and rationale, the evidence such tests produced, the diagnostic results so indicated, any answers to related questions, and finally, treatment recommendations. In general, clients are most receptive when information is direct, specific, concise, and provided to them in an understanding and sensitive manner (Evans et al., 2017). This means that good attending skills facilitate the information-giving process, including appropriate use of eye contact, voice tone, body language and posture, and verbal skills. It is also important to encourage and thoroughly answer any questions clients may have regarding the test data and diagnostic conclusions on a level that renders the material readily comprehensible. Asking clients to repeat the information given can confirm the degree to which they have attended to and understood what was shared.

Reframing is another therapeutic microskill in which the examiner provides an alternative perspective that modifies, restructures, or affords new meaning to clients' perspectives. Such a microskill can be employed effectively to modify apparently negative findings into a potential for growth, positive change, hope, and optimism. Frequently, clients' distress can be significantly ameliorated when they are given a valid diagnostic explanation for their ongoing difficulties, along with assisting them in averting undeserved self-blame and guilt. For example, understanding that one has a SLD or ADHD and is not "lazy," "unmotivated," or "unintelligent," can be remarkably therapeutic in and of itself, along with the realization that once a problem is accurately identified, it can now be improved or "fixed." At other times, feedback can be shocking as in learning that one's neuropsychological test battery shows evidence of a probable major neurocognitive disorder of the Alzheimer's type. Here, additional therapeutic microskills such as *empathy*, and *reflection of content* and *reflection of feeling* can assist clients in understanding and accepting their diagnosis, and motivating them for discussing and acting upon recommended therapy irrespective of their prognosis.

The focus then becomes the treatment recommendations because this informs examinees and any collaterals what they can do to remedy the identified disorders and problems. Specific treatment recommendations should follow logically and clearly. Here, the psychologist is being directive in the form of advice giving, which involves prescribing or providing solutions or plans of action (Evans et al., 2017). That being said, ethically it should be left to clients to ultimately decide what to do with respect to the results, conclusions, and recommendations. Hence, the examiner should be prepared to elaborate upon the proffered treatment recommendations, including potential benefits and risks, any alternatives clients may consider, and the risks of not following through with them.

Referral Sources

If the case was referred by another clinician, the final report should be released to both that professional and the examinee (or collaterals) immediately subsequent to its completion. This may be done if the proper release of information (ROI) forms were completed and signed as recommended (see Form 3.2) at the point the testing case was opened (if an external referral) or when the case was initially referred (if an internal referral).

Although many referring clinicians are not well versed in psychometrics, the vast majority are sufficiently cognizant of the DSM–5 nosology in order to comprehend the essential diagnostic summary, answers to related referral questions, and especially, treatment recommendations. Furthermore, the obtained test scores are readily available in the body of the final report (viz., section titled, "Test Data and Interpretation"), which facilitates a more in-depth understanding of the results, along with the manner in which the diagnoses and answers to related referral questions were derived. Finally, referring clinicians should be encouraged to contact the testing psychologist directly with any follow-up questions. This will facilitate the continued use of the test results in a therapeutic manner, here being more consistent with the tenets of collaborative therapeutic assessment as defined previously (see Finn et al., 2012).

Other Third Parties

Pertinent additional *third parties* who should also receive a copy of the final report are most frequently identified during the assessment process, feedback, or even after the case is closed or discharged. In this case, additional ROI forms (viz., Form 3.2) must be completed for each third party that is to receive a copy of the report. All ROI forms should be made a formal part of the examinee's medical record, either via hard copy or scanning the documents into an electronic file. This practice creates a detailed and accurate written record of all entities who have requested and received a copy of the final report, along with any other portions of the examinee's medical record. This includes their identities and all needed contact information. In the alternative, the examinee or any pertinent collaterals (e.g., parents/guardians) have the legal authority to release their copy of the final (and initial) report if they so desire. Once communication is done, Stage 5 and the entire assessment and testing process is complete. Hence, the case is ready for termination in the form of transfer or discharge.

Closing the Case: Transfer or Discharge

At this point, there remains one more crucial step in the process. This is to formally and legally close the case. Why is it so important to show evidence that a previously active type of service or case has been officially and properly terminated? The answer relates to what is referred to as a duty of care. In general, the law imposes a duty for people to act with *due care* (i.e., a *duty of care*), defined as the manner in which a reasonably prudent person would act in the same or similar circumstances. For professionals, the duty of care is not only to that expected of a reasonable person, but also of a reasonable person with that type of specialized training. Hence, the more training, the more one's duty of care. As applied to this context, a *duty of care* essentially means that the psychologist must be competent when providing assessment and testing services (including remaining consistent with ethical principles); that is, what quality of services would be reasonable for a competently trained psychologist to provide in the circumstances of the case.

Okay, so what is the point. In addition to taking the opportunity to instruct regarding a psychologist's legal obligations, if the case has not been properly closed or terminated, and appears to remain an active case, this duty of care may continue unbeknownst to the psychologist. Therefore, if something untoward occurs to the client thereafter, for example, an attempted or completed suicide, that psychologist may be liable due to an alleged breach of the aforementioned duty that caused the damage and harm.[23] In short, the psychologist should show that (a) assessment and test results were properly communicated, (b) treatment recommendation were explained with assisted referrals to all advised follow-up treatments, (c) results were released as requested by the examinee, and (d) the case was properly closed with written documentation. Whether this means terminating the specific type of mental health service within or from the agency or practice depends upon the type of testing referral (i.e., internal or external).

Transfer

If the assessment case was an internal referral, then a *transfer* of services from one department to another within the agency or practice is typically required, especially if this is a more comprehensive community mental health services (CCMHS) facility. In such instance, mental health services are diverse, consisting of multiple departments as seen in large hospital settings. Within such a comprehensive organization of related services, *continuity of care* is maximized because the mental health record is typically shared and available to all clinicians involved in the client's treatment, especially if an electronic filing system is being used (which is becoming increasingly common).

An official transfer appearing in a client's medical record places all providers who remain active in the client's treatment on notice that such services have been closed, including the reason(s) for termination (e.g., "Psychological testing has been completed, all goals have been met"). It also signifies that the clinician who provided that service is no longer actively involved and tracking the case. Consequently, the terminating clinician is formally documenting that he or she is no longer continuing a duty of care. However, all clinicians still actively involved in the case (as representative of the facility) remain responsible for providing a reasonable standard of mental health care consistent with their specialty (e.g., psychiatry, clinical social work, psychotherapy). This is denoted by the term, "Transfer," appearing in Figure 2.1 without being enclosed by a box, and in proximity to the box titled, "Mental Health Clinician Assessment (and Treatment)," which in turn denotes the mental health clinician who initially made the internal referral.

As stated prior, most (if not all) contemporary mental health centers use an electronic medical records software system. Therefore, files are easily accessed by all clinicians in the agency who add to and remove their specialized mental health services as needed to maximize clients' progress. When services are removed, they must be terminated by means of transfer to the lead clinician, which is usually the one whom *admissions* (also known as *intake*) first referred to so as to begin treatment within the facility. In addition to a running record of all treatment interventions, such electronic records include all critical documents that are entered of record by means of scanning. These scanned documents include some of the following: (a) initial and final psychological assessment reports; (b) all consent forms; (c) assessment and testing service record forms; and (d) all ROIs. Practicing in such an organization is preferable because these aspects all contribute to quality care.

Discharge

If the assessment case is an external referral, however, then termination requires a formal *discharge* from the entire facility. This is denoted in Figure 2.1 by the solid-lined box titled, "Discharge." Although discharge may not be needed in the event of transfer for an internal referral, solid lines were used in Figure 2.1 to emphasize its mandated nature in the case of external referrals. In contrast to a transfer, a discharge renders the entire case inactive concerning the facility or practice in which psychological assessment and testing was provided. In order for discharges to properly show a discontinuation of the duty of care, the same tasks and documentation are required as in a transfer. The difference is that there are no other active mental health services being provided the client. Therefore, both the provider and the facility or practice is showing an end to their duty of reasonable mental health care.

Recapitulation

This chapter addressed the final two phases of the psychological assessment and testing process. Stage 4 began with strategies for scheduling test administration appointments, including recommended number and duration, order of test administration, and the use of available computer technology to minimize error variance and maximize reliability and validity. Similarly, recommendations were made regarding test scoring, with even greater emphasis on the utilization of computer software for performing the needed computations and data transformations both rapidly and accurately. The majority of the chapter, however, focused on delineating the steps involved in generating the "Final Psychological Assessment Report," beginning with use of the initial report as a guiding framework. The transformation of the initial into the final report was described in two primary phases. First, initial amendments to the report prior to entering any new sections were discussed. Second, a large focus was upon integrating the new sections, including assessment and test battery lists, test data and interpretation, summary of results, final diagnostic conclusions, and treatment recommendations. This process of generating a final version was illustrated by showing a neuropsychological sample case, using footnotes within the report to locate and describe the amendments and new sections that were added. Special attention was given to the practice of simultaneous test data reporting, interpretation, and integration, creating a summary of results, and contributing to a final diagnostic summary and treatment recommendations, hence bringing to a close Stage 4. The final portion of the chapter dealt with the intermediate billing issues, the communication of findings (Stage 5), and closing a case by means of either transfer or discharge. References were made to the Figure 2.1 flowchart throughout the chapter in order to closely track the assessment and testing sequence from test administration through termination; that is, Stages 4 and 5.

This completes Part I of this book, which was devoted to delineating the psychological assessment and testing process from the point of initial referral through the closing of a case. The stage has now been set for Part II, which is devoted to presenting all of the tests classified and thereafter enumerated in Table 1.1. Each chapter in Part II will present one class of tests, including their description, statistical features, administration procedures, scoring and data yield, forms that provide data tables for reporting test scores to be entered into the "Test Data and Interpretation" section of final reports, and interpretive excerpts and guidelines for how to interpret the test data. The e-resources on the Routledge website builds on this information by illustrating prototypical case examples analogous to the sample case presented in this chapter except in more detail. The sample cases illustrate how test data are reported, interpreted, and gradually integrated and summarized such that they ultimately contribute to accurate diagnostic summaries, effectively address all related questions, and finally, lead to logically related treatment recommendations.

Key Terms

- ability-achievement discrepancy analysis
- achievement test
- admissions (intake)
- attention-deficit/hyperactivity disorder (ADHD)
- autism spectrum disorder (ASD)
- borderline personality disorder
- collaborative therapeutic assessment
- conditional probability
- Conners Comprehensive Behavior Rating Scales (Conners CBRS)
- Conners Early Childhood (Conners EC)
- construct validity
- continuity of care
- Continuous Performance Test (CPT)
- convergent validity
- descriptive statistics
- diagnosis

- discharge
- due care
- duty of care
- dyslexia
- empathy
- false negative results
- false positive result
- false positive results
- feedback
- generalized anxiety disorder (GAD)
- historical diagnosis
- inductive reasoning
- inferential statistics
- information-giving
- intellectual disability (ID)
- intelligence test
- ipsative
- ipsative analysis
- Millon Clinical Multiaxial Inventory, Third Edition (MCMI–III)
- Mini–Mental State Examination, Second Edition, Brief Version, Blue Form (MMSE–2–BV–BF)
- Minnesota Multiphasic Personality Inventory–2 (MMPI–2)
- multitrait-multimethod
- NEO Personality Inventory, Third Edition (NEO–PI–3)
- NEPSY–II, Form Ages 5 to 16, Full Battery
- NEPSY–II, Full Battery
- NEPSY–II, General Battery
- neurocognitive disorder
- Neuropsychological Assessment Battery (NAB)
- neuropsychological testing
- non-autism developmental testing
- organic
- outliers
- posttraumatic stress disorder (PTSD)
- preauthorization (PA)
- principal diagnosis
- psychogenic
- psychotherapy
- reflecting content
- reflecting feeling
- reframing
- reliability
- serifs
- signs
- specific learning disorder in reading
- specific learning disorders (SLDs)
- Structured Interview of Reported Symptoms, Second Edition (SIRS–2)
- symptoms
- Test of Memory Malingering (TOMM)
- third parties
- Times New Roman
- traditional information gathering model
- transfer
- Trauma Symptom Inventory, Second Edition (TSI–2)
- 12-point font size
- utility
- validity
- Vineland Adaptive Behavior Scales, Third Edition (Vineland–3)

Notes

1. In the sample case, "Initial Psychological Assessment Report," becomes, "Final Neuropsychological Assessment Report."
2. The date listed should be changed to correspond to the month, day, and year the final report was finished and signed by the examiner so as to render it a legal document and formal part of the examinee's medical record.
3. Re-calculate the chronological age of the examinee in years and months (if early childhood, also in total months).
4. A new section of the final report titled, "Assessment and Test Battery," should be inserted immediately after the section, "Presenting Symptoms." The examiner should select the assessment and test battery list for the appropriate developmental period (see Forms 4.1, 4.2, 4.3, and 4.4), add the dates of completion or submission for each technique or test, and insert them in the order that they appear in the report (not according to the order of administration, which may be different).
5. The "Assessment and Test Battery" listing always begins with the initial clinical interview followed by the mental status examination and behavioral observations.
6. Screening tests used during the initial assessment are listed in alphabetical order after the "Mental Status Examination and Behavioral Observations," entry.
7. All tests used in a particular case are listed in the order presented within the report.
8. **S**erifs are small lines or strokes attached to the end of letters, which have been shown to facilitate reading. Essentially, the serifs assist the human eye in gliding from one letter to another and one word to another within a sentence. This is why Times New Roman has been selected as the primary font in all the forms and test data tables. Also selected is a 12-point font size, which is 1/6th inch in height, again with some exceptions of smaller font to fit the material on one page for ease of use. Both of these selections are in contrast to the default in Microsoft Word, which is Calibri (Body) at 11-point font size. Although this occasionally may present problems when inserting forms and tables into reports due to the software occasionally reverting back to default, it is worth the extra effort to render the report easier and inviting to read.
9. The screening test for neurocognitive impairment that was administered during the initial assessment should be inserted immediately following the mental status examination and behavioral observations section of the report. Here, these data are performance-based and represent additional signs of potential neurocognitive impairment, hence bolstering the case for the medical necessity of follow-up neuropsychological memory testing.
10. This screening test's full title, "Mini-Mental State Examination, Second Edition, Expanded Version, Blue Form (MMSE–2–EV–BF)," which would appear in the initial report because the assessment and test battery listing would not yet be added, should be reduced to its acronym because the full title now appears in the inserted test battery listing of the final report.
11. The optional section titled, "Initial Psychological Assessment Summary," which is used when the initial assessment is sufficient in addressing all of the diagnostic issues presented in the testing referral (see Forms 3.3–3.6), hence not requiring follow-up testing, should be deleted from the initial and thus this final report.
12. All of the comments in the section titled, "Initial Psychological Assessment Summary and Follow-Up Testing Plan," should be proofread for accuracy and changed to past tense to reflect the fact that it pertains to the test data and interpretation presented in the body of the final report.
13. All language following the selected list of tests up to the diagnostic summary section should be deleted and replaced by the title, "Test Data and Interpretation," which represents the body of the final report where the empirical data will be entered and interpreted (see Part II for data tables for all tests).
14. The first word of the diagnostic summary title should be modified from "Initial" to "Final." The document should then be saved as a final report file titled, "F_Smith, John J. 1234567," and saved in a subfolder, "Final Psychological Assessment Reports." Contrast this with the initial file title, "I_Smith, John J. 1234567," which would be saved in a subfolder, "Initial Psychological Assessment Reports."
15. Test administration narrative note is inserted prior to reported test data, which bolsters the validity of all subsequently reported performance-based test results.
16. Test administration narrative note inserted prior to interpreting test data in order to bolster validity.
17. The WMS–IV data table is inserted within the "Test Data and Interpretation" body of the final report. Because it is the only test within the battery, there is no issue regarding order of test presentation. Table numbers are labeled in the order they appear throughout the entire report. Hence, the WMS–IV's table is sequenced as number 2 behind the MMSE–2–BF table.
18. There are certainly many critics who argue against presenting test results in such a sequence (e.g., Cohen & Swerdlik, 2018). In fact, it was common in years past to train psychologists to proceed immediately to data integration and interpret all results within a narrative format. Typically, the only actual scores that were inserted into the report were full scale and relevant composite IQ scores, again without the use of tables. However, over the years of clinical testing practice, an increasing proportion of the test scores were being inserted in tabular format, some by request from referring clinicians, although further reinforced by consistent positive feedback from clinicians on the clarity and organization of the reports, including forensic referrals. Contemporary referral sources are much more savvy with numbers and very much want to see the data supporting the diagnostic results and conclusions. It also speeds the process of report generation and reduces the need for long narratives that most clinicians, with limited time, will cease reading prematurely. In short, people want both (a) the facts, and (b) succinct conclusions that make sense in light of the presented data. This recipe will sell in today's climate.
19. The "Summary of Results" section ties together the essential test results, diagnostic summary, and general treatment approach. The typical length is a concise one, perhaps two paragraphs. The content should address (a) the discovered or positive diagnoses and supporting evidence (i.e., most to least prominent), (b) diagnoses that were ruled out or negated (i.e., most to least prominent), (c) any unresolved issues and reasons therefore (including the consequential need for supplementary testing), (d) direct answers to referral questions with supporting evidence by reference, and (e) the advised overall treatment approach.
20. The final diagnostic summary is modified according to the results, beginning with mental health, neurodevelopmental, and personality disorders. The leading or foremost disorder is listed the principal diagnosis, followed by secondary disorders of progressively lesser significance. Specific notes are made to emphasize certain aspects of the test results (e.g., stating previously suspected diagnoses that were ruled out or negated by test data). Finally, do not overlook the addition of diagnostic specifiers, including creative ones that fit unique data patterns (e.g., borderline personality disorder, severe, with transient psychotic episodes).

21. Prognosis is modified from is deferral status to a more definitive designation, with an appended explanation that supports the decision.
22. Treatment recommendations should be consistent with the general approach first outlined in the summary of results, and be prioritized as are the listed diagnoses. That is, the treatment recommendations that are directed toward the principal diagnosis should be listed first, followed by those that address the remaining disorders from approximately most to least significant.
23. The *law of torts* or private wrongs, such as personal injury, define the elements of *negligence* as follows: (a) duty; (b) breach; (c) causation; and (d) damages. The duty is the due care legally imposed upon one individual to another, breach means the duty was violated, causation means that the breach was the direct cause without which the harm would not have occurred (i.e., proximate cause), and damages are the proven extent of the injuries or harm. This footnote is for readers who may be interested in the law.

References

American Psychiatric Association. (2013). *Diagnostic and statistical manual of mental disorders* (5th ed., DSM–5). Arlington, VA: Author.

American Psychological Association. (2020). *Publication manual of the American Psychological Association* (7th ed.). Washington, DC: Author.

Ben-Porath, Y. S., & Tellegen, A. (2008, 2011). *Minnesota multiphasic personality inventory–2–RF (MMPI–2–RF): Manual for administration, scoring, and interpretation.* Minneapolis: MN: University of Minnesota Press.

Bornstein, R. F. (1998). Interpersonal dependency and physical illness: A meta-analytic review of retrospective and prospective studies. *Journal of Research in Personality, 32,* 480–497.

Bornstein, R. F. (1999). Criterion validity of objective and projective dependency tests: A meta-analytic assessment of behavioral prediction. *Psychological Assessment, 11,* 48–57.

Briere, J. (2011). *Trauma symptom inventory, second edition (TSI–2): Professional manual.* Lutz, FL: Psychological Assessment Resources (PAR).

Campbell, D. T., & Fiske, D. W. (1959). Convergent and discriminant validation by the multitrait-multimethod matrix. *Psychological Bulletin, 56,* 81–105.

Citardi, M. (2009, December 11). *Current procedural technology: History, structure, process & controversies.* University of Texas, McGovern Medical School. Retrieved from https://med.uth.edu/orl/2009/12/11/current-procedural-technology-history-structure-process-controversies/

Conners, C. K. (2008). *Conners comprehensive behavior rating scales (conners CBRS): Manual and interpretive update.* North Tonawanda, NY: Multi-Health Systems (MHS).

Conners, C. K. (2009). *Conners early childhood manual (conners EC).* North Towanda, NY: Multi-Health Systems (MHS).

Evans, D. R., Hearn, M. T., Uhlemann, M. R., & Ivey, A. E. (2017). *Essential interviewing: A programed approach to effective communication* (9th ed.). Boston, MA: Cengage Learning.

Exner, J. E. (2001). *A Rorschach workbook for the comprehensive system* (5th ed.). Asheville, NC: Rorschach Workshops.

Exner, J. E. (2003). *The Rorschach a comprehensive system: Basic foundations and principles of interpretation* (4th ed., Vol. 1). Hoboken, NJ: John Wiley & Sons.

Finello, K. M. (2011). Collaboration in the assessment and diagnosis of preschoolers: Challenges and opportunities. *Psychology in the Schools, 48,* 442–453.

Finn, S. E. (2003). Therapeutic assessment of a man with "ADD". *Journal of Personality Assessment, 80,* 115–129.

Finn, S. E. (2007). *In our clients' shoes: Theory and techniques of therapeutic assessment.* New York, NY: Psychology Press.

Finn, S. E., Fischer, C. T., & Handler, L. (Eds.). (2012). *Collaborative/therapeutic assessment: A casebook and guide.* Hoboken, NJ: John Wiley & Sons.

Finn, S. E., & Martin, H. (1997). Therapeutic assessment with the MMPI–2 in managed health care. In J. N. Butcher (Ed.), *Objective psychological assessment in managed health care: A practitioner's guide* (pp. 131–152). New York, NY: Oxford University Press.

Finn, S. E., & Tonsager, M. E. (1997). Information-gathering and therapeutic models of assessment: Complementary paradigms. *Psychological Assessment, 9,* 374–385.

Finn, S. E., & Tonsager, M. E. (2002). How therapeutic assessment became humanistic. *The Humanistic Psychologist, 30,* 10–22.

Fischer, C. T. (1978). Collaborative psychological assessment. In C. T. Fischer & S. L. Brodsky (Eds.), *Client participation in human services: The Prometheus Principle* (pp. 41–46). New Brunswick, NJ: Transaction Books.

Folstein, M. F., Folstein, S. E., White, T., & Messer, M. A. (2010). *Mini–mental state examination, second edition: User's manual.* Lutz, FL: Psychological Assessment Resources (PAR).

Furr, R. M. (2018). *Psychometrics: An introduction* (3rd ed.). Thousand Oaks, California: Sage Publications.

Ganellen, R. J. (1996). Comparing the diagnostic efficiency of the MMPI, MCMI–II, and Rorschach: A review. *Journal of Personality Assessment, 67,* 219–243.

Ganellen, R. J. (2007). Assessing normal and abnormal personality functioning. *Journal of Personality Assessment, 89,* 30–40.

Hughes, T. L., Gacono, C. B., & Owen, P. F. (2007). Current status of Rorschach assessment: Implications for the school psychologist. *Psychology in the Schools, 44,* 281–291.

Huprich, S. K. (Ed.) (2006). *Rorschach assessment of personality disorders.* Mahwah, NJ: Lawrence Erlbaum Associates.

Irwing, P., Booth, & Hughes, D. J. (Eds.). (2018). *The Wiley handbook of psychometric testing: A multidisciplinary reference on survey, scale, and test development* (Vol. 1). Hoboken, NJ: John Wiley & Sons–Blackwell.

Ivancevich, J. M. (1983). Contrast effects in performance evaluation and reward practices. *Academy of Management Journal, 26,* 465–476.

Korkman, M., Kirk, U., & Kemp, S. (2007a). *NEPSY–II: Administrative manual.* San Antonio, Texas: The Psychological Corporation (PsychCorp)-Pearson.

Korkman, M., Kirk, U., & Kemp, S. (2007b). *NEPSY–II: Clinical and interpretative manual.* San Antonio, Texas: The Psychological Corporation (PsychCorp)-Pearson.

Maurer, T. J., Palmer, J. K., & Ashe, D. K. (1993). Diaries, checklists, evaluations, and contrast effects in measurement of behavior. *Journal of Applied Psychology, 78*, 226–231.

McCrae, R. R., & Costa, P. T., Jr. (2010). *NEO inventories for the NEO personality inventory, third edition (NEO–PI–3), NEO five factor inventory, third edition (NEO–FFI–3), NEO personality inventory, revised (NEO PI–R): Professional manual.* Lutz, FL: Psychological Assessment Services (PAR).

Meyer, G. J., & Archer, R. P. (2001). The hard science of Rorschach research: What do we know and where do we go? *Psychological Assessment, 13*, 486–502.

Meyer, G. J., & Handler, L. (1997). The ability of the Rorschach to predict subsequent outcome: Meta-analysis of the Rorschach prognostic rating scale. *Journal of Personality Assessment, 69*, 1–38.

Millon, T., Millon, C., Davis, R. D., & Grossman, S. D. (2006a). *Millon adolescent clinical inventory (MACI) manual* (2nd ed.). Minneapolis, MN: NCS Pearson.

Millon, T., Millon, C., Davis, R. D., & Grossman, S. D. (2006b). *Millon clinical multiaxial inventory manual* (3rd ed.; MCMI–III). Minneapolis, MN: NCS Pearson.

Pearson. (2020). *Q-Global: Better insights. Anytime. Anywhere.* Author. Retrieved from https://qglobal.pearsonclinical.com/

Price, L. R. (2017). *Psychometric methods: Theory into practice* (1st ed.). New York, NY: The Guilford Press.

Rogers, R., Sewell, K. W., & Gillard, M. S. (2010). *Structured interview of reported symptom, second edition (SIRS–2).* Lutz, FL: Psychological Assessment Resources (PAR).

Schuh, A. J. (1978). Contrast effect in the interview. *Bulletin of the Psychonomic Society, 11*, 195–196.

Smither, J. W., Reilly, R. R., & Buda, R. (1988). Effect of prior performance information on ratings of present performance: Contrast versus assimilation revisited. *Journal of Applied Psychology, 73*, 487–496.

Sparrow, S. S., Cicchetti, D. V., & Saulnier, C. A. (2016). *Vineland adaptive behavior rating scales, third edition (Vineland–3): Manual.* Minneapolis, MN: Pearson.

Stern, R. A., & White, T. (2003a). *Neuropsychological assessment battery (NAB): Psychometric and technical manual.* Lutz, FL: Psychological Assessment Resources (PAR).

Stern, R. A., & White, T. (2003b). *Neuropsychological assessment battery (NAB): Administrative, scoring, and interpretation manual.* Lutz, FL: Psychological Assessment Resources (PAR).

Tellegen, A., & Ben-Porath, Y. S. (2011). *Minnesota multiphasic personality inventory–2 restructured form: Technical manual.* Minneapolis: MN: University of Minnesota Press.

Tombaugh, T. N. (1996). *Test of memory malingering (TOMM).* North Tonawanda, NY: Multi-Health Systems (MHS) University Press.

Viglione, D. J. (1999). A review of recent research addressing the utility of the Rorschach. *Psychological Assessment, 11*, 251–265.

Wechsler, D. (2009a). *Wechsler Memory Scale, Fourth Edition (WMS–IV): Administration and scoring manual.* San Antonio, TX: The Psychological Corporation-Pearson.

Wechsler, D. (2009b). *Wechsler Memory Scale, Fourth Edition (WMS–IV): Technical and interpretative manual.* San Antonio, TX: The Psychological Corporation-Pearson.

Wechsler, D. (2014a). *Wechsler intelligence scale for children, fifth edition (WISC–V): Administration and scoring manual.* Bloomington, MN: The Psychological Corporation (PsychCorp)-Pearson.

Wechsler, D. (2014b). *Wechsler intelligence scale for children, fifth edition (WISC–V): Technical and interpretive manual.* Bloomington, MN: The Psychological Corporation (PsychCorp)-Pearson.

Wexley, K. N., Yukl, G. A., Kovacs, S. Z., & Sanders, R. E. (1972). Importance of contrast effects in employment interviews. *Journal of Applied Psychology, 56*, 45–48.

See Routledge's e-resources website for forms. (www.routledge.com/9780367346058)

Part II

The Psychological Tests

Test Data Tables and Interpretive Excerpts

Part II presents in detail the various tests listed in the book's inventory, including (a) the constructs they measure, (b) their structure and organization, (c) their history of development (if applicable), (d) their data tables, and (e) an interpretive strategy. The latter is supplemented by visual flowcharts for the more complex and intricately designed tests or test series, which are available for download on Routledge's e-resources website. Inserted into the data tables are narrative excerpts designed to guide interpretation and to increase test utility. The data tables are presented in both hard copy within the chapters for illustration, and in modifiable electronic word processing format for use in actual practice. Once again, the latter are available on the Routledge e-resources website. They are to be inserted into the "Test Data and Interpretation" section of the "Final Psychological Assessment Report," which is an updated extension of the "Initial Psychological Assessment Report." This material is further supplemented by case examples also available on Routledge's e-resources website, which illustrate how the psychological assessment and testing process outlined in Figure 2.1 works in actual practice.

More specifically, Chapter 5 begins the presentation of tests designed for the screening of psychopathology, two of which are multiscale instruments intended to cover an array of possible disorders and problems from age 2 years through adulthood. The remaining screening tests more narrowly target attention-deficit/hyperactivity disorder (ADHD) and neurocognitive impairment. Chapter 6 covers developmental disorders and delays, including the measurement of major developmental abilities and autism spectrum disorder (ASD). The ensuing three chapters cover the measurement cognitive abilities, including (a) intelligence or cognitive competence (Chapter 7), (b) achievement or the learning of fundament academic skills (Chapter 8), and (c) neurocognitive abilities or basic brain-behavior relationships (Chapter 9). The next sequence of three chapters turn the focus on measuring clinical disorders and personality disorders. First, the rating scales tests are covered in Chapter 10 and principally target clinical disorders. While two such measures are multidimensional in design, covering an age range from 2 years through 18 years, the majority are more narrowly focused upon sensory processing (integration) disorders, ADHD, ASD, and trauma-related disorders. Chapter 11 presents the major personality inventory tests, most of which emphasize the measurement of personality functioning, especially psychopathology, although also pertain to clinical disorders. Most are of the self-report variety, although one also includes an observer-report version. While the measures in Chapter 12 are also designed to principally measure personality functioning, along with secondary implications for clinical disorders, they do so by asking the examinee to perceive and interpret visual stimuli. This largest and core section of the book ends felicitously with Chapter 13, which presents two tests designed to detect the feigning of psychopathology for an identifiable reward, incentive, or personal gain (viz., malingering).

DOI: 10.4324/9780429326820-6

5   Screening Tests

Overview

This chapter presents an array of *screening tests* that are designed for use during an initial clinical interview. In contrast to the majority of other chapters in Part II where there are measures that are homogeneous in terms of format, the screening tests presented here consist of a heterogeneous group of three distinct designs, including (a) projective tests, (b) rating scales, and (c) neurocognitive tests. Projective methods are performance-based, largely unstructured, and open-ended, with a dual purpose of (a) engaging the examinee in the assessment and testing process, and (b) obtaining added clinical information pertaining to psychological functioning and clarifying key diagnostic issues. In contrast, the more structured and standardized rating scale and neurocognitive screens have as their principal objective determining the need and *medical necessity* for further more comprehensive testing. Next, this chapter presents these screening tests in the aforementioned order, with a focus on their general design (and history if relevant), intended population, administration, scoring, and interpretation process. Regarding the standardized measures, interpretation is facilitated by presenting the data tables that have been prepared for each screening test, including their design, which scores to report, and how they may be interpreted most efficiently and accurately.

Projective Tests Used for Screening

Projective tests present a series of relatively ambiguous stimuli, which are designed to elicit unique responses that reflect the examinee's emotions, thoughts, needs, conflicts, and personality characteristics. Two types of projective tests are employed during an initial clinical interview, including a projective drawing task and sentence completion test (SCT).[1] The former is best suited for examinees in early to middle childhood because of its greater association with play versus resembling a task that must be completed. In contrast, SCTs are more suitable for adolescents because of their more advanced cognitive abilities (see, e.g., Piaget, 1952). Examinees who are of intermediate age (i.e., older children and preadolescents) may be given a choice or provided either one depending upon their estimated cognitive abilities, social-emotional maturity, and purpose(s) of the assessment. The particular measures that are used are discussed next.

Kinetic Drawing System for Family and School

Synopsis

The projective drawing method used is the *Kinetic Drawing System for Family and School* (hereafter, *Kinetic Drawing System*; Knoff & Prout, 1985). Although the authors designed this method so as to integrate a child's psychological functioning across both home and school environments, the *Kinetic–Family–Drawing* (KFD) is principally used and the *Kinetic–School–Drawing* (KSD) is administered only when a child (a) strongly prefers the latter, or (b) provides a rapid and poor quality KFD. Clinical interpretation of such drawings was developed based on a sample ranging in age from 5 to 20 years, although this measure is more typically used with a somewhat younger age range from 4 to 18 years. A brief history of this method is in order prior to explaining how it is used during an initial clinical interview.

Succinct History of Family Projective Drawings

Initially, Hulse (1951) asked children to draw a picture of themselves and their families. The drawings were examined according to tone, quality, and its content (e.g., proximity of figures). This procedure became known as the *Draw–A–Family* (DAF) technique, although was limited by its static and noninteracting quality. Later, Burns and

DOI: 10.4324/9780429326820-7

Kaufman (1970, 1972) added a valuable kinetic aspect to the DAF by instructing children to draw themselves and their families, "doing something." This dynamic quality to children's drawings was believed to provide even greater insights as to their feelings and perceptions, along with the role of the family in influencing the child's functioning and development (Burns, 1982; Burns & Kaufman, 1970, 1972; Prout & Phillips, 1974). Later, Prout and Phillips (1974) applied the same approach to children's school environments, which resulted in the KSD. The latter was further developed by Sarbaugh (1982), who employed qualitative analyses, and Prout and Celmer (1984), who conducted qualitative analyses that demonstrated a significant relationship between the KSD and various aspects of psychological functioning (e.g., academic achievement).

Use During Initial Clinical Interviews

As stated prior, the FKD portion of the Kinetic Drawing System is routinely administered to younger examinees for purposes of (a) rapport building, (b) engaging them within the assessment process, and (c) information gathering. The latter includes both process (i.e., how they draw) and (b) content (i.e., what they draw). It also affords the examiner time to interview the primary caregiver regarding key developmental history information.

ADMINISTRATION

As originally designed, the Kinetic Drawing System consumes about 20 to 40 minutes of administration time, although this includes both KFD and KSD, along with advised prompts and follow-up inquiries. Because use of this drawing system is typically limited to the KFD, and only an initial instruction is provided with limited follow-up inquiry, administration time is most frequently between 10 and 15 minutes. This method proceeds in two phases; that is, the Performance Phase and Inquiry Phase, analogous to the Rorschach (see Chapter 12).

The Performance Phase begins by handing examinees a sheet of plain white paper and pencil with eraser, then asking them to simply draw of picture of everyone in their family, "doing something" (Knoff & Prout, 1985, p. 4). The instruction is intended to emphasize the kinetic aspect of the task and additionally encourages the drawing of whole people versus stick figures. For very young examinees, crayons may also be afforded in order to add a color component to the analysis and to make the task more engaging and enjoyable. It is important for the examiner to discourage any assistance from other family members who may be present; for example, a parent who reminds the child to add a family member who until then has been omitted.

The Inquiry Phase is initiated when examinees indicate that they are done, with their drawing, either by stating this verbally or by nonverbally laying the picture and pencil down. Then the examinee is simply asked to identify everyone in the picture, describe what is happening generally, and then what each character is doing more specifically (see Knoff & Prout, 1985, pp. 4–5). Depending upon time and context, queries can be made as to what some of the main characters are thinking and feeling. Remember that this measure is only being used here as a screening tool, hence to assist in developing general impressions and hypotheses about examinees' functioning in the context of their primary object-relations and attachments. In lieu of, or following a poor quality KFD, the Performance Phase of the KSD can be initiated with the instruction to draw a school picture, which includes the teacher, examinee, and one or two friends once again, "doing something." The Inquiry Phase is identical to that of the KFD, with the exception of the different context and people.

SCORING

The Kinetic Drawing System consists of a fairly elaborate qualitative scoring system, facilitated by use of the Scoring Booklet associated with the Handbook (Knoff & Prout, 1985). The qualitative scoring categories include the following: (a) Actions of and Between Figures; (b) Figure Characteristics; (c) Position, Distance, and Barriers; (d) Style; and (e) Symbols. The pictures are analyzed in terms of the frequency of certain scores within each category. Such a system is much too detailed and time consuming for use as a screening measure. However, if one can avoid the temptation to over-interpret, there are certain scores that are capable of assisting in hypothesis testing. In fact, a "hypothesis-generating and hypothesis-testing model" is espoused by the authors, which regards the issue of interpretation; a topic to which the discussion now turns.

INTERPRETATION

For screening purposes, the analytic guidelines proposed by Burns (1982) is followed. In particular, he advises that examiners proceed through the following general interpretive sequence: (a) consider the drawing in broad terms, including its tone, general quality, and salient actions and emphases; (b) evaluate all individuals and animate representations (e.g., pets) in terms of their interactions, expressions, and activities; (c) evaluate all inanimate representations (e.g., tree, sun, clouds, balls) in terms of their interactions, expressions, and activities. Develop hypotheses about how these broad aspects of the drawing assist in accounting for the presenting symptoms and what kinds of psychopathology may be present in this case (e.g., oppositional and defiant themes, anxiety, aggressive themes and content). These hypotheses, in turn, should facilitate the choice of follow-up psychological testing that are indicated.

Next, time permitting, the examiner can scan Table 5.1 for any identifiable characteristics and, using clinical judgement, determine if any of the associated interpretations apply to the case facts. Here, listed are those characteristics that have been found to be most useful over the years of the author's testing experience in developing hypotheses, especially those pertaining to the presence of various types of individual and family systems psychopathology. They are taken from four of the five aforementioned diagnostic categories. The omitted category is Symbols, which have never really been very reliable in predicting and explaining meaningful human behavior or traits (e.g., buttons representing dependency (DiLeo, 1983). The majority are keyed towards identifying psychopathology (e.g., general blackening indicating potential depression or dysphoria), although in many cases their absence or opposing result can negate various types of psychopathology (e.g., an absence of excessive attention to detail can help rule out *obsessive-compulsive disorder* or *OCD*). Additionally, they tend to be the ones most easily identified even with a cursory-style search. This was intentional considering that time is such a precious commodity when conducting an initial clinical interview. Lastly, many of these same characteristics can be applied to KSD drawings for purposes of screening psychopathology.

A succinct case example is provided in Figure 5.1. This drawing was done by a boy age 7 years 3 months, who was referred by his pediatrician for acting out behavioral problems. When asked to draw a picture of him and his family doing something together, he initially refused and crossed his arms in defiance. His father acquiesced while his

Table 5.1 Family Kinetic Drawing (FKD) Interpretation for Screening Purposes

Diagnostic Category	Characteristic	Interpretation
Actions of and Between Figures	Ball playing isolated to one figure	Difficulties relating to the environment; loner[a]
Actions of and Between Figures	Hanging, falling, unstable figures	Tension or anxiety[ab]
Actions of and Between Figures	Dirt themes	Dysphoric feelings[ab]
Actions of and Between Figures	Figure in dangerous position	Tension, turmoil, and anxiety[c]
Figure Characteristics	General blackening	Depression or dysphoria[ab]
Figure Characteristics	Barriers between figures	Emotional distancing[d]
Figure Characteristics	Transparencies (visible internal organs)	Tenuous reality testing; psychosis; low IQ[c]
Figure Characteristics	Omission of self	Poor self-concept; feeling left out; feeling insignificant[eg]
Figure Characteristics	Greater relative height of figures	Perceived as having greater psychological importance[e]
Figure Characteristics	All stick figures	Low IQ[c]
Figure Characteristics	Large person	Significant object relation[g]
Figure Characteristics	Small person	Insecurity[g]
Position, Distance, and Barriers	Lack of interaction between figures	Poor communication or relating among figures[af]
Position, Distance, and Barriers	Distant	Feelings of isolation and rejection[c]
Position, Distance, and Barriers	Compartmentalization	Lack of communication[g]
Position, Distance, and Barriers	Small figures near lower edge	Feeling insecure, inadequate, depression[g]
Position, Distance, and Barriers	Figures drawn in upper half	Optimism, narcissism[g]
Position, Distance, and Barriers	Underlining	Instability; desire for stability[abg]
Style	Heavy, overworked line quality	Anxiety; impulsivity; aggression[c]
Style	Light, broken, or uneven line quality	Insecurity, inadequacy, fear[c]
Style	Excessive attention to details	Compulsiveness; insecurity[c]
Style	Erasures	Compulsiveness; insecurity[ac]
Style	Asymmetric drawing	Poor organization; impulsivity[c]
Style	Ordering of figures	Relative importance within the family structure[c]
Style	Proximity between figures	Strong identification between figures; wish to be closer[abe]

Source. Knoff, H. M., & Prout, H. T. (1985). *Kinetic Drawing System for Family and School: A handbook*. Los Angeles, CA: Western Psychological Services (WPS), pp. 8–20.

Note. Compartmentalization = separation of members by frames.

[a]Burns & Kaufman, 1972; [b]Burns, 1982; [c]Reynolds, 1978; [d]Brannigan, Schofield, & Holtz, 1982; [e]Klepsch & Logie, 1982; [f]Burns & Kaufman, 1970; [g]DiLeo, 1983.

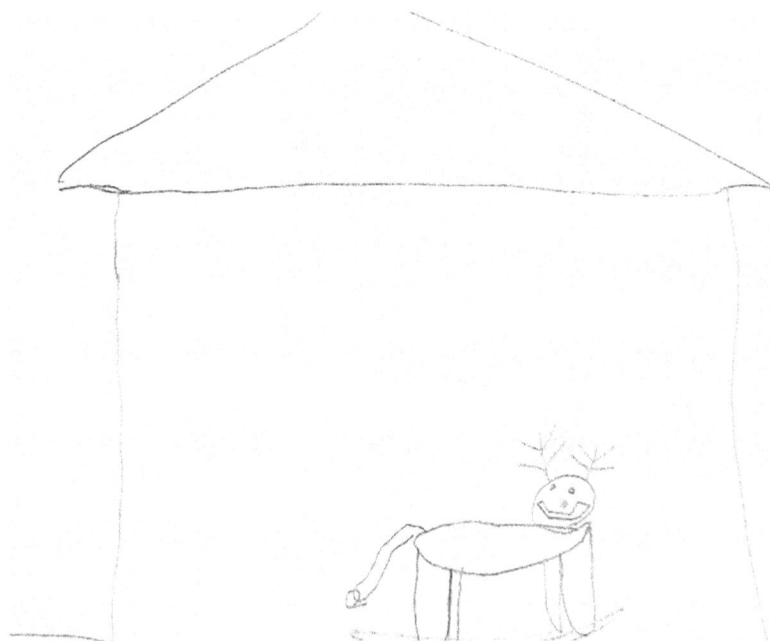

Figure 5.1 Kinetic Family Drawing (KFD) Case Example

Note. Family kinetic drawing by a 7 year, 3-month-old male. The omission of self and family symbolizes the poignant feelings of rejection experienced by this child. The scribbled lines he drew beneath the reindeer symbolize his anxiety associated with the unstable nature of the family relationships and circumstances.

mother scolded him ineffectually for not complying. After five minutes of ignoring his defiance, he spontaneously drew the picture in Figure 5.1 of a "reindeer" in an empty house with scribbled underlining immediately beneath the reindeer. The following characteristics are notable with interpretations in parentheses: (a) drawing a reindeer versus his family (overtly oppositional and defiant); (b) omission of self and family (feelings of rejection regarding self and family); (c) underlining the reindeer (emotionally unstable home environment and desire for stability); and (d) ambivalent facial expression on the reindeer that appears more human in character (projection of the boy as the reindeer with a tenuous smile, hence repressing underlying anxiety).

Indeed, the assessment information indicated that the intimacy within the marital dyad had decompensated and the parents were proceeding through marital dissolution. The family system, which also included two sisters, was marked by vacillations between overt conflict and emotional distance among the members. Considering both the drawing and the family system dynamics, it was hypothesized that the boy's acting out behaviors were functioning to unite his mother and father within a parental role and thus attempt to maintain an intact family system. However, the boy's symptoms were also a manifestation of his own underlying feelings of rejection, and likely resultant anxiety and depression. To conclude, both the process and content of this boy's drawing was of remarkable diagnostic use in addition to its interpretation being done with notable efficiency.

Finally, having children briefly describe their drawings provides them with an opportunity to show and explain what they have produced. The attention alone can be reinforcing, although what they reveal can lead to extremely informative hypotheses. For example, a 7-year-old boy drew a total of five individuals that comprised his family in proximity to a large square shaped object that represented a pool. When asked which figure he was, he stated, "Nowhere because I forgot to draw myself." The tenor of the drawing included a general blackening by heavy use of a lead pencil. What hypothesis would one infer from these facts and his statement of "forgetting" to draw himself? Both experience and research indicates that children of this age tend to have very high self-esteem (Butler, 1990; Diehl, Youngblade, Hay, & Chui, 2011). This typically is evidenced by a proclivity to draw themselves first. Certainly, forgetting to draw himself is significant, if for no other reason that it contravenes the instruction to, "draw you and your family doing something together, some activity." Such data leads to hypotheses of low self-esteem, feeling ignored in the family, feeling left-out or unacknowledged, and a potential depressive disorder, which is rather impressive for a quick screening activity.

The most reliable and valid hypotheses are those which are most proximate to the facts presented within a particular case, especially if organized by theoretical principles. The aforementioned child may be lacking in empathy or mirroring from his parents, hence leading to an empty feeling or sense of self, which is exemplified by his "forgetting" to draw himself (see Kohut, 1971, 1977). Note that this salient KFD response and associated interpretation can be made swiftly and efficiently, and can be justified as long as it represents a hypothesis to be tested with more comprehensive test data. For a more thorough description of this measure and its use in clinical assessment, the reader is referred to the Kinetic Drawing System Handbook (Knoff & Prout, 1985). Another more comprehensive source that predated this system and significantly contributed to the interpretation of kinetic family drawings in assessing children is the book by Burns and Kaufman (1970).

Sentence Completion Test

Synopsis

The *Sentence Completion Test* (SCT) consists of a list of beginning partial sentences, usually referred to as *stems*, and asks the respondent to finish them in any manner that makes them full and understandable statements. This technique[2] is based upon the assumption that the open-ended responses will reveal the individual's thoughts, feelings, and unresolved conflicts perhaps more effectively than by direct questioning (Weiner & Greene, 2008). Consistent with this assumption, the SCT is employed to achieve the same objectives as delineated for the KFD, including: (a) rapport building; (b) engaging the examinee within the assessment process; and (c) information gathering. As was done for the Kinetic Drawing System, a succinct history of this method will be offered prior to explaining how it is used during a clinical interview.

Succinct History of Sentence Completion Tests

The memory investigator Hermann Ebbinghaus (1885, 1913) is usually credited with the first SCT in 1879, which he created in order to measure intelligence and reasoning capacity in German school children (Hersen, 2003). Next, Carl Jung was the first to consider using sentences to assess personality functioning (Hersen, 2003). From Jung's original interest, he developed his *word association test* in which people were asked to say the first thing that came into their mind to a list of target words. This method promoted the belief that intrapsychic functioning could be analyzed by means of word associations. Later, word association techniques expanded into different versions, including words of varying content and degrees of abstraction (Rhode, 1957). Gradually, clinicians began to realize that single word responses were limited in terms of the amount and quality of assessment information that was yielded. Therefore, the technique expanded from one word to the use of brief phrases, and finally to complete sentences. By the late 1920s, SCTs began to proliferate (Rhode, 1957).

In 1928, Arthur Payne employed the SCT to assess specific career-related personality traits (Schafer, Rotter, & Rafferty, 1953), while Alexander Tender investigated various emotional reactions, including fears, aversions, and emotional attachments (Schafer et al., 1953). However, it was Amanda Rhode who developed the SCT as a formal measure of personality, hence using it to reveal people's unconscious or latent motives, needs, sentiments, emotions, and attitudes of which they were not completely aware (Weiner & Greene, 2008). The majority of contemporary SCTs emulate the approach employed by Rhode, which is classified by many experts in projective testing as a *completion technique* versus an association technique (Walsh & Betz, 2001). Although the SCT has never really benefitted from a well validated standardized scoring system (Silverstein, 1999), for screening purposes this is fortunately not necessary.

Use During Initial Clinical Interviews

Providing older children and adolescents an open-ended activity in which they can express their feelings and perceptions, rather than inundating them with direct and potentially intrusive questions, can be an effective use of SCTs during an initial clinical interview (Oster, 2016). Following a review of the presenting symptoms, examinees can feel somewhat self-conscious and potentially defensive. After all, discussing the number and type of symptoms, especially externalizing behaviors that are associated with disciplinary procedures (e.g., episodes of emotion dysregulation and temper outbursts), can be stressful. Therefore, they are typically asked to complete an SCT early in the interview process, either during the latter stages of the presenting symptoms, or more frequently soon thereafter, in order to ensure that they have been given an opportunity to offer their opinions regarding the key difficulties. There are a multitude of SCT forms available in the public domain. They can be readily found by simply typing in the search terms, "*Sentence Completion Test–Child*" and "*Sentence Completion Test–Adolescent*."

Again, typically after discussing the presenting symptoms, including both onset and course, examinees are provided with a copy of a SCT selected for their particular developmental period, a clipboard, and a sharpened pencil with eraser. This permits them to remain comfortably in their seat while they complete the form. They are then provided with the following brief step-by-step instructions. First, they are asked to print their names and record the date at the top of the form in the blanks provided. Second, they are informed that each item presents the first part of a sentence and that they are to finish it so that it makes a complete sentence. Third, it is emphasized that there are no right or wrong answers, but that they should try and do their best writing and to print so that it can read later.

In terms of item stem content, the younger childhood form tends to contain wishes (e.g., I wish I could be. . .), basic emotions, (e.g., angry, happy), fundamental relationships (i.e., mother, father, teacher, self), common types of behaviors (e.g., bad, good), likes and dislikes, animal content, and peer relations (e.g., friends). The older adolescence form tends to have briefer stems (i.e., less structure), and addresses more intense and complex emotions (e.g., worry, regret, frustration) futuristic goals and hopes (e.g., potential jobs), attitudes towards the same and opposite sex, relationships towards authority and with peers, and finally, all principal family relationships (i.e., father, mother, sister, brother, self).

INTERPRETATION

For screening purposes, an empirical scoring system is unnecessary. Rather, the approach here may be described as a subjective-intuitive analysis of underlying motives or issues projected into the examinee's responses. More specifically, after the examinees and their families have exited the office, the SCT responses can be perused for any of the following: (a) repetitive themes (e.g., pessimistic thoughts, feelings of rejection); (b) perception of self (e.g., low self-esteem); (c) perception of major attachment figures (e.g., attitudes towards mothers, fathers); (d) any clarifications or additions to the presenting symptoms (e.g., pessimistic thoughts, evidence of dyslexia, such as phonetic misspellings and continuing letter reversals); or (e) any other responses that may provide clues as to what is associated with, causing, or aggravating the presenting symptoms, or new information that was not divulged during the course of the interview (e.g., thoughts of self-harm).

Rating Scales Tests Used for Screening

The screening tests in this section are both multidimensional and unidimensional. The former consists of two measures that complement each other in the sense that they cover the majority of the lifespan, which is an extremely convenient feature for an examiner charged with selecting an age-appropriate comprehensive screening test. The latter are by design more targeted toward detecting *attention-deficit/hyperactivity disorder* (ADHD) symptomatology. Therefore, this section begins with the more inclusive screens in terms of detecting a range of psychopathologies and move to the more narrowly defined ADHD instruments.

Multidimensional Screening Tests

As stated prior, there are two multidimensional screening tests that cover first from age 2 to 18 years, and then again continuing from 18 years through adulthood; hence, an overlap at age 18 years. Together, these are intended for screening a variety of potential problems and disorders most common within the respective broad age ranges. They are especially useful when interviewees have significant difficulty delineating the presenting symptoms due to lack of introspection or psychological mindedness, suffer from *alexithymia*, and/or are poor historians. This section will next proceed in chronological order.

Clinical Assessment of Behavior, Parent Form

SYNOPSIS

The *Clinical Assessment of Behavior*, (*CAB*; Bracken & Keith, 2007) is a reliable observer-based rating scale for objectively identifying the presence of a variety of behavioral and emotional disorders in children and adolescents ages 2 years 0 months through 18 years 11 months. The CAB is easy to administer, score, and interpret, and comes with computer scoring software to further expedite the process and enhance test utility. Items are patterned after disorders in the *Diagnostic and Statistical Manual of Mental Disorders, Fourth Edition, Text Revision* (*DSM–IV–TR*; American

Psychiatric Association, 2000), although as a screening device are easily adaptable to the *Diagnostic and Statistical Manual of Mental Disorders, Fifth Edition* (*DSM–5*) nosology (American Psychiatric Association, 2013).

The entire instrument actually consists of three rating forms, including (a) the CAB Parent Extended Rating Form (CAB–PX), (b) the CAB Parent Form (hereafter CAB Parent Form; CAB–P), (c) the CAB Teacher Rating Form (CAB–T), and (d) the *Clinical Assessment of Behavior Scoring Program* (*CAB–SP*; Bracken, Keith, & PAR Staff, 2007). The CAB–PX includes 170 items and takes about 30 to 40 minutes to complete, thus being prohibitively long for purposes of screening during an initial assessment. Use of the CAB–T is precluded by non-availability of the respondent. Therefore, the *Clinical Assessment of Behavior, Parent Form* (*CAB–P*; Bracken & Keith, 2007) is the form to be employed during an initial clinical interview screen for various types of child and adolescent psychopathology.

NORM REFERENCE SAMPLE

The CAB's *norm reference sample* comprised 2,114 individuals ranging in age from 2 years 11 months through 18 years 11 months, including both genders, a large range of racial and ethnic backgrounds, and gathered from all major geographical regions of the United States. More specifically, the norm reference sample demographic characteristics were based upon the U.S. Bureau of the Census March 2001 data (U.S. Bureau of the Census, 2001). The sample was well matched to the population parameters of gender, race/ethnicity, and age, along with the four major U.S. geographic regions Midwest, Northeast, South, and West. However, the norm reference sample contained parent households that were somewhat more educated than that of the corresponding population.

In developing the norms for all forms, including the CAB–P, few if any significant differences were found among the various demographic groups. However, to reflect expected developmental and gender differences among some of the key psychological constructs measured by the CAB, different norms were created for each of the two genders among three age groups, including 2 to 6 years, 7 to 12 years, and 13 to 18 years. Hence, the CAB essentially consists of six groups of norms (Bracken & Keith, 2007, p. 37, Table 4.5).

ADMINISTRATION

The CAB–P can be administered in 10 to 15 minutes, hence rendering it a viable screening measure to be used during a 60-minute initial assessment appointment. The items require an 8th grade reading level and thus should be comprehensible to most respondents without added assistance. The form asks for the examinee's identifying information and basic information regarding the respondent, including relationship to the examinee. The demographic portion of the measure can be rapidly entered as such information is readily available during the interview process. Respondents are asked to answer all items and to rate how often the examinee engages in the described behavior "lately," using a Likert-type rating scale, generally involving the following response options: 1 = *Always or Very Frequently*; 2 = *Often*; 3 = *Occasionally*; 4 = *Rarely*; and 5 = *Never*. If the respondent expresses uncertainty on any of the items, the examiner may encourage the use of "best guesses" as being more accurate than that of prorating.

SCORING

All scoring is accomplished through the CAB–SP software. The examiner first enters the demographic information, ensued by the numbered responses to each of the 70 items on the CAB–P. Based upon clinical experience, this consumes as little as minutes. The CAB–SP provides the standardized data instantly on various types of scales and clusters. These include more general areas of functioning, more specific areas of functioning, both problems and adaptive strengths, and finally, validity scales, here termed *Veracity Scales*.

All of these scales can be seen in Form 5.1, which will be introduced here and expanded upon in the ensuing interpretation section. First, the respondent's relation to the examinee is identified as this may vary depending upon the family context and circumstances. This is ensued by two tables of data. The first (i.e., Table 1) presents the Veracity Scales, which is the logical starting point for interpretation as they pertain to our confidence in the diagnostic results. The second (i.e., Table 2) presents the actual diagnostic screening data.

Regarding Table 1 Veracity Scale interpretation, it was found that about 95% of all Cluster profiles in the norm reference sample yielded 0 or 1 *T*–scores of 70 and greater or 30 and lesser. Between 5% and 1% of the Cluster profiles yielded 2 to 5 *T*–scores of 70 and greater or 30 and lesser. Lastly, less than 1% yielded 6 to the maximum 10 *T*–scores in these extreme ranges. Hence, The CAB–P has two Veracity Scales, one for too many extremely high *T*–scores of 70 and above, and one for too many extremely low *T*–scores of 30 and below (see Form 5.1, Table 1, Respondent Veracity Scale). Because these results were based upon a normative sample, versus a clinical sample, and considering that comorbidity is common among the latter, the most conservative less than 1% criterion seemed to be the most reasonable threshold to use to interpret a possible invalid profile due to a negative impression of the youth (i.e., too many *T*–scores of 70 or above) or a positive impression of the youth (i.e., too many scores of 30 or lower).

Moving to the diagnostic information, the overall CAB Behavioral Index and Clinical Clusters (see Form 5.1, Table 2) are most relevant for screening purposes as they provide data regarding the potential presence of mental and behavioral disorders and symptoms may indicate the need for more comprehensive follow-up testing depending upon the pattern of results. More specifically, the Clinical Clusters represent groups of symptoms associated with educational problems (viz., Mental Retardation, hereinafter Intellectual Disability, Learning Disability), behavioral problems (viz., Anger, Aggression, Bullying), and mental and developmental disorders (viz., Anxiety; Depression; Conduct Problems, hereinafter Conduct Disorder; Attention-Deficit/Hyperactivity, hereinafter Attention-Deficit/ Hyperactivity Disorder; Autistic Spectrum Behaviors, hereafter Autism Spectrum Disorder).

For each of the Clinical Clusters, the CAB–SP provides the following data: (a) raw score; (b) *T*–score (*mean* = 50, *standard deviation* = 10); (c) *percentile rank (PR)*; (d) *90% confidence interval (CI)*; and (e) *qualitative classification*. If missing or omitted responses on any scale do not exceed 10%, the CAB–SP prorates the standard scores by multiplying the obtained raw score by the number of scale items, divided by the number of items completed. Omissions exceeding 10% result in no score for that scale; hence, invalid results for that particular scale. Again, omitted responses should not be a problem since the measure is being administered during the course of a face-to-face initial clinical interview, which provides an opportunity for examiners to prompt for needed answers.

INTERPRETATION

As stated before, interpretation should begin with the Veracity Scales (see Form 5.1 Table 1). Recall that the veracity-related data were collected from a non-clinical norm reference sample. Because comorbidity can be expected among clinical samples, the more conservative 1% criterion for excessive responding seems to be the most reasonable to employ. Thus, typical (i.e., valid) profiles are those with 5 or less *T*–scores equal to or above 70 (i.e., no exaggeration of symptoms), and those with 5 or less *T*–scores equal to or below 30 (i.e., no minimization of symptoms).

Three narrative interpretation options follow Table 1 and provide both efficiency and flexibility in interpreting the validity of the CAB–P Behavioral Index and Clinical Cluster data. They are easily identified by italics font label and number (i.e., *Interpretation #*), along with a single italicized lead word that describes the gist of the drafted version (e.g., *Valid*). Therefore, *Interpretation 1* should be used when data for the Veracity Scales are typical, and hence inferred as being valid. The latter two are contingent upon the qualitative observations of the testing psychologist. For example, if all ten scores are above 70 and such severe and pervasive psychopathology is clearly incongruent with the mental status examination data and referral information, such results can be deemed summarily invalid and the diagnostic scores thereafter not reported as being misrepresentative (see *Interpretation 3*). In contrast, if there are six *T*–scores above 70 that are consistent with other assessment data, the second statement suggesting that the data are to be interpreted with caution is perhaps a more inference (see *Interpretation 2*). Note that the italicized words and phrases are intended to be deleted from the final draft of the assessment report, along with the alternate two narrative versions that do not apply.

Considering that the complete initial assessment, including semi-structured clinical interviewing, mental status examination and behavioral observations, and the CAB–P must all be completed within 60 minutes, interpretation must proceed rapidly toward the most important Clinical Clusters. Table 2 in Form 5.1 begins with the CAB Behavioral Index, which virtually represents an aggregation of all 70 CAB–P items (Bracken & Keith, 2007, p. 19). Compared to all other scores provided by this measure, this index represents the most accurate estimate of clinical risk for general maladjustment and *psychological disorder*. This is because it relies upon the greatest number of items compared to any other Clinical Clusters. Proceeding then from general to specific, all Clinical Clusters in Table 2 are listed in the order they appear in the CAB–SP printout in order to facilitate data entry. It should be noted, however, that the percentile rank (PR) and 90% confidence interval (90% CI) columns are reversed in order to afford greater priority to the analysis of measurement error. Also, the examiner has the flexibility to report only the most relevant scales or results in order to speed the process of reporting (e.g., conveying only extremely high-risk scores or only those scales most germane to the differential diagnostic issues).

Note that the *T*–score mean, standard deviation, and range are reported in the general notes to Table 2, ensued by the interpretive guide employed in determining the degree of clinical risk for each Clinical Cluster. The reported range was identified by scrutinizing the full *T*–score ranges reported for the CBI and all Clinical Clusters for the CAB–P (Bracken & Kieth, 2007, Appendix B). Increasing risk of a disorder or behavior problem is also explicitly denoted by an accumulating presence of appended asterisks (i.e., one for *mild clinical risk*, two for *significant clinical risk*, and three for *very significant clinical risk*). The resulting classification for each reported *T*–score is also listed in the final column for those readers who may find it difficult to interpret quantitative data.

By utilizing all of the condensed information proffered in Table 2, the reader is able to discern the meaning of scale elevations, including scores that may be deemed threshold or bordering between two interpretive ranges. This information effectively integrates the dimensional nature of determining risk as opposed to relying exclusively upon categorical risk analysis. Lastly, the Mental Retardation (MD) Clinical Cluster antiquated label was supplanted with Intellectual Disability (ID) to be consistent with contemporary nomenclature, including a specific note acknowledging that this relabeling was done along with its rationale. Lastly, the general table notes include the full label for all table abbreviations, a cross (†) symbol denoting that any data with this appendage have been prorated as indicated prior, and a double-dash (--) symbol denoting the absence of a score also as indicated prior.

Narrative interpretation of Table 2 results should immediately follow, proceeding from general (i.e., addressing the CBI Behavioral Index) to more specific (i.e., describing the Clinical Cluster profile). The number and type of Clinical Clusters showing varying degrees of clinical risk should be summarized, with the greatest emphasis upon the relatively highest statistically significant elevations (if any). To facilitate such interpretation, a pre-drafted narrative excerpt follows Table 2, moving from the general CAB Behavioral Index to the more specific Behavioral Index/Clinical Cluster data.

Positive results can be used to indicate either that (a) further testing is *medically necessary*, or that (b) a diagnosis has been confirmed (i.e., if the referral source simply desires a screening result). In the alternative, negative results may contribute to the conclusion that further testing is unnecessary. Finally, the assessment and standardized screening test data may effectively narrow the diagnostic issues and thus reduce the number and type of follow-up tests needed. Insurance carriers that identify examiners who dexterously use standardized screening data to reduce or eliminate the need for follow-up testing will gain credibility concerning future requests for psychological testing services. That is, future preauthorization (PA) requests submitted by that psychologist will be more likely deemed to be legitimate and not an attempt to increase billable hours.

Personality Assessment Screener

SYNOPSIS

The *Personality Assessment Screener* (*PAS*; Morey, 1997) is a brief 22-item self-report inventory that provides standardized screening data for a wide range of psychological symptoms, issues, and pathology for ages 18 years through adulthood. This questionnaire's items form a hierarchy resulting in a PAS Total score, along with ten "element" scores, with each representing a cluster or domain of clinical problems or issues. These elements comprise those domains that define the more comprehensive Personality Assessment Inventory (PAI; Morey, 1991), which is identified as the "parent" or full-length instrument of the PAS, although the latter being designed as a more rapid screening instrument. As is illustrated subsequently, these elements also relate to key psychopathological constructs relevant to clinical psychology practice with adults.

NORM REFERENCE SAMPLE

The PAS was normed on 2,631 individuals ranging in age from 18 years through adulthood, using approximately equal numbers of those from community (N = 1,385) and clinical (N = 1,246) settings, and stratified according to 1995 U.S. census projections in terms of age, race, and gender (U.S. Bureau of the Census, 1988). This standardization sample completed both the PAS and the full-length PAI (Morey, 1991) in order to compute PAS to PAI probability estimates. That is, based upon each individual's PAS score, probability estimates for PAI scores were computed. Of note, the sample showed the full range of parent PAI scores. Hence, there was no evidence of range restriction which would otherwise distort such estimates.

ADMINISTRATION

The PAS Response Form HS is designed to be manually administered and scored. It consists of a two-part carbonless form in which examinees' answers to statements (e.g., I am talkative) are recorded on an underlying scoring grid. In general, examinees are instructed as follows: "Read each statement and decide whether it is an accurate statement about you" (Morey & PAR, 1997, PAS Response Form HS, first page). This is done by use of a four-point *Likert-type scale* with the following *response anchors* (i.e., response alternatives whose meaning is denoted by verbal descriptors and assigned location on a physical continuum without using numbers): (a) *False, Not At All True* (*F*); (b) *Slightly True* (*ST*); (c) *Mainly True* (*MT*); and (d) *Very True* (*VT*). Examiners are to emphasize the need for the respondent to provide answers to all items. They may also assist in providing dictionary-type definitions to words not adequately understood. Administration time averages about five minutes.

SCORING

PAS items are those found to be maximally sensitive in detecting the symptom clusters that comprise each of the ten elements on the full-length PAI. The elements themselves were derived by successive factor analyses (Morey, 1991). The PAS is hand-scored by first separating the two pages that comprise the PAS Response Form HS. On the bottom page, the examinee's responses appear in an underlying soring grid as *raw scores* 0, 1, 2, and 3, which are associated with the aforementioned four response anchors in this respective order. These raw scores are then manually transferred by the examiner to blank spaces aligned in columns under each element. They are next totaled and transformed into exact P values (hereafter *P–scores*) by using a table in the manual (i.e., Morey, 1997, Table A2, p. 69). Element raw scores are then summed for a total raw score, which is again transformed into an exact *P–score* by using another appendix table (i.e., Morey, 1997, Table A1, p. 68). A profile of all these scores can then be created on the bottom sheet to facilitate interpretation.

The PAS may also be computer-scored by utilizing the PAI Software Portfolio (Morey & PAR Staff, 2008). This software permits the examiner to provide examinees with the PAS Response Form, render their answers to each item orally, while the examiner enters their responses electronically into the scoring software data entry screen. This procedure ensures that all items are given a response, minimizes scoring errors, and yields all needed scores immediately with interpretative summary statements for each scale. It also conserves PAS Response Form HS scoring sheets for use in the event computer scoring is hindered or unavailable. However, since hand-scoring consumes no more than five minutes of time (per clinical experience), this method is also sufficient for screening purposes. To reduce scoring time further, profiling the *P–scores* on the PAS Response Form HS is unnecessary if using the PAS data table described subsequently (see Form 5.2).

INTERPRETATION

The *P–score* measures the probability that an examinee would produce a deviant protocol on the more comprehensive parent PAI (i.e., the probability that one or more particular clinical problems are present). Of course, this assumes that the PAI is both a reliable and valid instrument for diagnostic purposes, a statement that has more than sufficient empirical support (see, for example, Morey, 1991). Therefore, a *P–score* that exceeds 50 indicates that the examinee is more likely than not to manifest a clinically significant psychological disorder; the greater the score, the greater the likelihood. Recall that *sensitivity* is the ability of a measure to identify the presence of a psychological construct if it actually exists (see Chapter 3), here psychopathology. Within a clinical screening context, it is frequently recommended that cutoff scores be employed so that they maximize sensitivity such that actual clinical problems are detected and not missed, hence avoiding the cost of false negatives (i.e., people with severe psychological problems neither being identified nor treated).

With these considerations in mind, interpretation of this screening measure proceeds as is customary; that is, from general to specific. At the most general level is the PAS Total (PAS–T) raw score and its corresponding *P–score* (see Form 5.2, Table 1). Proceeding from lowest to highest, *P–score* ranges and their associated degree of risk descriptive labels are as follows: (a) 0.00 to 14.99 is a *low risk*; (b) 15.00 to 29.99 is a *normal risk*; (c) 30.00 to 47.99 is a *mild risk*; (d) 48.00 to 74.99 is a *moderate risk*; (e) 75.00 to 99.81 is a *marked risk*; and (f) 99.81 to 99.99 is an *extreme risk*. If the PAS–T does not fall into the moderate risk range or higher (i.e., PAS Total raw score ≥ 19, *P–score* ≥ 48.00), then the interpretation process should terminate with a negative result. As stated in the professional manual, "Interpretation of an individual PAS element should only be attempted if the PAS Total score reveals an elevation (i.e., PAS Total raw score ≥ 19) because in the absence of an elevated Total score, an isolated element is considerably less likely to reflect a problem" (Morey, 1997, p. 10). Furthermore, this threshold has been empirically shown to achieve the greatest balance between sensitivity and specificity. In particular, a PAS–T *P–score* of 48.00 correctly identifies 84.7% of those who show clinically significant symptoms upon more thorough evaluation, while accurately classifying 78.7% of those not showing clinically significant symptoms. This was shown to be the most advantageous balance between correct positive and negative decisions (Morey, 1997, Table 3, p. 9).

Proceeding from left to right, Table 1 in Form 5.2 presents columns for the PAS–T name, *P–score*, and qualitative description, respectively. The general note to this table defines the meaning of the *P–score*, while the first specific table note shows the qualitative descriptions associated with each score range. Note that the low, normal, and mild risk ranges are integrated as they all signify an insufficient degree of risk for follow-up analyses, while the remaining three score ranges are denoted by greater numbers of appended asterisks. Therefore, should the PAS–T *P–score* show negative results, the examiner merely retains the non-significant narrative explanation and deletes all of Table 2. In the case of positive data, the significant result narrative interpretation is selected and the analysis moves to Table 2, which comprises all of the Element *P–scores*. Of note, the italicized wording should be deleted from the final report it is meant as instructional versus substantive.

Table 2 is designed to show the profile of Element *P*–scores in order to determine what particular symptom clusters or disorders are likely to be present and at what degree of risk. Respectively from left to right, the table columns show the Element names, *P*–scores, qualitative descriptions, and succinct explanations of measured symptoms and traits. Table notes mirror those displayed in Table 1 by including a definition of the *P*–score, Element, and qualitative descriptions associated with *P*–score ranges. All such information is also readily available on the PAS score sheet.

Regarding the Element *P*–scores, interpretation is as follows: (a) 0.0 to 39.9 is a *normal risk*; (b) 40.0 to 49.9 is a *mild risk*; (c) 50.0 to 74.9 is a *moderate risk*; and (d) 75.0 to 100.0 is a *marked risk*. The Element scores do not have as great a raw score range and thus do not discriminate as effectively at the extreme ranges. In result, *P*–scores for the 10 elements have two fewer interpretive intervals at the most extreme ends (i.e., no low and extreme ranges). Hence, it is advised that moderate elevations and above be recommended for further testing in order to achieve acceptable levels of sensitivity within a clinical practice setting. The descriptions of measured symptoms and traits found in the final column of Table 2 are based upon those provided by the professional manual (Morey, 1997, pp. 10–15). Specific recommendations for more comprehensive formal testing can be drafted contingent upon the number and type the *P*–score elevations found in Table 2.

Two narrative paragraphs designed for Table 2 interpretation are provided. The first represents a stem designed to infer what types of psychopathology may be present and in need of further testing. The second consists of language that infers a negative screening result for the remaining clusters and domains of psychopathology that were measured by this screening test.

Summary

This section reviewed two multidimensional screening tests of standardized rating scale format. Together, they are capable of providing a rapid measure of risk for an array of common types of psychopathology for the majority of the lifespan, which includes virtually all clientele that would be referred for testing in a mental health practice setting. Next, are unidimensional measures designed to detect a risk for ADHD symptomatology across a broad age spectrum.

Unidimensional Screening Tests

As covered in preceding chapters (see, e.g., Chapter 3), *unidimensional tests* measure a single psychological construct, frequently in a good deal of depth and detail. ADHD is one of the most common neurodevelopmental disorders encountered in mental health. It affects an estimated 5% to 7% of children (Barkley, 2014; Frick & Nigg, 2012; Kieling et al., 2010), which is considered to be an underestimate (Voort, He, Jameson, & Merikangas, 2014) due to the age of onset being relaxed from 7 to 12 years in the DSM–5 (American Psychiatric Association, 2013). In fact, some estimate the prevalence of ADHD to be as high as 11% (Visser, S. et al., 2014), including a 4.4% rate in U.S. adults (Kessler et al., 2006) also considered to be an undervalue as the criteria were developed primarily for children (Chung et al., 2019). The high frequency of testing referrals for ADHD in testing practice continues to be consistent with these data. Therefore, it is extremely useful to have three unidimensional screening tests for ADHD that cover the majority of the lifespan, all of which are covered in this section. They will be reported in chronological order beginning with an early childhood version and ending with an adult form.

Conners Early Childhood, Behavior, Short Version, Parent Form

SYNOPSIS

The *Conners Early Childhood, Behavior, Short Version* (*Conners EC–BEH–S*) is an abridged edition of the full-length Conners Early Childhood (Conners EC; Conners, 2009a; see also Chapter 14). It was developed by taking a subset of items that manifested maximum correlations with the complete Behavioral Scales from which they were culled. There are six of these abridged Behavioral Scales that comprise the short version, including Inattention/Hyperactivity, Defiant/Aggressive Behaviors, Social Functioning/Atypical Behaviors, Anxiety, Mood and Affect, and Physical Symptoms. Of most relevance here is the Inattention/Hyperactivity Behavioral Scale. If more than ADHD is suspected in this age range, then the abovementioned CAB–P is the more felicitous choice.

The six items that constitute the Inattention/Hyperactivity Behavioral scale short version are displayed in Form 5.3, Table 2. The items are not numbered in a typical numerical sequence (i.e., 1–6) because they reflect the number in which they appear on the actual Response Form. This permits the examiner to locate the items rapidly on the Response Form for rapid data entry into this table for purposes of item analysis (i.e., precisely what symptoms are being rated). These six items were found to produce the desired maximum and highly significant correlation with the full-length version of this Behavior scale ($r = .97$, $p < .001$; Conners, 2009a, p. 149). Because this curtailed measure is intended to be used during an initial clinical interview for screening purposes, only the parent form is of interest here; that is, the *Conners Early Childhood, Behavior, Short Version, Parent Form* (*Conners EC–BEH–SP*).

NORM REFERENCE SAMPLE

The standardization sample for the Conners EC–BEH–SP is the same one used for the full-length version of this rating scale. Briefly, it consisted of 800 children ages 2 to 6 years with equal numbers of boys and girls ($Ns = 400$). Additionally, the demographic distribution was matched according to the 2000 U.S. Census figures (U.S. Bureau of the Census, 2000).[3]

ADMINISTRATION

The Conners EC–BEH–SP Response Form contains 47 brief items and requires a minimum 6th grade English reading level (Conners, 2009a, p. 19). The latter was determined by using the Flecsh-Kincaid Grade Level Formula (Flesch, 1948; Kincaid, Fishburne, Rogers, & Chissom, 1975). It takes on average only 10 minutes for the respondent to complete. The instructions are to rate each item to the extent it is true (or frequent) in the past month of the examinee as follows: (a) 0 = *Not true at all (Never Seldom)*; (b) 1 = *Just a little true (Occasionally)*; (c) 2 = *Pretty much true (Often, Quite a bit)*; and (d) 3 = *Very much true (Very often, Very frequently)*. Although there are also two open-ended items regarding other concerns or skills of the child, both of which are listed last, the examiner may request that these be omitted in the interest of time.

SCORING

The Conners EC has optional unlimited computer software scoring that applies to both short and full-length versions of this measure. Raw scores can be inputted, computer-scored, and entered into Form 5.3, Tables 1 and 2, within a span of five minutes. Table 2 is designed to show the raw scores (i.e., 0–3 as keyed above) for each of the items that load on the Inattention/Hyperactivity scale. The item numbers listed in Table 2 are those assigned on the Response Form. This permits the examiner to quickly locate the raw scores on either the Response Form or the computer-scored printout. In fact, the latter can be programmed to print the item raw scores organized by scale. In either case, listing the item numbers in this manner permits cross-referencing between the report and raw data for purposes of feedback. This also facilitates an item analysis of which ADHD symptom clusters are present and to what degree. Table 1 is designed for standard score entry, including *T*–score (mean = 50, standard deviation = 10), 95% CI, and PR, along with a succinct description of the measured symptoms.

INTERPRETATION

The principal focus is on the dimensional *T*–score because it is based upon all six items, rendering it significantly more reliable than any other reported scores. It is also standardized, meaning that it is a uniform score and adjusted for age and gender (see Chapter 3). This is why the analysis begins with these data, which is also consistent with a more general to specific (i.e., deductive) approach to test interpretation. Therefore, any *T*–scores falling between 60 and 69 are more than one standard deviation above the mean with a very high PR in the 80s, and are considered statistically *elevated*. Those 70 and above are statistically *very elevated*. Either statistical elevation should be interpreted as a positive screening result and ensued by item analysis to comment on the apparent type of presentation; that is, inattentive, hyperactive, or both. Such positive results support a recommendation for follow-up testing while negative results can help rule out such diagnosis. The associated confidence interval can assist interpretation in close cases by referencing the margin of error as commonly reported in polling data. Finally, interpreting the PR is in many cases easier for parents to comprehend. For example, if a *T*–score of 87 is associated with a PR of 98, the examiner can simply state that their child's screening result shows potential ADHD symptoms that are higher than 98 percent of other children of similar gender and age, which supports the need for follow-up testing.

A narrative written interpretation should immediately follow Table 1. Due to the limits of time, it should be no longer than two or three sentences. To facilitate such interpretation, a succinct pre-drafted excerpt is provided. First, the *T*–score elevation should be addressed in terms of whether or not it is statistically elevated. If not, the results are interpreted as negative and the analysis typically stops. If it is close but not significant, an item analysis can be done to determine the reason for the sub-threshold elevation. If it is positive, a brief summary of the item profile can be done to supplement the need for follow-up testing. This is done by reporting the item raw score data in Table 2. Once again, a pre-drafted narrative excerpt is provided to expedite the interpretive process.

Conners 3rd Edition, ADHD Index Version, Parent Form

SYNOPSIS

The *Conners 3rd Edition* (*Conners 3*; Conners, 2009b) is a behavioral rating scale instrument for measuring the presence of attention-deficit/hyperactivity disorder (ADHD), along with common co-occurring problems and disorders in individuals ranging in age from 6 to 18 years. It is essentially a multi-informant assessment system that consists of forms for parents and teachers, along with a self-report form for ages 8 to 18 years. It consists of four principal components, including full length versions, short versions, ADHD Index versions, and Global Index versions.

Once again, the *Conners 3rd Edition, ADHD Index Version* (*Conners 3–AI*; Conners, 2009b) is of most relevance as it provides screening data for this specific disorder as applied to an older group of minors up to the age of majority. It is an extremely brief measure with the purpose of determining whether or not a more complete formal evaluation for ADHD is warranted. Hence, this form was selected for use during an initial psychological assessment in cases where an individual was referred precisely for the purpose of ruling in or out the presence of ADHD. More specifically, in an effort to select the one most useful version available in this system for ADHD screening administration, the *Conners 3, ADHD Index Version, Parent Form* (*Conners 3–AI–P*; Conners, 2009b) was prioritized over the teacher and self-report forms. This choice was based upon the logic that a parent or caregiver would be (a) immediately accessible during the interview process (versus a teacher), (b) more objective (versus self-report), and (c) able cover the entire 6- to 18-year age range (versus self-report). Hence, this form and version is described next.

NORM REFERENCE SAMPLE

Two standardization samples are of concern here. First, the normative data for all Conners 3 versions were collected over an 18-month duration and consisted of 3,400 individuals ranging in age from 6 to 18 years. This overall sample was stratified by age, gender, and race/ethnicity according to the 2000 Census Bureau data (U.S. Bureau of the Census, 2000). The Conners 3–AI–P was standardized on two samples ranging in age from 6 to 18 years, the first termed a derivation sample ($N = 158$) used to develop the measure's items, and the second called a confirmatory sample ($N = 180$) used to measure its statistical appropriateness. The samples included twice as many males as females, and the vast majority were Caucasian, along with some Hispanic, African American, and an Other category. Finally, 50% of each sample had a confirmed ADHD diagnosis while 50% were from a general nonclinical population.

The final measure included the 10 items on the long-form that best differentiated ADHD from the nonclinical population. For example, considering sensitivity (i.e., correctly detecting ADHD cases), *specificity* (i.e., correctly identifying nonclinical cases), *positive-predictive power* (*PPP*) (i.e., the percentage of youth identified by the Conners 3–AI–P as having ADHD who actually do have the disorder), and *negative-predictive power* (*NPP*) (i.e., the percentage of youth identified by the Conners 3–AI–P as nonclinical who actually do not have ADHD), the overall average *Kappa statistic* (k) ranged from .78 to .88 (with 1.00 representing perfect prediction and 0.00 representing less than chance prediction) (Conners, 2009b, p. 27).

ADMINISTRATION

The Conners 3–AI–P contains ten brief items with a Likert-type rating scale. Similar to the Conners EC, the respondent is asked to rate the degree of truth (or frequency) of certain ADHD symptoms shown by the child or adolescent within the previous month as follows: 0 = *Not true at all* (*Never, Seldom*); 1 = *Just a little true* (*Occasionally*); 2 = *Pretty much true* (*Often, Quite a bit*); and 3 = *Very much true* (*Very often, Very frequently*).

The measure requires a grade equivalent reading level of 5.5 (or halfway through 5th grade), which represents an approximate age level of 10 years. This captures a generous minimum reading level while ensuring that all relevant ADHD symptoms are accurately described; that is, the item wording can be understood by most respondents without oversimplifying the symptom descriptions. The average time to complete the Conners 3–AI–P is five minutes. Because this measure is used during a live face-to-face interview, the examiner can help ensure that all items are answered by the respondent by contending that "best guesses" are more accurate than item omissions, which would necessitate prorating and thus a much less precise scoring method. Further, the demographic portion of the measure is rapidly completed as such information is readily available in all clinical interviews. Of course, this fact can be applied to all screening measures that are employed during clinical interviews.

SCORING

This measure is sufficiently brief such that manual scoring is accomplished within 5 minutes. In consequence, computer scoring is needless. As the respondent circles the desired ratings on the response sheet, which is a two-part carbonless form as described for the PAS earlier, this automatically imprints into an underlying grid scoring sheet as item raw scores. Parent ratings of 3, 2, 1, and 0 record as raw scores of 2, 1, 0, and 0, respectively. These point reductions are due to total raw scores above 11 reaching a ceiling maximum *T*–score of 90, hence not providing any additional discriminatory power. The examiner simply adds the scores on the underlying grid for a "Total Raw Score."

There are two scoring and interpretation tables available; in Form 5.4 they are enumerated as Table 1 and Table 2. The psychologist may use both tables for maximum information or, if time is short, simply the first table. Table 1 contains all of the transformed standard scores. The dimensional *T*–score is determined by entering the Total Raw Score into a table located on the scoring sheet based upon the examinee's gender and age. The *T*–score (mean = 50, standard deviation = 10) is first reported, followed by the confidence interval (CI) and percentile rank (PR). The 95% CI is determined by the reported standard error of measurement (SEM) in the manual. Specifically, the Conners 3 reports the SEM Total in Table K.30 (Conners, 2009b, p. 458) as 3.16; hence, 3 when rounded to the nearest whole number. Therefore, to compute the 95% CI, the examiner simply subtracts and adds 6 points (i.e., 2 SEMs) to the obtained *T*–score. The PR can be derived by referring to any standard normal distribution table, which can be found on various sources on the internet (see, e.g., MedFriendly, 2020).

For readers of this book, however, a standard score to percentile rank conversion guide has been designed, which is located in Appendix A, Table A.1. In particular, this table lists a number of different standard score linear transformations in successive columns, including *z–scores*, *standard scores*, *scaled scores*, and *T–scores*, and how values of each metric are interrelated, along with associated PR area transformations in the final column. These values are adapted from three different sources (McCrae, & Costa, 2010, Appendix F, p. 136; MedFriendly, 2020; Meyer, Viglione, Mihura, Erard, & Erdberg, 2011, Appendix E, p. 498), along with the use of *interpolation*, all of which effectively filled in gaps in the table while being as precise as possible (in many cases, providing values from one to two decimal places for all *z*–scores, and including some *T*–scores and PRs). This table provides a convenient guide for examiners to make rapid conversions for purposes of the accurate and inclusive reporting of psychological test data. By using the data tables to facilitate data entry for each test, along with the abovementioned conversion guide, examiners have the capability of providing readers with thorough and informative test data, which help facilitate interpretation of the results. Lastly, the probability of an ADHD diagnosis is determined by entering the Total Raw Score into a separate "Probability Score Table," also located on the underlying scoring sheet, then finding the associated probability.

Table 2 enables the psychologist to enter all of the item raw scores, which are summarized in terms of their content and tallied in the order they appear on the response sheet, followed by a Total Raw Score. This affords an idea of exactly what symptoms (i.e., items) contributed to the total, hence addressing the type of ADHD that may be present, in addition to the overall score. Of note, this was also done on the Conners EC.

INTERPRETATION

Table 1 data determines the Conners 3–AI–P ADHD screening result. First, if the *T*–score falls within either the *elevated* (i.e., 60–69) or *very elevated* (i.e., 70–90) range, this indicates a positive screen for ADHD. The CI and PR can supplement the interpretation, especially the latter as it is easier to understand for the layperson. A bonus feature here, however, is the probability estimate. Specifically, Total Raw Scores of about 5 and higher tend to result in statistically elevated *T*–scores complemented by an increasingly higher odds of an ADHD diagnosis. For example, a Total Raw Score of 9 for an 8-year-old male is associated with a *T*–score of 86 (i.e., very elevated) and an 87% probability of having ADHD. These data would be interpreted as a positive screening result for ADHD, which justifies a recommendation for more comprehensive follow-up testing. In contrast, a less than 50% probability would be aa unequivocal example of a negative screen.

A pre-drafted narrative excerpt follows Table 1, which interprets the overall screening data results. If the data are elevated and indicative of ADHD, then Table 2 item raw scores can be reported and interpreted so as to analyze the symptom clusters present and which are most apparent or elevated. Once again, a pre-drafted excerpt follows Table 2 to expedite this interpretative process.

Conners' Adult ADHD Rating Scales, Screening Version, Self-Report Form

SYNOPSIS

The *Conners' Adult ADHD Rating Scales* (CAARS; Conners, Erhart, & Sparrow, 1999) is actually a versatile instrument that consists of long, short, and screening versions, all of which come in both self-report and observer-report forms for assistance in determining a diagnosis of ADHD in adulthood. The longer self-report and observer-report forms are presented in Chapter 10. Here, because an increasing number of insurance carriers are requiring screening data for purposes of preauthorizing more in-depth adult ADHD testing, the *Conners' Adult ADHD Rating Scales, Screening Version, Self-Report Form (CAARS–S–SR;* Conners et al., 1999) is of most relevance for potential inclusion initial assessments. It is an extremely brief measure with the principal objective of determining whether or not a more complete formal evaluation for ADHD in a person 18 years and older is justified (i.e., medically necessary).

NORM REFERENCE SAMPLE

The CAARS self-report forms for all three versions (i.e., full-length, short, and screening) were standardized on 1,026 adults located in the United States and Canada, including 466 males and 560 females ranging in age for 18 to 80 years. This initial large sample was used to develop the items. A second confirmatory sample ($N = 180$) was used to measure these items' statistical appropriateness. However, the two ADHD symptom subscales Inattentive and Hyperactive-Impulsive consisted of smaller confirmatory sample sizes ($N = 144$) for ages 18 to 39 years, and ($N = 82$) for ages 40 and older, with females somewhat outnumbering males. Separate norms were provided for age and gender as described in the scoring section later. This was necessary due to significant age and gender effects found among the CAARS scores in the norm reference data.

ADMINISTRATION

The CAARS–S–SR contains 30 items with a Likert-type rating scale, generally involving the following now familiar response options: (a) 0 = *Not at all, never;* (b) 1 = *Just a little, once in a while;* (c) 2 = *Pretty much, often;* and (d) 3 = *Very much, very frequently.* The instructions do not provide a specific numerical time frame except to ask how much or frequently the items describe the respondent, "recently." This measure requires a grade equivalent reading level of 4, which represents an approximate age-level of 9 years. Average time to complete this measure is 10 minutes. Because the CAARS–S–SR is used during a live face-to-face interview, it ensures that all items will be answered as the examiner can encourage "best guesses" as better than providing no answer. Further, the demographic portion of the measure is rapidly completed as such information is readily available during all clinical interviews.

SCORING

Scoring is accomplished manually in 5 minutes, hence obviating the need for computer scoring. As the respondent circles answers on the response sheet, this prints into an underlying scoring sheet in the form of item raw scores. The examiner then transfers the raw scores into empty boxes located under one of three scales as follows: (a) DSM Inattentive; (b) DSM Hyperactive-Impulsive; and (c) ADHD Index.[4] The sums of the raw scores for each scale are then computed. Next, a fourth "DSM Total Scale" is computed based upon the sum of the total raw scores for the DSM Inattentive Scale and DSM Hyperactive-Impulsive Scale. Lastly, the total raw scores for each of the four previously mentioned scales are transferred to a profile sheet for the purposes of transforming the total raw scores into standardized *T*–scores (mean = 50, standard deviation = 10, range 26 to 90). Such transformations are based upon gender-specific norms (i.e., male or female) and four age groups as follows: (a) 18 to 29 years; (b) 30 to 39 years; (c) 40 to 49 years; and (d) 50 and older.

Referring now to Form 5.5, there is one scoring and interpretation table available (i.e., Table 1), which includes all four ADHD scales beginning with the scale name, *T*–score, 95% CI, and PR. The 95% CI can be determined by the reported standard error of measurement (SEM). In particular, the CAARS Technical Manual reports the SEMs for the self-report forms, including all ages together, although separately for men and women, and for the four pertinent scales on the screening form (Conners et al., 1999, Table 6.11, p. 63). Considering that there are four scales and two genders, this results in a grand total of 8 SEMs as follows: 2.53; 2.45; 1.73; 1.78; 2.38; 2.44; 3.04; and 3.08. Taking the average SEM and rounding to the nearest whole number seemed the most logical and efficient manner of computing a confidence interval for this screening test; hence, 2.43 rounded to 2. The 95% CI is then calculated by simply adding and subtracting 2 SEMs to the obtained *T*–score (i.e. ± 4 points). Once again, the PR can be derived by referring to the standard score conversion Table A.1 (see Appendix A).

INTERPRETATION

Interpretation is accomplished by considering the pattern of standard scores in Table 1 (Form 5.5). On this particular screening measure, the *T*–score elevations on each of the four scales govern the analysis. Specifically, *T*–scores above 65 are considered to be statistically *elevated* and those above 70 are *very elevated*. Respectively, one and two asterisks are appended to statistically elevated and very elevated scores, hence visually depicting positive screening results.

Once it is determined that there exist statistical elevations, profile analysis should be conducted as follows. First, the ADHD Index is probably the most useful scale in determining the need for follow-up testing as it consists of the 12 items from the full-length version that best discriminate between those adults with and without a diagnosis of ADHD. Second, especially if the ADHD Index is positive, the other three scales can be interpreted together to develop hypotheses as to which type of presentation is most likely to be present; that is, inattentive, hyperactive/ impulsive, or combined. Again, the results do not need to be definitive as they represent screening data. A pre-drafted excerpt that summarizes the various possible outcomes of this screening measure follows Table 1 (Form 5.5), which is designed to expedite the interpretive process. This language may be used in whole or part to effectively summarize the screening test results.

Neurocognitive Tests Used for Screening

Neurocognitive disorders are characterized by declines in cognitive abilities that interfere with an individual's daily functioning (see also Chapter 9). There is an array of etiologies, ranging from disease, to chronic substance abuse, and *traumatic brain injury* (*TBI*). Many diseases, such as Alzheimer's dementia, manifest in different subtypes and degrees of severity (American Psychiatric Association, 2013; Bajenaru, Tiu, Antochi, & Roceanu, 2012; Visser, F. et al., 1997). Many are also progressive with an insidious onset. *Cognitive* declines can begin with occasional memory lapses, repeating questions asked previously, or frequently misplacing items. As neurocognitive disorders progress, affected people may become lost in familiar contexts or become irritated when they cannot provide answers to simple questions. They may even intentionally or inadvertently make up answers (termed *confabulation*) to fill in gaps in memory. With continued deterioration in neural functioning, there are notable declines in higher-order intellectual abilities, including difficulties thinking abstractly and potential problematic changes in personality; for example, paranoia, aggression, depression, and even psychotic symptom (See, e.g., La Rue, 2015; Lyketsos, 2009).

While early detection is vital for purposes of early treatment intervention, clinicians have difficulty detecting neurocognitive disorders due to their frequent gradual onset and overlapping symptoms with standard psychiatric *clinical syndromes*, including *major depressive disorder* (*MDD*) and *generalized anxiety disorder* (*GAD*), both of which can hinder memory and other cognitive abilities. *Neurocognitive screening tests* can play a vital role both in (a) detecting the need for more comprehensive *neuropsychological testing* (see also Chapter 9), and (b) providing evidence supporting the medical necessity for such testing. In fact, some insurance carriers require screening evidence of neurocognitive impairment in order to provide PA for both neuropsychological and standard psychological testing.

This section presents two types of performance-based neurocognitive screening tests. One is extremely flexible in that it consists of three versions depending upon how much evidence of impairment is needed. The other covers a somewhat wider age range down to age 16 years whereas the former covers from 18 years through adulthood. The one shortcoming is that there are no empirical neurocognitive screening tests for examinees under 16 years of age. Therefore, for such cases the *Stanford-Binet Intelligence Scales, Fifth Edition, Abbreviated Battery IQ* (*ABIQ*) (*SB5–ABIQ*; see Roid, 2003a, 2003b, 2003c) is recommended, although the initial assessment will likely have to be extended to 90 minutes so as to make administration, scoring, and interpretation viable. However, adding 30 minutes to an initial assessment can be a more propitious alternative versus having all requested testing services denied for want of medical necessity.

First to be covered is the more versatile Mini-Mental State Examination, Second Edition (MMSE–2; Folstein, Folstein, White, & Messer, 2010) because it is used most frequently for adult neurocognitive testing referrals. This will be followed by the Wechsler Memory Scale, Fourth Edition, Brief Cognitive Status Exam (WMS–IV, BCSE; Wechsler, 2009a, 2009b), which has a lower age range of 16 years.

Mini-Mental State Examination, Second Edition

Synopsis

The *Mini-Mental State Examination, Second Edition (MMSE–2*; Folstein et al., 2010) is designed primarily as a screening instrument for neurocognitive impairment and secondarily to track an individual's progress or course over time. It is an improvement of the original *Mini-Mental State Examination* (*MMSE*; Folstein, Folstein, & McHugh, 1975), which itself was one of the most widely employed screening measures of neurocognitive impairment (Lezak, How-ieson, & Loring, 2004). It was also used to monitor progression and patients' response to treatment over time (see, e.g., Christiensen, Hadzi-Pavlovic, & Jacomb, 1991), as well as screening large populations for neurocognitive dysfunction (see, e.g., Crum, Anthony, Basset, & Folstein, 1993).

Building upon the MMSE, the MMSE–2 retains the original structure of the examination, while (a) replacing problematic items, (b) adding items such that three versions of varying length and cut-offs for positive screening results are available, and (c) creating an alternate form to guard against the confounding effect of practice in the event retesting is desired. Hence, the MMSE–2 has three versions and two forms. The three MMSE–2 versions differ in length and cut-off scores, with the latter determining screening results as positive or negative for the presence of neurocognitive disorder. The alternate Blue and Red Forms contain items of comparable content and difficulty level (i.e., they may be considered to be *parallel forms* or *equivalent forms*).

In determining which version to administer, the following guidelines are to be considered. The longer the version, the more responsive it is to changes associated with the aging process, the more sensitive it is to detecting subcortical dementias, and the more effective it is at obviating *ceiling effects* caused by including items that are insufficiently difficult to detect neural dysfunction. The main disadvantage of using longer versions include increased time of administration and added invasiveness due to progressively complex and challenging items. The shortest version is useful in detecting more probable cases of neurocognitive impairment in the briefest amount of time.

Versions of the Mini-Mental State Examination, Second Edition

The three versions are summarized next in order of increasing length because they build upon each other in a natural sequence or hierarchical fashion. Because the Blue Form and Red Form are equivalent, they will be discussed together.

MINI-MENTAL STATE EXAMINATION, SECOND EDITION, BRIEF VERSION, BLUE/RED FORM

The *Mini-Mental State Examination, Second Edition, Brief Version, Blue/Red Form* (*MMSE–2–BV–BF/RF*; Folstein et al., 2010) assesses the first four cognitive functions in the original MMSE (Folstein, Folstein, & Fanjiang, 2001), with updated norms (see below) including registration (i.e., immediate repetition of three unrelated words), orientation to time and place, and recall (i.e., repeating the same words with delay and interference of rehearsal). These items are listed in Form 5.6, Table 1. A caveat is that items comprising the brief version are relatively easy to pass, which offsets to some degree the aforementioned high detection threshold and risks a ceiling effect (i.e., being insufficiently difficult such that individuals with true neurocognitive disorder pass the screening test criteria). Also, administration of fewer items is less reliable as compared to more items (see e.g., Miller, Lovler, & McIntire, 2013). Thus, the brief version should be administered only in cases where examinees are already showing severe symptoms that are likely to be detected even with fewer items of less difficulty.

MINI-MENTAL STATE EXAMINATION, SECOND EDITION, STANDARD VERSION, BLUE/RED FORM

The *Mini-Mental State Examination, Second Edition, Standard Version, Blue/Red Form* (*MMSE–2–SV–BF/RF*; Folstein et al., 2010) assesses all of the cognitive functions included in the MMSE predecessor, with updated norms (see below) and some revised items for greater reliability and validity. These items are enumerated in Form 5.7, Table 1. Thus, it adds attention and calculation (i.e., *serial sevens*), naming objects, repetition of a phrase, comprehending and reproducing three commands in sequence, reading a sentence and reproducing its instruction, writing a sentence, and copying a partial overlapping two-dimensional figure. While the standard version is more accurate than the brief version, ceiling effects continue to be possible especially if the examinee has a reputable educational background. Therefore, to maximize the chances of a true positive screening decision and to justify the ordering of a full neuropsychological test battery, administering the longest version presented next is advised.

MINI-MENTAL STATE EXAMINATION, SECOND EDITION, EXPANDED VERSION, BLUE/RED FORM

The *Mini-Mental State Examination, Second Edition, Expanded Version, Blue/Red Form* (*MMSE–2–EV–BF/RF*; Folstein et al., 2010) contains two newly developed items added to the aforementioned standard version, including "Story Memory," which measures both verbal explicit learning and verbal free immediate recall, and "Symbol–Digit Coding," which measures both perceptual-motor speed and incidental learning (Folstein et al., 2010). These and all previous items are listed in Form 5.8, Table 1. The greater number of points available on these two items reflect their increased complexity. Together, they significantly reduce the odds of ceiling effects and resulting incorrect screening decisions.

Norm Reference Sample

The *standardization sample* included a total of 1,531 cognitively healthy individuals ranging in age from 18 years through 100 years. Data was collected between November 2007 and November 2008 by 57 examines across 26 U.S. states. The sample was comprised of 54% females and 46% males, an educational range from about 6 to 16 years (the majority having 12–15 years of education), a range of ethnic groups consistent with the U.S. proportions (i.e., whites, blacks Hispanics, other), and from all regions of the U.S. Exclusion criteria included significant hearing loss or visual impairment, inability to read English of at least 4th grade level, dementia, and acute/severe psychiatric disorder.

Two clinical samples ($N = 232$) were also collected in order to assist in determining the degree to which the MMSE–2 items discriminated between normal healthy individuals and those with established neurocognitive disorders. The clinical samples were apportioned into those with diagnosed Alzheimer's disease and those with subcortical dementia (viz., Parkinson's disease, Huntington's disease, and vascular dementia).

Administration

The MMSE–2–EV administration form should be used for all screenings that employ this measure. This is because all three versions are incorporated into this administration form. Hence, the examiner may terminate administration at any one of the three versions contingent upon the ongoing results, the case facts, the time available, and the particular objectives of screening. This obviates the need of making an a priori decision as to which version to administer; a key advantage when attempting to predict human behavior. This fact that each shorter version is incorporated into the longer version is adduced by scrutinizing the items listed on Forms 5.6, 5.7, and 5.8. Here, one can note that each longer version merely adds items to the data table while retaining all previous items.

The administration process per se begins by obtaining permission from examinees if they may be asked questions about their memory as part of the clinical assessment. Considering that this is a performance-based test, it is imperative that others in the room be prohibited from assisting the examinee in answering any of the questions. Moving the examinee closer to the examiner's desk and keeping others in the background and out of sight can help prevent any interference or distraction. Items are organized and named by virtue of the neurocognitive function it is designed to measure (e.g., Recognition). While some are single items worth one-point each, most are multi-step items worth one-point for each step and response (e.g., counting backwards from 100 by 7 in five steps worth a total of 5 points). Administration times for the brief, standard, and expanded versions are 3 to 5 minutes, 10 minutes, and 20 minutes, respectively. These estimated times also include scoring and interpretation because they both occur simultaneously with administration. Finally, the examiner should note the form that is being used by retaining its respective initials; namely, Blue Form (BF) or Red Form (RF).

Scoring

Scoring is done by hand as the single- and multi-step items are administered and responded to by the examinee. While most of the scoring is straightforward and recorded as pass or fail, there are two remarkably complex multi-step items on the expanded version that resemble subtests seen on actual neuropsychological test batteries. These include Story Memory and Processing Speed, which will next be briefly described. Regarding Story Memory, a brief narrative account is read orally to the examinee, who is asked to repeat back as much of the facts as possible using the same words as did the examiner. Examinees earn credit for each target word or phrase listed on the record form for up to a maximum of 25 points. Processing Speed is timed for 30 seconds and measures how rapidly examinees learn a system of numerical and figural codes, earning up to a maximum raw score of 35 by writing in as many correct number–symbol pairs as possible. A template is provided to facilitate scoring.

The principal analysis is based upon (a) the pattern of neurocognitive function item raw scores, and (b) the Total Raw Score. These data are located in the lone table (i.e., Table 1) shown in Forms 5.6, 5.7, and 5.8 for reporting the screening results of each version. There are three columns as follows: (a) the neurocognitive function item names; (b) the examinee's obtained raw score for each item; and (c) the maximum possible score for each item. The Total Raw Score in boldface represents an aggregate or summation of all the raw scores earned by the examinee during the simultaneous administration and scoring process (i.e., the second or middle column). Although the MMSE–2 provides standardized *T*–scores that are adjusted for age and education, they are extremely restricted in range for both the brief and standard forms, and there is no consistent guide as to when a *T*–score is to be considered clinically elevated. Second, the process of finding the *T*–score value associated with the examinee's Total Raw Score, age, and education in the appropriate manual tables, after which they must be incorporated into the table and report, would consume an additional amount of time that is not justified by the little additional diagnostic information provided. Therefore, the use of the MMSE–2 *T*–scores is a useful practice in this infrequent case. That is, the raw score data and cut-offs discussed subsequently are of sufficient import.

Interpretation

The manual provides tables that report the sensitivity, specificity, *positive predictive power* (PPP), negative predictive power (NPP), and *percent-correct classification* (PCC) of specific MMSE–2 raw scores for various clinical samples (e.g., dementia). In the manual, it is again advised that sensitivity and NPP should be emphasized for purposes of screening the presence of potential neurocognitive dysfunction. That is, the priority in screening for such serious neuropathology is to error on the side of not missing a true case, which practically means that there is more of a willingness to risk proceeding with comprehensive testing when such was ultimately not necessary. Thus, if a false positive case happens to be selected for comprehensive testing, one is willing to accept the lost time, effort, and finances consumed in doing so. On the other hand, the cost of a false negative is that of a lost opportunity for early detection and intervention, which can be critical in improving quality of care and treatment progress in many neurocognitive cases.

Therefore, for each version, brief, standard, and expanded, the cut-off Total Raw Score that would provide a NPP of .97 was found in the manual tables for a sample of individuals with general dementia. By applying this NPP value, 97% of all cases not tested would be truly negative, hence a correct decision. This also means that there is only a 3% likelihood that an individual with dementia would have somehow produced a negative screen (i.e., a score higher than the cut-off, equivalent to passing a test); hence an error rate of 3%. Extending this logic to failing scores that fall below the stated *cut-off score*, one can be 97% confident that an individual with dementia was indeed correctly referred for more comprehensive testing. A caveat is that one cannot argue that the MMSE–2 correctly identifies 97% of those with dementia as that constitutes sensitivity. Such characteristic would be vital for a full-length neuropsychological test battery rather than a screening test. For screening purposes, the goal is to minimize the odds of failing to test a case that ultimately needed it, which is what NPP assists in doing. Therefore, a high NPP rate such as 97% reasonably minimizes errors in deciding not to test when testing should have been done (here 3%). From this analysis, it should be apparent how this decision rule succeeds in erring on the side of doing testing rather than not.

In order to communicate this in the screening results, a statement is made within a specific table note that using the aforementioned cut-off, there is 97% confidence that an actual case of dementia is indeed being referred for more comprehensive testing. Irrespective of the result, this should provide reassurance to the examinee and any collaterals present that a responsible decision is being made, although it should be emphasized that a positive screen does not mean that there is a 97% chance that an examinee actually has a neurocognitive disorder. If examinees and any collaterals continue to misinterpret this statement despite reasonable efforts to explicate its meaning, it is better off deleted as in such instance it obfuscates the point.

As can be seen in Forms 5.6, 5.7, and 5.8, listed are both the maximum score and cut-off score for each version that would provide this 97% confidence rate. Specifically, they are as follows: (a) the MMSE–2–BV–BF has a maximum score of 16 with a cut-off score of 14 or less showing a positive screen (b) the MMSE–2–SV–BF/RF has a maximum score of 30 with a cut-off score of 27 or less being positive; and (c) the MMSE–2–EV–BF/RF has a maximum score of 90 with a cut-off score of 50 or less being positive. Immediately following the table and its notes, the "Screening Result" appears in italics font. After the item raw scores and Total Raw Score have been entered by the examiner, the applicable negative or positive screening result label should be retained. Thereafter, the most accurate qualitative "Level of Consciousness" descriptor should be selected and followed by a brief summary interpretation of the screening results. This summary should reiterate the overall screening results.

In order to facilitate an interpretation of said results, a succinct pre-drafted excerpt immediately follows the table and qualitative descriptor. It can be modified to summarize negative or positive results, and if positive, whether more circumscribed memory testing or more comprehensive neuropsychological testing is indicated (see also Chapter 9). In addition, positive results can be ensued by a rapid profile analysis delineating which neurocognitive functions showed the most potential dysfunction (i.e., time permitting), although is not vital because screening results are usually intended to be brief and item analysis has very questionable reliability.

The Wechsler Memory Scale, Fourth Edition, Brief Cognitive Status Exam

Synopsis

The *Wechsler Memory Scale, Fourth Edition, Brief Cognitive Status Exam* (*WMS–IV–BCSE*; Wechsler, 2009a, 2009b) is designed to identify examinees that manifest significant neurocognitive deficits or that are low functioning. It is an optional subtest to the full-length *Wechsler Memory Scale, Fourth Edition* (*WMS–IV*), which is presented in Chapter 9. The WMS–IV–BCSE measures orientation to time, incidental recall, mental control, planning and visual perceptual processing, inhibitory control, and verbal productivity. These items are enumerated in Form 5.9, Table 1. Because this subtest has the ability to discriminate between normal healthy controls and those with neurocognitive disorder (see below), it can also be used as a viable screening measure for this variety of psychopathology.

Norm Reference Sample

The WMS–IV–BCSE was standardized based upon the normative sample used for the full-length WMS–IV. In particular, this standardization sample consisted of 1,400 adults, including 100 in each of 14 age bands ranging from 16 years to 90 years. Because the WMS–IV has both an Adult Battery (ages 16–69 years) and an Older Adult Battery (ages 65–90 years), the total sample was apportioned into two subgroups. Specifically, 900 were utilized for the Adult Battery whereas 500 were used for the Older Adult Battery, which is expected as the latter covers a smaller age range. Those from ages 16 to 64 contained an equal number of males and females, although those greater than 65 years contained more women than men so as to be consistent with the 2005 U.S. Census data (U.S. Bureau of the Census, 2005). The racial/ethnic composition of the normative sample was also consistent with the U.S. population according to the 2005 U.S. Census data (U.S. Bureau of the Census, 2005). Finally, the normative sample was stratified according to five educational levels as follows: (a) elementary school only; (b) some high school; (c) high school graduate; (d) some college; and (e) college degree and more. The impressive number of age bands and educational levels play a vital role in establishing WMS–IV–BCSE criteria that effectively discriminate between normal and clinical cases of neurocognitive disorder. This is due to the facts that the scores are corrected for varying levels of these two variables, yielding comparable or more accurate information when compared to the first edition of the MMSE (cited above).

Administration

The same WMS–IV–BCSE subtest appears near the front of both the Adult Battery and Older Adult Battery record forms, where examinee's responses and scores are entered manually by the examiner. As can be seen by reference to Form 5.9, Table 1, each item contains multiple questions or steps and thus varying quantities of maximum scores (comparable to the majority of MMSE–2 items). In general, the examinee is asked to perform tasks that are relatively straightforward for a normal healthy population, including orientation to time, mental control, clock drawing, incidental recall, automaticity and inhibitory control, and verbal production.

Clinical practice using this subtest indicates that it typically takes about 15 minutes to administer, score, and interpret for a normal healthy adult who performs perfect or near perfect outcomes. Orientation to time moves quickly due to its rather terse and direct questions. However, an aspect of WMS–IV–BCSE administration that should not be overlooked is its requirement of quite a few materials. In addition to the record form, the following are needed: (a) response booklet (upon which the examinee draws a clock); (b) pencil without eraser; (c) stopwatch; (d) clock or wristwatch; (e) administration and scoring manual; and (f) scoring template. More specifically, the stimulus book is required for all item instructions and the stimuli for examinee performance on two items. The latter include (a) showing a sequence of four object drawings for later verbal recall (i.e., "Incidental Recall"), and (b) having the examinee twice read a series of four rows of shapes as quickly as possible without making errors; that is, first reading the shape names correctly and then the opposite shape names (viz., "Inhibition").

Timing contributes to credit earned on three items (versus one for the MMSE–2). These include (a) "Mental Control" wherein the examinee is asked to recite a series of numbers and words in reverse sequence, (b) "Inhibition" wherein the examinee names shapes correctly and oppositely (cited prior), and (c) "Verbal Reproduction" wherein the examinee states as many words as possible that represent a particular category within 30 seconds. In all instances, examinees are afforded more credit for faster times to completion or total number of correct responses. As will become apparent, because this screening measure is more reliant upon processing speed and reaction time, there is a concomitant increase in the need to correct for age effects. Finally, the WMS–IV Response Booklet and pencil without eraser is required for Clock Drawing (also cited prior). Here, the examinee is asked to draw by freehand an *analog clock*, which displays an approximate time by means of hands that spin around a dial and point to particular locations (a device that is becoming increasingly supplanted by the *digital clock*, which is numeric and displays a more exact time). The more detailed instructions are to draw the face then numbers, followed by accurately depicting a specifically designated time by means of drawing in the minute and hour hands.

Scoring

While the majority of examinees' responses are initially recorded as typical raw scores (i.e., 1 = correct, 0 = incorrect), all of the scores that contribute to the total and used for interpretation are weighted raw scores. *Weighted raw scores* are the first of two additional corrections made to maximize diagnostic accuracy, and are quantitatively defined by the percentage of examinees that score within a particular raw score range. For example, for many WMS–IV–BCSE items, a weighted raw score of 0 is associated with a cumulative percentage of 0–1%, followed by a weighted raw score of 1 for 2–4%, 2 for 5–9%, 3 for 10–24%, and 4 for 25% and higher. Although the weighted raw scores may change in value both within and across items (e.g., 0, 2, 4, 8 or 0, 5, 8), along with the cumulative percentages, this example provides an idea of how the weighting process generally works; that is, adjusting raw scores such that they reflect the percentile rank of an individual's performance compared to the norm reference sample, which in turn represents the normal population of adults. Another way to define weighted raw scores is that they reflect the base rate of normal healthy individuals that obtain various raw scores on these screening items. Ultimately, then, the total weighted raw score will inform as to where an individual falls in rank with the normal population (see below when discussing interpretation). It is these weighted raw scores that are reported in the WMS–IV–BCSE data table shown in Form 9.9. A general table note defines weighted raw scores and their principal objective (i.e., to enhance diagnostic discrimination and accuracy).

Delineating the design of Table 1 in Form 5.9, there exist three columns as follows: (a) neurocognitive function item name; (b) examinee's weighted raw score for each neurocognitive function item; and (c) maximum possible weighted raw score for each neurocognitive function item. The final row is devoted to the "Total Weighted Raw Score" name, the examinee's total weighted raw score, and the maximum possible grand total score, which are all in boldface in order to emphasize their diagnostic import. Analogous to the MMSE–2, all scoring is done by hand. However, a key disadvantage is that scoring is significantly more involved in several aspects as contrasted with the MMSE–2. First, all raw scores must be converted into weighted raw scores. Although the necessary conversions of raw scores to weighted raw scores are conveniently juxtaposed, this extra step being required of all items accumulates and together adds precious time to its use, in addition to increasing the odds of human error. Of even greater import is the rather complex scoring for Clock Drawing, which requires the use of a translucent Scoring Key template with a clock face outline and circular shapes in premeasured units of millimeters. The precision this device affords the examiner is required to reliably quantify the examinee's performance, including a total 13 facets of the clock drawing that receive raw scores each ranging from 0 to 1 or 2 (e.g., numbers, contour, hands). Remember that this all must be done in the presence of the examinee and any collaterals in to order interpret the results and provide feedback during the initial assessment. Although this measure can and should be ready in reserve as a secondary neurocognitive screening measure, it is prudent to prioritize the MMSE–2 and use the WMS–IV–BCSE only in exigent circumstances (e.g., in the event the MMSE–2 administration was invalid or was very recently given by another mental health clinician, hence risking added error variance due to practice effects).

Interpretation

Once the "Total Weighted Raw Score" is computed, it is entered into a classification table located on the WMS–IV Record Form. It is at this juncture where the WMS–IV Ages 16 to 69 Years Record Form and Ages 65 to 69 Years Record Form differ. On the former form, this classification table is apportioned into three age groups, 16 to 29 years, 30 to 44 years, and 45 to 69 years, which is further partitioned into the aforementioned five age groups. On the latter form, there are only two age groups, 65–69 years and 70–90 years, each of which is again further divided into the above-mentioned five educational groupings. The body of both tables consist of five columns of classification levels and total weighted raw score ranges for each combination of age group and education level. From least to most impaired, the classification level labels are *average, low average, borderline, low,* and *very low.*

According to the technical and interpretive manual, these classification levels are defined by the *base rate (BR)* of performance as shown by the norm reference sample, which is representative of the population of normal healthy individuals. Only 2% to 4% of healthy controls fall within the low classification range whereas less than 2% fall in the very low classification level (i.e., respective BRs of 2–4% and < 2%). Therefore, the low and very low classifications are both interpreted as significant cognitive impairment, which best discriminate between a normal healthy population and a clinical neurocognitive population (Wechsler, 2009b, pp. 172–173). Although the manual does not discriminate between the low and very low levels in terms of interpretation, the statistical base rate data indicates that more confidence can be stated when a screening result falls within the very low classification. In consequence, this discrimination is made in Table 1 of Form 5.9.

Specifically, the classification level and its five labels are listed in boldface in the last row and two respective columns of Table 1. The examiner merely deletes the classification levels that do not apply and retains the one indicated by the data. One asterisk is appended to the *low* classification to show positive screening results associated with a 2% to 4% BR, while two asterisks are attached to the *very low* level at a BR of less than 2%. Below Table 1 and its notes is the screening result line in italics font as was done for the MMSE–2. The examiner merely retains the correct result (viz., negative or positive), which is ensued by a succinct narrative summary of the screening results. In the case of positive results, a pithy item analysis can assist in hypothesizing what specific neurocognitive deficits are present, which in turn facilitates follow-up test selection.

One final consideration, the WMS–IV Technical and Interpretative Manual (Wechsler, 2009b) reports the NPP associated with using the low and very low class levels together to be .81. This means that 81% of all individuals performing at borderline, low average, and average levels, and who are consequently interpreted as a negative screening result, are correctly healthy normal individuals who do not have a neurocognitive disorder. Stated alternatively, about 19% of individuals performing in these three higher levels will actually have a neurocognitive problem (also known as a false negative). Using the same logic as for the MMSE–2, these criteria have an 81% degree of confidence that people with a neurocognitive difficulty will be correctly referred for follow-up testing. Comparatively speaking, this means that the MMSE–2's NPP of .97 also tends to outperform that of the WMS–IV–BCSE; another reason to favor the former as a first choice for neurocognitive screening with the latter playing a secondary role. Also, because base rate figures are easier for many people to comprehend and therefore more informative, the confidence information is not reported as was done for the MMSE–2. Rather, it is focused exclusively on the BR interpretation in the table notes. Lastly, a succinct pre-drafted narrative excerpt follows the table comparable to that provided for the MMSE–2. This can be used to expedite interpretation of the screening results.

Recapitulation

This chapter initiated Part II of this book, which is devoted to presenting all of the major psychological tests listed in Table 1.1 that are used in resolving diagnostic issues and related questions in contemporary mental health practice. More specifically, the focus of Chapter 5 was on psychological tests that can be used as screening measures during initial clinical interviews to achieve various objectives, including developing rapport, acclimating the examinee to the assessment and testing process, ruling out suspected disorders, and providing evidence for the medical necessity of follow-up testing for suspected disorders. Screening tests were presented in three classes, including projective techniques, standardized rating scales, and performance-based neurocognitive tests. Each class of tests was discussed in terms of some or most of the following: test design, brief history of development (if applicable), norm reference sample, administration, scoring, and interpretation. Interpretation of the standardized screening tests was explained within the context of tables designed by me, which organize and report the primary data in such a manner that useful diagnostic inferences can be established. The remainder of Part II employs a similar organization, hence instructing the reader not merely what these tests are and what they measure, but also how these tests may be used effectively in clinical practice. The ensuing Chapter 6 covers developmental tests, which focus on the early detection of delays in various domains, including motor, cognitive, social, and adaptive behavior skills.

Key Terms

- alexithymia
- analog clock
- attention-deficit/hyperactivity disorder (ADHD)
- base rate (BR)
- Clinical Assessment of Behavior (CAB)
- Clinical Assessment of Behavior Scoring Program (CAB–SP)
- Clinical Assessment of Behavior, Parent Form (CAB–P)
- clinical syndrome(s)
- cognitive
- completion technique
- confabulation
- confidence interval (CI).
- Conners 3, ADHD Index Version, Parent Form (Conners 3–AI–P)
- Conners 3rd Edition (Conners 3)
- Conners 3rd Edition, ADHD Index Version (Conners 3–AI)

- Conners Early Childhood, Behavior, Short Version (Conners EC–BEH–S)
- Conners' Adult ADHD Rating Scales (CAARS)
- Conners' Adult ADHD Rating Scales, Screening Version, Self-Report Form (CAARS–S–SR)
- cut-off score
- Diagnostic and Statistical Manual of Mental Disorders, Fifth Edition (DSM–5)
- Diagnostic and Statistical Manual of Mental Disorders, Fourth Edition, Text Revision (DSM–IV–TR)
- digital clock.
- Draw–A–Family (DAF)
- equivalent forms
- generalized anxiety disorder (GAD)
- interpolation
- Kappa statistic (k)
- Kinetic Drawing System for Family and School (Kinetic Drawing System)
- Kinetic–Family–Drawing (KFD)
- Kinetic–School–Drawing (KSD)
- major depressive disorder (MDD)
- mean (M or $\overline{X}$)
- medical necessity
- medically necessary
- Mini-Mental State Examination (MMSE)
- Mini-Mental State Examination, Second Edition (MMSE–2)
- Mini-Mental State Examination, Second Edition, Brief Version, Blue/Red Form (MMSE–2–BV–BF/RF)
- Mini-Mental State Examination, Second Edition, Expanded Version, Blue/Red Form (MMSE–2-EV–BF/RF)
- Mini-Mental State Examination, Second Edition, Standard Version, Blue/Red Form (MMSE–2-SV–BF/RF)
- negative-predictive power (NPP)
- neurocognitive disorders
- neurocognitive screening tests
- neuropsychological testing
- norm reference sample
- obsessive-compulsive disorder (OCD)
- parallel forms
- percent-correct classification (PCC)
- percentile rank (PR)
- Personality Assessment Screener (PAS)
- positive predictive power (PPP)
- projective tests
- *P*–score (probability score)
- psychological disorder/s
- qualitative classification
- rating scales
- raw score(s)
- response anchors
- scaled scores
- screening tests
- sensitivity
- Sentence Completion Test (SCT)
- Sentence Completion Test–Adolescent (SCT–A)
- Sentence Completion Test–Child (SCT–C)
- specificity
- standard deviation (*s* or *SD*)
- standard score(s)
- standardization sample
- Stanford–Binet Intelligence Scales, Fifth Edition, Abbreviated Battery IQ (SB5–ABIQ)
- stems
- traumatic brain injury (TBI)
- *T*–score

- unidimensional tests
- Veracity Scales
- Wechsler Memory Scale, Fourth Edition (WMS–IV)
- Wechsler Memory Scale, Fourth Edition, Brief Cognitive Status Exam (WMS–IV–BCSE)
- weighted raw scores
- word association test
- *z*–score

Notes

1. It is instructive to point out that there has been disagreement on whether or not to even classify SCTs as projective in nature. In particular, some experts believe that SCTs provide too much structure to be considered truly projective. Rather, it is contended that they are better conceived of as open-ended self-report inventories (see, e.g., Semeonoff, 1976, p. 301)
2. Perhaps "technique" or "method" are more felicitous terms when referring to most SCTs rather than as tests, which connotes a more formal, uniform process of administration, including an appropriate standardization sample to facilitate scoring and interpretation. This is especially true when referring to the more informal manner in which the SCT is being used here; that is, as a screening device.
3. The Conners EC will be discussed in more detail in Chapter 10 where the full-length form is presented.
4. The precise names for the first three scales are DSM–IV Inattentive Symptoms, DSM–IV Hyperactive/Impulsive Symptoms, and DSM–IV Symptoms Total. However, the IV was dropped in order to help (a) abbreviate the table for ease of use, and (b) reduce any confusion that might occur by including outdated DSM edition numbers. In any case, the item content is sufficiently close to the criteria used in the updated DSM–5 so as to yield valid results for screening purposes. Additionally, the acronym for this screening test varies slightly from that in the manual, which is labeled CAARS–Self-Report: Screening Version (CAARS–S:SV). It seems that preference should be given to the version of the test instrument, followed by the respondent form (e.g., self-report, parent, other, and teacher). Of greater importance, this order of "version type–respondent form" is consistent with most other rating scales listed in this book. Hence, this order made the most sense.

References

American Psychiatric Association. (2000). *Diagnostic and statistical manual of mental disorders* (4th ed., text rev., DSM–IV–TR). Washington, DC: Author.

American Psychiatric Association. (2013). *Diagnostic and statistical manual of mental disorders* (5th ed., DSM–5). Arlington, VA: Author.

Bajenaru, O., Tiu, C., Antochi, F., & Roceanu, A. (2012). Neurocognitive disorders in DSM 5 project–Personal comments. *Journal of the Neurological Sciences, 322*, 17–19.

Barkley, R. A. (2014). *Attention-deficit hyperactivity disorder: A handbook for diagnosis and treatment* (4th ed.). New York, NY: Guilford Press.

Bracken, B. A., & Keith, L. K. (2007). *Clinical assessment of behavior (CAB): Professional manual.* Lutz, FL: Psychological Assessment Resources (PAR).

Bracken, B. A., Keith, L. K., & PAR Staff. (2007). *Clinical assessment of behavior scoring program (CAB-SP; CD-ROM).* Lutz, FL: Psychological Assessment Resources (PAR).

Brannigan, G. G., Schofield, J. J., & Holtz, R. (1982). Family drawings as measures of interpersonal distance. *The Journal of Social Psychology, 117*, 155–156.

Burns, R. C. (1982). *Self-growth in families: Kinetic family drawings (K–F–D) research and applications.* New York, NY: Brunner/Mazel.

Burns, R. C., & Kaufman, S. F. (1970). *Kinetic family drawings (K–F–D): An introduction to understanding children through kinetic drawings.* New York, NY: Brunner/Mazel.

Burns, R. C., & Kaufman, S. F. (1972). *Actions, styles, and symbols in Kinetic family drawings (K–F–D): An interpretive manual.* New York, NY: Brunner/Mazel.

Butler, R. (1990). The effects of mastery and competitive conditions on self-assessment at different ages. *Child Development, 61*, 201–210.

Christiensen, H., Hadzi-Pavlovic, D., & Jacomb, P. (1991). The psychometric differentiation of dementia from normal aging: a meta-analysis. *Psychological Assessment, 3*, 147–155.

Chung, W., Jiang, S-F., Paksarian, D., Nikolaidis, A., Kathleen, R., Merikangas, K. R., & Milham, M. P. (2019). Trends in the prevalence and incidence of attention-deficit/hyperactivity disorder among adults and children of different racial and ethnic groups. *Journal of the American Medical Association (JAMA), 2*, e1914344.

Conners, C. K. (2009a). *Conners early childhood manual (Conners EC).* North Towanda, NY: Multi-Health Systems (MHS).

Conners, C. K. (2009b). *Conners third edition manual (Conners 3).* North Towanda, NY: Multi-Health Systems (MHS).

Conners, C. K., Erhart, D., & Sparrow, E. P. (1999). *Conners' adult ADHD rating scales (CAARS).* North Towanda, NY: Multi-Health Systems (MHS).

Crum, R. M., Anthony, J. C., Basset, S. S., & Folstein, M. F. (1993). Population-based norms for the mini-mental state examination by age and educational level. *Journal of the American Medical Association (JAMA), 269*, 2386–2391.

Diehl, M., Youngblade, L. M., Hay, E. L., & Chui, H. (2011). The development of self- representations across the life span. In K. L. Fingerman, C. A. Berg, J. Smith, & T. C. Antonucci (Eds.), *Handbook of life-span development.* New York, NY: Springer.

DiLeo, J. H. (1983). *Interpreting children's drawings.* New York, NY: Brunner/Mazel.

Ebbinghaus, H. (1885). *Memory: A contribution to experimental psychology.* New York, NY: Dover Publications.

Ebbinghaus, H. (1913). *Memory: A contribution to experimental psychology*. New York: Teachers College Press. (Translated from the 1885 German original.)

Flesch, R. (1948). A new readability yardstick. *Journal of Applied Psychology, 32*, 221–233.

Folstein, M. F., Folstein, S. E., & Fanjiang, G. (2001). *Mini–mental state examination: Clinical guide*. Lutz, FL: Psychological Assessment Resources (PAR).

Folstein, M. F., Folstein, S. E., & McHugh, P. R. (1975). "Mini–Mental State": A practical method for grading the cognitive state of patients for the clinician. *Journal of Psychiatric Research, 12*, 189–198.

Folstein, M. F., Folstein, S. E., White, T., & Messer, M. A. (2010). *Mini–mental state examination, second edition (MMSE–2): User's manual*. Lutz, FL: Psychological Assessment Resources (PAR).

Frick, P. J., & Nigg, J. T. (2012). Current issues in the diagnosis of attention deficit hyperactivity disorder, oppositional defiant disorder, and conduct disorder. *Clinical Psychology, 8*, 77–107.

Hersen, M. (2003). *Comprehensive handbook of psychological assessment volume 2: personality assessment*. Hoboken, NJ: John Wiley & Sons.

Hulse, W. C. (1951). The emotionally disturbed child draws his family. *Quarterly Journal of Child Behavior, 3*, 152–174.

Kessler, R. C., Adler, L., Barkley, R., Biederman, J., Conners, C. K., Demler, O., Faraone, S. V., Greenhill, L. L., Howes, M. J., Secnik, K., Spencer, T., Ustun, T. B., Walters, E. E., & Zaslavsky, A. M. (2006). The prevalence and correlates of adult ADHD in the United States: Results from the national comorbidity survey replication. *American Journal of Psychiatry, 163*, 716–723.

Kieling, C., Kieling, R. R., Rohde, L. A., Frick, P. J., Moffitt, T., Nigg, J. T., . . . Castellanos, F. X. (2010). The age at onset of attention deficit hyperactivity disorder. *American Journal of Psychiatry, 167*, 14–16.

Kincaid, J. P., Fishburne, R. P., Rogers, R. L., & Chissom, B. S. (1975). *Derivation of new readability formulas (automated readability index, fog count and Flesch reading ease formula) for Navy enlisted personnel* (Research Branch Rep. No. 8–75). Memphis, TN: Naval Air Station.

Klepsch, M., & Logie, L. (1982). *Children draw and tell: An introductionto the projective uses of children's human figure drawings*. New York: Brunner/Mazel.

Knoff, H. M., & Prout, H. T. (1985). *Kinetic drawing system for family and school: A handbook*. Los Angeles, CA: Western Psychological Services (WPS).

Kohut, H. (1971). *The analysis of the self*. New York, NY: International Universities Press.

Kohut, H. (1977). *The restoration of the self*. New York, NY: International Universities Press.

La Rue, A. (2015). Dementia: A health care team perspective. In P. A. Lichtenberg, B. T. Mast (Eds. In Chief), B. D. Carpenter, & J. L. Wetherell (Assoc. Eds.), *APA handbook of clinical geropsychology: Vol. 1. History and status of the field and perspective on aging* (pp. 515–547). Washington, DC: American Psychological Association.

Lezak, M. D., Howieson, D. B., & Loring, D. W. (2004). *Neuropsychology assessment* (4th ed.). New York, NY: Oxford University Press.

Lyketsos, C. G. (2009). Dementia and milder cognitive syndromes. In D. G. Blazer & D. C. Steffens (Eds.), *The American psychiatric publishing textbook of geriatric psychiatry* (4th ed.). Washington, DC: American Psychiatric Publishing.

McCrae, R. R., & Costa, P. T., Jr. (2010). *NEO inventories for the NEO personality inventory, third edition (NEO–PI–3), NEO five factor inventory, third edition (NEO–FFI–3), NEO personality inventory, revised (NEO PI–R): Professional manual*. Lutz, FL: Psychological Assessment Services (PAR).

MedFriendly. (2020). *Standard score to percentile conversion*. Retrieved June 26, 2020, from www.medfriendly.com/standardscoretopercentileconversion.html

Meyer, G. J., Viglione, D. J., Mihura, J. L., Erard, R. E., & Erdberg, P. (2011). *Rorschach performance assessment system (R–PAS): Administrative, coding, interpretation, and technical manual*. Toledo, OH: Rorschach Performance Assessment System, L.L.C.

Miller, L. A., Lovler, R. L., & McIntire, S. A. (2013). *Foundations of psychological testing* (4th ed.). Thousand Oaks, CA: Sage Publications.

Morey, L. C. (1991). *Personality assessment inventory (PAI): Professional manual*. Odessa, FL: Psychological Assessment Resources (PAR).

Morey, L. C. (1997). *Personality assessment screener (PAS): Professional manual*. Lutz, FL: Psychological Assessment Resources (PAR).

Morey, L. C., & PAR Staff. (2008). *Personality assessment screener (PAI) software portfolio (CD-ROM)*. Lutz, FL: Psychological Assessment Resources (PAR).

Oster, G. D. (2016). *Using drawings in clinical practice enhancing intake interviews and psychological testing*. New York, NY: Routledge.

Piaget, J. (1952). *The origins of intelligence in children*. New York, NY: W. W. Norton.

Prout, H. T., & Phillips, P. D. (1974). A clinical note: The Kinetic school drawing. *Psychology in the Schools, 11*, 303–306.

Prout, H. T., & Celmer, D. S. (1984). School drawings and academic achievement: A validity study of the Kinetic school drawing technique. *Psychology in the Schools, 21*, 176–180.

Reynolds, C. R. (1978). A quick-scoring guide to the interpretation of children's Kinetic Family Drawings (KFD). *Psychology in the Schools, 15*, 489–492.

Rhode, A. (1957). *The sentence completion method: It's diagnostic and clinical application to mental disorders*. New York, NY: The Ronald Press.

Roid, G. H. (2003a). *Stanford-Binet intelligence scales, fifth edition*. Itasca, IL: Riverside.

Roid, G. H. (2003b). *Stanford-Binet intelligence scales, fifth edition, examiner's manual*. Itasca, IL: Riverside.

Roid, G. H. (2003c). *Stanford-Binet intelligence scales, fifth edition, technical manual*. Itasca, IL: Riverside.

Sarbaugh, M. E. A. (1982). Kinetic drawing–school (KD–S) technique. *Illinois School Psychologists' Association Monograph Series, 1*, 1–70.

Schafer, R., Rotter, J., & Rafferty, J. (1953). Test of personality: Word techniques. In R Schafer (Ed.), *Contributions toward medical psychology* (pp. 577–598). New York, NY: Ronald Press.

Silverstein, M. L. (1999). *Self psychology and diagnostic assessment: Identifying selfobject functions through psychological testing*. New York, NY: Routledge.

U.S. Bureau of the Census. (1988). *Educational attainment in the United States: March 1987 and 1986* (Population Report Series P–20, no. 148). Washington, DC: Author.

U.S. Bureau of the Census. (2000). *Profile of general demographic characteristics, 2000* [PDF File]. Washington, DC: Author.

U.S. Bureau of the Census. (2001). *Current population survey, March 2001* [Data File]. Washington, DC: U.S. Department of Commerce.

U.S. Bureau of the Census. (2005). *Current population survey, October 2005: School enrollment supplement file* [CD-ROM]. Washington, DC: Author.

Visser, F. E., Aldenkamp, A. P., van Huffelen, A. C., Kuilman, M., Overweg, J., & van Wijk, J. (1997). Prospective study of the prevalence of Alzheimer-type dementia in institutionalized individuals with Down syndrome. *American Journal on Mental Retardation, 101,* 400–412.

Visser, S. N., Danielson, M. L., Bitsko, R. H., Holbrook, J. R., Kogan, M. D., Ghandour, R. M., Perou, R., & Blumberg, S. J. (2014). Trends in the parent-report of health care provider-diagnosed and medicated attention-deficit/hyperactivity disorder: United States, 2003–2011. *Journal of the American Academy of Child & Adolescent Psychiatry, 53,* 34–46.

Voort, J. L. V., He, J. P., Jameson, N. D., & Merikangas, K. R. (2014). Impact of the DSM–5 attention-deficit/hyperactivity disorder age-of-onset criterion in the US adolescent population. *Journal of the American Academy of Child & Adolescent Psychiatry, 53,* 736–744.

Walsh, W. B., & Betz, N. E. (2001). *Tests and assessment* (4th ed.). Upper Saddle River, NJ: Prentice Hall.

Wechsler, D. (2009a). *Wechsler memory scale, fourth edition (WMS–IV): Administration and scoring manual.* San Antonio, TX: The Psychological Corporation (PsychCorp)-Pearson.

Wechsler, D. (2009b). *Wechsler memory scale, fourth edition (WMS–IV): Technical and interpretative manual.* San Antonio, TX: The Psychological Corporation (PsychCorp)-Pearson.

Weiner, I., & Greene, R. (2008). *Handbook of personality assessment.* Hoboken, NJ: John Wiley and Sons.

See Routledge's e-resources website for forms. (www.routledge.com/9780367346058)

6 Developmental Tests

Overview

There are various causal models of psychopathology that have been proposed. Of most relevance to tests in this chapter is the *developmental psychopathology model*, which conceptualizes abnormality as resulting from *adaptational failures* arising from delay, fixation, regression, and/or deviance (Mash & Dozois, 1996; Mash & Wolfe, 2013). *Delay*, *fixation*, and *regression* especially consider the departure of an ability, characteristic, or behavior from *developmental norms* (i.e., typical skills and achievement expected at a particular age) as key to understanding the onset, course, and treatment of psychological disorders. *Deviance* considers both the presence of abnormal signs (e.g., rigid and repetitive behaviors) and associated absence of abilities that should be present when considering an individual's age (e.g., lack of social interest). In other words, in all of the aforementioned instances, *chronological age (CA)* is of prime consideration in defining and treating psychopathology.

Consistent with this model, all four tests presented in this chapter principally measure the presence of abnormality by the degree to which an individual manifests deviations from established norms; that is, statistically different scores than expected based upon CA. In most cases, lower scores are diagnostically meaningful in that they show evidence of delay, fixation, or regression. These tests include the following: (a) Bayley Scales of Infant and Toddler Development, Third Edition (Bayley–III; Bayley, 2006a, 2006b) and its recent successor Bayley Scales of Infant and Toddler Development, Fourth Edition (Bayley–4; Bayley & Aylward, 2019a, 2019b); (b) Adaptive Behavior Assessment System, Third Edition (ABAS–III; Harrison & Oakland, 2015a); and (c) Vineland Adaptive Behavior Scales, Third Edition (Vineland–3; Sparrow, Cicchetti, & Saulnier, 2016). The fourth and final test focuses mostly upon detecting the presence of deviance in the form of qualitative impairments in social and behavioral functioning. Here, higher scores detect the greater presence of deviance. It has been considered by many experts in the field to be the gold standard in detecting signs of autism (Maye, Kiss, & Carter, 2017) and is titled the Autism Diagnostic Observation Schedule, Second Edition (ADOS–2; Lord, Luyster, Gotham, & Guthrie, 2012; Lord, Rutter, Dilavore, Risi, Gotham, & Bishop, 2012). Prior to examining these tests in detail in such sequence, they will next be briefly compared and contrasted for context.

To begin, two similarities are noteworthy. First, all four tests can be administered in infancy through early childhood. Hence, they are ideally designed for the early detection of delay, fixation, regression, and/or deviancy. Second, they all actively involve primary caretakers within the assessment process, either by providing ratings based upon their familiarity with, and observations of, the examinee, and/or assisting in the administration of actual test items (e.g., prompting the caregiver to call the child's name to observe an interpersonal response).

Next, they differ in two essential ways, including age range and test format. Regarding the former, the Bayley–III concentrates upon the first 3.5 years (i.e., 1–42 months), while the remainder cover virtually the entire lifespan. The term "virtually" was used because the ADOS–2 begins at 12 months. This is due to the fact that, except in profoundly disturbed or delayed cases, an insufficient amount of development has occurred to permit the reliable detection of *autism spectrum disorder (ASD*; Luyster et al., 2009; Osterling, Dawson, & Munson, 2002; Ozonoff et al., 2008, 2010; Zwaigenbaum et al., 2005). As will be covered subsequently, the ADOS–2's standardization sample does not exceed 40 years 11 months, despite its claim to be "through adulthood." Furthermore, these developmentally based tests differ in format. Most uniquely, the Bayley–III employs a combination of two formats, including (a) performance-based items targeting cognitive, language, and motor skills, and (b) observer-based ratings measuring more real-world social-emotional and adaptive behavior. In contrast, the ABAS–3, Vineland–3, and ADOS–2 rely on one format only; that is, the former two being observer-based while the latter performance-based.

With these considerations in mind, the chapter will present these four measures beginning with the Bayley–III, which is uniquely specialized for measuring early developmental departures from developmental norms. This will be ensued by the two lifespan measures of adaptive behavior. The chapter ends with the ADOS–2, which is a

DOI: 10.4324/9780429326820-8

performance-based measure uniquely designed for the detection of signs of autism down to age 12 months and thereafter through to middle adulthood. The presentation of each test follows a similar organization for pedagogical purposes. That is, information is more easily learned and recalled when presented within an organized and predictable framework (Collins & Quillian, 1969). As the chapter unfolds, these tests will increasingly coalesce around a clear developmental theme.

Bayley Scales of Infant and Toddler Development, Third Edition

Synopsis

The *Bayley Scales of Infant and Toddler Development, Third Edition* (Bayley–III; Bayley, 2006a, 2006b) is an individually administered test with observer-based rating scales designed to evaluate the functioning of examinees in infancy and early childhood ranging in age from 1 month to 42 months. Its cardinal objective is to identify early developmental delays in major domains of functioning, along with providing information regarding treatment intervention.

The test consists of five content domains, three of which are performance-based scales. First, the Cognitive Scale measures a uniform *mental development* construct that includes sensorimotor abilities, exploration and object manipulation, object-relations, concept formation, and memory. In order to retain its uniform focus on mental tasks, the Cognitive Scale minimizes the use of language. Second, the Language Scale measures two facets of communication, including both receptive and expressive language. Receptive language items assess preverbal behaviors, including the ability to recognize sounds, receptive vocabulary (e.g., identifying objects and pictures), and morphological development and markers (e.g., plurals). Expressive communication consists of preverbal communication (e.g., babbling), vocabulary use (e.g., naming), and *morposyntactic development* (e.g., two-word phrases).

Third, the Motor Scale assesses both fine (i.e., small muscle movements) and gross (i.e., large muscle movements) motor skills. Fine motor skill items measure the extent to which children use their eyes, fingers, and hands, including *prehension* (e.g., grasping), perceptual-motor integration (e.g., building simple structures), motor planning and speed (e.g., tracing), reaching, functional hand skills, and response to tactile information (e.g., discrimination of objects using touch). Gross motor items generally measure how well children control and move their bodies, including head control, stepping, standing, walking, climbing, and running. The focus here is on movement of the limbs and torso, static positioning, dynamic movement, balance, and motor planning.

The final two domains include the Social-Emotional Scale and Adaptive Behavior Scale. Both employ an observer-report format because they are designed to answer not what children are able to do, but what children actually show what they are capable of doing in the real-world environment. Such a question can best be measured by a primary caretaker who is quite familiar with the child on a daily basis. The Social-Emotional Scale is designed to identify social and emotional developmental milestones by means of a structured caregiver questionnaire. This particular scale is a derivative of the *Greenspan Social-Emotional Growth Chart: A Screening Questionnaire for Infants and Young Children* (Greenspan, 2004). Its items focus upon functional emotional skills, including self-regulation, interest in the world, ability to communicate needs and establish relationships, using emotions in a purposeful manner, and utilizing emotional signals to solve problems.

Lastly, the Adaptive Behavior Scale assesses a child's age-appropriate use of independent skills requisite for effective daily living. Particular skills measured by this questionnaire include communication, community use, health and safety, leisure, self-care, self-direction, functional pre-academics, home living, socialization, and motor skills. Prior to delving further into the details of the Bayley–III, a brief history of this measure is provided next for useful context.

History of the Bayley Scales

The Bayley Scales have thus far proceeded through several iterations. Its historical evolution is instructive of both the developmental constructs that it measures and parallel advances in child developmental research that guide assessment and treatment. Therefore, this section is devoted to tracking the evolution of the Bayley Scales with the most detailed focus on the current edition. This provides valuable context on the key developmental constructs measured by this test, and therefore how it may be most effectively employed diagnostically.

Bayley Scales, First Edition

The original *Bayley Scales of Infant and Toddler Development* (BSID; Bayley, 1969) was derived from three theoretically eclectic scales of infant development, along with a wide array of infant and early childhood research. Because this measure was based upon a variety of sources, it offered a flexible measure with diverse viewpoints that was not restricted to any one developmental theory (e.g., psychoanalytic, cognitive). These included, *The California First-Year Mental Scale* (Bayley, 1933), *The California Preschool Mental Scale* (Jaffa, 1934), and *The California Infant Scale of Motor Development* (Bayley, 1936).

The BSID was instrumental in introducing a unique approach to testing this very young population. Specifically, Nancy Bayley believed that the strict administration and scoring procedures characteristic of analogous cognitive tests for older children, adolescents, and adults were much too inflexible for infants and young children. At the same time, some degree of standardized administration and scoring was needed in order to develop age-based norms from which the appropriateness of young children's development could be measured. In consequence, the 1969 BSID integrated flexibility into the typical standardized administration and scoring process. In particular, although items were carried out according to explicit instructions, their order and rate of completion varied contingent upon a number of factors, including CA, temperament, and rate of success.

In addition to a more flexible standardized administrative process, items presented infants and toddlers with situations, tasks, and stimuli that successfully attracted and maintained their interest, and upon which an observable set of behavioral responses were produced that formed the basis of the BSID's developmental norms for ages 2 through 30 months. This more flexible administration and scoring approach notwithstanding, the BSID was classified by the experts as a *power test*, which is one in which the items form a sequence of increasing difficulty and complexity, including those that are extremely difficult to pass (Anastasi & Urbina, 1997). All subsequent editions of this test are similar in design in that items are administered in a modified power sequence; that is, items are administered in an approximate rather than an exact order of difficulty.

Bayley Scales, Second Edition

The *Bayley Scales of Infant and Toddler Development, Second Edition* (*BSID–II*; Bayley, 1993) made several improvements to the BSID. These included the following: (a) updating the norm-reference sample; (b) modernizing and improving the stimulus materials to be increasingly engaging; (c) refining content validity; and (d) enhancing the psychometric quality of the test (i.e., increased *reliability*, *validity*, and *utility*). Further, the flexible administration format was preserved, which was a notable achievement considering the improved reliability and validity correlation coefficients (i.e., increased administrative flexibility tends to reduce such correlations, all things being equal). Next, the Bayley–III (Bayley, 2006a, 2006b) benefitted from a vast body of child developmental research that was conducted since the BSID–II published in 1993. In particular, many of the core constructs measured by the earlier Bayley Scales were elaborated upon such that the Bayley–III items tap behaviors that more accurately represent developmental abilities associated with the psychological adjustment of infants and young children.

Bayley Scales, Third Edition

This section is apportioned according to the five scales that comprise the Bayley–III test structure. The principal constructs measured by each scale are delineated so that the diagnostic usefulness of this test becomes more clearly apparent. One will notice an emphasis on the Cognitive and Language Scales that benefitted most significantly from updated research and are both performance-based.

COGNITIVE SCALE

One of the most notable modifications of the Bayley–III was the addition of an independent Language Scale (discussed subsequently). This allowed the BSID–II Mental Scale to be expanded so that more purely defined cognitive constructs that impacted cognitive development could be measured, hence the change in this scale's name. A description of the cognitive constructs measured by this scale follow.

Play is defined as including activities that are freely sought and pursued solely for the sake of enjoyment (American Psychological Association, 2015, p. 802). Although play as defined was focused upon obtaining enjoyment, it was also proposed as a natural activity that facilitated cognitive growth (Bruner, 1972; Piaget, 1952; Singer, 1973; Vygotsky, 1978). For example, Piaget believed that play promotes cognitive development by helping children integrate information into existing mental structures or schemes, while Vygotsky proposed that play provided children with the means for establishing meaning and thus facilitating symbolic thinking. These hypotheses ultimately received significant empirical support (see, e.g., Johnson, 1976).

Thus, a sequence of increasingly sophisticated play items was developed for inclusion in the Bayley–III, which was designed to measure infants' and young children's cognitive functioning. This sequence consisted of the ability to play with a single object at 6 months (Piaget, 1952), combining or relating objects at about 8 months, engaging in relational actions at 9 months (e.g., placing a lid on a pot; Fenson, Kagan, Kearsley, & Zelaso, 1976), showing *symbolic* or *pretend play* (i.e., permitting one object to be used to represent another object) by 24 months (Belsky & Most, 1981), and thereafter manifesting increasingly complex symbolic play in the form of integrating substitutions and fantasy in pretense at 36 months (e.g., using the hand with thumb in the ear and pinky finger pointing at the mouth as a telephone and having a conversation).

Information processing was discussed previously in Chapters 2 and 7 in the context of conceptualizing human memory and its assessment during a mental status examination. More generally, *information processing tasks* manipulate data in order to accomplish some kinds of objectives or goals, including such things as problems-solving, learning, and recalling information previously stored. Since publication of the BSID–II, the proliferation of neuroscientific theory and research increasingly established that information processing also played a major role in cognitive development, including a number of tasks in infancy and early childhood that were found to be capable of predicting cognitive functioning in later life (Colombo & Frick, 1999). These tasks included preference for novelty, habituation, paired comparison, memory, reaction time, and anticipation of patterns (Bornstein & Sigman, 1986; Colombo & Frick, 1999; Dougherty & Haith, 1997; Kail, 2000; Scatz, Kramer, Ablin, & Matthay, 2000). Hence, some of these information processing type tasks were added to the Bayley–III Cognitive Scale, including those that measure attention to novelty, habituation, memory, speed of processing, and problem-solving. As will become apparent, these are inter-related abilities and will be delineated next.

Attention to novelty is operationally defined as how long an infant focuses upon a new stimulus. As the same stimulus is repeatedly presented to the infant, the length of attention dissipates, which is a robust and predictable phenomenon termed *habituation*. Habituation in infants has been interpreted as evidence for learning, more specifically learning to be bored. That is, once infants learn a stimulus, they become "bored" and naturally search for new items, which is in turn referred to as *preference for novelty*. The faster the rate at which habituation occurs, the faster the learning and more cognitively competent the infant. Habituation has also been used efficaciously as an indication of memory.

In particular, imagine an infant learns and habituates to a picture of a novel design (i.e., Stimulus A). After an interval of 15 minutes, that same picture (i.e., Stimulus A) and a picture of a new design (i.e., Stimulus B) is shown to the infant. If the infant spends more time attending to the novel design (i.e., Stimulus B), this indicates that the infant has recognized the first design (i.e., has remembered it) by remaining habituated (or bored) in response to it. In contrast, if the infant attends to both designs equally, the inference is that there is no recall or memory as the infant has *dehabituated* to the first design (i.e., Stimulus A). Habituation (and its counterpart dishabituation) has been shown to be one of the most reliable predictors of later intelligence, which is why it is incorporated into various Cognitive Scale items on the Bayley–III. For instance, speed of habituation in infancy was found to be negatively correlated with intellectual functioning at age 8 years (Sigman, Cohen, Beckwith, & Parmelee, 1986). To elaborate here, Bayley–III items measure infant memory and ability to habituate to both visual and auditory stimuli. Specifically, subsequent to habituation, infants are tested as to whether they spend more time attending to the prior familiar stimulus or a second novel stimulus. If they look longer at the latter, this is evidence of a preference for novelty and thus greater memory (Bornstein & Sigman, 1986; Fagan, 1970, 1982).

Speed of processing is a related information processing task measured by the Bayley–III items, which is operationally defined as the rate of habituation. More specifically, items here measure the number of trials it takes the examinee to complete a task; that is, the lesser number of trials, the faster the habituation and speed of processing. It is interesting to note that the speed or rate of habituation also reflects the maturation of the infant's *central nervous system (CNS; Rovee-Collier, 1987)*. The more readily an infant habituates to stimuli, the more intact the CNS. On a neurobiological level, processing speed is mirrored by increases in the number of inter-neural synapses or connections between neurons, along with increases in *myelination* (Berthier, DeBlois, Poirier, Novak, & Clifton, 2000).

Finally, *problem-solving* represents a more complex higher-order type of information processing that involves thinking, reasoning, memory, and the synthesis of information (Aylward, 1988). Items specifically tap increasingly sophisticated skills, including retrieving an object that is part hidden at age 6 months, retrieving an object that is completely hidden at age 9 months, and finding a hidden toy after being displaced from its original point of disappearance at age 24 months (Dunst, 1982).

Finally, number concepts and counting were incorporated into the Bayley–III Cognitive Scale in recognition that these abilities are also central to cognitive development (Silverman & Rose, 1980; Gelman & Tucker, 1975; Wynn, 1990). These skills form a hierarchy a difficulty in the first three years of life, beginning with *one-to-one correspondence* (i.e., counting each object in a set only once, sometimes facilitated by one touch per object), *counting* (i.e., the act of determining the total number of objects in a set or group), *subitizing* (i.e., identifying a number of objects in a set rapidly without counting), and *cardinality* (i.e., the measure of elements of a set). Cardinality is shown by age 3.5 years, hence the oldest age covered by this test (Mix, 2009). As an aside, many Bayley–III items form such a hierarchy. Hence, if a young child passes a more difficult item within such a set (e.g., building a tower of 5 blocks), prior items are afforded automatic credit (e.g., building a tower of 3 blocks). Additionally, many items on the Bayley–III can be scored by means of incidental observation (e.g., screwing the lid on a jar or pretending to feed a doll during free play, both of which are actual items). These aspects improve test utility because not all items must be formally given, hence curtailing administration time.

LANGUAGE SCALE

Language is a communication system in which a limited number of signals (i.e., sounds, letters, gestures) can be integrated according to rules, which are capable of generating an infinite number of messages. To master English, for example, one must learn a sound-symbol system. Language is believed to be vital to an individual's development because it permits one to communicate with others. Furthermore, analogous to the Cognitive Scale items, increases in language and communication skills are accompanied by concomitant advances in cognitive development (Hoff, 2014).

The Bayley–III measures both receptive and expressive language in separate subtests because they are thought to require different abilities that develop independently of each other. The Receptive Communication subtest begins with items that measure auditory acuity (i.e., sharpness in discerning sounds), including responding to a person's voice, and discriminating and localizing sounds (Clifton, Rochat, Robin, & Berthier, 1994; Litovsky & Ashmead, 1997). Later items measure the ability to comprehend and respond appropriately to words and requests. Language comprehension precedes language production by several months, including a receptive vocabulary of about 50 words at 12 months (Bates et al., 1988; Chapman, 2000; Oviatt, 1980). It is important to note that these items are administered in the absence of contextual cues as these can spuriously increase the young child's true receptive vocabulary.

As stated prior, Expressive Communication items are listed in a separate subtest and focus on the young examinee's ability to produce language. Although many of the ensuing language abilities are informally assessed during an initial psychological assessment by means of caregiver report, here they are measured more precisely by direct prompting and performance on the part of the examinee; that is, prompting, observation, and scoring are standardized. More specifically, items here begin with basic vocalizations, including *cooing* (i.e., repeated vowels), *babbling* (i.e., single consonant and vowel sounds), and stringing together longer sounds. Later items measure the ability to use single words and subsequently longer and more sophisticated sentences for purposes of communicating with others. For example, infants' the first words are typically objects (i.e., 12 months; Nelson, 1973), which are ensued by actions performed by oneself and then by others (Huttenlocher, Smiley, & Charney, 1983). Thereafter, between the ages of 12 to 24 months, there manifests a quadrupling in the number of words comprehended and produced (Bates et al., 1988; Bloom & Markson, 1998). By age 3 years, children can produce simple sentences (Owen, 2001). Other items in this subtest measure children's ability to combine words and gestures.

MOTOR SCALE

The Bayley–III Motor Scale items generally measure quality of movement, sensory integration, perceptual-motor integration, prehension, and locomotion. The latter two represent basic developmental milestones. Analogous to the Language Scale, the Motor Scale is apportioned into Fine Motor and Gross Motor subtests as these represent sufficiently independent abilities. *Gross motor skills* collectively include whole-body movements that are controlled by large muscles in the torso, arms, and legs, while *fine motor skills* refer to small muscle movements in the hands and wrists. Consistent with the *cephalocaudal* (i.e., head to toe) and *proximodistal* (i.e., from near-to-far or from inward to the outward periphery) principles of development, gross motor skills tend to precede fine motor skills (e.g., children can run before they can write their names).

Fine Motor subtest items in part measure coordination and control of eye movements as they become more controlled and accurate with age (Aslin & Salapatek, 1975). Infants can track slow-moving objects at 2 months (Dayton & Jones, 1964), and more rapidly moving objects from 2 to 4 months (Aslin, 1981). Reaching and grasping become more controlled with increasing age (Berk, 1998). Newborns generally swipe or swing their arms toward objects, although rarely make contact (Bertenthal & Clifton, 1998), ensued by more intentional reaching at 3 to 4 months and successful reaching for moving objects at 5 months (Robin, Berthier, & Clifton, 1996). Grasping objects also follows a measurable trend by Bayley–III items. Specifically, infants use a whole hand grasp by 3 to 4 months (Bertenthal & Clifton, 1998). By 5 months, they can hold and transfer objects from hand to hand (Rochat & Goubet, 1995). By 12 months, infants can grasp small objects between the thumb and opposing forefinger.

The Gross Motor subtest items measure head control, trunk control, locomotion, and motor planning. Many of these items measure various milestones in motor development, including the development of locomotion that has been well researched. Examples include movement to prone (e.g., rolls from back to stomach), sitting (e.g., sits without support), precursors to walking (e.g., moves from sitting to hands and knees, stands alone), and walking (e.g., walks backward two steps). Because the quality of a child's movement has been shown to be a reliable indicator of motor dysfunction (Bly, 1983; DeGangi, Berk, & Valvano, 1983), this facet can be gauged using the Behavior Observation Inventory and Developmental Risk Indicators as part of the Bayley–III (see Bayley–III, 2006b, Appendix B).

SOCIAL-EMOTIONAL SCALE

The Social-Emotional Scale is to be completed by the child's primary caregiver and is designed to measure *functional emotional milestones (FEMS)*, which are also known as *functional emotional developmental capacities (FEDCS)* (Interdisciplinary Council on Development and Learning Disorders [IDCLD], 2000). FEMS are defined as fundamental affective patterns that represent healthy psychological adjustment and provide purpose to an array of mental processes. Generally, they consist of the following abilities: (a) to engage in a variety of emotions (e.g., happiness, sadness); (b) to experience, express, and understand a broad range of emotional signals (e.g., smiling); and (c) to expound upon feelings using words and symbols (e.g., engaging in pretend play).

The Bayley–III Social-Emotional Scale was founded upon the *Greenspan Social-Emotional Growth Chart: A Screening Questionnaire for Infants and Young Children* (Greenspan, 2004). This growth chart delineates the functional emotional milestones identified by Greenspan, including six stages (or capacities) for children from birth through 42 months, which not coincidently mirrors the age range of the Bayley–III standardization sample. They are depicted in Table 6.1. Each stage or capacity is associated with an age-range within which they are most characteristically mastered. Those presented in Table 6.1 are based upon more contemporary evidence garnered subsequent to the publication of the Bayley–III. It is important to emphasize that these milestones are distinct from the mere development of emotions (e.g., happiness, sadness, surprise) in that they are much more implicated in children's psychological adjustment and ability to adapt (Greenspan & Shanker, 2004; Greenspan, 1997, 1989; Greenspan, DeGangi, & Wieder, 2001). Although some items in the Social-Emotional Scale address selected sensory processing patterns, which have been shown to impact children's emotional functioning, there are much more thorough measures of this construct available in the selected inventory (see Table 1.1 and Chapter 10). Hence, they will not be further discussed here.

ADAPTIVE BEHAVIOR SCALE

Analogous to the prior scale, the Bayley–III Adaptive Behavior Scale was founded upon the *Adaptive Behavior System, Second Edition (ABAS–II;* Harrison & Oakland, 2003), which incidentally is the predecessor to the next developmental test presented in this chapter; namely, the Adaptive Behavior System, Third Edition (see subsequently). This scale is also observer-based and is designed to measure children's functional skills necessary for attaining increased degrees of autonomy and independence. The items are behavioral in content and focus, and measure what children (a) actually do, and (b) may be able to do on their own (i.e., without assistance). More specifically, *adaptive skills* are defined as, "those practical, everyday skills required for children to function and meet environmental demands,

Table 6.1 Fundamental Emotional Milestones

Stage #	Age Range	Title	Ability
1.	0–3 months	Self-Regulation and Interest in the World	Becoming calm, attentive, and interested in the world.
2.	2–7 months	Engaging and Relating	Displaying positive emotions with primary caregivers; engaging in human relationships.
3.	3–10 months	Purposeful Two-Way Communication	Opening and closing circles of communication; engaging in dialogue.
4.	9–18 months	Complex Communication and Shared Problem Solving	Engaging in a series of interactive emotional signals or gestures to communicate.
5.	18–48 months	Using Symbols and Creating Emotional Ideas	Using symbols or ideas to convey intentions or feelings.
6.	36–54 months	Logical Thinking and Connecting Ideas	Building bridges between ideas

Sources. Adapted from Bayley, N. (2006a). *Bayley Scales of Infant and Toddler Development, Third Edition (Bayley–III): Administrative manual.* Bloomington, MN: Pearson (PsychCorp).; retrieved July 16, 2020 by Interdisciplinary Council on Development and Learning (ICDL), *Functional emotional development.* Bethesda, MD: Author, www.icdl.com/dir/fedcs

Note. Once children master these six milestones, they have the tools for communicating, thinking, and emotional coping, including the ability to distinguish fantasy from reality.

including effectively and independently taking care of oneself and interacting with other people" (Bayley, 2006b, p. 10). The specific scales are presented subsequently.

Norm Reference Samples

Because the Bayley–III is essentially and three-part measure of infant and early childhood development, it consists of as many norm reference samples. They are presented in the same order outlined prior.

Cognitive, Language, and Motor Scales

The Bayley–III standardization sample for the three performance-based scales was selected according to the U.S. Bureau of the Census data garnered in October 2000 (U.S. Bureau of the Census, 2000). The total sample size was 1,700, which consisted of 17 age groups of approximately equal numbers of males and females ranging in age from 16 days to 43 months 15 days. In addition to age, the sample was stratified according to parent education level, race/ethnicity, and geographic region. There were five levels of parental education as follows: 0–8 years; 9–11 years, 12 years; 13–15 years; and 16 years or more. The proportions of Whites, Blacks, Hispanics, Asians, and Other matched the U.S. Census figures within each of the aforementioned age groupings. Lastly, the United States was apportioned into four major regions, including Northeast, South, Midwest, and West. In order to most accurately represent the population of children ages 1 month through 42 months, approximately 10% of the norm reference sample included children with Trisomy 21, cerebral palsy, autism spectrum disorder (ASD), preterm birth, *language disorder*, and at risk for developmental delay.

Social Emotional Scale

As alluded to prior, the Bayley–III Social Emotional Scale employed the Greenspan Social-Emotional Growth Chart standardization data to generate its own norms. The sample consisted of 456 children ranging in age from 15 days to 42 months, once again based upon the U.S. Bureau of the Census data collected in October 2000 (U.S. Bureau of the Census, 2000). The sample had approximately equal numbers of males and females and was stratified according to parent education level, race/ethnicity, and geographic region. Here, there were eight age cohorts as follows: 0–3 months; 4–5 months; 6–9 months; 10–14 months; 15–18 months; 19–24 months; 25–30 months; and 30–42 months. There were four parent education levels, including less than 12 years, 12 years, 13 to 15 years, and 16 years and greater. Race/ethnicity proportions and regions of the country were comparable to those reported for the Bayley–III performance-based scales above.

Adaptive Behavior Scale

The Bayley–III Adaptive Behavior Scale used the standardization sample of the ABAS–II Parent/Primary Caregiver Form, which covered children from birth to 5 years of age. This norm reference sample totaled 1,350 children of approximately equal numbers of males and females, distributed among 13 age groupings as follows: 0–3 months; 4–7 months; 8–11 months; 12–15 months; 16–19 months; 20–23 months; 24–19 months; 30–35 months; 36–41 months; 42–47 months. All age groups had subsamples of 100, with the exception of the oldest including 150. Children older than 42 months were dropped from this sample in order to remain within the age limits of the Bayley–III. Parent educational level, race/ethnicity, and geographic regions were all comparable to those of the former two standardization samples (e.g., there were five parent educational levels ranging from less than 8 years to 16 years and higher).

Administration

The Bayley–III is comprised of five scales, three of which are performance-based and done via individual administration between the examiner and examinee, and two being observer-based and completed by a caregiver via questionnaire format. The former consists of the Cognitive, Language, and Motor Scales while the latter includes the Social-Emotional Scale and Adaptive Behavior Scales in questionnaire format. The two require different administration approaches. First, the individually administered performance-based portion entails a single 2-hour appointment with the testing psychologist to be scheduled at a later date. Second, the questionnaire can be given to the caregiver with instructions regarding completion and submission immediately after the Bayley–III has been selected as part of the test battery and in proximity to the adjournment of the initial assessment. Although this practice may seem somewhat risky considering that Bayley–III administration would technically begin prior to obtaining *preauthorization (PA)* from the examinee's insurance company, recall that this being a developmental test, the appropriate test services codes *Current Procedural Technology (CPT) Code 96112* and *CPT Code 96113* refer to developmental testing, which are routinely approved without PA (see Chapter 3). Therefore. The risk is typically minimal and testing can be initiated rapidly and at a propitious time.

More specifically, as the examinee and family are exiting the office following the initial interview, and with instructions fresh in mind, the caregiver should be asked to complete the questionnaire in in the waiting area with pen and clip board, then submitting the completed form prior to leaving the facility. In this manner, this portion of the Bayley–III is done and can be reviewed for compliance with instructions and even scored time permitting. Generally speaking, this is an auspicious time to ask relevant individuals to complete test-related forms as clients tend to be remarkably motivated at this incipient juncture in the assessment process, just having completed an initial interview with the hope of obtaining valuable answers to diagnostic questions and the opportunity for effective treatment. If there are any problems in the way the form has been completed, they can be easily corrected later in the assessment process (e.g., when the performance-based aspects of the Bayley–III are being administered in a scheduled two-hour session).

Following the aforementioned administration procedure, discussion of Bayley–III administration begins with the observer-based tests, ensued by the individually administered performance-based tests. However, prior to discussing the major Bayley–III scales, computing the examinee's age at testing is delineated because this impacts administration both on this test and all other standardized tests that rely upon age-based norms.

Computing Age at Testing

A unique feature of the Bayley–III is an optional adjustment of children's computed testing age for their estimated degree of prematurity. Upon reflection, this may be a variable worth controlling considering that this type of testing is more proximate to examinees' DOB than the majority of other available standardized psychological tests (see Table 1.1). More specifically, the *Bayley–III adjustment for prematurity age* (CA_{adj}) is simply a second subtraction of the length of prematurity from an examinee's computed *chronological age* (*CA*; see Chapter 3).

Table 6.2 illustrates the steps employed when computing an examinee's CA for purposes of most kinds of standardized testing that relies upon age norms. Hence, this procedure can be generalized to all standardized tests presented in this Part II. The Bayley–III, however, is unique in offering an optional adjustment for an examinee's degree of prematurity. In the hypothetical, the examinee's DOB is 03/15/2019 and she is being tested on 07/18/2020. For the Bayley–III, her resulting CA is presented in two ways. The first uses a years:months:days format (i.e., 1 year, 4 months, and 3 days). This format is the one most frequently espoused by standardized psychological tests that rely upon norms defined principally by age, although without reporting the number of days and without rounding up the months. The second is the months:days format in which the number of years is converted to months and added to the month's column. Here, the child's 1 year is converted to 12 months, which is subsequently added to 4 months and resulting in an age of 16 months 3 days. This is the format most conducive to following age cut-offs and start-points reported in the Bayley–III administrative materials. Remember the computational steps illustrated in Table 6.2 for deriving an examinee's CA as they are generally used by most other standardized tests.

Being a test of early development, however, the Bayley–III goes further in adjusting for an examinee's duration of prematurity, although note that it is not to be used for those older than 24 months (i.e., 2 years) as the effects of prematurity usually dissipate over time and do not require adjustment. In the hypothetical, the child is premature

Table 6.2 Computing Chronological Age (CA) and Chronological Age Adjusted for Prematurity (CA_{adj})

	Years	Months	Days
Date Tested	20	07	18
Date of Birth (DOB)	19	03	15
Chronological Age (CA) (years:months:days)	**01**	**04**	**03**
Chronological Age (CA) (months:days)	—	**16**	**03**
Modified CA for Subtraction	—	15	33
Estimated Duration of Prematurity	—	02	15
CA Adjusted for Prematurity (CA_{adj})[a]	—	**13**	**18**

Note. The hypothetical regards an examinee undergoing standardized testing that relies upon age norms. DOB is March 15, 2019. Date of testing is July 18, 2020. She is estimated to be premature by 2.5 months. For purposes of computation: 1 years = 12 months; 1 month = 30 days. Computed age values are never rounded up. -- = not applicable.

[a] Adjustments for prematurity are reserved for examinees who are of 1 to 24 months CA at testing.

by 2½ months. Considering that each month is 30 days, this child is 2 months and 15 days premature. In order to subtract this from her computed CA of 16 months 3 days, 1 month had to be converted to 30 days and added to the day's column, resulting in 15 months 33 days (CA) minus 2 months 15 days (prematurity duration), which ultimately equals 13 months 18 days. It is the discretion of the examiner as to which group this child should be compared, including either (a) those with whom she was born (i.e., her CA at 15 months 33 days), or (b) those with whom she shares the same biological gestation age (i.e., her CA_{adj} at 13 months 18 days). The manual advises using the latter as these are the child's true peers. After 24 months or 2 years, this issue becomes moot and only the CA is employed both on the Bayley–III and all other standardized tests that are normed on the basis of age cohorts.

Social-Emotional and Adaptive Behavior Questionnaire

As the name indicates, the *Social-Emotional and Adaptive Behavior Questionnaire* consists of both of these scales in one booklet and in such order. The questionnaire is to be completed only by caregivers who are reasonably familiar with the child, which is typically one or both parents together or parent surrogates. The Social-Emotional Scale instructions indicate to respondents that this measure's objective is to learn how their children interact with them according to how they meet certain social-emotional milestones. For each item, they are to indicate how often they observe the behavior as described in declarative statements as follows: 0 = *Can't tell*; 1 = *None of the time*; 2 = *Some of the time*; 3 = *Half the time*; 4 = *Most of the time*; and 5 = *All of the time*. There is a grand total of 35 items ordered by increasing levels of sophistication, which generally require less than 10 to 15 minutes' administration time for the entire measure. However, stop points are indicated among the sequence of items, including 0 to 3 months, 4 to 5 months, 6 to 9 months, 10 to 14 months, 15 to 18 months, 19 to 24 months, 25 to 30 months, and 31 to 42 months. Therefore, respondents are to complete items until they reach the appropriate stop point associated with their child's age. As such, administration time can vary depending upon the child's CA, with lesser times associated with younger age examinees.

The Adaptive Behavior Scale immediately follows the Social-Emotional Scale as being part of the same booklet. This scale is self-described as measuring what daily skills their children display that help them adapt in various real-world environments, including home, school, and other settings. In total, the scale addresses ten skill areas, including Communication, Community Use, Functional Pre-Academics, Home Living, Health and Safety, Leisure, Self-Care, Self-Direction, Social, and Motor. Only seven of these apply to examinees younger than 12 months whereas all 10 apply to older children. Respondents are to rate their children in terms of how often they correctly perform each behavior when it is needed as follows: 0 = *Is Not Able*; 1 = *Never or Almost Never When Needed*; 2 = *Sometimes When Needed*; and 3 = *Always or Almost Always When Needed*. Items are again ordered by increasing levels of difficulty, although here there are no stop points. Rather, the respondent is cautioned that some items may be excessively easy or difficult but to continue to rate all of them as instructed.

Next to each item, there is a *Check if you guessed* box, which should be marked if the rating is estimated, never observed in the proper circumstance, or the behavior has never had an opportunity to be demonstrated. More than two guesses per skill area requires the examiner to prompt the respondent to resolve the estimate, otherwise the score is deemed questionably valid and in need of supporting independent evidence. Because the form is asked to be completed immediately after the initial assessment, an opportunity for resolution is made possible either the day it is completed or, more commonly, prior to or immediately after the performance-based portion of the Bayley–III has been administered. The ten subscales range from 22 to 27 items totaling 241 in all. There are no stop points, thus all items are to be completed within a subscale. Because the items are shorter in length than the Social-Emotional Scale, they can be completely in less time. Based upon clinical experience with parents, the ten subscales take about 20 minutes to complete, hence about 30 to 45 minutes for the entire questionnaire (less time for children younger than 12 months).

Cognitive, Language, and Motor Scales

The Cognitive, Language, and Motor Scales, are all individually administered. This includes the Receptive and Expressive Communication subtests that comprise the Language Scale, and the Fine and Gross Motor subtests that comprise the Motor Scale. The most efficacious arrangement during administration consists of the examiner, child, and one of the primary caregivers in the assessment room, along with the test stimulus materials arranged in an organized manner such that they are easily found and accessible yet hidden from the child's view to prevent distraction.

Developmental test items contain some features that require some adaptation on the part of the examiner who may be more accustomed to traditional psychological testing, including some disadvantages and some advantages. On the one hand, each item typically requires an increased quantity of stimulus materials (e.g., set of different colored pegs and a peg board), more time to set up, added prompts to elicit a scorable response, and perhaps above all patience. On the other hand, some items can be counted when a child shows scorable responses spontaneously in free play, when a more difficult item in a series is observed thus automatically crediting all easier forms and being able to score responses elicited by the caretaker according to directions. The latter facets together exemplify the flexibility that is incorporated into the Bayley–III test design. Additionally, the Record Form summarizes each item's key features, the needed materials, and the scoring criteria.

Each of these scales and subtests have strict start points, reversal rules, and discontinue rules designed to abbreviate administration time and administer items most likely to be within the young child's capabilities. This also maintains the child's interest and motivation by averting the administration of items that are excessively difficult or easy. Items are ordered by increasing levels of difficulty. Start points are set by using either the computed CA or CA_{adj} for those 24 months and younger (see Table 6.2). If the child fails any of the first three items given from the start point, the examiner is to reverse to the prior set point and move forward from there and in the same manner. Thus, the examiner must keep reversing back to prior set points until the child passes the first three items, then moving forward from that point. A scale or subtest is discontinued when the examinee fails five consecutive items, after which it is assumed that no more items would be passed.

Administration time varies depending upon the examinee's age and extent of developmental delays. The reported average time to complete this portion of the Bayley–III is 50-minutes for examinees younger than 12 months and 90 minutes for those 12 through 42 months (Leaders Project, 2013).

Scoring

The Bayley–III yields an impressive quantity of data and hence potential types of analyses. The ones that are presented subsequently are most useful in terms of diagnosis and treatment planning for this age group in mental health practice. This test comes with the *Bayley Scales of Infant Development, Third Edition, Scoring Assistant* (Pearson, 2006), which is an unlimited scoring software CD ROM. It is indispensable in transforming raw scores into all of the various standard scores to be reviewed subsequently. It is one of the few remaining unlimited scoring programs published by Pearson as they have transitioned to internet scoring, along with charging per requested score or interpretive report.

Form 6.1a includes all of the data tables employed when scoring and reporting the relevant Bayley–III output. It is used as a point of reference throughout the next two sections on Bayley–III scoring and interpretation. In delineating the Bayley–III data tables, the discussion is apportioned into (a) reporting the examinee's age at testing, (b) primary data analysis, (c) secondary data analysis, and (d) tertiary data analysis. This scheme is analogous to reporting the results of an empirical study and provides a familiar and convenient framework.

Reporting the Examinee's Testing Age

Prior to the first data table there are entries that indicate whether an age adjustment for prematurity has to be done and, if so, what the adjusted age is in months and days. The CA of the child is reported at the beginning of the final report and does not need to be repeated here as it is redundant. In the event an adjusted age was not employed, the examiner retains the "no" alternative and deletes the adjusted age line or may simply delete both lines; the latter choice especially if the child is older than 24 months such that the adjusted age is summarily precluded.

Primary Data Analysis

Table 1 (Form 6.1a) presents the data for the five principal scales. In order, the six columns include the scale name, composite score, 95% confidence interval (CI), percentile rank (PR), qualitative description, and a synopsis of the abilities measured by each scale. The composite score metric is the same as that used by major intelligence tests (i.e., mean = 100, standard deviation = 15; range 40–160; see also Chapter 11), hence permitting direct comparisons between developmental and IQ scores especially if a child happens to be retested when older to determine response to treatment or progression. Although the 90% CI as a more felicitous balance between confidence and precision (see Wechsler, 1975), the 95% confidence is employed here to be consistent with the subtest scaled scores where this must be estimated manually (see Form 6.1a, Table 2). In cases where the subtest scores are not reported (i.e., Form 6.1a, Tables 2 & 3), the software can be programmed to compute 90% Cis to be inserted into Table 1. The software computes PRs based upon the theoretical standard normal curve, hence this fact is reported in a specific table note. These are included because they are easier for laypeople to interpret when reading the report.

Qualitative descriptions are nominal categories that facilitate test interpretation. Although the software reports these automatically, a convenient table is provided that associates both composite score and scaled score ranges with (a) standard deviation ranges from the mean, and, most significantly here, (b) qualitative descriptions suggested by the technical manual (Bayley, 2006b, pp. 113, 114). The final column presents a succinct description of the abilities measured by a particular scale to facilitate interpretation. Notice that selected target words are italicized and defined in a specific table note to further assist test interpretation and for the reader (see also subsequently).

Table 1 (Form 6.1a) notes define all abbreviations reported in the table, provide composite score metrics, and denotes which scales are performance-based, observer-based, and derived from a single subtest score. The latter are referred to as *composite equivalent scores* because the single subtest scaled score is converted directly into a composite score metric by means of linear transformation (i.e., a simple conversion of units). Hence, The Cognitive Scale and Social-Emotional Scale are technically subtest scores that are converted into composite scores via linear transformation. Finally, there is a symbol (i.e., "—") for scores that are not reported for various reasons, including such reasons as invalid administration. This symbol is routinely used in these test data tables. Also note that after each table, the word interpretative in italics appears underneath where excerpts appear that guide test interpretation.

Secondary Data Analysis

Tables 2 and 3 (see Form 6.1a) provide the data for the Language and Motor subtests, both of which contribute to their respective composite scores reported in Table 1.[1] The tables are designed in analogous fashion to the composite score data table, including subtest name, scaled score, 95% CI, theoretical PR, qualitative description, and a summary of measured abilities. Scaled scores have a mean of 10 and standard deviation of 3 (range 1–19). Neither the software scoring assistant nor the manual provide Cis, PRs, or qualitative descriptions for these subtest scaled scores directly. Thus, added investigation was needed in order to include these important scores in the data tables.

In order to compute the desired Cis, the stability coefficients reported in the technical manual for both the Language and Motor subtests were found and their standard errors of measurement (*SEM*) were computed using the formula $SEM = SD\sqrt{1 - r_{xx}}$, where r_{xx} is the average stability coefficient, and *SD* is 3 (see, e.g., Furr, 2018, p. 127, equation 5.16). Rounding to the nearest whole number, both were 1. Hence, to manually estimate the 95% confidence band, the examiner merely needs to add and subtract 2 *SEM*s from the obtained score, which is explained in the table notes. This kind of *SEM* estimation is done when other standardized tests in this Part II do not report the needed *SEM*s to permit the reporting of Cis. This is a critical part of test interpretation as it (a) indicates relative differences (i.e., ipsative analyses) within an examinee's protocol rapidly and efficiently, and (b) correctly recognizes error in measurement.

Concerning the PRs, the Bayley–III technical manual affords a listing of composite scores associated with both scaled scores and PRs, the latter according to the theoretical standard normal distribution (Bayley, 2006b, Table 6.1, p. 109). The scaled scores and their associated PRs are listed in an adapted table (see Table 6.3). The examiner

Table 6.3 Composite/Standard Score to Scaled Score to Percentile Rank Conversion Guide

Composite/ Standard Score	Scaled Score	Percentile Rank
145	19	99.9
140	18	99.6
135	17	99
130	16	98
125	15	95
120	14	91
115	13	84
110	12	75
105	11	63
100	10	50
95	9	37
90	8	25
85	7	16
80	6	9
75	5	5
70	4	2
65	3	1
60	2	0.4
55	1	0.1

Source. Adapted from Bayley, N. (2006b). *Bayley Scales of Infant Development, Third Edition (Bayley–III): Technical manual.* San Antonio, Texas: The Psychological Corporation-Pearson, Table 6.1, p. 109.

Note. Composite/Standard score mean = 100, standard deviation = 15; scaled score mean = 10, standard deviation = 3; percentile rank (PR) median = 50; range = 1–99. PRs are based upon the theoretical standard normal distribution.

Table 6.4a Bayley Scales of Infant and Toddler Development, Third Edition (Bayley–III) Qualitative Description Classification Guide

Composite (equivalent) Scores	Scaled Scores	SDs from the Mean	Qualitative Description
130 to 160	16 to 19	+2 to +4	Very superior
120 to 129	14 to 15	+1⅓ to +1⅔	Very high
110 to 119	12 to 13	+⅔ to +1	High average
90 to 109	8 to 11	−⅔ to +⅓	Average
80 to 89	6 to 7	−1⅓ to−1	Low average
70 to 79	4 to 5	−2 to−1⅔	Borderline
40 to 69	1 to 3	−3 to−2⅓	Extremely low

Source. Adapted from Bayley, N. (2006b). *Bayley Scales of Infant Development, Third Edition (Bayley–III): Technical manual.* San Antonio, Texas: The Psychological Corporation-Pearson, Inc., Tables 6.1, p. 109, 6.2 and 6.3, p. 113, & 6.4, p. 114.

Note. *SDs* = standard deviations.

merely references this table to locate the scaled score and the associated PR. If this table is for some reason temporarily inaccessible, the examiner can also reference Table A.1 (see Appendix A), which also provides this information although in a less efficient manner because it entails some estimation; that is, because PRs are more discriminating in one-hundredths of a unit (i.e., a *centile*), the same scaled score is associated with a range of PRs, thus requiring the examiner to find the PR that falls at the approximate center of the list of such scaled scores.[2] In terms of providing qualitative descriptions for the scaled scores, the examiner may reference Table 6.4a, which associates the scaled score ranges with the appropriate qualitative descriptions. Finally, the measured abilities incorporate key developmental concepts, which are defined in terse manner in specific tabular notes.

Table 4 (Form 6.1a) provides a scale score summary of all 10 adaptive behavior subtests that contribute to the Adaptive Behavior Composite reported in Table 1. The table is designed as a mirror image of Tables 2 and 3 as they are on the exact same metric, including scaled scores, Cis, PRs, qualitative descriptions, and succinctly defined measured abilities. For purposes of manually computing the 95% Cis, which again is not provided by the scoring software, the *SEM* was computed in similar fashion, here inputting into the aforementioned formula the average of all ten subtests' stability coefficients, resulting in a somewhat larger *SEM* of 2. This is not surprising in that the coefficients are based upon untrained laypersons' ratings of observed behavior. Here, the examiner adds and subtracts 4 points (i.e., 2 *SEMs*) to the obtained score for the 95% CI. The *SEM* and its computation method is entered into a specific table note. Also signified in a specific table note are the three subtests that are not administered to children younger than 12 months.

Tertiary Data Analysis

Finally, Table 5 (Form 6.1a) provides a formal statistical analysis of relative differences between all pairwise comparisons of subtest scores, there being 15 in total. This table consists of six columns, including the subtest comparison names, score for the first listed name, score for the second listed name, the computed difference (i.e., 1st listed score minus 2nd listed score), the critical value i.e., (the difference score) that occurred in the norm reference sample at a 5% rate, and the base rate. The critical value deserves some elaboration because it entails hypothesis testing. Here, the critical value is the difference between the listed scores that occurred at a 5% rate in the norm reference sample. This is denoted by the .05 that follows the label "Critical value," which is the heading for this column. Therefore, if the obtained difference score equals or exceeds the listed critical value difference score, this means that it occurs only 5% or less of the time assuming a true null hypothesis of no significant difference. This is of sufficiently low probability to reject the null hypothesis of no difference. In such case, an asterisk is appended to the obtained difference score in the table and the pertinent subtest scores are interpreted to be meaningfully discrepant.

Some may consider not reporting the critical value and simply report whether or not the obtained difference was significant. If so, the critical value column can be deleted. However, that critical value difference score is preferred because (a) the reader can determine the degree of difference between the obtained difference score and the difference showing statistical significance (which is especially important considering the dichotomous decision inherent in hypothesis testing), and (b) it represents an exercise in proofreading for the examiner. When reporting so many numbers, it becomes increasingly likely that an error will be made. Therefore, actually reporting the critical value vis-à-vis or juxtaposed with the obtained difference is an effective "double-check" on the report.

Finally, the base rate of the obtained difference is much easier to comprehend. It is essentially the percentage of the norm reference sample that obtained such a difference. Of course, the norm reference sample represents the population of the examinee's same-aged peers. According to the technical manual, anything lower than 10% is considered abnormal (Bayley, 2006b). However, this is a more complex and debatable issue, as will become apparent in the sections that follow.

Interpretation

Interpretation should generally proceed according to the order of tables in Form 6.1a. Further, interpretation should follow each table independently. This is denoted by an italicized heading, "Interpretation," followed by a series of narrative excerpts designed to guide the examiner through the interpretation, moving from general to increasingly specific. The interpretation of data in subsequent tables may integrate those from previous tables in an orderly sequence. However, the data in the immediate table are to be afforded precedence. If the examinee is (a) younger than 24 months, and (b) the result of a premature delivery, the CA_{adj} should be selected for purposes of transforming raw scores into standard scores. Of course, to be consistent, this same age should have been employed during administration in determining start and stop points. The chief analyses regard a comparison of the examinee with same-aged peers; that is, norms-based comparisons. Therefore, the composite scores in Table 1 (Form 6.1a) initiate the interpretation process.

Composite Score Summary

The Cognitive and Social-Emotional composites both measure a single construct and are not the outcome of two or more subtests. Therefore, their composite (i.e., equivalent) scores, CIs, PRs, and qualitative descriptions represent the primary focus. In contrast, the Language, Motor, and General Adaptive Behavior data are true composite scores and are based upon a series of subtest scores, especially the latter. Therefore, if any of these show extremely low scores, the subtests that contributed to that composite should be reported, analyzed, and interpreted. In contrast, if these scales are all measured to be within normal limits, then reporting the subtest scores may not be needed. Specifically, if scrutiny of the subtest scores also show (a) an absence of impairment, and (b) remarkable CI overlap, then the examiner can save time and space in the report by simply noting in the Table 1 interpretation that the composite is measured to be within normal limits and is an accurate measure of that overall ability. Borderline composite scores can be interpreted as indicating a risk of impairment in that area of functioning in the future, which should be ensued by a reporting of the subtest scores to show which were responsible for lowering the composite. The PRs are most apposite in communicating the results to laypersons. However, the examiner must recall that PRs exaggerate differences in the middle of the distribution and minimize those in the extremes.

The narrative excerpts following Table 1 first regard the performance-based data, then proceed to the observer-based results. The interpretive process moves from norm-based comparisons, highlighting overall functioning as indicated by the qualitative descriptions, then examining whether the profile indicates or rules out any developmental delays or disorders. If so, then there is an option to recommend further analysis of the subtest results for a more detailed investigation of delays or problems.

Next, ipsative analysis of Table 1 data can be done by comparing the degree of overlap or separation among the CIs. Care must be taken here not to prematurely conclude that there is no meaningful difference between any two composite scores. Recall that these are 95% CIs, which can lead to false negative decisions due to the imprecision that accompanies such a high degree of confidence (i.e., concluding that there is no difference when there exists one in reality). Certainly, if there is no overlap between two composites, this would indicate the need for a more formal subtest scaled score discrepancy analysis (see Table 5, Form 6.1a). On the other hand, the testing referral might not need such an in-depth analysis of relative differences. If diagnosis is all that is being requested, then the norm-based analysis is sufficient with a discretionary brief ipsative analysis using the CIs.

Subtest Scaled Score Summary

Tables 2, 3, and 4 (Form 6.1a) present the subtests that contribute to the true composite scores Language, Motor, and Adaptive Behavior. Notice that they are in the same sequence as they appear in Table 1 (Form 6.1a). Because these tables mirror the design of Table 1, they are to be analyzed in similar manner beginning with norm-based comparisons; that is, how the examinee compares to same-aged peers. The only difference is that the subtests use a scaled score metric (mean = 10, standard deviation = 3; range = 1–19), which is smaller, with less variability, and with less discriminatory capability. Fortunately, the remainder of the analysis is the same. During the normative analysis, it should be noted which subtest had the greatest Impact upon the associated composite score, which would generally be more extreme high or low score, operationally defined as one or more standard deviations from the mean. Each of the tables including subtest data have their own interpretive excerpts that are designed to guide the examiner through the process. Each begins with an analysis of where the subtests generally fall in terms of descriptive category, then determining if there are any low scores or weaknesses. Thus, the first considerations are norm based.

Next, ipsative analysis can be done by examining the degree of overlap among the 95% cIs. For Language and Motor subtests, this is straightforward considering that there are only two subtests to compare. Again, if diagnosis is all that is being requested, CI comparisons are sufficient. However, if added detail is being sought concerning treatment recommendations, more formal discrepancy analyses are required. A follow-up narrative excerpt is drafted for ipsative comparisons, noting whether there is overlap or separation among the cIs. If there is separation, then the focus is on identifying weaknesses as these require the greatest need for intervention.

Subtest Scaled Score Discrepancies

Table 5 (Form 6.1a) is strictly designed for formal ipsative analyses, which are primarily employed for facilitating specific treatment recommendations. That is, the data analyses here are intended to detect an examinee's relative strengths and weaknesses in order to (a) target interventions for those areas most in need of improvement, while (b) exploiting an examinee's areas of achievement and growth as a catalyst for treatment progress. The first four columns in Table 5 are descriptive and show (a) which two subtests are being compared, (b) the direction the subtraction, and (c) the resulting difference score with directional sign (i.e., + or –). However, it is the final two columns of data in Table 5 that are essential to interpretation.

The critical value column sets the criteria for determining whether chance can be ruled out as an explanation for the obtained difference. The Bayley–III offers two criteria, including .05 and .15. The former requires that the obtained difference occurs less than 5 times in 100 by chance to consider it a meaningful difference whereas the latter requires a 15 times in 100 chance. This means that for any one decision, there is a 5% and 15% chance of making a wrong decision. However, if an examiner makes all 15 pairwise comparisons in Table 5, this increases the chance of making at least one wrong decision by approximately 15 times. This is referred to as the *familywise* or *experiment-wise* error rate (see, e.g., Howell, 2014; Gravetter & Wallnau, 2017; Warner, 2021). Such mistakes in judgment are technically termed *Type I errors* (Howell, 2014; Gravetter & Wallnau, 2017; Warner, 2021), and result in claims that there are meaningful effects or differences when in fact this is not the case. Because this can result in unnecessary or poorly designed treatment, such Type I errors can have a deleterious effect in mental health practitioners' attitude towards psychological testing.

Two points are to be made here, both of which focus on minimizing this decision-making error rate. First, in such circumstances it is prudent to use the more conservative critical value offered by a standardized test, such as here using .05 with the Bayley–III. Second, make only those comparisons that are absolutely vital. The latter supports the rationale for initially making relative comparisons in the previous tables using the CI column. The gist here is that Table 5 pairwise comparisons should be done judiciously. Comparisons should be limited to those most crucial for treatment planning and intervention. Therefore, it should be rare that all pairwise comparisons in Table 5 are employed.

For those comparisons that are indicated, the first analysis is whether no not the critical value has been reached or surpassed. If not, the analysis ends because the obtained difference could have resulted merely by chance factors. This renders the ensuing base rate moot. If, on the other hand, the difference is deemed to be statistically significant, then the discrepancy is meaningful as being beyond chance factors. *Base rate* is the percent of time that the obtained difference occurred in the norm reference sample, which represents the population of same-aged peers. This datum represents a more practical *effect size* estimate in that it illustrates how often an event or outcome occurs in a representative normal population. There is debate as to how low a base rate should be in order to interpret it as "abnormal" or an "aberrant" event or outcome. Many experts believe it should be based upon case facts and clinical judgment.

For example, the Bayley–III technical manual states as follows: "Users must decide what level of occurrence can be considered rare. This decision depends on clinical judgement, the purpose of assessment, and the degree of risk the user is willing to assume" (Bayley, 2006b, p. 119). However, it is convenient to have a more particular criterion. In researching recommendations as to such a standard, Sattler (2001) initially advised using a base rate of 10% and lower as representing a large effect and thus being, "abnormal." Later, Sattler (Sattler, 2014; Sattler & Ryan, 2009) added to this position somewhat and suggested that a 15% base rate can be considered "unusual," whereas the most conservative 5% base rate can be considered a "rarity." Therefore, these three criteria are entered into a specific table note as a reminder to the examiner that all three may be used together as a continuum or degree of aberration rather than a dichotomous decision and denoted as follows: $n \leq 15\%$ = unusual; $n \leq 10\%$ = abnormal; and $n \leq 5\%$ = rare and profoundly abnormal. This seems to be a most effective balance between clarity of decision-making and flexibility in diagnostic practice. To facilitate this analysis, narrative excerpts are inserted. The first describes results that show an absence of significant differences. The ensuing excerpt is designed to list the significant differences along with their effect sizes in parentheticals.

Bayley Scales of Infant and Toddler Development, Fourth Edition

Synopsis

The *Bayley Scales of Infant and Toddler Development, Fourth Edition* (*Bayley–4*; Bayley & Aylward, 2019a, 2019b) is an individually administered test that measures the developmental functioning of both infants and young children from ages 1 months to 42 months. Hence, it covers the exact age range as does the Bayley–III. The cardinal objective of the Bayley–4 is to detect the presence and degree of developmental delays (or deficits) in this young population, which again remains consistent with that of the Bayley–III.

In identifying developmental delays, the Bayley–4 incorporates the following associated components: (a) administration of standardized test items (e.g., problem solving, stacking blocks); (b) direct observation of behaviors and developmental milestones; and (c) the active involvement of the primary caregiver in item administration, the provision of pertinent historical information, and behavioral ratings (Aylward, 2018; Bagnato, Neisworth, & Pretti-Frontczak, 2010).

Test Structure

The overall test structure is virtually identical to that of the Bayley–III, although there are some modifications at the item level that bear identifying. First, the Bayley–4 consists of three performance-based scales whose items are found in the Administrative Manual (Bayley & Aylward, 2019a) and Record Form as follows: (a) Cognitive; (b) Language; and (c) Motor. The Cognitive Scale is comprised of only one subtest, while the latter two are dichotomized into two subtests. In particular, the Language Scale contains both the Receptive Communication and Expressive Communication subtests, while the Motor Scale is apportioned into the Fine Motor and Gross Motor subtests. Second, the Bayley–4 is also comprised of two observer-report measures that are administered by means of the *Social-Emotional and Adaptive Behavior Questionnaire*. Similarities and modifications to the Bayley–4 content are summarized next such that its data yield can be interpreted accurately. The ensuing sections begin with the three performance-based scales followed by the two observer-based scales.

Cognitive Scale

The information processing tasks from the previous edition are largely continued in the Bayley–4, such as novelty preference, habituation, memory, anticipation of patterns, and reaction time. This is because such abilities correlate best with later intelligence test scores (Rose, Feldman, Jankowski, & Van Rossem, 2012), and also *executive functioning* measures (Carlson, 2005; Cuevas & Bell, 2014; Turk-Brown, Scholl, & Chun, 2008). Also similar to the Bayley–III are items that measure play (Thibodeau, Gilpin, Brown, & Meyer, 2016; Yogman et al., 2018) and quantitative reasoning, including one-to-one correspondence, stable number order, and cardinality (Geary & vanMarie, 2018; Izard, Streri, & Spelke, 2014).

In terms of modifications, the measurement of processing speed has been augmented by including more timed tasks, due to evidence that this ability is highly related to young children's underlying neurological maturation, learning, and executive functioning (Cohen et al., 2016). The measurement of higher-order problem-solving has also been bolstered, which involves reasoning, memory, and especially synthesis of information (Aylward, 1988, 2009; Grieiff et al., 2015). Finally, some items from the Bayley–III have been either deleted or combined to reduce redundancy and the duration of administration.

Language Scale

As stated prior, the Language Scale is comprised of Receptive Communication and Expressive Communication subtests, although items are added to more directly measure communication developmental milestones in this area (e.g., estimated percentage of intelligible speech production). More specifically, the Receptive Communication subtest measures the comprehension of nonverbal communication, vocabulary development, morphological development (e.g., understanding the use of pronouns), grasping morphological markers (e.g., tenses and possessives), social referencing (i.e., the ability to use an adult's affective reactions in order to regulate one's own emotions and behaviors), and verbal comprehension. This is especially important during the first year of life when infants should be becoming attuned to patterns and rhythms of speech, including the ability to respond to words and short phrases at 9 months, and a vocabulary of about 50 words at age 12 months (Pence Turnbull & Justice, 2017).

The Expressive Communication subtest continues to focus measurement upon preverbal communication (including especially babbling, gesturing, turn-taking, and joint referencing), vocabulary development, (e.g., naming objects and attributes, such as colors and size), and syntactic (i.e., word order) and morphological (i.e., word form) development. Such preverbal abilities are vital because they facilitate the phonological learning of our sound-symbol language system (Goldstein & Schwade, 2008). Note that some of these measured language skills help detect both communication disorders (e.g., language disorder; *social pragmatic communication disorder*, and autism spectrum disorder). Although the Bayley–III items are comparable, the Bayley–4 items are more pertinent to detecting signs of autism and certainly relate to many of the developmental milestones covered in the initial psychological assessment forms (see Chapter 3, Forms 3.3–3.5). As in the Cognitive Scale, some items from the Bayley–III were deleted and/or combined to avoid redundancy. Other items were added to expand the age range on this scale.

Motor Scale

The Bayley–4 Motor Scale also continues to consist of two subtests, including the Fine Motor and Gross Motor versions. In contrast to the Bayley–III, however, the Bayley–4 contains newer items that relate to neurodevelopmental functioning; that is, the gradual increase of upper brain control over lower brain centers (Amiel-Tison & Gosselin, 2008; Aylward, 2010). This line of development refers to the increase of cortical control by the cerebral hemispheres and basal ganglia over the more primitive brainstem and cerebellum. More specifically, the Fine Motor subtest measures prehension (i.e., the ability to grasp and seize), perceptual-motor integration (e.g., object manipulation), motor planning (e.g., reaching), and motor speed (e.g., visual tracking). The Gross Motor subtest measures *proximal stability* and the movement of both the limbs and torso, including static positioning (e.g., sitting, standing) and dynamic movement (e.g., locomotion, coordination, balance, motor planning). Here, new items are added to measure neurodevelopmental functioning (e.g., integration of reflexes), and other items from the Bayley–III were deleted or combined to reduce redundancy, shorten test duration, and integrate a polytomous scoring model (see subsequently). As in the Language Scale, items are also added to expand the age range on this scale.

Social-Emotional Scale

The Social-Emotional Scale is again a modification of the aforementioned Greenspan Social-Emotional Growth Chart: A Screening Questionnaire for Infants and Young Children (Greenspan, 2004). It is designed in the exact manner as in the Bayley–III; namely, to measure attainment of the major social and emotional developmental milestones in this young population. Of particular focus are functional emotional skills, including self-regulation, interest in the world, communicating needs, engaging with people and establishing relationships, employing emotions effectively, and using emotional signals and gestures to resolve problems. The items, response format, and instructions are virtually identical to that found in the Bayley–III version. Hence, no further comments here are needed.

Adaptive Behavior Scale

Finally, although the Adaptive Behavior Scale content and focus has remained essentially the same as in the Bayley–III, it has borrowed items from an alternative measure; that is, the Vineland Adaptive Behavior Scales, Third Edition (Vineland–3; Sparrow et al., 2016), which is reviewed in its entirety later in this chapter. in consequence, this aspect of the Bayley–4 measures overall adaptive behavior according to the organizational structure of the Vineland–3, which, in addition to offering more updated norms, is somewhat different in content than that of the ABAS–II (Harrison & Oakland, 2003). Specifically, the Bayley–4 Adaptive Behavior Scale consists of the following domains and subdomains (the latter in parentheses): (a) Communication (Receptive and Expressive); (b) Daily Living Skills (Personal); and (c) Socialization (Interpersonal Relationships, and Play and Leisure). Finally, the three domains contribute to a General Adaptive Behavior Scale score, which represents the examinee's overall adaptive behavior functioning.

Summary

The purpose of this section was to (a) provide an overview of the structural organization of the Bayley–4, (b) compare and contrast it to the Bayley–III; and (c) highlight some item-level changes and modifications to the adaptive behavior scale. Because of the great deal of similarity between the two editions, the remaining sections proceed directly into the updated standardization sample, some changes in administration that affect scoring, the data yield, and interpretation of the Bayley–4 scores by presenting the test data tables that have been prepared for reporting results from this measure within a developmental or psychological assessment report. Additionally, a flowchart has been prepared that outlines interpretation of the Bayley–4 (which can also be applied to the Bayley–III with some modifications).

Norm Reference Sample

The standardization sample for the performance-based Cognitive, Language, and Motor Scales consisted of 1,700 children, ranging in age from ages 1 month to 42 months, which were apportioned into 17 age groups each containing 100 individuals. The youngest 7 groups (i.e., from 1 to 7 months) each covered an interval of 30 days or 1 month. From 8 months through 28 months, the intervals were doubled in duration to 2 months. Finally, the oldest three cohorts were 90 days or 3 months long (i.e., 29–32 months; 33–38 months; and 39–42 months). Thus, the youngest ages had the smallest age intervals because this is where development proceeds at its most rapid pace.

This sample was stratified according to the data garnered by the U.S. Census Bureau (2014, 2017) across the following categories: (a) age; (b) sex; (c) race/ethnicity; and (d) parent educational level. Regarding sex, the sample consisted of approximately equal numbers of girls and boys. In terms of race/ethnic groups, the sample was distributed according to reported population percentages, including Whites, African Americans, Asians, Hispanics, and Other. Parental education was divided into four levels as follows: 0–11 years; 12 years (i.e., high school diploma or equivalent); 13–15 years (i.e., some college through associate degree); and 16 plus (i.e., college or graduate degree). Finally, the U.S. was apportioned into four major geographic regions as follows: Northeast, South, Midwest, and West. Although, exclusionary criteria eliminated all children with clinical conditions that could impair performance on the Bayley–4, the standardization sample included 34 children (i.e., 2%) with documented Down syndrome in order to intentionally increase the variance at the lower end of the normal distribution.

Concerning the Social-Emotional Scale, the Greenspan Social-Emotional Growth Chart was administered to the caregivers of 320 children. The sample was selected according to the 2017 U.S. Census statistics (U.S. Census Bureau, 2017) and was apportioned into 8 groups ($n = 40$) ranging in age from 1 to 42 months, and further stratified according to parental education, race/ethnicity, region, and sex. Finally, the Vineland–3 norm reference sample for the Bayley–4 age range (i.e., 1–42 months) was used to generate norms for the Adaptive Behavior Scale (see subsequent description of the Vineland–3 in this chapter).

Administration

The Bayley–4 is similar to that of the Bayley–III in many of its administrative aspects. These include the following: (a) caregiver participation in administration of the performance-based scales; (b) caregiver observer-report format for the Social-Emotional and Adaptive Behavior Questionnaire; (c) behavioral frequency observer-report items and age-defined stop points for the Social-Emotional Scale; (d) series items (i.e., items with identical directions but varying performance criteria that can be scored simultaneously); (e) related items (i.e., items with different instructions but same materials to speed administration); (f) determining age at testing and optional adjustment for prematurity; (g) subtests and items to be administered in order with some discretionary flexibility; and (h) *adaptive testing* using start points, reverse rules, and discontinue rules.

Although the similarities between the third and fourth editions of the Bayley are numerous, there are three principal differences worthy of mention. The first alteration refers to the significantly shorter administration time on the Bayley–4 performance-based scales. Although such duration depends upon several factors, the examinee's age is the most reliable predictor and are as follows: (a) ages 0 to 12 months = 35 minutes; (b) ages 13 to 24 months = 63 minutes; (c) ages 25 to 42 months = 68 minutes. Notice that these estimates are about 30 minutes briefer than that for the Bayley–III (see prior).

There are two reasons for this reduction. First, items that were highly inter-correlated were either dropped or combined because they did not contribute unique variance to the overall subtest and scaled scores. Second, and perhaps the most influential reason, is the inclusion of *Caregiver Questions* in 51 of the performance-based item instructions. *Caregiver Questions* are those items in which, when the child refuses to respond or otherwise does not provide a scorable response to an item question or prompt, the caregiver can be asked to rate the frequency with which the examinee can successfully perform the task or provide a passing answer as follows: (a) *Almost every time* or *at least 75% of the time* (2 points); (b) *Some of the time* or *less than 75% of the time* (1 point); and (c) *None of the time* or *0% of the time* (0 points). Therefore, these items are scored based upon the caregiver's direct observations of such behavior across a variety of environments.

This rather significant modification in item administration rules is based upon empirical research showing that garnering data in this manner can be extremely helpful in developmental screening measures and is now routinely done in such venues (American Academy of Pediatrics, 2006; Aylward & Verhulst, 2008). This includes the assessment of children who are at medical risk for some disease or disorder (Blaggan et al., 2014; Johnson, Wolke, & Marlow, 2008; Martin et al., 2013). This modified feature is designed to reduce frustration for all involved and maintains a brisk administrative process. Additionally, the examinee's abilities are measured based upon his typical performance across a variety of settings (versus a one-time clinical observation) and minimizes missing data due to examinees' refusal to respond.

A second principal difference in Bayley–4 administration is the new (at least to this measure) *polytomous scoring approach*, which is now applied to all of the performance-based items (i.e., Cognitive, Language, and Motor Scales). *Polytomous models* of measurement possess more than two possible scores. The most commonly known examples of such models include Likert-type 5-point scales and partial credit items on essay type examinations (e.g., 0 to 10 points). Polytomous models are contrasted with dichotomous models that have only two possible scores (e.g., 0 and 1, True or False). The Bayley–III performance-based items are dichotomous wherein the examiner scores "1" for passing and "0" for failing an item. The problem with dichotomous scoring is that it does not capture an examinee who is beginning to manifest a particular skill, although does not do so consistently.

Because development is constant, dynamic, and irregular, a dichotomous scoring system may either miss an emerging skill or erroneously score such skill as being absent, both of which contribute to error variance. To remedy this situation and build into the performance-based items more discriminatory power, yet avoid making the scale too cumbersome to use, the Bayley–4 now uses a 3-point polytomous scale. Although the item content varies, the scale can be generally summarized as follows: 0 = *Absence of a skill or ability* (i.e., the skill is not yet present); 1 = *An emerging skill* (i.e., the skill is present to some degree but is inconsistent and present only some of the time); 2 = *Successful mastery of a skill* (i.e., the skill occurs consistently or almost all of the time). A score of "0" (i.e., not present) may either indicate a delay or a deficit. A score of "1" (i.e., emerging) implies an expectation that full mastery will eventually manifest itself. Finally, a score of "2" (i.e., mastery) represents successful mastery of a skill. It can be plainly seen that this scale effectively captures a skill that is in the process of emerging, although is not yet complete or consistent in its current state of development.

A third variance is the changed format of the Adaptive Behavior Scale, which is the direct consequence of deriving its items from an alternative adaptive behavior measure; namely, the Vineland–3. The Bayley–4 Adaptive Behavior Scale now consists of five sections, including (a) Receptive, (b) Expressive, (c) Personal, (d) Interpersonal Relationships, and (e) Play and Leisure. For each item, caregivers are to circle the score that best describes what their children do independently or autonomously as follows: 0 = *Never*; 1 = *Sometimes*; and 2 = *Usually or often*. A score of 2 also includes situations in which the child has outgrown the behavior. There is also a check box that should be marked if the caregivers estimated their score. Finally, the caregiver is instructed to discontinue a section after a sequence of 5 scores of "0." Of note, start points are always at Item 1.

Scoring

This section reviews the various scores available on the Bayley–4, with emphasis on those that are utilized in the data tables for reporting these test results within a psychological assessment report. Additional scores that are not used are briefly reviewed to provide a more comprehensive description of what this version of the Bayley Scales has to offer. As a brief note that does indirectly affect the data, the examinee's CA, along with a discretionary adjustment for prematurity, are computed as done when using the Bayley–III.

Scores Employed in the Bayley–4 Data Tables

Standard scores (*SSs*) have a mean of 100 and standard deviation (*SD*) of 15, with a range of 45 to 155. These may be seen in Table 1 of Form 6.1b, with the metric defined in the general table notes. The 95% confidence interval (CI) is selected such that the examinee's true score has a 95% certainty of falling within the reported range (note that a 90% CI is also an option). Percentile ranks (*PRs*) are area transformations that show the examinee's ordinal position compared to same aged peers. The PR ranges for these data are provided in the Administrative Manual (Bayley & Aylward, 2019a) and computer scoring program (see below). Consistent with the polytomous scoring model (see prior), lower scores denote a greater degree of either deficit or delay, which is defined in all general table notes.

Table 6.4b Bayley Scales of Infant and Toddler Development, Fourth Edition (Bayley–4) Qualitative Description Classification Guide

Standard Scores	Scaled Scores	SDs from the Mean	Descriptive Classification
130 to 160	16 to 19	+2 to +4	Extremely high
120 to 129	14 to 15	+1⅓ to +1⅔	Very high
110 to 119	12 to 13	+ ⅔ to +1	High average
90 to 109	8 to 11	–⅔ to +⅓	Average
80 to 89	6 to 7	–1⅓ to –1	Low average
70 to 79	4 to 5	–2 to –1⅔	Borderline
40 to 69	1 to 3	–3 to –2⅓	Extremely low

Source. Adapted from Bayley, N., & Aylward, G. P. (2019b). *Bayley Scales of Infant Development, Fourth Edition (Bayley–4): Technical manual.* Bloomington, MN: NCS Pearson, Table 5.1, p. 62.

Note. *SD*s = standard deviations.

The descriptive classification scheme has changed both its own label from the prior "qualitative description" (see Form 6.1a), along with its various categories. Table 6.4b shows a descriptive classification guide for the Bayley–4 data, including standard score ranges, scaled score ranges, SDs from the mean, and descriptive classification labels. Immediately after the aforesaid classifications in Table 1 (Form 6.1b) is a column for reporting age equivalent (AE) scores, which are available for all performance-based subtests. Because the Cognitive Scale is based on only one subtest, it has only one AE score. However, the Language and Motor scales consist of two subtests, hence two AE scores. Therefore, initials follow these AE scores to identify the respective subtest to which it applies. They are incorporated here in the event only Table 1 is reported within a psychological report, which is not infrequent given the limitations of clinical testing time. Additionally, their positioning here is more felicitous in terms of interpretation. Although they have limitations, these can be easily clarified, especially when reported in the context of all the other test scores enumerated in the table.

The Bayley–4 subtests are reported in a scaled score metric, including a smaller mean of 10, *SD* of 3, and a range of 1 to 19. These are reported in Table 2 for the Language subtests (i.e., Receptive Communication and Expressive Communication) and Table 3 for the Motor subtests (i.e., Fine Motor and Gross Motor); both in Form 6.1b. Because the 95% CIs are not available for these subtests, the respective *SEM*s for the Language and Motor subtests (see Bayley & Aylward, 2019b, Table 3.7, p. 34) were averaged by me for each scale independently and reported in the specific table notes to the nearest whole number such that they can be rapidly computed and entered into the data table. As all subtest *SEM*s are just under a value of 1.00, this represents a convenient value to enter into the specific notes for both Table 2 and 3. The PR values can be referenced in Table 6.3, while descriptive classes can be found in Table 6.4b.

Difference scores are available for the scale SSs to determine if the main performance-based scales are statistically significant either at the .10 or .05 level of significance. Furthermore, base rates are computed as effect size measures for each of the difference scores, which again represent the percent of the norm reference sample that manifest that difference score.

Scores Not Employed in the Bayley–4 Data Tables

Growth scale values (GSWs) are available on the Bayley–4, which have a mean of 500 and a *SD* of 25. GSWs permit the measurement of an examinee's progress compared to previous administrations; hence, the degree of a child's progress in an absolute sense (versus relative to same aged peers). These are not typically used due to the general infrequency with which retesting is requested in the mental health field. Considering the relatively small age range for this test, the odds of requested retesting are even lower. These types of scores are more likely to be employed by a Head Start early intervention program with ages out at age 3 years.

Another score not used is unique and actually can be integrated into the narrative interpretation of the test data tables. It is referred to as *Percent Delay*, which some school systems require for eligibility of special services. *Percent Delay* is the amount of delay shown by a child as a proportion (or percent) of chronological age (CA). It is computed as follows:

$$\text{Percent Delay} = 100\% - \frac{\text{AE}}{\text{CA}} \times 100 \qquad \text{Equation 6.1}$$

where AE is the examinee's age equivalent score, CA is the examinee's age from birth (or adjusted for prematurity) and multiplying by 100 transforms the proportion into a percent delay. Hence, a child with a Cognitive Scale AE of 30 months, who is 35 months old would have an approximate 14% delay (i.e., 30/35 = 0.8571 x 100 = 85.71 ≈ 86%;

100%–86% = 14%). Because Table 1 provides the AEs, and the CA (or adjusted CA) is already known, the Percent Delay can be easily computed and reported in the narrative interpretation.

Finally, the subtest scaled score differences are also available for analyzing pairwise comparisons for all performance-based subtests and Adaptive Behavior subdomains. These analyses include hypothesis tests on the difference scores and base rates as done for the SS differences. Such detailed analyses are not typically done on the subtest or subdomain levels. Therefore, tables are not included for such comparisons.

Computer Scoring for the Bayley–4

Computer scoring for the Bayley Scales is now done on the Pearson internet website Q–global (Pearson, 2021) platform. There is a charge for each Score Report. Further, there are separate reports for (a) the performance-based Cognitive, Language, and Motor Scales, and (b) the Social-Emotional and Adaptive Behavior Questionnaire. When both are scored, they can be integrated into one report and downloaded or printed in hard copy format.

Interpretation

To facilitate the interpretive steps of the Bayley–4 data, Figure 6.1 on the Routledge e-resources website provides a flowchart of both the required and optional analyses, which should be downloaded and referenced for the following immediate discussion. Once again, a core tenet of effective and rewarding testing practice is knowing what to emphasize and what to minimize or eliminate in terms of reporting and interpreting the data yield. The first component of Figure 6.1, which should be immediately conspicuous, is the large degree of discretion afforded the examiner in interpreting the data. This is denoted by the many broken-lined boxes in the figure.

Basic Bayley–4 Scales

The fundamental data is comprised of what can be referred to as the basic or fundamental Bayley–4 scales. These include the three performance-based scales (viz., Cognitive, Language, and Motor) and two observer-based scales (viz., Social-Emotional and Adaptive Behavior). The first and principal interpretations should consist of normative or age-corrected comparisons with the examinee's peers (including adjustments for prematurity). If there are no delays or deficits noted in this principal data, the analysis may end here because several major neurodevelopmental disorders have been successfully and simultaneously ruled out, including *intellectual disability* (*ID*), language disorder, and *developmental coordination disorder*.

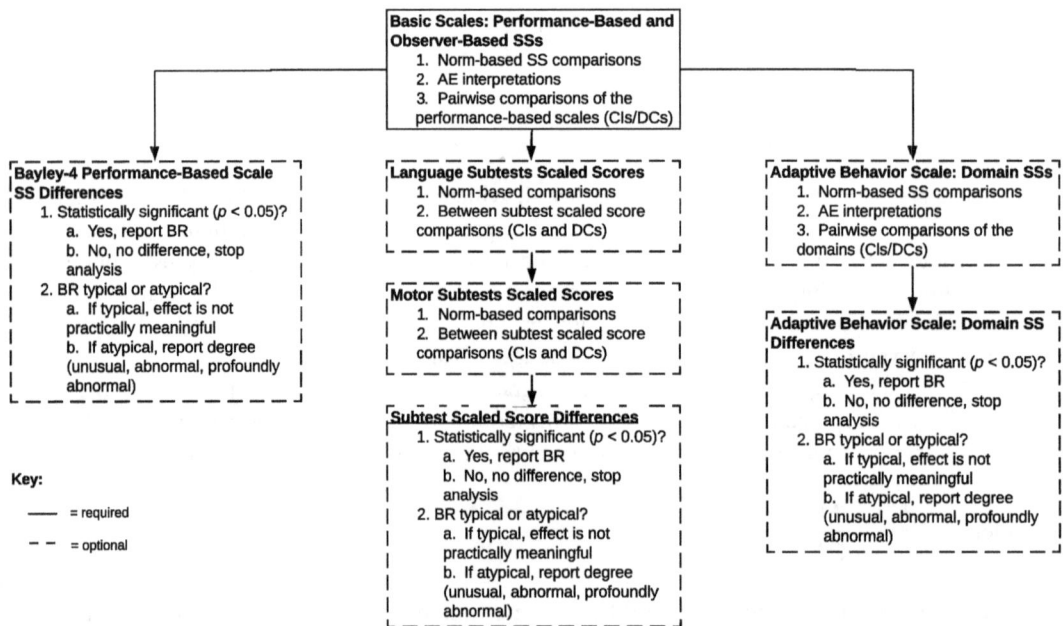

Figure 6.1 Bayley Scales of Infant and Toddler Development, Fourth Edition (Bayley–4) Interpretative Process

In Form 6.1b, there is a series of pre-drafted interpretive statements immediately following Table 1 with two versions; that is, one that summarizes the presence of negative results (i.e., no evidence of deficits or delays) and a more detailed version describing the presence of one or more delays or deficits. The terminology *deficits* and *delays* are both used so that the examiner may choose which she wants to emphasize. Both versions focus first on norm-based comparisons with descriptive categories, followed by PRs and AE interpretations. Note that the AE interpretations ensure that the inferences are phrased in terms of the typical age who obtained the same raw score as the examinee. Following the identification of impairments, the interpretation moves to the remainder of scores and abilities that were measured to be within normal limits (if any).

The remainder of the required analyses comprises an informal inspection of any between scale differences by examining the extent of overlap among the respective CIs (i.e., an informal within-subject analysis of personal strengths and weaknesses). Large overlap indicates no difference whereas increasing degrees of separation shows evidence of concomitant degrees of variance among the measured abilities. A lack of any overlap between any two CIs indicates likely differential functioning. If confirming such differences carries significant diagnostic or treatment weight, then more formal scale pairwise comparisons can be done among the performance-based scales.

Formal Analysis of Performance-Based Scale Differences

This discretionary analysis involves pairwise comparisons between all possible combinations of the performance-based scales, which total three given that there are three scales. It is advised that time should be devoted to these analyses only under the following conditions: (a) scale differences will help complete needed differential diagnosis and/or critical treatment recommendations; and (b) the informal CI analysis showed one or more likely discrepancies (i.e. little or no overlap). Otherwise, the examiner is simply filling space that can only serve to obfuscate the key findings.

This analysis is completed in three steps as shown in Table 2 (Form 6.1b; see also Figure 6.1, left box). First, only those comparisons that are needed should be selected to help minimize the familywise error rate. Second, hypotheses tests are done on each comparison or difference score. Third, only statistically significant tests should be followed with base rate analyses to report and interpret the effect sizes of the differences as shown in the Table 2 specific notes. Those differences that are statistically significant (i.e., are real differences) and unusual (i.e., rare in the normal population) have diagnostic and treatment implications. Pre-drafted interpretive statements immediately follow Table 2 and serve to guide the examiner through the inferential process.

Performance-Based Subtest Scaled Score Analyses

The Language and Motor performance-based scales are each comprised of two subtests. In the ideal circumstance, the subtests that contribute to each scale would be equivalent, which would in turn mean that the overall scale is a good overall representative measure. In contrast, when there exists a discrepancy between the subtests, it means that the overall score is no longer an accurate summary of the examinee's overall ability on that scale. In such instance, reporting and interpreting the more specific subtest scores is recommended. Figure 6.1 shows this line of analysis in the middle sequence of boxes, beginning with the Language subtests, then followed by the Motor subtests as enumerated within Table 1.

For both Language and Motor Scale subtests, the analytic steps mirror those in Table 1 (Form 6.1b; top middle box in Figure 6.1). In particular, the norm-based comparisons are done with the scaled scores and their associated descriptive classifications, followed by PRs, and finally, an ipsative comparison of the two CIs to informally examine a potential discrepancy. Note that AE scores are not reported and interpreted here because they already appeared in Table 1. This decision was made because Table 1 data are required, hence guaranteeing that the AEs will be involved in the core portion of the Bayley–4 results. Pre-drafted interpretive statements follow Tables 3 and 4 (see Form 6.1b), which guide the examiner through the process.

If more formal ipsative analyses are needed or desired, the investigation moves to Table 5 (see Form 6.1b), which makes two pairwise comparisons; namely, one between the two Language subtests and one between the two motor subtests. Subtests that contribute to different scales are not compared because at this level they do not add to differential diagnosis and treatment planning and originate from conceptually dissimilar categories of skills. This analysis mirrors that of formally examining SS differences among the performance-based scales. That is, hypothesis tests are done on the scaled score differences, with follow-up base rate effect size analyses done only when the difference is statistically significant. Finally, pre-drafted interpretive statements following Table 5, which again takes the examiner through the inferential process.

Adaptive Behavior Scale Domains

In the event the General Adaptive Behavior Scale is showing very or extremely low functioning, hence showing the presence of deficit or delay, the three domain scores that contributed to it should be reported, even if it appears that they are equivalent. This is because they are not reported in any of the other tables and it is important to show their levels of functioning to determine their unique impact upon the general score. In the event the General Adaptive Behavior Score is showing within-normal limits functioning, the domains should still be reported if one or more of them are showing impairment in functioning. In such cases, by definition there must be significant variability among the domains because one or more must be higher in order to offset the low score(s). Hence, the only instance in which the domain scores need not be reported and interpreted is when all scores are showing an absence of deficit or delay.

Table 6 in Form 6.1b is designed for reporting and interpreting the adaptive behavior domain scores (see also Figure 6.1, top box on right-hand side). The first step is to make norm-based *SS* comparisons and interpreting the associated categories of functioning. If the examinee scores close to two categories, this should be noted as the following example: "from very low to extremely low functioning." Interpreting the associated PRs and AE scores are easier for laypeople to understand and provide and more comprehensive (yet still fairly succinct) description of the examinee's functioning. This should be ensued by ipsative informal pairwise comparisons among the CIs, examining and interpreting the degree of overlap. CIs with little or no overlap should be Interpreted as likely showing discrepant functioning, hence portraying relative strengths and weaknesses. If these have significant diagnostic or treatment implications, follow-up formal relative comparisons should be done, otherwise the Bayley–4 analyses can now be considered complete. Pre-drafted excerpts follow Table 6, which guide the examiner through the interpretive process (see also Figure 6.1, top right box). These statements end with integrating the conclusions with diagnostic implications.

Adaptive Behavior Scale Domain Standard Score Differences

This final discretionary phase in Bayley–4 interpretation provides formal relative comparisons among the three measured adaptive behavior domains. This two-step process parallels that done among the performance-based *SS* differences, beginning with a hypothesis test on the difference *SS* at the .05 level of probability, and a base rate effect size interpretation contingent upon a statistically significant prior result. If the hypothesis test is not significant, a double dash symbol should be inserted in lieu of a base rate value. The base rate interpretive scheme is inserted in a specific table note, with atypical conclusions denoted by one to three cross symbols (i.e., †) depending upon the degree of abnormality. Again, the base rate indicates how uncommon the result is in the normal population.

Adaptive Behavior Assessment System, Third Edition

Synopsis

The *Adaptive Behavior Assessment System, Third Edition* (*ABAS–3*; Harrison & Oakland, 2015a) is a norm-referenced, comprehensive, standardized measure of adaptive behavior necessary to function autonomously and effectively in terms of self-care, interpersonal responding and communicating, and meeting environmental demands; the latter including home, school, work, and community. *Adaptive behavior* is defined as the performance of daily activities required for personal and social sufficiency (Sparrow, Cicchetti, & Balla, 2005, p. 6), and which directly affects the quality of one's life. The adaptive domains and skill areas that comprise this measure are based upon criteria as defined by the *American Association on Intellectual and Developmental Disabilities* (*AAIDD*, 2010), *American Association on Mental Retardation* (*AAMR*, 2002), American Psychiatric Association (2000, 2013), *Individuals with Disabilities Education Improvement Act* (2004), and *World Health Organization* (*WHO*, 2001, 2007). This measure is clinically useful in that it effectively identifies a person's functional limitations often observed in neurodevelopmental disorders, such as intellectual disability (ID) and autism spectrum disorder (ASD). The age range spans from birth to 89 years 11 months (i.e., 0 to 89:11). Therefore, it is also useful in measuring the degree to which these adaptive behaviors have deteriorated due to neurocognitive dysfunction.

Norm Reference Sample

The ABAS–3 was standardized on a nationally representative sample of 4,500 individuals ranging in age from 0 to 89 years 11 months. The sample was stratified in terms of gender, race/ethnicity, and socioeconomic status (SES; defined by education level) according to proportions reported in the 2010 U.S. Census (U.S. Bureau of the Census, 2010). Further, both typically developing people and those with disabilities were included as the latter are also expected to be present in the general population in various proportions. Because the ABAS–3 consists of five different forms of overlapping age ranges, a total of 7,737 forms were completed on individuals in the norm reference sample.

Administration

The ABAS–3 contains a total of five forms, each differentiated by (a) type of respondent, (b) type of environment or setting, and (c) age of the target individual to be rated. They include the following: (a) Parent/Primary Caregiver Form, Ages 0 to 5; (b) Parent Form, Ages 5 to 21; (c) Teacher/Daycare Provider Form, Ages 2 to 5; (d) Teacher Form, Ages 5 to 21; and (e) Adult Form, Ages 16 to 89. The latter may be either observer-rated or self-rated. All forms require a 6th grade reading level. Average time to complete each of the forms is about 20 minutes.

All potential observer-respondents are advised to have, "frequent, recent, prolonged contact," concerning the individual they are rating (Harrison & Oakland, 2015a, p. 9). Operationally, this means having observed the examinee for several recent months, most days, for several hours per day, within settings that require the adaptive skills to be rated. In outpatient settings, standardized measures of adaptive behavior are most commonly employed when testing for suspected ID and ASD. Hence, the single respondent who is the most felicitous match with the aforementioned operational definition of an appropriate observer-respondent is typically selected. This will most frequently be a parent figure who has raised the child since birth or soon thereafter and has observed adaptive behaviors manifested across both time and an array of environments. This means that the Parent/Primary Caregiver Form, Ages 0 to 5, and the Parent Form, Ages 5 to 21, will be the two most frequently used forms for a testee 21 years and under, while the Adult Form, Ages 16 to 89, to be completed by an observer-respondent parental figure, would most probably be used for older examinees.

In other circumstances, the selection may be less apparent as between a teacher, guardian, and/or foster parent, each of whom have observed the individual for a more limited time and in more circumscribed situations. Again, it is most efficacious to select the one individual who best fits the operational definition of an observer respondent, as opposed to selecting two respondents and performing an optional interrater analysis. Although this measure permits a test user to perform a quantitative interrater comparison, it must be done by manual computation via a "Rater Comparison Worksheet," which is both labor intensive and lacking reliable criteria for interpreting significant interrater discrepancies. If the Adult Form is to be self-rated, the individual must be deemed intellectually and psychologically capable of completing such a task. Separate norms are employed for self- versus other-ratings.

Once the respondent is selected, the proper form is given with complete instructions, including the admonition to answer all items. Respondents are to rate examinees, or themselves as examinees, in terms of how often each behavior is correctly performed when needed as follows: 0 = *Is not able*; 1 = *Never (or almost never) when needed*; 2 = *Sometimes when needed*; and 3 = *Always (or almost always) when needed*. An added column is included that indicates whether the respondent guessed or estimated the particular rating. If this seems familiar it is because these are the same alternatives afforded by the Bayley–III Adaptive Behavior Scales items, which adopted them from the pertinent portions of the ABAS–II introduced previously.

More specifically, a score of 0 indicates the presence of an *ability deficit*, defined as a behavior being absent because the person lacks the necessary skills. The person may not have developed the skills needed for age-appropriate functioning in the environment due to delay or disability, or may simply be of insufficient age or simply too young. Scores of 1 and 2 constitute a more and less *performance deficit*, respectively, denoting an individual who has acquired the ability yet does not display the behavior consistently or reliably within the environment and to varying degrees; that is, the behavior is not always used when needed. A score of 3 indicates that the behavior is not showing a performance deficit. Lastly, the option to indicate that the response was based upon conjecture is actually intended to encourage the respondent to answer all items, ostensibly by communicating that guesswork is an acceptable strategy in making a reply. However, the outcome may be the antithesis of this strategy's intent because the computer software (discussed subsequently) will suppress the scoring of a skill area if three or more items are marked as being estimated. On the other hand, it will also terminate the scoring process if four or more items are omitted. Both result in catastrophic consequences because all subsequent scores dependent upon that skill area will also fail to yield data.

Therefore, three particularly helpful rules of administration are as follows. First, as advised when discussing the Bayley–III questionnaire administration, instruct the primary caregiver to complete the ABAS–3 immediately after it is selected as part of the targeted test battery (i.e., if the primary caregiver is present, able, and willing). Any omissions or errors in responding to the form can thereafter be corrected at a later point in time, such as during a subsequently scheduled testing appointment. The form may also be administered orally by the examiner, in whole or in part, the responses then recorded and aggregated, and finally entered into the computer software. Second, inform respondents that when they have had no opportunity to observe the behavior in question, they can use their ratings to similar behaviors on the form to assist their selection. Third, scores should be based upon observed successful performance, even if the examinee uses a support device to complete the behavior (e.g., a walker to ambulate or use of a magnifying glass to read).

The immediate issues that must be resolved at this juncture are (a) how many respondents are to be chosen, and (b) which respondent(s) will provide this data. A principal reason for choosing the ABAS–3 as part of the test inventory is the vast array of forms and potential respondents that may be employed in garnering such data. In total, there are five forms covering as many different age ranges, along with a minimum of three types of respondents (i.e., caregiver, teacher, self). The answer to the first issue is one respondent. The reason is that this measure is much too long and comprehensive so as to make analyzing more than one respondent unwieldy. If only one is selected, this renders the choice of respondents even more critical. In such instances, precedence is afforded to a primary caretaker as such an individual has usually observed the examinee across the greatest number and variety of situations, and across the longest uninterrupted duration of time. If adaptive behavior abilities are conceptualized as analogous to personality traits (i.e., relatively consistent patterns of behavior across time and to some extent situations), then such a selection makes logical sense. If there are two primary caregivers (e.g., mother and father), then the option is given to them in (a) choosing the one that is most familiar with the child, or (b) completing the form together and resolving discrepancies in the process of choosing responses to items.

Occasionally there are circumstances in which someone other than a primary caregiver (i.e., teacher; self) is the most felicitous choice. First, the most cogent reasons for selecting a teacher for a respondent is as follows: (a) when the primary caregiver is relatively new to the child (e.g., a new foster parent) such that the particular teacher actually has more familiarity with the examinee; and (b) when the parent shows signs of *alexithymia*, low intelligence, lack of *psychological mindedness*, resistance, indecisiveness, or other response biases that will likely skew the results. If the ABAS–3 is being used to assess an adult, and there are no viable primary caregiver choices (e.g., a parent who is continuing to provide needed care, staff within a residential treatment facility), the Adult Form, Ages 16 to 89 can be used as a self-report form if the examinee possesses the requisite reading comprehension ability (i.e., minimum 6th grade) and self-awareness.

Finally, it may have already been apparent that there are some overlapping ages among the forms, hence providing a choice of two viable forms based upon chronological age alone. In such circumstances, it is advisable to use the form that possesses the greatest chance of effectively covering the examinee's estimated range of skills and living circumstances. For example, a severally impaired 5-year-old with suspected ID and ASD would probably be most accurately measured by the Parent/Primary Caregiver Form because it covers skills of individuals down to infancy versus the Parent Form. Likewise, a 20-year-old who has completed high school, is living semi-independently, and is working a part-time job would be more accurately measured by the Adult versus Parent Form.

Scoring

The *Adaptive Behavior Assessment System, Third Edition (ABAS–3) Scoring Assistant* (Harrison & Oakland, 2015b), affords this measure with invaluable unlimited computer scoring capability. Utilizing this tool is strongly advised for purposes of (a) enhancing clinical utility and (b) reducing human error associated with hand scoring. Manual scoring as an option is probably best reserved for training purposes. Therefore, the scoring steps discussed in this section is based upon use of the ABAS–3 Scoring Assistant.

Steps in Computer Scoring

First, the respondent is instructed to submit the completed ABAS–3 form to the examiner as soon as is practical. If the respondent is a primary caregiver available during the initial assessment, a request should be made that it be completed that same day or soon thereafter and submitted to the front desk or other support staff when done. Second, a cursory examination of the form is done to ensure that all pages have been completed. Third, if there exist one or two item omissions within any one adaptive skill area, despite explicit written instructions on the form to complete all items, the examiner is permitted to estimate a rating based upon other ratings made by the respondent associated with comparable behaviors, including a score of "0" indicating an inability (Harrison & Oakland, 2015a, p. 15). Three or more item omissions within an adaptive skill area precludes further scoring, including all subsequent scores contributed to by that adaptive skill area. In particular, lack of a score for any one adaptive skill area would also inhibit scoring for adaptive domain score to which it contributes, along with the overall composite score. Hence, sufficient responses can be given either based upon the respondent's answers to comparable items or based upon information garnered during the mental status examination and behavioral observations.

Fourth, the "total guessed" box for each adaptive skill area is examined. As stated prior, if there are four or more guesses within an adaptive skill area, the computer software will not yield a score. Therefore, they are not entered formally. However, a note is made to interpret the data cautiously and this is ultimately included in the report. Fifth, raw scores are aggregated for each skill area, then entered into the ABAS–3 scoring software to obtain the needed standard score transformations. Forms 6.2, 6.3, 6.4, 6.5, and 6.6 represent the data tables for all five ABAS–3 forms.

Because they may be considered *alternate forms* (i.e., different versions of the same test), they are discussed simultaneously while noting any special differences as they arise.

Primary Data Analysis

Proceeding from general to specific, Table 1 (see Forms 6.2–6.6) presents the score data, including the General Adaptive Composite (GAC), the three domains or contributors to the GAC (viz., Conceptual, Social, and Practical), and a fourth optional Adaptive Skill Area that is elevated to standard score status due to its key role in development (i.e., Motor skills and Work skills). There are six columns that list the following: (a) scale name; (b) standard score (mean = 100; standard deviation = 15); (c) 95 % CI; (d) PR (i.e., based upon the theoretical standard normal distribution; see Chapter 3); (e) nominally defined descriptive category; and (f) a succinct description of the abilities and skills measured. Of note, the range 120 down to 40 is heavily weighted toward the lower or impaired range. This was done by design considering that the most frequent reason adaptive abilities are measured is to detect degrees of impairment. In fact, the DSM–5's decision to elevate the adaptive behavior measure to be the determining factor in designating the degree of ID, versus the IQ score as was done historically, is consistent with the ABAS–3 design.

The computer scoring software provides all of the information needed for reporting data in Table 1 (Forms 6.2–6.6), including the descriptive class. Table 1 notes define the standard score metric, the directional meaning of lower scores indicating greater impairment (hence in the pathological direction), table abbreviations, the domains that contribute to the overall measure, and information needed to define the unique characteristics of the optional adaptive skill area. Although the content of the optional adaptive skill areas may differ (i.e., motor skills versus work skills), many of their inherent components are comparable. First, they both contribute significantly to an individual's autonomy and independence; that is, motor skills for early childhood and work skills for adolescence and adulthood. Second, they are conversions from the scaled score metric, which represents their point of origin. In order to report their standard equivalent score, the examiner would proceed through the following steps: (a) refer to Table 6.3; (b) find the proper scaled score value in the middle column; and (c) move over to the first column to find the associated standard score. For example, if the examinee's Motor Adaptive Skill Area scaled score was 11, the standard equivalent score would be 105.

Because the computer scoring assistant does not compute the CI or the PR for the optional Adaptive Skill Areas, they must be estimated. Regarding the CI, the analysis began by finding all of the *internal consistency reliability coefficients* for both the Motor and Work Adaptive Skill Areas in the technical manual (see Harrison & Oakland, 2015a, p. 74, Table 5.7). These reliability coefficients were chosen because (a) they illustrate that these skill areas clearly measure a homogeneous construct, and (b) they are quite impressively high. Therefore, they contribute to greater validity, smaller *SEM*s, and greater precision in our estimates of examinees' true scores on these scales. Second, average of these coefficients for each skill area was computed. Third, the average coefficients were entered into the formula $SEM = SD\sqrt{1 - r_{xx}}$, where r_{xx} is the average reliability coefficient and SD equals 15 on a standard score metric. The latter computes an *SEM* based upon a standard score *SD* and not the smaller scaled score *SD* of 3. Finally, the result was rounded to the nearest whole unit. To compute a 95% CI, the examiner merely adds and subtracts two *SEM*s to the obtained standard equivalent score. Finally, the PR can be found quickly by referring back to Table 6.3 and finding the PR value in the third column that is associated with the obtained standard equivalent score (or its correspondent scaled score). In the example being used, the standard equivalent score would have a 95% CI of 105 ± 6 (i.e., 2 x 3) = 99 to 111, along with a PR of 63. Hence, there is 95% confidence that the examinee's true Motor Adaptive Skill Area standard equivalent score is as low as 99 and as high as 111, which traverses largely the average to possibly high average range. Additionally, the examinee scores equivalent to or higher than 63% of the population of same aged peers.

While the younger-age Forms 6.2 and 6.3 offer the Motor Adaptive Skill Area as an optional standard equivalent score, the three older-age Forms, 6.4, 6.5, and 6.6 include an optional Work Adaptive Skill Area, which requires the examinee to be employed either part- or full-time. The Work standard equivalent score and PR are determined in like fashion by use of Table 6.3. Further, the *SEM* was similarly computed by use of $SEM = SD\sqrt{1 - r_{xx}}$, again using the average of the reported internal consistency coefficients for this skill area. In this case, the correlations were somewhat higher, which translates into a smaller *SEM* or error rate. Hence, the *SEM* was 2 rather than 3, including rounding to the nearest whole number. However, other than content, this is the only difference between the two optional skill areas.

Secondary Data Analysis

While Table 1 data consist of norm-based comparisons, Table 2 in Forms 6.2 through 6.6 provides an opportunity to conduct ipsative analyses with regard to the domain scores. These are relative comparisons that determine whether or not there are statistically significant difference among the adaptive behavior domains. These hypothesis tests are conducted in the same manner as done with the Bayley–III data (see Table 5, Form 6.1a). In this instance, there are three pairwise comparisons. Thus, Table 2 consists of 4 columns, including the following: (a) the domain comparison by name; (b) the computed or obtained difference (i.e., the first minus the second listed test); (c) the difference value associated with a 5% chance in 100 of occurring assuming a null hypothesis of no difference; and (d) the base rate of the obtained difference (i.e., the percentage of the norm-reference sample that obtained that difference score). The third column in this listing labeled "c" again deserves some elaboration, especially if this analysis among the Bayley–III data was recondite.

The computer software reports the difference score that had only a 5% chance of occurring assuming that there actually is no difference between the respective two domains. This difference score is referred to as the "Critical value" in the Table 2 third column. The .05 value represents the 5% chance criterion, sometimes referred to in statistics as the *alpha level* or confidence level selected to rule out chance as an explanation for the obtained difference score. For example, assume that the ABAS–3 computer scoring software reports 5.88 as the critical value for the Social minus Practical domain difference. This means that if the obtained difference score was 5.88 or larger, this difference would occur less than 5 times in 100 due to chance factors. This is such a low probability that the chance explanation for the obtained difference can now be rejected (i.e., the null hypothesis of no difference is rejected). Hence, the conclusion is that the two domains are meaningfully different. A typical way of saying this is that the difference between the Social and Practical domains is *significantly significant*; that is, the examinee's social and practical skills are significant different. If as in this example the critical value is significant (i.e., the obtained difference is equal to or greater than the critical value), an asterisk is to be appended to the obtained value in the "Difference" column. Again, recall that virtually the same analysis was done in the Bayley–III Table 5 data (see Form 6.1a).

Finally, the computer scoring routinely lists base rates of both 15% and 5%, with boxes placed just prior to each value designed to be computer checked if the obtained difference score meets the smaller or more conservative of the two criteria. Hence, if neither is met the check-boxes for both remain empty. If both are met, the software will check the smaller or more conservative of the two (i.e., the 5% criterion). Therefore, both criteria are listed in the final base rate column, one with a greater than or equal sign juxtaposed with 15%, and a less than or equal sign juxtaposed with both 15% and 5% base rate criteria. Recall that Sattler (2001) considers the 15% and 5% base rates to be unusual and abnormally rare, respectively. Because these are the only two alternatives reported by the computer scoring assistant, they are the only ones included in the data table. The cross symbols (i.e., †) are appended to emphasize the degree of aberration indicated by a particular base rate.

Tertiary Data Analysis

Each domain is broken down into adaptive skill areas, which function as subtests that measure more narrowly defined constructs. This reflects the hierarchical structure of the ABAS–3, which mirrors that of the Bayley–III and a host of other ability tests. These adaptive skill areas are measured in scaled score units (mean = 10; standard deviation = 3) being that they have less items and discriminatory power. In Forms 6.2 through 6.6, the three adaptive skill area data tables are enumerated as Table 3 (viz., Conceptual Adaptive Domain), Table 4 (viz., Social Adaptive Domain), and Table 5 (viz., Practical Adaptive Domain). The tables are prepared comparable to that of Table 1, including six columns as follows: (a) scaled scores; (b) 95% CIs; (c) PRs; (d) descriptive classification; and (e) measured abilities. Similar to many computer software scoring programs, CIs, PRs, and descriptive categories are not provided for the more narrowly defined subscales (e.g., subtests, subdomains). This is unfortunate because they are vital to the analysis of test data. However, typically test publishers' technical manuals provide the information needed such that these statistics can be reasonably estimated. The pertinent facts are reviewed next.

The ABAS–3 technical manual reports the *SEM*s for all adaptive skill areas, domains, and composites for each of the five forms, including separate *SEM*s for both observer- and self-report respondents on the Adult form. Therefore, the average *SEM* was simply computed for each adaptive skill area, rounded to the nearest whole number, and reported this as the *SEM* value to utilize when computing the 95% CI.[3] In all cases, the *SEM* values were between 0.40 and 0.86 (see Harrison & Oakland, 2015a, p. 74, Table 5.7). Therefore, all SEMs were computed as 1 after being rounded to the nearest whole number. Although rounding to the nearest half number could have been done for greater precision, this did not seem worth the extra effort. Therefore, the examiner can simply add and subtract 2 points to the obtained scaled score values for all adaptive skill areas when estimating the 95% CIs. In order to be consistent, this is why the 95% CIs in Table 1 was selected as applied to the domain standard scores rather than the alternative 90% CI.

Moving to PRs, these values may be quickly identified by referencing Table 6.3. In order to find the correct nominal descriptive classification, Table 6.5 was created. This is an adaptation of Table 3.1 in the ABAS–3 technical manual, which is actually an integration of two tables (see Harrison & Oakland, 2015a, p. 35, Table 3.1). Scrutiny

Table 6.5 Adaptive Behavior Assessment System, Third Edition (ABAS–3) Description Classification Guide

Composite/Adaptive Domain Standard (equivalent) Score	Adaptive Skill Scaled Score	Descriptive Classification
120	15–19	High
110–119	13–14	Above average
90–109	8–12	Average
80–89	6–7	Below average
71–79	4–5	Low
40–70	1–3	Extremely low

Source. Adapted from Harrison, P. L., Oakland, T. (2015a). *Adaptive Behavior Assessment System, Third Edition (ABAS–3)* [Manual]. Torrance, CA: Western Psychological Services (WPS)., Table 3.1, p. 35.

Note. Standard score mean = 100, standard deviation = 15; range = 40–120; scaled score mean = 10, standard deviation = 3; range = 1–19.

of Table 6.5 also unequivocally illustrates the intentional favoritism of the ABAS–3 scores toward the lower end of the scale, the purpose of which adds discriminatory power toward increasing degrees of dysfunction. Although this increases the risk of *ceiling effects*, they are considered less potentially problematic because adaptive behavior measures are typically done in order to detect impaired rather than superior functioning.

The chief difference among the five ABAS–3 booklets regards the Adult Form (Form 6.6), Table 5 (both observer- and self-report respondents). Note the appearance of the Work Adaptive Skill Area in this location in scaled score format, which also appears in Table 1 as a standard equivalent score (see prior). The reason is that this adaptive skill area, when administered and scored, contributes to both the GAC and Practical Adaptive Doman score. Specific table notes to that effect are inserted into both the Table 1 and Table 5 notes. So why choose to report these data in both tables? In reporting test data, the following logic is pursued; (a) when more narrowly defined skill areas are being reported (i.e., adaptive skill areas), and (b) they contribute to a score on a more broadly defined area that has already been reported (i.e., adaptive domains), then (c) all such narrowly defined areas should be reported. The purpose is to provide a balanced or more complete profile analysis (i.e., the pattern of scores among the more narrowly defined skills areas) in order to clarify or explain more fully that particular broadly based score (i.e., the Practical Adaptive Domain score). If such clarification of the broadly based score is not needed (e.g., diagnosis is sufficiently accomplished by merely reporting the more broadly based score), then none of the more specific scores are needed. The rule applies to all tests that possess a hierarchical structure or design. To conclude, this is the reason why the Work Adaptive Skill Area has been included in both Tables 1 and 5, as the latter provides the examiner with the option of reporting this skill area in either or even both locations.

Interpretation

As indicated in the latter portion of the previous section, the ABAS–3 has a hierarchical test design, proceeding as follows: (a) GAC; (b) adaptive domains; and (c) adaptive skill areas. The more broad-based scores have greater degrees of reliability and validity because more items contribute to their standard score transformations. At the same time, the more narrowly defined scales can provide valuable supplementary information, especially in identifying specific targets of treatment. Therefore, Table 1 in Forms 6.2 through 6.6 represents the beginning and cardinal focus for test interpretation. That is, Table 1 contains the core data and is the minimum to be reported and interpreted. If psychodiagnosis is the chief objective for the testing case, it frequently is sufficient in terms of test interpretation.

Composite and Standard Score Summary

Proceeding from general to specific in terms of test structure and constructs contained therein, the GAC should be interpreted first as all inclusive, especially noting the standard score and descriptive class. Next, the three primary domains should be scrutinized in terms of standard score, 95% CI, and classification. Interpretive excerpts follow Table 1 (Forms 6.2–6.6). The first paragraph guides the examiner through interpretation of the GAC, including its descriptive class, CI, and PR, all based upon test norms. The next question to address is how comparable are the domains to (a) the GAC, and then (b) to each other? Here, analysis of the 95% CIs is useful. If any have either no or very little overlap with the CI of the GAC, then these are the domains responsible for moving the GAC either higher or lower. On the other hand, if all overlap quite well with the CI of the GAC, then the GAC is a reliable and valid measure of the examinee's overall adaptive behavior. Next, examine the degree of overlap among the CIs of the three primary domains. Again, those that overlap are comparable and those that do not are likely to be significantly different. If there are no apparent differences, the ABAS–3 analyses are complete as typically this is sufficient to render key diagnostic conclusions for disorders such as ID and autism, the latter with its qualitative impairment in social relationships. The continuing interpretive statements following Table 1 guide the examiner through both the norm-based and ipsative informal domain comparisons. The final statement in the interpretive excerpt gives the option of either moving on to formal domain pairwise comparisons or declining to do so because the discrepancies are not diagnostically relevant to the case.

For the youngest examinees, the Motor Adaptive Skill Area standard equivalent score is reported. Low and extremely low scores contribute to ASD diagnoses and motor disorders (see Chapter 4 and Form 4.1). Analogously, the Work Adaptive Skill Area standard equivalent score is reported when the examinee is employed as this is a good prognostic sign of growing autonomy and independence.

Adaptive Domain Standard Score Comparisons

If there appear to be significant difference among the domains as evidenced by non-overlapping CIs, and it is vital diagnostically to confirm these differences in order to show an examinee's relative strengths and weaknesses, then Table 2 (Forms 6.2–6.6) can be used for more formal ipsative analyses among the principal domains. This is accomplished by using hypothesis testing principles and pragmatic base rates as *effect sizes* (i.e., how large is the effect). Of note, Table 2 is only reported when knowing the presence of relative differences has vital treatment implications. Otherwise, the CI analysis is sufficient for analyzing variability; that is, it is rapid and of reasonable accuracy. Once again, to facilitate test interpretation, two sets of narrative statements follow Table 2 (Forms 6.2–6.6). The first is drafted for results in which there are no significant differences found among the reported pairwise comparisons. In contrast, the second narrative lists the pairwise differences that are significant, with effect sizes to be reported in parentheticals.

Adaptive Skill Area Scaled Score Summary

Tables 3 through 5 (Forms 6.2–6.6) are important to report if (a) a particular domain is low or especially extremely low, and/or (b) treatment planning is heavily dependent upon the pattern of an examinee's specific skills. When a domain is particularly low, it may be important to profile the adaptive skill areas to show which are responsible for lowering the adaptive domain. If such is done, a similar comparison and contrast of their 95% CIs can be useful to interpret which represent relative strengths and weaknesses for purposes of treatment planning.[4]

Lastly, parallel narrative statements follow each of the adaptive skill area data tables. As typical, their purpose is to increase the rate and efficiency of score reporting and interpretation, while ensuring that all key aspects of the data are diligently interpreted. There are three paragraphs drafted in similar fashion. The first addresses the general norm-based elevations of the subtest scores in terms of their descriptive class or descriptive class range in the event there is variability among them. The second paragraph addresses the lowest and highest scores according to norms in order to address strengths and weaknesses compared to same aged peers. The last paragraph is drafted for analysis of any ipsative or intraindividual differences. These may be used in whole or part or modified as needed. If examiners follow these interpretive excerpts, such ensures that nothing will be overlooked in terms of test interpretation, and anything omitted will have been done so in order to effectively abbreviate the report.

Vineland Adaptive Behavior Scales, Third Edition

Synopsis

The *Vineland Adaptive Behavior Scales, Third Edition* (*Vineland–3*; Sparrow et al., 2016) is an individually administered test of adaptive behavior. There are three administration forms, including the (a) Interview Form, (b) Parent/Caregiver Form, and (c) Teacher Form, all of which can be done electronically online or by hard copy booklet. Each form comes in two versions as follows: (a) a comprehensive version that provides all available scores, including an overall score, domain scores, and subdomain scores; and (b) a domain version, which is circumscribed to the overall score and domain scores.

This discussion will be emphasizing the on-line Interview Form because it is the most efficient, accurate, comprehensive, and cost-effective. The norm reference sample for the Vineland–3 Interview Form, Comprehensive Version, is comparable to its predecessor the *Vineland Adaptive Behavior Scales, Second Edition* (*Vineland–II*; Sparrow et al., 2005), ranging from birth (i.e., 0) to age 90+ years. The Interview Form, Domain-Level version begins at age 3 years 0 months through 90+ years. The Parent/Caregiver Form has the same test structure, versions, and age ranges as the Interview Form. Lastly, the Teacher Form consists of the same structure and versions, although includes a much narrower age range from 3 years 0 months to 21 years 0 months (although the 18:0 year norms are used for 19:0–21:11 years).

Compared to the Vineland–II, the Vineland–3 has retained certain core features while modifying others so as to improve the test. As indicated prior, the following three components have been retained: (a) three basic administrations; (b) test structure; and (c) norm reference sample age ranges. The most essential changes consist of the following: (a) Domain-Level brief versions; (b) updated item content; (c) extended age range to 9 years 11 months for the Motor Skills Domain, although is no longer included in the overall Adaptive Behavior Composite (ABC); (d) basal and ceiling rules applied automatically based upon the respondent's answers to previous items when using the comprehensive on-line computerized administrations of all three forms; (e) added item-specific probes on the Interview Form to elicit more accurate responses from respondents and perhaps reduce overall administration time; (f) item rating of 1 label has changed from *Sometimes or Partially* to *Sometimes* for greater simplicity and consistency (i.e., including only a frequency dimension on all scores); (g) eliminating the *Don't Know* and *No Opportunity* options and supplanting them with an *estimate the frequency* probe in order to reduce the number of item omissions; and (h) a more appropriate and later starting age of 3 years 11 months for the Domestic and Community subdomains.

Because the Vineland–3 is in many respects identical to that of the Vineland–II, a more detailed historical section is deemed unnecessary. In fact, if one compares the data tables that have been designed for the two editions, they are virtually identical except for the name of course. Of note, many of the newer editions of tests and psychology-related publications are employing Arabic numerals rather than Roman numerals as being more contemporary (in addition to being easier to read and interpret).

Norm Reference Samples

The Vineland–3 norm reference samples were designed to be representative of the U.S. population within the aforementioned age range covered by each form; that is, Interview Form, Parent/Caregiver Form, and Teacher Form. More specifically, the samples were constructed according to the American Community Survey 2014 done by the U.S. Census Bureau (Ruggles, Genadek, Goeken, Grover, & Sobek, 2015). Samples were stratified according to (a) mother's (or father's) educational level as a proxy for socioeconomic status (viz., 0–12 years, no diploma, high school diploma, some college/associate degree, bachelor's degree or more); (b) race/ethnicity (viz., African American, Asian, Hispanic, White, Other); and (c) geographic region (northeast, south, north central, west).

Norm reference sample sizes were 2,560 individuals each for the Interview Form and Parent/Caregiver Form, ranging in age from birth through the late-90s, and 1,415 individuals for the Teacher Form, ranging in age from 3 years 0 months to 18 years 11 months, and applying the 18-year-old norms through age 21 years 11 months. In addition, each sample was broken down into age bands of equal numbers of males and females, with narrower age bands used for younger individuals due to their more rapid rates of growth as compared to older individuals though age 70 years (i.e., 3-month intervals across 1-year-olds, 6-month intervals for 2- to 4-year-olds, 1-year intervals for 5- to 11-year-olds, 2-year-intervals for 12- to 20-years-olds, and 20-year-intervals from 20- to 70-year-olds). After 70 years, age intervals were decreased to 10 years. Approximately 11.9% of the norm reference samples were those in various special education categories (e.g., autism, emotional disturbance, ID), which was considered a reasonable match to the 12.9% rate noted in the population. Taken together, the norm reference samples for the three forms were considered to be a sufficient representation of major demographic variables in the population.

More specifically, norms were first developed for the v–scale scores, which are used at the most specific subdomain level (see subsequent). They were developed by a common process referred to as inferential norming (Wilkins, Rolfhus, Weiss, & Zhu, 2005). *Inferential norming* is a common process in which key statistical indexes or *moments*, here including the mean (*M*), standard deviation (*SD*), and measures of skewness, were calculated for each of the 28 age bands as indicated prior (Sparrow et al., 2016, pp. 93–94). These were then plotted across age groups using linear regression and polynomial regression equations (i.e., regression formulas with predictors to the 2nd, 3rd, and 4th power) to derive predictions or estimates of age group midpoint population moments (hence the term *inferential norming* or statistical procedure that estimates population parameters from representative sample statistics). The linear and polynomial regressions were needed to account for different patterns of growth observed across the age bands (e.g., faster development at younger ages). From these prediction formulas, the test developers were able to derive theoretical distributions of development for each age group, which yielded percentiles for each raw score. Finally, the percentiles were converted to the v–scale standard score, which has a mean of 15 and standard deviation of 3, and a rather large range from 1 to 24; that is, compared to the more typical scaled score metric used in many standardized tests (i.e., mean = 10; standard deviation = 3; range 1–19). This larger range metric, which was also employed by the predecessor Vineland–II (Sparrow et al., 2005), more effectively captures the extremes of development at both ends of the score distribution; that is, not simply at the lower end. At this point, *v–scale score* norms were created for each subdomain.

Next, in order to derive domain standard scores, the v–scale subdomain scores assigned to each domain were summed or aggregated for each individual in the norm reference sample. Age bands were created by combining adjacent groups, and statistical tests (e.g., analysis of variance or ANOVA) were done to ensure that the mean v–scale scores and variances were not significantly different across the age groupings. The v–scale score distributions were then used to compute percentiles, which were converted to domain standard scores with a mean of 100 and standard deviation of 15, and an impressively large range of 20 to 140. Finally, the ABC was derived by aggregating the domain standard scores in the same manner as the v–scale scores were summed to create the domain standard scores. However, the ABC has the same standard score metric (mean = 100, standard deviation = 15) as domain standard scores. One other note is needed for the Domain-Level Form norms. Here, raw scores were converted directly into domain standard scores in an analogous manner that the aforementioned v–scale scores were derived from raw score conversions into percentiles.

Contrasting the Two Adaptive Behavior Measures: Vineland–3 Versus the ABAS–3

This section of the Vineland–3 adduces why two standardized tests of adaptive behavior which are extremely similar in design, content, and format, are included in the book's inventory. When psychologists are in the process of building an inventory of psychological tests, they should consider (a) the populations they are servicing, (b) the kinds of psychopathology they most frequently encounter, (c) the types of referral questions they are or will likely receive, and (d) the rate of recurrence of each of the initial three characteristics. The latter characteristic helps determine how and where financial resources will be most effectively distributed. Furthermore, it is prudent to avoid unnecessary redundancy in constructing a test inventory, which may be defined as possessing two or more measures that perform the same function. So, why have two adaptive behavior measures in the book's test inventory that appear to be so equivalent?

The primary dissimilarity between the Vineland–3 and ABAS–3 is that the former possesses a convenient structured interview format for both its comprehensive and domain level versions. Such format provides two components that may be more desirable in certain cases, including: (a) increased accuracy of responses due to both (i) available interview probes, and (ii) the ability to otherwise clarify the respondent's ratings; and (b) the increased likelihood third party payers will reimburse for the time needed to administer the interview. That is, some managed care companies (e.g., in the state of Indiana, the Healthy Indiana Plan or HIP) will not reimburse for the use of any measure that can be considered a pure "rating scale," which unfortunately includes measures such as the ABAS–3. In contrast, even the most stringent insurance companies will afford preauthorization (PA) testing services to cover the time for required face-to-face administration. Therefore, use of either the Vineland–3 Comprehensive Interview Form or Domain-Level Interview Form would be eligible for PA of testing services units, which means being reimbursed for one's legitimate work in providing valuable psychological testing services.

Then why not just use the Vineland? In point of fact, the Vineland–3 hard copy forms do not discriminate as well among the various age groups, and do not have an adult form that doubles as both observer-based data and self-report data as does the ABAS–3. Thus, the ABAS–3 can be superior depending upon the case facts if paper forms must be used. An added reason to use the ABAS–3 if paper forms are required regards its unlimited scoring software. In contrast, the Vineland–3's computer scoring is internet-based and the psychologist is charged for each score report (see subsequently). Therefore, if the use of paper forms will be needed (e.g., the respondent is not able to attend assessment sessions; insurance PA for rating scales is afforded), it is advantageous to have the ABAS–3 as part of the test inventory, especially if adaptive behavior measures are frequently used in a psychologist's testing practice as this exploits the unlimited scoring feature of the ABAS–3 computer scoring software.

Administration

The discussion here will focus on the Interview Form, which consists of both the Comprehensive version and the Domain-Level version. Again, this is because the main advantage of this measure over the ABAS–3 is the availability of the structured interview format, which permits the use to clarifying probes and other interventions by the interviewer so as to improve accuracy in ratings.

In comparing the two interview alternatives, the Domain-Level version tends to be more pragmatic because the primary focus in mental health testing practice is on diagnosis, for example, ruling in a diagnosis of intellectual disability (ID). Therefore, the Domain-Level Interview Form is typically sufficient for mental health testing objectives and it is much more efficient. As evidence, the Domain-Level Interview Form contains 135 core items, along with an additional 25 items for the optional Motor Domain and 35 items for the optional Maladaptive Behavior Domain, hence totaling a maximum of 195 items. This is compared to the 381 core items and 502 total items on the Comprehensive version, which renders the Domain-Level Interview Form to be only 1/4th as long and therefore most cost effective.

Prior to initiating the interview, there are two options given to include a Motor Skills Domain (up to age 9 years), and a Maladaptive Behavior Domain (ages 3 years and older), the latter consisting of Internalizing, Externalizing, and Critical Items categories. Neither of these domains are included in the Adaptive Behavior Composite (ABC), which is why they are both optional. The Motor Skills Domain is normed on individuals from birth through age 9 years 11 months. Although it does not contribute to the ABC, it does provide useful information regarding a child's development and should be included when possible. In contrast, the Maladaptive Behavior Domain is significantly less useful compared to other rating scales, which are much more detailed and discriminating for purposes of differential diagnosis. Therefore, this option and can be skipped for purposes of efficiency unless only screening for behavior problems is desired.

The semi-structured interview should be done individually and face-to-face (versus via telephone). The manual refers to the administrative approach as the *Vineland semistructured interview technique* (Sparrow et al., 2016, p. 19). By this, it is meant that the interviewer is to ask a "suggested interview question" for a particular topic, each containing two to six items; for example, "What safety precautions within the home environment does Joe follow?" This question is open ended and designed to potentially elicit answers to several of the items in that particular topic, which are presented in list form on the computer screen below the interview question; for this example, the Daily Living Skills: Home Safety cluster. Each item appearing in the content cluster has a selection below it labeled *Probe*, which when clicked upon opens a recommended prompt, such as, "What about . . . ?" This probe is designed to acquire information necessary to score a particular item not yet scorable with the given information from the suggested question. Finally, there is a second selection for an item labeled *Scoring Criteria*, which when clicked provides specific scoring instructions; for example, "Give credit if individual names the actions when asked . . ."

Due to its much greater length, the Comprehensive Interview employs start points based upon the examinee's CA, along with basal (i.e., *four consecutive items* yielding maximum scores of 2) and ceiling (i.e., *four consecutive items* yielding failing scores of 0) rules. The computer software automatically applies the start points, basal, and ceiling rules so that the interviewer can focus on the accurate scoring of items. The Domain-Level Interview is sufficiently abbreviated such that all items must be given. The scoring options for most items are as follows: (a) when the behavior is needed or appropriate, the individual *usually* performs it without help or prompting (score = 2); (b) when the behavior is needed or appropriate, the individual *sometimes* performs it without help or prompting (score = 1); or (c) the individual *never* performs the behavior, or *never* performs it without help or prompting; succinctly, 2 = *Usually*; 1 = *Sometimes*; 0 = *Never*. However, some items (e.g., Says at least 22 words.) are binary as follows: 2 = *Yes*; 0 = *No*. The interviewer enters in the scores based upon the respondent's answers to the suggested interview question and any clarifying probes. All items must be scored or the computer software will prohibit advancing to the next screen. The scoring criteria assists in determining the final score for an item. When the respondent is unsure, for example, there has been no opportunity for the behavior to be observed, the proper instruction should be "guess," and the adjacent *Estimated* box should be checked (replacing the *No Opportunity* or *Don't Know* options in the Vineland–II). Once all of the items have been scored, an Assessment Complete screen appears and scoring can now be done.

Scoring

The computer software scoring for the Vineland–3 is more complex in that it provides a significant amount of data that are not very useful. Therefore, first provided is a description of the Vineland–3 score report formats for the two different interview versions discussed prior: that is, the Comprehensive and Domain-Level Interview Form Reports. This is ensued by the data tables that have been designed for reporting the Vineland–3 test results within a psychological assessment report.

Q–Global Computer Score Reports

The internet-based Q–global program (Pearson, 2021) provides a both a Comprehensive and Domain-Level Interview Form Report immediately subsequent to successful administration. Essential portions of the Comprehensive Report are as follows: (a) ABC and Domain Score Summary; (b) Subdomain Score Summary; (c) Domain Pairwise Differences Comparisons; (d) Subdomain Pairwise Differences Comparisons; and (e) Maladaptive Behavior Results. The former provides the composite and domain standard scores ($M = 100$; $SD = 15$), 95% CI (which can be changed to 90%), PR, and a difference score for each domain computed as follows; the domain standard score (*SS*) minus the mean or average of the examinee's standard scores (*Mean SS*). The examinee's *Mean SS* is provided in a table note. Therefore, minus scores indicate that such domain was lower than the examinee's own average domain score while positive scores indicate the opposite. Although these difference scores are useful for relative comparisons (i.e., ipsative analysis), the norm-based comparisons are most essential for making accurate diagnoses. Finally, the base rate for the difference score is reported as equal to, or less than, the lowest of 25%, 15%, 10%, 5%, and 2%. Of note, descriptive classifications (here termed adaptive levels) are not reported by the scoring software and must be referenced in the manual (Sparrow et al., 2016, Table 4.1, p. 68).

The Subdomain Score Summary reports the subdomains using the *v*–scale score metric (mean = 15; standard deviation = 3). However, it fails to report other statistics that are routinely used in this book in analyzing test results, such as CIs, PRs, and adaptive levels. The computer scoring also reports the *v*–scale score differences from the examinee's mean *v*–scale score and associated base rates, analogous to the domain score summary discussed prior. However, these are not used in the test data tables because they are unnecessarily detailed.

The ensuing two tables of the output respectively show (a) all possible pairwise domain and subdomain comparisons, (b) their computed or obtained differences, (c) whether or not these differences are statistically significant at the .05 level of probability (i.e., whether the differences would occur 5 times in 100 or less due to chance factors) or .10 level (i.e., whether the differences would occur 10 times in 100 or less due to chance factors), and lastly, (d) the base rate of these obtained differences.

Vineland–3 Data Tables for Psychological Assessment Reports

The Vineland–3 data tables for reporting test results are presented in Form 6.7. They are designed for reporting both the Comprehensive and Domain-Level Interview data by including tables that accommodate the ABC, domain-level standard scores, and the subdomain-level *v*–scores.

PRIMARY ANALYSES

In order of presentation, Table 1 (Form 6.7) consists of the ABC, all three domains contributing to the ABC (viz., Communication, Daily Living Skills, and Socialization), and the optional Motor Skills domain. The essential data include the composite and domain standard scores (*M* = 100; *SD* = 15), 95% CIs (which can be changed to 90%), PRs, adaptive levels, and measured skills. General table notes delineate the metrics, define the summary notations, and indicate that the lead data are presented in bold font. This includes the no score denotation (i.e., --) in instances where the optional Motor Skills domain is not used, or when a domain becomes invalid due to greater than 25% of a domain's items being estimated (see Sparrow et al., 2016, p. 47).

An analysis of relative domain differences can be done most efficiently by considering the CIs and their degree of overlap. Percentile ranks can be more emphasized if the anticipated reading audience consists mostly of those unfamiliar with standard scores. Lastly, the qualitative interpretations are defined by a combination of the following: (a) those used in the updated Vineland–3 for adaptive levels in order of increasing impairment *high, moderately high, adequate, moderately low,* and *low;* and (b) those used in the Vineland–II for apportioning the bottommost adaptive level *low* into degrees of deficit. That is, rather than having an excessively large single most impaired range from 70 down to 20 being designated as *low,* it is preferable to continue to employ the Vineland–II scheme that offers more discrimination. This should make sense since it exploits the Vineland–3's attempt to sufficiently cover both high and low extremes of functioning.

The combined Vineland–3 and Vineland–II adaptive levels can be seen in Table 6.6. As can be observed, these ranges mirror those of the DSM–5 degree of ID severity and can be very useful in providing more accurate differential diagnosis. Note that the higher range in the new Vineland–3 is lowered somewhat to 140 versus 160, and

Table 6.6 Vineland–3 Adaptive Level Guide

Standard Scores	v–Scale Scores	Adaptive Level
130–140	21–24	High
115–129	18–20	Moderately high
86–114	13–17	Adequate
71–85	10–12	Moderately low
50/55–70	8–9	Mild deficit★
35/40–50/55	5–7	Moderate deficit★
25–35/40	4–6	Severe deficit★
20–25	1–3	Profound deficit★

Sources. Adapted from (a) Sparrow, S. S., Cicchetti, D. V., & Balla, D. A. (2005). *Vineland Adaptive Behavior Scales, 2nd Edition (Vineland–II): Survey forms manual.* Minneapolis, MN: Pearson, Tables 4.1 and C.4, pp. 65 and 253; (b) Grossman, H. J. (Ed.). (1983). *Classification in mental retardation.* (1983 rev.). Washington DC: American Association on Mental Deficiency, p. 13. (Cited in Sparrow, S. S., Cicchetti, D. V., & Balla, D. A. (2005). *Vineland Adaptive Behavior Scales, 2nd Edition (Vineland–II): Survey forms manual.* Minneapolis, MN: Pearson, p. 253.); Sparrow, S. S., Cicchetti, D. V., & Saulnier, C. A. (2016). *Vineland Adaptive Behavior Rating Scales, Third Edition (Vineland–3): Manual.* Minneapolis, MN: Pearson, Table 4.1, p. 68.

Note. ★ denotes a *low* classification in the Vineland–3 adaptive level scheme.

therefore must now be scaled down 20 standard score points. The remaining score ranges and adaptive levels are the same. The Domain-Level computer score report provides a table for suggested qualitative descriptors for various standard score ranges as does the manual, which also includes the ν–scale score ranges and qualitative descriptors (Sparrow et al., 2016, p 68, Table 4.1). However, neither provides a breakdown of the large 50-point *low* range into more discriminatory deficit categories, hence reference to Table 6.6 is needed for such information.

SECONDARY ANALYSES

Table 2 provides the data for an ipsative analysis of any significant differences among all pairwise comparisons of adaptive domains that have been measured, including the optional Motor Skills domain. The table contains five columns as follows: (a) domain names in the order subtracted; (b) first standard score; (c) second standard score; (d) obtained difference score, including an appended asterisk (i.e., ★) if such is statistically significant at the 5% level; and (e) the base rate of the norm reference sample that manifested the obtained difference score. It should be here noted that, in contrast to the ABAS–3 computer scoring, the critical value difference scores for the Vineland–3 are not reported; simply whether or not the obtained difference was statistically significant. However, these values are available in Appendix B of the manual, which is actually an online resource for the Vineland–3 (see Sparrow et al., 2016, Appendix B, p. 303). In any case, preferable to simply list the information reported by the computer scoring output as such information is not vital when balanced against the precious time that would be consumed in locating these values. Lastly, this computer scoring software does enumerate the base rates of the obtained difference scores as the lowest of one of the following: > 25%; ≤ 25%; ≤ 15%; ≤ 10%; ≤ 5%; and ≤ 2%. Therefore, the significance scheme endorsed by Sattler (2001) was inserted and denoted in Table 2 by cross symbols (i.e., †), which as can be recalled was also employed in the Bayley–III subtest scaled score discrepancy analysis.

TERTIARY ANALYSES

Tables 3, 4, and 5 (Form 6.7) are designed to report the subdomain ν–scale score data. They are in the same order in which they appear in Table 1; that is Communication, Daily Living Skills, Socialization, and Motor Skills (if given). As stated prior, the computer software does not print out the CIs, PRs, and adaptive levels that are essential in analyzing test data. Therefore, in order to report the CIs, the subdomain standard errors of measurement (*SEM*s) were securitized in the manual. More specifically, the *SEM*s for the subdomains using the interview form are reported in Table 6.2 in the manual (Sparrow et al., 2016, p. 119), and are based upon internal consistency reliability coefficients, hence comparable to the one's selected for the ABAS–3 when estimating *SEM*s for the adaptive domain scaled scores. Of particular interest is the reported *SEM* averaged over all of the age bands for each subdomain. For example, the *SEM* averaged over all age bands for the Receptive Subdomain is 1.07. Therefore, regardless of age, if an examinee's Receptive Subdomain score is 15, then the 95% confidence interval would be 15 ± 2.14 (i.e., 1.07 x 2) or 13 to 17 (rounding to the nearest whole number). However, to render it even more efficient while not sacrificing accuracy, one would be justified in averaging all the average subdomain *SEM*s; that is, computing a grand mean. This is readily done because they are all very close to 1.00 (i.e., with a range 0.72 to 1.30). The overall average turned out to be 0.99, which is conveniently rounded to 1.00 as the nearest whole number; a common practice when estimating CIs. In the end, for all subdomain Tables 3, 4, 5, and 6 (Form 6.7), the *SEM* is the average of all average subdomain *SEM*s reported in the Vineland–3 manual, which turns out to be an even 1.00. This information is reported in the special tabular notes to each of the subdomain Tables 3 through 6).

The PRs for the more esoteric ν–scale scores are expectedly different than for the more common scaled scores. In particular, the ν–scale score is five points higher than the typical scaled score. Again, the intent was to expand the range of the lower scores to 4.66 *SD*s below the mean. Therefore, their associated PRs are different from the more typical scaled score ($M = 10$; $SD = 3$) used in the vast majority of standardized tests (e.g., ABAS–3, IQ tests). Therefore, a ν–scale score to PR conversion chart has been prepared and is available in Table 6.7. This was easily done by using a standard normal distribution table available in most introductory statistics texts (see, e.g., Field, 2018, pp. 725–728). The lowest two scores surpass four standard deviations below the mean and had to be done by means of interpolation. They may not be exact, although are reasonably accurate, especially when considering how little differences there are at the extremes of a distribution of scores.

Note that Table 6.7 is deliberately formatted in non-APA style format (see American Psychological Association, 2020) in terms of including the internal vertical and horizontal lines so that it is easier for the reader to correctly find the obtained ν–scale score and its associated PR value. This was especially needed because of the alternating ν–scale score and PR columns that were required to obviate the table from becoming excessively long, especially when attempting to include the tabular general notes.

Table 6.7 v–Scale Score to Percentile Rank Conversion Guide

v–Scaled Score	Percentile Rank	v–Scaled Score	Percentile Rank	v–Scaled Score	Percentile Rank
24	99.86	16	63	8	1
23	99.60	15	50	7	.4
22	99.01	14	37	6	.1
21	98	13	26	5	.04
20	95	12	16	4	.01
19	91	11	10	3	.003
18	84	10	6	2	.0008
17	75	9	2	1	.0002

Note. The *v*–scale scores were first converted to *z*–score units, which were then used to estimate the associated percentile rank using a table of the standard normal distribution (e.g., see Field, 2018) and/or a *z*–score to percent calculator available on various internet sites (e.g., see Z–Score to Percentile Calculator, used March 21, 2019). Sufficient decimal places were used to best differentiate the PR values associated with various *v*–scale scores.

Interpretation

Form 6.7 may be used irrespective of the Interview Form version used during administration. If the Comprehensive version was administered, then potentially all tables may be utilized in interpretation. In such instance, the "Domain-Level" words in the major heading should be deleted. In contrast, if the shorter Domain-Level version was given, then the word "Comprehensive" in the major heading should be deleted, along with Tables 3 through 6 as there are no subdomain data to interpret. Irrespective of the Interview Form version employed, Vineland–3 interpretation begins with the composite and domain data.

Finally, note that each table is designed to be interpreted independently. This is denoted by the italicized "Interpretation" heading following each table. As will be seen, Table 1 offers two pre-drafted narrative interpretations while the remaining tables include only a terse prompt due to the innumerable permutations that can result among these data.

Composite and Domain-Level Standard Score Summary

Interpretation proceeds from general to specific; here from the composite, to the three primary domains contributing to the composite, and ending with the optional Motor Skills Domain (if administered). The ABC frequently determines or impacts diagnoses within the neurodevelopmental category, especially ID. Analysis of the domains and their influence upon the ABC follows the diagnostic meaning of the ABC. The remaining interpretive strategy mirrors that of the ABAS–3. Hence, in the interests of brevity, the reader is referred to the interpretive section of the ABAS–3 for Table 1 (Forms 6.2–6.6).

Feedback from first edition readers indicated that common narrative excerpts following the tables were very useful. Therefore, immediately following Table 1 are two interpretive summaries of characteristic results as follows: (a) a no-impairment profile; and (b) a clear impairment profile with follow-up. The latter is succeeded by bullet-points, the first of which confirms an ID diagnosis with an estimation of degree. This is consistent with DSM–5 advising that adaptive behavior standard scores supplant the IQ score in determining degree or level of impairment. The second bullet point uses language indicating that the Table 1 results are consistent with the presence of neurodevelopmental psychopathology, including a recommendation for formal pairwise comparisons among the domains to further clarify the symptom pattern (see Table 2, Form 6.7). Again, use of Table 2 is unnecessary if adequately addressed when discussing the Table 1 CIs and their degrees of overlap.

Domain Pairwise Difference Comparisons

Table 2 (Form 6.7) also mirrors that of the ABAS–3 in terms of providing all pairwise comparisons of measured domains, here including the optional Motor Skills domain. This statistically detailed analysis is needed largely in cases where the referral source is relying upon a relative strengths and weaknesses profile interpretation for purposes of treatment planning. Interpretation of Table 2 results may also be done if the profile of domain scores is highly variable, hence having potentially diagnostic implications. Otherwise, the more efficient CIs analysis be done. To be more precise, CIs comparisons can proceed as follows (especially at 95% confidence): (a) no overlap means a significant difference; (b) partial overlap means a possible or cautiously interpreted significant difference; and (c) little or no overlap means no significant difference. The ordinal PRs can be emphasized in interpretation if the reading audience consists of those unfamiliar with standard scores.

Subdomain v–Scale Score Summary

Tables 3, 4, 5, and 6 are optional in that they focus exclusively upon the subdomain profile. First, if the Domain-Level Interview was administered, these data can simply be deleted as they were not measured by this version of the test. Second, even in cases where the Comprehensive Interview Form was used, reporting these data depends upon the following two factors: (a) the presence of deficit scores at the domain standard score level; and (b) the referral source's need for detailed treatment recommendations that target specific skills that are most in need of improvement or rehabilitation. If neither of these factors are manifest, then these data may be considered nonessential and thus not interpreted in the interests of focusing the report upon the most vital issues rather than inundating the reader with excessive details that obfuscate the main points.

If these data are reported, providing the reader with the meaning of the v–scale scores, along with their CIs, PRs, and adaptive levels is important so as to be complete yet efficient. The associated adaptive levels may be found in Table 6.6, which is the same guide used for the standard scores. Although the Q–global (Pearson, 2021) computer scoring software provides pairwise comparisons for all subdomains, the faster CIs analysis should suffice.

Autism Diagnostic Observation Schedule, Second Edition

Synopsis

The *Autism Diagnostic Observation Schedule (ADOS–2;* Lord, Luyster, Gotham, & Guthrie, 2012; Lord, Rutter et al., 2012) is a semi-structured, standardized, performance-based measure, principally designed to detect signs of ASD in individuals ranging in age from 12 months through adulthood, who can walk independently, and who are otherwise free of motor and sensory impairments (including especially vision and audition). Stated more succinctly, the objective of the ADOS–2 is to provide standardized contexts in which to directly observe and measure any social and communicative signs of autism in individuals across the majority of the lifespan. The ultimate objective is to facilitate the reliable and valid diagnosis of ASD in those who have the disorder.

In particular, the ADOS–2 test format includes a series of pre-planned structured and unstructured activities, which serve to organize the interaction during which an examinee's social interactions, communications, and various behaviors are elicited and observed for signs of autism. ADOS–2 items represent the distinct aspects of the examinee's behavior that are targeted for observation. Items, materials, and prompts are organized into units called modules that are based upon combinations of CA and language abilities. Observations made during test administration are subsequently coded according to standardized criteria, and then transformed into empirically based algorithm scores in order to render decisions regarding an autism diagnosis. If the result is positive, a comparison score can also be computed that measures severity level, and which permits comparing the examinee to others with documented autism who is of the same CA and language ability.

Put succinctly, the ADOS–2 is a performance-based test specifically designed to measure signs of autism and to make informed decisions regarding such diagnosis. Its immediate predecessor is the *Autism Diagnostic Observation Schedule (ADOS;* Lord, Rutter, DiLavore, & Risi, 1999). The ADOS–2's revisions and updates, including improved guidelines for administration, coding and interpretation, more sophisticated scoring and algorithms, and a new component for the assessment of toddlers, has contributed to this measure being referred to as, "the gold standard" for diagnosing autism (Kanne, Randolph, & Farmer, 2008; Ozonoff, Goodlin-Jones, & Solomon, 2005).

Testing for the presence of autism requires mastery of multiple key terms and concepts. In fact, once sufficiently trained in the use of this test, one develops a much deeper understanding and appreciation of this disorder. Although key terms are identified and defined throughout this book, an even greater emphasis on semantics is required here. Therefore, a special table is offered in which a range of key words are listed in alphabetical order and clearly defined. The reader is now referred to Table 6.8 and encouraged to become intimately familiar with its terms and their meaning. This will expedite the learning process and mastery of this complex yet extremely useful measure in diagnostic testing practice.

Table 6.8 Autism Diagnostic Observation Schedule, Second Edition (ADOS–2) Key Terms and Definitions

Term	Definition
Complex sentence	Utterance with two or more clauses.
Distal	Refers to pointing to objects sufficiently far from the individual so that such behavior denotes either (a) an attempt to direct the attention of another to the object, and/or (b) coordinate gaze to an object and person; as opposed to touching or attempted touching.
Gesture	An action of the hands or body that is used to communicate a message to another person; the action does not include holding an object (e.g., pretending to fly an airplane).^
Gesture–conventional	Action that has a standard social meaning within a particular culture.[†]
Gesture–descriptive	Pantomime actions used when trying to describe or represent an action, object, or event for communicative purposes (e.g., waving index finger across teeth as demonstrating tooth brushing).[†]
Gesture–emotional	Action that expresses affect or situation-elicited feeling (e.g., thumbs up to mean approval or satisfaction).[†]
Gesture–emphatic	Action that involves hand movements or beats that are integrated into an individual's speech in order to provide emphasis when talking; special consideration is afforded to (a) how well the gestures are timed with speech, and (b) the degree to which gestures are exaggerated or muted.[†]
Gesture–informational	Action used to convey specific types of facts or knowledge (e.g., holding up four fingers to mean, "I am four years old").[†]
Gesture–instrumental	Action that is intended to achieve a goal (e.g., waving arm means "come here") or holding one's hand out to obtain something (e.g., begging).[†]
Giving	Handing objects to another person across a range of *pragmatic contexts*.
Joint-attention	Giving or showing an object to another person for shared enjoyment or interest.
Neologism	A new word or word combinations, the meaning of which is understood only by the user.
Phrase speech	Flexible use of non-echoed, three-word utterances that sometimes involve a verb, and are spontaneous, meaningful word combinations.
Play–functional	The use of toys or objects in the manner in which they were intended.[†]
Play–imaginative	The use of toys or objects which involves pretending or symbolism, including using one object to represent a different object (e.g., using dolls as independent agents of action or yarn as spaghetti).[†]
Pragmatic context	The purpose or intention of a given vocalization or utterance evinced within a particular situation (e.g., making a request, sharing enjoyment, directing attention, seeking emotional comfort).
Pronoun error across person	The incorrect use of pronouns across first, second, and third person perspectives; (e.g., you, she, or he to mean I).
Requesting	A conventional indication (e.g., gesture, eye contact, vocalization, facial expression) of an individual's desire for a particular action or object.
Response to name	Orienting to and making eye contact with the person who calls his/her name.
Showing	Deliberately orienting or placing an object where it can be seen by another person with no identifiable purpose of getting help or participating in a routine.
Simple phrase	One-word utterance that is associated with a gesture (aka holophrases) or two-word utterance that excludes filler words (e.g., "My ball," or "You go"); one step less sophisticated than phrase speech.
Social overture	Any behavior initiated by the individual that is directed to another person for the purpose of communicating intent (e.g., making eye contact, directing a facial expression, touching, addressing verbally).★
Social response	Same as *social overture* (e.g., making eye contact, directing a facial expression, touching, addressing verbally), but the individual shows these behaviors in response to another person's actions or to the social situation.^
Three-point gaze shift	Sequence in which (a) individual looks at an object, (b) then looks at a person in order to catch his/her gaze and direct it to the object, and finally (c) looking back at the object; alternate sequence is looking at person–object–person.
Toy–miniatures	Reduced-size model of real-life object (e.g., toy telephone or car); aka representational toy.[†]
Toy–cause-effect	Requires an action in order to produce a particular effect (e.g., jack-in-the-box).[†]
Toy–construction	Principal purpose is building or stacking (e.g., letter blocks).[†]
Toy–non-meaningful placeholder	Ambiguous object, such as a rectangular wooden block, which is used to test whether an examinee can use such object as a representation of a real-life object recently seen (e.g., to represent a recently seen toy car that moves) or not previously seen; a test for functional and symbolic imitation.
Verbal fluency	Consists of (a) producing a range of flexible sentence types and grammatical forms, (b) using language to provide information about events beyond the immediate context, and (c) describing logical connections within a sentence (e.g., using "but" or "though").

Note. ★ denotes that the definition was obtained from Lord, Rutter et al. (2012, p. 19); ^ denotes that the definition was obtained from Lord, Rutter et al. (2012, p. 20); † denotes that the definition was obtained from Lord, Rutter et al.(2012, p. 21). Italicized words provided in definitions are themselves key terms that are defined within the table.

Norm Reference Samples and Standardization

Being a performance-based test that purportedly detects the presence of autism and measures its severity, this norm reference section is expanded in order to discusses the manner in which this instrument was standardized. In particular, the ADOS–2 was standardized on a sequence of three validation samples, including individuals ranging in age from 14 months to 40 years. Furthermore, these samples consisted of individuals who were without significant sensory or motor impairments, including normal and intact vision and hearing, along with being able to walk independently. In general, participants were classified as follows: (a) autism (i.e., those meeting full criteria for the disorder); (b) *autism spectrum disorder* or *ASD–A*[5] (i.e., those meeting partial criteria, including *Asperger's disorder* and *pervasive developmental disorder, not otherwise specified* or *PDD–NOS*); and (c) non-autism disorders (e.g., *oppositional defiant disorder, communication disorder*). It is noteworthy that the non-autism group included very few normally developing individuals because the principal objective was the differential diagnosis among groups with various forms of confirmed psychopathology (as opposed to simple abnormal versus normal control comparisons). Standardization of such a diagnostic instrument focused upon its reliability and validity in samples most likely to be the target of testing; that is, (a) is it precise and stable, and (b) does it measure what it claims to measure and is it justified in its use.

The initial validation sample included 381 referrals, ranging in age from 15 months to 40 years, who were used in standardizing the ADOS (Lord et al., 1999). Many were subsequently used in the ensuing extended validation sample, which was used in both reliability and validity analyses for the new ADOS–2. This was possible because the ADOS–2 items were functionally identical to those of the ADOS. The final extended validation sample consisted of 912 assessments as follows: (a) 57% autism; (b) 27% ASD–A; and (c) 17% non-spectrum. Lastly, an ADOS–2 replication sample was used to determine the reliability of the algorithms. This third sample included individuals aged 18 months to 16 years, the rationale being that this age range would capture the majority of cases being assessed by this measure.

The majority of reliability and validity studies referenced immediately subsequent focus on three principal scores that contribute directly to test interpretation, the latter including (a) a diagnostic classification, and (b) a dimensional measure of degree or level of autism signs. These scores are particular labels employed in this book and generally include: (a) Social Affect (SA) Algorithm Score Total; (b) Restricted and Repetitive Behavior (RRB) Algorithm Score Total; and (c) Overall Algorithm Score Total (SA + RRB). The labels for the domain scores vary somewhat for some modules, although for purposes of reviewing the ensuing reliability and validity studies, they are reasonable accurate. As alluded to by the labels, the domain scores are aggregated into the final total, which, in turn, is employed in both types of interpretation. These scores will be explained in sufficient detail in the scoring section. More immediately, this brief introduction of ADOS–2 scores was needed in order to better understand the reliability and validity evidence, which for the most part focuses on these scores, along with some analyses being conducted at the item-level (e.g., factor-analytic and internal consistency statistics). The first round of analyses involves the reliability and validity of the ADOS–2 classification.

Reliability and Validity of ADOS–2 Classification

Reliability studies that investigated consistency and accuracy of the ADOS–2 included the following types of analyses: (a) internal consistency; (b) interrater reliability; and (c) test-retest reliability. These are reviewed first because it is axiomatic that without reliability there can be no validity (see, e.g., Furr, 2018). Regarding internal consistency, intra-class correlations for the Social Affect and Restricted and Repetitive Behaviors domains were typically within the mid-.90s, hence showing that items within these domains are strongly related to or resemble each other. Interrater reliability for the ADOS–2 is also vital, considering that items are rated using a sequence of codes, which are ultimately used to classify an examinee as either autism, ASD–A, or non-spectrum. Such data shows a typical range of 92% to 98% interrater agreement on examinees' ultimate ADOS–2 classification, depending on the unit or module used. In addition, individual items showed similar levels of interrater agreement, ranging from 83% to 100% (see Lord, Rutter et al., 2012, Tables D1–D4, pp. 256–259). Lastly, test-retest reliability coefficients over an average 10-month period for the Overall Algorithm Score Total, SA Algorithm Score Total (SA domain), and RRB Algorithm Score Total (RRB domain) were within the following ranges, respectively: (a) .94–.99; (b) .92–.98; and (c) .79–.91. These ADOS–2 scores ultimately determine both the classification and degree of autism signs (see subsequent). Such data indicate that these key scores are sufficiently stable over time.

Moving to validity, does the ADOS–2 actually measure signs of autism, and, if so, can it be used to (a) classify an individual as either autism, ASD–A, or non-spectrum, and (b) measure the level of autism signs while controlling for the effects of expressive language ability and CA? First, exploratory and confirmatory factor analyses consistently show the expected two-factor structure, forming the SA and RRB domains. In addition, while factor analyses show that the two domains SA and RRB are independent, they are also sufficiently correlated to justify their aggregation into an overall total.

Table 6.9 Specificity and Sensitivity of ADOS–2 Algorithms: Autism Versus Non-Spectrum

Sensitivity	Specificity
91–98	50–94
82–94	80–100

Note. Sensitivity = the statistical probability that the ADOS–2 algorithm will correctly identify an examinee who has autism (versus a non-spectrum disorder). Specificity = the statistical probability that the ADOS–2 algorithm will correctly identify an examinee as having a non-spectrum disorder (versus autism). Data reported in Lord, Rutter et al., 2012, Table 9, p. 243).

Table 6.10 Specificity and Sensitivity of ADOS–2 Algorithms: Autism Spectrum Versus Non-Spectrum

Sample Type	Sensitivity	Specificity
ADOS–2 Extended Validity Sample ($N = 685$)	77–95	19–83
ADOS–2 Replication Sample ($N = 238$)	60–95	65–88

Note. Sensitivity = the statistical probability that the ADOS–2 algorithm will correctly identify an examinee who has an autism spectrum disorder (versus a non-spectrum disorder). Specificity = the statistical probability that the ADOS–2 algorithm will correctly identify an examinee as having a non-spectrum disorder (versus an autism spectrum disorder). Data reported in Lord, Rutter et al., 2012, Table 10, p. 245).

Predictive validity is also vital for such a diagnostic measure. Here, can the ADOS–2 significantly predict examinees' classification as autism, ASD–A, or non-spectrum? First, *logistic regression* analyzes whether several continuous variables (e.g., the Vineland–3 ABC score) can accurately predict an individual's classification within a nominal type variable (e.g., diagnostic class: normal; behavior disorder; developmental disorder). Such analyses were done to determine how effective selected ADOS–2 continuous scores (i.e., Overall Algorithm Score Total, SA Algorithm Score Total) were in predicting an examinee's actual classification (i.e., autism, ASD–A, non-spectrum). Succinctly, such analyses continuously showed that the Overall Algorithm Score Total was the best at predicting examinees' classification. Supplemental mean differences analyses using the *F*-ratio also demonstrated that examinees in each of the three ADOS–2 classes manifested significantly different mean overall total scores, SA domain scores, and RRB domain scores.

Lastly, and probably most important are the following: (a) *sensitivity*, or the statistical probability that an individual who does have autism will be correctly identified as such by the ADOS–2 (i.e., calculated as the number of true positive results divided by the number of true positive and false negative results); and (b) *specificity*, or the statistical probability that an individual who does not have autism will be correctly identified as negative by the ADOS–2 (i.e., computed as the proportion of true negative results to the total of true negative and false positive results). Such analyses were done on both the ADOS–2 extended validity sample and the ADOS–2 replication sample. Also, because there are three classes, such analyses were done on autism versus non-spectrum and on autism spectrum versus non-spectrum. Recall that for the purpose of these studies, autism spectrum was defined as including Asperger's syndrome and pervasive developmental disorder not otherwise specified (PDD-NOS).

Sensitivities and specificities are summarized in Table 6.9 (viz., autism vs. non-spectrum) and Table 6.10 (viz., autism spectrum vs. non-spectrum) for each class discrimination. Both sensitivities and specificities are quite high for the ADOS–2's ability to correctly classify examinees into autism versus non-spectrum. Considering that these categories are furthest from each other symptomatically, these results are both expected and vital to its validity. Indeed, the sensitivities and specificities are lower for the more difficult discrimination between autism spectrum and non-spectrum classification, although still quite impressively high.

Reliability and Validity of ADOS–2 Degree of Autism Signs

As will be discussed in the ensuing section concerning scoring, subsequent to classification, for most units or modules the Overall Algorithm Score Total (SA + RRB) is transformed into a dimensional score, ranging from 1 to 10, that is adjusted for expressive language level and CA. Standardization of such a score was done in a rather complex manner but will be delineated here using a more succinct and straightforward style.

The standardization sample comprised 1,118 individuals with ASD–A, including 1,807 ADOS–2 assessments due to some providing repeat testing, and ranging in age from 2 to 16 years. ASD–A cases were selected because this sample was expected to provide the greatest variability in severity of symptoms and therefore the most apposite measure of symptom degree or level. That is, including only fully developed autism cases would likely have produced a ceiling effect, hence causing range restriction and artificially reducing any resulting measures of relationship. Similarly, including only non-spectrum cases would risk a floor effect, causing range restriction at the lower end of the scale.

Next, the ASD assessments were divided into four expressive language levels, which "were divided further into narrowly defined age groups" (Lord, Rutter et al., 2012, p. 246). This created a matrix of 18 (language x age) cells. Finally, the Overall Algorithm Score Total scores (hereinafter in this section *total scores*) within the cells were "mapped" onto a 10-point continuous equal interval scale as follows: (a) 1 to 3 representing total scores associated with a non-spectrum ADOS–2 classification; (b) 4 to 5 representing total scores with an ASD–A ADOS–2 classification; and (c) 6 to 10 representing total scores within the autism ADOS–2 classification assigned by quintiles (i.e., 5 equal portions).

Initial reliability studies indicate that the Comparison score is reasonably stable within a range of 1.5 points over a two-year period and including a standard error of measurement (SEM) of 0.08. Other data have demonstrated that this score is reasonably independent of CA and verbal IQ.

Summary

These reliability and validity statistics on key ADOS–2 algorithm scores, and their use in deriving both a classification and comparison score (i.e., degree or severity of symptoms), represent only a partial sampling of those available in the manual. However, they do provide a succinct and comprehensible description of the structure, design, and quality of this unique measure. They also provide a rapid review of this test's accuracy and construct validity such that this information can be employed within a test report or test feedback situation.

Administration

ADOS–2 administration is a rather complex undertaking for two principal reasons: (a) it is designed to detect deviations representative of an extremely intricate type of psychopathology; and (b) it covers all major developmental periods (i.e., virtually the entire lifespan). Therefore, this section is divided into general administrative aspects and considerations and more specific item activities and observations.

General Administrative Aspects and Considerations

The ADOS–2 uses a series of standardized structured and unstructured activities designed to elicit certain social interactions and communications from the examinee, referred to as *presses* (but compare with Murray, 1938; see also Chapter 16). Activities represent pre-planned tasks administered by the examiner, which permit standardized observations of the examinee's reactions and behaviors. Thus, "activities serve to structure the interaction; they are not ends in themselves" (Lord, Rutter et al., 2012, p. 13). In complementary fashion, ADOS–2 items target aspects of an examinee's behavior that is to be observed and recorded in written summary form by the examiner during the administration for later scoring and interpretation. Typical administration times range from 40 to 60 minutes, depending upon many factors, including most especially the module used and the degree to which the examinee adapts to the testing circumstances.

Many ADOS–2 items consist of a hierarchy of presses or prompts, which are to be followed in sequence until the examinee either provides a satisfactory response or has proceeded through the hierarchy to completion in the absence of such a response. Items also differ in terms of (a) summary versus single observation, and (b) majority of examples versus the best example. *Summary ADOS–2 items* require that the examiner consider all such behaviors observed during the entire administration, while *single ADOS–2 items* limit consideration to that one observation. The *majority of examples ADOS–2 items* stipulate that the examiner consider behaviors that dominate, as opposed to the *best ADOS–2 item* (i.e., the most sophisticated response). In this sense, the ADOS–2 differs from developmental and cognitive tests whose items are typically limited to the single observation, best example variety.

The ADOS–2 manual (Lord, Rutter et al., 2012) provides specific step-by-step instructions regarding the process for each unit or module in separate sections. Such description begins with a listing of all the required materials for each module (e.g., Lord, Rutter et al., 2012, Figure 6.3, Materials Used with Module 1, p. 26), which is useful for efficient preparation. Next provided are detailed and summary descriptions of single presses, press hierarchies, verbal and nonverbal prompts, interview questions, and most critically, the focus of observation (i.e., the target behaviors to note for scoring).

The ADOS–2 consists of five modules, each with its own protocol and schedule of activities. Modules differ largely in terms of the required (a) level of expressive language skills, and/or (b) chronological age (i.e., the relevance of tasks and objects that best match various cohorts). Together, they cover examinees ranging from age 12 months with no expressive language to adults who are verbally fluent.

Briefly, the Toddler Module (hereinafter Module T) is designed for children ages 12 to 30 months, who are either preverbal or who use *holophrases* (i.e., single word utterances). Module 1 Pre-Verbal/Single Words is designed for children ages 31 months and older (usually up to age 3 years), who do not yet consistently use *phrase speech* (i.e., the flexible use of non-echoed, three-word utterances, which occasionally involve a verb and are spontaneous, meaningful word combinations). Therefore, Module 1 essentially matches the language skills of those for the Toddler Module (i.e., ranging from no speech to inconsistent phrase speech), but who are older in chronological age. Module 2 Phrase Speech is designed for examinees who consistently use three-word utterances, although are not yet *verbally fluent*; that is, the ability to produce a range of flexible sentence types and grammatical forms, using language in order to provide information about events beyond the immediate context, and describing some logical connections within a sentence (e.g., using "but" or "though").

Whereas Modules T, 1, and 2 are generally best matched for use with examinees ranging in age from early childhood through middle childhood, Modules 3 and 4 are typically used for examinees ranging in age from late childhood through adulthood; that is, for individuals who are verbally fluent as defined prior. Module 3 Child/Adolescent differs from Module 4 Adolescent/Adult primarily in the types of tasks and relative emphasis on interviewing. In particular, Module 3 is best matched for verbally fluent older children and young adolescents (typically under 16 years) who still use action-figure toys in play with some mixed interview questions and conversation, while Module 4 is much more heavily reliant upon interview questions and interpersonal conversation, and thus is typically most appropriate for individuals aged 16 years and older.

There are two rare but notable exceptions to these general module descriptions and criteria. First, a rare verbally fluent child who is younger than three years of age is best matched with Module 2, although the examiner may wish to substitute some of the younger-age toys from Modules T and/or 1. Second, adults and adolescents who use phrase speech or who are nonverbal can be administered Modules 1 or 2, although interpretation should be done with caution due to these modules not including (a) adolescents and adults in their norm reference samples, and (b) standardized toys and activities appropriate for older individuals (thus requiring substitutions borrowed from Modules 3 and 4). The latter results in the standardized administration of Modules 1 and 2 being necessarily modified, therefore requiring qualified scoring and interpretation of the data. Other than these two special considerations, the examiner can make a reliable estimate as to the proper module to use for any particular examinee. Of course, the examiner can and should change modules if a mismatch becomes apparent early on in the administration. Next, the modules are discussed in more detail supplemented by a table to help guide the proper selection of a module for a particular examinee. This table is used frequently, especially to resolve cases falling at the threshold between two potential modules.

Specific Activities and Observations

Selection of the proper module is vital for reliable and valid results. It also obviates the disconcerting need to restart an administration after realizing that the chosen module is a poor fit for the testee. Each of the aforementioned modules has a protocol booklet that is color coded for ease of selection. The five modules are listed succinctly in Table 6.11, including their names, required expressive language ability, CA recommendation, and booklet color. Included in the specific table notes are key definitions of the meanings of *simple phrases*, *phrase speech*, and *fluent speech*, which are principal criteria for Modules 2, 3, and 4. Note that various combinations of expressive language ability and CA determine module selection. Table 6.11 was designed as a succinct guide to help an examiner select which module to employ for any particular examinee, especially in borderline or threshold cases. Such a pithy guide is not available in the manual.

For example, a non-verbal child would be eligible for either Module T or 1, with age being the final determinant. Analogously, an individual who is verbally fluent would be eligible for Module 3 or 4, once again with CA as the tie breaker. One notable exception to these fairly straightforward criteria is the aforementioned exceptional precocious young child who possesses fluent speech. Because the materials and activities for Modules 3 and 4 are most appropriate for middle adolescence through adulthood, including sequences of interview questions, Module 2 is advised in the ADOS–2 manual. Similarly, the examiner is encouraged to borrow materials and activities from

Table 6.11 Autism Diagnostic Observation Schedule, Second Edition (ADOS–2) Module Selection Guide

Module Name	Expressive Language Ability	Age Recommendation	Protocol Booklet Color
Toddler Module	Pre-verbal/simple phrases[a]	12–31 months	Purple
Module 1	Pre-verbal/simple phrases[a]	31 months and older	Green
Module 2	Phrase speech[b]	Any age; 3-year-olds with fluent speech[b]	Yellow
Module 3	Fluent speech[c]	Child/adolescent; up to 15 years	Blue
Module 4	Fluent speech[c]	Adolescent/adult; 16 years & older	Blue

Note. [a]*Simple phrases* = one-word utterances that are associated with a gesture (aka holophrases) or two-words utterances that exclude filler words (e.g., "My ball," or "You go"). [b]*Phrase speech* = the flexible use of non-echoed, three-word utterances that sometimes involve a verb, and are spontaneous, meaningful, word combinations. [c]*Fluent speech* = producing a range of flexible sentence types and grammatical forms, using language to provide information about events beyond the immediate context, and describing some logical connections within a sentence (e.g., using *but* and *though*).

other modules so as to better match them with the age of the examinee, especially in cases where expressive language ability is significantly discordant from that expected for CA (e.g., non-verbal adults and verbally fluent 6-year-olds (Lord, Rutter et al., 2012, p. 11).

The protocol booklets are organized into three sections, including (a) Observation, (b) Coding, and (c) Algorithm. Observation pertains to administration and will be the focus of this section. The Coding and Algorithm sections of the protocol booklets are both relevant to scoring and, hence, will be discussed in earnest in the ensuing scoring section, with an emphasis on use of the ADOS–2 computer scoring software (consistent with the theme of efficient and accurate testing practice).

The Observation portion of the protocol booklet consists of the following: (a) listing the name of each activity (within a recommended order); (b) delineating an activity's hierarchy of presses (if applicable); (c) enumerating a list of interview questions (if applicable); and, most importantly, (d) describing the target behaviors to be observed and assessed. Succinctly, a *hierarchy of presses* refers to a multiphasic item subdivided into a ranked step-wise series of related-activities, which together are designed to elicit progressively more sophisticated or complex communications or social interactions on the part of the examinee. Examinees who show complete mastery of all these ranked steps receive more adaptive code ratings, whereas those showing partial or absent mastery receive increasingly maladaptive code ratings.

In addition, some of the items refer to making observations across a variety of pragmatic contexts. A *pragmatic context* is defined as the purpose or intention of a given vocalization or utterance within a particular situation. Examples include making a request, sharing enjoyment with another, directing the attention of another, and seeking emotional comfort. From this, it becomes clear that what is being emphasized is the examinee's ability to communicate on a social and emotional level, both in terms of frequency and flexibility. As a general rule, more credit is given for such vocalizations that are spontaneous; that is, the less prompting, the more favorable the score (i.e., lower scores denote more adaptive functioning, higher scores more maladaptive functioning).

Although the protocol booklets aid the examiner in giving the items, they do not include many of the specific instructions needed for standardized administration. Such detailed information is provided in the ADOS–2 manual and must be committed to semantic, episodic, and procedural long-term memory by the examiner by means of simple repetition and elaborative rehearsal, supplemented by supervised practice. As noted in the manual, however, this type of administration differs significantly from what most psychologists are accustomed to, which is administering items from a manual and/or record form, with sufficiently structured verbal instructions, prompts, and questions that are readily available (typically in bold colored font for easy detection and reciting), and thereafter recording specific responses in written form for later scoring and interpretation. Even the Bayley–III, with its more flexible format, provides more structure, including a record form with start and stop points. Indeed, examiners' first several administrations of the ADOS–2 can be experienced as extremely alien to what they are accustomed to in practice. Therefore, to help new examiners adapt to this unique test, personal administrative guides can be created for each separate module. Next, discussion focuses on how such personal guides can be creatively organized.

ADMINISTRATION GUIDES

Although the publisher declined to grant permission to share personality created notes as succinct administration guides for readers, it is permissible to generally outline their format and cite their sources. In this manner, it can be illustrated how examiners can be active in their learning how to administer a new, unique, and intricate test. Similar strategies in years past have been successful in assisting this author how to use other complex measures, such as the Rorschach Inkblot Test using three different systems. The general strategy is to place only the core administrative instructions succinctly in a format where the needed information can be located quickly and easily while working with an examinee (and perhaps also a parent or caregiver).

More specifically, the module administration guide (i.e., Form 6.8) is designed as a sample outline in tabular form with three columns as follows: (a) Activity; (b) Instructions, presses, and prompts; and (c) Focus of clinical observation for code rating. The first identifies the item number-letter designation and brief title of the associated activity to be administered in that module, and in the advised (although modifiable) order. By the design of this test, there is no one-to-one correspondence between an item activity and an item score. This is because the activities are intended to evoke examinee behaviors and reactions that can apply to multiple items. This is referred to as *double-coding* and its effect is to significantly decrease or speed up administration time.

The second column includes a summary of instructions (e.g., needed materials, preparation), *presses* (i.e., activities designed to evoke certain social interactions and communications from the examinee), and *prompts* (i.e., verbal cues to be used by the examiner when the examinee shows no further response and/or needs encouragement). Here, another factor that reduces administration time is that some of the target behaviors are low incidence occurrences, which require only one or two brief observations for accurate scoring. By implication, once the examiner has sufficient observational data to score all of the relevant items for interpretation, the administration can be effectively terminated.

Also included in the second column are verbatim instructions, which should appear in a distinct font (here, bold and italics), hence resembling standardized test administrative manuals to which testing psychologists are inured, commonly utilize, and are most familiar with, especially because these components are an integral part of training in general standardized testing practice. Lastly, the ADOS–2 administrative manual includes a figure that effectively summarizes the materials needed for each particular module. Hence, this figure is cited within the table notes such that the examiner can quickly reference this information.

The third and final column indicates the target behaviors that are to be observed and ultimately quantified by use of numerical codes. Also included in parentheticals and italicized font are the recommended administration times. These are based upon a combination of logic, and a pragmatic objective of maintaining administration times proximate to or under 45 total minutes (not including time for setting and cleaning up the testing room). If working on an hourly schedule, this would afford 15 minutes for coding, which is to be done immediately after test administration per ADOS–2 guidelines. This last tenet is effective in increasing both the speed and accuracy of making the necessary code ratings.

SPECIALIZING IN MODULE ADMINISTRATION

A final administration issue to address whether or not a testing psychologist can choose to be trained in some, but not all five modules; analogous to psychologists choosing to specialize in working with individuals within delimited age ranges. In this instance, best practice answer is "no." That is, it is advised that one be trained in the use of all modules, with the single possible exception of excluding the Toddler Module. Why? There are three cogent arguments. The first concerns the variables that must be considered when assigning an examinee to a particular module. Specifically, the applicability of all five modules is based upon an interaction of the dual dimensions (a) degree of expressive language ability, and (b) CA (see Table 6.11). In result, any particular case that is referred for autism testing may be initially considered for one of several modules, the determination of which will not be made until completion of a thorough clinical interview, including a review of presenting symptoms, developmental history, mental status examination, and behavioral observations. If the psychologist conducting the initial assessment is not trained in all of the modules, there is a risk that the case will need to be referred out to another agency and provider, or at minimum, an alternate provider within the same agency, either of which can be disconcerting to the prospective examinee and any involved family members.

Second, it is extremely useful and informative to compare and contrast the various activities across the modules, including the necessary adjustments for various language levels and chronological ages. Such cognizance also enhances comprehension of both autism-related manifestations, many of which are expressed in degrees of severity (e.g., echolalia), and the manner in which they are prompted for observation and measurement.[5] Third, as stated prior, the examiner may need to borrow materials and activities from other modules in instances where expressive language ability is discordant from CA (e.g., verbally advanced young children or nonverbal adults). Being adept at administering all five modules would facilitate such use of clinical judgment in making such decisions.

Scoring

For each module, the items to be scored are organized into comparable groupings as follows: (a) Language and Communication; (b) Reciprocal Social Interaction; (c) Play/Imagination; (d) Stereotyped Behaviors and Restricted Interests; and (e) Other Behavior/Abnormal Behaviors. The total number of items vary somewhat among the modules, ranging from 29 (viz., Modules 2 and 3) to 41 (viz., Module T).

Two general scoring rules apply for all modules. First, scoring the items is to be done immediately ensuing administration, which is in accord with effective general testing practice. Second, scoring is to be based exclusively upon behaviors observed during ADOS–2 administration, not upon verbal report or by inference. In this manner, scoring accuracy and objectivity is intended to be maximized. In actuality, ADOS–2 scoring is a two-step process, including (a) making ratings for each item on a dimensional coding scheme, and (b) transforming the ratings into algorithm scores to be used for interpretation. These steps are done within the Coding and Algorithm sections of the protocol booklet, respectively. These steps will next be delineated.

Code Ratings

First, scoring begins by making what the manual refers to as *code ratings*. That is, the examiner uses the ADOS–2 *codes* to make initial *ratings*.[6] Therefore, examiners render their ratings of examinees' behavior using the ADOS–2 code system. Most items have codes that include a dimensional rating scale consisting of three alternatives (i.e., 0–1–2) or as many as four alternatives for increased discrimination (i.e., 0-1-2-3), hence representing a continuous equal interval scale of measurement.[7] These code ratings form the basis of the ADOS–2 scoring, and their conventions are as follows: 0 = *no evidence of abnormality*; 1 = *mildly abnormal or slightly unusual*; 2 = *definitely abnormal*; and, when available, 3 = *markedly abnormal*. Therefore, higher codes indicate more autism-related signs. Items that consist of four alternatives (versus three) are considered to be in need of increased clarity, along with a greater opportunity to measure change in autism-related signs over time. A minority of items have codes that are technically dichotomous (i.e., alternatives of 0 or 2), although practically speaking are incorporated into the aforementioned dimensional rating scale by means of aggregation.

There are other special codes that can be rated on selected items. However, these do not add autism-related signs to the final scoring because they are transformed into algorithm scores of 0 (to be discussed subsequently). Briefly, they include the following: 4 = *non-verbal through entire administration*; 7 = *abnormal behavior not captured by other items*; 8 = *the behavior to be coded did not or could not occur*; 9 = *the behavior was not coded due to examiner error or by item omission*. Technically, these special codes represent nominal data because they define categories of responses identified by a number.[8], [9] Because they do not contribute to the quantitative analysis (i.e., being converted into scores of 0), their principal use is to add qualitative information to the assessment. For example, a Code 7 can be used to document the presence of hyperactivity, which can later be noted during test interpretation as the need to empirically examine the possible co-existence of ADHD.

Algorithm Scores

Second, the rated codes are then transformed into algorithm scores that are used for test interpretation. If done manually, such transformations are made on the inside cover of the last page of the respective protocol booklet. Whether by hand or computer, the code ratings are transformed into item algorithm scores as follows: (a) code ratings of 3 are converted to 2; (b) code ratings of 7, 8, and 9 are converted to 0; and (c) code ratings of 1 and 2 remain the same value. The item algorithm scores are thereafter aggregated into domain total algorithm scores, typically the two domains of social affect (SA), and restricted and repetitive behavior (RRB), which in turn are once again aggregated into an Overall Algorithm Score Total. The final computation integrates the Algorithm Score Total with Chronological Age to obtain a dimensional Comparison Score with a range of 0 to 10, with higher scores indicating greater degrees of autism-related symptoms (i.e., empirically observed signs). It is the Overall Algorithm Score Total that comprises the basis for test interpretation for all five modules, in addition to the Comparison Score for Modules 1, 2, and 3.

As stated prior, the ADOS–2 fortunately possesses the *Autism Diagnostic Observation Schedule, Second Edition (ADOS–2) Unlimited-Use Computer Scoring Software* (Western Psychological Services, 2012), which is an unlimited use computer scoring software CD ROM. Thus, if done by computer scoring, which again is enthusiastically encouraged for reasons stated earlier, the code ratings are simply entered into the program, which performs the transformations when prompted. *ADOS–2 algorithms* are sequences of specified items and quantitative rules designed to maximize the accuracy of the ultimate test result; that is, the ADOS–2 classification as either (a) non-spectrum, (b) autism-spectrum (i.e., as specially defined by this test), and (c) autism. The proper algorithm to employ in a particular case is contingent upon the (a) the module used (i.e., all modules), (b) chronological age (CA) of the examinee (i.e., Modules T, 1, 2), and (c) expressive language ability of the examinee (i.e., Modules T, 2).

Code Rating Sheets for Data Entry

In order to further facilitate test utility, code rating sheets were created for this author's personal use based upon experience in inputting the data into the computer software. Again, the publisher denied a request to share them, which is regrettable because they effectively increase the speed and accuracy of data input. However, a very attenuated outline with only the elementary components can be shared in order to illustrate the strategy used in creating them. To begin, the prime objective of such a code rating sheet was considered, which was to minimize the amount of time needed to obtain the ADOS–2 classification result and comparison score (if applicable). Hence, certain minimal demographic information was required, along with a subset of items needed for the computer to effectuate the specified algorithm for that module and examinee characteristics. Once this information was identified, a code rating summary sheet for each module was designed and, if also applicable, the CA and expressive language ability of the examinee within a particular module (see Form 6.9). For example, two code rating sheets were designed for Module 1 because it consisted of two algorithms as follows: (a) Few to No Words Algorithm; and (b) Some Words Algorithm.

In terms of organization, it was determined that each coding sheet should begin with entries for the examinee's name, file or record number, and date, along with a table consisting of four columns, including (a) the item letter–number designation, (b) the item title/name, (c) a summary description of the item and associated activity, and (d) the available codes for each item (which can vary). The demographics should be limited to those for simple identification and to initiate computer scoring. The first row in Form 6.9 represents the aforesaid column headings, while the second row illustrates a hypothetical item. To help maximize the rate and ease of scoring, the alpha-numeric order of items in these code rating forms should match that of the computer software. Note that in the hypothetical example, Item X-1 determines the type of algorithm employed but is not considered in the algorithm per se. Therefore, this is the special kind of item that can be found for example in Module 1 of the ADOS–2. All other listed items ought to contribute directly to the algorithm and ultimate results for purposes of brevity. The summary description in the third column should be circumscribed to the target behavior(s) that directly influenced the code ratings. That is, it should serve only as a quick memory aid to the examiner in recalling and referencing the more detailed scoring criteria that is available in the 446-page manual and module protocol booklets.

For instance, a summary description may indicate that the target behaviors include repetitive movements of the hands, fingers, arms, or body, across a minimum two tasks or activities, but does not state exactly what code to select if the target behavior occurs only once or partially. Hence, immediately after administration, examiners can best use such code rating sheets by, first and foremost, being well prepared and practiced, then reviewing each item, its summary description, and circling the most appropriate code rating until all items have been completed. Of course, references to the protocol booklet and manual are to be done as needed. Important notes should be added following the table to remind the examiner of how the coding sheet is to be used and the information to be gained.

Before concluding this section, a critical facet of the ADOS–2 scoring process needs to be emphasized here because it is most responsible for reducing the time needed to obtain the essential results. As stated prior, not all ADOS–2 items are used in the algorithms for subsequent interpretation; that is, only those items that gained empirical support for maximizing diagnostic precision were included within the scoring algorithms (Lord, Luyster et al., 2012, p. 7; Lord, Rutter et al., 2012). Algorithms were initially developing in the first edition of the ADOS, although were updated for the ADOS–2 Modules 1 through 3 using a larger and more heterogeneous sample in order to maximize both test sensitivity and specificity. Module T is new to the ADOS–2 and thus has its own originally developed algorithm, while Module 4 continues with the algorithm used in the first edition due insufficient sample sizes for the updated edition.

In any case, in order to further increase the utility of this test using the computer scoring software, the aforementioned coding sheets were circumscribed to those items essential to completing the applicable algorithm. Table 6.12

Table 6.12 Number of Total and Required Items for Algorithm Process as a Function of Module and Module Algorithm

Module Name	Algorithm	Total Items	Required Items
Module T	All Younger/Older With Few to No Words	41	15
Module T	Older With Some Words	41	15
Module 1	Few to No Words	34	15
Module 1	Some Words	34	15
Module 2	Younger Than 5 Years	29	14
Module 2	Aged 5 Years or Older	29	14
Module 3	Child/Adolescent	29	14
Module 4	Adolescent	32	16[a]

Note. Module T = Toddler Module. Total items = all items included in the particular module. Required items = items that need to be scored in the ADOS–2 computer software scoring system in order for it to compute an autism classification according to the selected algorithm.

[a]Five of these 16 items required by the ADOS–2 computer software scoring system are not actually part of the Module 4 algorithm; the reason they are required by the computer software but not part of the algorithm is not explained.

was created to illustrate the degree to which test utility is enhanced when data entry is curtailed in such manner. Briefly, this table shows the total number of items per module if all were code rated juxtaposed with only those items required to run the algorithm for an autism classification and comparison (i.e., severity) dimensional score. As can be seen, the number of items can generally be reduced from about 33% to as much as 50%. Clearly, then, this practice effectively shortens test scoring time and emphasizes objective actuarial test interpretation. Hence, one must consider the time savings if relying exclusively upon the items empirically shown to be the best predictors of autism, especially when classification and degree are the cardinal objectives of testing.

Time permitting, and especially in borderline cases, the examiner can also enter in and generate codes for items not included in the algorithm scoring, both for supplemental quantitative and (most especially) qualitative clinical judgment. The key words here refer to available time. When time must be prioritized, greater reliance on empirically supported actuarial analysis is preferred versus subjective clinical judgment. However, even in instances where there is more available time, *actuarial assessment* (also known as *statistical method* or actuarially based psychodiagnosis) has proved to be consistently superior when compared to *clinical assessment* (also known as *clinical judgment*; Hanson, 2005, 2009; Meehl, 1954). Further, if desired, the examiner can always augment the assessment based upon the non-algorithm items, hence enriching the diagnosis in a manner consistent with *structured clinical judgment*, a practice which integrates actuarial data with clinical-based inference.

Summary

In order to effectuate a visual image of the ADOD–2 process, which summarizes everything that has been presented thus far, the reader is referred to Figure 6.2, which should be downloaded from Routledge's e-resources website and referenced for the ensuing discussion. Although a more comprehensive flowchart of the assessment and testing process was presented in Figure 2.1 and discussed in detail throughout Part I, the ADOS–2 is sufficiently complex that it justifies its own visual flowchart. The first three boxes symbolize the steps in module selection, administration (including the needed supplementary materials), and scoring. The two key scores that form the basis of test interpretation are in bold font, as well as the two types of test interpretation; one categorical and the other dimensional to be discussed immediately subsequent. Because the ADOS–2 scoring is so involved, presentation of the tables used for

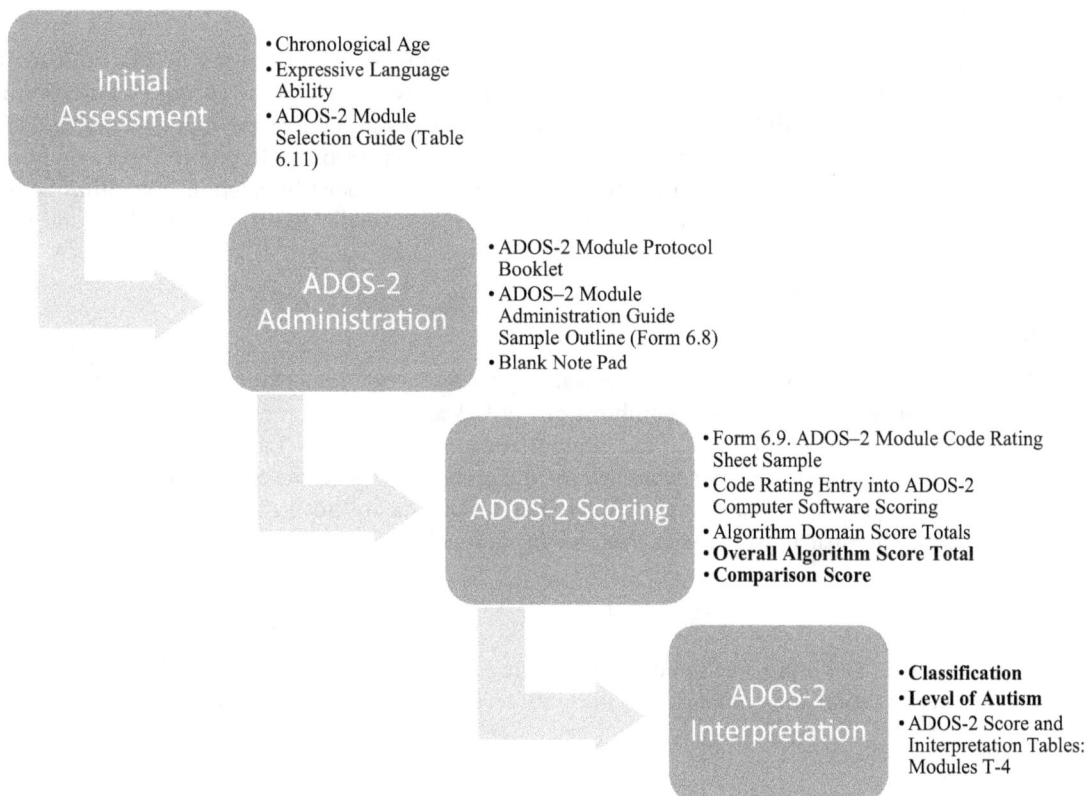

Figure 6.2 ADOS–2 Administration, Scoring, and Interpretative Process

reporting ADOS–2 results in psychological testing reports is deferred until the next interpretation section. ADOS–2 interpretation is portrayed by the final box of Figure 6.2 and is presented in detail immediately subsequent.

Interpretation

In order to report and interpret the ADOS–2 data yield most efficaciously in assessment reports, an independent set of test data tables was diligently designed for each of the eight algorithms that comprise this complex measure. Eight was necessary because, although there are only five modules, recall that three were dichotomized into two algorithms, each of which utilize somewhat alternate code ratings and diagnostic thresholds. They are presented in Forms 6.10, 6.11, 6.12, 6.13, 6.14, 6.15, 6.16, and 6.17.

In each case, the sequence of data tables is not to be interpreted until after the final diagnostic table in the series. That is, the tables proceed in a logical sequence with sufficient detail to clearly delineate the meaning of the data as the reader progresses through the sequence. There is a clear trend in that the initial tables provide summaries for each domain separately, which is ensued by an integration of the data into the algorithm score total summary, the resulting classification, and lastly, the dimensional comparison score. Hence, as will become apparent, all that is needed is a narrative interpretation subsequent to the final table that simply summarizes and integrates the chief findings. Modules 1, 2, and 3 are identical in organization and include all mentioned data. Hence, they will form the basis of the ensuing section. Concerning Modules T and 4, special modifications were required and will be identified at felicitous points in the discussion.

Social Affect (SA) Domain Item Summary

Referring to Forms 6.10 through 6.17, Table 1 presents the data for the Social Affect (SA) domain, including (a) the item title and number-letter, (b) possible code rating range, (c) examinee's obtained code rating, (d) possible adjusted algorithm score, and (e) the examinee's adjusted algorithm score. A summary Algorithm Score Total for the SA domain is presented at the bottom of the table and is on bold font for emphasis. One difference here is that Module 4 does not consist of social affect items. In its stead is a Communication (COM) domain, although with the identical type of score data.

Restricted and Repetitive Behavior (RRB) Domain Item Summary

Table 2 presents the same data as in Table 1 but for the Restricted and Repetitive Behavior (RRB) domain. Table 2 in Module 4 presents a diagnostic summary for the COM domain, showing which the autism classification is indicated by the data in Table 1. This difference is because the RRB items in Table 4 are supplemental and not part of the algorithm. Table 2 in Module 4 is not in bold font because it represents only one of three components in deriving an overall final autism classification; the other two being the (a) Social Interaction Algorithm Score Total and its associated classification, and then the (b) combined COM + SI Overall Algorithm Score Total and its related autism classification.

Module Algorithm Score Total Summary

Table 3 combines the SA and RRB scores into an Overall Algorithm Score Total. Modules T, 1, and 2 employ one of two algorithms, contingent upon different combinations of CA and level of expressive language. These data are presented in bold font as they form the basis of the interpretation summarized in Table 4. For Module 4, however, Table 3 presents the same data as in the first table, except the scores pertain to the SI domain, ensued by Table 4, which presents the SI diagnostic summary. Again, these diagnostic data are not in bold font because there is one more step in completing the final autism classification for Module 4.

Module Diagnostic Summary

Table 4 in Modules T, 1, 2, and 3 presents the diagnostic summary, which is internally all highlighted in bold font. Here, the ADOS–2 classification and comparison score with level (i.e., degree of severity) is shown.

ADOS–2 CLASSIFICATION

The Overall Algorithm Score Total determines the ADOS–2 classification, including either non-spectrum, autism spectrum, or autism. This is determined either manually by reference to (a) Table 4 notes, (b) the ADOS–2

Classification table on the back of the final page of the protocol booklet, and/or (c) the computer automated scoring output. It is important to recall that the autism spectrum construct (i.e., ASD–S), as defined by this measure, consists of such diagnoses as Asperger's disorder and the previously termed PDD–NOS diagnosis. Technically, the autism classification represents a scale of measurement most consistent with an ordinal category (Stevens, 1946). That is, the greater the aggregated algorithm score, the greater the classification in terms of consisting of autism signs. However, precisely how much greater is not addressed.

ADOS–2 COMPARISON SCORE

The Comparison Score is a dimensional measure that is adjusted for CA and expressive language ability. It is determined by use of an ADOS–2 Comparison Score table found on the back side of the final page of the protocol booklet. This table enumerates categories of increasing age ranges across the top, a far left and right column of comparison scores listed from 10 down to 1, and overall algorithm score totals in the body of the table. The Comparison Score is found by entering the examinee's Overall Algorithm Score Total in the proper age column, then moving to the far right or left row to identify the corresponding Comparison Score. This score represents the level or degree of autism-related signs, as manifested by the examinee during test administration, compared to individuals with documented ASD of comparable language ability and CA. The computer software does this automatically during the process of transforming the code ratings into algorithm scores, computing aggregated Algorithm Domain Scores, and lastly the Overall Algorithm Score Total. Table 4 general notes indicate the scores associated with various autism classification assignments and levels of severity.

Toddler Module Special Classification Scheme

Module T presents a modified, more conservative classification scheme based upon, "degrees of concern," that the examinee will at a later point in development meet the criteria for an autism-spectrum diagnosis; namely (a) little-to-no concern, (b) mild-to-moderate concern, and (c) moderate-to-severe concern. Further, Module T does not yield a comparison score.

Module 4 Adolescent/Adult Algorithm Special Classification Scheme

The Module 4 final autism classification is uniquely determined by various combinations of the COM classification result, SI classification result, and combined COM + SI classification result. These permutations are presented in Table 6 of the Module 4 tabular series and are in internal bold font because this represents the ultimate test outcome and interpretation. As Module T, Module 4 does not offer a comparison score. For this reason, if there are equal reasons for administering Module 3 or Module 4 to an examinee, the advice of the authors is to administer the former because it yields both a classification and accompanying comparison score.

Concluding Comments

Although the ADOS–2 is extremely complex, the creation of personal administration guides (see, e.g., Form 6.8) and code rating sheets (see, e.g., Form 6.9) by the examiner as illustrated previously, along with use of the data reporting tables (Forms 6.10–6.17) and ADOS–2 testing flowchart (Figure 6.2 on Routledge's e-resources website) reviewed prior, should all make the process much more viable in terms of both learning, mastering, and using this measure. Taken together, they will also assist in obtaining accurate and meaningful results, and in terms of reporting them in an efficient and comprehensible manner. All told, this unique test is a performance-based instrument that directly measures signs of autism in a standardized quantitative manner. It can also be used to measure response to treatment via test-retest procedures as it applies to individuals over their lifespans. As such, it should be part of every assessment that is attempting to detect the presence of this neurodevelopmental disorder.

Recapitulation

This chapter delineated fours standardized tests, each of which measured constructs that have an affinity to the developmental process. They included the Bayley–III, ABAS–3, Vineland–3, and ADOS–2. By espousing a developmental focus, all four tests can be used in the first three years of an examinee's life, three of which can be used in proximity to birth. However, three of the tests cover all major developmental periods, from infancy through adulthood, while two cover virtually the entire lifespan. All of these facets further support the rationale for placing them together in one chapter emphasizing the topic of development, both normal although especially abnormal. Finally, all of these tests embrace a developmental psychopathology model wherein age is a principal variable in defining what constitutes abnormality. The ensuing chapter begins a trilogy of topics concerning the measurement of various kinds of cognition (e.g., competence, achievement, neurocognition), and continue to be extremely relevant in the diagnosis of neurodevelopmental and neurocognitive disorders. The first of these regards the measurement of intelligence, which is a felicitous selection considering that such tests are considered to be the major impetus for the growth of psychological testing practice.

Key Terms

- ability deficit
- actuarial assessment
- actuarially based psychodiagnosis
- adaptational failures
- adaptive behavior
- Adaptive Behavior Assessment System, Third Edition (ABAS–3)
- Adaptive Behavior Assessment System, Third Edition (ABAS–3) Scoring Assistant
- Adaptive Behavior System, Second Edition (ABAS–II)
- adaptive skills
- adaptive testing
- ADOS–2 algorithms
- alexithymia
- alternate forms
- American Association on Intellectual and Developmental Disabilities (AAIDD)
- American Association on Mental Retardation (AAMR)
- attention to novelty
- Autism Diagnostic Observation Schedule (ADOS)
- Autism Diagnostic Observation Schedule, Second Edition (ADOS–2) Unlimited-Use Computer Scoring Software
- autism spectrum disorder (ASD)
- babbling
- base rate
- Bayley Scales of Infant and Toddler Development (BSID)
- Bayley Scales of Infant and Toddler Development, Fourth Edition (Bayley–4)
- Bayley Scales of Infant and Toddler Development, Second Edition (BSID–II)
- Bayley Scales of Infant and Toddler Development, Third Edition (Bayley–III)
- Bayley Scales of Infant Development, Third Edition, Scoring Assistant
- best ADOS–2 item
- California First-Year Mental Scale
- California Infant Scale of Motor Development
- California Preschool Mental Scale
- cardinality
- Caregiver Questions
- central nervous system (CNS)
- cephalocaudal
- chronological age (CA)
- clinical assessment
- clinical judgment
- code ratings
- composite equivalent scores
- cooing
- counting
- Current Procedural Technology (CPT) Code 96112
- deficits
- delay
- developmental coordination disorder
- developmental norms

- developmental psychopathology model
- deviance
- double-coding
- effect size
- fine motor skills
- fixation
- fluent speech
- functional emotional developmental capacities (FEDCS)
- functional emotional milestones (FEMS)
- Greenspan Social-Emotional Growth Chart: A Screening Questionnaire for Infants and Young Children
- gross motor skills
- habituation
- hierarchy of presses
- holophrases
- Individuals with Disabilities Education Improvement Act (2004)
- inferential norming
- information processing
- information processing tasks
- intellectual disability (ID)
- internal consistency reliability coefficients
- ipsative analysis
- language
- logistic regression
- majority of examples ADOS–2 items
- mental development
- moments
- morposyntactic development
- myelination
- one-to-one correspondence
- Percent Delay
- performance deficit
- phrase speech
- play
- polytomous models
- polytomous scoring approach
- power test
- pragmatic context
- preauthorization (PA)
- preference for novelty
- prehension
- presses
- pretend play
- probe
- problem-solving
- prompts
- proximal stability
- proximodistal
- psychological mindedness
- regression
- reliability
- sensitivity
- simple phrases
- single ADOS–2 items
- social pragmatic communication disorder
- Social-Emotional and Adaptive Behavior Questionnaire
- specificity

- speed of processing
- statistical method
- subitizing
- summary ADOS–2 items
- symbolic play
- utility
- validity
- verbally fluent
- Vineland Adaptive Behavior Scales, Second Edition (Vineland–II)
- Vineland Adaptive Behavior Scales, Third Edition (Vineland–3)
- Vineland semistructured interview technique
- v–scale score
- World Health Organization (WHO)

Notes

1. It should be noted that the Bayley–III computer scoring assistant calculates and provides all of the subtest scaled scores, including those for the Cognitive Scale and Social-Emotional Scale. These scaled scores are redundant with the composite equivalent scores because they have merely been converted from the scaled score metric into a composite score metric. Because this renders the scaled scores to these scales superfluous, they need not be included again anywhere in the Bayley–III data tables in Form 6.1a.
2. You will note a composite/standard score first column in Table 6.3, which will be required later when reporting scores for the ABAS–3. For this next instrument, there are two subtests that are principally measured in scaled score units (i.e., mean = 10, standard deviation = 3), which necessitate conversion into standard score units (mean = 100, standard deviation = 15). For this purpose, columns 1 and 2 of Table 6.4a (or Table 6.4b) will be needed. Again, Table A.1 (see Appendix A) can also be used for this purpose, although due to its greater length and comprehensiveness, it is more cumbersome to use.
3. Those most familiar with *SEM*s and CIs may pause to ask why the average *SEM* was not used when computing the Motor and Work Adaptive Skill Areas. The answer is that these *SEM*s are based upon standard deviations of 3 and not 15 as used in the formula *SEM* = *SD*; that is, five times as small. Hence, such SEMs would be much too small and there was uncertainty in how to adjust for this difference. Therefore, the internal reliability coefficient for these two adaptive skill areas was used with a *SD* of 15 in said formula to be consistent with a standard equivalent score metric, which would ensure that the estimates were of proper proportion. Here, using the adaptive skill areas, the *SEM*s were already based upon a *SD* of 3 and thus could simply be averaged.
4. The ABAS–3 scoring assistant actually performs ipsative statistical analyses to determine is any of the adaptive skill areas are different from the computed average scaled score. Again, the difference score is considered statistically significant if it exceeds the critical value that occurs 5% of the time assuming a null hypothesis of no difference. It also lists the base rate compared to 15% and 5%. Such analyses are not used as they are much too detailed and time consuming to justify interpreting.
5. The DSM–5 published contemporaneously with the ADOS–2. In result, the ADOS–2 was standardized according to the prior pervasive developmental disorders nosology, which included autism, Asperger's disorder, Rett's disorder, childhood disintegration disorder, and pervasive developmental disorder not otherwise specified (American Psychiatric Association, 2000). Therefore, the ADOS–2 considered the autism diagnosis as the complete disorder, symptomatically speaking, and conceptualized an atypical class consisting of Asperger's and PDD–NOS as partial autism manifestations, thus assigning the label autism spectrum disorder. Because this label is identical to that of the DSM–5 for the complete autism diagnosis, the ASD–A abbreviation is being used to denote the ADOS–2 class of atypical or partial autism, and ASD for the DSM–5 designation for autism, hence differentiating the two in the main text. The implication in the ADOS–2 approach is that the complete autism diagnosis is defined as the most severe form, while Asperger's and PDD–NOS represent less pathological or healthier forms. Finally, the non-autism class is listed in the ADOS–2 as the third class as on a continuum from more to less severe. Although these are debatable issues, it is important to understand the ADOS–2 measurement approach.
6. As alluded to before in the main text, comprehension of autism and its various manifestations at different ages and degrees of expressive language ability increases exponentially subsequent to learning the ADOS–2 activities, target behaviors, and coding scheme.
7. These terms are used interchangeably within the ADOS–2 manual, which can lead to confusion.
8. Technically, many would argue that this is an ordinal scale. However, using accepted practice and by convenience, as in a Likert-type scale, the ADOS–2 code ratings will be considered here as an equal-interval scale (see, e.g., Howell, 2014; Gravetter & Wallnau, 2017; Field, 2018).
9. This designation is moot, however, since these codes are in due course transformed into scores of 0 for purposes of interpretation, here denoting a lack of autism-related signs.

References

American Academy of Pediatrics. (2006). Identifying infants and young children with developmental disorder in the medical home: An algorithm for developmental surveillance and screening. *Pediatrics, 118*, 405–420.

American Association on Intellectual and Developmental Disabilities (AAIDD). (2010). *Intellectual disability definition, classification, and systems of supports* (11th ed.). Washington, DC: Author.

American Association on Mental Retardation (AAMR). (2002). *Mental retardation: Definition, classification, and systems of supports* (9th ed.). Washington, DC: Author.

American Psychiatric Association. (2000). *Diagnostic and statistical manual of mental disorders* (4th ed., text rev., DSM–IV–TR). Washington, DC: Author.

American Psychiatric Association. (2013). *Diagnostic and statistical manual of mental disorders* (5th ed., DSM–5). Arlington, VA: Author.

American Psychological Association. (2015). *American psychological association (APA) dictionary of psychology* (2nd ed.). Washington, DC: Author.

American Psychological Association. (2020). *Publication of the American psychological association: The official guide to APA style* (7th ed.). Washington, DC: Author.

Amiel-Tison, C., & Gosselin, J. (2008). The Amiel-Tison and Gosselin neurological assessment from birth to 6 years of age. In P. J. Accardo (ed.), *Capute and Accardo's neurodevelopmental disabilities in infancy and childhood* (3rd ed., pp. 321–332). Baltimore, MD: Paul H. Brookes Publishing.

Anastasi, A., & Urbina, S. (1997). *Psychological testing* (7th ed.). Upper Saddle River, NJ: Prentice Hall.

Aslin, R. N. (1981). Development of smooth pursuit in human infants. In D. F. Fisher, R. A. Monty, & J. W. Senders (Eds.), *Eye movements: Cognition and visual perception* (pp. 31–51). Hillsdale, NJ: Erlbaum.

Aslin, R. N., & Salapatek, P. (1975). Saccadic localization of visual targets by the very young human infant. *Perception and Psychophysics, 17*, 293–302.

Aylward, G. P. (1988). Infant and early childhood assessment. In M. G. Tramontana & S. R. Hooper (Eds.), *Assessment issues in child neuropsychology* (pp. 225–248). New York, NY: Plenum Press.

Aylward, G. P. (2009). Developmental screening and assessment: What are we thinking? *Journal of Developmental & Behavioral Pediatrics, 30*, 169–173.

Aylward, G. P. (2010). Neuropsychological assessment of newborns, infants, and toddlers. In A. Davis (Ed.), *Handbook of pediatric neuropsychology* (pp. 201–212). New York, NY: Springer.

Aylward, G. P. (2018). Issues in neurodevelopmental testing of infants born prematurely. The Bayley Scales of Infant Development third edition and other tools. In H. Needleman & B. J. Jackson (Eds.), *Follow-up for NICU graduates: Promoting positive developmental and behavioral outcomes for at-risk infants* (pp. 241–253). Cham, Switzerland: Springer International.

Aylward, G. P., & Verhulst, S. J. (2008). Comparison of caretaker report and hands-on neurodevelopmental screening in high-risk infants. *Developmental Neuropsychology, 33*, 124–136.

Bagnato, S. J., Neisworth, J. T., & Pretti-Frontczak, K. (2010). *Linking authentic assessment and early childhood interventions: Best measures for best practices* (2nd ed.). Baltimore, MD: Paul H. Brooks Publishing.

Bates, E., Bretherton, I., Snyder, L., Beeghly, M., Shore, C., McNew, S., et al. (1988). *From first words to grammar: Individual differences and dissociable mechanisms*. New York, NY: Cambridge University Press.

Bayley, N. (1933). *The California first-year mental scale*. Berkeley, CA: University of California Press.

Bayley, N. (1936). *The California infant scale of motor development*. Berkeley, CA: University of California Press.

Bayley, N. (1969). *Manual for the Bayley scales of infant development*. San Antonio, TX: The Psychological Corporation.

Bayley, N. (1993). *Bayley scales of infant development* (2nd ed.). San Antonio, TX: The Psychological Corporation.

Bayley, N. (2006a). *Bayley scales of infant and toddler development, third edition (Bayley–III): Administrative manual*. Bloomington, MN: Pearson (PsychCorp).

Bayley, N. (2006b). *Bayley scales of infant and toddler development, third edition (Bayley–III): Technical manual*. Bloomington, MN: Pearson (PsychCorp).

Bayley, N., & Aylward, G. P. (2019a). *Bayley scales of infant and toddler development, fourth edition (Bayley–4): Administrative manual*. Bloomington, MN: NCS Pearson.

Bayley, N., & Aylward, G. P. (2019b). *Bayley scales of infant and toddler development, fourth edition (Bayley–4): Technical manual*. Bloomington, MN: NCS Pearson.

Belsky, J., & Most, R. K. (1981). From exploration to play: A cross-sectional study of infant free play behavior. *Developmental Psychology, 17*, 630–639.

Berk, L. E. (1998). *Development through the lifespan*. Boston, MA: Allyn & Bacon.

Bertenthal, B. I., & Clifton, R. K. (1998). Perception and action. In D. Williams (Ed.), *Handbook of child psychology* (5th ed., Vol. 2, pp. 51–102). New York, NY: John Wiley & Sons.

Berthier, N. E., DeBlois, S., Poirier, C. R., Novak, M. A., & Clifton, R. K. (2000). Where's the ball? Two- and three-year-olds reason about unseen events. *Developmental Psychology, 36*, 394–401.

Blaggan, S., Guy, A., Boyle, E. M., Spata, E., Manktelow, B. N., Wolke, D., & Johnson, S. (2014). A parent questionnaire for developmental screening in infants born late and moderately preterm. *Pediatrics, 134*, e55–e62.

Bloom, P., & Markson, L. (1998). Capacities underlying word learning. *Trends in Cognitive Sciences, 2*, 67–73.

Bly, L. (1983). *The components of normal movement during the first year of life and abnormal motor development* (Monograph of the Neuro-Developmental Treatment Association). Birmingham, AL: Pittenger Associates, Pathway Press.

Bornstein, M. H., & Sigman, M. D. (1986). Continuity of mental development from infancy. *Child Development, 57*, 251–274.

Bruner, J. S. (1972). Nature and uses of immaturity. *American Psychologist, 27*, 687–708.

Carlson, S. M. (2005). Developmentally sensitive measures of executive function in preschool children. *Developmental Neuropsychology, 28*, 595–616.

Chapman, R. S. (2000). Children's language learning: An interactionist perspective. *Journal of Child Psychology and Psychiatry, 41*, 33–54.

Clifton, R. K., Rochat, P., Robin, D. J., & Berthier, N. E. (1994). Multimodal perception in the control of infant reaching. *Journal of Experimental Psychology, 20*, 876–886.

Cohen, A. H., Wang, R., Wilkinson, M., MacDonald, P., Lim, A. R., & Takahashi, E. (2016). Developmentof human white matter fiber pathways: From newborn to adult ages. *International Journal of Developmental Neuroscience, 50*, 26–38.

Collins, A. M., & Quillian, M. R. (1969). Retrieval time from semantic memory. *Journal of Verbal Learning and Verbal Behaviour, 8*, 240–247.

Colombo, J., & Frick, J. (1999). Recent advances and issues in the study of preverbal intelligence. In M. Anderson (Ed.), *The development of intelligence* (pp. 43–71). Hove, England: Psychology Press.

Cuevas, K., & Bell, M. A. (2014). Infant attention and early childhood executive function. *Child Development, 85*, 397–404.

Dayton, G. O., & Jones, M. H. (1964). Analysis of characteristics of fixation reflex in infants by use of direct current electrooculography. *Neurology, 14*, 1152–1156.

DeGangi, G. A., Berk, R. A., & Valvano, J. (1983). Test of motor and neurological functions in high-risk infants: Preliminary findings. *Developmental and Behavioral Pediatrics, 4*, 182–189.

Dougherty, T. M., & Haith, M. N. (1997). Infant expectations and reaction times as predictors of childhood speed of processing and IQ. *Developmental Psychology, 33*, 146–155.

Dunst, C. J. (1982). The clinical utility of Piagetian-based scales of infant development. *Infant Mental Health Journal, 3*, 259–275.

Fagan, J. F. (1970). Memory in the infant. *Journal of Experimental Child Psychology, 9*, 217–226.

Fagan, J. F. (1982). New evidence for the prediction of intelligence from infancy. *Infant Mental Health Journal, 3*, 219–228.

Fenson, L., Kagan, J., Kearsley, R. B., & Zelaso, P. R. (1976). The developmental progression of manipulative play in the first two years. *Child Development, 47*, 232–236.

Field, A. (2018). *Discovering statistics using SPSS: IBM SPSS statistics* (North American Edition, 5th ed.). Los Angeles, CA: Sage Publications.

Furr, R. M. (2018). *Psychometrics: An introduction* (3rd ed.). Thousand Oaks, CA: Sage Publications.

Geary, D. C., & vanMarie, K. (2018). Growth of symbolic number knowledge accelerates after children understand cardinality. *Cognition, 177*, 69–78.

Gelman, R., & Tucker, M. E. (1975). Further investigation of the young child's conception of number. *Child Development, 46*, 167–175.

Goldstein, M. H., & Schwade, J. A. (2008). Social feedback to infants' babbling facilitates rapid phonological learning. *Psychological Science, 19*, 515–523.

Gravetter, F. J., & Wallnau, L. B. (2017). *Statistics for the behavioral sciences* (10th ed.). Boston, MA: Cengage Learning.

Greenspan, S. I. (1989). *The development of the ego: Implications for personality theory, psychopathology, and the psychotherapeutic process.* Madison, CT: International Universities Press.

Greenspan, S. I. (1997). *The growth of the mind and the endangered origins of intelligence.* Reading, MA: Addison–Wesley Publishing.

Greenspan, S. I., & Shanker, S. (2004). *The first idea: How symbols, language, and intelligence evolved from our primate ancestors to modern humans.* Reading, MA: Perseus Books.

Greenspan, S. I., DeGangi, G. A., & Wieder, S. (2001). *The functional emotional assessment scale (FEAS) for infancy and early childhood: Clinical research applications.* Bethesda, MD: Interdisciplinary Council on Developmental and Learning Disorders.

Greenspan, S. L. (2004). *Greenspan social-emotional growth chart: A screening questionnaire for infants and young children.* San Antonio, TX: Harcourt Assessment.

Grieiff, S., Wüstenberg, S., Goetz, T., Vainikainen, M.-P, Hautamäki, J., & Bornstein, M. H. (2015). Longitudinal study of high-order thinking skills: Working memory and fluid reasoning in childhood enhance complex problem solving in adolescence. *Frontiers in Psychology, 6*, 1060.

Hanson, R. K. (2005). Twenty years of progress in violence risk assessment. *Journal of Interpersonal Violence, 20*, 212–217.

Hanson, R. K. (2009). The psychological assessment of risk for crime and violence. *Canadian Psychology, 50*, 172–182.

Harrison, P. L., & Oakland, T. (2003). *Adaptive behavior assessment system, second edition (ABAS–II)* [Manual]. San Antonio, TX: The Psychological Corporation.

Harrison, P. L., & Oakland, T. (2015a). *Adaptive behavior assessment system, third edition (ABAS–3)* [Manual]. Torrance, CA: Western Psychological Services (WPS).

Harrison, P. L., & Oakland, T. (2015b). *Adaptive behavior assessment system, third edition (ABAS–3), Unlimited scoring software* [CD-ROM & USB Key]. Torrance, CA: Western Psychological Services (WPS).

Hoff, E. (2014). *Language development* (5th ed.). Belmont, CA: Wadsworth.

Howell, D. C. (2014). *Fundamental statistics for the behavioral sciences* (8th ed.). Belmont, CA: Wadsworth, Cengage Learning.

Huttenlocher, J., Smiley, P., & Charney, R. (1983). Emergence of action in the child: Evidence from verb meanings. *Psychological Review, 90*, 72–93.

Individuals with Disabilities Education Improvement Act of 2004, Pub. L. No. 108–446, § 2, 40 Stat. 118 (2004).

Interdisciplinary Council on Development and Learning Disorders (IDCLD). (2000). *Clinical practice guidelines: Redefining the standards of care for infants, children, and families with special needs.* Bethesda, MD: Author.

Izard, V., Streri, A., & Spelke, E. (2014). Toward exact number: Young children use one-to-one correspondence to measure set identity but not numerical equality. *Cognitive Psychology, 72*, 27–53.

Jaffa, A. S. (1934). *The California preschool mental scale.* Berkeley, CA: University of California Press.

Johnson, J. E. (1976). Relations of divergent thinking and intelligence test scores with social and nonsocial make-believe play of preschool children. *Child Development, 47*, 1200–1203.

Johnson, S., Wolke, D., & Marlow, N. (2008). Developmental assessment of preterm infants at 2 years: Validity of parent reports. *Development Medicine & Child Neurology, 50*, 58–62.

Kail, R. (2000). Speed of information processing: Developmental change and links to intelligence. *Journal of School Psychology, 38,* 51–61.

Kanne, S. M., Randolph, J. K., & Farmer, J. E. (2008). Diagnostic and assessment findings: A bridge to academic planning for children with autism spectrum disorders. *Neuropsychology Review, 18,* 367–384.

Leaders Project. (2013). *Test review: Bayley–III.* Teachers College Columbia University. Retrieved from www.leadersproject. org/2013/11/25/test-review-bayley-iii/#:~:text=Bayley%2DIII%20administration%20time%20is,children%20older%20than%20 13%20mos

Litovsky, R. Y., & Ashmead, D. H. (1997). Development of binaural and spatial hearing in infants and children. In R. H. Gilsky & T. R. Anderson (Eds.), *Binaural and spatial hearing in real and virtual environments* (pp. 571–592). Hillsdale, NJ: Lawrence Erlbaum Associates.

Lord, C., Luyster, R. J., Gotham, K., & Guthrie, W. (2012). *Autism diagnostic observation schedule, second edition (ADOS–2) [Manual: Toddler Module].* Torrance, CA: Western Psychological Services (WPS).

Lord, C., Rutter, M., Dilavore, P. C., & Risi, S. (1999). *Autism diagnostic observation schedule: manual.* Los Angeles, CA: Western Psychological Services (WPS).

Lord, C., Rutter, M., Dilavore, P. C., Risi, S., Gotham, K., & Bishop, S. L. (2012). *Autism diagnostic observation schedule, second edition (ADOS–2) [Manual: Modules 1–4].* Torrance, CA: Western Psychological Services (WPS).

Luyster, R., Gotham, K., Guthrie, W., Coffin, M., Petrak, R., Pierce, K., . . . Lord, C. (2009). The autism diagnostic observation schedule–toddler module: A new module of a standardized diagnostic measure for autism spectrum disorders. *Journal of Autism and Developmental Disorders, 39,* 1305–1320.

Martin, A. J., Darlow, B. A., Salt, A., Hague, W., Sebastian, L., McNeill, N., & Tarnow-Mordi, W. (2013). Performance of the parent report of children's abilities–revised (PARCA–R) versus the Bayley scales of infant development III. *Archives of Disease in Childhood, 98,* 955–958.

Mash, E. J., & Dozois, D. J. A. (1996). Child psychopathology: A developmental-systems perspective. In E. J. Mash & R. A. Barkley (Eds.), *Child psychopathology* (pp. 3–60). New York, NY: The Guilford Press.

Mash, E. J., & Wolfe, D. A. (2013). *Abnormal child psychology* (5th ed.). Belmont, CA: Wadsworth, Cengage Learning.

Maye, M. P., Kiss, I. G., & Carter, A. S. (2017). Definitions and classification of autism spectrum disorders. In D. Zager, D. F. Cihak, & A. Stone-MacDonald (Eds.), *Autism spectrum disorders: Identification, education, and treatment* (pp. 1–22). New York, NY: Routledge, Taylor & Francis Group.

Meehl, P. E. (1954). *Clinical versus statistical prediction: A theoretical analysis and a review of the evidence.* Minneapolis: University of Minnesota Press.

Mix, K. S. (2009). How spencer made number. First uses of the number words. *Journal of Experimental Child Psychology, 102,* 427–444.

Murray, H. A. (1938). *Explorations in personality.* New York, NY: Oxford University Press.

Nelson, K. (1973). Structure and strategy in learning to talk. *Monographs of the Society for Research in Child Development, 38* (1–2, Serial No. 149), 1–135.

Osterling, J. A., Dawson, G., & Munson, J. A. (2002). Early recognition of 1-year-old infants with autism spectrum disorder versus mental retardation. *Development and Psychopathology, 14,* 239–251.

Oviatt, S. L. (1980). The emerging ability to comprehend language: An experimental approach. *Child Development, 51,* 97–106.

Owen, R. E. (2001). *Language development: An introduction* (5th ed.). Boston, MA: Allyn & Bacon.

Ozonoff, S., Goodlin-Jones, B. L., & Solomon, M. (2005). Evidence-based assessment of autism spectrum disorders in children and adolescents. *Journal of Clinical Child and Adolescent Psychology, 34,* 523–540.

Ozonoff, S., Iosif, A.–M., Baguio, F., Cook, I. C., Hill, M. M., Hutman, T., . . . Sigman, M. (2010). A prospective study of the emergence of early behavioral signs of autism. *Journal of the American Academy of Child and Adolescent Psychiatry, 49,* 256–266.

Ozonoff, S., Macari, S., Young, G. S., Goldring, S., Thompson, M., & Rogers, S. J. (2008). Atypical object exploration at 12 months of age is associated with autism in a prospective sample. *Autism, 12,* 457–472.

Pearson. (2006). *Bayley scales of infant and toddler development, third edition: Scoring assistant and PDA* (Version 2.0.2) [Computer software, CD ROM]. Author.

Pearson. (2021). *Q–global: Better insights. Anytime. Anywhere.* [Internet Web-Based Computer Scoring]. https://qglobal.pearsonclinical. com/qg/login.seam.

Pence Turnbull, K. L., & Justice, L. M. (2017). *Language development from theory to practice* (3rd ed.). Upper Saddle River, NJ: Pearson Education.

Piaget, J. (1952). *The origins of intelligence in children.* New York, NY: International University Press.

Robin, D. J., Berthier, N. E., & Clifton, R. K. (1996). Infants' predictive reaching for moving objects in the dark. *Developmental Psychology, 32,* 824–835.

Rochat, P., & Goubet, N. (1995). Development of sitting and reaching in 5- to 6-month-old infants. *Infant behavior and Development, 18,* 53–68.

Rose, S. A., Feldman, J. F., Jankowski, J. J., & Van Rossem, R. (2012). Information processing from infancy to 11 years: Continuities and prediction of IQ. *Intelligence, 40,* 445–457.

Rovee-Collier, C. (1987). Learning and memory in infancy. In J. D. Ososky (Ed.), *Handbook of infant development* (2nd ed., pp. 98–148). New York, NY: John Wiley & Sons.

Ruggles, S., Genadek, K., Goeken, R., Grover, J., & Sobek, M. (2015). *Integrated public use microdata series: Version 6.0* [Machine-readable database]. Minneapolis, MN: University of Minnesota.

Sattler, J. M. (2001). *Assessment of children: Cognitive applications* (4th ed.). San Diego, CA: Jerome M. Sattler Publisher.

Sattler, J. M. (2014). *Foundations of behavioral, social, and clinical assessment of children* (6th ed.). LaMesa, CA: Jerome M. Sattler Publisher.

Sattler, J. M., & Ryan, J. J. (2009). *Assessment with the WAIS–IV*. San Diego, CA: Jerome M. Sattler Publisher.

Scatz, J., Kramer, J. H., Ablin, A., & Matthay, K. K. (2000). Processing speed, working memory and IQ: A developmental model of cognitive deficits following cranial radiation therapy. *Neuropsychology, 14*, 189–200.

Sigman, M., Cohen, S. E., Beckwith, L., & Parmelee, A. H. (1986). Infant attention in relation to intellectual abilities in childhood. *Developmental Psychology, 22*, 788–792.

Silverman, I. W., & Rose, A. P. (1980). Subitizing and counting skills in 3-year-olds. *Developmental Psychology, 16*, 539–540.

Singer, J. L. (1973). *The child's world of make-believe: Experimental studies of imaginative play*. New York, NY: Academic Press.

Sparrow, S. S., Cicchetti, D. V., & Balla, D. A. (2005). *Vineland adaptive behavior scales, second edition (Vineland–II): Survey forms manual*. Minneapolis, MN: Pearson.

Sparrow, S. S., Cicchetti, D. V., & Saulnier, C. A. (2016). *Vineland adaptive behavior rating scales, third edition (Vineland–3): Manual*. Minneapolis, MN: Pearson.

Stevens, S. (1946). On the theory of scales of measurement. *Science, 103*, 677–680.

Thibodeau, R. B., Gilpin, A. T., Brown, M. M., & Meyer, B. A. (2016). The effects of fantastical pretend play on the development of executive functions: An intervention study. *Journal of Experimental Child Psychology, 145*, 120–138.

Turk-Brown, N. B., Scholl, B. J., & Chun, M. M. (2008). Babies and brains: Habituation in infant cognition and functional neuroimaging. *Frontiers in Human Neuroscience, 2*, 16.

U.S. Bureau of the Census. (2000). *Current population survey, October 2000: School enrollment supplemental file* [CD ROM]. Washington, DC: U.S. Bureau of the Census (Producer/Distributor).

U.S. Bureau of the Census. (2010). *Census 2010 summary file 1 United States*. Washington, DC: Author.

U.S. Census Bureau. (2014). *American community survey, 2014 1-year period estimates*. Washington, DC: Author.

U.S. Census Bureau. (2017). *American community survey, 2017 1-year period estimates*. Washington, DC: Author.

Vygotsky, L. S. (1978). *Mind in society: The development of higher psychological processes*. Cambridge, MA: Harvard University Press.

Warner, R. M. (2021). *Applied statistics I: Basic bivariate techniques* (3rd ed.). Los Angeles, CA: Sage Publications.

Wechsler, D. (1975). *The collected papers of David Wechsler*. New York, NY: Academic Press.

Western Psychological Services (WPS). (2012). *Autism diagnostic observation schedule (ADOS–2): Unlimited computer scoring software*. (Version 1.210) [Computer software, CD ROM]. Torrance, CA: Author.

Wilkins, C., Rolfhus, E., Weiss, L., & Zhu, J. (2005). *A simulation study comparing continuous and traditional norming with small sample sizes*. Paper presented at American Educational Research Association Annual Conference, Montreal, Canada.

World Health Organization (WHO). (2001). *International classification of functioning, disability, and health*. Geneva: Author.

World Health Organization (WHO). (2007). *International classification of functioning, disability, and health: Children and youth version*. Geneva: Author.

Wynn, K. (1990). Children's understanding of counting. *Cognition, 36*, 155–193.

Yogman, M., Garner, A., Hutchinson, J., Hirsh-Pasek, K., Golinkoff, R. M., Committee on Psychosocial Aspects of Child and Family Health, & Council on Communications and Media. (2018). The power of play: A pediatric role in enhancing development in young children. *Pediatrics, 142*, 1–17.

Zwaigenbaum, L., Bryson, S., Rogers, T., Roberts, W., Brian, J., & Szatmari, P. (2005). Behavioral manifestations of autism in the first year of life. *International Journal of Developmental Neuroscience, 23*, 143–152.

See Routledge's e-resources website for forms. (www.routledge.com/9780367346058)

7 Intelligence Tests

Overview

Intelligence is a complex construct that requires clear terminology so as to avoid unnecessary obfuscation when delineating its measurement (Bartholomew, 2004). In particular, intelligence, intelligence quotient, and g will be referenced routinely throughout this chapter. Although they may be used as synonyms, they really do have subtle yet meaningful differences that will be made that this early juncture before proceeding any further.

First, *intelligence* is a term that is used in ordinary discourse and is defined as IRT (American Psychological Association, 2015; Ciccarelli & White, 2020; Sternberg & Kaufman, 1998; Wechsler, 1975). Fundamentally speaking, this definition espouses the *aptitude view* of intelligence that emphasizes the ability to learn (also referred to as mental competence), in contrast to the *achievement view* that is more associated with educational attainment (Larsen & Buss, 2021; see also Chapter 8). This definition is readily understood and effectively communicates to readers to what this ability trait refers. This definition is employed, in part or whole, among the data tables for each of the tests presented in this chapter. However, this definition is insufficient for measurement purposes. In other words, it falls short of being an acceptable operational definition wherein intelligence is defined in the manner in which it is either measured or manipulated.

Second, *intelligence quotient* (*IQ*) is a quantitative index or composite that is computed by the use of scores obtained from a set of items. The items used are typically those that have been judged by experts as representing the construct of intelligence (also known as content validity). Additionally, these items should also have some empirical support, such as being correlated with other constructs that would be expected if they truly measured intelligence (e.g., academic grades). Together, these issues address construct validity. In any case, when *IQ* is used in this chapter, it refers to a quantitative index or score showing how much of this construct an examinee possesses, either by means of mental age (MA) or number of deviations from the mean when compared to same-aged peers.

Third, and finally, g (or g factor) represents a hypothetical construct that is employed to explain a pattern of responses obtained by calculating the IQ. That is, g is based upon the assumption that there exists a single latent dimension that is able to account for the variance in multiple specific cognitive abilities; that is, g represents a single complex cognitive ability or general intelligence. It may also potentially describe a single major dimension of brain structure or function (see, e.g., Gardner, 1999, 2006).

Now that these related terms have been delineated, the discussion can proceed with the chapter's chief focus. The measurement of intelligence has a long and informative history, and remains a central component of contemporary testing in mental health practice. This chapter includes four individually administered intelligence tests that many would agree are the best psychology has to offer, including the three Wechsler versions that together cover the majority of the lifespan, and the Stanford-Binet. They should be part of every psychologist's test inventory as they complement each other in several key facets related to their structure and design. They are as follows: (a) the Wechsler Preschool and Primary Scale of Intelligence, Fourth Edition (WPPSI–IV; Wechsler, 2012a, 2012b); (b) the Wechsler Intelligence Scale for Children, Fifth Edition (WISC–V; Wechsler, 2014a, 2014b); (c) the Wechsler Adult Intelligence Scale, Fourth Edition (WAIS–IV; Wechsler, 2008a, 2008b); and (d) Stanford–Binet Intelligence Scales, Fifth Edition (SB5; Roid, 2003b, 2003c, 2003d).

Prior to discussing each of these tests individually, it is important to review some theoretical and measurement issues regarding intelligence because it relates to the issue of how they can be most favorably used in practice. This will serve as a natural segue into describing some of the principal diagnostic reasons they should be included within a targeted test battery. When these tests are later reviewed individually, they will be compared and contrasted at various strategic points when deemed useful such that the reader is thereafter able to make informed decisions about which to select in various case circumstances.

DOI: 10.4324/9780429326820-9

Theoretical and Measurement Issues

Implicit Versus Explicit Theories

The conceptualization of intelligence can be dichotomized into implicit and explicit theories. *Implicit theories* are personal or subjective definitions of intelligence developed by laypeople based upon their experience and perception of how the world works, along with their cultural background (Baral & Das, 2004). Implicit theories can emphasize a range of characteristics as being part of intelligence, such as verbal abilities and academic success (especially reading), although also including non-ability traits as politeness and respect depending upon culture (Baral & Das, 2004). In contrast, *explicit theories* of intelligence are promulgated by psychologists, which are based upon hypotheses that are tested and refined by empirical research. It is these theories that represent the principal focus.

Explicit Theories

Explicit or scientific theories of intelligence can be further apportioned into those that are non-psychometric and those that are psychometric. *Non-psychometric theories* are qualitative in nature and view intelligence from a theoretical perspective. For example, Piaget conceptualizes intelligence as evolving within a stage-like sequence, hence changing in quality or form as the result of biological maturation and experience (Piaget, 1952, 1970). Another example is Howard Gardner's theory of *multiple intelligences* where he argues that there exist nine independent types of abilities, many of which are not measured by formal tests and are based upon or controlled by different brain regions (Gardner, 1998, 1999). They include verbal, logical-mathematical, musical, visual-spatial, movement, interpersonal, intrapersonal, existential, and natural (Gardner, 1999; Gardner & Moran, 2006).

In contrast, *psychometric theories* endeavor to explain the components or structure of intelligence by attempting to quantify the relationships among items and tests of various narrowly defined abilities. Clusters of items and specific tests that form factors represent hitherto latent variables, which in turn signify essential components of intelligence. It is these types of theories that are emphasized in the ensuing sections this chapter.

Psychometric Theories

The g Factor

The first most pertinent psychometric theory is that of Spearman (1904). He conceived of intelligence as comprised of two abilities, including a *g factor* that represented a complex type of *general intelligence*, and *s factors* that represented a related series of narrowly defined tasks or *specific intelligences* (*s factors*; *e.g.*, vocabulary, math). The implication was that the *g* factor would effectively predict how well an individual would perform on all of the *s* factors. For example, if a person possessed superior general intelligence, she would predictably tend to be superior in all or most of the measured specific abilities. The reason Spearman's theory is most applicable to this chapter is that traditional intelligence tests, such as the ones to be discussed, measure the *g* factor as exemplified by the full scale or overall test score, which as stated in the introduction to this chapter, is commonly referred to as the intelligence quotient (or IQ). Indeed, Spearman found significant correlations among various specific tests of ability, which he interpreted as providing empirical evidence for a global *g* factor construct.

Primary Mental Abilities

Later, Louis Thurstone (1938) proposed a multifactor theory including seven *primary mental abilities*, which he initially believed were independent. They included reasoning, comprehension, perceptual speed, word fluency, numerical ability, spatial visualization, and associative memory, which were published in the *Chicago Tests of Primary Mental Abilities* (Thurstone & Thurstone, 1941). Later, Thurstone acknowledged that these abilities did overlap sufficiently to consider *g* as a higher-order factor.

Hierarchical Model of Intelligence

Also relevant was Philip Vernon (1965) who integrated Spearman's *g* factor and Thurstone's primary mental abilities into a more comprehensive *hierarchical model of intelligence*. His primary contribution was to review and summarize an extensive volume of research on intelligence and propose a unified structure for this complex construct (Aiken, 1996). Specifically, at the base of the model (i.e., the first level) were the most specifically defined abilities, all of which were subject to being measured empirically. Those in proximity were thought to be most highly correlated such that they formed minor group factors. These minor group factors represented the second level of the hierarchy. The third level was comprised of two clusters of minor group factors, which were labeled major group factors. Lastly, the two major group factors were considered to be moderately correlated and formed the pinnacle of the hierarchy, here presenting a global summary of intelligence or Spearman's *g* factor (Gustafsson, 1989).

The proposal of a hierarchical conceptualization of intelligence was a watershed moment because measurement could now be focused upon the level required by the testing referral question or issue. That is, it was now possible to measure or quantify specific abilities, aggregate them to form more broadly defined domains, and lastly, integrate the domains to form a general or global level of intelligence. This hierarchical structure and levels analysis for each of the intelligence tests reviewed in this chapter shall become readily apparent, which is why it is being emphasized here. Additionally, the emergence of a hierarchical perspective on intelligence and its measurement served to resolve much of the controversy associated with the nature and definition of this complex and vital construct. In that sense, Vernon's work had significant heuristic value despite the fact he did not contribute much empirical work.

Two-Factor Theory: The Gf-Gc Model of Intelligence

Raymond Cattell and John Horn both proposed that intelligence was comprised of two principal factors rather than a single *g* factor (Horn, 1991; Schneider & McGrew, 2012). By means of *factor analysis*, Cattell and Horn corroborated Thurstone's multiple intelligences, although also discovered two second-order factors (i.e., on a higher second level immediately under the first level *g* factor). These second-order factors were fluid intelligence and crystalized intelligence. In particular, *fluid intelligence* is a fundamental mental capacity that controls abstract problem solving and reasoning, which is considered culture-free, independent of acquired knowledge, and genetically influenced. Succinctly, it represents one's capacity to learn and comprehend new information; essentially one's virtual brain-acumen. Alternatively, *crystalized intelligence* consists of one's fund of acquired knowledge, vocabulary, and skills based upon experience, education, and learning. This two-factor theory is consistent with a hierarchical model in that crystalized and fluid intelligence are comprised of quantifiable lower-level or more specific abilities. This theory is also known as the *Gf-Gc model of intelligence*. Additionally, they are interrelated and contribute to the global *g* factor. Again, the intelligence tests covered in this chapter possess factor structures that incorporate aspects of this model.

Extensions of the Gf-Gc Model of Intelligence

In addition to the *Gf-Gc* model, Horn proposed further abilities based upon visual and auditory processing, memory, processing speed, reaction time, quantitative abilities, and reading-writing abilities (Flanagan & Dixon, 2013). By means of additional factor analyses, he discovered a number of other second-order factors. The complete enumeration of the Cattell-Horn broad factors, considered on a level just beneath the *g* factor, was as follows: (a) Gf–fluid intelligence; (b) Gq–quantitative knowledge; (c) Gc–crystallized intelligence; (d) Grw–reading and writing ability; (e) Gsm–short-term memory; (f) Gv–visual processing; (g) Ga–auditory processing; (h) Glr–long-term retrieval; (i) Gs–processing speed; (j) CDS–correct decision speed. This listing denotes their measured rank-order strength of association with the *g* factor. Thus, fluid intelligence yielded the strongest correlation with global intelligence whereas correct decision speed manifested the weakest association (Flanagan, Ortiz, Alfonso, & Mascolo, 2002). This extended model was known as the Cattell-Horn Gf-Gc theory of intelligence (McGrew, 1997).

Later in 1993, John Carrol argued that intelligence was comprised of three levels or *strata* (*stratum* the singular form), which were differentiated according to the degree to which the assessed ability was specific or more general. His *three stratum hierarchical model of intelligence* resulted from his reanalysis of more than 461 data sets and was commended by many in the field (see, e.g., Horn, 1998; Jensen, 2004). According to this theory, Spearman's broadest and most complex *g* factor was at the top, which was labeled Stratum III. One level below, Stratum II consisted of broad intellectual abilities, including the Gf-Gc main factors and many of Horn's added broad factors. Specifically, they included (a) Gf'–fluid intelligence, (b) Gc–crystallized intelligence, (c) Gy–general memory and learning, (d) Gv–visual perception, (e) Gu–auditory perception, (f) Gr–retrieval ability, (g) Gs–cognitive speed, (h) Gt–decision reaction time. There is some disagreement at this juncture that is worthy of noting. Whereas Carroll particularly included a Stratum III *g* factor, Cattell and Horn seemed to devalue this concept (Alfonso, Flanagan & Radwan, 2005).

The Cattell-Horn-Carroll Theory of Intelligence

During the middle to latter 1990's, psychologist Kevin McGrew proposed an integration of the Cattell-Horn Gf-Gc model and the Carroll three stratum theory (McGrew, 1997), which was a viable project given their similarities. The new integrated theory became known as the *Cattell-Horn-Carroll (CHC) theory of intelligence* (Alfonso et al., 2005;

Flanagan & Dixon, 2013; McGrew, 2008; Schneider & McGrew, 2012). The 2012 version of the CHC theory retains the Stratum III global *g* factor, although expands the Stratum II broad factors to a total of 16 as compared to 10 for the Cattell-Horn Gf-Gc model and 8 for the Carrol three stratum model. More specifically, the added Stratum II factors were as follows: (a) Gkn–domain specific knowledge; (b) Gps–psychomotor speed; (c) Go–olfactory abilities; (d) Gh–tactile abilities; (e) Gk–kinesthetic abilities; and (f) Gp–psychomotor abilities (Schneider & McGrew, 2012).

The CHC Theory and the Intelligence Tests

The objective of reviewing the aforementioned psychometric theories and empirical research is that one will find the same hierarchical structure and three level strata in all of the ensuing contemporary intelligence tests. That is, the most narrowly defined Stratum I abilities are measured quantitatively by what are typically referred to as subtests. Stratum II abilities are epitomized by the more broadly defined factor indexes or domains, which are derived by combinations of subtest scores. Finally, the Stratum III global *g* factor is represented by the full scale IQ (FSIQ) score, which is derived by a combination of all pertinent index scores (hence occasionally referred to as a composite). One will also see among the stratum II factors many of the same kinds of more general abilities (e.g., verbal comprehension, fluid intelligence, processing speed, and visual-spatial processing). Why is this so?

The early versions of the major individually administered IQ tests were based upon idiosyncratic theoretical ideas and historical precedents of what people thought constituted the structure of intelligence (Alfonso et al., 2005). In fact, the majority of intelligence tests in publication prior to 2000 measured very few Stratum II abilities. As science has progressed through the 21st century, the CHC theory has gained increasing empirical support as a comprehensive account of human intelligence. In result, it has become the primary impetus for the development and continued revision of the major intelligence tests (Keith & Reynolds, 2010). Next, some of the principal reasons for including an intelligence test within a targeted test battery in mental health practice is discussed. Thereafter, independent presentations of the three Wechsler tests and the most recent edition of the Stanford-Binet form the basis of the remainder of this chapter.

Reasons for Intelligence Testing in Mental Health Practice

When considering the use of an intelligence test, the examiner must consider whether such a measure is capable of addressing the key diagnostic issues presented by the case facts and circumstances (e.g., is an individual competent to stand trial). This question actually addresses the issue of *construct validity*, which is defined as the degree to which a test measures the psychological characteristic or trait it purports to measure (Messick, 1989). Another way to word this definition is to ask, "Does this test perform in a manner consistent with its stated objectives?" In this case, the question is whether formal intelligence tests actually measure this construct as defined prior (i.e., the aptitude version). Recall that this definition focuses essentially upon the ability to think, reason, learn, and use knowledge in adapting to the environment. Thus, such tests should be correlated with, or predictive of, learning, reasoning, and adapting.

Examining the literature, construct validity for tests that measure *g* or IQ has been most consistently provided by robust and reliable predictions of academic performance and educational attainment spanning over 100 years (Binet, 1903; Deary & Johnson, 2010; Dreary, Strand, Smith, & Fernandes, 2007; Elshout & Veenman, 1992; Gagne & St. Pere, 2001; Johnson, Dreary, & Iacono, 2009; Kaufman, Reynolds, Liu, Kaufman, & McGrew, 2012; Sternberg & Kaufman, 1998; Terman, 1916; Willingham, 1974). Additional corroborating and cogent evidence of the adaptive nature of intelligence is provided by a wealth of predictive positive correlations between IQ and occupational performance (Hunt & Madhyastha, 2012; Hunter, 1983; Hunter & Hunter, 1984; Kuncel, Ones, & Sackett, 2010), mental and physical health, health behaviors, and longevity (Deary, Whalley, & Starr, 2003; Gottfredson, 2004; Gottfredson & Deary, 2004; Johnson, Corley, Starr, & Dreary, 2011), and, at least in part, social mobility (Capron & Duyme, 1989; Mackintosh, 1998). In fact, there are indications that intellectual ability or IQ may have commensurate or greater impact upon many real life outcomes as opposed to stylistic non-cognitive personality traits (e.g., see Gottfredson, 2004). This brief review indicates that that such tests truly measure the construct of intelligence as here defined.

Now that some evidence has been presented that these measures perform as desired, the next step is to review some of the most frequent uses of intelligence tests in mental health practice. First, and most obviously, intelligence tests are required when assessing for *intellectual disability* (*ID*). Irrespective of the DSM–5 elevating the adaptive behavior measure to be the factor that determines the degree of ID, this diagnosis continues to require an IQ test score approximately two standard deviations below a normative mean.

Second, they are also useful as part of a neuropsychological battery in which the focus of testing is on memory ability and an *ability–memory discrepancy analysis* is diagnostically desired or indicated (see also Chapter 9). In such analyses, the measured *g* factor (typically the FSIQ) is used to estimate what an individual's memory scores should be assuming normal functioning. If the individual's memory scores fall significantly below what is expected based upon the measured overall IQ score, this indicates significant impairment and is evidence for a neurocognitive disorder. Such comparisons are useful if an examinee falls at either extreme end of the intelligence test score distribution. Thus, imagine a hypothetical in which a 35-year-old male possesses gifted intelligence and is being referred for memory testing for suspected neurocognitive disorder. Assume that he does have such neuropsychological disorder, although in the hypothetical this is not known. If only the memory test is administered, it is likely he will score well within the normal range due to his high levels of intelligence, thus masking the underlying neuropathology. However, administering an IQ test would effectively adjust our expectations upward on the memory test as the high IQ scores would predict better than average performance on the memory test, hence averting a false negative decision (i.e., this male looks normal but he is not, relatively speaking).

Third, intelligence tests are useful in analogous situations in which testing is being done for a suspected specific learning disorder (SLD). If an examinee possesses gifted intelligence, she may score normal or above on an achievement test, which again may mask an underlying SLD. Similarly, if she possesses very low or extremely low intelligence, she may show spuriously low scores on the achievement test, hence making it appear as if she has multiple SLDs whereas the more accurate diagnosis would be either borderline intellectual functioning or ID. The second and third uses of intelligence tests are delineated in more detail in Chapters 9 and 8, respectively, including tables that assist in the discrepancy analyses. In the author's experience, use of intelligence tests in neuropsychological test batteries is more frequent than in testing for SLDs, which is why they are listed here in such order.

Fourth, intelligence tests are extremely useful when testing for *autism spectrum disorder* (ASD). For one, approximately 31% of individuals with diagnosed ASD have comorbid ID. Two, scrutiny of the DSM–5 autism-related nosology shows the need to address multiple specifiers as part of the diagnosis, including with or without intellectual impairment and language impairment. Even in autism testing cases where intelligence is estimated to be within normal limits, such measurement is useful in order to identify relative strengths and weaknesses. For instance, a 9-year-old female who tested positive for autism manifested a 31-point differential between her verbal comprehension and visual-spatial (i.e., nonverbal) abilities. Hence, despite having a global IQ test score within normal limits, her verbal abilities clearly were impaired, both in a normative comparison and in a relative or ipsative sense. This is why the measuring the intelligence should be routinely considered when testing for autism.

Fifth, intelligence tests may be employed independently as a screening tool for a host of disorders and as supporting evidence for non-cognitive disorders. This primarily regards both a normative and especially *ipsative* (i.e., intra-individual) profile analysis. For example, statistical differences between verbal and nonverbal abilities can be used to screen for SLDs and disruptive behavioral problems. In addition, certain patterns of IQ scores can be supportive of other disorders that deserve further attention. For example, verbal IQ has been shown to be consistently lower than nonverbal IQ in cases of *conduct disorder* (CD) in children, indicating a specific and pervasive deficit in language (Gremillion & Martel, 2013; Jaffee & D'Zunlla, 2003; Zadeh, Im-Bolter, & Cohen, 2007). It has been further hypothesized that such verbal deficiencies contribute to severe conduct disturbances by hindering the development of self-control, emotion regulation, and the labeling of emotions, which in turn causes a lack of empathy for others' feelings and needs (Hastings, Zahn-Waxler, Robinson, Usher, & Bridges, 2000; Peterson et al., 2013). Garnering such data within a testing case would be vital because it leads directly to treatment recommendations that target such language deficits, hence helping to improve the likelihood of effective therapy.

The most likely related referral questions that can be addressed by intelligence tests include (a) estimating the likely success of an individual matriculating through a training or educational program, (b) suggesting the level and types of training indicated by the results, (c) addressing issues of mental competence, and (d) recommending adjustments in psychological interventions based upon an examinee's measured degree of intelligence. The most likely referral sources that may directly or indirectly request or require intelligence testing as part of the assessment include (a) welfare programs to assist in determining eligibility for disability benefits, (b) vocational rehabilitation programs to assist in career development, (c) court referrals to determine issues of competency and insanity, (d) mental health therapists such that they may modify treatment intervention accordingly, and (e) adults or parents whose child is experiencing significant difficulties in academic performance.

There are many other uses of intelligence tests in mental health practice. More will undoubtedly become apparent as the specific tests are presented, including their data tables to be employed in reporting test results. The review begins with the Wechsler series, which will proceed in order of examinee *chronological age* (CA). The chapter will conclude with the Stanford-Binet. Comparisons will be made between the two to assist the reader in determining the cases and circumstances for which they are better suited.

The Wechsler Tests

The initial *Wechsler-Bellevue Intelligence Scale* (Wechsler, 1939) was developed as a measure of global intellectual ability, although the test structure also permitted one to obtain scores on more specific skills. In contrast to its then major competitor, the Stanford-Binet (Terman, 1916; Terman & Merril, 1937), its items were specifically designed for a target population of adults. This was in construct to later editions of the Stanford-Binet that initially used childlike items on adults. It also deemphasized speed of performance, which Wechsler believed unfairly disadvantaged older test takers. With this initial test, Wechsler also instituted the *point scale* wherein examinees were awarded one point for each correct answer, which supplanted the age norms used in the Stanford-Binet. The employment of point scales was a major modification because it permitted the use of the *deviation IQ*, which is based upon the assumption that intelligence is normally distributed throughout the population. When such tests are normed on different age groupings, examinees' test scores can be compared to their same age peers in the form of standard deviation units from the mean or central tendency. Virtually all major intelligence tests today utilize point scales, including the contemporary Stanford-Binet (although as will become apparent, the latter further subdivides subtest into clusters of six items of increasing difficulty, referred to as testlets).

Wechsler was principally viewed as a *g* theorist due to his emphasis on a single summary dimensional score that represented a general complex factor of intelligence (Kaufman, Flanagan, Alfonso, & Mascolo, 2006). Items were organized into groupings based upon content, which Wechsler viewed simply as different manifestations of overall intelligence. Currently, there is robust empirical evidence for a *g* factor representing general intelligence at the top of a hierarchical model, with broad-based abilities at the mid-level, and narrow abilities at the lowest level (Carroll, 1993, 2012; Horn & Blankson, 2012; Johnson, Bouchard, Krueger, McGue, & Gottesman, 2004; Salthouse, 2004).

This review began with the three *Wechsler* intelligence tests because of several advantages they have over the Stanford-Binet. These include greater efficiency in administration and scoring, a more felicitous overall match between test items and stimuli with their target populations, an empirically-based factor structure consistent with CHC theory (although so also is the Stanford-Binet), and being co-normed with the Wechsler tests of achievement and memory. The latter permits statistical ability-achievement and ability–memory discrepancy analyses when needed (see Chapters 8 and 9, respectively). The order in which these tests will be presented is from younger to older, hence beginning with the preschool version and ending with the adult test.

Wechsler Preschool and Primary Scale of Intelligence, Fourth Edition

Synopsis

The *Wechsler Preschool and Primary Scale of Intelligence, Fourth Edition* (*WPPSI–IV*; Wechsler, 2012a, 2012b) is designed as a measure of intelligence for those of preschool age and into the early primary grades. Its age ranges extend downward to age 2 years 6 months to 7 years 7 months, inclusive. There are two versions, one for ages 2 years 6 months through 3 years 11 months, and the other for ages 4 years 0 months through 7 years 7 months. The WPPSI–IV is a modification of the immediate predecessor, the *Wechsler Preschool and Primary Scale of Intelligence, Third Edition* (*WPPSI–III*; Wechsler, 2002), which represented a major revision of this scale. It is therefore prudent to provide a succinct history of this scale's development as part of the initial summary.

HISTORICAL DEVELOPMENT

In the 1950s through early 1960s, there was an increasing need for preschool assessment of intelligence. In response, the *Wechsler Preschool and Primary Scale of* (*WPPSI*; Wechsler, 1967) was developed for children ranging in age from 4 years 0 months through 6 years 6 months. It included the subtests Information, Comprehension, Arithmetic, Vocabulary, Similarities, Sentences, Geometric Design, Block Design, Mazes, Picture Completion, and Animal House. Next, the *Wechsler Preschool and Primary Scale of Intelligence, Revised Edition* (*WPPSI–R*; Wechsler, 1989) retained all of the original subtests and added Object Assembly. Furthermore, the age range was expanded to 3 years 0 months through 7 years 3 months. Hence, easier and more difficult items were required to avoid basal and ceiling effects. For both editions, factor analytic studies demonstrated a two-factor model of intelligence, including verbal and performance (non-verbal) factors (Carlson & Reynolds, 1981; Gyurke, Stone, & Beyer, 1990; Liu & Lynn, 2011; Schneider & Gervais, 1991; Silverstein, 1969; Stone, Gridley, & Gyurke, 1991).

However, the WPPSI–III was the major revision, extending the age range down further to 2 years 6 months and apportioning the scale into two age bands or versions as delineated above for the WPPSI–IV. Each version contained different subtest batteries, which were most conducive to that particular age band. The WPPSI–IV continues with a very comparable structure, including the two versions for younger and older examinees. The following subtests are continued from the WPPSI–III: Information, Similarities, Vocabulary, Comprehension, Receptive Vocabulary, Picture Naming, Block Design, Object Assembly, Matrix Reasoning, and Picture Concepts. Further, five new subtests were added and include Picture Memory, Zoo Locations, Bug Search, Cancellation, and Animal Coding. The subtest item content was revised to decrease the emphasis on speed and fine motor skill demands, and to incorporate features that are more developmentally fitting and pleasing to young children. The specific abilities measured by these subtests will be presented shortly. Based upon experience, children really do enjoy the manipulatives and materials, including an ink dauber versus pencil, which makes it easy to present the test as akin to play, which effectively fosters their attention, cooperation, and motivation. The factor structure of the WPPSI–IV follows.

WPPSI–IV FACTOR-STRUCTURE

Because there are two versions of the WPPSI–IV, there are essentially two factor-structures. For ages 2 years 6 months through 3 years 11 months, a three-factor hierarchical model demonstrated the best fit of the data for the inter-item correlations, including the following: (a) a full scale *g* factor; (b) three primary factors (viz., Verbal Comprehension, Visual Spatial, and Working Memory) with very high g-*loadings* (i.e., correlation-like indicators of the degree to which each factor measures general intelligence); and (c) seven subtests at the lowest level measuring specific abilities. The older age band evinced a five-factor hierarchical model, with a full scale *g* factor again at the top, with Verbal Comprehension, Visual Spatial, Fluid Reasoning, Working Memory, and Processing Speed representing brood-band mid-level factors with very high g-loadings, and 15 subtests at the lowest level. These results are consistent with the CHC theory of intelligence, including the following: (a) a Stratum III level complex *g* factor at the top; (b) Stratum II level factors (i) Verbal Comprehension–Crystalized Ability, (ii) Visual Spatial–Visual Processing, (iii) Fluid Reasoning–Fluid Reasoning, (iv) Working Memory–Short-Term Memory, and (v) Processing Speed–Processing Speed; and (c) a Stratum I series of subtests that measures narrowly defined and quantifiable specific abilities.

Norm Reference Sample

The WPPSI–IV norm reference sample consisted of 1,700 children who were apportioned into nine age groups. For the youngest seven groups, age intervals were measured in 6-month timeframes, whereas the oldest two groups were measured in 12-month intervals. All groups contained 200 children with the exception of the oldest, which contained only 100 children. All groups consisted of equal numbers of males and females. Finally, the standardization sample was stratified to match the 2010 U.S. Census (U.S. Bureau of the Census, 2010) proportions according to race/ethnicity, parental education level, and geographic region.

Administration

Test administration is contingent upon two principal considerations, including (a) CA of the examinee, and (b) the degree and kind of IQ score information desired. If the examinee is between 2 years 6 months and 3 years 11 months, then the younger age band version would be selected. If the examinee is 4 years 0 months to 7 years 7 months, then the older age-band version would be chosen. Irrespective of the age band, however, the test is individually administered, including both the examiner and examinee. With the exception of the youngest children under the age of three years, parents and collaterals are asked to remain in the waiting area while the child is escorted into the testing room for administration. Those younger than 3 years of age may need to have a family member in the room to minimize anxiety, although they should be required to sit behind the child and asked to remain quiet.

Both versions use recommended start points, reversal rules, and discontinue rules in an attempt to abbreviate test administration and maintain motivation on the part of the examinee. The items are ordered in increasing degrees of difficulty. As such, *start points* are associated with computed CA and are designed to be passed rather easily to bolster effort, confidence, and motivation. *Reversal rules* revert to easier items when start point tasks are failed until two correct responses are obtained. The *discontinue rules* have become quite brief relative to earlier Wechsler editions, with most subtests now imposing a three consecutive failure rule, along with two subtests that require more time for administration using a two consecutive failure rule (e.g., Block Design). The objective here is to reduce administration time and to prevent discouragement from repeated failures. It is advisable to begin with easier items prior to the advised start point for examinees who will likely obtain significantly impaired levels of intelligence. Next, a decision needs to be made regarding what intellectual information is desired. The potential information available to the examiner is somewhat different depending upon which version is used.

YOUNGER AGE BAND VERSION

This version contains three potential levels of analysis as follows: (a) full scale; (b) primary indexes; and (c) ancillary indexes. If only a full scale IQ score is desired, the administration can be circumscribed to core subtests Receptive Vocabulary, Information, Block Design, Object Assembly, and Picture Memory. This would minimize administration time to about 27 minutes.

However, the manual advises that sufficient subtests should be administered in order to yield a full scale IQ and all three primary index IQ scores Verbal Comprehension, Visual Spatial, and Working Memory. This would require six subtests, including all of the aforementioned five core subtests, plus Zoo Locations. Administration time for such analysis is still only about 32 minutes on average. Finally, there are ancillary scales that are theoretical as opposed to empirical, which include Vocabulary Acquisition, Nonverbal, and General Ability. Nonverbal can be computed using four of the six subtests required for the full scale and primary indexes. Hence, this would not add any subtests to the administration as it simply combines the subtests used for Visual Spatial and Working Memory. The Picture Naming subtest would need to be added to compute the other two. Of these, the full scale and primary indexes provide, "a comprehensive description and evaluation of a child's cognitive abilities" (Wechsler, 2012b, p. 16). Therefore, the data table for the younger age band (see Form 7.1) includes the full scale, three primary indexes, and the six required subtests.

OLDER AGE BAND VERSION

The 4 years 0 months to 7 years 7 months' age band version of the test affords the same three-level analysis, although with an increased number of broad-based Stratum II empirically supported factors, consistent with the notion that the structure of intelligence becomes more complex and differentiated with age (see, e.g., Piaget, 1952, 1970). If an examiner simply desires a full scale IQ score (e.g., to rule in ID), then six core subtests are required, including Information, Similarities, Block Design, Matrix Reasoning, Picture Memory, and Bug Search. Estimated administration time is 31 minutes, hence the same as for the younger version within the margin of error. However, in typical cases the preference is to measure and report both the complex *g* factor at the top of the hierarchy, along with all of the empirically backed primary scales, which also has CHC theoretical parallels. If sufficient time for intelligence testing has received insurance preauthorization (PA), typically a 2-hour duration, it would seem a waste to simply measure and report the full scale IQ score.

In order to report the full scale and five primary scales, 10 subtests are required. These consist of all the subtests contributing to the full scale, plus the following four: Object Assembly; Picture Concepts; Zoo Locations; and Cancellation. Total estimated administration time is an even 60 minutes, which is extremely efficient for an individually administered test of human intelligence.[1] The theoretical ancillary index scales are also greater in number, including Vocabulary Acquisition, Nonverbal, General Ability, and Cognitive Proficiency. However, unless there is a clearly specified reason justifying the employment of one or more of these supplemental indexes, these should not be included in the analysis as the number of required subtests and the time needed for their administration are prohibitive when balanced with the information yielded.

Scoring

Consistent with Wechsler's point scale approach (see prior), the WPPSI–IV core data yield linearly transformed scores that measure how far examinees' fall from the average of same-aged peers in standard deviation units; that is, examinees' raw scores are *age corrected*. The two linearly transformed scores are the subtest scaled score and the index and full scale standard scores. These can be observed in Forms 7.1 and 7.2, Table 1 general notes. Because these scores represent the core data, they will be delineated in the subsequent two sections in such order.

STANDARD SCORES

Beginning at the top of the intelligence construct hierarchy, the full scale IQ score (representing the *g* factor) has a mean of 100 and standard deviation of 15, along with an impressively large range from 40 to 160. The index scores carry the same metric, although with a somewhat smaller range of 45 to 155. This is not apparent from the general table notes because it has been incorporated into the larger full scale IQ range for brevity. That is, the small difference did not seem sufficiently important to include a separate general note for the index score range.

Table 1 (Forms 7.1, 7.2) contains six columns, including the scale name, standard score, 95% *confidence interval* (*CI*), *percentile rank* (*PR*), *qualitative descriptor*, and a succinct summary of the abilities measured by that scale. Each row represents a separate full scale or index scale. Beginning with the first row is the full scale IQ, which appears in bold for emphasis properly accorded to the general *g* factor. The subtests that contribute to the FSIQ score are identified in a specific table note to alert the reader to this fact. This also permits the examiner to use this table if only those subtests were used to compute the FSIQ. In that case, only the FSIQ information would be entered into the table with the remaining entries having the double dash symbol entered (i.e., --) for no score or simply deleting these non-used rows. The CI informs readers of the error rate and also provides a rapid means of estimating likely differences among indexes. The PR represents an areas transformation showing the percent of the norm reference group the examinee performed equal to or better than. However, it should be noted that the reported PRs are based upon the theoretical standard distribution and not those of the standardization sample. Both the CI and PR are defined for the reader in general table notes.

Table 2 provides formal analyses of all pairwise index standard score comparisons that mirrors that of the Bayley–III and other tests reviewed in Chapter 6. Essentially, hypotheses tests are run on each of the difference scores, the null hypothesis being that the two indexes are not statistically different. The critical value column shows the difference score that begins the rejection region for the hypothesis test. Hence, any difference score that is equal to or greater than the obtained difference is statistically significant at the .01 *alpha level*. In other words, if significant, this alpha level indicates that the obtained difference score would occur less than 1 time in 100 due to chance factors, which can easily be ruled out at such a low probability. These analyses can be run at a more liberal .05 level, but recall that the *familywise error rate* (also known as the *experimentwise error rate*) exponentially increases as more hypothesis tests are done. For example, if three hypothesis tests are run at .05, the familywise error rate is now approximately 15% (not exactly but the point is made). Hence, only those hypothesis tests that are necessary should be done and at the most conservative .01 level.

Finally, the base rate of the difference score should be reported as both an effect size and a practical explanation of the result if the difference was significant, appending one, two, or three cross symbols (i.e., †) to denote unusual, abnormal, and profoundly abnormal results, respectively. Recall the *base rate* is the percentage of the norm reference sample that manifested the obtained difference score; the lower the percent, the more aberrant the result. If the difference is not significant, the base rate can be left with a double dash symbol (i.e., --).

SCALED SCORES

The remaining tables in Forms 7.1 and 7.2 report the subtest scaled score metric, which is comparatively smaller with a mean of 10, standard deviation of 3, and a range of 1 to 19. Each table is devoted to reporting the two subtest scores that contributed to one of the primary indexes enumerated in Table 1. Note that they appear in the same sequence as the indexes in Table 1. The tables are deliberately organized to mirror that of Table 1, including the subtest name, scaled score, 95% CI, PR, qualitative descriptor, and measured abilities. The CIs for scaled scores are not reported in either the manual or computer scoring output and thus can be computed from the average of the pertinent subtest SEMs for that index, then rounded to the nearest whole number. The PRs are also not reported but can be rapidly referenced in the scaled score to PR conversion guide provided in Table 7.1, which was adapted from the parallel Bayley–III Table 6.3 in Chapter 6 (Bayley, 2006b, p. 109).

Table 7.1 Scaled Score to Percentile Rank Conversion Guide

Scaled Score	Percentile Rank
19	99.9
18	99.6
17	99
16	98
15	95
14	91
13	84
12	75
11	63
10	50
9	37
8	25
7	16

(*Continued*)

Table 7.1 (Continued)

Scaled Score	Percentile Rank
6	9
5	5
4	2
3	1
2	0.4
1	0.1

Source. Adapted from Bayley, N. (2006). *Bayley Scales of Infant Development, Third Edition (Bayley–III): Technical and interpretive manual.* San Antonio, Texas: The Psychological Corporation-Pearson, Table 6.1, p. 109.

Note. Scaled score mean = 10; standard deviation = 3; percentile rank (PR) median = 50; range = 1–99. PRs are based upon the theoretical standard normal distribution.

OTHER SCORES

Briefly, it should be mentioned that other data are available among the WPPSI–IV data that are not used for various reasons, among them being to emphasize the core results in order to focus the assessment report on the most vital findings. One includes the *age equivalent score*, which represents the age in years and months that the examinee's raw score typifies. Its weaknesses are lack of equal intervals (similar to PRs) and most especially, the examinee is not being compared to same-aged peers; that is, this score is not age-corrected. Second are *process scores*, which are more qualitative in nature. They are based upon some modification in administration that provides unique information about the examinee's performance and ability. One example of a process score includes *testing the limits* wherein for instance an examinee is permitted to keep working on a puzzle until completion despite being over the time limit for a valid raw score. The process score in this case would represent the examinee's performance controlling for the effects of speed. Process scores are interesting but such information can be captured more efficiently merely through making selective test observations.

COMPUTER SCORING

The same internet-based Q–global (Pearson, 2021) software that currently provides computer scoring for the Bayley–4 and Vineland–3 offers WPPSI–IV computer scoring. There are basically two types of reports: score and interpretive. The score report provides all of the core data, including composite score summary and graphic profile, scaled score summary and graphic profile, all pairwise comparisons, and all ancillary scores. The interpretive report goes further and provides comprehensive interpretations of all data provided in the score report, which can fill 17 pages of single-spaced narrative interpretations, tables, and graphs, and concluding with a brief parent report summary. There is a charge for each score and interpretative report.

In this case, however, the manual scoring is faster, more efficient, and personalized, although admittedly there is a greater risk for human error. The main argument for purchasing and having a few score and interpretive reports in reserve is in the event an extremely complex case must be completed, including multiple ipsative comparisons. However, if score reporting and interpretation focuses on the full scale IQ and the primary indexes, and the data tables in Forms 7.1 and 7.2 are used, manual scoring and interpretation should be satisfactory.

Interpretation

Interpretation for both the younger and older age band versions will be discussed together, with discriminations made when needed. Interpretations should proceed from general to specific, following the three-tiered hierarchical model of intelligence demonstrated by means of factor-analysis and theory. Figure 7.1 is available for download on Routledge's e-resources website and has been created to assist in tracking the interpretive process for all Wechsler tests, which is possible considering their comparable test structures. In addition, pre-drafted narrative excerpts follow each Wechsler test data table. These include language that guides the examiner through the advised interpretative process. They may be modified or deleted as determined by the particular case facts and objectives.

FULL SCALE IQ AND THE PRIMARY INDEXES

Table 1 in Forms 7.1 and 7.2 should initiate test interpretation beginning with the full scale IQ score, followed by norm-based analyses among the primary index scores (see also Figure 7.1). For laypeople, the PRs and qualitative interpretations are important, especially the latter for diagnostic purposes. The publication of the *Wechsler Intelligence Scale for Children, Fifth Edition* (Wechsler, 2014a, 2014b) introduced an updated qualitative descriptor scheme that is advised for all Wechsler IQ tests. This can be seen in Table 7.2. In actuality, only the two highest or most favorable descriptions changed from "very superior" and "superior" to "extremely high" and "very high," respectively. The chief rationale was to better match the wording of the three highest and lowest categories such that parallel form was

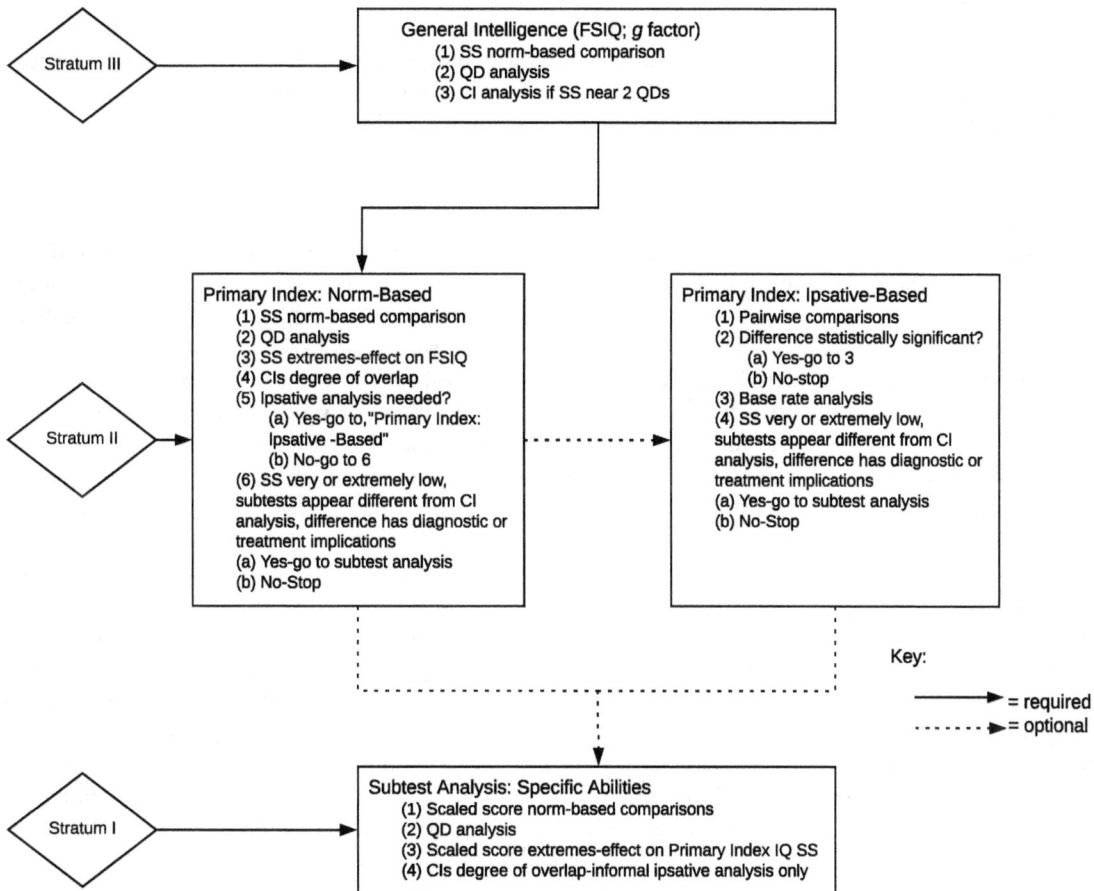

Figure 7.1 Wechsler Intelligence Tests Interpretive Process

Table 7.2 Wechsler Intelligence Tests Qualitative Description Guide

Standard Scores	Scaled Scores	Standard Deviations from the Mean	Qualitative Description
130 and above	16 to 19	+2 to +3	Extremely high
120 to 129	14 to 15	+1⅓ to +1⅔	Very high
110 to 119	12 to 13	+⅔ to +1	High average
90 to 109	8 to 11	−⅔ to +⅓	Average
80 to 89	6 to 7	−1⅓ to −1	Low average
70 to 79	4 to 5	−2 to −1⅔	Very low (borderline)
69 and below	1 to 3	−3 to −2⅓	Extremely low

Source. Adapted from Wechsler, D. (2014). *Wechsler Intelligence Scale for Children, Fifth Edition (WISC–V): Technical and interpretive manual.* Bloomington, MN: Pearson Education, Inc. (PsychCorp), Tables 6.1, 6.2, & 6.3, pp. 150, 151, & 153, respectively.

achieved (e.g., very low paired with very high). Also, it was believed that this language was more neutral in terms of connotation or informal meaning. A "borderline" term is added in a parenthetical with the very low class in order to make it compatible with a DSM–5 diagnosis of borderline intellectual functioning (see Chapter 4). This may be deleted if not applicable to a particular case.

Note that the measured abilities of each scale included in the final column of Table 1 (see Forms 7.1 and 7.2) are judiciously worded in order to facilitate test interpretation and ensure that what has been stated to be measured is clear. Also note that the lay definition of intelligence offered at the beginning of this chapter is used for summarizing the meaning of the Full Scale IQ (i.e., FSIQ) in Table 1. The primary indexes are similarly summarized in terms of the essential abilities measured by each scale.

After the norm-based comparisons, index comparisons should be analyzed first by examining the relative positions of the CIs. Indexes which have little or no overlap should be suspected as significantly different. If more formal analysis of this issues is needed, then Table 2 hypothesis tests on the difference can be made, but the examiner must be selective due to the familywise error rate increasing chances of a *Type I error* (i.e., concluding that there is a difference when in fact there is not). As a rule, compare only those indexes in which the CIs have little or no overlap. Also, a verbal versus nonverbal comparison has always had diagnostic relevance. Hence, Verbal Comprehension versus Visual Spatial and Verbal Comprehension versus Fluid Reasoning could both be done routinely.

SPECIFIC SUBTEST ABILITIES

Interpretations at the most specific Stratum I level are most relevant when (a) the broad primary index scale to which the subtests contribute is significantly low, and/or (b) the subtests show an apparent significant difference or gap with one being low or very low (see also Figure 7.1). First, if the index to which the subtests contribute is low or extremely low, then at least one or both of the associated subtests are also likely to be impaired, in which case they should be reported and interpreted. Second, irrespective of the index score, if there appears to be a significant gap between subtests and one subtest is low or very low, and such difference is key to diagnosis and/or treatment, then they should be reported in order to identify the underlying weakness. This can be easily done by noting the degree of separation or overlap between the 95% CIs using the aforementioned scheme first reported in Chapter 10: (a) no overlap means a significant difference is present; (b) moderate overlap means a possible difference is present; and (c) complete or nearly complete overlap means an absence of difference. Interpreting the subtest scaled scores and relative differences here avoids reporting an apparent "normal" primary index scale that inadvertently masks an underlying more specific weakness that affects diagnosis or treatment recommendations.

On the other hand, if in the examiner's clinical judgment, the underlying specific weakness is peripheral to the diagnostic issues or questions, then reporting the subtest score profile is unnecessary and can be skipped in the interests of brevity. Interpreting the qualitative descriptor for the reported subtests can be done by referencing Table 7.2, including possibly noting the number of standard deviations from the mean the scaled score falls. In most cases, it suffices to report the full scale and primary indexes, including normative analyses, and if needed, ipsative analyses, even if there are some possible differences at the subtest level. This is because subtests are typically less reliable and valid due to having less items, and principal diagnostic issues infrequently depend upon the consideration of narrowly defined abilities.

Wechsler Intelligence Scale for Children, Fifth Edition

Synopsis

The *Wechsler Intelligence Scale for Children, Fifth Edition* (*WISC–V;* Wechsler, 2014a, 2014b) is a comprehensive, individually administered intelligence test for examinees who range in age from 6 years 0 months through 16 years 11 months inclusive. As such, it overlaps at the younger end of the age range with that of the afore-described WPPSI–IV from 6 year 0 months to 7 years 7 months. If an examinee falls within this interval, clinicians should choose the test that is most likely to avert floor effects or ceiling effects. Thus, if an examinee's level of intelligence is suspected to be impaired, using the WPPSI–IV is indicated as such test is capable of yielding lower scores. In contrast, a child with suspected gifted intelligence would match better with the WISC–V because there would be no artificial limitation imposed at the higher end of the ability score spectrum. As there have been remarkably frequent revisions of this version of the Wechsler IQ test series, brief review will be provided for context as was done for the WPPSI–IV.

HISTORICAL DEVELOPMENT

The *Wechsler Intelligence Scale for Children* (*WISC*; Wechsler, 1949) was actually a modification of the Wechsler Bellevue Intelligence Scale (Wechsler, 1939) for adults. In particular, the following subtests were adapted for use by children ages 5 years to 15 years, inclusive: Information; Arithmetic, Similarities; Vocabulary; Digit Span; Comprehension; Picture Completion; Picture Arrangement; Block Design; Object Assembly; and Coding. These 12 subtests contributed to two index scores that were theoretically based, including Verbal IQ and Performance (or nonverbal) IQ, both of which were combined for the Full Scale IQ or *g* general intelligence factor. Again, this clearly placed Wechsler within the *g* factor genre of intelligence theoreticians.

The *Wechsler Intelligence Scale for Children, Revised Edition* (*WISC–R*; Wechsler, 1974) primarily updated the norms and shifted the age range up one year on both extreme ends, hence 6 to 16 years. The test structure continued with the full scale IQ (FSIQ), theoretical verbal IQ (VIQ) and performance IQ (PIQ), and the 12 subtests at the lowest level, 6 of which contributed to each index score. It was the *Wechsler Intelligence Scale for Children, Third Edition* (*WISC–III*; Wechsler, 1991) that introduced the empirically based primary index scores, including the Verbal Comprehension Index (VCI), Perceptual Organization Index (POI), Freedom from Distractibility Index (FDI), which could be scored and interpreted along with the more traditional FSIQ, VIQ, and PIQ. The latter was retained due to test consumer demand. That is, many psychologists utilized this structure for diagnostic purposes and naturally resisted the move to the new empirically-based primary indexes.[2]

Cotemporaneous with the WISC–III publication was the discovery that intelligence levels had been rising over the past 100 years (Flynn, 1987). More specifically, it was estimated that IQ scores increase about 3 points every decade (Flynn, 1984, 1987, 1999, 2007; Flynn & Weiss, 2007; Matarazzo, 1972). This phenomenon subsequently received a good deal of research support and was duly titled the, "*Flynn effect*" (see, e.g., (Fletcher, Stuebing, & Hughes, 2010; Flynn, 2006, 2009; Neisser, 1998). More to the point, it was found that testing with the WISC–III would result in an average 5-point drop in IQ compared to testing with the WISC–R due to the former adjusting for the population increase in intelligence (Kanaya, Scullin & Ceci, 2003). The impact of the Flynn effect on the WISC and all similar comprehensive intelligence tests was to strongly encourage an updating of their norms approximately every 5 to 10 years, this to avoid over-estimating examinees' intelligence by comparing them to an older generation with "easier norms." That is, using an outdated IQ test risks overestimating an examinee's IQ by 3 to 5 points for each decade it is out of date. Thus, thereafter the WISC series and intelligence tests in general have been published more frequently.

Next, the *Wechsler Intelligence Scale for Children, Fourth Edition* (*WISC–IV*; Wechsler, 2003) was published about 12 years later, which was a much more rapid updating than for previous versions. This edition dropped some of the subtests that were more traditional, including Object Assembly and Picture Arrangement. This was somewhat disconcerting to many psychologists because they employed these subtests for diagnostically important information. For example, the Picture Arrangement subtest required examinees to place cards within a social sequence that made sense, hence tapping into social intelligence. What was occurring was a gradual transition of all the Wechsler IQ tests from the more theoretical FSIQ, VIQ, and PIQ test structure to a more empirically based test structure that was increasingly consistent with the CHC theory of intelligence.

Hence, five new subtests were developed for the WISC–IV. First, Word Reasoning was a new measure of verbal comprehension. Second, Matrix Reasoning and Picture Concepts were new measures of fluid reasoning. Third, Letter–Number Sequencing was an added measure of Working Memory. Fourth, and finally, Cancellation was added as a measure of processing speed. At this juncture, one should now be able to discern the increasing references to the CHC theory of intelligence, which symbolizes the increasing move of the Wechsler test structure to that of this theory.

Of perhaps most significance, the theoretical VIQ and PIQ dichotomy was dropped in its entirety, hence becoming an historical footnote. However, this is the manner in which scientific inquiry is intended to work, continually improving theoretical constructs as they are tested by empirical data. Also, because some of the new subtests contained somewhat different measured specific abilities, the WISC–IV also modified some of the names of the empirically based primary indexes to which they contributed in order to more accurately reflect the abilities measured. Specifically, the POI was renamed the Perceptual Reasoning Index (PRI), and the FDI was renamed the Working Memory Index (WMI).

At this point, the WISC–IV was comprised of a four-factor structure, including the complex *g* factor at the top, followed by four primary indexes, including Verbal Comprehension, Perceptual Reasoning, Working Memory, and Processing Speed. A number of independent studies had confirmed this four-factor structure for both the WISC–IV and for the adult version discussed below (see, e.g., Bodin, Pardini, Burns, & Stevens, 2009; Ward, Bergman, & Herbert, 2012; Watkins, 2010; Watkins, Wilson, Kotz, Carbone, & Babula, 2006). This discussion has now reached the WISC–V, which continues the trend toward a factor-analytically defined test structure and increasing consistency with the CHC theory of intelligence.

WISC–V FACTOR STRUCTURE

Subsequent to the WISC–IV being published, researchers began to garner evidence for a five-factor structure (see Benson, Hulac, & Kranzler, 2010; Keith, Fine, Taub, Reynolds, & Kranzler, 2006; Weiss, Keith, Zhu, & Chen, 2013a, 2013b). In essence, verbal comprehension and processing speed remained unmodified, while perceptual reasoning and working memory were distributed across three factors. These three factors represented visual spatial abilities, fluid reasoning, and working memory abilities. Recall that this same five-factor model was evinced for the older age-band version of the WPPSI–IV (Wechsler, 2012a, 2012b). The WISC–V internal test structure was consequently investigated in light of this new data and the incorporation of three new subtests, each of which was designed to strengthen one of the primary factors. The latter included Visual Puzzles (i.e., a mental rotation task without a motor component), Figure Weights, and Picture Span, which were associated with visual spatial abilities, fluid reasoning, and working memory, respectively.

The development of the WISC–V was based upon the theoretical assumption that the test measures general intellectual ability (i.e., a *g* factor), which manifests itself among five domains of cognitive abilities, including Verbal Comprehension, Visual Spatial, Fluid Reasoning, Working Memory, and Processing Speed. Interestingly, this comports with David Wechsler's initial conceptualization of intelligence (Wechsler, 1939). Results showed that the expected five-factor model provided an excellent fit of the data and significantly better than that of any four-factor models that were attempted. These results endured (a) when done for all age groupings that comprised the norm reference sample (discussed subsequently) and (b) when delimiting the analysis to only the primary subtests (i.e., the subtests that contribute to each empirically supported primary index score).

Examining the particular factor loadings, Fluid Reasoning manifests clearly the strongest correlation with the second or higher order *g* factor, being perfect or nearly perfect (Wechsler, 2014a, 2014b, p. 83). Recall that a *factor loading* is the measured degree of association and percent of variance explained between a variable (here Fluid Reasoning) and its factor (here the *g* factor). This result is consistent with independent researchers (see, e.g., Kaufman & Kaufman, 2004; Keith et al., 2006; Wechsler, 2008b, 2012b; Weiss et al., 2013a, 2013b). This indicates that the Fluid Reasoning factor can be used as an abbreviated estimate of an individual's general intellectual ability if limited time and expense prohibits administration of the complete test. Additionally, this five-factor structure is consistent with the CHC theory of intelligence as was that of the WPPSI–IV older age band version. The ensuing sections present the standardization sample, administration, scoring, and interpretation, the latter which defines the specific and broad-based abilities measured by this test.

Norm Reference Sample

The WISC–V standardization sample consisted of 2,200 children distributed across 11 age cohorts at one-year intervals, beginning at 6 years 0 months through 16 years 11 months. Each age group was comprised of 200 individuals. Within each age group, the sample was stratified by sex, race/ethnicity, parent education level, and geographic region such that they proportionally matched those reported by the 2012 U.S. Census Bureau statistics (U.S. Bureau of the Census, 2012). There was a list of exclusionary criteria employed in selecting the normative sample. Some of these criteria included primary language not English, lack of verbal ability, significantly oppositional behavior during testing, having completed any intelligence testing within 6 months of the current testing, identical twins, manifesting a sensory or motor impairment (i.e., visual, auditory, motor), diagnosis of a condition that may affect cognitive performance, and taking a medication that may compromise cognitive functioning.

Administration

Administering the WISC–V is similar to that of the WPPSI–IV, although there is less dependence upon brightly colored stimulus materials and manipulatives (e.g., ink stamper). Administration time ranges from 45 to 65 minutes, contingent upon the desired data yield, age of the examinee, and varying patterns of performance by examinees. For example, while the majority of examinees proceed rather smoothly from the recommended start point to a series of consecutive misses once a certain level of difficulty has been reached, there are those whose performance is inconsistent and vacillates continuously from correct to incorrect responses thus protracting administration time.

Like the WPPSI–IV (especially the older age band version), the WISC–V is individually administered in all cases including examiner and examinee, and incorporates start, reversal, and discontinue rules to abbreviate the time needed to complete the required items and to maintain motivation. Start rules are based upon CA and are designed to be passed rather easily to bolster the examinee's confidence and encouragement. Reversal rules are imposed such that the child passes two consecutive items prior to once again progressing to more difficult tasks. Discontinue rules work the same as in the WPPSI–IV.

Scoring

Scoring for the WISC–V largely parallels that of the WPPSI–IV. As such, commentary here will be more abbreviated in the interests of preserving space for other relevant material. Form 7.3 contains all of the data tables for reporting WISC–V results within a psychological assessment and test report. It has virtually the same organization as the WPPSI–IV tables (see Forms 7.1 and 7.2). As with previous tests, only the most psychometrically sound data are used with supplementary scores that are more comprehensible to laypeople. This provides a felicitous balance between precision and accuracy on the one hand and pragmatism on the other hand. Scores are not typically employed will be briefly noted.

STANDARD SCORES

The core data of the WISC–V is analogous to that of the WPPPS–IV older age band version, including standard scores (mean = 100, standard deviation = 15, range = 40–160), ensued by 95% CI, PR, qualitative descriptor, and a conceptual definition of all reported scales. These are incorporated into Table 1 of Form 7.3, which begins with the scale name followed by the core data. Even a cursory inspection of Table 1 shows a mirror image to Table 1 of Form 7.2, showing that both the foundational structure of intelligence and the principal scores are equivalent from age 4 years 0 months through 16 years 11 months. That is, scores are age-corrected (i.e., compared to same-aged peers) and are based upon deviations from the mean. Of course, items within each subtest are order by increasing levels of difficulty, proceeding from simpler and concrete to more complex and abstract. However, the factorial structure is the same. The advantage of this comparable factorial structure is that longitudinal comparisons become easier and more straightforward when retesting is done in clinical practice.

The CI is set at 95% in order to make it compatible with any subsequent reporting of the subtest scaled scores, which use plus and minus two SEMs in reporting their CIs at the 95% level. If the subtest data are not reported, the examiner can report the standard score CIs at 90%, which some psychologists prefer, including David Wechsler himself (Wechsler, 1939). The reported PRs are based upon the theoretical standard normal distribution and not that of the norm reference sample. Table 1 general notes outline the standard score metric, define abbreviations, inform the reader which subtests contribute to the FSIQ, and provide references for the provided definition of intelligence. They also define the meaning of a CI and PR principally for the benefit of laypeople. Note that the table begins with the FSIQ data, which are emphasized in bold font. The examiner does have the option of reporting only the FSIQ data and either deleting the rest or inserted the double-dash (i.e. --) no score symbol.

Formal pairwise primary scale comparisons are provided in Table 2 (Form 7.3). Hypothesis tests are run on the obtained differences at the .01 level of probability (i.e., less than 1 in 100), although can be done at the more liberal 0.5 level if desired. If the obtained difference is equal to or greater than the listed critical value, this means that the probability of the obtained difference is less than .01 and hence statistically significant. That is, chance has been ruled out as an explanation for the obtained difference. Due to the accumulating familywise error rate with each hypothesis test, the more conservative .01 level should be used and restricting the pairwise comparisons to those that are diagnostically germane to the case. For all statistically significant results, the base rate is to be reported as an effect size measure (i.e., how large is the effect practically speaking). Again, the base rate is the percent of the normative sample that obtained that score difference; the smaller the base rate, the larger the effect.

SCALED SCORES

Tables 3, 4, 5, 6, and 7 in Form 7.3 report the scaled scores for the subtests that contributed to the full scale and primary index scores enumerated in Table 1. Again, they are listed in the order that they appear in Table 1, hence making it easier to reference if needed. The table organization parallels that of Table 1, beginning with the subtest name, scaled score (mean = 10, standard deviation = 3, range = 1–19), 95% CIs, PRs, and qualitative descriptors. As in the WPPSI–IV test, the CIs are not provided for the scaled scores but can be estimated using SEMs. The technical and interpretive manual reports the average SEM for each subtest across all 11 age groupings (see Wechsler, 2014b, Table 4.4, p. 61). Here, the average SEM for each of the 10 subtests that contributed to the Table 1 (Form 7.3) core data set were culled, then summed, and a grand average was computed. This grand average was 1.09, which turned out to be 1 when rounding to the nearest whole number. This means that 2 points should be added and subtracted from the obtained scaled score to compute the subtest 95% CI in Tables 3 through 7. Although PRs are also not provided, they can be referenced in Table 7.1 as was done for the WPPSI–IV. Finally, the qualitative descriptors, which are technically nominal or categorical data, may be referenced in Table 7.2.

OTHER SCORES

Wechsler IQ tests are well known for providing a wealth or abundance of score types to help describe an individual's intellectual functioning. First, an age equivalent score informs us what age is typical of an examinee's raw score. Age equivalent scores are available for each subtest. As stated prior, age equivalent scores are used with caution because they are not age corrected and are between age group comparisons.

Second, standard, scaled, and raw process scores are available. These scores do not contribute to the FSIQ or index scores, but are intended to provide more detailed information about an examinee's cognitive processes. For example, one of the 10 process scores is *Block Design Partial Score* (i.e., *BDp*). This scaled process score is based upon the total number of correctly placed single blocks across all items including any time bonus. Such alternative scoring gives at least partial credit for any blocks assembled within the time limit versus giving credit only when the entire design is completed. Hence, this can provide a more valid estimate of cognitive performance in children who may be extremely impulsive or careless and consistently fail to persevere until the entire design is completed (e.g., those with ADHD). The major problem with process scores is that they are time consuming both to score and interpret, in addition to all of the essential data that must be garnered and interpreted.

Third, there are error scores available to employ on the WISC–V. Succinctly, *error scores* are simply process scores that are based upon particular types of mistakes manifested by the examinee. One type of error score is called, *Block Design Rotation Errors*. These are instances in which the internal design is accurately assembled as a gestalt, but receives no credit due to the design being improperly rotated by 45 degrees or more for example. Such errors may be diagnostically informative and indicate a type of neurocognitive processing difficulty. Another type of interesting error score is called *Coding Rotation Errors*, wherein the examinee repeatedly writes the code under the number that is an exact reversal of the correct code symbol, analogous to young children writing letter reversals, such as "b" for "d." If observed in older children, this particular error is a sign of *dysgraphia* and potentially *dyslexia*. Most psychologists are trained to make general test observations which, although are more informal, are as helpful as when such *error scores* are done by design. Thus, these are not employed on a formal basis but more informally under the rubric of test administration observations.

COMPUTER SCORING

Internet-based Q–global (Pearson, 2021) software provides computer score reports and interpretive reports for the WISC–V. Again, there is a charge for each report. As for the WPPSI–IV, manual scoring and the data tables are typically used for the WISC–V for reporting and interpretation. The psychologist may want to purchase a limited number of score reports to have in reserve in the event of an unusually complex case that must be completed with extremely limited time. Unfortunately, unlimited computer scoring via CD-ROM was discontinued after the WISC–IV was replaced.

Interpretation

As with the majority of test interpretations, analysis should proceed from general to increasingly specific as the case demands. Consistent with a *g* factor approach, interpretation begins at Stratum III or the top of the intelligence construct hierarchy, through Stratum II, and possibly Stratum I. The latter depends upon the diagnostic issues in the case and on how much importance is placed upon describing the examinee's specific abilities. Again, please refer to Figure 7.1 on the Routledge e-resources website, which presents an interpretive flowchart that effectively summarizes the steps delineated below in the narrative. In addition, once again pre-drafted narrative excerpts follow each data table. These include language that guides the examiner through the advised interpretative process. They may be modified or deleted as determined by the particular case facts and objectives.

FULL SCALE IQ AND THE PRIMARY INDEXES

Interpretation begins with Table 1 (Form 7.3) focusing on the FSIQ standard score and its nominal ability descriptor, usually in search for diagnostic implications (e.g., borderline intellectual functioning). If the FSIQ falls in proximity to a particular diagnostic threshold, then reference to the 95% CI is useful in order to analyze the degree to which the interval straddles two categories (e.g., very low or borderline and extremely low). The PR is useful for laypeople as a supplement to the qualitative descriptor. For this reason, both the CI and PR are defined in general table notes. Of course, analyzing the FSIQ is a normative comparison.

Next, the primary index scores should be analyzed primarily in terms of norm-based comparisons. Hence, analysis should focus on the overall pattern of primary index scores, including especially where they fall in terms of standard scores and qualitative categories, especially if there exist any extreme scores. Extreme scores are most responsible for impacting the FSIQ, hence they should be afforded priority. Next, relative or ipsative comparisons should be done by examining the 95% CIs as delineated previously; that is, no overlap shows a significant difference, moderate overlap a possible difference, and large overlap no difference or equivalent ability. If there appear to be significant differences and such will impact diagnosis and/or treatment, formal pairwise comparisons are indicated, thus moving to Table 2.

Interpreting primary index standard score differences should be done judiciously due to the cumulative effects of the familywise error rate when running multiple pairwise comparisons. Ideally, such comparisons should be selected in an a priori manner; that is, preceding any data scoring and based upon conceptual reasons. For example, a treatment-related diagnostic issue may be determining whether there is a significant verbal-nonverbal discrepancy due to suspicion of a specific learning disability. In such case, two pairwise comparisons could be preplanned, including that between the Verbal Comprehension Index (VCI) and Visual Spatial Index (VSI), along with the VCI and Fluid Reasoning Index (FRI). Although less ideal, other comparisons could be analyzed if unexpected differences appear among the CIs that may be of diagnostic interest. Note that Table 1 and Table 2 in Form 7.3 are meant to be interpreted independently, although results should be integrated gradually when appropriate.

As in the case of the WPPSI–IV, the WISC–V yields ancillary index scales, along with complementary index scales. They are optional and intended for unique referral questions. Because there have been many instances in which these data have not been useful, they are not computed, reported, or interpreted. They are likely most useful in school psychological testing cases in which psychoeducational interventions must be developed within the context of an *Individualized Education Program (IEP)*. For example, the Quantitative Reasoning Index (QRI) is an indicator of a child's mathematics reasoning skills, which in turn is closely related to general intelligence (Flanagan & Kaufman, 2009; Lichtenberger & Kaufman, 2013; Weiss et al., 2013a, 2013b). Thus, such data are more pertinent to academic achievement and educational matters and unnecessarily redundant for mental health testing practice. Finally, complementary index scales provide more of the same overly specific information that tends not to be useful in mental health testing practice.

SPECIFIC SUBTEST ABILITIES

Many psychologists argue against reporting subtest scaled score results due to such data being less reliable as the result of fewer items (cf., Flanagan & Kaufman, 2009). It is the author's opinion that the primary subtest score results should be interpreted under the following conditions: (a) the primary index to which they contribute is very low or extremely low; (b) there appears to be a significant discrepancy between the two subtests contributing to that index, as evidenced by a lack of overlap among the 95% CIs; and (c) the significant difference has clear diagnostic or treatment implications. If none of these three criteria are met, there is usually no need to report subtest results. The tables are available, however, for those who believe that providing a subtest scaled score analysis is important in all instances and thus should be routinely done (see also Figure 7.1). Finally, the WISC–V provides a number of secondary subtests that may be used independently or in particular combinations so as to compute Ancillary Index Scales. These do not appear in the WISC–V data tables in Form 7.3 because they have not been found to be useful for mental health testing purposes.

Wechsler Adult Intelligence Scale, Fourth Edition

Synopsis

The *Wechsler Adult Intelligence Scale, Fourth Edition* (*WAIS–IV*; Wechsler, 2008a, 2008b) represents a valid and reliable measure of global or general adult intelligence (i.e., a *g* factor), along with clusters of higher-order cognitive ability domains (Carrol, 1993; Keith, 1990). This test is normed on individuals ranging in age from 16 years 0 months through 90 years 11 months, inclusive. Of the three Wechsler tests, the WAIS–IV covers the most expansive age range of 75 years, a spectrum that involves profound variations in cognitive abilities (Kaufman & Lichtenberger, 2006; Lezak, Howieson, & Loring, 2004; Salthouse, 2004). For instance, age-related declines in cognitive test performance can manifest as early as ages 20 to 29 years, although the most salient changes are exhibited after 55 years of age (Kaufman, 2000; Salthouse, 2004).

Modifications in test performance depend upon the type of cognitive domain. For example, verbal abilities increase at 16 years of age, peak at age 50, and show a gradual decline beginning at age 55 years (Kaufman, 2000; Ryan, Sattler, & Lopez, 2000; Salthouse, 2004). In contrast, performance on perceptual reasoning, visual spatial abilities, and fluid intelligence begin to show deterioration during the middle 30s (Kaufman, 2000; Kaufman & Lichtenberger, 2006; Ryan et al., 2000), with rapid declines between the ages of 50 and 60 years (Salthouse, 2004). Working memory starts to gradually decrease at age 45 years, while processing speed begins to wane much earlier at age 20 years, ensued by a more rapid deterioration at age 35 years (Kaufman, 2000; Kaufman & Lichtenberger, 2006; Ryan et al., 2000). The latter appear to be associated with parallel declines in fluid reasoning and working memory (Lindenberger, Mayr, & Kliegl, 1993; Salthouse, 1996, 2000; Salthouse & Ferrer-Caja, 2003). The point of this review is to illustrate how the development of the WAIS–IV focused upon minimizing the potential confounding impact of these cognitive changes upon the measurement of adult intelligence across this expansive age-range. Also, this review was to emphasize the importance of age-related comparisons to avoid dire errors in interpretation. In other words, the norm-based data of the WAIS–IV should be employed such that the examinee's performance is controlled for the effects of age or is age-corrected (see, e.g., Lezak et al., 2004). This will be illustrated in the norm reference sample section, along with follow-up sections concerning administration and especially scoring and interpretation.

Not surprisingly, the WAIS–IV test possesses an organizational structure comparable to those of the more recently published WISC–V (Wechsler, 2014a, 2014b) and WPPSI–IV (Wechsler, 2012a, 2012b), which were presented in previous sections. However, because it was published prior to the discovery of the aforementioned five-factor model of intelligence, the WAIS–IV has only four-factors; hence, more equivalent to that of the WISC–IV. As such, a brief history will be reviewed to clarify its point in development compared to the more contemporary Wechsler IQ tests for younger age bands.

HISTORICAL DEVELOPMENT

The WAIS–IV evolved directly from the *Wechsler-Bellevue Intelligence Scale* (*WB*; Wechsler, 1939), beginning with the original *Wechsler Adult Intelligence Scale* (*WAIS*; Wechsler, 1955). The WAIS retained all 11 WB subtests, including Information, Comprehension, Arithmetic, Similarities, Digit Span, Vocabulary, Digit Symbol, Picture Completion, Block Design, Picture Arrangement, and Object Assembly, although deleted and replaced many items and scoring rules to simplify matters. The *Wechsler Adult Intelligence Scale, Revised Edition* (*WAIS–R*; Wechsler, 1981) was published almost 30 years later, which is a much longer time interval since the discovery and resulting impact of the Flynn effect (Flynn, 1987). This edition again retained the 11 subtests of the WB and WAIS, although incorporated many newer items, and devised more administration and scoring rules in order to enhance both reliability and validity. For example, bonus points were awarded for perfect performance and more teaching prompts were added to ensure that the examinee understood test instructions when beginning scorable items. The test structure retained the FSIQ, which represented the *g* factor, and VIQ–PIQ dichotomy. Additionally, the older age groups in the standardization example (viz., 65–69 years and 70–74 years) were more closely matched to the Census Bureau figures than in previous editions.

Next, the *Wechsler Adult Intelligence Scale, Third Edition* (*WAIS–III*; Wechsler, 1997) introduced three new subtests to the previous 11, including Matrix Reasoning, Letter–Number Sequencing, and Symbol Search. First, Matrix Reasoning required nonverbal logic, including the ability to identify the pattern in a visual-spatial array. Second, Letter–Number Sequencing asked the examinee to recall an increasingly large series of letters and numbers in alphabetical and counting order, respectively, which was a measure of working memory ability. Third, Symbol Search was a straightforward measure of processing speed wherein the examinee was asked to find and mark target symbols within a large group that were first presented within a smaller group. As a consequence of integrating the three new subtests with those of the 11 prior subtests (hence, 14 total), the WAIS–III created four new empirically supported primary index scores each representing independent domains of cognitive functioning as follows: (a) Verbal Comprehension Index (VCI); (b) Perceptual Reasoning Index (PRI); (c) Working Memory Index (WMI); and (d) Processing Speed Index (PSI). These were added to the prior traditional FSIQ and VIQ–PIQ test organization, which is delineated next.

FACTOR-STRUCTURE

In review, the statistical procedure of factor analysis produces intercorrelated clusters of items called factors. A core part of the analysis consists of what are termed factor loadings, which again are simply correlation coefficients (i.e., 0 to ±1.00) that represent the degree and direction of the relationship among items and the factors to which they are related. Larger factor loadings mean that items possess greater relationships with their factors, including a larger percentage of the variance explained and more influence. A factor analysis output is solely dependent upon its input. Hence, the aforementioned empirical indexes were produced due to the intercorrelations computed among the 11 prior subtests and especially the three new subtests, which is the main point here.

In particular, a series of confirmatory factor analyses were done on the norm reference sample as a whole (i.e., 16–90 years; N = 2,200), and for each of five age groupings (i.e., 16–19 years, n = 400; 20–34 years, n = 600; 35–54 years, n = 400; 55–69 years, n = 400; 70–90 years, n = 400). *Confirmatory factor analyses* determine how well a data pattern fit a previously specified factor-structure using quantitative logic analogous to the chi-square (i.e., χ^2) statistic. This is contrasted with *exploratory factor analyses*, which is designed to discover what factors best account for all of the inter-item correlations. In all cases, the four-factor model produced the best fit, with evidence of a second-order model separating out a higher-order g factor, with four-factors at a lower level, including Verbal Comprehension, Perceptual Reasoning, Working Memory, and Processing Speed. Factor loadings with the g factor ranged from .70 for Processing Speed to .90 for Working Memory.

Referring back briefly to the WISC–V and WPPSI–IV will be instructive because we can essentially predict what the as yet unpublished WAIS–V will essentially look like. Recall that in each of the WISC–V and WPPSI–IV cases, a five-factor model was evinced by the factor analyses. In effect, the perceptual reasoning domain was apportioned into a visual spatial ability and a fluid reasoning ability, which we explore in more detail using the most recently published WISC–V. The subtests Block Design and Visual Puzzles (a new subtest) clustered on one factor whereas Matrix Reasoning and Figure Weights (a new subtest) loaded most strongly on a separate factor. Whereas the Block Design, Matrix Reasoning, and some older subtests that were dropped loaded on a factor called the Perceptual Reasoning Index, the most recent factor analyses comprising the new combination of subtests demonstrated that the prior perceptual reasoning ability was, in actuality, two independent abilities.

In particular, the PRI was apportioned into the two domains named the Visual Spatial Index (VSI) and the Fluid Reasoning Index (FRI), both of which are increasingly consistent with the CHC theory of intelligence (refer back to Form 7.3, Table 1, VSI and FRI measured abilities). The VSI measures visual spatial reasoning, integration and synthesis of part-whole relationships, attentiveness to visual detail, and finally, visual motor integration. Notice the reliance upon spatial processing, visual discrimination, visual attention, and visual-motor integration; the common thread being visual spatial reasoning and logic. In contrast, the FRI applies more to the identification and application of conceptual relationships, and requires the use of inductive logic, quantitative reasoning, simultaneous processing, and abstract thinking. Although both are related to nonverbal reasoning, *fluid reasoning* ability is more linked to general visual intelligence and the ability to learn novel concepts.

As new subtests are developed and incorporated into the Wechsler IQ tests, the following two trends for the WAIS–V are predicted: (a) a five-factor second-order model will be revealed that mirrors that of the WISC–V; and (b) the current PRI will be apportioned into a visual spatial ability and fluid reasoning ability, hence ever more consistent with the CHC theory of intelligence. Indeed, a Figure Weights subtest was added to the WAIS–IV in a secondary role to bolster the measurement of fluid reasoning ability. This was in response to the greater role *fluid reasoning* was being afforded in several prominent theories of intelligence, including that of the CHC model (Carroll, 1997; Cattell, 1943, 1963; Cattell & Horn, 1978) and Sternberg's triarchic theory (Sternberg, 1995). Specifically, tasks that required fluid reasoning included the process of, "manipulating abstractions, rules, generalizations, and logical relationships" (Carroll, 1993, p. 583).

Norm Reference Sample

The WAIS–IV was normed on a national sample of U.S. English-speaking individuals aged 16 years 0 months through 90 years 11 months. The sample of 2,200 individuals was stratified by age, sex, race/ethnicity, education level, and geographic region according to the October 2005 U.S. Bureau of the Census (U.S. Bureau of the Census, 2005). More specifically, the sample was apportioned into 13 age cohorts as follows: 16–17; 18–19; 20:24; 25–29; 30–34; 35–44; 45–54; 55–64; 65–69; 70–74; 75–79; 80–84; and 85–90. All age groups had equal numbers of females and males, except for the five older age groups that consisted of proportions that matched those of the census data (viz., more females to males). Racial proportions matched those of the census data, including Whites, African Americans, Hispanics, Asians, and Other. Educational levels were defined as 8 years or less, 9–11 years, 12 years, 13–15 years, and 16 years or more. For examinees that were 16 to 19 years of age, parental education was used. If the 16- to 19-year-old examinee was living with two parents, the average of the two was used. Lastly, the United States was apportioned into four major regions, including Northeast, Midwest, South, and West.

Administration

The WAIS–IV administration process had to be carefully designed to accommodate many of the aforementioned sensory, psychomotor, and cognitive changes that occur across the remarkably large age range covered by this IQ test (Kaufman & Lichtenberger, 2006; Lezak et al., 2004; Storandt, 1994). These include declines in sustained attention, auditory discrimination, working memory, and processing speed.

First, in order to minimize the confounding effects of declining attentional resources in older adults (Kaufman & Lichtenberger, 2006), subtest instructions were made as explicit as possible, including both demonstration items and sample items. *Demonstration items* are done by the examiner and are designed to explain and illustrate via modeling the manner in which the items are completed. For example, the Visual Puzzles subtest is essentially a mental rotation task in which the examinee must identify three of six pieces below that fit next to each other to create the puzzle located at the top of the stimulus book page. The examiner explains the instructions and then completes the first task while the examinee observes. *Sample items* are extremely easy items that are completed by the examinee. They typically do not count toward the final subtest score and are intended for providing the examinee a mockup of what is to follow.

Some subtests employ both types of items to ensure that examinees know what is expected of them. For instance, the Visual Puzzles initial sample item is ensued by a second, easy item, wherein the examinee is asked to find the three pieces that fit together to make the target puzzle at the top of the stimulus page. It is a simple task in which three of the six selections match exactly the shape and orientation of the sections of the target puzzle, with the single exception of one shape that must be rotated 90 degrees (i.e., from horizontal to vertical) to make it fit. This example illustrates how a brief sequence of demonstration and sample items can actively and efficiently engage older adult examinees in order to minimize the confounding effects of deteriorating attention and concentration.

Second, an overemphasis on rapid task performance was deemed to be especially problematic for older adults due to decreases in their motor functioning and slowed cognitive processing (Armour-Thomas & Gopaul-McNicol, 1997; Lezak et al., 2004; Salthouse, 2004). Therefore, although the implementation of time limits was needed to reduce overall testing time and examinee frustration, the emphasis on time bonuses was reduced somewhat to reduce the potential confounding effects of slower motor processing speed associated with aging. For example, the number of timed items with bonus points was significantly reduced on Block Design and eliminated completely on Arithmetic.

Third, it was recognized that similar sounding numbers on Digit Span (e.g., 5 and 9) and Letter–Number Sequencing could cause confounds due to problems in auditory discrimination. An example of an auditory confound is when the examinee incorrectly reports a 5 due to failure to differentiate that sound from 9, rather than that being caused by a true lapse in memory. The incorrect score here was thus due to a sensory-perceptual limitation and not a memory limitation, which is a clear example of a confounding variable contributing to error variance and an ultimate deleterious effect on test validity. To minimize such effects, phonetically similar numbers were reduced in Digit Span and complexly eliminated in Letter–Number Sequencing.

Fourth, analogous to auditory discrimination, the WAIS–IV was designed to reduce demands upon visual acuity. This was accomplished by effectively enlarging all of the stimulus book artwork (e.g., Block Design pictures). In addition, Symbol Search and Coding symbols were simplified and enlarged. Fifth, excessive motor demands risk underestimating the intelligence of older adults with coordination and other physical difficulties (e.g., rheumatoid arthritis and tremors). To adapt the WAIS–IV materials such that the effects of motor skills were reduced, Picture Arrangement and Object Assembly were supplanted by two subtests that measured pure visual spatial reasoning without the need for fine motor abilities; namely, Visual Puzzles (i.e., a mental rotation task) and Figure Weights (i.e., inductive logical reasoning, quantitative reasoning, and visual spatial reasoning).

Test administration time was also effectively reduced. As will become apparent subsequently, the WAIS–IV requires 10 subtests in order to produce both the FSIQ and four-factor primary indexes for an estimated 67 minutes' administration time. In comparison, the WAIS–III required 13 subtests for an estimated 80 minutes' administration time. The shorter time interval obviously places reduced demands upon examinees' attentional capacities.

In addition to fewer requisite subtests, the use of reduced discontinue rules effectively shorten testing time. That is, most subtests terminate subtest administration following three consecutive scores of "0," this compared to many of the WAIS–III discontinue rules using six consecutive scores of "0" as the termination criterion. On some subtests that require more time to instruct and complete (e.g., Block Design), the discontinue rule is even more diminutive (i.e., two consecutive scores of "0"). Finally, many of the test materials were modified in order to ease and increase the rate of administration and scoring. Stimulus book pages are turned toward the examinee, which reduces the reaching distance for the examiner. Furthermore, the norm reference tables are placed in a logical order such that raw scores can be easily found and transformed into age-corrected data and subsequent interpretation.

Scoring

The WAIS–IV data yield is essentially the same as for the WPPSI–IV and WISC–V. These consist of standard scores, scaled scores, CIs, PRs, qualitative descriptors, difference scores, hypothesis testing on the difference scores, and base rates. Once again, CIs, PRs, and nominal qualitative categories are not directly available, although can be estimated with data provided in the technical manual (Wechsler, 2008b). The ensuing sections present these scores in addition to some that are not routinely used in mental health practice. The score types that are employed may be seen in Form 7.4.

STANDARD SCORES

As previously discussed, standard scores are fundamental to norm-based comparisons, which are vital when measuring intelligence among such a large age range of 75 years. Table 1 (see Form 7.4) presents these scores, along with all of their supporting data. More specifically, Table 1 contains six columns, including scale name, standard score (mean = 100, standard deviation = 15, range = 40 to 160), 95% CI, PR, qualitative descriptor, and measured abilities. The metrics are reported in general table notes, along with abbreviations of other scores, notation that full scale data are in bold font, and the double-dash symbol (i.e., --) for no score being reported. Notice that the full scale IQ is summarized using the layperson's definition proposed near the beginning of this chapter. The standard score range applies to the full scale IQ, although the primary index score range is somewhat smaller (viz., 50–150). The latter is incorporated into the larger full scale for purposes of brevity. The CIs show the likely value of the examinee's true score with 95% certainty. Lastly, the PRs are based upon the theoretical standard normal distribution and are not on the norm reference group numbers. The CI and PR are defined in the general table notes. Thus, if they are not interpreted in the narrative, the reader who may be a layperson will still be able to discern their meaning.

Table 2 in Form 7.4 presents all pairwise comparisons among the primary indexes, along with the obtained difference score, the critical value that begins the rejection region of the null hypothesis predicting no difference between the scores (i.e., at the .01 level of probability), and the base rate. The most conservative .01 level was chosen to help minimize a Type I error caused by an accumulating familywise error rate caused by multiple hypotheses tests in one analysis (i.e., spuriously concluding a significant difference). The base rate interpretive scheme proposed by Sattler and Ryan (2009) is denoted by appended crosses, which is defined in the specific table notes. Two rules apply here as follows: (a) report only those pairwise comparisons that have vital diagnostic and/or treatment implications; and (b) report base rate data only for those difference scores that are statistically significant, otherwise insert the double-dashed no score symbol that is defined in general table notes.

SCALED SCORES

Tables 3 through 6 in Form 7.4 are designed for reporting all of the subtest scaled scores and their supporting data yield. Again, they are reported in the same order that their respective primary indexes are listed in Table 1. They are all designed analogous to Table 1 to assist the interpretive process and the reader of the data, including six columns as follows: (a) scale name; (b) scaled score (i.e., mean = 10, standard deviation = 3, range = 1–19); (c) 95% CI; (d) PR; (e) qualitative descriptor; and (f) a succinct definition of the abilities being measured by that scale. The CIs can be estimated by adding and subtracting two SEMs from the obtained scaled score. The SEM was estimated by taking an average of all subtest SEMs reported in the technical and interpretive manual (Wechsler, 2008b, Table 4.3, p. 45), which turned out to be 0.99 and rounded to 1 as the nearest whole number. Although only those subtests that contribute to the full scale IQ and four primary indexes were used, the same result was reached when including all subtests (i.e., primary and secondary) in the WAIS–IV battery and subsequently rounding to the nearest whole number. The scaled score PRs may be found by reference to Table 7.1, whereas the qualitative descriptors are reported in Table 7.2. Note that the latter are the new updated qualitative descriptors most recently reported in the WISC–V (Wechsler, 2014b, Table 6.3, p. 153). To reiterate, their strengths are parallel form and minimizing any negative connotation.

OTHER SCORES

Other than those reviewed in the prior two sections, the only other type of score provided by the WAIS–IV that are not used are the aforementioned process scores. Because this is the single type of added score, a succinct history is provided. These were first proposed for the Wechsler IQ tests by Edith Kaplan (1988), who generalized them from their use in neuropsychological testing where qualitative interpretation of test performance, analysis of errors, and testing the limits were routinely employed in formulating diagnostic impressions. The WAIS–R was the first edition where such scores were incorporated (Kaplan, Fein, Morris, & Delis, 1991), specifically to modify its focus to be used effectively as part of a neuropsychological test battery versus more traditional psychological testing.

Block Design and Digit Span are two primary subtests that possess process scores, which are derived using a scaled score metric. These subtests have been shown to measure abilities that when impaired suggest the presence of brain dysfunction. They can be computed without modifying standardized administration procedures, which is an advantage because computing such scores does not interfere with the core data, both in terms of administration and scoring. For Block Design, the process score is computed without the time bonus points. Such score controls for the effects of processing speed and provides a measure of an examinee's performance in the absence of such influence. Digit Span yields six process scores, including separate scores for digits forward, backward, and sequencing (i.e., reporting the numbers from lowest to highest). The standard score for the Digit Span subtest regards all of these in the aggregate, thus hindering more detailed analysis of performance if relevant to diagnosis. For example, although all Digit Span tasks require the storage and retrieval of auditory information, the backwards version requires more working memory resources because the information must be retained in memory until it has been reworked and reported in a form different from its initial presentation (de Jong & de Jong, 1996; MacDonald, Almor, Henderson, Kempler, & Anderson, 2001; Sattler, 2008; Werheid et al., 2002).

COMPUTER SCORING

This version of the Wechsler IQ tests can be scored on the Q–global (Pearson, 2021) website in the same manner as the WPPSI–IV and WISC–V. For those fortunate enough to have purchased the previously available WAIS–IV Scoring Assistant (Pearson, 2008), which is loaded into the PsychCorp Center II build or framework on the psychologist's personal computer, unlimited scoring for the duration of this published edition is available. This will be replaced by the Q–global (Pearson, 2021) web-based scoring whenever the WAIS–V is published. This test, however, can be easily scored manually, especially for purposes of mental health. Without the CD-ROM version, it is prudent to purchase a limited number of the more reasonably priced score reports for extremely complicated cases and score the majority manually, facilitated by use of this test's data tables (see Form 7.4).

Interpretation

At this juncture, the similarity of the Wechsler IQ test structure across all three versions should be apparent. This is the reason Figure 7.1 on the Routledge e-resources website was created for download, which affords a visual flow-chart of the recommended interpretive process for all Wechsler IQ tests designed specifically for mental health practice. Consistent with the thesis of this book, test score reporting and interpretation must be judiciously selective so as to remain succinct, relevant, and comprehensive for a particular case. In other words, each testing case should have clearly identified diagnostic and treatment objectives which effectively delimit the scope of the analyses and reporting of the results. Excessively long reports with seemingly incessant data will only discourage readers from perusing the entire report. With these prelusory comments in mind WAIS–IV test interpretation will follow Figure 7.1 in general and Form 7.4 in particular. Hence, the former should be downloaded for reference.

FULL SCALE IQ AND THE PRIMARY INDEXES

As typical, the interpretive process is initiated at Stratum III, the top of the hierarchical structure of intelligence (i.e., the FSIQ representing the general intelligence or *g* factor). At this level, a norm-based comparison using the examinee's standard score reflects the core of the analysis because it is age-corrected. This would be reflected by the data in Table 1 of Form 7.4. The associated qualitative descriptor should also be reported. Because this represents nominal or categorical data, which also has ordinal features, it should be noted whether the standard score falls well-within a category, or whether it is sufficiently proximate to a higher or lower category such that it straddles more than one. If the latter circumstance is present, special emphasis should be afforded the CI and the degree to which it overlaps adjacent categories. This is especially important if there are consequential diagnostic implications. For example, a FSIQ score of 70 is technically within the "very low" qualitative descriptor. However, examination of the CI would show significant overlap into the extremely low range of functioning, which should be mentioned in the overall interpretation.

Figure 7.1 (see e-resources) displays a solid arrow toward the "Primary Index: Norm-Based" box, denoting the required progression to comparable norm-based comparisons across the four-factor primary index standard scores. These data are reported in Table 1 (Form 7.4). The analysis should mirror that for the FSIQ, noting the standard scores and their associated qualitative descriptors. Extreme standard scores and their effects on the FSIQ should be interpreted. Next, informal primary index score comparisons should be done by examining the degree of overlap among the 95% CIs; no overlap indicates a significant difference, moderate overlap a possible difference, and little or no overlap no difference. If there appear to be differences among very low or extremely low scores, and these differences have important diagnostic or treatment implications, formal ipsative analysis should then be pursued. In Figure 7.1 (e-resources), the broken arrow extending from the "Primary Index: Norm-Based" box to the "Primary Index: Ipsative-Based" box, denotes this being an optional step, which is done in Table 2 of Form 7.4.

If conducting a formal analysis of primary index scores, only those pairwise comparison with diagnostic or treatment relevance should be done to avoid a cumulative effect of the familywise error rate. Furthermore, only differences that are statistically significant should provide a base rate analysis. Otherwise, the no report double-dash symbol should be inserted.

SPECIFIC SUBTEST ABILITIES

As portrayed in Figure 7.1 (e-resources), the "Primary Index: Norm-Based" box, the listed item 6 refers to whether or not subtest score analysis is indicated. Again, some experts disavow the interpretation of specific abilities at this level (i.e., Stratum I) because of the reduced degree of reliability associated with these scores (McDermott, Fantuzzo, & Glutting, 1990). Even among those who believe such analysis should routinely be done do typically caution that such interpretation should not be done in isolation, but within the context of clinical interview information, mental status examination data and behavioral observations, medical and educational histories, and supplementary test data (Kaufman, 1994; Matarazzo, 1990, 1999; Prifitera & Saklofske, 1998). A middle ground here is assumed by interpreting subtest scores only under certain well-defined circumstances, which are outlined in Figure 7.1, box "Primary Index: Norm-Based," item 6. Specifically, the following conditions must be satisfied to justify the time, writing space, and effort to pursue a subtest analysis: (a) the particular primary index standard score is "very low" or "extremely low"; (b) the subtests loading on that primary index appear to be significantly different (i.e., there is very little or no overlap among the 95% CIs); and (c) the difference has important diagnostic or treatment implications. If these conditions are not all met, the interpretive process can be terminated at this point.

The Stanford Binet Tests

The original developer of this series of intelligence tests, and intelligence tests in general, was Alfred Binet, a trained attorney by trade. However, he was fascinated with psychological measurement as evidenced by his frequently practicing on his two daughters. He began his investigations by measuring more simplistic skills such as reaction time, which was in concert with the then emphasis on measuring psychophysical variables. However, he quickly moved to measuring more complex variables, including language, memory, and reasoning. At this juncture, he observed that these higher-order abilities produced greater between-subject variability and were more associated with age-related changes (Goodenough, 1949). In 1895, Binet and colleague Victor Henri published *La psychologie individuelle* (Binet & Henri, 1895), which proffered one of the first models of intelligence. In particular, this model proposed that intelligence consisted of a number of more complex, "mental faculties," including memory, comprehension, attention, and concentration, along with less sophisticated psychomotor abilities, such as eye-hand coordination and hand strength, all of which could be measured by developing the appropriate tasks. Ten years thereafter, Binet and Theodore Simon produced the first formal intelligence test felicitously titled the Binet-Simon Intelligence Scale (Binet & Simon, 1905).

Binet-Simon Intelligence Scale

Binet-Simon Intelligence Scale (Binet & Simon, 1905) was designed to diagnose learning disorders in children within the French school system. It consisted of 30 items intended to measured higher-order mental abilities and were ranked in increasing order of difficulty. The test's norm reference sample was comprised of five age cohorts ranging from 3 to 11 years who were appraised by the school system as having average or normal ability. Thus, testees who were able to solve items typical of their age group were measured as having average intelligence. If they could solve items less or more than their age group, they were measured as having below and above average intelligence, respectively.

In 1908, the test was revised to include a larger age range from 3 to 15 years, an increased number of items to 58, a larger standardization sample ($N = 203$), and most especially, grading performance based upon age levels (Binet & Simon, 1908). In particular, examinees were graded on the highest age level they could pass with 75% mastery, which represented the incipience of the *mental age (MA)* concept. Next, the 1911 revision of the Binet-Simon added age levels for a total of 11 and for the first time included both adult items and adults in the norm reference sample (see Binet & Simon, 1916). Up to this point, the Binet-Simon Intelligence Scale claimed to be a measure of general intelligence (i.e., a *g* factor), which was comprised of abstract thinking and reasoning, memory, and judgment (Matarazzo, 1990, 1999).

Simultaneously with the evolution of the Binet-Simon Intelligence Scale, the statistician Charles Spearman was utilizing factor analysis to effectuate scale development. This technique was the primary impetus for further intelligence test development because it was able to reduce immense amounts of data (i.e., items) into more manageable chunks called factors. These factors represented latent (i.e., hitherto hidden) variables or constructs that could help explain human behavior. When Spearman applied this technique to investigate the structure of intelligence, he discovered an underlying mental ability factor that he called, "*psychometric g,*" abbreviated "*g.*" More specifically, he found numerous correlations between *specific ability tests* (i.e., narrowly defined subtests) that loaded onto a single statistical factor; viz., a *g* factor. Hence, Spearmen's theory of intelligence was comprised of various specific abilities (e.g., quantitative reasoning, visual-spatial ability, and verbal reasoning), wherein about 50% of its variance could be accounted for by a general *g* factor, and the remaining 50% by variance attributed to (a) specific abilities and (b) measurement error. Succinctly, Spearman's model was referred to as a two-factor theory of intelligence, including "*g*" and "*s,*" with the remainder due to "*e.*" The point here is to illustrate how two lines of development, the Binet-Simon and factor analysis, merged to contribute to the advancement of intelligence and its measurement.

Stanford-Binet Intelligence Scale

The Binet-Simon test was eventually translated into English in the United States in 1908. Thereafter, it was extensively revised in 1916 by Louis Terman of Stanford University, thus becoming the *Stanford-Binet Intelligence Scale* (Terman, 1916). This edition retained the concept of a global intelligence by claiming to measure a general mental ability. Items also continued to be clustered by age levels. Hence, items in which two-thirds to three-fourths of an age group could successfully pass defined each age level. Furthermore, the test length was nearly doubled to that of 90 and the standardization sample was superior in terms of size; namely, 100 children and 400 adults.

In terms of metrics, this edition introduced the *intelligence quotient* (IQ) concept, which was founded upon a ratio between mental age (MA), which represented the highest age-level of items an examinee mastered by the aforementioned specified proportion, and chronological age (CA), which represented an individual's actual age in years since birth, multiplied by 100 in order to remove any decimals.

Subsequent Editions: 1930s Through 1970s

During the ensuing two decades, Terman collaborated with Maud Merrill who initially was his student, to create two parallel forms of the test in 1937 using many of the same items as in the 1916 edition. These parallel versions of the test were published as Form L (for Lewis) and Form M (for Maud), each possessing 129 items and a new standardization sample of 3,200 subjects ranging in age from 18 months through 18 years (see Goodenough, 1942). The proclaimed improvements were (a) providing two scales versus only one, (b) being capable of measuring a larger range of functioning, (c) utilizing more adequate representative sampling, and (d) drafting clearer procedures for administration and scoring (Terman & Merrill, 1937). During the 1950s, Merrill became the principal test developer and integrated the best items from Forms L and M to publish a combined Form L–M in 1960 (Terman & Merrill, 1960), which represented the third edition of the test. The principal revision was the adoption of the deviation IQ analogous to that introduced by Wechsler (1939; see prior). However, the metric differed slightly in variability, including the same central tendency mean of 100, although with a standard deviation of 16 versus 15 points. The deviation IQ had by this juncture in the history of intelligence testing become the preferred method of measuring this construct. This is because individuals across various age groups could be measured by a uniform scale. Hence, from this point the Stanford-Binet tests emphasized the point-scale format which continues presently. The 1960 third edition was subsequently re-normed in 1973 along with the addition of alternate items at all age levels (Terman & Merrill, 1973).

Stanford-Binet Intelligence Scale, Fourth Edition

The *Stanford-Binet Intelligence Scale, Fourth Edition* (SB4; Thorndike, Hagen, & Sattler, 1986) afforded three major modifications. First, this test featured a point-scale format again following that of the Wechsler tests, which superseded the prior age-scale format utilized by Binet. Recall that point scales organize items by type or kind into subtests (e.g., all block design items ordered from least to most difficult) and are conducive to computing the degree of various kinds of intelligence by the amount of deviation from the average performance of same-aged peers. In contrast, an *age scale* groups items principally by age level (i.e., the age group that can master a specified proportion of items of a particular degree of difficulty) and provides a direct translation of an examinee's performance into a MA. In actuality, the Stanford-Binet has more of a hybrid format in which items are principally groups by kind into subtests, although are ordered by increasing difficulty consistent with age levels. For example, the routing subtests of the current edition provide start points that are defined by CA.

Second, scores for several factors were made available in addition to that of the global IQ. These included Verbal Reasoning, Abstract/Visual Reasoning, Quantitative Reasoning, and Short-Term Memory. Although prior editions included items related to such factors (McNemar, 1942; Sattler, 1965), they were not quantified and associated with scores. Now that a point-scale subtest format was in use, items of similar content and abilities could now be measured. These subtest scores clustered together via factor analysis to form the aforementioned factors, which could now be quantified by aggregating total raw scores and transforming them into age-based uniform standard scores that showed an examinee's degree of deviation from the mean.

Third, this test introduced the practice of *routing* in which performance on a core subtest determined the proper start points on other subtests. This practice is alternately referred to as *multi-stage testing* or *adaptive testing* (Reckase, 1989), and is designed to abbreviate test administration time and maximize examinees' effort by having them complete items that are neither excessively easy nor difficult.

Stanford–Binet Intelligence Scales, Fifth Edition

The remainder of this section delineates the current edition of the Stanford-Binet, following the same organization as the Wechsler tests to effectively structure the presentation.

Synopsis

The *Stanford–Binet Intelligence Scales, Fifth Edition* (SB5; Roid, 2003b, 2003c, 2003d) is an individually administered assessment of intelligence and cognitive abilities for people aged 2 years 0 months through 85 years and older. The Full Scale IQ (FSIQ) consists of 10 subtests, 5 nonverbal and 5 verbal. This composite score represents the *g* factor (i.e., a complex general ability factor), further apportioned into Nonverbal IQ (NVIQ) and Verbal IQ (VIQ), along with five cognitive factor indexes, the latter including Fluid Reasoning (FR), Knowledge (KN), Quantitative Reasoning (QR), Visual-Spatial Processing (VS), and Working Memory (WM) (Roid, 2003b, 2003c, 2003d).

This hierarchical factor structure possesses both theoretical and empirical support. First, the five SB5 factors are equivalent to those in the leading research-based CHC theory of intellectual abilities that have the highest *g* loadings (see Flanagan, 2000; Evans, Floyd, McGrew, & Laforgee, 2001). The SB5 and CHC counterparts are respectively as follows: (a) Fluid Reasoning (FR)–Fluid Intelligence (Gf); (b) Knowledge (KN)–Crystalized Knowledge (Gc); (c) Quantitative Reasoning (QR)–Quantitative Knowledge (Gq); (d) Visual-Spatial Processing (VS)–Visual Processing (Gv); and (e) Working Memory (WM)–Short-Term Memory (Gsm) (Roid, 2003d, p. 8–9). Three of these SB5-CHC factor pairings have proven particularly effective in predicting school achievement, including the following: (a) KN-Gc; (b) WM-Gsm; and (c) QR-Gq. Second, the SB5 IQ composites and factor indexes are supported by confirmatory factor analyses for both the five-factor model, and the nonverbal and verbal domains (see Roid, 2003d).

Norm Reference Sample

The SB5 was normed on a nation-wide representative sample of 4,800 people ranging in age from 2 years 0 months through 85 years and older. The sample was stratified by age, gender, ethnicity, geographic region, and socioeconomic stats (SES) based upon the U.S. Census Bureau (2001). The data was garnered during a one-year duration from 2001 to 2002. Subjects were obtained from four regions of the United States, including Northeast, Midwest, South, and West. The sample was stratified into 23 age groupings. From ages 2 through 4, the age groupings were divided into half-year intervals each of which consisted of 200 subjects. From ages 5 through 16, groupings were apportioned into one-year durations, which also included 200 subjects each. Finally, ages 17 to 20 years formed a grouping of 122 individuals. Thereafter, age groupings were of 10-year intervals and included between 100 and 200 subjects each. Finally, the 80 and older grouping included 200 subjects.

Socioeconomic levels were measured by years of education completed for adults aged 18 years and older, and years of education completed by parents for those younger than 18 years, both according to the 1999 Census Bureau (U.S. Bureau of the Census, 1999). Proportions of males and females were approximately equal for all age groupings, with the exception of the older age cohorts who had a larger proportion of women. Finally, categories of race/ethnicity consisted of White, Black, American Indian, Alaskan Native, Asian, and Native Hawaiian or Other Pacific Islander, here in proportions according to the 2001 U.S. Census Bureau (U.S. Bureau of the Census, 2001).

Administration

Administration time for the FSIQ is estimated to be 45 to 75 minutes, including approximately 30 minutes each for the NVIQ and VIQ (Roid, 2003b). A unique attribute of this IQ test is that each cognitive factor consists of nonverbal and verbal subtest counterparts, hence permitting a nonverbal IQ-verbal IQ comparison that informs the degree to which the FSIQ is representative of the examinee's overall intellectual functioning. Discrepancies between the NVIQ and VIQ that are statistically significant at the .05 level, along with an accompanying base rate of 15% or less as unusual in the population (Sattler, 1988, 2001; Sattler & Ryan, 1998, 2009), indicate that the FSIQ may be supplanted by one of these alternative composites as a more reliable and valid representation of the examinee's overall level of intelligence. Such decision would be based upon both clinical judgment and the purposes of testing. In such instances, although all ten subtests would have been administered, only those five subtests that contributed to the selected replacement IQ composite score (i.e., the VIQ or NVIQ) would be reported and interpreted. An accompanying rationale as to why such selection was made would also be required.

Another unique administrative feature of the SB5 is that the NVIQ subtest oral instructions are remarkably succinct and thus require only a minor amount auditory ability on the part of the examinee. Therefore, in cases where the examinee manifests a neurocognitive impairment in language (e.g., aphasia) or other communication disorder (e.g., receptive language disorder), is an English language learner, or suffers from some type of auditory handicap, the examiner has the option of administering only the nonverbal subtests and computing a NVIQ as a representative of overall intellectual functioning. In complementary fashion, the verbal subtests and the associated VIQ can be strategically utilized in cases involving a visually impaired examinee. Lastly, in instances where a brief measure of intelligence is desired, for example if general cognitive ability is only in need of screening or testing time is extremely limited, an Abbreviated Battery IQ (ABIQ) composite score is available. In particular, this composite only consists of the nonverbal and verbal routing subtests (viz., Object Series/Matrices and Vocabulary, respectively), and requires an efficient 15 to 20 minutes of administration time.

Finally, as just stated, the SB5 employs adaptive testing in the form of two routing subtests, one which determines the start points on the four remaining nonverbal subtests (viz., Object Series/Matrices), and one which determines the start points on the four remaining verbal subtests (viz., Vocabulary). Items are grouped by the following: (a) subtest content (e.g., Quantitative Reasoning); (b) Levels 1 to 6 ordered in terms of increasing difficulty; and (c) groupings of six items per level called *testlets*. The routing subtests indicate which testlet an examinee will begin administration for the ensuing verbal and nonverbal subtests. The beginning levels may be the same or different for the nonverbal and verbal subtests, depending upon the examinee's performance on the particular routing subtest.

Basal rules dictate when an examinee is to be dropped back to a prior testlet level. For example, if the examinee receives 2 or fewer points out of 6 possible on Level 3 of Quantitative Reasoning, he is to drop back to testlet Level 2 of Quantitative Reasoning. Similarly, *ceiling rules* are imposed to direct which testlet level an examinee is to discontinue administration. For example, if an examinee receives 2 or fewer points on testlet Level 4 of Knowledge, she is to discontinue the Knowledge subtest administration. Administration continues until all nonverbal and verbal subtests have reached their ceiling testlet level; nonverbal subtests are administered first followed by the verbal subtests. The routing, basal, and ceiling rules work to condense test administration and maintain examinee motivation, consistent with the tenets of adaptive testing.

Scoring

The SB5 continues to employ the point-scale format, deviation IQ, standard scores, scaled scores, CIs, and PRs as the core data comparable to the Wechsler tests. Hence, this section is organized similar to that of the Wechsler scoring sections, beginning with the standard scores, follows by scaled scores, and finishing with brief comments regarding additional scores not typically employed, along with computer scoring software. However, there will also be inserted a section on the SB5 abbreviated IQ, which is a special feature built into this test. These scores are presented in Form 7.5, which provides the data tables for reporting SB5 results within the context of a psychological assessment report.

STANDARD SCORES

The SB5 is unique in the sense that it not only yields a general ability FSIQ deviation composite score as does the Wechsler series, but it also provides a direct comparison between overall nonverbal and verbal intellectual functioning. Therefore, the SB5 is ideal if the examiner suspects a significant differential between the two very general abilities. This comparison is made possible by the fact that each of the five factors are the result of both a nonverbal and verbal version of that primary ability. In terms of a hierarchical model, the FSIQ, VNIQ, and VIQ would be located at the top or Stratum III.

Table 1 in Form 7.5 is designed for two chief objectives: (a) a typical norm-based analysis of the FSIQ, NVIQ, and VIQ composites; and (b) analysis of whether or not the FSIQ represents an accurate overall summary of an individual's intellectual functioning, as evidenced by a single pairwise comparison of the NVIQ and VIQ. As such, Table 1 lists the three composites beginning with the FSIQ in bold font for emphasis, followed by the NVIQ and VIQ. The table follows the same organization as the Wechsler data tables, beginning with the standard score, 95% CI, PR, ability category, and measured abilities. The standard score metrics are listed in the general table notes, including a mean of 100, standard deviation of 15, and a generous range from 40 to 160. CIs are again at the 95% degree of certainty to be consistent with subtest scores if presented. PRs are based upon the standard normal distribution. Both are defined in the general table notes for the benefit of laypeople and especially if not interpreted within a narrative format of the report.

The principal pairwise comparison consists of a hypothesis test that is run on the obtained difference between the VNIQ and VIQ at the .05 or 5% level of probability. This is accompanied by the examining the base rate of this difference in the norm reference sample. Rather than including an entire new table to report this single analysis, these data are simply reported in the narrative following Table 1, which is much briefer and to the point. The interpretative manual advises that the NVIQ and VIQ differential is to be deemed remarkably discrepant if the hypothesis test of no difference is rejected and the base rate is 15% or less (Roid, 2003c).

Table 2 provides the standard score summary for the five factors that contribute to the FSIQ as follows: (a) Fluid Reasoning (FR); (b) Knowledge (KN); (c) Quantitative Reasoning (QR); (d) Visual Spatial Processing (VS); and (e) Working Memory (WM). It should be reported subsequent to Table 1 if the FSIQ is to represent the examinee's general intellectual functioning. It is organized in the same manner as Table 1, including five columns beginning with the factor index name, standard score, 95% CI, PR, ability category, and measured abilities.

These scores are the same deviation-type standard scores as reported in Table 1, again which have a mean of 100 and a standard deviation of 15.

SCALED SCORES

Scaled scores employ the same metric as in the Wechsler tests, including a mean of 10, standard deviation of 3, and a range from 1 to 19. Recall that each of the five factors have a nonverbal and verbal version. Tables 3 and 4 report the NVIQ subtests and VIQ subtests for each factor reported in Table 2, respectively. Both tables afford the same scheme as that of Table 2, except that the scales are now more narrowly defined subtests, with scaled scores, 95% CIs, PRs, ability category, and measured symptoms. The 95% CIs are derived by taking the reported SEMs for each subtest averaged across all age groupings (Roid, 2003d, Table 3.2, p. 66) and rounding to the nearest whole number; which happens to be 1 in all cases.

Here, it is important to report that both the Stanford-Binet and Wechsler series are beginning to compute the CIs for the FSIQ and factors (i.e., Strata III and II) using (a) the examinee's estimated *true score* (versus the obtained score), and the *standard error of estimation* (*SEE*) to calculate the CIs versus the SEM. What does this do? It is argued that this method is more accurate because (a) we are attempting to estimate an examinee's true score (not obtained score), (b) the true score will always be regressed toward the mean to a greater or lesser extent, therefore, (c) the interval should be asymmetrical such that the estimated true score falls towards the less extreme direction (Dudek, 1979; Glutting, McDermott, & Stanley, 1987). Because the formulas for the estimated true score and SEE are cumbersome to do manually for a test report, the CIs are reported for the scaled scores using the SEM and obtained scores. The added work is not justified by the minor increase in precision using the estimated true score and SEE method. When computer scoring software begins reporting the CIs for subtest data using the latter method, they should be readily reported. PRs for the subtest data can be found in Table 7.1, which reports the scaled score to PR conversions. Both CIs and PRs are defined in general tabular notes for the benefit of laypeople reading the report.

Before moving on to the abbreviated IQ, it should be noted that the subtest data are only be reported under the following conditions: (a) the IQ composite to which they contribute is selected by the examiner to represent the general *g* factor; or (b) (i) that IQ composite is showing significant levels of impairment *and* (ii) the associated specific abilities have independent and vital diagnostic or treatment implications. The reason this approach is recommended refers to the metric used and the degree of test reliability when reporting data at this specific level of analysis.

First, consider that average reliabilities for the three IQ scores range from .95 to .98. Similarly, the factor index reliabilities range from .90 to .92. In contrast, the available subtest scores use a less precise metric (mean = 10;

standard deviation = 3) and possess lower reliabilities into the middle to low .80s. According to the experts, reliability coefficients in the .90s are excellent, whereas those within the .80s are only adequate to marginally good (see Charter, 2003; Groth-Marnat, 2009; Hogan, 2015; Hunsley & Mash, 2008; Kaplan & Saccuzzo, 2013; Murphy & Davidshofer, 2001; Nunnally & Bernstein, 1994). When it comes to measuring one's intelligence, it is prudent to be as accurate as possible. Hence, score reporting for the SB5 should be limited to the IQ scores and factor indexes, which possess the greatest degree of reliability and thus accuracy. Additionally, as will become apparent subsequently, these scores yield a significant amount of interpretative information about an examinee's intellectual functioning.

ABBREVIATED IQ SCORE

The abbreviated IQ composite (ABIQ) uses the same metric as the aforesaid IQ scores and factor indexes. Not surprisingly, its reliability is somewhat lower, although sufficiently respectable to be utilized as a *screening measure* of overall IQ functioning (i.e., reliabilities range from .80 to .88) (Roid, 2003c, 2003d). As stated previously, the ABIQ is useful when a quick screening measure of intellectual functioning is needed. Form 7.6 provides a tabular format for reporting the data of a *Stanford-Binet Intelligence Scales, Fifth Edition, Abbreviated Battery (SB5–ABIQ)*. The table is itself abbreviated, and includes columns for its label, standard score, 95% CI, PR, ability category, and its succinct definition focused upon the limited specific abilities measured by the two routing tests, Object Series/Matrices and Vocabulary. General table notes summarize its metric, define table abbreviations, the directional meaning of scores, identification of the routing subtests that contribute to this measure, and definitions of CI and PR.

OTHER SCORES

In addition to the aforementioned core data, the SB5 offers an age-equivalent score that is derived from *item response theory (IRT)*. The particular IRT model used (i.e., Rasch) calibrates the likelihood of an examinee passing an item as a ratio of ability level over item difficulty level (De Ayala, 2009; Embretson & Reise, 2000). The actual metric that converts to an age-equivalent score is referred to as the *W* scale, with a middle-most score of 500 anchored at 10 years 0 months (i.e., 10:0) (see Roid, 2003c, pp. 19–22). The age equivalent is most useful in intellectual disability cases in which estimating a mental age is useful; for example, a court of law attempting to determine competency or insanity of a criminal defendant. Although the SB5 offers additional scores, such as *change-sensitive scores (CSS)* that have the ability of measuring an examinee's degree of change in various cognitive abilities, and an Extended IQ that estimates extreme IQ scores (i.e., below 40 and above 160), such data are either rarely used in mental health services and/or are too unstable or precarious in their computations.

COMPUTER SCORING

Currently, the SB5 can be computer scored by means of an online scoring system (see Roid, 2016). Here, purchasers can obtain one-year of unlimited scoring. Previously, this scoring system was available on CD-ROM (Roid, 2003a), which was loaded onto the psychologist's personal computer and provided unlimited scoring for an unlimited duration. As with the WAIS–IV, this is no longer available. Look for all or most major psychological tests to have computer scoring via an online web-based service, including either charging a fee per score report or purchasing a license for unlimited scoring for a time-determined period. Use of such computer services is strongly advised when scoring is complex or an extended analysis is required. Pertaining to the SB5, if one possesses the CD-ROM Scoring Pro, it may be used simply because it is convenient and of no charge. If the only option was use of the current online scoring, it would be prudent to use it only when time was very limited or an extended analysis was needed.

Interpretation

Interpretation should proceed in a sequence from general to increasingly specific until all of the diagnostic issues are addressed. Figure 7.2 is available for download on Routledge's e-resources website and was created in order to portray the interpretive process as a visual flowchart, analogous to what was done for the Wechsler tests presented previously. Form 7.5 contains the tables for reporting the SB5 data within the context of a psychological test report.

COMPOSITE SCORES

SB5 interpretation begins with the IQ composites, FSIQ, VIQ and NVIQ, respectively (see Table 1, Form 7.5; Figure 7.2). Hence, the FSIQ should first undergo a norm-based analysis, including its ability category and examining whether the 95% CI falls within or between two categories. Immediately following Table 1 (Form 7.5), there appears a pre-drafted narrative norm-based interpretation of the FSIQ. For purposes of deriving a DSM diagnosis, including borderline intellectual functioning and intellectual disability (ID), the FSIQ should be the default selection for the following reasons: (a) it is the most reliable score available due to it being based upon all 10 subtests; (b) it is conceptually most consistent with the idea of a single overall cognitively based diagnosis; and (c) it can be effectively qualified by simply adding differential verbal-nonverbal information to the final diagnostic workup if there exists a significant discrepancy between the two abilities.

The VIQ or NVIQ should only supplant the FSIQ for diagnostic purposes under the following conditions: (a) when only one of the two is administered due to an examinee's special needs (e.g., the examinee is nonverbal); or (b) when only one of the two is deemed to be valid due to unusual circumstances occurring during test administration (e.g., the examinee's responses reveal a hitherto disguised nonverbal learning disability such that the VIQ represents a more accurate measure of cognitive competence). In such circumstances, the NVIQ or VIQ should represent the general intelligence *g* factor and be employed for diagnostic purposes (e.g., ID). Furthermore, the ensuing interpretation would focus only upon the subtests contributing to that IQ composite. That is, both the FSIQ and non-utilized IQ composite should neither be reported nor interpreted.

Figure 7.2 (see Routledge's e-resources) illustrates this by the solid arrow proceeding from the top box to the "Factor Index: Norm-Based" box toward the middle left of the flowchart. This denotes that the FSIQ should be the prime representative of overall intelligence unless an exceptional circumstance is present. If the exception occurs,

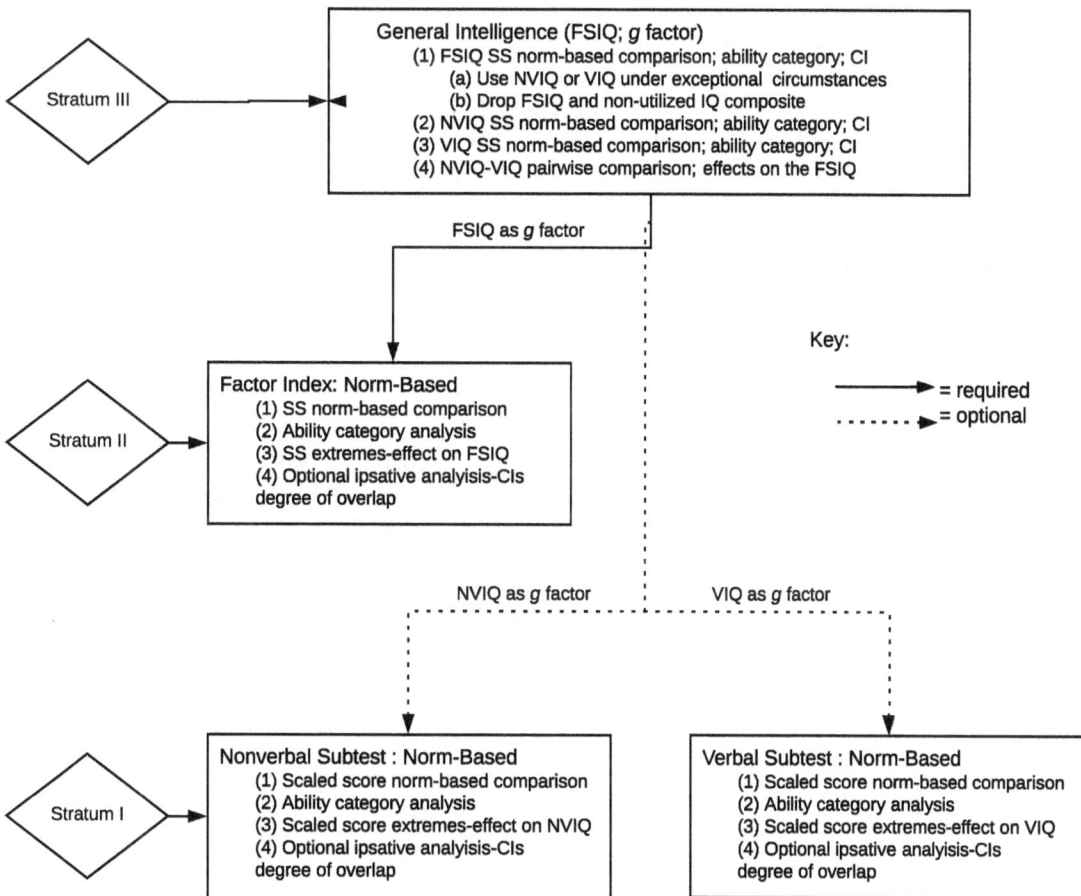

Figure 7.2 Stanford-Binet Intelligence Scales, Fifth Edition (SB5) Interpretive Process

then the broken arrow should be followed to either (a) the "Nonverbal Subtest: Norm-Based" box if the NVIQ is representing the *g* factor, or (b) the "Verbal Subtest: Norm-Based" box if the VIQ is representing *g* factor. In Form 7.5, there are narrative interpretations explicating the use of both the NVIQ and VIQ as replacements for the FSIQ, whichever befits the case circumstances.

Next, the NVIQ and VIQ should undergo a norm-based interpretation analogous to that done for the FSIQ, including the ability categories and CIs. There are pre-drafted norm-based narrative interpretations of both the NVIQ and VIQ, including language analogous to that drafted for the FSIQ. This examination leads naturally into the NVIQ–VIQ pairwise comparison. For such comparison, there is a final narrative summarizing such analysis, including the hypothesis test interpretation and meaning of the base rate effect size. These excerpts are inserted to speed the process of the SB5 test interpretation. The next natural step in the interpretive process is to focus upon the factor indexes, assuming that the FSIQ score is being used as representing the *g* factor.

FACTOR INDEXES

Once the overall intellectual functioning results have been inferred, analysis shifts to the SB5 factor index scores, first for a norm-based investigation, followed by an ipsative analysis (see Table 2, Form 7.5; Figure 7.2, see Stratum II box). Here, the examinees norm-based strengths and weaknesses can inform which factors were responsible for the FSIQ result. Scrutinizing the positioning of the factor index CIs represents the basis of the ipsative or intra-individual comparisons, which should be considered optional and done only if there is significant variance among the standard scores and associated diagnostic and/or treatment implications. Note the pre-drafted narrative interpretation following Table 2, Form 7.5, which covers all of the norm-based analyses and ends with the relative comparisons.

SPECIFIC SUBTEST ABILITIES

Both the nonverbal and verbal subtest norm-based analyses mirror that of the factor index score data, and are presented in Tables 3 and 4 of Form 7.5, respectively. They are at Stratum I within the hierarchical structure of this construct, hence represent the most specific abilities. They also use the less discriminatory scaled score metric with a much smaller range from 1 to 19 and are the least reliable of all the data due largely to relying on the smallest number of items. For these reasons, they should only be interpreted under either of the following conditions: (a) their associated IQ composite has supplanted the FSIQ; or (b) (i) there was a remarkable difference in the NVIQ–VIQ comparison according to the previously stated criteria (i.e., statistical significance at .05 and base rate ≤ 15%), (ii) one of the IQ composites falls within the impaired range, and (c) the discrepant abilities have diagnostic and/or treatment implications. If they are interpreted, the ability categories can be referenced in Table 7.3, which juxtaposes both the standard scores and scaled scores with both the detailed and succinct labels.

ABBREVIATED IQ

The ABIQ should be interpreted only as a screening measure of an individual's estimated overall intelligence. The ability category can be referenced in Table 7.3. Scores falling within the impaired range should be qualified by a recommendation that follow-up intelligence testing with a full battery of subtests is needed to confirm that impairment is indeed present. In other words, a diagnosis should not be afforded based upon these results; only

Table 7.3 Stanford-Binet Intelligence Scales Ability Category Guide

Standard Scores	Scaled Scores	Detailed Description	Succinct Description
145 to 160	19 to 19	Very gifted or highly advanced	Highly advanced
130 to 144	16 to 18	Gifted or very advanced	Very advanced
120 to 129	14 to 15	Superior	Superior
110 to 119	12 to 13	High average	High average
90 to 109	8 to 11	Average	Average
80 to 89	6 to 7	Low average	Low average
70 to 79	4 to 5	Borderline impaired or delayed	Borderline impaired
55 to 69	2 to 3	Mildly impaired or delayed	Mildly impaired
40 to 54	1 to 1	Moderately impaired or delayed	Moderately impaired

Source. Adapted from Roid, G. H. (2003d). *Stanford-Binet Intelligence Scales, Fifth Edition (SB5), Interpretive manual: Expanded guide to the interpretation of the SB5 test results*. Rolling Meadows, IL: Riverside Publishing, Table 2.2, p. 22.

a recommendation that complete testing is warranted due to a positive screening result for possible cognitive impairment. Following Table 1, Form 7.6, there are two pre-drafted narrative interpretations. The first advises follow-up testing due to a screen-positive result for possible intellectual impairment, while the second associates the screening result with that of the mental status examination that likely preceded the screening. The latter is appropriate if follow-up testing is not being pursued and the assessment is examining the reliability of the screening outcome.

Recapitulation

This chapter was devoted to the construct of intelligence and the major individually administered tests that measure this human cognitive ability trait. It began with a review of the alternate definitions used for this construct, including a layperson's narrative version, an IQ test score quantitative format, and the concept of a latent variable g factor. Next, the primary reasons for using an intelligence test in mental health practice were delineated. The core sections of the chapter involved a detailed review of the Wechsler series of IQ tests and the Stanford-Binet. Data tables for each individual test were presented, which show how the test results can be reported and interpreted within a psychological assessment report. Furthermore, flowcharts of the interpretive process for each series of tests were presented and reviewed to facilitate learning how to effectively derive diagnostic and treatment-related meaning from the data yield. Supplementary tables were also provided that facilitate use of the data tables, for example, tables for converting test data into an alternate metric and finding the proper ability categories for standard scores. The ensuing Chapter 8 on achievement continues the general subject of testing cognitive characteristics, although this refers to measuring the degree to which an individual has learned skills in the academic classroom. Because this type of testing is less emphasized in mental health practice and much more common in the educational field, the following chapter includes only two major tests.

Key Terms

- ability-memory discrepancy analysis
- achievement view
- adaptive testing
- age equivalent score
- age scale
- alpha level
- aptitude view
- autism spectrum disorder (ASD)
- basal rules
- base rate
- Binet-Simon Intelligence Scale
- Block Design Partial Score (BDp)
- Block Design Rotation Errors
- Cattell-Horn-Carroll (CHC) theory of intelligence
- ceiling rules
- change-sensitive scores (CSS)
- Chicago Tests of Primary Mental Abilities
- chronological age (CA)
- Coding Rotation Errors
- conduct disorder (CD)
- confidence interval (CI)
- confirmatory factor analyses
- construct validity
- crystalized intelligence
- demonstration items
- deviation IQ
- discontinue rules
- dysgraphia
- dyslexia
- error scores

- experimentwise error rate
- explicit theories
- exploratory factor analyses
- factor analysis
- factor loading
- fluid intelligence
- fluid reasoning
- Flynn effect
- g (g factor)
- general intelligence
- Gf-Gc model of intelligence
- hierarchical model of intelligence
- implicit theories
- Individual Education Program (IEP)
- intellectual disability (ID)
- intelligence
- intelligence quotient (IQ)
- ipsative
- IQ
- item response theory (IRT)
- La psychologie individuelle,
- mental age (MA)
- multiple intelligences
- multi-stage testing
- non-psychometric theories
- percentile rank (PR)
- point scale
- primary mental abilities
- process scores
- psychometric g
- psychometric theories
- qualitative descriptor
- reversal rules
- routing
- s factors
- sample items
- screening measure
- specific ability tests
- specific intelligences
- standard error of estimation (SEE)
- Stanford-Binet Intelligence Scale
- Stanford-Binet Intelligence Scale, Fourth Edition (SB4)
- Stanford–Binet Intelligence Scales, Fifth Edition (SB5)
- Stanford-Binet Intelligence Scales, Fifth Edition, Abbreviated Battery (SB5–ABIQ)
- start point/s
- stratum (*pl.* strata)
- testing the limits
- testlets
- three stratum hierarchical model of intelligence
- true score
- Type I error
- Wechsler Adult Intelligence Scale (WAIS)
- Wechsler Adult Intelligence Scale, Fourth Edition (WAIS–IV)
- Wechsler Adult Intelligence Scale, Revised Edition (WAIS–R)
- Wechsler Adult Intelligence Scale, Third Edition (WAIS–III)

- Wechsler Intelligence Scale for Children (WISC)
- Wechsler Intelligence Scale for Children, Fifth Edition (WISC–V)
- Wechsler Intelligence Scale for Children, Fourth Edition (WISC–IV)
- Wechsler Intelligence Scale for Children, Revised Edition (WISC–R)
- Wechsler Intelligence Scale for Children, Third Edition (WISC–III)
- Wechsler Preschool and Primary Scale of (WPPSI)
- Wechsler Preschool and Primary Scale of Intelligence, Fourth Edition (WPPSI–IV)
- Wechsler Preschool and Primary Scale of Intelligence, Revised Edition (WPPSI–R)
- Wechsler Preschool and Primary Scale of Intelligence, Third Edition (WPPSI–III)
- Wechsler-Bellevue Intelligence Scale (WB)

Notes

1. This is not an understatement considering that IQ tests 30 to 40 years ago required somewhere between 2 to 2½ hours to administer.
2. Psychological testing works like any other business; that is, the consumer must like and be satisfied with the product. Test publishers are occasionally faced with dilemmas involving whether to make changes in test structure that are empirically sound yet may not be popular with consumers. The publishers at Pearson faced this dilemma in transitioning from the theoretical scales to the empirical indexes. By the late 1980s, factor analytic studies were increasingly showing that a move toward the empirically supported CHC theory of intelligence for all Wechsler IQ tests was indicated. Simultaneously, many practitioners were so accustomed to the FSIQ, VIQ, and PIQ structure that there was a palpable risk that many would transition to other IQ tests who were competitors with this system. The way the publishers at Pearson dealt with this situation was to make such transition gradual over two editions, which ultimately was a sagacious choice.

References

Aiken, L. R. (1996). *Assessment of intellectual functioning.* New York, NY: Plenum Press.

Alfonso, V. C., Flanagan, D. P., & Radwan, S. (2005). The impact of Cattell-Horn-Carroll theory on test development and the interpretation of cognitive abilities. In D. P. Flanagan & P. L. Harrison (Eds.), *Contemporary intellectual assessment: Theories, tests and issues* (2nd ed.; pp. 185–202). New York, NY: Guilford Press.

American Psychological Association. (2015). *American psychological association (APA) dictionary of psychology* (2nd ed.). Washington, DC: Author.

Armour-Thomas, E., & Gopaul-McNicol, S. A. (1997). Bio-ecological approach to cognitive assessment. *Cultural Diversity and Mental Health, 3,* 131–141.

Baral, B. D., & Das, J. P. (2004). What is indigenous to India and what is shared? In R. J. Sternberg (Ed.), *International handbook of intelligence* (pp. 270–301). New York, NY: Cambridge University Press.

Bartholomew, D. J. (2004). *Measuring intelligence: Facts and fallacies.* Cambridge, UK: Cambridge Iniversity Press.

Bayley, N. (2006b). *Bayley scales of infant and toddler development: Technical manual* (3rd ed.). Bloomington, MN: Pearson (PsychCorp).

Benson, N. Hulac, D. M., & Kranzler, J. H. (2010). Independent examination of the wechsler adult intelligence scale (WAIS–IV): What does the WAIS–IV measure? *Psychological Assessment, 22,* 121–130.

Binet, A. (1903). *Experimental study of intelligence.* Paris: Schleicher.

Binet, A., & Henri, V. (1895). La psychologie individuelle. *L'Année psychologique, 2,* 411–465.

Binet, A., & Simon, T. (1905). Méthodes nouvelles pour le diagnostic du niveau intellectuel des anormaux. *L'Année psychologique, 11,* 191–336.

Binet, A., & Simon, T. (1908). Le development de l'intelligence chez les enfants. *L'Année psychologique, 14,* 1–94.

Binet, A., & Simon, T. (1916). *The development of intelligence in children.* Baltimore, Williams & Wilkins. (Reprinted 1973, New York: Arno Press; 1983, Salem, NH: Ayer Company).

Bodin, D., Pardini, D. A., Burns, T. G., & Stevens, A. B. (2009). Higher order factor structure of the WISC–IV in a clinical neuropsychological sample. *Child Neuropsychology, 15,* 417–424.

Capron, C., & Duyme, M. (1989). Assessment of the effects of socioeconomic status on IQ in a full cross-fostering design. *Nature, 340,* 552–553.

Carlson, L., & Reynolds, C. R. (1981). Factor structure and specific variance of the WPPSI subtests at six age levels. *Psychology in the Schools, 18,* 48–54.

Carroll, J. B. (1993). *Human cognitive abilities: A survey of factor-analytic studies.* Cambridge, UK: Cambridge University Press.

Carroll, J. B. (1997). The three-stratum theory of cognitive abilities. In D. P. Flanagan & P. L. Harrison (Eds.), *Contemporary intellectual assessment: Theories, tests, and issues* (pp. 122–130). New York, NY: Guilford Press.

Carroll, J. B. (2012). The three-stratum theory of cognitive abilities. In D. P. Flanagan & P. L. Harrison (Eds.), *Contemporary intellectual assessment: Theories, tests, and issues* (3rd ed., pp. 883–890). New York, NY: Guilford Press.

Cattell, R. B. (1943). The measurement of intelligence. *Psychological Bulletin, 40,* 153–193.

Cattell, R. B. (1963). Theory of fluid and crystalized intelligence: A critical experiment. *Journal of Educational Psychology, 54,* 1–22.

Cattell, R. B., & Horn, J. L. (1978). A check on the theory of fluid and crystalized intelligence with description of new subtest designs. *Journal of Educational Measurement, 15,* 139–164.

Charter, R. A. (2003). A breakdown of reliability coefficients by test type and reliability method, and the clinical implications of low reliability. *The Journal of General Psychology, 130,* 290–304.

Ciccarelli, S. K., & White, J. N. (2020). *Psychology* (6th ed.). Hoboken, NJ: Pearson Education.

De Ayala, R. J. (2009). *The theory and practice of item response theory.* New York: Guilford Press.

de Jonge, P., & de Jonge, P. F. (1996). Working memory, intelligence and reading ability in children. *Personality and Individual Differences, 21,* 1007–1020.

Deary, I. J., & Johnson, W. (2010). Intelligence and education: Causal perceptions drive analytic processes and therefore conclusions. *International Journal of Epidemiology, 39,* 1362–1369.

Deary, I. J., Whalley, L. J., & Starr, J. M. (2003). IQ at age 11 and longevity: Results from a follow-up of the Scottish mental survey 1932. In C. E. Finch, J. M. Robine, & Y. Christen (Eds.), *Brain and longevity: Perspectives in longevity* (pp. 153–164). Berlin: Springer.

Dreary, I. J., Strand, S., Smith, P., & Fernandes, C. (2007). Intelligence and educational achievement. *Intelligence. 35,* 13–21.

Dudek, F. J. (1979). The continuing misinterpretation of the standard error of measurement. *Psychological Bulletin, 86,* 335–337.

Elshout, J., & Veenman, M. (1992). Relation between intellectual ability and working method as predictors of learning. *Journal of Educational Research, 85,* 134–143.

Embretson, S. E., & Reise, S. P. (2000). *Item response theory for psychologists.* Mahwah, NJ: Lawrence Erlbaum Associates.

Evans, J. J., Floyd, R. G., McGrew, K. S., & Leforgee, M. H. (2001). The relations between measures of Cattell-Horn-Carroll (CHC) cognitive abilities and reading achievement during childhood and adolescence. *School Psychology Review, 31,* 246–262.

Flanagan, D. P. (2000). Wechsler-based CHC cross-battery assessment and reading achievement: Strengthening the validity of interpretations drawn from Wechsler test scores. *School Psychology Quarterly, 15,* 295–329.

Flanagan, D. P., & Dixon, S. G. (2013). The Cattell-Horn-Carroll theory of cognitive abilities. In C. R. Reynolds, K. J. Vannest, & E. Fletcher-Janzen (Eds.), *Encyclopedia of special education* (pp. 368–382). Hoboken, NJ: John Wiley & Sons.

Flanagan, D. P., & Kaufman, A. S. (2009). *Essentials of WISC–IV assessment* (2nd edition). Hoboken, NJ: John Wiley & Sons.

Flanagan, D. P., Ortiz, S. O., Alfonso, V. C., & Mascolo, J. T. (2002). *The achievement test desk reference (ADTR): Comprehensive assessment and learning disabilities.* Boston, MA: Allyn & Bacon.

Fletcher, J. M., Stuebing, K. K., Hughes, L. C. (2010). IQ scores should be corrected for the Flynn effect in high stakes decisions. *Journal of Psychoeducational Assessment, 28,* 469–473.

Flynn, J. R. (1984). The mean IQ of Americans: Massive gains 1932 to 1978. *Psychological Bulletin, 95,* 29–51.

Flynn, J. R. (1987). Massive IQ gains in 14 nations: What IQ tests really measure. *Psychological Bulletin, 101,* 171–191.

Flynn, J. R. (1999). Searching for justice: The discovery of IQ gains over time. *American Psychologist, 54,* 5–20.

Flynn, J. R. (2006). Tethering the elephant: Capital cases IQ, and the Flynn effect. *Psychology, Public Policy, and Law, 12,* 170–189.

Flynn, J. R. (2007). *What is intelligence? Beyond the Flynn effect.* New York: Cambridge University Press.

Flynn, J. R. (2009). Searching for justice: The discovery of IQ gains over time. *American Psychologist, 54,* 5–20.

Flynn, J. R., & Weiss, L. G. (2007). American IQ gains from 1932 to 2002: The WISC subtests and educational progress. *International Journal of Testing, 7,* 209–224.

Gagne, F., & St. Pere, F. (2001). When IQ is controlled, does motivation still predict achievement? *Intelligence, 30,* 71–100.

Gardner, H. (1998). Are there additional intelligences? The case for naturalist, spiritual, and existential intelligences. In J. Kane (Ed.), *Education, information, and transformation* (pp. 111–131). Upper Saddle River, NJ: Merrill-Prentice Hall.

Gardner, H. (1999). *Intelligence reframed: Multiple intelligences for the 21st century.* New York, NY: Basic Books.

Gardner, H. (2006). *Five minds for the future.* Boston, MA: Harvard Business School Press.

Gardner, H., & Moran, S. (2006). The science in multiple intelligences: A response to Lynn Waterhouse. *Educational Psychologist, 41,* 227–232.

Glutting, J. J., McDermott, P. A., & Stanley, J. C. (1987). Resolving differences among methods of establishing confidence limits for test scores. *Educational and Psychological Measurement, 47,* 607–614.

Goodenough, F. L. (1942). Studies of the 1937 revision of the Stanford-Binet scale. I. Variability of the IQ at successive age-levels. *Journal of Educational Psychology, 33,* 241–251.

Goodenough, F. L. (1949). *Mental testing: Its history, principles, and applications.* New York, NY: Rinehart.

Gottfredson, L. S. (2004). Intelligence: Is it the epidemiologists' elusive "fundamental cause" of social class inequalities in health? *Journal of Personality and Social Psychology, 86,* 174–199.

Gottfredson, L. S., & Deary, I. J. (2004). Intelligence predicts health and longevity, but why? *Current Directions in Psychological Science, 13,* 1.

Gremillion, M. L., & Martel, M. M. (2013). Merely misunderstood? Receptive, expressive, and pragmatic language in young children with disruptive behavior disorders. *Journal of Clinical Child & Adolescent Psychology, 43,* 765–776.

Groth-Marnat, G. (2009). *Handbook of psychological assessment* (5th ed.). New York, NY: John Wiley & Sons.

Gustafsson, J. E. (1989). Broad and narrow abilities in research on learning and instruction. In R Kanfer, P L Ackerman & R Cudek (Eds.), *Abilities, motivation and methodology: The Minnesota symposium on learning and individual differences* (pp. 203–232). Hillsdale, NJ: Erlbaum.

Gyurke, J. S., Stone, B. J., & Beyer, M. (1990). A confirmatory factor analysis of the WPPSI–R. *Journal of Psychoeducational Assessment, 8,* 15–21.

Hastings, P. D., Zahn-Waxler, C., Robinson, J., Usher, B., & Bridges, D. (2000). The development of concern for others in children with behavior problems. *Developmental Psychology, 36,* 531–546.

Hogan, T. P. (2015). Reliability. In R. L. Cautin & S. O. Lilienfeld (Eds.), *Encyclopedia of clinical psychology* (pp. 1–9). Hoboken, NJ: John Wiley & Sons.

Horn, J. L. (1991). Measurement of intellectual capabilities: A review of theory. In K. S., McGrew, J. K. Werder, & R. W. Woodcock (Eds.), *WJ–R technical manual* (pp. 197–232). Chicago, Il: Riverside Publishing.

Horn, J. L. (1998). A basis for research on age differences in cognitive capabilities. In J. J. McArdle & R. Woodcock (Eds.), *Human cognitive abilities in theory and practice* (pp. 57–91). Chicago, IL: Riverside Press.

Horn, J. L., & Blankson, A. N. (2012). Foundations for better understanding of cognitive abilities. In D. P. Flanagan & P. L. Harrison (Eds.), *Contemporary intellectual assessment: Theories, tests and Issues* (3rd ed., pp. 73–98). New York, NY: Guilford Press.

Hunsley, J., & Mash, E. J. (Eds.). (2008). *A guide to assessments that work.* New York, NY: Oxford.

Hunt, E., & Madhyastha, T. M. (2012). Cognitive demands of the workplace. *Journal of Neuroscience, Psychology, and Economics, 5,* 18–37.

Hunter, J. E. (1983). *Test validation for 12,000 jobs: An application of job classification and validity generalization analysis to the General Aptitude Test Battery (GATB)* (Test Research report No. 45). Washington, DC: US Employment Service, US Department of Labor.

Hunter, J. E., & Hunter, R. F. (1984). Validity and utility of alternate predictors of job performance. *Psychological Bulletin, 96,* 72–98.

Jaffee, W. B., & D'Zunlla, T. J. (2003). Adolescent problem solving, parent problem solving, and externalizing behavior in adolescents. *Behavior Therapy, 34,* 295–311.

Jensen, A. R. (2004). Obituary-John Bissell Carroll. *Intelligence, 32,* 1–5.

Johnson, W., Bouchard, T. J., Jr., Krueger, R. F., McGue, M., & Gottesman, I. I. (2004). Just one *g*: Consistent results from three test batteries. *Intelligence, 32,* 95–107.

Johnson, W., Corley, J., Starr, J. M., & Dreary, I. J. (2011) Psychological and physical health at age 70 in the Lothian birth cohort 1936: Links with early life IQ, SES, and current cognitive function and neighborhood environment. *Health Psychology, 20,* 1–11.

Johnson, W., Dreary, I. J., & Iacono, W. G. (2009). Genetic and environmental transactions underlying educational attainment. *Intelligence, 37,* 466–478.

Kanaya, T., Scullin, M. H., & Ceci, S. J. (2003). The Flynn effect and US policies: The impact of rising IQ scores on American society via mental retardation diagnosis. *American Psychologist, 58,* 778–790.

Kaplan, E. (1988). A process approach to neuropsychological assessment. In T. J. Boll & B. K. Bryant (Eds.), *Clinical neuropsychology and brain functions: Research, measurement, and practice* (pp. 129–167). Washington, DC: American Psychological Association.

Kaplan, E., Fein, D., Morris, R., & Delis, D. C. (1991). *WAIS–R as a neuropsychological instrument.* San Antonio, TX: The Psychological Association.

Kaplan, R. M., & Saccuzzo, D. P. (2013). *Psychological testing: Principles, applications, and issues* (8th ed.). Belmont, CA: Wadsworth/ Thomson Learning.

Kaufman, A. S. (1994). *Intelligent testing with the WISC–III.* New York, NY: John Wiley & Sons.

Kaufman, A. S. (2000). Seven questions about the WAIS–III regarding differences in abilities across the 16 to 89 year life span. *School Psychology Quarterly, 15,* 3–29.

Kaufman, A. S., & Kaufman, N. L. (2004). *Kaufman assessment battery for children* (2nd ed.). Bloomington, MN: NCS Pearson.

Kaufman, A. S., & Lichtenberger, E. O. (2006). *Assessing adolescent and adult intelligence* (3rd ed.). Hoboken, NJ: John Wiley & Sons.

Kaufman, A. S., Flanagan, D. P., Alfonso, V. C., & Mascolo, J. T. (2006). Test review: Wechsler intelligence scale for children, fourth edition (WISC–IV). *Journal of Psychoeducational Assessment, 24,* 278–295.

Kaufman, S. B., Reynolds, M. R., Liu, X., Kaufman, A. S., & McGrew, K. S. (2012). Are cognitive *g* and academic *g* one and the same thing? An exploration on the Woodcock–Johnson and Kaufman tests. *Intelligence, 40,* 123–138.

Keith, T. Z. (1990). Confirmatory and hierarchical confirmatory analysis of the different ability scales. *Journal of Psychoeducational Assessment, 8,* 391–405.

Keith, T. Z., & Reynolds, M. R. (2010). Cattell-Horn-Carroll abilities and cognitive tests: What we've learned from 20 years of research. *Psychology in the Schools, 47,* 635–650.

Keith, T. Z., Fine, J. G., Taub, G. E., Reynolds, M. R., & Kranzler, J. H. (2006). Higher order, multisample, confirmatory factor analysis of the Wechsler intelligence scale for children–fourth edition: What does it measure? *School Psychology Review, 35,* 108–127.

Kuncel, N. R., Ones, D. S., & Sackett, P. R. (2010). Individual differences as predictors of work, educational, and broad life outcomes. *Personality and Individual Differences, 49,* 331–336.

Larsen, R. J., & Buss, D. M. (2021). *Personality psychology: Domains of knowledge about human nature* (7th ed.). New York, NY: McGraw-Hill.

Lezak, M. D., Howieson, D. B., & Loring, D. W. (2004). *Neuropsychological assessment* (4th ed.). New York, NY: Oxford University Press.

Lichtenberger, E. O., & Kaufman, A. S. (2013). *Essentials of WAIS–IV assessment* (2nd ed.). Hoboken, NJ: John Wiley & Sons.

Lindenberger, U., Mayr, U., & Kliegl, R. (1993). Speed and intelligence in old age. *Psychology and Aging, 8,* 207–220.

Liu, J., & Lynn, R. (2011). Factor structure and sex differences on the Wechsler Preschool and Primary Scale of Intelligence in China, Japan and United States. *Personality and Individual Differences, 50,* 1222–1226.

MacDonald, M. C., Almor, A., Henderson, V. W., Kempler, D., & Anderson, E. S. (2001). Assessing working memory and language comprehension in Alzheimer's disease. *Brain and Language, 78,* 17–42.

Mackintosh, N. J. (1998). *IQ and human intelligence.* Oxford: Oxford University Press.

Matarazzo, J. (1990). Psychological assessment versus psychological testing: Validation from Binet to the school, clinic, and courtroom. *The American Psychologist, 45,* 999–1017.

Matarazzo, J. D. (1972). *Wechsler's measurement and appraisal of adult intelligence* (5th ed.). Baltimore: Williams & Wilkins.

Matarazzo, J. D. (1999). Psychological assessment versus psychological testing: Validation from Binet to the school, clinic, and courtroom. *American Psychologist, 45*, 999–1017.

McDermott, P. A., Fantuzzo, J. W., & Glutting, J. J. (1990). Just say no to subtest analysis: A critique on Wechsler theory and practice. *Journal of Psychoeducational Assessment, 8*, 290–302.

McGrew, K. S. (1997). Analysis of the major intelligence batteries according to a proposed comprehensive Gf–Gc framework. In D. P. Flanagan, J. L. Genshaft & P. L. Harrison (Eds.), *Contemporary intellectual assessment: Theories, tests, and issues* (pp. 151–179). New York, NY: Guilford.

McGrew, K. S. (2008). *The Australian standardization of the Woodcock Johnson III Cognitive and Achievement Battery.* Paper presented at the Conference of the Australian Psychological Society, Hobart, Tasmania, Australia.

McNemar, Q. (1942). *The revision of the Stanford-Binet Scale: An analysis of the standardization data.* New York, NY: Houghton Mifflin.

Messick, S. (1989). Validity. In R. Linn (Ed.), *Educational measurement* (3rd ed., pp. 13–103). New York, NY: MacMillan.

Murphy, K. R., & Davidshofer, C. O. (2001). *Psychological testing: Principles and applications* (5th ed.). Upper Saddle River, NJ: Prentice-Hall.

Neisser, U. (1998). *The rising curve: Long-term gains in IQ and related measures.* Washington, DC: American Psychological Association.

Nunnally, J. C., & Bernstein, I. H. (1994). *Psychometric theory* (3rd ed.). New York: McGraw-Hill.

Pearson. (2008). *WAIS–IV scoring assistant.* [PsychCorp Center II framework; CD-ROM computer software]. San Antonio, TX: Author.

Pearson. (2021). *Q–global: Better insights. Anytime. Anywhere.* [Internet Web-Based Computer Scoring]. Retrieved from https://qglobal. pearsonclinical.com/qg/login.seam.

Peterson, I. T., Bates, J. E., D'Onofrio, B. M., Coyne, C. A., Lansford, J. E., Dodge, K. A., . . . Van Huile, C. A. (2013). Language ability predicts the development of behavior problems in children. *Journal of Abnormal Psychology, 122*, 542–557.

Piaget, J. (1952). *The origins of intelligence in children.* New York, NY: International Universities Press.

Piaget, J. (1970). Piaget's theory. In P. H. Mussen (Ed.), *Carmichael's manual of child psychology* (Vol. 1). New York, NY: John Wiley & Sons.

Prifitera, A., & Saklofske, D. (1998). *WISC–III: Clinical use and interpretation.* San Diego, CA: Academic Press.

Reckase, M. D. (1989). Adaptive testing: The evolution of a good idea. *Educational Measurement: Issues & Practice, 8*, 11–15.

Roid, G. H. (2003a). *Stanford-Binet intelligence scales, fifth edition: SB5 Scoring Pro.* [CD-ROM computer software]. Rolling Meadows, IL: Riverside Publishing.

Roid, G. H. (2003b). *Stanford-Binet intelligence scales, fifth edition (SB5), examiner's manual.* Rolling Meadows, IL: Riverside Publishing.

Roid, G. H. (2003c). *Stanford-Binet intelligence scales, fifth edition (SB5), interpretive manual: Expanded guide to the interpretation of the SB5 test results.* Rolling Meadows, IL: Riverside Publishing.

Roid, G. H. (2003d). *Stanford-Binet intelligence scales, fifth edition (SB5), technical manual.* Rolling Meadows, IL: Riverside Publishing.

Roid, G. H. (2016). *Stanford-Binet intelligence scales, fifth edition (5th ed.): Online scoring and reporting system user's guide* [Internet Web-Based Computer Scoring]. Austin, TX: Pro-Ed. Retrieved September 4, 2020, from www.proedinc.com/Downloads/14462%20 SB-5_OSRS_UserGuide.pdf

Ryan, J. J., Sattler, J. M., & Lopez, S. J. (2000). Age effects on Wechsler Adult Intelligence Scale–III subtests. *Archives of Clinical Neuropsychology, 15*, 311–317.

Salthouse, T. A. (1996). The processing speed theory of adult age differences in cognition. *Psychological Review, 103*, 403–428.

Salthouse, T. A. (2000). Aging and measures of processing speed. *Biological Psychology, 54*, 35–54.

Salthouse, T. A. (2004). Localizing age-related individual differences in a hierarchical structure. *Intelligence, 32*, 541–561.

Salthouse, T. A., & Ferrer-Caja, E. (2003). What needs to be explained to account for age-related effects on multiple cognitive variables? *Psychology and Aging, 18*, 91–110.

Sattler, J. M. (1965). Analysis of functions of the 1960 Stanford-Binet intelligence scale, form L-M. *Journal of Clinical Psychology, 21*, 173–179.

Sattler, J. M. (1988). *Assessment of children* (3rd ed.). San Diego, CA: Author.

Sattler, J. M. (2001). *Assessment of children* (4th ed.). San Diego, CA: Author.

Sattler, J. M. (2008). *Assessment of children: Cognitive foundations* (5th ed.). San Diego, CA: Author.

Sattler, J. M., & Ryan, J. J. (1998). *Assessment of children: Revised and updated third edition WAIS–III supplement.* San Diego, CA: Author.

Sattler, J. M., & Ryan, J. J. (2009). *Assessment with the WAIS–IV.* La Mesa, CA: Author.

Schneider, B. H., & Gervais, M. D. (1991). Identifying gifted kindergarten students with brief screening measures and the WPPSI–R. *Journal of Psychoeducational Assessment, 9*, 201–208.

Schneider, W. J., & McGrew, K. S. (2012). The Cattell-Horn-Carroll model of intelligence. In D. P. Flanagan & P. L. Harrison (Eds.), *Contemporary intellectual assessment: Theories, tests, and issues* (3rd ed., pp. 99–144). New York, NY: Guilford Press.

Silverstein, A. B. (1969). An alternative factor analytic solution for Wechsler's intelligence scales. *Educational and Psychological Measurement, 19*, 763–767.

Spearman, C. (1904). "General intelligence" objectively determined and measured. *American Journal of Psychology, 15*, 201–293.

Sternberg, R. J. (1995). *In search of the human mind.* Fort Worth, TX: Harcourt Brace College Publishers.

Sternberg, R. J., & Kaufman, J. C. (1998). Human abilities. *Annual Review of Psychology, 49*, 479–502.

Stone, B. J., Gridley, B. E., & Gyurke, J. S. (1991). Confirmatory factor analysis of the WPPSI–R at the extreme of the age range. *Journal of Psychoeducational Assessment, 9*, 263–270.

Storandt, M. (1994). General principles of assessment of older adults. In M. Storant & G. R. VandenBos (Eds.), *Neuropsychological assessment of dementia and depression in older adults: A clinician's guide* (pp. 7–32). Washington, DC: American Psychological Association.

Terman, L. M., & Merrill, M. A. (1937). *Measuring intelligence*. Boston: Houghton Mifflin Harcourt.

Terman, L. M. (1916). *The measurement of intelligence: An explanation of and a complete guide for the use of the Stanford revision and extension of the Binet-Simon Intelligence Scale*. Boston, MA: Houghton Mifflin.

Terman, L. M., & Merrill, M. A. (1960). *Stanford-Binet intelligence scale: Manual for the third revision form L–M* (1972 Norm Tables by R. L. Thorndike). Boston: Houghton Mifflin.

Terman, L. M., & Merrill, M. E. (1973). Sample items from Stanford-Binet Scale. In F. Rebelsky & L. Dorman (Eds.), *Child development and behavior*. Alfred A. Knopf.

Thorndike, R. L., Hagen, E. P., & Sattler, J. M. (1986). *Stanford-Binet intelligence scale: Fourth edition*. Itasca, IL: Riverside Publishing.

Thurstone, L. L. (1938). Primary mental abilities. *Psychometric monographs* (Vol. 1). Chicago, IL: Chicago University Press. Cited in H. H. Harman (1960). *Modern factor analysis*. Chicago, IL: University of Chicago Press.

Thurstone, L. L., & Thurstone, T. G. (1941). *The Chicago tests of primary mental abilities*. Chicago, IL: Science Research Associates.

U.S. Bureau of the Census. (1999, March). *Current population survey, 1999* [Data file]. Washington, DC: Author.

U.S. Bureau of the Census. (2001). *Census 2000 summary file 1 United States*. Washington, DC: Author.

U.S. Bureau of the Census. (2005). *Current population survey, October 2005: School enrollment supplement file* [CD-ROM]. Washington, DC: Author.

U.S. Bureau of the Census. (2010). *Current population survey, October 2010: School enrollment supplement file* [CD-ROM]. Washington, DC: Author.

U.S. Bureau of the Census. (2012). *Current population survey, October 2012: School enrollment supplement file* [CD-ROM]. Washington, DC: Author.

Vernon, P. E. (1965). Ability factors and environmental influences. *American Psychologist, 20*, 723–733.

Ward, L. C., Bergman, M. A., & Herbert, K. R. (2012). WAIS–IV subtest covariance structure: Conceptual and statistical considerations. *Psychological Assessment, 24*, 328–340.

Watkins, M. W. (2010). Structure for the Wechsler intelligence scale for children–fourth edition among a national sample of referred students. *Psychological Assessment, 22*, 782–787.

Watkins, M. W., Wilson, S. M., Kotz, K. M., Carbone, M. C., & Babula, T. (2006). Factor structure of the Wechsler intelligence scale for children–fourth edition among referred students. *Educational and Psychological Measurement, 66*, 975–983.

Wechsler, D. (1939). *Wechsler-Bellevue intelligence scale*. New York, NY: The Psychological Corporation.

Wechsler, D. (1949). *Wechsler intelligence scale for children; manual*. The Psychological Corp.

Wechsler, D. (1955). *Wechsler adult intelligence scale*. New York: NY: The Psychological Corporation.

Wechsler, D. (1967). *Wechsler preschool and primary scale of intelligence (WPPSI)*. New York, NY: The Psychological Corporation (PsychCorp).

Wechsler, D. (1974). *Wechsler Intelligence scale for children, revised edition (WISC–R):* San Antonio, TX: The Psychological Corporation (PsychCorp).

Wechsler, D. (1975). *The collected papers of David Wechsler*. New York, NY: Academic Press.

Wechsler, D. (1981). *Wechsler adult intelligence scale–revised (WAIS–R)*. New York: NY: The Psychological Corporation.

Wechsler, D. (1989). *Wechsler preschool and primary scale of intelligence, revised edition (WPPSI–R)*. San Antonio, TX: The Psychological Corporation (PsychCorp)-Pearson.

Wechsler, D. (1991). *Wechsler intelligence scale for children, third edition (WISC–III)*. San Antonio, TX: The Psychological Corporation (PsychCorp).

Wechsler, D. (1997). *Wechsler adult intelligence scale, third edition (WAIS–III)*. New York: NY: The Psychological Corporation.

Wechsler, D. (2002). *Wechsler preschool and primary scale of intelligence, third edition (WPPSI–III)*. San Antonio, TX: The Psychological Corporation (PsychCorp)-Pearson.

Wechsler, D. (2003). *Wechsler intelligence scale for children–fourth edition (WISC–IV): Administration and scoring manual*. San Antonio, TX: The Psychological Corporation-Pearson.

Wechsler, D. (2008a). *Wechsler adult intelligence scale, fourth edition (WAIS–IV): Administration and scoring manual*. San Antonio, TX: The Psychological Corporation (PsychCorp)-Pearson.

Wechsler, D. (2008b). *Wechsler adult intelligence scale–fourth edition (WAIS–IV): Technical and interpretive manual*. San Antonio, TX: The Psychological Corporation (PsychCorp)-Pearson.

Wechsler, D. (2012a). *Wechsler preschool and primary scale of intelligence, fourth edition (WPPSI–IV): Administration and scoring manual*. Bloomington, MN: The Psychological Corporation (PsychCorp)-Pearson.

Wechsler, D. (2012b). *Wechsler preschool and primary scale of intelligence, fourth edition (WPPSI–IV): Technical and interpretive manual*. Bloomington, MN: The Psychological Corporation (PsychCorp)-Pearson.

Wechsler, D. (2014a). *Wechsler intelligence scale for children, fifth edition (WISC–V): Administration and scoring manual*. Bloomington, MN: The Psychological Corporation (PsychCorp)-Pearson.

Wechsler, D. (2014b). *Wechsler intelligence scale for children, fifth edition (WISC–V): Technical and interpretive manual*. Bloomington, MN: The Psychological Corporation (PsychCorp)-Pearson.

Weiss, L. G., Keith, T. Z., Zhu, J., & Chen, H. (2013a). WAIS–IV clinical validation of the four- and five-factor interpretive approaches [Special edition]. Journal of *Psychoeducational Assessment, 31*, 94–113.

Weiss, L. G., Keith, T. Z., Zhu, J., & Chen, H. (2013a). WISC–IV clinical validation of the four- and five-factor interpretive approaches [Special edition]. *Journal of Psychoeducational Assessment, 31,* 94–113.

Werheid, K., Hoppe, C., Thöne, A., Müller, U., Müngersdorf, M., & von Cramon, D. Y. (2002). The adaptive digit ordering test: Clinical application, reliability, and validity of a verbal working memory test. *Archives of Clinical Neuropsychology, 17,* 547–565.

Willingham, W. W. (1974). Predicting success in graduate education. *Science, 183,* 273–278.

Zadeh, Z. Y., Im-Bolter, N., & Cohen, N. J. (2007). Social cognition and externalizing psychopathology: An investigation of the mediating role of language. *Journal of Abnormal Child Psychology, 35,* 141–152.

See Routledge's e-resources website for forms. (www.routledge.com/9780367346058)

8 Achievement Tests

Overview

The construct of *achievement* is generally defined as the degree of previous learning or accomplishment in various types of subject matter or specifically defined academic areas (Gregory, 2011; Miller, McIntire, & Lovler, 2011). Hence, achievement tests measure past learning or the amount of learning that has already been attained as the result of exposure to a defined instructional experience. That is, it represents a test of developed skill or knowledge. This is contrasted with *intelligence*, which was previously defined as an aptitude; that is, a potential or ability to learn in the future (see also Larsen & Buss, 2021). Recall that this represents a more general and stable cognitive ability trait. Considering this broad definition, achievement tests are innumerable in terms of kind. As long as the test is measuring how much an individual has learned, whether it be in a formal classroom (e.g., mathematics), a trade (e.g., welding), or demonstrating a skill for licensure (e.g., driving examination), it aptly falls under the category of an achievement test.

More specifically, in mental health practice, achievement tests most commonly measure fundamental academic skills requisite for success in education. The objective is to detect impairments, delays, or dysfunctions that may hinder academic success, and thereby be associated with or cause later maladjustment. For instance, the *Individuals with Disabilities Education Improvement Act of 2004* (IDEA, 2004) identifies the following eight areas of achievement to be assessed for a diagnosis of *learning disabilities*:[1] oral expression, listening comprehension, written expression, basic reading skills, reading comprehension, reading fluency, mathematics calculation, and mathematics problem solving. In fact, the organizational structure of the two achievement measures presented in this chapter are modeled after this law, in whole or in part, and are designed to principally detect *specific learning disorders* (SLDs) and related *communication disorders* (e.g., *language disorder*). Note that all of these areas are taught in the formal classroom, and thus are derived principally by instruction and practice. As defined, it is not surprising that achievement tests are primarily the purview of the educational field. Many health insurance companies attest to this by denying *preauthorization* (PA) of any requested testing that is principally psychoeducational in nature (see Chapter 7 regarding issues of PA).

It would be a grave error, however, to conclude that such testing is not relevant to mental health practice. First, testing referrals for learning disorders and related academic problems, which by definition require achievement testing, have been steadily increasing in the author's own practice over the past 10 years. Second, unlike medical disorders that are palpable and can be observed, learning disabilities are latent and frequency go undetected (Lewandowski & Lovett, 2014). Symptoms also vary tremendously and affect many areas of functioning, including mastering the fundamental skills of reading, writing, and mathematics, along with deleteriously affecting work, family relationships, daily routines, and even friendships (Beitchman & Brownlie, 2014). Third, there is significant comorbidity among learning problems and other psychological disorders. For instance, children with learning difficulties are three times as likely to have significant behavioral problems by age 8 years (i.e., 32% to 9%; Benasich, Curtiss, & Tallal, 1993).

Furthermore, a review of 150 studies showed that about 75% of children with academic delays also (a) had significant deficits in social skills (Kavale & Forness, 1996) and (b) tend to make negative impressions on others (Mok, Pickles, Durkin, & Conti-Ramsden, 2014). These findings show that there is an unequivocal link between learning disorders and other types of psychopathology, hence rendering the diagnosis of academic-related and learning disorders integral to mental health practice and not circumscribed to academia. Finally, ensuring academic success is vital to career productivity, advancement, and success (Roth, Bevier, Switzer, & Schippmann, 1996) and ultimately to one's ongoing psychological adjustment (Kaplan, Damphous, & Kaplan, 1994). In all of these ways, achievement testing is exceptionally relevant to mental health practice and thus warrants its own independent chapter in this book.

Two of the most commonly used individually administered achievement tests are presented later, and represent the core sections of this chapter, including data tables for presenting their results within the context of a psychological assessment report. They include the following: (a) Wechsler Individual Achievement Test, Third Edition (WIAT–III;

DOI: 10.4324/9780429326820-10

PsychCorp-Pearson, 2009a, 2009b); and (b) Woodcock–Johnson, Fourth Edition, Tests of Achievement (WJ IV ACH; Mather & Wendling, 2014; Schrank, Mather, & McGrew, 2014a). Prior to this, a brief history of achievement tests is provided, the purpose of which is to create a useful framework for the more specific tests. Next, the primary diagnostic reasons for including such measures within a targeted test battery in mental health practice are presented, along with some unique insurance coverage issues.

A Succinct History of Achievement Tests

It has been proposed that achievement testing began as far back as 2200 B.C. in China (DuBois, 1966, 1970). These tests were used to select which applicant would be selected for various government positions. Like many standardized achievement tests today, these early tests required a good deal of instruction and training in order to pass. In the United States (U.S.), the accountability movement and standards-based education has had significant impacts upon how achievement tests have been developed, employed, and interpreted in this country. Hence, these will next be discussed.

Accountability means that school systems are responsible for their product, which refers to student learning. In turn, student learning is frequently measured by achievement tests. Therefore, these kinds of tests are an inherent component of assessing the accountability of schools. The incipience of accountability occurred during the 1960s and was influenced by three events. First, the Union of Soviet Socialist Republics (U.S.S.R.; now Russia) was the first to launch a successful orbital space flight, to the chagrin of the U.S. In response, there were clarion calls for educational reform in the U.S., including demands for improvement in science, technology, and education in general. Second, there was a significant increase in funding for education, which tripled from the 1950s through the 1970s (National Center for Education Statistics, 2001). Third, the *Elementary and Secondary Education Act (ESEA)* was passed by the U.S. Congress in 1964, which increased federal funding of an array of educational initiatives. These developments led to the *No Child Left Behind Act*, which was technically a revision of the ESEA that increased further the requirement of standardized testing to ensure that all children's educational needs were being met, and the aforementioned *Individuals with Disabilities in Education Act of 2004*, which delineated the skill sets to be assessed for the detection of *specific learning disorders (SLDs)*. As stated, that latter has had a direct and continuing influence on both the content and organizational structure of the two achievement tests discussed later in this chapter.

The accountability movement has since evolved into a *standards-based education* approach to teaching in the schools (see Cizek, 2001; Thurlow & Ysseldyke, 2001). Such approach requires (a) an unequivocal delineation of course content and subjects to be learned at each grade level, (b) a clear definition of the required levels of performance so that they could be measured, and (c) a guarantee that all students will be afforded the opportunity according to their needs to learn the material. Hence, the major impetus for achievement testing the various academic subjects was to ensure that the school systems in the U.S. were performing according to their primary function. For this reason, such tests are typically group administered in classrooms or via online testing in order to determine if the desired proportion of students were learning at an acceptable rate. A good example is the *Iowa Assessments* (previously known as the *Iowa Test of Basic Skills*; Hoover et al., 2007).

In slight contrast, when achievement tests are employed within the context of mental health practice, the focus shifts to the individual examinee rather than large samples of students within the education system. For this reason, the tests in this chapter possess two key characteristics as follows: (a) individually administered; and (b) measures of general achievement. First, the one-on-one nature of administration renders possible the observation and recording of test behaviors that are useful to diagnosis (e.g., responding impulsively, giving up prematurely, making the same phonetic errors when pronouncing nonsense words). Second, the overall test surveys learning across and array of academic skills and subjects. This is usually done by apportioning the various skills and subjects into more narrowly defined subtests (e.g., word reading, mathematics problem solving), which accounts for these measures sometimes being referred to as *achievement batteries*.

This completes the very brief summary of the evolution of achievement tests that measure academic skills in mental health practice. Next is a recitation of the various reasons why a psychologist would include a measure of general achievement within a targeted test battery for mental health purposes.

Diagnostic Reasons for Using an Achievement Test in Mental Health Practice

In mental health practice, the principal reason for requesting an achievement test is to rule out one or more SLDs or communication disorders listed in the *Diagnostic and Statistical Manual of Mental Disorders, Fifth Edition (DSM–5*; American Psychiatric Association, 2013). Recall that SLDs may be present when reading, written expression, and/ or mathematics are well below average (i.e., a *standard score* [SS] of 78 and below, along with a *percentile rank (PR)* of

7 for the "greatest diagnostic certainty"; American Psychiatric Association, 2013, p. 69), intelligence is estimated to be normal, sensory-perceptual dysfunction and other psychopathology (e.g., anxiety, depression) is ruled out, and the provisions of sufficient educational opportunity has been substantiated. The DSM–5 criteria continue to permit the use of an *ability achievement discrepancy* (*AAD*) to identify a SLD, although has simplified testing to the aforementioned SS and PR range. In either case, standardized testing is an inherent component of making such diagnosis. The remaining rule out variables are typically handled in a satisfactory way by means of clinical interview and mental status examination. If there remains a question of whether intellectual functioning may be impaired, then an IQ test should also become part of the test battery.

Of note, an IQ test should also be included if there is a suspicion that an individual may possess gifted intelligence (i.e., full scale IQ of 120 and above or "very high" to "extremely high" intellectual functioning). This is because there is a reasonable risk that an individual of such high mental competence can score within the normal range of achievement when compared to the population of same-aged peers. A more valid test of SLDs in such cases is to include an intelligence test and perform and AAD analysis to determine if individuals' achievement scores are lower than expected according to their measured IQ. In effect, this controls for their atypically high IQ and informs the examiner whether they are not performing commensurate with their cognitive ability. This type of analysis will be clearer when discussed within the context of using the WIAT–III.

In terms of formal diagnosis, recall that DSM–5 has technically consolidated all previously recognized learning disorders into one general class, then has subtyped them into four versions by type of general academic skill or domain. These include the following: (a) with impairment in reading (i.e., F81.0); (b) with impairment in written expression (i.e., F81.81); and (c) with impairment in mathematics (F81.2). Furthermore, each of these subtypes enumerates more detailed skills (which are referred to as subskills in the DSM–5) that can be identified as individually problematic and thus targets for intervention. A fourth mixed category is found in the ICD–10 (mixed disorder of scholastic skills, F81.3), which can be useful in cases where an atypical academic skill or combination of skills have been revealed by standardized testing, although this can risk insurance companies refusing to cover such atypical diagnoses because there is no clear counterpart in DSM–5. Therefore, it is advised that this diagnosis be avoided if possible, at least if practicing in the U.S.

Also relevant to achievement testing are cases of suspected communication disorders. Most especially, these include language disorder and *speech sound disorder* (previously *phonological disorder*). Language disorder now includes impairment in receptive and/or expressive skills whereas in previous DSM editions they were separate (see, e.g., American Psychiatric Association, 2000).

There are psychologists who utilize designated achievement tests and subtests to assist in ruling out attention-deficit/hyperactivity disorder (ADHD). However, selected neuropsychological subtests that measure the more fundamental and diagnostically relevant abilities of attention and executive functioning are far superior in directly and more accurately detecting the existence of ADHD symptoms (see Chapter 9).

Although infrequent in practice, a potential use of an achievement test is to address any referral questions which simply request a measure of an individual's mastery of identified fundamental academic subjects. The most likely referral sources in mental health practice include (a) vocational rehabilitation programs to assist in determining educational needs and to foster alternative career development, (b) mental health professionals such that they may adjust treatment intervention accordingly, (c) university student support services departments to test for one or more suspected SLDs regarding one of their students, and (d) adults or parents who believe that they or their child may have an undiagnosed SLD.

Unique Insurance Coverage Issues for Achievement Testing in Mental Health Practice

There are unique insurance preauthorization (PA) issues for achievement testing in mental health. They are all related to the premise that for clients under the age of 18 years and matriculating through compulsory formal education, academic achievement testing is the purview of the school system and not a mental health issue. Therefore, for minor clients, only the most comprehensive commercial health insurance policies will cover such testing, most especially those that do not require PA for psychological testing services. For adults, however, such testing is actually more likely to be approved because (a) such services are not provided by law by an alternative source (i.e., a school system), (b) academic achievement is more immediately pertinent to carrier advancement, and (c) lack of career advancement more directly impacts overall functioning, including mental health.

Therefore, for most insurance policies covering a minor client, the testing psychologist must do one or more of the following during an initial psychological assessment interview in an attempt to increase the odds of obtaining PA for achievement testing: (a) demonstrate a temporal association between academic difficulties or delay and mental disorder (e.g., depression, anxiety); (b) indicate repeated attempts by the parents to petition the academic system for psychoeducational assessment and subsequent refusals of the latter to do so, outlining the school's reasoning for lack of action; (c) show that the parents have engaged in repeated efforts to assist the child in improving the problematic academic skills without significant improvement; and (d) create a connection between diagnosis of a strongly suspected SLD or communication disorder and the clear impact it will have on modifying the treatment regimen. In essence, the odds of obtaining PA improve as the academic problem is increasingly linked to a mental health issue, especially if the latter has become sufficiently severe to be listed as the principal disorder. This demonstrates that the mental health issue has become the primary concern, although the academic issue continues to require resolution for sufficient treatment progress to become a viable objective.

Finally, some community-based referrals will cover such achievement testing for mental health clients. First, the Department of Child Services (DCS; or equivalent in other jurisdictions) typically will cover such testing for minors, especially in cases of neglect in which the child lacked any cognitive or emotional stimulation, or was exposed in utero to an array of psychoactive drugs that represent *teratogens*. Scrutiny of Form 3.13 in Chapter 3 outlines typical objectives listed by DCS in the state of Indiana, which includes providing a psychiatric diagnosis and assessing the client's learning. Second, vocational rehabilitation services will frequently refer an adult client for cognitive testing, which includes achievement testing to assist in ascertaining the learning needs of the client. Third, pediatricians and family medical practitioners have been a fairy frequent referral source for "LD testing," which increases the chances of obtaining medical necessity although certainly does not guarantee PA. Fourth, some university systems will cover such testing for their students through their psychological or counseling services centers as part of general student services, which is used to determine if students should be afforded accommodations as they matriculate through their major areas of study. Although it is possible that neurological patients will be referred for achievement testing to determine the effects of disease or brain trauma on such skills for purposes of rehabilitation, such referrals usually require more basic neuropsychological testing to determine the functioning of more basic brain-behavior relationships, and/or intelligence testing to determine the nature and extent of more high-order cortical functioning (see Chapter 7).

The Major Achievement Test Batteries

This begins the core information of this chapter; namely, the presentation of the two major, individually administered, general achievement test batteries in the book's inventory. First covered is the WIAT–III (Pearson-PsychCorp, 2009a, 2009b) because it has been co-normed with all of the current Wechsler intelligence tests (see Chapter 7). This facet is vital because it permits an AAD analysis if one is needed. While the *Woodcock–Johnson, Fourth Edition, Tests of Achievement* (*WJ IV ACH*) is co-normed with the *Woodcock–Johnson, Fourth Edition, Tests of Cognitive Abilities* (*WJ IV COG*; Schrank, McGrew, & Mather 2014b), the latter is not part of this book's inventory. Again, when building a test inventory, decisions must be made in order to minimize unnecessary redundancy as a cost control measure. Both achievement tests complement each other sufficiently to justify having both in the inventory, although only one set is needed for a less commonly needed AAD analysis.

Using only one for an AAD is especially prudent considering that the DSM–5 has made LD testing much simpler with their *SS* and *PR* as subaverage criteria, hence rendering a much more involved and complex AAD analysis discretionary and based upon unique case facts (see Chapter 4). In particular, the Wechsler series was chosen because they are much more generally involved in testing cases, including IQ, neuropsychological, and achievement. For example, co-normed Wechsler tests also appear in Chapter 9 when *ability memory discrepancy* (*AMD*) analyses are discussed. Therefore, psychologists who perform more psychoeducational services may choose the *Woodcock–Johnson, Fourth Edition* (*WJ IV*; Schrank, McGrew, & Mather 2014a) battery of instruments as their measure for conducting AAD analyses.

Wechsler Individual Achievement Test, Third Edition

Synopsis

The *Wechsler Individual Achievement Test, Third Edition* (*WIAT–III*; Pearson, 2009a, 2009b) is an individually administered, general achievement test, originally designed for students aged 4 years 0 months through 19 years 11 months, although later with an expanded range from 20 years 0 months through 50 years 11 months. In terms of grade range, the test's academic coverage is from preschool (i.e., pre-kindergarten) through grade 12. The use of age norms is advised for use with college students who have graduated from high school and for mental health populations in general, the latter because grade norms can include older individuals who are repeating grade levels.

The WIAT–III is co-normed on the WPPSI–IV, WISC–V and WAIS–IV for purposes of an AAD analysis if that is the approach desired for the diagnosis of a SLD. As stated prior, the newly published DSM–5 criteria no longer require such a laborious testing approach. If one is desired, however, prepared data tables have been prepared that facilitate the analysis and reporting of such results.

The WIAT–III is designed to incorporate the most effective facets of both its predecessors, the original *Wechsler Individual Achievement Test* (*WIAT*; PsychCorp, 1992) and *Wechsler Individual Achievement Test–Second Edition* (*WIAT–II*; Pearson, 2005), in addition to being increasingly compatible with current federal laws on the detection of learning disabilities (see IDEA, 2004) and with improved items, administrative and scoring rules, *utility*, *reliability*, and *validity*. For instance, easier and more difficult items were added to increase the floor and ceiling of the test to maximize the diagnosis of learning disabilities and gifted students, respectively. Next is a section describing the structural organization of this test, which is actually a test battery considering the array of subtests available, each of which measures a more specific skill set. This is ensued by a section delineating some diagnostically related revisions made for this edition of the test, which will facilitate test interpretation discussed later in this chapter.

Test Structure

The WIAT–III is comparable in structure to the Wechsler intelligence tests, possessing a three-tier hierarchical structure as follows (from general to specific with the number of each in parentheses): (a) total achievement composite (1); (b) broad academic area composites (7); and (c) subtest scores (16). This organization is largely supported by expected intercorrelations among the WIAT–III subtest and composites scores reported in the technical manual (Pearson, 2009b, pp. 40–43) as opposed to factor analytic data observed so frequently with other cognitive standardized tests (e.g., intelligence tests covered in Chapter 7).

Although some of the subtest composite scores are the result of two sub-components (e.g., the Sentence Composition subtest is the result of Sentence Combining and Sentence Building raw scores), these are not transformed into interpretable SSs and therefore do not technically represent a level. However, they may be qualitatively analyzed for purposes of planning intervention. In general, the test battery covers from pre-kindergarten (PK) through 12th grade. Adults who complete the WIAT–III are assigned the highest grade completed up to 12th grade as a maximum, which determines subtest start points when using age-based norms as done with a mental health population. The subtests are somewhat staggered according to grade levels to which they pertain, with some being relevant only to a circumscribed number of grades contingent upon the skill being assessed. Hence, the broad domains to which the subtest contribute also are pertinent to somewhat varying grade levels, which is discussed at several points below.

Beginning at the top of the hierarchy (i.e., Stratum III; Carrol, 1993) the Total Achievement composite is the result of 13 of 16 subtests. In addition, some subtests do not contribute to the Total Achievement at all grade levels. For example, the Spelling subtest is administered for grades kindergarten (K) through 12, but contributes to the total only for grades K through 2. There are too many other permutations for this review, hence the discussion will move to Stratum II or the broad academic areas or domains. Grade levels pertinent to each broad domain are in parentheses, although this information is not provided as applied to the subtests to avoid excessive detail.

First, Oral Language (Grades PK–12) consists of Listening Comprehension and Oral Expression. Listening Comprehension consists of two components, including Receptive Vocabulary (i.e., listening vocabulary) and Oral Discourse Comprehension (i.e., making inferences about oral sentences). Oral Expression consists of three components, including expressive vocabulary, oral word fluency (i.e., word retrieval), and sentence repetition (i.e., oral syntactic knowledge).

Second, there are three domains related to reading, which share different combinations of reading-related subtests. Total Reading (Grades 1–12) includes Word Reading (i.e., simply sounding our single words of increasing difficulty), Pseudoword Decoding (i.e., pronouncing non-words), Oral Reading Fluency (i.e., reading passages for rate and accuracy), and Reading Comprehension (i.e., reading passages for understanding). Basic Reading (Grades 1–12) is comprised of the former two subtests whereas Reading Comprehension (Grades 2–12) consists of only the latter two subtests.

Third, Written Expression (Grades K–12) includes Sentence Composition (i.e., combining sentences to convey the same meaning as in original form and creating sentences using a target word), Essay Composition (i.e., compositional writing with organization and productivity), and for some grades, Spelling (i.e., writing letters and words within the context of a sentence) and Alphabet writing Fluency (i.e., the ability to write as many letters of the alphabet as possible within a 30-second time limit).

Fourth, and finally, Mathematics (Grades K–12) consists of Math Problem Solving (i.e., answering untimed math word problems using basic concepts, daily applications, geometry, and algebra with discretionary scratch paper), and Numerical Operations (i.e., completing math calculation problems involving basic skills and operations, geometry, algebra, and calculus). Optional Math Fluency Addition, Subtraction, and Multiplication subtests are available for measuring speed and accuracy in each of these operations. These are timed at 60 seconds each and measure fluency, which is not done with the aforementioned subtests that contribute to the Mathematics composite.

This section provided an overview of how the WIAT–III is generally structured. Next the major revisions to this edition are reviewed that are most pertinent to diagnosis, which prepares the way for the data tables that have been prepared for reporting and interpreting WIAT–III results.

General Diagnostically Related Revisions

The following paragraphs highlight the major diagnostically related changes made to the WIAT–III. Understanding them will facilitate the interpretation of results yielded by this rather complex measure of achievement, including helping readers to become familiar with achievement testing concepts and language. They will also supplement the data tables that have been created for reporting and interpreting WIAT–III scores within a psychological assessment report.

ORAL LANGUAGE SUBTESTS

First, relevant to the Oral Language composite of this test evidence indicates that oral language can affect the acquisition of both reading and writing skills, hence should be measured together (Kavanagh, 1991). Because inner language and experience forms the foundation for oral language, it may be concluded that the latter also forms the basis for developing both reading and writing (Johnson & Myklebust, 1967; Myklebust, 1973). Therefore, relationships among these three skill sets should be measured and analyzed (Johnson, 1982; Gregg & Mather, 2002). Research also shows that oral language is highly correlated with early reading skills as many lower level readers are delayed in various language skills (Mann, Cowin, & Schoenheimer, 1989), including repeating spoken sentences (Holmes & McKeever, 1979; Jorm, 1979, 1983; Mann, Liberman, & Shankweiler, 1980). Furthermore, individuals with difficulties in written expression possess problems in oral language skills, including problems in written syntax (Gregg & Hafer, 2001) and spelling, the latter being associated with a *phonological processing* deficit (Moats, 2001). Hence, the WIAT–III Oral Language subtests were revised such that they were linked more closely with reading and writing tasks.

Second, an Oral Discourse Comprehension subtest was added to the WIAT–III, which measures listening comprehension skills needed in the classroom. More specifically, these items test the skill of understanding both single sentences and extended discourse, the latter requiring the individual to create logical connections between ideas and making judgements of which ideas are more or less important (Carlisle, 1991). Listening comprehension can also be related to reading problems. In particular, reading comprehension has been proposed to require listening comprehension, word reading, and decoding (Gough & Tunmer, 1986). If a person does poorly on reading comprehension, it could be due to any one or more of these skills. Therefore, a comprehensive achievement test must measure all three components (Carlisle, 1991).

Third, the Expressive Vocabulary subtest from the WIAT–II was retained but moved to the Oral Language composite in order to complement the Listening Comprehension subtest that contributes to that same composite. Because the Listening Comprehension subtest measures Receptive Vocabulary and the Expressive Vocabulary subtest measures expressive vocabulary, the Oral Language composite now contains both aspects of language ability. The Oral Language composite can now be analyzed as a whole or broken down into expressive and receptive language. This is consistent with the DSM–5, which integrates both receptive and expressive impairments into the single diagnosis versus separate receptive language disorder and receptive–expressive language disorder in the *Diagnostic and Statistical Manual of Mental Disorders, Fourth Edition, Text Revision* (DSM–IV–TR; American Psychiatric Association, 2000).

Fourth, an Oral Word fluency subtest was retained from the WIAT–II with somewhat modified scoring rules. It is a timed subtest that asks examinees to report as many words as possible from a common category. It is designed to tap *word retrieval* (i.e., lexical access), cognitive flexibility, and working memory, especially the former considering that a common category is selected. Both word retrieval and a phonological processing difficulty may account for low scores, which can be elucidated by examining other scores, including Word Reading Speed, Pseudoword Decoding Speed, and Oral Reading Fluency.

READING-RELATED SUBTESTS

There are also a number of reading-related subtests now available on the WIAT–III that facilitates diagnosis and will now be addressed. To begin, an Early Reading Skills subtest was created in order to provide a measure of both pre-reading and early reading skills. Such skills consist of *phonological awareness* (i.e., the capability of manipulating word sounds (e.g., rhyming), and awareness of *phonological-orthographic relationships* (e.g., how word sounds are presented in written form). Measuring these related skills are vital because impairments in them have been frequently associated with reading disabilities (Catts, Gillispie, Leonard, Kail, & Miller, 2002; Bradley & Bryant, 1978; Gough & Tunmer, 1986). Furthermore, early detection of these skills prior to formal reading instruction has been found to be a robust predictor of later reading disorders (Puolakanaho et al., 2008), including letter naming (Adams, 1990; Lennon & Slesinski, 1999), which is also measured by the Early Reading Skills subtest.

Also concerning reading is the Word Reading subtest, which was actually retained from the WIAT–II, although updated to include a broader range of spelling-sound patterns more conducive to item-level skills analyses. Additionally, a timed component was added such that this subtest is now capable of measuring both speed and accuracy as part of the word reading process. The timed component was needed due to research showing that speed limitations in reading both words and *pseudowords* (i.e., nonsense words) was correlated with *dyslexia* (i.e., neurologically caused disability in reading, spelling, and writing words (van der Leij & van Daal, 1999). When an individual's reading pace is slow and labored due to either lack of familiarity or impairment, increased cognitive resources must be utilized, thus leaving a paucity of remaining resources for purposes of comprehension (Berninger, 1998). Therefore, slow reading rate can also cause reduced reading comprehension (Katzir, Kim, Wolf, Morris, & Lovett, 2008). For this reason, although the Word Reading subtest is timed, the administration instructions do not reference this so that examinees read at their typical pace and without compromising either rate or accuracy.

Another important reading subtest is Pseudoword Decoding, which was also retained from that of the WIAT–II. Decoding these non-words requires examinees to recode spelling into pronunciation (i.e., the phonology–orthography connection), which is a learning mechanism referred to as *phonological recoding* (Rayner, Foorman, Perfetti, Pesetsky, & Seidenberg, 2001). Impairment in this ability has been shown to be a defining characteristic of dyslexia (Lyon, Shaywitz, & Shaywitz, 2003) and accounts for a signification portion of the variation in reading comprehension skill (Braze, Tabor, Shankweiler, & Mencl, 2007). Briefly, the WIAT–II Reading Comprehension was also retained but updated with a lower floor to better identify impairments at the more impaired end of the scale, with revised passages and questions.

A final reading subtest here worthy of mention is Oral Reading Fluency, which is part of the WIAT–III battery in response to both empirical research and legislative criteria that emphasize the importance of reading fluency as part of the education curriculum. Three core characteristics of a highly skilled reader include the abilities to read rapidly, accurately, and with understanding (National Institute of Child Health and Human Development, 2000). This subtest yields SSs that permit the comparison of rate with accuracy, thus being capable of determining all combinations of these two dimensions (i.e., slow but accurate; slow and inaccurate; fast but inaccurate, and fast and accurate). It has been proposed that an individual with an *accuracy disability* shows impairment in both speed and correctness whereas an individual with a *rate disability* has intact word recognition (i.e., accuracy) but is impaired in terms of reading rate (Lovett, 1987). Thus, Oral Reading Fluency addresses these all of these issues. Although Reading Comprehension is not measured here, it is measured elsewhere and examinees are informed that they will be asked a question about the passage, hence encouraging them to read here for understanding.

WRITTEN EXPRESSION SUBTESTS

Writing skills evolve from ordered patterns of random scribbling through the following predictable steps: (a) the formation of true letters; (b) writing meaningful words; (c) forming a series of related words; and (d) composing meaningful sentences that each incorporate a complete thought (Traweek & Berninger, 1997). Consistent with this developmental sequence, the WIAT–III is comprised of subtests that measure the ability to write graphemes (e.g., word parts), whole words, sentences, and discourse, including tasks that range from low-level (i.e., letter writing, spelling) to higher level skills (i.e., composing sentences and an essay). This range of tasks is deemed vital due to the fact that the various skills can affect each other in reciprocal fashion. That is, an examinee can perform poorly at higher level tasks primarily due to difficulties with lower-level tasks (Berninger, Cartwright, Yates, Swanson, & Abbott, 1994; Whitaker, Berninger, Johnston, & Swanson, 1994). Therefore, both must be measured independently to adequately diagnose what variables underlie an examinee's writing problems.

Students with writing disabilities have shown a variety of skill problems, including impairments in word productivity, *syntax* (i.e., rules that guide the proper formation of sentences, including grammar, word order, and punctuation), *semantics* (i.e., vocabulary), and mechanics (Gregg, Coleman, Davis, & Chalk, 2007; Houck & Billingsley, 1989; Moran, 1981; Thomas, Englert, & Gregg, 1987). For example, it was found that 75% of all word omissions were manifested by students with writing disabilities (Houck & Billingsley, 1989). In order to detect such a wide array of writing problems, the WIAT–III writing subtest was revised to provide an expanded depth of skill coverage. These include Alphabet Writing Fluency and Spelling for more basic skills (i.e., spelling letter sounds, alphabet letters, and single words), along with Sentence Composition and Essay Composition for more advanced skills (i.e., composing complete sentences, linking and organizing sentences to form paragraphs, writing correct grammar and mechanics).

More specifically, the Alphabet Writing Fluency consists of timed alphabet writing, which has proven to be a strong predictor of later reading, spelling, and writing skills (McCutchen et al., 2002; Berninger et al., 1992, 1994) and accounts for the majority of unique variance in writing ability in early childhood (Berninger et al., 1992). By about 2nd grade (i.e., age 7 years), children's alphabet writing should become automatic. When this is delayed, special assistance is indicated (see Berninger, 1998). This is why the Alphabet Writing Fluency subtest extends through 3rd grade.

Similarly, the Spelling subtest has been refined to consist of a greater number of levels of morphological knowledge, along with a greater variety of morphological features. Spelling from dictation requires *phonological abilities* (i.e., word sounding), *orthographic skills* (i.e., writing letters and graphemes), and awareness of *phoneme–grapheme correspondence*. Because a vast majority (if not all) individuals with dyslexia have significant difficulties these underlying abilities, they demonstrate extremely poor spelling (Lyon et al., 2003). In fact, spelling is considered to be more difficult to learn than reading, and is more persistent when delays are manifested (Moats, 2001). In part, this is because spelling requires more accurate memory of letter patterns and rules governing letter positions and semantics (Bailet, 2001). Hence, the improvement in the WIAT–III Spelling subtest was deemed to be vital.

Moving to the higher-level writing subtests, Sentence Composition consists of two components, Sentence Combining and Sentence Building. The former requires the integration of separate sentences into one that retains the meaning of the original sentences, while the latter asks examinees to construct sentences using a target word. Together, these components require the composing of well-formulated sentences, a skill that is remarkably difficult for people with writing disorders. In result, individuals with writing disorders perform poorly on these component tests as evidenced by much shorter sentences of very low quality (Houck & Billingsley, 1989). That being said, compositional writing has been shown to be the most problematic skill for student with writing disabilities (Mayes, Calhoun, & Lane, 2005), including repeated errors in spelling, punctuation, capitalization, and handwriting legibility, along with poor organization, limited productivity, and weak theme development (Houck & Billinglsey 1989; Lane & Lewandowski, 1994; Myklebust, 1973; Poplin, Gray, Larsen, Banikowski, & Mehring, 1980; Poteet, 1978; Thomas et al., 1987). For these reasons, the Essay Writing subtest was revised so as to measure word count, theme development and text organization, and grammar and mechanics (i.e., grammar, spelling, capitalization, and punctuation skills). Because these subtests measure high-level skills, the examiner's manual provides a detailed scoring rubric that assists in reliable scoring when an examiner is properly trained and practiced (see Pearson, 2009a, pp. 44–46).

MATHEMATICS SUBTESTS

Research has found that individuals with mathematics disorder generally have difficulties in the following three areas: (a) multistep problem solving; (b) regrouping and renaming; and (c) remembering number facts automatically (Bryant, Bryant, & Hammill, 2000). The Math Problem Solving, Numerical Operations, and Math Fluency subtests were designed to tap all three areas and provide a more in-depth skills analysis by classifying certain types of problems. The latter was deemed to be important because those with math disabilities tend to show wide variability in their strengths and weaknesses of specific skills (Geary, 2004).

More specifically, Math Problem Solving requires a wide variety of math reasoning skills, which was deemed to be vital because individuals with math disabilities employ immature and improper math logic and solution strategies, resulting in slower rates of solving problems and increased errors (Geary, 2004). They also continue to rely on procedure-based versus memory-based solutions, from which it may be inferred that there are underlying difficulties in storage and retrieval of math facts (Geary, 2004). The Numerical Operations subtest is designed to measure calculation skills and is an adaptation from the WIAT–II with a higher ceiling and lower floor. This subtest taps the weaknesses in math fact retrieval, counting, and selection and application of procedures that those with math disabilities manifest (Geary, 2004).

Finally, *math fluency* is defined as showing rapid and accurate methods for computing numbers (see National Council of Teachers of Mathematics, 2000). This skill has been found to be associated with the later development of more complex math skills as measured by the Math Problem Solving and Numerical Operations subtests. In result, math fluency skill has been added to curriculum standards and has become an instructional standard for grades K through 8. A high number of individuals with math disorder manifest weaknesses in the recall of math facts, along with counting and procedural skills (Geary, 2004), which tend to persist into secondary education (Calhoon, Emerson, Flores, & Houchins, 2007). In order to detect significant weaknesses in these skills, the WIAT–III added three optional Math Fluency subtests that involve the following basic operations: addition, subtraction, and multiplication.

SUMMARY

The objective of this section was to provide readers with the major revisions done in this edition of the Wechsler achievement test that are based upon the latest empirical research and that are diagnostically important. Secondarily, it was to acquaint readers with essential features of the WIAT–III subtests so as to facilitate the reporting and interpretation of the data yield, which is delineated in more detail in subsequent sections.

Norm Reference Samples

There was a total of four standardization samples for the WIAT–III. Three were included when the test battery was first published in 2009 (Pearson, 2009b). They were comprised of two grade-based samples, one for fall ($N = 1,400$) and one for spring ($N = 1,375$), both ranging from grades PK through 12. The third sample was based on age ($N = 1,826$), ranging from 4 years 0 months through 19 years 11 months. In 2010, an adult standardization sample was added based upon age, ranging from 20 years 0 months through 50 years 11 months (Pearson, 2010). Which of the four norms are applied depends upon (a) examinee age, and (b) whether the examiner selects age-based or grade-based norms. Note that only age-based norms are available for adults, although as stated prior, such norms are more appropriate for testing within the mental health field. Finally, which of the two grade-based norms to be applied are determined by when during the year testing is done. More specifically, fall norms apply between August and December, inclusive, whereas spring norms apply from January through July, inclusive (see Pearson, 2009a, p. 33). Breakdowns of the various norms will be done next by dichotomizing them into younger (ages 4–19 years; grades PK–12) and older cohorts (ages 20–50 years).

YOUNGER NORMS

The age-based norms will be discussed first since they are most appropriate in mental health cases. The 1,826 students were apportioned into 14 age cohorts. Ages 4 through 13 years were divided into 4-month intervals, while ages 14 through 16 were broken down into longer 12-month intervals, and finally, ages 17 through 19 years formed one 3-year interval. Each group contained 128 participants with the exception of the oldest, which contained 190 individuals. The fall and spring grade-based norms were distributed into 14 groups PK through 12th grade, each of which consisted of 100 students except for the spring PK class, which included only 75 children.

Other than age and grade, the younger norms were stratified according to the proportions of sex, race/ethnicity, parent education level, and geographic region reported by the October 2005 U.S. Bureau of the Census (U.S. Bureau of the Census, 2005). Regarding sex, the groupings were comprised of approximately equal numbers of males and females. Race/ethnic grouping included Whites, African Americans, Asians, Hispanics, and Other, again according to the aforementioned population. Parental education was allocated as follows: 0 to 11 years; high school diploma or equivalent; 13 to 15 years; and 16 or more years. Regions of the country included Northeast, South, Midwest, and West.

OLDER NORMS

The older standardization sample was stratified according to the March 2008 Census Bureau population figures utilizing virtually the same variables except grade as follows: age, sex, race/ethnicity, parent- or self-education, and geographic region. The sample totaled 225 adults that were apportioned into three age cohorts, including 20 to 25 years, 26 to 35 years, and 36 to 50 years, with each group containing 75 individuals. Sex was again allocated evenly and the same race/ethnic groupings were employed. Although the same education intervals were employed as for the younger norms, the actual level for each participant was derived differently depending upon age group. In particular, parental or guardian education was used for the youngest 20- to 25-year group. If two parents or guardians were listed, the average was used. For the remaining groups, self-education level was used.

Administration

Administrative considerations for the WIAT–III include subtest selection, item sets, start points, reverse rules, discontinue rules, and stop points. Sample and practice items are also provided as on the intelligence tests to help ensure that the examinee knows how to perform on the various subtests. Together, all of these help ensure that the examinee is given items that are moderately challenging and contribute to enduring motivation to perform at maximum or near maximum capability.

First, subtest selection regards administering the proper subtests that (a) address the referral issues, and (b) are appropriate for the individual's grade level. Hence, the individual is to be administered subtests that pertain to the most recent grade level attended, applying to both grade-based norms and age-based norms. For example, Alphabet Writing Fluency applies to PK through grade 3, whereas Essay Composition is given to examinees enrolled in grades 3 through 12.

Once the proper subtests have been selected, most possess start points. Subtest items are generally ordered by increasing levels of difficulty. *Start points* represent the recommended item (and its difficulty level) to begin administration, which are denoted by appended grade level numbers in the Record Form. These indicate the most current or recent grade level attended by the examinee. Start points were determined to have a 99% pass rate in the norm reference sample. For adults, grade 12 is advised for start points, although the examiner do have some discretion to begin at earlier or later items but only if compelling evidence so indicates. Two subtests employ what are referred to as *item sets*, which are clusters of items of a particular difficulty level, including Reading Comprehension and Oral Reading Fluency. These work similarly to the individual items except that these are groupings of stimuli and item questions of about the same difficulty level.

Reverse rules provide instructions to revert to prior easier items in the event the examinee misses one or more of the first three items at the start point; that is, unless the start point was the first item in the subtest. Typically, the reversal criterion is three consecutive correct answers, then all previous items are all given credit. The antithesis is represented by *discontinue rules*, which instruct the examiner at which point to stop subtest administration and provide no further credit for subsequent items; that is, unless the last item in the subtest is reached. Discontinue rules were established empirically when its application permitted 93% of the norm reference sample to maintain the same raw score PR (i.e., the percent of the standardization sample that the examinee scored equal to or better than). For item sets, reverse rules apply when the examinee scores under a specified cut-off score within a beginning item set (e.g., earning 2 or less points out of 6 total in the set). The examiner is then instructed to reverse one grade level and to apply this reversal rule a maximum of two more times (i.e., reversing a maximum of three times).

Finally, *stop points* instruct the examiner when to terminate subtest administration irrespective of examinee performance. There are two kinds of stop points: timed and grade level difficulty. First, timed subtests end when the indicated duration elapses (e.g., Oral Word Fluency, which is a component of the Oral Expression subtest). Second, Reading Comprehension and Oral Reading Fluency both end when the determined item set has been completed. For example, each grade level item set for Oral Reading Fluency consists of two reading passages. Once those two passages that make-up the item set are completed, the subtest is completed. Of note, stop points are much more common in achievement tests as compared to intelligence testing because certain skills in the latter are much easier to measure in groups of equivalent difficulty level (e.g., reading entire passages with accompanying questions each representing a different difficulty level).

Scoring

The section will outline the data yield from the WIAT–III, focusing on the scores that are most frequently relied upon and generally the manner in which they are derived. This information will facilitate test interpretation. Many of the scores and computations are comparable to those of the intelligence tests discussed in Chapter 7. Hence, much of this will be review for those who perused the prior chapter topic.

RAW SCORES AND WEIGHTED RAW SCORES

First, most scoring begins with subtest raw score totals, most of which are derived by aggregating the total number correct. This includes all items prior to the start point or reversal rule that did not require administration due to the examinee passing the required items. Total raw scores for the aforementioned item sets are not directly comparable. Therefore, vertical scaling was done in order to transform the original raw scores into equal intervals that can be added so as to reflect consistently increasing mastery; that is, each raw score point is equivalent to any other raw score point in the subtest so that aggregating them represents consistent improvement. Complex statistical programs that are beyond the purview of this book assist in such vertical scaling, such as WINSTEPS (see, e.g., Linacre, 2005) to which the interested reader is referred. Such scaling result in weighted raw scores for subtests that employ item sets (viz., Reading Comprehension and Oral Reading Fluency), which are subsequently transformed into standard scores.

STANDARD SCORES

Once the subtest raw scores and weighted raw scores are obtained, they are converted into subtest standard scores (SSs; mean 100, standard deviation = 15, range = 40–160). SSs were derived by *inferential norming* (Wilkins, Rolfhus,

Weiss, & Zhu, 2005), which is a statistical process in which various *moments* or basic calculations are used to derive a score distribution's mean, variance, skewness, and other pertinent characteristics. These statistics are then used to compute estimates of the corresponding population moments. From these, theoretical distributions are derived for each of the norm reference samples discussed prior, which yield percentiles for each raw score. Finally, the percentiles are converted to the aforesaid SSs.[2] This was the process used to derive the *SS* norms for the WIAT–III.

Next, in order to compute the WIAT–III composite scores, the appropriate subtest SSs were aggregated. Then for each scale, the distribution of the sum of subtest SSs were normalized and smoothed to represent a standard normal distribution, again with a mean of 100, standard deviation of 15, and range from 40 to 160. Therefore, the WIAT–III is unique in the fact that its subtests, composites, and the total are all on the same *SS* metric.[3]

CONFIDENCE INTERVALS

Confidence intervals (*Ci*s) for the WIAT–III are available for both 90% and 95% degree of certainty. They were derived by use of the formula,

$$SEM = SD\sqrt{1 - r_{xx}}$$

Equation 8.1

where *SEM* is the *standard error of measurement* (*SEM*), and r_{xx} represents the split-half reliability coefficients computed for the WIAT–III subtests, composites, and total score reported in the technical manual (Pearson-PsychCorp, 2009b, pp. 27–36). Here, the *SEM* represents the standard or average deviation of the error in a test; here, the WIAT–III. When two *SEM*s are added to and subtracted from the obtained score, that creates a 95% CI; that is, it can be stated with 95% certainty that an individual's true score falls with that range. This is the CI that is usually selected, although this is left to the discretion of the examiner. Certainly, the ones offered by the WIAT–III are the most commonly selected. The technical manual does not state why the split-half coefficients were selected for derivation of the WIAT–III Cis, although because they are higher, they result in being more precise.

PERCENTILE RANKS

Percentile ranks (or percentiles) indicate the proportion of the norm reference sample, which represents the population of same-aged (or graded) peers, who the examinee scored equal to or better than. Stated another way, it is the percentage of the standardization sample that falls below the examinee. Hence, an examinee whose PR is 50 scored equal to or better than 50% of the norm reference sample. The PR has a median (or average) of 50 and a range from 0 to 99 (i.e., it does not extend to 100 because an individual cannot score better than herself). Although easy to comprehend, PRs represent an ordinal scale (Stevens, 1946) and do not represent equal intervals. Thus, only more or less can be determined; how much is left unaddressed. In addition, because they are area transformations, they cluster toward the middle of the distribution where changes in SSs magnify or exaggerate changes in associated PRs. For this reason, it is preferable to first list SSs and their Cis, followed by their associated PRs.

DESCRIPTIVE CLASSIFICATIONS

As for the intelligence tests, nominal categories that also have an inherent order of increasing function, are reported for the purpose of placing a student's performance within a general class. Although more imprecise, this classification provides a general idea as to the level of functioning the examinee is showing in various areas of achievement. In cases where the examinee falls close the boundary between classes, the descriptive classification should be qualified as such.

DIFFERENCE SCORES

This section covers two kinds of difference scores that are important to be cognizant of in achievement testing: (a) differences between composite scores; and (b) ability achievement discrepancy (AAD) analyses. The former regards intra-individual (or ipsative) comparisons and contributes to analyzing the presence of any relative strengths or weaknesses among the broad achievement areas, in addition to any further differences among the most narrowly defined subtest achievement skills. This issue of difference scores has two facets: (a) statistical significance of the difference score (i.e., is it due to error or chance, or is it a true or real effect); and (b) the frequency or base rate of the difference score (i.e., is it clinically meaningful; Groth-Marnat, 2003; Kaufman & Lichtenberger, 1999; Matarazzo & Herman, 1985; Silverstein, 1981). Although both of these have appeared in the two previous chapters, they assume even greater importance here because they can be used to assist in corroborating the presence of learning disabilities and guiding intervention.

AAD analyses pertain to the complex and potentially controversial issue of diagnosing SLDs. As stated previously, the DSM criteria has been modified from a more complex AAD-type conceptualization to a more straightforward subaverage approach. For example, the *DSM–IV–TR* (American Psychiatric Association, 2000) generally considered learning disorders to represent achievement as being *substantially below* that of ability or aptitude, which causes significant dysfunction in academic accomplishment and related areas of daily living. The key term, "substantially below" was further defined as, "a discrepancy of more than 2 standard deviations between achievement and IQ; American Psychiatric Association, 2000, p. 49). In contrast, the DSM–5 (American Psychiatric Association, 2013) now conceptualizes SLDs as achievement being, "well below average for age" (p. 69). Although it also went further by establishing quantitative guidelines for what constitutes, "well below average" (see subsequently) there is no longer a requisite direct comparison with IQ. The only mention of IQ in DSM–5 is to note that ID and SLDs can coexist. In particular, if learning difficulties are in clear excess of those expected by one's assessed degree of intellectual impairment, then a SLD–IQ comorbidity is established.

So, how does the DSM–5 quantify well below average? It specifically states that, in order to achieve, "the greatest diagnostic certainty," an achievement score within an academic domain must be "at least 1.5 standard deviations [*SD*] below the population mean for age, which translates into a *SS* of 78 or less, which is below the 7th percentile" (American Psychiatric Association, 2013, p. 69). Although technically a *SS* of 78 is equivalent to and below rather than only below the 7th percentile (see, e.g., MedFriendly, 2020; McCrae & Costa, 2010; Appendix A) this would be a conservative and objectively defined criterion to espouse, which will be seen subsequently in the data tables for the WIAT–III.

Federal law is also trending away from an AAD conceptualization of learning disabilities. For example, the IDEA (2004) all but eliminated an AAD from the list of eligibility requirements for special education services, hence rendering such test data as irrelevant. Specifically, although IDEA 2004 regulations permit the use of an AAD analysis for making a learning disability diagnosis, "a local education agency *shall not* be required to take into consideration whether a child has a severe discrepancy between achievement and intellectual ability (Sec. 614(b)(6)(A), italics added)). The words "shall not" in legal parlance represents mandatory language. Taking both the clinical approach of the DSM–5 and legal approach, then, a psychologist practicing such testing within the mental health field is free to employ an AAD analysis if the case facts so indicate; however, these results have only clinical meaning and are not legally binding.

So where does one stand with AAD analyses? There remains a clear role for AAD. In particular, if an examinee is known or suspected to have ID, then administration of both an IQ test and achievement test, along with an AAD analysis is warranted; this includes the stated need to rule out both SLD and ID. At the other end of the intellectual spectrum, if an examinee is likely to possess *intellectual giftedness* (i.e., an IQ of about 130 or above), or such has been established by past formal intelligence testing, then it would again be advisable to compute an AAD, here to avert a false negative result. That is, an individual with gifted intelligence is likely to obtain achievement test scores significantly above a *SS* of 78 (PR 7 or less) and yet this may be significantly below their personally measured aptitude. Although it would be challenging to find a school system that would classify such a student with a SLD, the child's parents may want to know this information so that their child performs to their true potential.

For these reasons, a number of data tables are presented for reporting and interpreting AAD analyses using the WIAT–III in the section that discusses interpretation. This comports with many researchers in the field who continue to recommend such an approach as an aid to diagnosing learning disabilities (see, e.g., Kavale & Forness, 1995; Kavale, Holdnack, & Mostert, 2005).

OTHER SCORES

As can be imagined, the WIAT–III offers additional scores that are typically not used in formal reports. In addition to *age-equivalent* (*AE*) scores, this test also provides *grade-equivalent* (*GE*) scores. In review, the former represents the raw score average for a particular age, typically expressed in years:months. For example, an AE of 5:10 on Numerical Operations indicates that the examinee's raw score was equivalent to the raw score average for those in the norm reference sample who were aged 5 years 10 months. If the examinee's *chronological age* (*CA*) is 6:7, it means that his numerical skills are equivalent to individuals 9 months younger than himself. Analogously, a GE of 7.4 on Numerical Operations means that the examinee's raw score equals the average raw score for students in the 4th month of 7th grade. Ges are more felicitous when grade-based norms are being used. Hence, Aes are more suitable for achievement testing in the mental health field.

Normal curve equivalent (NCE) scores have a mean of 50, standard deviation of 21.06, and range from 1 to 99. They are derived from the formula $50 + 21.063 \times z$, where z is a standardized z–score with a mean of 0.00 and standard deviation of 1.00. Their primary advantage is possessing an equal interval measurement scale, although only 1, 50, and 99 correspond to PRs. They were developed for the U.S. Department of Education by the RMC Research Corporation in 1976 to assess the effectiveness of the Title I Program (Mertler, 2002), and refined later by Tallmadge and Wood (1978). However, these scores are more conducive to measuring the progress of groups of students versus individual examinees and are not pertinent in the mental health testing venue.

Stanines are also available on the WIAT–III, both grade based and age-based. *Stanine* is short for "standard nine," which is a score that results from the conversion of a grade- or age-based score into a 9-point scale, ranging from 1 to 9, with a mean of 5 and standard deviation of 2. These scores are frequently used in the field of education because student performance can be facilely compared over a normal distribution. The formula for a stanine is as follows:

$$\text{stanine} = \frac{\text{obtained Raw Score} - \text{Mean}}{\text{Standard Deviation}} \qquad \text{Equation 8.2}$$

where the z–score ranges are associated with stanine scores. For example, a z–score below −1.75 (e.g., −2.00) translates to a stanine of 1. A z–score ranging from −0.25 to +0.25 translates to a stanine of 5 (i.e., the average or mean). Hence, raw test scores can be converted to a one-digit whole number in order to greatly simplify test interpretation, usually for parents of students.

Growth Scale Values (GSVs) permit the examiner to compare an examinee's performance on a single subtest across multiple administrations. These scores are ideal for tracking an individual's progress on particular skills over time (i.e., over grades or ages). GSV values are arbitrary, although they are considered to be an equal interval metric. For example, for 1st grade the mean GSV could be 340 whereas for 12th grade it is 500. GSVs can be tracked over time to measure an examinee's ongoing change in skill level. In the mental health field, retesting is not as common as in the education field, and when it does occur, the test-retest interval tends to be extremely long such that the tests are typically in new editions. Hence, GSVs are not frequently useful in mental health psychological testing.

COMPUTER SCORING

The WIAT–III can currently be computer scored only on the Q–global (Pearson, 2021) website in the same manner as the Wechsler intelligence tests. For those fortunate enough to have purchased the previously available WIAT–III Scoring Assistant (Pearson, 2009c), which is loaded into the PsychCorp Center II framework on the psychologist's personal computer, unlimited scoring for the duration of this published edition is available. This will be replaced by the Q–global (Pearson, 2021) web-based scoring whenever the WIAT–4 is published. Pearson is estimating that the WIAT–4 will be published later in the fall of 2020 as evidenced by their advertising for advanced copy purchases. Both the WIAT–III Scoring Assistant (Pearson, 2009c) and web-based Q–Global (Pearson, 2021) scoring provides rapid and efficient computer scoring, including all relevant difference score comparisons such as the AAD analyses.

Next discussed are the data tables for reporting and interpreting WIAT–III score results within a psychological assessment report. First reviewed are the reporting and interpreting of the achievement test results independently without the addition of intelligence test data so as to (a) most effectively familiarize readers with this instrument, and (b) show its most common uses. Subsequently, the application of the WIAT–III within the context of AAD analyses is illustrated, which may be necessitated when testing for SLDs in individuals with exceptional aptitudes.

Interpretation

The WIAT–III is a complex test battery in the sense that it contains multiple subtests that are applicable to different grade ranges. This is due to the fact that the narrowly defined subtest skills may not be part of the formal curriculum at different grade levels. For example, students do not typically begin to compose essays and complete multiplication in earnest until the 3rd grade. Therefore, Essay Composition and Math Fluency–Multiplication are not administered to children in pre-kindergarten (PK) through 2nd grade. Similarly, the majority of children are capable of writing the entire alphabet within 30 seconds by 3rd grade (Pearson-PsychCorp, 2009b, p. 43). Therefore, the Alphabet Writing Fluency subtest is not administered to students enrolled in 6th grade for example due to likely ceiling effects, which contributes little to diagnosis.

Fortunately, the organization of the subtests and composite scales are such that they may be dichotomized into data tables for examinees at the following two levels: (a) PK (see Form 8.1a); and (b) Kindergarten (K) through 12th grade (see Form 8.2a). Consistent with manual recommendations, adults are to be classified in the latter grouping and at the 12th grade (Pearson-PsychCorp, 2009/2010, Appendix l., p. 551). The ensuing two sections present the WIAT–III data tables for each of these grade levels as opposed to the type of score as was done for the intelligence tests in the prior chapter. To expedite description of the process, a flowchart outlining the major phases in the process is presented in Figure 8.1, which is available on Routledge's e-resources website for download and reference thereafter. Notice that the structural organization of the achievement construct mirrors that for the intelligence construct discussed in Chapter 7. In fact, the same three strata levels can be used, with Total Achievement at Stratum III, the broad-based achievement composites at Stratum II (which are accordant with DSM–5 learning disorder subtypes), and the narrowly defined subtest skills at Stratum I (which are accordant with the DSM–5 learning disorder subskills). The overall process is also virtually the same with the single exception of an option to engage in formal analysis of intraindividual subtest scores. This is because a *pattern of strengths and weaknesses (PSW)* supplemental approach to detecting learning disabilities is an acceptable practice, especially in the field of education (see IDEA, 2004; McGrew, LaForte, & Schrank, 2014; see also later in this chapter).

WIAT–III ACHIEVEMENT TEST (PRE-KINDERGARTEN)

The data tables in Form 8.1a are intended for reporting and interpreting the WIAT–III achievement scores for examinees at the PK level, irrespective of whether or not they are actually matriculating through a pre-academic program. Table 1 provides rows for the Total Achievement scale and the Oral Language composite, which are the

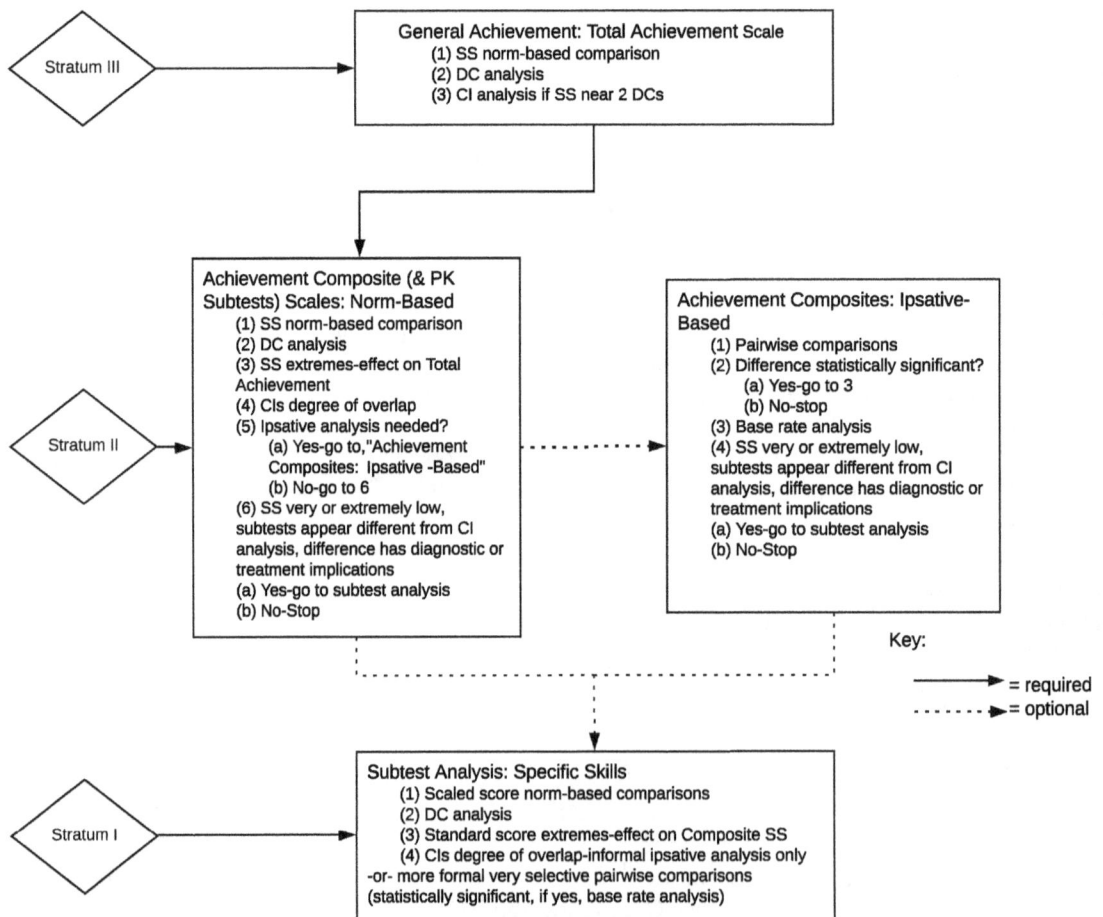

Note. SS = standard score; DC = descriptive classification (i.e., nominal categorical data); CI = confidence interval (i.e., the likelihood of an examinee's true score falling within a specified range); PK = pre-kindergarten. Norm-based = an examinee's scores compared to a representative sample of same-aged peers (i.e., age-corrected scores). Stratum (pl. = strata) = levels of a complex construct that form a hierarchical model, proceeding from most general at the top (i.e., Stratum III) to most specific at the bottom (i.e., Stratum I). Ipsative-based = intraindividual or within person comparisons of an examinee's scores that identify relative strengths and weaknesses.

Figure 8.1 Wechsler Individual Achievement Test, Third Edition (WIAT–III) Basic Interpretive Process

only two available at this grade level. There are six columns going across Table 1 (see Form 8.1a), including scale name, SS, 95% CI, PR, descriptive classification, and the measured skills. Proceeding from general to specific and in a norm-based fashion (see Figure 8.1, Stratum III, top box), the overall achievement descriptive classification that is associated with the SS should be interpreted first, including the 95% CI and PR. The pre-drafted narrative statements that follow Table 1 can be used to guide this interpretive process. Of vital importance is the diagnostic threshold for a SLD; namely a SS equal to or less than 78, with an associated PR equal to or less than 7. This can be located in each table that enumerates any WIAT–III scale's SS, CI, and PR (see Tables 1–2, Form 8.1a). If the Total Achievement data reaches the diagnostic threshold, this should be emphasized by stating the likelihood of finding one or more SLDs among the subsequent data. In other words, although a diagnostically low Total Achievement score does not specify in which and how many academic areas are affected due to its being excessively broad, it does indicate that one or more SLDs are most likely to be detected as the data are successively interpreted.

Next, the Oral Language composite should be interpreted in the same manner, followed by an added comparison with the Total Achievement score. Note that the SS range, PR, standard deviation units from the mean, and associated descriptive classifications are listed in Table 8.1 in order to facilitate test interpretation, although the aforementioned computer scoring automatically provides such information, along with the examiner's manual (Pearson, 2009a). Again, if the OL composite reaches the diagnostic threshold for a SLD, this is sufficient for a diagnosis of a learning-related disorder because these data come from a composite score and thus at the domain level. This interpretation should be highlighted with a recommendation to investigate the subtests that contributed to it; this for identifying specific subskills that describe the disorder in more detail (see Table 2). In terms of DSM–5 psychopathology, the correct diagnosis here would be a language disorder (see Chapter 4).

Next, Table 2 presents the PK subtests, including the first two listed that contribute to the OL composite. These are designated with the initials "OL" appended to the subtest name. In Figure 8.1 (see Routledge's e-resources website), this refers to the solid arrow proceeding from the top box at Stratum III to the left-middle box at Stratum II. Notice that in Figure 8.1, the PK subtests are in parentheses and enter the process at this early juncture because there are so few broad-based and narrow achievement skills available for measuring at this pre-academic level. The fact that all WIAT–III scales use the same score metrics also makes analysis of both composites and subtests in the same table possible. In any case, Table 2 scores should principally be interpreted in a norm-based manner, noting the functioning level of each skill by its descriptive classification, then determining if any skill area reaches or exceeds the diagnostic threshold for a SLD. After all, this is the primary reason for administering an achievement test. Because these are subtests, they represent specific skill areas (i.e., subskills using DSM–5 language) versus broad-based, Stratum II, academic domains. Therefore, a SLD would not be diagnosed on the basis of a subtest alone, although the impairment and risk for later SLD in that area should be noted. For example, if a 4-year-old examinee earned a SS of 75 on Math Problem Solving, the impairment in that subskill would be noted, along with the risk for a SLD in mathematics later in development. As will become apparent subsequently, SLDs should be made when one or more of the WAIT–III composite scales are below the diagnostic threshold because they are the most felicitous representatives of a specified academic area of impairment as set out in the DSM–5.

Next, ipsative analysis can be done informally among the subtests by examining the degree of overlap among the various CIs. It is most efficient to begin with the subtests that are most discrepant from each other and work toward those with increasing degrees of overlap. Because PSWs analyses are more relevant to interpreting achievement test

Table 8.1 Wechsler Individual Achievement Test, Third Edition (WIAT–III) Descriptive Classification Guide

Standard Scores	Percentile Rank Range[ab]	Standard Deviations from the Mean[c]	Descriptive Classification
146 to 160	99.89 to 99.99	+3.05 to +3.75	Very superior
131 to 145	98.00 to 99.87	+2.05 to +3.00	Superior
116 to 130	86.00 to 98.00	+1.05 to +2.00	Above average
85 to 115	16.00 to 84.00	−1.00 to +1.00	Average
70 to 84	2.00 to 14.00	−2.00 to−1.05	Below average
55 to 69	0.13 to 2.00	−3.00 to −2.05	Low
40 to 54	0.01 to 0.11	−3.70 to −3.05	Very low

Source. Adapted from Pearson-PsychCorp. (2009a). *Wechsler Individual Achievement Test–Third Edition (WIAT–III): Examiner's manual.* San Antonio, TX: Author, Table 4.1, p. 81.

Note. Standard score mean = 100, standard deviation = 15, range 40 to 160. [a]Derived from the theoretical standard normal distribution. [b]Gaps and tied values due to rounding error. [c]Rounded up when the same standard score was associated with different values.

data in search of potential learning disabilities, formal pairwise comparisons are more frequently done especially between any two subtests that appear to be discrepant upon initial examination (i.e., Cis with little or no overlap). Although there are too many permutations to cover all potential data patterns, some pre-drafted narrative excepts following Table 2 have been inserted that can help guide some of the most common interpretive outcomes, especially those pertinent to whether or not the data reach the DSM–5 diagnostic threshold for SLDs.

Finally, Table 3 in Form 8.1a is designed for reporting and interpreting subtest level scores differences. Each row presents an independent and specific pairwise comparison. In the aggregate, all possible pairwise comparisons are presented in the table. Therefore, the examiner can selectively interpret only those that are most pertinent to the case, either according to the stated diagnostic issues and/or the unfolding data pattern, and either deleting or entering double dashes within the unused portions. As can be seen, the table is organized as in previous tests, including the first score, second score, obtain or computed difference (with or without an appended asterisk to denote significance status), the critical value (i.e., the number designating the threshold for a significant result), and base rate (i.e., the percent of the norm reference sample that manifested the obtained difference score). In Figure 8.1, the focus now is at the juncture in which the broken arrow proceeds from the left box at Stratum II down to the "Subtest Analysis: Specific Skills" box. Most of the directives in that lowest box (viz., 1, 2, and 3) have already been done by virtue of the PK subtests being analyzed at Stratum II due to the paucity of broad-based composite scales and specific subtests. Hence, the only directive that applies is (4) where it instructs the reporting and interpreting of selective formal pairwise comparisons among the subtests.

Although the WIAT–III permits the use of either .05 or .01 as the critical value to rule out chance as an explanation for the score differences (i.e., the hypothesis test alpha level), it is preferable to use the more conservative .01 as a guard against the accumulating *familywise* (or *experimentwise*) *error rate* for multiple hypotheses tests done in the same overall analysis. The base rates are designed to record values with up to one decimal place, with "greater than or equal to" and "less than or equal to" signs to insert quickly. The interpretation scheme for the base rates continues to employ the evolving criteria proposed over the years by Sattler (2001, 2014 and Sattler & Ryan, 2009) as follows: $n \leq 15\%$ = unusual; $n \leq 10\%$ = abnormal; and $n \leq 5\%$ = rare and profoundly abnormal. Recall that they should only be interpreted when statistically significant, otherwise the examiner will be interpreting an effect size that does not reflect a true or real difference, which violates statistical logic and should not be done.

WIAT–III ACHIEVEMENT TEST (KINDERGARTEN THROUGH GRADE 12 AND ADULTHOOD)

This analysis concerns any examinee who is enrolled in Kindergarten through Grade 12, and thereafter extending through adulthood to age 50 years 11 months. For such analysis, all of Figure 8.1 now applies (see Routledge's e-resources), with many more measured broad-based and more narrowly defined skills being measured as part of the formal curriculum. It is extremely consistent with the Wechsler intelligence test organizational structure and analysis, with the exception of norm-based comparisons with the DSM–5 diagnostic threshold for designating the presence of a SLD, and (b) more emphasis on ipsative score differences. Before delving into all of the interpretive facets, the principal focus is on whether or not each (a) broad-based academic composite, and (b) specific subtest area exhibit a *SS* of 78 or less, and an accompanying PR of 7 or less; the former for making a SLD diagnosis and the latter for listing specific subskills that are especially showing significant levels of impairment. Because all of the competing variables that could explain low average achievement should have been ruled out by previous assessment information (e.g., clinical interview, mental status examination, previous test scores), the single remaining criteria are the aforementioned *SS* and PR scores. Of course, it can rapidly become much more complicated considering all of the data and the various approaches for detecting whether or not a learning disability is present. That is why it is imperative to remain focused on the rather parsimonious quantitative threshold promulgated by the DSM–5, at least from a mental health perspective.

Thus, starting at the top of Figure 8.1 with the Total Achievement, and Table 1 in Form 8.2a, is the *SS* 78 or below and PR 7 or below? If yes, the interpretation should reflect the likely presence of one or more SLDs among the remaining data. If negative, this should be interpreted as such, although this fact alone does not necessarily rule out SLDs, especially if there exists remarkable variability among the composite scores. Hence, this possibility should be left open. A beginning narrative paragraph has been drafted in Form 8.2a following Table 1, which guides the examiner through interpretation of the Total Achievement, including whether the threshold for a suspected learning disorder was exceeded. If there is a shortage of time for report generation, reporting and interpreting the Total Achievement score can actually be deleted so that interpretation can immediately begin with the Stratum II domain composite scores that are the prime focus of diagnosis.[4]

Once the Total Achievement has been interpreted (or omitted), analysis moves to Stratum II; that is, the norm-based analysis of each composite scale. Hence, in Figure 8.1 (see Routledge's e-resources), progress is from the top box down the solid arrow to the box titled, "Achievement Composite (& PK Subtests) Scales: Norm-Based". Here, it must be determined if any of the composites fall below threshold. In Form 8.2a, interpretive statements that immediately follow Table 1 address any composites that exceeded or did not exceed the diagnostic threshold for SLD, which can be copied and repeated for as many composites that manifested the same result. Asterisks are to be appended to any SSs that are significant for a SLD in order to aid interpretation (including that for the Total Achievement if included). In the event all composites result in normal functioning, an interpretive statement has been composed to that effect following the positive result versions. Note that Table 1 provides key definitions for many of the reported statistics, including the meaning of CI and PR, which is also explained in the narrative interpretation. Hence, the table is drafted for individuals of varying degrees of sophistication. For example, laypeople will likely rely upon the descriptive classifications and narrative interpretations while other psychologists will likely rely only upon the numbers within the table, especially the SSs and CIs.

Ipsative differences among the composites are more pertinent when dealing with achievement scores. Hence, the criteria for making formal pairwise comparisons among the composites are relaxed and easier to meet. More specifically, such comparisons should be pursued even if Cis are only moderately separated. This examination is portrayed in Figure 8.1 (e-resources) by the broken arrow proceeding from the left box at Stratum II to the right box at the same level titled, "Achievement Composites: Ipsative-Based." Table 2 in Form 8.2a is designed for all possible pairwise comparisons, although there should be some discretion as to which are the most relevant to the case in order to keep the familywise error rate to a minimum. This table is organized exactly like Table 3 in Form 8.1a, thus the reader can refer back to this discussion for specifics. The only difference is that the comparisons are among composite scores versus subtest scores, although they work the same. Pre-drafted narrative statements are offered after Table 2 to help structure the interpretation. Remember that base rates are not to be reported for score differences that are not deemed to be statistically significant.

Finally, the examiner has the option of reporting and interpreting data at the most specific level of analysis at Stratum I, the WIAT–III subtests that contribute to the broad-based composite academic areas. The reason these data are not frequently reported and interpreted is that they are not necessary for a DSM–5 diagnosis. Recall that the DSM–5 has integrated all prior subtypes of learning disorders into one unified category (viz., specific learning disorder), with the subsequent need to (a) specify the academic domain that is impaired for a diagnostic code (viz., F81.0 with impairment in reading; F81.81 with impairment in written expression, and F81.2 with impairment in mathematics), along with (b) the subskills within each domain that are compromised. (e.g., spelling accuracy). This diagnostic hierarchy has direct parallels with the structural organization observed in Figure 8.1 showing the WIAT–III levels. Specifically, the DSM–5 unified or single diagnostic class of specific learning disorder symbolizes the WIAT–III Total Achievement scale, the DSM–5 specified academic domains symbolize the WIAT–III composite scales (e.g., Mathematics), and the DSM–5 subskills symbolize the WIAT–III subtests specific skills (e.g., Reading Comprehension). The principal point is that the WIAT–III composite scales are sufficient for identifying the specific DSM–5 academic domain that is impaired for purposes of diagnosis. Going further in order to enumerate the subskills that are showing dysfunction no doubt assists in treatment planning, although is not requisite to make the diagnosis. Because testing time in mental health is so very limited, the focus tends to be on making an accurate diagnosis.

The major exception to this rule is when (a) there exists no overlap between the Cis of two subtests, (b) the subtests contribute to the same composite scale, and (c) the composite scale is below threshold and therefore positive for a SLD. In such case, only certain specific skills within a composite may be impaired. Therefore, reporting the SSs, PRs, and Cis of these subtests for both norm-based and ipsative comparisons can avert over-diagnosis; that is, stating that a broad academic domain is impaired when, in fact, the dysfunction is more limited to a subclass of academic skills within that domain. Other than this, however, identifying the general domain of academic dysfunction is typically sufficient. For such reporting and interpretation, Tables 3 (Oral Language subtests), Table 4 (Reading subtests), Table 5 (Written Expression subtests), Table 6 (Mathematics subtests), and Table 7 (Math Fluency subtests) are provided. Note that they are in the same order that their companion composites appear in Table 1. Also, each table has narrative excerpts following each table in order to facilitate the interpretive process. Next examined are the data tables that have been prepared in the event an AAD analysis is desired.

ABILITY ACHIEVEMENT DISCREPANCY (AAD) ANALYSIS: GENERAL COMMENTS

As indicated prior, the most frequent use of an achievement test within mental health practice would be to rule out DSM–5 SLDs and language disorder, the latter being classified under the communication disorders. Although DSM–5 has simplified the criteria for such diagnosis (i.e., $SS \leq 78$, $PR \leq 7$), an AAD should be done when an examinee is assessed as likely possessing either extreme of intellectual functioning; in particular, about 2 standard deviations or more above or below the mean of 100, hence, with a *SD* being 15 points, that would be SSs of 70 and 130 (i.e., $100 \pm [15 \times 2]$). In the case of low IQ, an examinee can score below the SLD criteria due to the presence of impaired cognitive function, hence resulting in a false positive learning disorder interpretation. At the other extreme, the examinee can score significantly above the SLD criteria due to gifted intelligence, hence appear to have no such learning difficulties. Both erroneous results are termed false negative interpretations. In either case, a fallacious decision has been made.

Elsewhere, achievement testing has been referred to as "high stakes" assessment (see, e.g., Vars, 2001) due to the fact that quite frequently major decisions are made based upon outcomes. For example, having a diagnosis of a SLD makes a student eligible for special interventions and accommodations without which academic underachievement or failure is a likely outcome. Therefore, all reasonable strategies should be undertaken to avoid such costly errors in this area of psychological testing. It is advisable to add a co-normed IQ test to the achievement test battery so as to perform an AAD as a control for the possible confounding effects of extreme intellectual functioning (either high or low). *Co-norming* is a process whereby two different measures are administered and standardized as one unit on the same norm reference sample. Co-norming eliminates error associated with comparing scores from two different samples. Stated another way, co-norming yields difference scores (i.e., achievement minus intelligence) that are based upon the same sample of individuals, hence rendering them as more accurate compared to being derived from two independent samples.

The WIAT–III is co-normed with all of the most recently published Wechsler intelligence tests presented in Chapter 7. Namely, they consist of the following: (a) *Wechsler Preschool and Primary Scale of Intelligence, Fourth Edition* (*WPPSI–IV*; Wechsler, 2012a, 2012b); (b) *Wechsler Intelligence Scale for Children, Fifth Edition* (*WISC–V*; Wechsler, 2014a, 2014b); and (c) *Wechsler Adult Intelligence Scale, Fourth Edition* (*WAIS–IV*; Wechsler, 2008a, 2008b). Because the WPPSI–IV has two forms (i.e., ages 2 years 6 months to 3 years 11 months [younger version], and 4 years 0 months to 7 years 7 months [older version]), there are a total of four AAD data tables.

More specifically, the following four results and interpretation tables are reviewed in this section in detail: (a) WPPSI–IV (younger version)/WIAT–III Ability Achievement Discrepancy Analysis (Form 8.3); (b) WPPSI–IV (older version)/WIAT–III Ability Achievement Discrepancy

Analysis (Form 8.4); (c) WISC–V/WIAT–III Ability Achievement Discrepancy Analysis (Form 8.5); and (d) WAIS–IV/WIAT–III Ability Achievement Discrepancy Analysis (Form 8.6). For purposes of brevity, these forms will be discussed simultaneously while inserting comments on germane differences when warranted. This is made possible due to both their data and analytic process being so similar. In fact, a flowchart has been designed in Figure 8.2 that takes the reader through the AAD interpretive procedure using the co-normed Wechsler tests. Again, this figure is available for download on Routledge's e-resources website for reference through the ensuing discussion.

Some prelusory comments are in order. Note that all of these results and interpretation tables include the entire complement of tests, composites, and subtests necessary to indicate whether or not a SLD or language disorder exists. This obviates the need to search for and insert additional tables from separate report forms. However, the testing psychologist may delete some of the auxiliary data for purposes of brevity. Such data are identified in the ensuing discussion. Additionally, succinct narrative excerpts have been inserted between tables as done in previous report forms, which serve to guide interpretation of the tabular score results. Of course, these can be modified or deleted depending upon the case facts.

THE AAD DATA TABLES FOR CO-NORMED WECHSLER TESTS

The analysis begins by selecting the intelligence test composite score which most accurately measures an examinee's cognitive competence. This score is used to quantitatively compute an examinee's expected level of achievement across the academic abilities measured. The Full Scale IQ (FSIQ) score as representative of the *g* factor is the most frequently utilized for this purpose. In fact, because there has yet to be an instance where an alternate IQ score would be a more felicitous choice (e.g., the Verbal Comprehension Index or VCI), the added tables previously used have been dropped to assist in making such decisions (see Spores, 2012, pp. 76–79). Even in cases where there is a significant verbal-nonverbal discrepancy, the FSIQ is the most reliable, valid, and stable measure that the intelligence test has to offer. Hence, one would be hard pressed not to select this score as the single predictor of an individual's level of expected achievement. In Figure 8.2 (see e-resources), this initial decision is denoted at "Step 1," wherein the FSIQ as representing the *g* factor is reported and interpreted in the typical norm-based manner.

In Forms 8.3 through 8.6, Table 1 is designed to begin such preliminary analysis of the intelligence test data, although only including the bolded FSIQ score results. If the examiner finds occasion to supplant the FSIQ with an alternative IQ score, it can be inserted here in lieu of the former. In such instance, however, the measured ability and some of the table notes must be modified. Narrative excerpts of Table 1 follow to help guide the norm-based interpretive process. Note that no other IQ scores are reported. Although it seems somewhat of a waste not to include more results here, it will become apparent that the AAD analysis yields an extremely large set of numbers that can rapidly become unwieldy for the reader and detract from the core results. Hence, continued efforts should be made to maintain as much brevity as possible when interpreting an AAD.

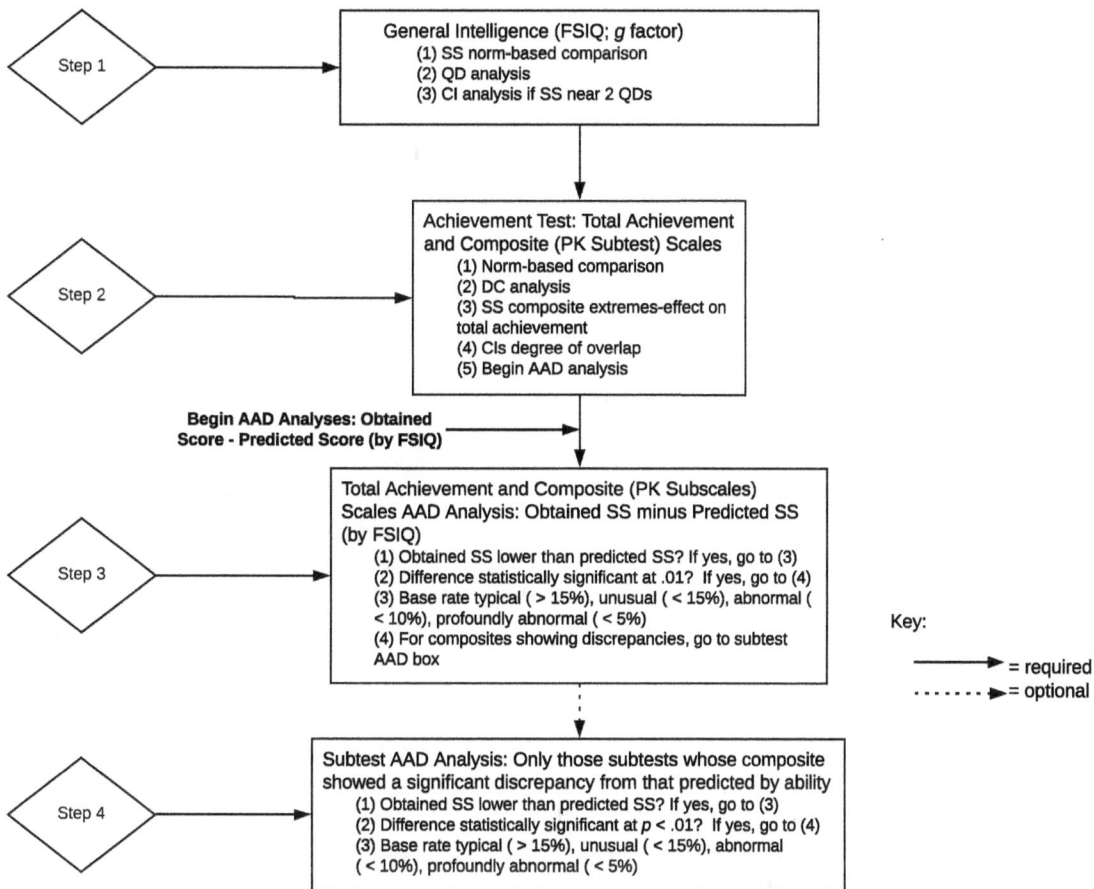

Figure 8.2 Wechsler Ability-Achievement Discrepancy (AAD) Analysis

Following Figure 8.2, the analysis moves to "Step 2," where the WIAT–III Total Achievement and composite scales are reported and interpreted in a typical norm-based manner. The purpose is to provide an inquiry of how the examinee's achievement in broad domains of functioning compare to same age peers, which sets the framework for subsequent ability-achievement comparisons. Of course, the PK structure is somewhat different in that the Oral Language composite is reported with the Total Achievement in Table 2, and a Table 3 has been added so as to include the PK subtests that are properly separated from the more broad-based scores. Recall that PK subtests are reported simply due to the paucity of academic skills that are not yet part of the preschool curriculum. The subtests could be listed with the Total Achievement and Oral Language composite in the same table to reduce the sheer number of tables in the report form, although conflating the two was to be avoided due to the fact that a discrepant specific skill area is in itself insufficient for a SLD diagnosis. Note that the AAD analysis has not yet begun at this juncture, although the preliminary data has prepared the way for such analyses. Following Table 2, pre-drafted interpretive statements have once again been inserted that guide the achievement total and composite norm-based interpretations.

In Figure 8.1 (see e-resources), "Step 3" initiates the AAD analysis in earnest. In actuality, the WIAT–III employs two statistical methods in computing the AAD analyses as follows: (a) simple difference; and (b) predicted difference. First, *simple difference discrepancy analyses* are obtained by subtracting the selected intelligence test composite score from each *actual* (or obtained) WIAT–III standard score. Because it is a more straightforward analysis, it is most easily comprehended by those unfamiliar with psychometrics and statistical analyses. However, the major problem with this method is that it does not adjust for regression to the mean; hence, it contains a larger error component. Briefly, regression to the mean is a well-known phenomenon in statistics in which an individual's subsequent score is most likely to move (or regress) toward the center of the distribution where most scores are located (i.e., at the mean or central tendency). Simply taking an individual's FSIQ does not adjust for this tendency to regress; that is, it is taken at face value. After all, an attempt is being made here to predict an individual's subsequent score by using one that is already completed. However, the linear regression formula does make predictions that tend to fall toward the distribution center, especially for extreme scores. As a consequence, although the simple difference method was previously included in the forms as an option, it has been omitted in favor of accuracy.

Predicted difference discrepancy analyses are computed by subtracting each WIAT–III standard score *predicted* by the selected intelligence test composite score from the *actual* WIAT–III standard score earned by the examinee. In Forms 8.4, 8.5, and 8.6, Table 3 begins the predicted difference analysis concerning the WIAT–III Total Achievement and composite scores. The PK AAD begins at Table 4, including only the Total Achievement and Oral Language composite. The organization of these tables represents the key facets of the predicted difference AAD method and will be explicated in a fair amount of detail. First, the tabular organization is comparable in many respects to tables that examine statistically significant differences and base rates for composite and subtest pairwise comparisons, although there are some differences. There are six columns in all going across the table. The first column identifies the scale being analyzed. The second column lists the actual score obtained by the examinee during testing. The third column lists the WIAT–III score predicted by means of the examinee's selected ability score; most frequently the FSIQ or the general intelligence *g* factor. Column four is the difference score resulting from the obtained score minus the predicted score. This order of subtraction was chosen because the sign indicates whether or not the obtained score is above or below the predicted score. For example, if the difference score is positive or a value of "0" resulting in no sign, it means that the obtained score is above or equal to the predicted score, which automatically rules out a discrepancy diagnostic of a SLD. In contrast, a negative difference score indicates that the obtained score is below the predicted score, which means that the result is in the direction of a possible SLD. What remains is a hypothesis test on the negative difference, which was chosen to be at the most conservative .01 level to minimize the familywise error rate due to multiple hypotheses tests done within the same study or case. The value that begins the rejection range for the hypothesis test is listed in the fifth column. Lastly, if the negative difference is statistically significant, a base rate should be reported and interpreted according to the scheme used for all previous base rate analyses. Lastly, for nonsignificant results, a double-dash should be entered into the base rate column, which is defined in the general table notes.

Immediately following the table, narrative statements have been inserted that guide interpretation of the tabular data. The first version is for interpreting consistent negative results; that is, interpreting no significant results in the negative deficit direction. The second version lists all of the significant negative differences between the obtained and predicted WIAT–III total and composite scores, including the base rate result in order to communicate effect sizes (i.e., how severe is the deficit). Because these are broad-based composite scales, significant deficits may be interpreted as positive for a SLD in that academic domain. Base rates should not be reported where the difference is not statistically significant in the negative direction. Rather, a double dash symbol (i.e., —"--") should be inserted, which is defined in the general table notes. Any comparisons not in need of reporting should simply be deleted, although typically they are not all reported.

Finally, Step 4 in Figure 8.2 is an optional AAD for the WIAT–III subtest standard scores. The AAD for the PK subtests are listed in Table 5 of Form 8.3, whereas for the older three Forms 8.4, 8.5, and 8.6, they are listed in Table 4. The difference in table number is due to the added PK table that is designed for subtest norm-based analyses, which is not necessary for the older forms due to the much greater number of academic domain composite scales that are available. In any case, this AAD subtest table is designed in the exact same manner as is done for the AAD academic composite scales. It is important to recall that any significant differences here do not constitute SLDs in and of themselves because they represent narrowly defined skills or subskills. Although the DSM–5 encourages embellishing the SLD diagnosis with a listing of impaired subskills (i.e., as symbolized by deficits manifested among the WIAT–III subtests), they are not mandatory and can be listed in their absence.

It should be reiterated that the three older AAD Forms 8.4 through 8.6 do not include tables for norm-based subtest analyses. The objective here is to curtail the report and help focus the analysis on the composites and the AAD. Consider that if all the subtest score tables were incorporated into the report, it would add four tables of data for a grand total of seven, including the lengthy AAD tables that present a voluminous set of scores. Of course, these tables can always be rapidly inserted into the report at the discretion of the examiner by copying them from Form 8.2a and pasting them into any of the older ADD Forms 12.4, 12.5, and 12.6.

SUMMARY

This section reviewed the manner in which the WIAT–III achievement data can be reported and interpreted within a psychological assessment and testing report. The initial focus was on analyzing whether the data surpassed the quantitative threshold established by the DSM–5 for diagnosing a SLD. This was done by dichotomizing the data into a PK version and a K through Grade 12 version (with adults up to age 50 years 0 months being assigned to the latter). However, the DSM–5 takes the position that a SLD can be diagnosed as comorbid with ID when the learning difficulties clearly exceed that which can be accounted for by the assessed degree of impaired intelligence. This indicates the continuing need for an AAD analysis in cases where the examinee's intelligence is evaluated as likely falling at either extreme end of the intellectual functioning spectrum. For this reason, Four Forms were presented for purposes of reporting and interpreting an AAD analysis, which covered the entire age range of the WIAT–III (i.e., 4 to 50 years, inclusive). The predicted-difference method was selected for all such analyses because it adjusts for regression to the mean, hence making the computed difference score more accurate.

Next introduced is the Wechsler Individual Achievement Test, Fourth Edition (WIAT–4; Breaux, 2020a, 2020b, 2020c; NCS Pearson, 2020), which published during the final months of preparing this manuscript. Because there has been a relative paucity of research on this newest edition of the WIAT, only its most fundamental data will be presented. For comprehensive and in-depth analyses, such as cases that require AAD examinations, it is advisable to continue with the WIAT–III, at minimum for 6 to 12 months in order to afford sufficient time for some research to be completed concerning the qualities of the WIAT–4, including reliability, validity, and utility.

Wechsler Individual Achievement Test, Fourth Edition

Synopsis

The *Wechsler Individual Achievement Test, Fourth Edition* (*WIAT–4*; Breaux, 2020a, 2020b, 2020c; NCS Pearson, 2020) is an individually administered test designed to measure the academic skills of people ranging in age from 4 years 0 months to 50 years 11 months. This covers a grade range from preschool (PK) through 12th grade and is a revision of the WIAT–III covered in detail prior.

The entire instrument consists of 20 subtests that together measure reading, written expression, and mathematical skills, along with listening and speaking skills. However, the examiner has wide discretion in selecting which of the available areas of achievement and related skill areas to measure. Of diagnostic relevance, the WIAT–4 continues to cover all eight specific learning disability domains specified by IDEA (2004) and the three disorders enumerated in the DSM–5. Next, the organizational structure of the WIAT–4 is covered, which identifies the core and supplemental data.

Test Structure

The WIAT–4 can be divided by type of data (i.e., core versus supplemental) and grade (i.e., PK versus K–12). First, the core data are comprised of Total Achievement, Reading, Written Expression, and Mathematics, while the supplemental data include reading-related skills (e.g., Decoding), Academic Fluency, Language Processing, and a new Dyslexia Index. The core data pertain to detecting SLDs. The supplemental data are relevant to skills that are associated with the major academic areas of achievement, most especially communication and language disorders.

For preschoolers, the WIAT–4 offers three core subtests that measure narrowly defined skills in reading, written expression, and mathematics, and that contribute to a Total Achievement score. They are Word Reading, Alphabet Writing Fluency, and Math Problem Solving. Because there is only one subtest per basic academic skill area, this leaves room for adding some potentially informative supplemental data when testing this young population. First, adding the Phonemic Proficiency (see below) subtest permits the computation of a *Dyslexia Index*, which functions as a screening measure for such neurodevelopmental problem. Furthermore, adding Listening Comprehension and Oral Expression subtests provides an Oral Language composite for the detection of a language disorder. Hence, a total of six subtests permit the early detection of potential disorders in reading writing, mathematics, language (i.e., expressive and receptive communication), and dyslexia. When testing preschoolers, all six of these subtests are typically administered to maximize the utility of this measure, although if time is circumscribed, then administering the three core subtests is a viable alternative.

Regarding Grades K through 12 (and adulthood; hereafter simply K–12), the core data consist of a Total Achievement score, three composites (i.e., Reading, Written Expression, and Mathematics), and seven subtests. The Reading composite includes Word Reading and Reading Comprehension, both of which are also found on the WIAT–III. The Written Expression composite is comprised of Spelling, Sentence Composition (Grades 2–12), and Essay Composition (Grades 4–12), along with Alphabet Writing Fluency (Grades K–1). Auxiliary data for this older group are much more diverse and include the following supplemental composites: Basic Reading, Decoding, Reading Fluency, Math Fluency, Writing Fluency, Oral Language, Phonological Processing, Orthographic Processing, and the Dyslexia Index. Next reviewed is the core and supplemental composites for this older group. Thereafter, the WIAT–4 will be presented as the other tests in terms of the standardization sample, administration, the data yield, and interpretation.

First, the Reading composite supplants the Total Reading composite of the WIAT–III, which is more straightforward and yields a more effective balance between word-level and text-level reading skills. Second, the Written Expression composite measures overall written expression skills by employing more age-appropriate subtests, including various combination of spelling, building sentences, combining sentences, alphabet writing accuracy and speed, and essay writing, each depending on the examinee's grade level. Third, the Mathematics composite is unmodified from that of the WIAT–III, which includes math reasoning and computational skills. All three contribute to an Achievement Total composite, which is used to measure PSWs in comparison to the three contributing composites. Therefore, for both the PK and K–12 versions, the Total Achievement composite represents a balance among reading, writing, and math skills.

Concerning the older-age WIAT–4 version, if case facts and insurance preauthorization (PA) permit, the Dyslexia Index and Oral Language composites may be added to the core battery. First, the Dyslexia Index composite can be added, which consists of Word Reading and Phonemic Proficiency for Grades K through 3, and Word Reading, Pseudoword Decoding, and Orthographic Fluency for Grades 4 through 12. These subtests were chosen by the developers because were best at discriminating individuals with and without a confirmed diagnosis of dyslexia within these grade-level cohorts (Breaux, 2020c, p. 114). The Oral Language composite consists of the Listening Comprehension and Oral Expression subtests. The former is comprised of both receptive vocabulary and oral discourse comprehension, hence understanding language at the level of the word, sentence, and contextual passages. It is a composite that is directly pertinent to diagnosing a DSM–5 language disorder and is conceptualized as representing a vital foundation for building basic literacy skills despite it not representing a core area of achievement. Oral language also has been found to effectively estimate crystalized intelligence and is distinct from academic skills variables (see, e.g., Kaufman et al., 2012; Pearson. (2009b).

Concerning the other supplementary composites, Basic Reading measures phonological skills, phonic decoding, and single-word reading skills, analogous to the definition of basic reading provided in IDEA (2004). Decoding measures detextualized phonic decoding and word reading skills. Reading, Writing, and Math Fluency all measure speed within each subject area, with ancillary focus on accuracy. Phonological Processing measures two skills deemed to be necessary for *orthographic mapping*; that is, the formation of letter-sound connections needed to read words by sight, spell words from recall, and for building vocabulary. These include phonemic proficiency and *phonic decoding* (i.e., responding orally to items that require the manipulation of sounds within words).

Norm Reference Sample

Standardization was initiated in October 2018 and continued through February 2020. Exclusionary criteria were those which were expected to deleteriously affect test performance and hence confound the normative data. These included lack of English as a primary language, uncorrected visual and hearing impairment, current hospitalization, neurological disorder, taking medications that could affect performance, and having taken an achievement test within the past 6 months.

The sample was stratified according to grade (i.e., for developing grade-based norms), age (i.e., for developing age-based norms), sex, race/ethnicity, education level, and geographic region; the latter three categories according to proportions reported in the 2018 U.S. Bureau of the Census (Ruggles et al., 2018). The grade-based norms consisted of 2,100 examinees enrolled in Grades PK through 12, including 150 students within each grade level. This sample was further apportioned into fall (i.e., August through November) and spring norms (i.e., March through July), each comprised of 1,050 students. Winter norms (i.e., December through February) were interpolated. Age-based norms consisted of 1,832 examinees aged 4 years 0 months through 50 years 11 months. Students were apportioned by 4-month age intervals between ages 4 through 12 years, 6-month intervals for age 13 years, 12-month intervals between 14 and 16 years, 3-year-intervals for ages 17 through 19 years, and multi-year intervals for the 20- through 30-year and 31- through 50-year cohorts. A total of 120 individuals were in each age group from 4 through 19 years, along with 100 and 52 people in the two oldest age groups, respectively.

Sex was distributed evenly among all apportioned grade and age groups. Race/ethnicity consisted of five groups, including African American, Asian, Hispanic, White, and Other. For examinees aged 4 through 19 years, education level was determined by the number of completed years of education earned by parents or guardians. If two parents were available, the average was computed and rounded up to the nearest average age levels. For examinees 20 through 50 years, self-educational level was used. Education level was apportioned as follows: (a) [1]2th grade or less; (b) high school graduate or equivalent; (c) some college or associate degree. Finally, the United States was divided into the following four geographic regions: Midwest; Northeast; South; and West. Hence, the WIAT–4 norm reference sample was stratified very much akin to that of the WIAT–III, of course with the major exception that the new norms are updated to match the U.S. population of individuals Grades PK though 12 and ages 4 through 50 years. Of note, use of the WIAT–4 in the mental health field should routinely use age-based norms because grade norms can include older students who have been retained, thus potentially increasing the average age for any particular grade level.

Administration

From the previous description, the fact that the WIAT–4 offers a multitude of subtests and composites to choose from in measuring various aspects of achievement should be conspicuous, especially for the older K–12 version. In fact, if an examiner were to administer all grade level subtests appropriate for an older student, it would take an estimated 130 minutes. This would require a 2½ to 3-hour testing appointment and would work to exceed the typical amount of units insurance carriers would approve for such testing. The point is that the examiner should be selective in the number of subtests and composites administered to an examinee when using this new instrument. Hence, this section first discusses which subtests and composites to select for younger and older clients, along with the underlying rationale. This is ensued by discussing some general administrative rules, many of which are used for the WIAT–III such that this part can be condensed in the interests of saving space.

Subtest and Composite Selection

Each WIAT–4 core or supplemental composite consumes about 10 to 20 minutes depending upon the examinee's grade level, ability, and test-taking style, along with the examiner's style and experience. As will become apparent subsequently, all grade appropriate subtests should be administered when testing preschoolers with the PK version of the WIAT–4. This will yield a Total Achievement score, one subtest for each of the core academic areas (viz., Reading, Written Expression, and Mathematics), a Dyslexia Index composite, and an Oral Language composite. The administration manual estimates that this all will require about 45 minutes (Breaux, 2020a). Thus, a one-hour testing appointment should suffice when testing a preschooler with the WIAT–4 according to the above strategy.

As regarding the older WIAT–4 version (i.e., Grades K–12), at a minimum, the subtests required for computing the following core composites should be done: (a) Total Achievement; (b) Reading; (c) Written Expression; and (d) Mathematics. This will result in a data yield sufficient for detecting the three subtypes of DSM–5 SLDs, including the more specific skills within each of these areas. Applying the 10-to-20-minute estimated duration for each composite, this battery of subtests should take anywhere from 30 to 60 minutes (mean duration = 45 minutes). Again, a one-hour testing appointment should suffice.

If there are additional diagnostic issues related to possible dyslexia, which is commonly listed by referral sources, and/or language disorder, then the subtests required for the Dyslexia Index composite and the Oral Language composite should be incorporated, which will add 20 to 40 minutes to the core composites for a grand total of 50 to 100 minutes (mean duration = 75 minutes). In such case, a two-hour testing appointment would be needed. Although the WIAT–4 possesses many other supplemental composites and their more specific subtests, these measure constructs that are less relevant to making mental health diagnoses, at least from their initial description. As more gain experience using the WIAT–4, it is likely that more of its data will be found to be useful in addressing various types of referral questions.

Administrative Rules

The WIAT–4 espouses an *adaptive testing* approach in like manner to that of the WIAT–III, including start points, reverse rules, basals and ceilings, discontinue rules, and item sets with stop points. Start points are determined by the most recent grade level enrolled in or completed by the examinee. Reverse rules revert back toward easier items in the event the examinee has unexpected difficulty with the grade-level start point. A basal is established when the examinee obtains a predetermined number of consecutive passes, resulting in moving forward toward increasingly difficult items with the assumption that all previous items would be likewise passed and thus automatically awarded credit. Discontinues rules define a preselected number of consecutively failed items after which the subtest is terminated, again with the complementary assumption that all subsequent items would likewise be failed. This is known as a ceiling.

An item set represents a fixed grouping of items of approximate equal difficulty that are determined by grade-level start and stop points. Item sets are placed in order of increasing difficulty as is done for individual items on the more typical subtests, which is more conducive for testing certain skills; for example, the Reading Comprehension subtest wherein each passage is associated with a set of items of equivalent difficulty level, and subsequent passages increase in complexity.

Stop points instruct the examiner to terminate the subtest irrespective of the examinee's performance. This is because the total raw score for each item set must be weighted to account for the gradual increase in difficulty among the item sets.

To this point, the WIAT–4 should sound much like that of the WIAT–III. However, there are some notable differences. First, there is an increase in the number of subtests that are timed so as to emphasize the measurement of fluency within the major subject areas. In fact, nine subtest possess strict time limits. This is because fluency has been increasingly shown to represent a vital factor in various academic skills. For instance, contextual reading fluency uniquely accounts for a significant amount of the variance in reading comprehension, over and above that contributed to by both word reading and listening comprehension (Kim & Wagner, 2015). It is thought that being able to read at a rapid and smooth rate frees up information processing resources for understanding what one is reading. That is, if too much energy is being devoted to reading words, there is insufficient focus upon deciphering the meanings of the words in context, which reduces contextual reading comprehension.

Another difference is the design of the Record Form. In particular, the WIAT–III Record Form contains much of the verbatim administrative instructions to be given the examinee, while the new WIAT–4 Record Form no longer includes such information. Although this results in a cleaner looking Record Form (i.e., less congested with information), this precludes the ability to administer the test without continued reference to the Administrative Manual. There is also a significant increase in the number of audio files needed for WIAT–4 administration. Although these are all provided on a flash drive, they must be copied onto either a computer or smart phone and played for the examinee. This requires the repeated starting and stopping of the audio device, and the constant moving to different audio files for rapid and smooth administration, which can become cumbersome and tedious. Subtests that require playback as part of the administration process include Phonemic Proficiency, Listening Comprehension-Oral Discourse Comprehension, Pseudoword Decoding, and Decoding Fluency; the latter two for knowing the correct pronunciation to an item response, which facilitates accurate scoring.

In addition, Pseudoword Decoding and Word Reading previously listed the nonwords and words, respectively, on one plasticized card (front and back) for administration to the examinee. They are now printed in smaller groupings within the stimulus book, which actually requires more page turning that tends to hinder a smooth administration process. Finally, many of the subtests can now be administered electronically, including one of the supplementary subtests in which this is the only method of administration (i.e., Orthographic Choice). Electronic administration must be purchased from the publisher on the Q-Global (Pearson, 2021) platform.

Scoring

Not surprisingly, the WIAT–4 data yield is comparable to that of the WIAT–III (see Forms 12.1b and 12.2b), so much so that only a summary of the scores employed will be here provided, with some added focus on the qualitative descriptors that have been amended. First, standard scores (SS) are used for both the composites and subtests, with a mean of 100, standard deviation (SD) of 15, and range of 40 to 160. Confidence intervals (CIs) are the typical 90% and 95% degrees of certainty while percentile ranks (PRs) have a median of 50 and range of 1 to 99. Concerning descriptive categories, the WIAT–4 offers both a 10-point and 15-point system with varying facets, both of which vary from that of the WIAT–III, to which the discussion now focuses upon.

The 10-point system is the traditional scheme that affords increased discrimination towards the middle of the distribution of SSs. According to this scheme, approximately 50% of the sample falls at the center of the distribution and should be preferred when the examinee's scores largely fall between −2 and +2 SDs from the mean. Table 8.2 displays the 10-point classification system in the first two columns. It should be obvious that this is the exact scheme currently espoused by the Wechsler IQ tests (see Chapter 11, Table 11.2). In contrast, the 15-point system relies upon the 15-point SD to define its categories wherein the average range spans from 85 to 115 and captures the middle 68% of the score distribution. This scheme may be favored if the examinee's scores fall at either extreme of the score distribution, and can be applied to the Wechsler ability tests due to these measures using the same SS metric. Of note, the WIAT–4 can be scored manually by using the scoring manual (Breaux, 2020b) and technical and interpretative manual (Breaux, 2020c), or by computer software on Q-global (Pearson, 2021). At this point, properly credentialed psychologists can purchase one year of an unlimited number of score reports, which is strongly recommended as manual scoring is extremely tedious with an attendant high risk for human error when referencing so many scores among various tables.

Interpretation

Figure 8.3 is available for download on Routledge's e-resources website, and is especially designed as an interpretive guide for reporting the WIAT–4 results for both the PK and K–12 versions. Forms 8.1b and 8.2b represent the data

Table 8.2 Wechsler Individual Achievement Test, Fourth Edition (WIAT–4) Descriptive Category Guide: 10-Point and 15-Point Systems

Standard Scores	10-Point System Descriptors	Standard Scores	15-Point Descriptors	Alternate 15-Point Descriptors
130–160	Extremely high	146–160	Very high	Upper extreme
120–129	Very high	131–145	High	
110–119	High average	116–130	Above average	Above average
90–109	Average	85–115	Average	Average
80–89	Low average	70–84	Below average	Below average
70–79	Very low	55–69	Low	Lower extreme
40–69	Extremely low	40–54	Very low	

Source. Adapted from Breaux, K. C. (2020c). *Wechsler Individual Achievement Test, Fourth Edition (WIAT–4): Technical and interpretive manual.* Bloomington, MN: NCS Pearson, Tables 3.2 & 3.3, p. 67.

Note. Standard score mean = 100, standard deviation = 15, range 40 to 160.

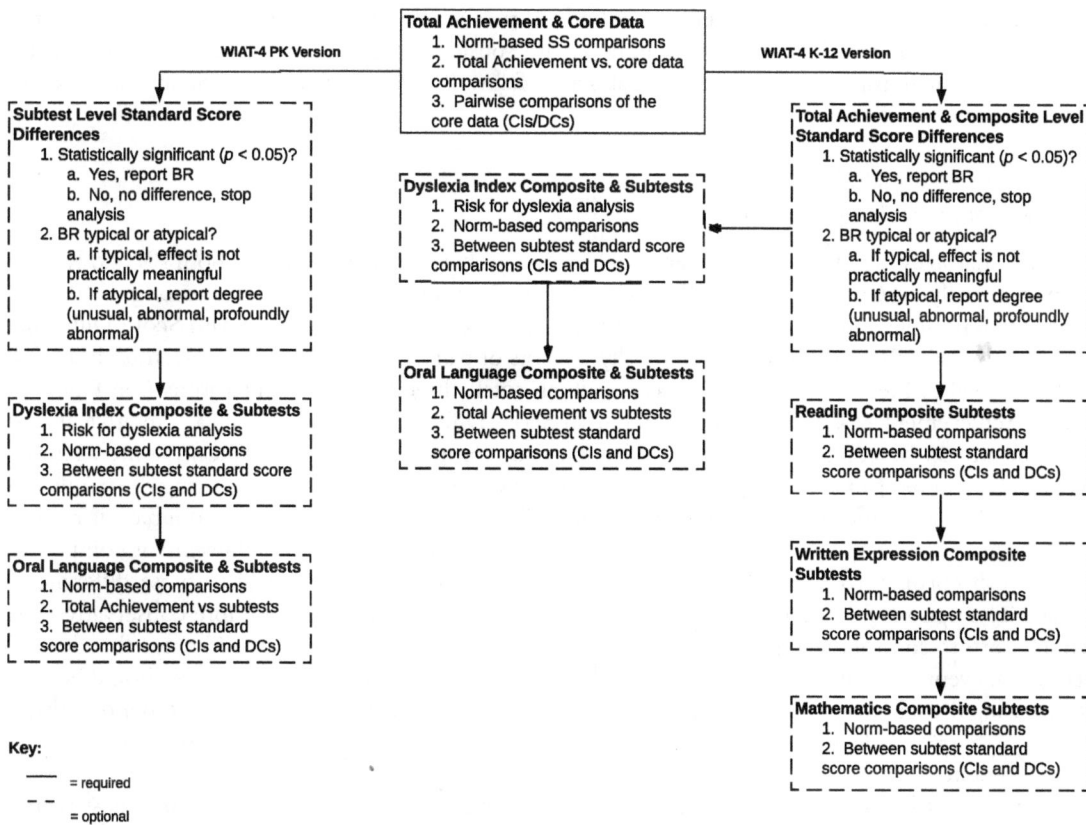

Figure 8.3 WIAT-4 Interpretive Process

tables for the WIAT–4 PK and K–12 versions, which mirror those created for the WIAT–III (see Forms 8.1a and 8.2a). This section follows both Figure 8.3, and Forms 8.1b and 8.2b, in the process of explicating the reporting and interpreting of the WIAT–4 data yield.

WIAT–4 Core Data Norm-Based and Informal Ipsative Analyses

Starting at the top box of Figure 8.3 titled, "Total Achievement & Core Data," interpretation focuses first on norm-based interpretations. The core data differ depending upon the version. The PK data focus on the core subtests, one in each academic area representing reading, written expression, and mathematics. The K–12 data focus upon core composites, once again each representing the aforementioned three academic areas. The analysis begins with the typical norm-based comparisons, first concentrating on the Total Achievement composite, followed by the subtest or domain composite core data. Concerning the PK version, informal pairwise comparisons are then made among the core subtest CIs to determine if follow-up formal ipsative analyses are indicated. The older K–12 version takes a different tact, primarily comparing each composite to the Total Achievement. This is done because the Total Achievement is conceptualized as the examinee's overall average performance where significant discrepancies with the Reading, Written Expression, and Mathematics composites reflect the presence of relative strengths and weaknesses. Hence, if the composite CIs and associated descriptive categories manifest little or no overlap with the Total Achievement composite, follow-up formal ipsative analyses are indicated.

Moving to the data tables, Table 1 in both Forms 8.1b and 8.2b are designed to report and interpret the Total Achievement composite and core data for the PK and K–12 versions, respectively. As regarding the K–12 core data, SSs that are equal to or lower than the DSM–5 defined threshold for SLDs indicate the presence of such psychopathology in particular academic areas. This is because they present composite scores versus simple subtest scores. Thus, it follows that similar results for the PK version only suggest the presence of SLD because they are subtest scores that measure more narrowly defined skill sets. The CIs, PRs, and descriptive categories follow the SSs to facilitate the norm-based and informal ipsative analyses listed in the top middle box in Figure 8.3 (see e-resources). Pre-drafted interpretive statements follow Table 1 in both forms, which guides the examiner through interpretation of the tabular scores. All remaining analyses in Figure 8.3 are considered to be discretionary as denoted by the boxes with broken lines, which implies that, in the event all scores fall well within normal limits or above, the analysis may terminate for want of positive findings.

WIAT–4 Core Data Formal Ipsative Analyses

Assuming the initial analysis indicated the presence of learning problems, the next step for both PK and K–12 versions is formal ipsative analyses. Concerning the PK version, this involves pairwise comparisons among the three subtests, which totals three possible combinations (see Figure 8.3, box titled, "Subtest Level Standard Score Differences"). In contrast, the analysis for the K–12 version principally consists of pairwise comparisons between each domain composite and the Total Achievement composite, again which totals three pairwise comparisons (see Figure 8.3, box titled, "Total Achievement & Composite Level Standard Score Differences"). As an ancillary ipsative analysis, each domain composite can be compared with each other domain composite in a more typical manner. However, this would double the number pairwise comparisons from three to six, hence significantly escalating the family wise error rate. Because finding a significant difference due to chance (i.e., a Type I error) essentially doubles, it is advised that the analysis be circumscribed to that between the domain composites and the Total Achievement composite.

Table 2 in both Forms 8.1b and 8.2b is designed to report and interpret the formal pairwise differences among the core data. The options for selecting a critical value are 0.05 and 0.10. Hence, the more conservative 5% level is employed in efforts to control the Type I error (i.e., stating that there exists a significant difference that does not actually exist). In the event that statistical significance is achieved, then a base rate of the difference should be reported as an effect size using the scheme enumerated within a specific note to Table 2 as follows: no cross denotes that the base rate is typical (n > 15%), † denotes that the base rate is unusual (n ≤ 15%), †† denotes that the base rate is abnormal (n ≤ 10%), ††† denotes that the base rate is rare and profoundly abnormal (n ≤ 5%). A no-score double dash should be entered if the result is non-significant as reporting an effect size of a difference that does not exist is antithetical to logic. The presence of relative weaknesses within the context of low norm-based SSs bolsters a diagnosis of SLD, this according to IDEA (2004).

WIAT–4 K–12 Subtest Score Analysis

The third step concerns only the older K–12 version (i.e., Form 8.2b) because the subtest scores have already been reported and interpreted in the PK version. In the event that (a) one or more domain composites have reached the SS/PR threshold for SLD, (b) there appears to be a significant discrepancy between the contributing subtests, and (c) one of the contributing subtests is measured to be within normal limits, then reporting and interpreting these subtests scores is indicated. In such circumstances, this means that the composite *SS* does not adequately represent the examinee's learning problems and that a more detailed examination is needed to achieve maximum interpretive accuracy; hence, justifying the time and space consumed by adding this appraisal. In fact, if the composite score straddles the threshold between diagnosis and no diagnosis, and only one of the contributing subtests meets or exceeds the diagnostic threshold, then this may no longer be considered sufficient for diagnosing a SLD, especially if the subtest measures a remarkably narrow range of skills.

Specifically, Tables 3, 4, and 5 in Form 8.2b are designed to report and interpret the Reading, Written Expression, and Mathematics composite subtests, respectively. They are listed in the same order as they appear in Table 1 and follow a similar organization, including the SSs, CIs, PRs, descriptive categories, and measured skills in such order. Interpretive statements follow each table, which guides the examiner through the advised interpretive process. In Figure 8.3 (see e-resources), these analyses are depicted by final three boxes proceeding down the far right side titled, "Reading Composite Subtests," "Written Expression Composite Subtests," and "Mathematics Composite Subtests."

WIAT–4 Supplemental Composite Analyses

The WIAT–4 comes with a combination of subtests at the PK level, K–3 level, and 4–12 level, which together contribute to a Dyslexia Index Composite. By itself, it is designed as a screening for this type of learning problem. When presented with the Total Achievement composite and core data, it can effectively add important treatment-relevant information to the diagnosis of a SLD, especially the subtype with impairment in reading. The DSM–5 references dyslexia as an alternative term referring to problems in word recognition, decoding, and spelling. Thus, dyslexia as defined largely falls under specific skills associated with reading, although also crosses over into written expression in reference to poor spelling. Therefore, it is advised that sufficient subtests be added in order to compute a Dyslexia Index and effectively supplement the data needed for measuring reading, written expression, and mathematics disorders, especially when the diagnostic issues pertain to the former two types of learning impairment.

In Figure 8.3 (see e-resources), there are two boxes titled, "Dyslexia Index Composite & Subtests," one falling within the PK version on the far left, and one falling within the K–12 version located in the middle, immediately under the top box. The latter includes the somewhat different subtest-combination for the K–3 and 4–12 Dyslexia Index composites. More specifically, Phonemic Proficiency and Word Reading are the two subtests that contribute to the Dyslexia Index at the PK level (see Form 8.1b, Table 3) and K–3 level (see Form 8.2b, Table 6). The 4–12 Dyslexia Index consists of Word Reading, Orthographic Fluency, and Pseudoword Decoding (see Form 8.2b, Table 7). Because Word Reading is also part of examinees' measured performance for reading at all levels, the Dyslexia Index can be computed upon the addition of only one subtest for the PK version and only two subtests at the older levels, which is an astute decision. To add to efficiency, interpretive excepts follow each Dyslexia Index table that incorporate language consistent with this being a screening measure if utilized on its own. Therefore, examiners may choose to simply screen for dyslexia if that reflects the reason for referral. In such instance, only the dyslexia table would be reported and interpreted.

Finally, the WIAT–4 provides also provides the data necessary to examine the presence of a language disorder if such is part of the diagnostic issues to be resolved. As stated prior, although not technically considered a SLD or learning disability, oral language has been found to correlate significantly with later reading and writing skills (Kavanagh, 1991), along with representing a reasonable estimate of crystalized intelligence (Kaufman, Reynolds, Lin, Kaufman, & McGrew, 2012). Therefore, it is recommended that the Oral Language composite and its subtests be routinely added to the PK version, especially due to its potential as a predictor of later reading and writing skills and an estimate of overall IQ. Furthermore, the PK battery is relatively brief due to the young age of examinees and the fact that many academic skills have not yet been developed or taught. Therefore, supplementing such a battery in order to measure more skills and render the data yield more complete makes logical sense. As applied to the K–12 level, the Oral Language Composite and subtests should only be added if a language disorder represents a core part of the diagnostic issues to be resolved in the case, especially if the Dyslexia Index is already being added to the battery.

The Oral Language data are presented in Form 8.1b, Table 4 for the PK version, and in Form 8.2b, Table 8, for the older version. These are the final tables in both forms, which is actually a metaphor for affording these data least priority, especially regarding the K–12 version. The tables are organized in similar fashion to the SLD tables, including SS, CI, PR, and descriptive category. Pre-drafted interpretative statements follow each table, which guides the examiner through the inferential process on the way to detecting whether or not a language or other communication disorder is present.

Summary

Subsequently, the Woodcock–Johnson, Fourth Edition, Tests of Achievement (WJ IV ACH) will be presented, including data tables for presenting an interpreting its data within a psychological assessment and testing report.

Although this battery comes with a co-normed test of cognitive abilities such that an AAD analysis is possible, this aspect of the Woodcock–Johnson is not provided because the WIAT–III and the companion Wechsler IQ tests have been chosen for this purpose. This is because the Wechsler-line of cognitive tests possess features more conducive to mental health issues, including for example also co-norming between intelligence and neuropsychological memory tests (see Chapter 9), whereas the WJ IV ACH is a more felicitous match for psychoeducational assessments (i.e., school psychological testing), including the inclusion of a *relative proficiency index* (*RPI*), which yields interpretations about an examinee's predicted quality of performance on skills analogous to the one's measured on the test, along with an *instructional zone*, which produces a continuum along a developmental scale ranging from easy (i.e., the independent level) to difficult (i.e., the dependence on being taught or guided level).

This should make sense since David Wechsler, founder of the Wechsler series of cognitive tests, developed his inaugural test within a psychiatric clinical facility (Wechsler, 1939). In contrast, Richard Wesley Woodcock, was a psychometrician who practiced heavily in school psychology, as evidenced by his receiving the Senior Scientist in School Psychology Award from Division 16 of the American Psychological Association in 1993 (Wikipedia Contributors, 2020). It is also logically consistent that this book, which focuses on testing within the field of mental health, would place greater emphasis on tests that are more conducive to clinical testing practice. Therefore, the choice of the WIAT–III as the basis for conducting an AAD when needed is based upon sound and consistent logic, and is not meant to communicate that the WJ IV ACH is an inferior product in any absolute sense. Indeed, many readers of this book may select the WJ IV as their AAD test, or even possess both achievement tests for such purpose. However, once again it behooves the practicing psychologist to attempt to avoid redundancy in building a sound test inventory. Therefore, the ensuing WJ IV presentation will be limited to the achievement tests, including both the standard and extended batteries. The two achievement test batteries will also be compared and contrasted to further highlight their components.

Woodcock–Johnson, Fourth Edition, Tests of Achievement

Synopsis

The *Woodcock–Johnson, Fourth Edition* (*WJ IV*; Schrank, McGrew et al., 2014a) is actually a collection of three distinct, individually administered, co-normed batteries, each measuring a different but related complex cognitive construct. First, the *Woodcock–Johnson, Fourth Edition, Tests of Cognitive Abilities* (WJ IV COG; Schrank, McGrew et al., 2014b) is essentially a comprehensive intelligence test, which measures different specific abilities (i.e., Stratum I), broad-based abilities (i.e., Stratum II), and a *g* factor (Stratum III) consistent with the *Cattell-Horn-Carroll (CHC) theory* discussed in Chapter 11 (Alfonso, Flanagan & Radwan, 2005; Flanagan & Dixon, 2013; McGrew, 2008; Schneider & McGrew, 2012). Second, the *Woodcock–Johnson, Fourth Edition, Tests of Oral Language* (WJ IV OL; Schrank, Mather, & McGrew, 2014b) is a comprehensive measure of receptive and expressive oral language abilities that are related to academic achievement. Third, and most relevant to this chapter, is the *Woodcock–Johnson, Fourth Edition, Tests of Achievement* (*WJ IV ACH*; Schrank, Mather, & McGrew, 2014a), which measures a broad range of narrowly defined specific academic skills (i.e., DSM–5-type subskills), more broadly defined curricular areas or domains (i.e., comparable to WIAT–III composite scales), and cross-domain general achievement skills (i.e., comparable to the WIAT–III total score).

The fact that these three batteries are co-normed means that they may be used together or in different combinations in order to measure various facets of an individual's cognitive functioning, including ability achievement discrepancy (AAD) analyses, ability–oral language comparisons, and achievement–oral language comparisons, along with intra-cognitive, intra-oral language, and intra-achievement comparisons, depending upon the case facts and needs. Furthermore, the WJ IV has been normed upon an impressively large nationally representative sample in excess of 7,000 individuals ranging in age for 2 years 0 months through 90+ years, thus exceeding the WIAT–III on both counts. Finally, the WJ IV ACH has three Forms A, B, and C for their standard battery, which are designed in the event retesting must be done on a continuing basis. For purposes of this book, only Form A is referenced throughout the description of the WJ IV ACH. That is, all references to Tests 1 through 11 of the Standard Battery pertain only to Form A. However, because these are referred to as *parallel tests* (Mather & Wendling, 2014, p. 2), any comments pertaining to Form A would be expected to generalize well to Forms B and C.

As will become apparent, the data yield is truly impressive, not being limited to the typical norm-based scores. That is, the WJ IV ACH also provides criterion-based proficiency scores that are more particularly relevant to the percentage of academic tasks an individual is likely to be successful or unsuccessful at doing compared to age- or grade-level peers. In particular, a *criterion-based test* compares an individual against a predetermined standard, performance level, or learning objective while a *norm-based test* compares the individual to the performance of age- or grade-level peers. The point here is that the WJ IV Ach provides both types of scores in one test battery while the WIAT–III does not, which is considered a true asset. Finally, ipsative comparisons are available on the WJ IV ACH as on the WIAT–III, although are computed in an alternate manner, hence affording the examiner with a substitute means of analyzing within-subject variability for purposes of psychodiagnosis and intervention planning.

Because the WIAT–III has been selected as the achievement test to perform AAD analyses when needed, the focus here will be circumscribed to the WJ IV ACH. The WJ IV COG will be addressed when providing an informative history of the WJ IV, which is founded upon the CHC theory of intelligence almost from its incipience, in contrast to the Wechsler tests that incorporated CHC concepts more gradually and recently. Next, a history of the WJ IV is provided with special focus on the role of CHC theory and its influence on the achievement tests and their data.

Historical Development of the Woodcock–Johnson

The first edition of this comprehensive cognitive battery was published as the *Woodcock–Johnson Psycho-Educational Battery* (*WJ*; Woodcock & Johnson, 1977). It was developed based upon a pure pragmatic decision-making model and without an underlying theory (McGrew, 1986, 1994; Woodcock, 1984). A series of multivariate analyses were done to elucidate a number of functions measured by the test battery, ranging from lower mental processes or simple operations to higher or more complex operations (Woodcock, 1978).

The first revision of the test adopted John Horn's (1991) two-factor theory of intelligence, which consisted of *crystalized intelligence* (i.e., fund of acquired knowledge) and *fluid intelligence* (i.e., abstract mental capacity for learning new information, which is also known as the *Gf-Gc model of intelligence*). As a consequence, the *Woodcock–Johnson Psycho-Educational Battery–Revised* (*WJ R*) added new tests so that it measured broad cognitive and academic abilities proposed by the two factor theory (McGrew, 2005). A chief revision objective of the *Woodcock–Johnson, Third Edition* (*WJ III*; Woodcock, McGrew, & Mather, 2001) was an increase in the detailing and quality of human cognitive abilities, which was facilitated by Carrol's vast meta-analysis of 461 data sets that formed the basis of his *three stratum hierarchical model of intelligence* cited in Chapter 11 (Horn, 1991). Later, Carrol (1993) critiqued his three-stratum theory by offering the following two admonitions: (a) much of the theory was based upon subjective judgment in the process of categorizing the derived factors from the independent data sets; and (b) the constructs proposed from the psychometric test data lacked any efforts at *cross-validation*. *Cross-validation* is a process of determining if the factorial structure of a test is consistent with sample of different individuals.

The theory has since been consolidated as the CHC model of intelligence (Schneider & McGrew, 2012; see also Chapter 7) and continues to evolve with some portions becoming more simplified and other portions more complex. Currently, the WJ IV represents the most contemporary version of CHC theory. In particular, the most significant modifications to the fourth edition of the WJ were to incorporate the latest constructs of CHC theory (outlined in detail in Chapter 7), including those of working memory, speed of lexical access, and memory for sound patterns. Those most relevant to the WJ IV ACH will be identified next.

SHORT-TERM WORKING MEMORY (GWM)

Short-term working memory (*Gwm*) is a dynamic, transient storage system that permits information, including prior stored knowledge and new sensory inputs, to be held in immediate awareness and manipulated as needed or required (Goldman-Rakic, 1992; Miller, Galanter, & Pribram, 1960). Working memory differs from simple short-term memory in that it includes the active manipulation of material and the simultaneous use of other cognitive functions, such as memory and retrieval, and visualization processes to effectuate goal attainment.

How does this relate to academic achievement? Specifically, limited short-term working memory capacity has been proposed as a potential cause of learning disabilities in that, if impaired or dysfunctional, it can act as a bottleneck for acquiring new information (Gathercole, 2004; Gathercole, Lamont, & Alloway, 2006). To bolster this proposition, it has been found that many children with SLDs in reading, written expression, and mathematics show clear deficiencies in Gwm (Bull & Scerif, 2001; de Jong, 1998; Mayringer & Wimmer, 2000; Siegel & Ryan, 1989; Swanson, 1994; Swanson, Ashbaker, & Lee, 1996). Therefore, among the WJ IV ACH tests, those that load most heavily on this factor are most likely to be deleteriously affected by limited Gwm (e.g., Reading Recall; see below).

SPEED OF LEXICAL ANALYSIS (LA)

Speed of lexical analysis (LA) involves a covariance between the speed at which objects can be accurately named (e.g., the Rapid Picture Naming test) and name-generating facility (e.g., the Retrieval Fluency test). In the WJ III, the immediate predecessor to the WJ IV, the correlation between these tests was thought to be associated with a single naming factor (Woodcock et al., 2001). However, currently in the WJ IV, it is proposed that verbal efficiency (Perfettie, 1985) and automaticity of lexical access (LaBerge & Samuals, 1974; Neely, 1977) underlie both tasks. LA is relevant to a number of WJ IV ACH achievement tests that rely upon these abilities, especially Reading Fluency, Sentence Reading Fluency, Oral Reading, Written Expression, and Math Fluency Facts (see subsequently).

MEMORY FOR SOUND PATTERNS (UM)

Memory for sound patterns (UM) represents a narrower ability classified under auditory processing (Gu) and memory for non-speech sound patterns initially proposed by Carroll (1993). In a parallel line of research separate from CHC theory, a phonological storage ability or short-term memory for speech sounds was proposed (Gathercole & Baddeley, 1989; Gathercole, Willis, Emslie, & Baddeley, 1992, 1994). This latter research suggested that the CHC auditory memory for sounds factor should integrate a more specific memory for speech sound patterns. This factor is relevant to many of the reading achievement tests that are reviewed below when the WJ IV ACH tests and clusters are presented. Succinctly, these include any test or cluster that requires reading coding or decoding, and reading automaticity, fluency, and accuracy. This is because an individual must hold auditory input in memory until subsequent aural input is added and processed as a whole unit or word. If such units cannot be held in suspension, separate syllables cannot be integrated into meaningful words. Next, the WJ IV ACH achievement test battery will be reviewed in a sequence comparable to the WIAT–III, including the standardization sample, administration, scoring, and interpretation. The scoring section will include some new types of data not commonly familiar to clinical psychologists and thus their derivations will also be presented to enhance comprehension and their use in mental health testing practice.

Norm Reference Sample

All three components that comprise the WJ IV, including cognitive, oral language, and achievement test batteries, were standardized on a sample of 7,416 participants, ranging in age from 2 years 0 months through 90+ years. The data were garnered from December 2009 through January 2012, hence spanning 25 months. The sample was composed of four subsamples as follows: (a) preschool sample of 664 children ranging in age from 2 years through 5 years; (b) 3,891 students from kindergarten through 12th grade; (c) 775 undergraduate and graduate students; and (d) 2,086 adults. Notice that the sample numbers favor the years in which the greatest amount of development in fundamental academic skills are realized.

Participants were randomly selected within a stratified sampling design as follows: (a) region of the country (i.e., Northeast, Midwest, South, and West); (b) sex (i.e., male and female); (c) country of birth (i.e., U.S. and Other); (d) race (i.e., White, Black, American Indian, Alaska Native, Asian, Native Hawaiian, Other Pacific Islander, Other); (e) ethnicity (Hispanic, Not Hispanic); (f) community type (i.e., preschool, K–12, and adult samples only)–Metropolitan (areas with population ≥ 50,000 plus adjacent outlying counties), Metropolitan (areas with population between 10,000 and 49,999 plus adjacent outlying counties, and (Rural (population < 10,000); (g) parent education (i.e., preschool, K–12, and adult samples only)—less than high school diploma, high school diploma, and greater than high school diploma; (h) type of school (K–12 sample only)—less than 9th grade, less than high school diploma, high school diploma, 1 to 3 years of college, Bachelor's degree, and Master's degree or higher; (i) employment status (adult sample only)—employment, unemployed, and not in the labor force; (j) occupation level of adults in the labor force—management/professional, service occupations, sales and office occupations, natural resources, construction, and maintenance occupations, production, transportation, and material moving occupations. The norming data were tracked closely throughout the aforesaid data gathering period in order to ensure that the final proportions reasonably matched those reported according to the 2010 U.S. population census projections (U.S. Bureau of the Census, 2010).

Administration

The majority of the WJ IV ACH standardized administration procedures are comparable to those employed in the WIAT–III achievement test battery. Therefore, this discussion will focus mostly upon the dissimilarities between the two measures and secondarily point out some chief similarities. To open, the general test administration process emphasizes two components; that is, accuracy and fluency. First, analogous to the WIAT–III, test instructions emphasize discipline on the part of the examiner in remaining true to the standardized administrative rules, referring to ideal objective of maintaining *exact administration*. This means providing commands to the examinee that are "identical" to those provided in both the Test Book (also known as a stimulus book), Record Form (upon which examinee responses and raw scores are entered by the examiner), and in the Examiner's Manual (Mather & Wendling, 2014, pp. 53–74).

Second, *brisk administration* specifies that the pace should be steady, consistent, and smooth, with an absence of unnecessary hiatuses or gaps during which time examinees can become bored, distracted, or impatient. In fact, these two facets of administration are applicable to virtually all standardized tests, which means that the examiner must be well practiced prior to administering the first live test. This does not necessarily mean that training for a new test, or new edition to a previously familiar test, must be intense, grueling, and of long duration. Skills generalize from test to test reasonably well, especially for newer editions of familiar tests, and many come with examiner's manuals that provide excellent detail regarding all aspects of standardization, principal changes from the earlier edition, case examples, and occasionally practice scoring items. Some also come with training videos, which can be purchased with the test and can be extremely useful by learning effectively through observation and imitation.

Even prior to administering the first item, the examiner must select the required tests to administer in order to properly address the referral issue(s). As stated prior, in mental health testing, achievement testing is primarily done to detect SLDs in reading, written expression, mathematics, and language skills, along with identifying the subskills that are particularly showing impairment or delay, and some information concerning degrees of severity. Therefore, typically selected is referred to as the WJ IV ACH *standard battery*, which includes the first 11 tests (i.e., 1 through 11) plus the first test in the *extended battery* (i.e., Test 12, Reading Recall). These may be perused in Forms 12.7 and 12.8, Table 2 (i.e., the reading-related tests), Table 5 (i.e., the written language-related tests), and Table 8 (i.e., the mathematics-related tests). Together, these tests yield sufficient data to determine whether any one or more of the three DSM–5 subtypes of learning and communication disorders (i.e., reading, written language, mathematics, language) are present, along with their fundamental subskills for purposes of diagnosis and treatment planning. As will become apparent, the additional Test 12 makes it possible to compute a Reading Comprehension domain cluster, which is a broad-based curricular area analogous to a Stratum level II factor in intelligence (e.g., Fluid Reasoning Index or FRI). In learning disability test referrals, reading difficulties are the most common complaints of the three subtypes, especially reading for understanding (i.e., comprehension). Therefore, including this one extra test is worth the extra 5 to 10 minutes its takes to administer it and yield the additional domain cluster score.

Speaking of duration, the manual estimates that it takes 40 minutes to administer the first 6 tests of the standard battery, which are referred to as the *core tests* because they make possible the pattern of strengths and weaknesses (PSW) analyses and some cross academic domain cluster scores (mentioned later). Each remaining test consumes 5 to 10 minutes depending upon how quickly the basals and ceilings are established. This means that administration of the recommended WJ IV ACH battery would take from 70 to 100 minutes, thus requiring a two-hour testing session assuming appointments are scheduled in hourly segments.

The tenor of the remaining administrative rules is meant more as guidelines rather than inflexible directives. Therefore, they tend to afford somewhat more discretion to the examiner when contrasted with the WIAT–III, which is somewhat surprising given the initial emphasis on exact administration. First, with the single exception of advising the examiner not to administer the three fluency tests in sequence, test order is completely discretionary, whereas the WIAT–III admonishes the examiner to stay true to subtest order as the battery was standardized. In addition, test starting points are merely "suggested," and can be moved back toward easier items if an examinee is struggling with the suggested start points, or even up toward more difficult items if start points appear to be excessively easy for an able examinee. Although the WIAT–III permits this, the evidence must be more than a simple preponderance and closer to a clear and convincing standard.

As in the WIAT–III, and as indicated prior, the WJ IV ACH uses *adaptive testing*, including basals and ceilings in an attempt to administer items of appropriate difficulty level and avoid examinee fatigue, frustration, and boredom. Basals and ceilings are specified sequences of items that examinees pass and fails, respectively. The assumption is that the examinee would have responded correctly to all items prior to the basal, and likewise would have responded incorrectly to all items following the ceiling. Therefore, such items do not need to be administered because it would not change an examinee's ultimate score and saves both time and effort. However, in contrast to the WIAT–III, the WJ IV ACH advises the examiner to "test by complete page," which means that the test should never be discontinued in the middle of a page on the Test Book. Therefore, if the discontinue rule is met (e.g., four consecutive incorrect responses) and there are three more items on the Test Book page, the remaining three items must still be given. If any of these remaining three are answered correctly, then the test must continue onto the next page. The rationale is that this will avoid giving negative feedback to examinees that they have likely failed because it is all too apparent that the test is being halted even when there are remaining items. The number of items needed to establish the basals and ceilings vary more significantly across the WJ IV ACH tests versus the WIAT–III subtests and also tend to be longer.

Another difference in administration relates to whom the tests should be administered, and again shows a tendency for the WJ IV ACH to afford more clinical judgment to the examiner. Specifically, in the WIAT–III, certain subtests are designated for only specified grade levels. Thus, an individual in 2nd grade is not to be administered Essay Composition, which begins at 3rd grade. Regarding the WJ IV ACH, all tests are to be administered again at the discretion of the examiner. If an examinee happens to fail all sample items, the test is to be immediately discontinued based upon the rationale that the individual's score would represent a skill that has not yet been taught versus a bona fide learning disability.

Three tests in the standard battery are timed, including Test 9–Sentence Reading Fluency, Test 10–Math Facts Fluency, and Test 11–Sentence Writing Fluency. The former two are 3-minute durations while the latter is 5 minutes. It is these tests that are recommended not to be administered in sequence and are analogous to some WIAT–III subtests that are also timed (e.g., Oral Word Fluency). Finally, also similar to the WIAT–III are the following: (a) use of sample items; (b) use of a Response Booklet for items that require writing or calculation; and (c) tests that require administration of a preselected block of items versus single items.

Scoring

The WJ IV ACH is a highly sophisticated instrument in terms of its psychometrics. this is a direct result of its founder's expertise as a trained psychometrician. Because of its psychometric erudition, the various types of scores available will be elucidated, how they are derived, and the ones that have been selected for use in mental health testing. This is important because some of these scores are typically unfamiliar to clinical psychologists and mental health professionals, and tend to be more acquainted to fields such as education. Therefore, definitions of key constructs will be provided throughout the ensuing discussion.

W SCORES

The *W score* is the foundational metric for all subsequently derived scores (e.g., standard scores, percentile ranks, relative proficiency indexes) available for the WJ III test batteries (McGrew & Woodcock, 2001). Woodcock and Dahl (1971) produced this measurement scale based upon a mathematical transformation of the Rasch model of data analysis, which is based on item response theory (IRT). IRT basically analyses the likelihood of an individual passing an item based upon two characteristics: (a) the amount of a particular ability possessed by the examinee; and (b) the difficulty level of the item. Without getting into the technicalities, the *W* scale is an *equal-interval scale*, meaning that the same amount of difference in the skill or ability is measured regardless of the interval's location along the scale, analogous to inches measured by a ruler except in the absence of an absolute zero.

More specifically, a person's ability level on a measured *trait* and the difficulty levels of all items are both represented on the *W* scale, therefore allowing both of these variables to be used as factors within the same mathematical calculations. A *trait* is here defined as any skill, ability, or area of knowledge. This characteristic "provides a particularly convenient set of predictive relationships based on the difference between a person's ability and item difficulty along the scale" (Woodcock, 1978, p. 77).

In norming the WJ, items are sorted by difficulty level; that is, the more individuals in the standardization sample that pass an item, the easier it is, and the fewer the individuals who pass the item, the more difficult its measurement. Next, a value is assigned to each item representing its difficulty level, which is called the *W difficulty* or *W score*. A *W* score is generated for every possible raw score. Thus, when a person obtains a raw score on a test, he earns a W score that represents both the difficulty level of the item, but perhaps more importantly, also his ability level on that test; hence, also termed *W ability*. This reflects the manner in which using IRT principles results in a *W* score metric that represents both the difficulty level of the item and the person's ability level on that particular trait as measured by the content of such item. Going further, the *W* ability for all WJ IV ACH tests is centered at 500, which estimates the average performance of a 10-year 0-month-old child using age equivalents (i.e., 10–0; see below) and the beginning of 5th grade (i.e., 5.0; see below) when applying grade norms. To provide context, the typical *W* range for WJ tests is 430 to 550 (McGrew & Woodcock, 1989). Hence, to emphasize this point, the *W* score represents *simultaneously* the individual's ability and item difficulty level. Higher *W* scores mean that the examinee has greater ability on that measured skill because she responded correctly to more difficult items as determined by the norm reference sample.

In complementary fashion, lower W scores mean that the examinee has lesser ability on that measured skill because she responded correctly only to the easier items. Next, it will be illustrated how the W score is used to show an individual's degree of development and then degree of proficiency, the latter being unique to this measure and extremely useful in treatment planning.

Continuing, the W scores are anchored or linked to both age and grade levels in intervals of years and months. For each age and grade grouping, the median W ability value is computed; that is, the level at which 50% of the sample responded correctly and 50% responded incorrectly. This level is termed the *reference W* because it represents the criterion score upon which examinees are compared (McGrew & Woodcock, 1989). Because the reference W for any age or grade group represents the median difficulty level, the individual scoring at a particular reference W has a 50% chance of responding correctly to any item of equivalent difficulty level. The more an examinee's ability level exceeds those of their peers (i.e., the reference W for that age or grade group), the more likely he will be successful on equivalent tasks for that measured skill. In contrast, the more an examinee's ability level is below those of his peers (i.e., the reference W for that age or grade group), the less likely he will be successful on equivalent tasks for that measured skill. The cardinal point here is that where individuals stand relative to the reference W, their success rate or degree of proficiency at tasks of equivalent difficulty level can be predicted (e.g., 40%, 70%, and 90%). One more step now in the measurement process using the W score.

The *W difference* (*W DIFF*) represents the discrepancy between (a) the examinee's obtained W score (i.e., measured ability), and (b) the age-based (or grade-based) reference W. The W DIFF is the value from which standard scores (SS), PRs, and relative proficiency indexes (RPIs; see below) are all derived. At this juncture, the fundamentals of the WJ IV ACH scoring metrics have been reviewed. Virtually all subsequent scores are derivatives of this W score metric. Therefore, it may behoove the reader to review this section again to ensure comprehension of at least the logic behind the W score.

THE MEASUREMENT OF GROWTH

Because the W scale is apportioned into equal intervals, it can measure the degree of growth upon retesting. That is, the W scale is constructed so that an increase of 10 W units represents the individual's ability to perform, with 75% success, tasks that he or she could previously perform with only 50% success. This is true for any 10-point increase on the W scale (Woodcock & Dahl, 1971; Woodcock, 1999). Norm-based comparisons do not show growth because they reflect group comparisons that are tied to rank order. If an examinee grows at the same rate as her peers, there will be no change in SS, PR, or qualitative category. However, the education system is highly interested in measuring growth or progress over time and by means of instructional intervention.

In mental health testing, the focus is more upon identifying the presence and degree of delay or impairment and not so much growth, with the exception of neuropsychological testing that can focus on measuring progression of disease or impairment. For some reason, there have been scant referrals for re-testing to determine if, and to what extent if any, mental health intervention has been successful in reducing symptoms, which is actually a valid use of testing resources. This may be due to lack of progress, premature termination, or planned termination because of successful symptoms remission. The few referrals for retesting have come in the form of neuropsychological retesting to determine any degree of disease progression. For this reason, the W score is not utilized for purposes of growth analysis, although it is available on the WJ IV ACH.

RELATIVE PROFICIENCY INDEX

The *Relative proficiency index* (*RPI*) is a measure of a person's *proficiency* (i.e., degree of expertise or capability) in a skill or area of knowledge compared with average age or grade level peers. It is a direct product of the W score discussed in the previous section. As stated previously, by virtue of placing an examinee's ability level (i.e., W ability) and item difficulty level (i.e., W difficulty) on the same scale (i.e., the W score), then the probability of passing items of varying levels of difficulty can be predicted on the basis of mathematical projections. For example, if an examinee's measured ability on Test 5 Calculation (i.e., W ability) is 500, and the median score for the examinee's age group on Test 5 Calculation (i.e., reference W) is 500, then the discrepancy between the two (i.e., W DIFF) is "0." This means that the examinee has a 50% likelihood (.500) of passing calculation items of equivalent difficulty. Furthermore, a W DIFF of +10 (W ability–reference W) shows a 75% likelihood of success, while a W DIFF of −10 is associated with a 25% chance of success (Woodcock, 1978; Woodcock & Dahl, 1971). Note that this is a *criterion-based approach* (versus norm-based approach) of examining an individual's skill level. Again, a criterion-based or referenced approach consists of measuring an individual's performance against is a pre-selected standard (e.g., a specified percentage of success in mastering the material). The criterion here is the median or a 50% proficiency rate. If this result were provided to the examinee's teacher, it would be predicted that this student would successfully pass about 50% of calculation items at his age or grade level.

Although using the median or 50% as a criterion is readily understood, it is much too low of a standard in the field of education. In the teaching of psychology courses, a 50% pass rate is typically failing whereas a 90% pass rate begins a grade of "A." Hence, from a teaching perspective, the criterion for proficiency is more typically 90%. As a consequence, to set the criterion for proficiency closer to 90%, the reference W in the WJ IV ACH is set at a difficulty level that is 20 units simpler than the median reference W (Woodcock, 1999). The outcome is a score that measures proficiency (i.e., mastery or expertise), called the *relative proficiency index* (*RPI*), which represents a criterion-referenced score describing the probability of an examinee's success in various academic tasks (e.g., oral reading) at the level of difficulty that 90% of average age or grade level peers can manage. The RPI is reported as a ratio, with the examinee's predicted degree of success in the numerator and the 90% criterion (which represents a constant) in the denominator. Thus, for Test 1–Letter-Word Identification, an RPI of 70/90 indicates that the examinee would pass 70% of task items that his average peers would pass at a 90% success or proficiency rate.

A useful analogy here are the Snellen charts that are used to measure visual acuity (i.e., the sharpness of one' vision). Here, 20/20 vision means that an individual can visually distinguish at 20 feet what people with normal vision distinguish at 20 feet (i.e., normal vision). Going further, an individual with 20/100 vision must be at 20 feet to distinguish what people with normal visual acuity can distinguish at 100 feet. Although the RPI modifies the numerator and not the denominator, it is the changing ratio and its interpretation that completes the analogy. The RPI ranges from 100/90 (i.e., W DIFF = +29 and above) to 0/90 (i.e., W DIFF =–69 and below), with a mean of 90/90 (i.e., W DIFF = 0) and increments in the numerator of 1% point. Note that by mathematical projections, each W DIFF score is associated with a particular ratio; for example, 88/90 = W DIFF of –2, 89/90 = W DIFF of–1, 91/90 = W DIFF of +1 and, 92/90–W DIFF of +2 (see Jaffe, 2009, Table 3, p. 9 for the entire RPI and associated W DIFF values).

Some sample interpretive statements are offered here to further demonstrate the RPI score, its meaning, and how it may be interpreted in testing cases. They are as follows: (a) "Steven's RPI on the Reading Recall test was 75/90, suggesting that, compared with typical age peers, his proficiency is at the lower end of the instructional range"; (b) "Linda obtained a SS of 87 on Passage Comprehension, which is within the low average range. Nevertheless, her RPI of 41/90 indicates that she is limited in her ability to comprehend brief passages, and this type of task will be very difficult for her"; (c) "On Auditory Memory Span, John's RPI is 65/90 and his SS is 85. Thus, regarding the ability to hold noncontextual information in short-term memory, John is predicted to retain only 65% compared with his typical grade peers' ability to retain 90%. Therefore, although his SS technically falls in the low average range of functioning, he is likely to show limited proficiency in this skill in the classroom"; (d) "Since Margaret was last tested, her RPI increased from 35/90 to 75/90. Therefore, whereas a year ago she was likely to handle grade-level reading material with only about 35% success, her current scores indicate that she would be about 75% successful."

A few comments about these interpretive statements are in order. The first example associates the RPI with an instructional zone, which is available on the Woodcock–Johnson online scoring and reporting program (Schrank & Dailey, 2014). The middle two interpretations (viz., "b" and "c") were designed to illustrate how the norm-based SSs can underestimate the degree of difficulty a student is having in the actual classroom. Specifically, in each case the SS of 85 (PR = 16) is clearly within the low average range, thus showing a degree of functioning that, although somewhat low, is still considered to be within normal limits. This SS result is also "normal" when compared to the DSM–5 definition, which is norm-based and set at a SS of 78 and below. However, the measured proficiency for both show much greater delay or impairment from a more pragmatic perspective; that is, what can this student manage in terms of percent of classroom proficiency. The point here is that the RPI and SS are based upon different derivations and communicate differing types of information. Therefore, it is vital to report and interpret both SS and RPI scores when they are available to avoid the risk of underestimating difficulties a student is experiencing inside the classroom while simultaneously damaging the perceived validity of standardized test score results. Again, this will be further explicated subsequently. The final interpretation was afforded in order to portray how effectively RPI scores can illustrate how much growth or progress a student has made based upon a longitudinal test–retest comparison of proficiency scores.

To conclude, the RPI describes the person's level of *proficiency* (i.e., expertise or competence) in the skill, ability, or area of knowledge based on the probability of his or her success on a specific level of task difficulty. It therefore represents the quality of an individual's performance. Descriptive classifications can also be used to supplement RPI interpretation. This topic discussed subsequently when comparing and contrasting RPI scores with the SSs. Next, the discussion moves into more familiar territory by examining norm-based peer-comparison scores, including standard scores (SS), percentile ranks (PRs), and descriptive categories. These all show an examinee's place in line or location in a distribution of same age or grade level peers in a norm reference sample.

STANDARD SCORES

In the WJ IV ACH, standard scores *SS*s are derived from calculations that are different from those of the RPI scores. It is composed of a two-step process, first transforming the examinee's *W* score (i.e., *W* difficulty or *W* DIFF) into a standardized *z* score, then applying a linear transformation, converting the *z* score into a *SS* with a mean of 100 and standard deviation of 15. The first formula is as follows:

$$z = \frac{W \text{ difference}}{SD}$$

Equation 8.3

where *z* is a standard score in standard deviation units ($\bar{x} = 0$, $SD = 1.00$), *W difference* is the discrepancy between an examinee's *W* ability score and the reference *W* for that test and age or grade level (i.e., *W* DIFF), and *SD* is the standard deviation of the *W* DIFF scores, which vary depending on the test and age or grade level. The second step is a linear transformation of the computed *z* score (computed from Equation 8.3) into a *SS* as follows:

$$SS = \bar{x} + (z \times SD)$$

Equation 8.4

where *SS* is the *SS* obtained by the examinee, is the selected mean value for the *SS* metric (i.e., 100), and *SD* is the selected standard deviation for the *SS* metric (i.e., 15). All of the *SS*s were computed in this manner from the *W* scores provided by the standardization sample.

An example will be provided here to (a) demonstrate the *SS* derivation, and (b) to compare this to the aforesaid RPI. The objective is to elucidate why these two scores can be so discrepant in terms of value and interpretation. Imagine Maria, age 8 years 1 month obtained a *W* score (*W* ability) of 495 on Test 1–Letter-Word Identification. If the reference *W* score is 510, then Maria's *W* DIFF is 495–510 = –15. If the *W* DIFF *SD* on this test happens to be 25, then Maria's z score is–15 ÷ 25 = –0.60. Her *SS* is then 100 + (–0.60 x 15) = 100 +–9 = 91 (see Chapter 3 for review of linear transformations). Therefore, two facets of the *SS* are portrayed. One, the WJ IV ACH *SS*s are all derived from the *W* scores yielded in the norm reference sample. Two, they represent norm-based comparisons. Next illustrated is why the *SS*s and RPIs can be so discrepant such that score interpretations can be both understood and explained.

Recall that RPIs are derived directly from the *W* DIFF scores and mathematical projections; for example, *W* DIFF of 0 = 90/90, *W* DIFF of –10 = 75/90, and *W* DIFF of –30 = 25/90 (see Jaffe, 2009, Table 3, p. 9). They do not involve *SD*s for the *W* DIFF as do the *SS*s. Because *W* DIFF *SD*s vary across the different WJ IV ACH tests and age or grade levels, *SS*s can also vary whereas RPIs remain constant. A continuing example that extends Maria's case will suffice. On the previous Test 1–Letter-Word Identification, recall that her *W* DIFF score was –15 (i.e., 495–510 = –15), which translates into an RPI of 63/90. This means that Maria is predicted to be 63% successful at word-letter identification skills when her same-aged peers are 90% successful, which places her at the lower end of the instructional range. Image now that Maria obtains a *W* ability score on Test 5 Calculation of 495, and its reference *W* is also 510 as on the previous test. Again, Maria will have a *W* DIFF score of–15 and an RPI of 63/90 (see Jaffe, 2009, Table 3, p. 9), which developmentally shows a mild delay (see Jaffe, 2009, Table 4, p. 10). However, the *SD* of the *W* DIFF score on Test 5–Calculation is only 16 (not 25), hence a much smaller variability. Her attendant z score now would be, $z = \frac{-15}{16} = -0.9375$, and her resulting *SS* would be, $100 + (-0.9375 \times 15) = 85.9375 \approx 86$.

There are two facets of these comparisons that need to be emphasized. One, Maria's RPIs are constant because they are based upon the same *W* DIFF scores that indicate identical proficiency prediction ratios (i.e., 63/90), while her *SS*s are discrepant due to varying *W* DIFF *SD*s (i.e., *SS*s = 91 and 86). Two, both *SS*s appear to overestimate what Maria is predicted to do in the classroom. While both *SS*s fall within normal limits (i.e., average and low average), her RPIs are indicating only 63% proficiency, which from an educational perspective reflects near failing work. That is, she is struggling with the material much more than her *SS*s reveal and can be misleading to teacher and educational professionals. This issue will be revisited in the ensuing interpretation section.

In conclusion, *SS*s have mean 100 and *SD* of 15, which are created by linear transformations of the *W* DIFF score, which itself is derived from the *W* score (i.e., *W* ability–reference *W*). They are also extended from 54 to 146, although the online program is reported to provide *SS*s from 0 to over 200. However, as will become apparent, only the *SS* range that covers the extended PRs as reported in the Examiner's Manual is included (see Mather & Wendling, 2014, Figure 5-1, p. 83).

CONFIDENCE INTERVALS

The *standard error of measurement* (*SEM*) is used to create *confidence intervals* (*CIs*) for the reported SSs. CIs give the reader an indication of the degree of certainty the examiner possesses in the reported SSs. Again, the optional 95%

degree of certainty is selected to be consistent with other similar tests (e.g., the WIAT–III). The Technical Manual indicates that internal consistency coefficients were used to compute SEMs for untimed subtests, while reliabilities for the remaining tests were computed according to information provided by the Rasch model underlying the computation of the aforementioned *W* scores (McGrew et al., 2014, pp. 90–91). This method basically provides a SEM for the *W* ability score for every participant in the standardization sample, hence is generally considered a more accurate estimate of error variance. In any case, the reported SEMs have the same meaning as those reported for all other tests previously presented.

PERCENTILE RANKS

Percentile ranks (PRs) or *percentiles* have the same meaning as in all previous standardized tests discussed in this book to this point. That is, they represent the proportion of the standardization sample (who in turn represent the population of same aged or grade level peers) that the examinee scored equal to or better than. PRs divide the scale into $1/^{10}$th intervals, hence centiles. The typical range is from 0 to 99, with an average in the form of a median of 50 (i.e., the 50th percentile). The only difference between a PR and a percentile is that the latter refers to a particular point (e.g., Billie scored at the 50th percentile) whereas the former refers to an interval (e.g., Billie's percentile rank was 50), although they essentially mean the same thing. That is, in either case, Billie scored equal to or better than 50% of the norm reference sample, which would typically be interpreted as average (viz., at the median).

The chief difference here is that the WJ IV ACH provides *extended percentile ranks* (Woodcock, 1987, 1998), which means that they provide a greater range and ability to discrimination at each extreme end of the distribution. Specifically, the scale reaches down to 0.1 (i.e., one tenth of one percent) and up to 99.9 (i.e., 999 out of 1,000, meaning that only 1 person out of 1,000 would have a score as high or higher). As a result, the extended PR scale adds a total of about 1.5 SDs discriminating power to the scale; that is, 0.75 of a *SD* at the extreme high end and 0.75 of a *SD* at the extreme low end. This is not unique, however, to this book as an extended PR is already provided in Appendix A with an equivalent PR of 99.99 at the top end (i.e., SS = 155) and a PR of 0.01 at the bottom end (i.e., SS = 45). A PR of 0.01 means that only 1 of 10,000 people would have a score as low or lower (McCrae & Costa, 2010; MedFriendly, 2020). The PRs are frequently reported due to their relatively straightforward definition, which can be readily understood by laypeople reading the test results. Again, a caveat is that they represent area transformations that tend to exaggerate differences in the middle of the distribution and minimize changes toward each extreme end. This is why extended PRs are important to report as they add discriminatory power to where it is needed on the scale.

WJ IV ACH CLASSIFICATIONS

The reported SSs are associated with descriptive classifications that represent a combination of nominal and ordinal measurement characteristics (Stevens, 1946). That is, SS ranges are associated with categories or classifications that are ranked in terms of degree of functioning. This is the traditional way SSs are apportioned and described in test data that measure various types of cognitive functioning. Table 8.3 presents the SS ranges and the suggested WJ IV classification labels in the first two columns, respectively. However, this is only one option.

Table 8.3 Woodcock–Johnson, Fourth Edition, Tests of Achievement (WJ IV ACH) Descriptive Class Guide

Standard Score (SS) Range	WJ IV Classification	Relative Proficiency Index (RPI)	Proficiency Classification
131 to 146	Very superior	98/90 to 100/90	Very advanced
121 to 130	Superior	95/90 to 98/90	Advanced
111 to 120	High average	82/90 to 95/90	Average
90 to 110	Average	67/90 to 82/90	Limited to average
80 to 89	Low average	24/90 to 67/90	Limited
70 to 79	Low	3/90 to 24/90	Very limited
54 to 69	Very low	0/90 to 3/90	Negligible

Sources. Adapted from (a) Mather, N., & Wendling, B. J. *(2014). Woodcock–Johnson, Fourth Edition, Tests of Achievement (WJ IV ACH): Examiner's manual.* Rolling Meadows, IL: Riverside Publishing, Table 5–4, p. 84; and (b) Jaffe, L. E. (2009). *Development, interpretation, and application of the W score and the relative proficiency index* (Woodcock-Johnson III Assessment Service Bulletin No. 11). Rolling Meadows, IL: Riverside Publishing. Explanation of the W score and RPI score metrics), Table 4, p. 10.

The alternative is to report the classifications based upon degrees of proficiency versus functioning. These are enumerated in the final column of Table 8.3. This means that the classifications are based upon RPI score ranges (not the *SS* ranges), and that the labels are modified to reflect degrees of success or mastery; namely (from less to increasingly greater), *negligible, very limited, limited, limited-to-average, average, advanced,* and *very advanced.* Note how the labels refer to degrees of mastering the academic skills or areas as opposed to functional labels such as low, average, and superior. Because of these two alternative classification schemes, two data tables have been created for reporting WJ IV ACH test scores, one that emphasizes functionality (i.e., Form 8.7) and one that emphasizes proficiency (i.e., Form 8.8). These forms will be reviewed in more detail in the ensuing interpretation section.

GRADE EQUIVALENTS

Grade equivalents (*GEs*) or *grade scores* represent the grade level in the norm reference sample wherein the median raw score corresponds to that of the examinee's raw score. It is reported in terms of grade and month of the academic year. Hence, a GE of 5.7 means that the examinee's raw score on a test or cluster is equivalent to the 7th month of 5th grade. GEs are the only scores that can be produced manually on the record form based upon a table adjacent to each test. The table provides three columns as follows: (a) examinee's raw score (i.e., total number correct); (b) age equivalent; and (c) GE. However, they are only estimates of the actual scores. The range is from < K.0 to > 12.9, which means less than the median for children beginning kindergarten and greater than the median for students in the 9th month of 12th grade. The online computer scoring program provides the exact GE, and uses the same "<" sign as the estimated GE at the lower end, although uses the ">" sign to denote GEs greater than the median score obtained by graduate students in their first year (i.e., > 17.9), or if scored by 2-year college norms, at the completion of the final year of those 2 years (i.e., > 14.9).

In addition to not reflecting equal interval scales of measurement, GE scores are interpretively problematic for tests that include a circumscribed range of difficulty level simply because the skill is taught primarily during the primary grades (e.g., Basic Reading). An example used in the Examiner's Manual (Mather & Wendling, 2014) is a third grade student earning a GE of 6.5 on a test intended to be administered at grade 3. A misinterpretation is to assume that this student will be successful on such tasks at a level of the 5th month of 6th grade. Rather, this indicates that such student has correctly answered a good deal of items at a 3rd grade level. That is, such circumstance reflects the degree of accuracy at the 3rd grade level because the skill does not practically extend to 6th grade. GE scores are most accurately reported when item difficulty level is evenly distributed over a wide array of difficulty levels and the test is properly normed. In mental health practice, this is typically not an issue because if a developmental-type score is wanted or needed, age equivalents are best to employ. The scores are next discussed.

AGE EQUIVALENTS:

Age equivalents (*AEs*) represent the median raw score on a test for a particular age group, typically reported in units of years and months. For example, a raw score of 9 on Test 1–Word-Letter Identification has an estimated AE of 4–6, which means 4 years 6 months. When an examinee of any chronological age (CA; e.g., 5 years 2 months) obtains that same raw score of 9 on Test 1–Letter-Word Identification, she will be assigned an AE of 4–6. As just indicated, AEs can also be estimated manually by means of tables juxtaposed to each test in the Test Record form. AEs range from < 2–0 to > 30, or less than 2 years 0 months to greater than 30 years, respectively. AEs are more relevant than GEs for (a) mental health testing, (b) young children not yet enrolled in formal schooling, and (c) adults who are not matriculating through a program of higher learning at the time of testing. Although the AEs have not routinely been reported in the past, at times they are listed in the narrative interpretation following each data table because, although not an equal interval measurement scale, they do communicate developmental level quite succinctly and effectively, which laypeople can understand if properly interpreted. However, at this point the SS and RPI trump the AE score because the former is a listed criterion for DSM–5 diagnoses of SLDs, and the RPI provides an extremely useful measure of proficiency in the classroom. However, adding yet another metric to the data tables risks inundating the reader of the report with an avalanche of numbers, which also can obfuscate the core results.

COGNITIVE-ACADEMIC LANGUAGE PROFICIENCY

According to Cummins (1984), there are two types of language proficiency. First, basic interpersonal communication skill (BICS) is capability in practical everyday communication, which is considered to be learned in the natural environment. In contrast, cognitive-academic language proficiency (CALP) is learned in the formal classroom, which also includes literacy skills (e.g., semantics). The online computer scoring software includes an option to report CALP levels. This information is not employed when testing for SLDs and language disorders in the mental health system and therefore will not be addressed further in this book.

The WJ IV ACH is one of the few measures that limits scoring to its online computer scoring program. Respectively, the home page title and address is (a) Riverside Score™ (2021), and (b) https://riversidescore.com/. Manual scoring is circumscribed to deriving AE and GE developmental-type scores, and even these are considered to be merely estimates of the actual scores provided by the online scoring program. Although computer scoring is typically advantageous due to its speed and accuracy, manual scoring should at minimum be an option in order to (a) provide an alternative method of scoring in the event internet access is precluded for any number of reasons, and (b) facilitate training. Regarding the latter, manually scoring a new test at least once is important for pedagogical reasons because the examiner learns the original derivation of various scores and their logic. This is another reason why using the WIAT–III is favored in most circumstances in mental health testing.

The Woodcock–Johnson program consists of separate data entry fields for the three batteries included in the WJ IV cognitive batteries (i.e., cognitive, oral language, and achievement). There is a fee for each case that is committed for scoring. Once the data have been entered and committed for scoring, there is a 90-day window of time provided for purposes of modifying the profile after which time the test can be rescored but with no further modifications. Because the achievement test battery is only being utilized, it is uncertain as to whether oral language and cognitive tests can be added to a protocol that is committed for scoring. However, an examiner can modify how many achievement tests are scored for the same case within this 90-day window. For example, a standard battery (Tests 1–11) was initially scored for a case, then later Test 12–Reading Recall of the extended battery was added in order to also include the Reading Comprehension Cluster score. This did not require and additional fee but was done within the 90-day window.

Also modifiable is the type of report that is scored and printed with a committed data set. The one that is most pertinent to providing data for the Woodcock–Johnson data tables is the Score Report, which provides the following basic data: (a) Cluster/Test name; (b) W score; (c) AE; (d) RPI; (e) SS and 95% C. Note that what is missing are PRs and interpretative classifications. Score reports can be printed in various types of organization and order of clusters and tests, although the simple numerical order of clusters and tests are most efficient because the data tables are already in an order most conducive to interpretation. In addition, intra-achievement variations are provided, which is an ipsative analysis that will be described in more detail in the ensuing interpretation section. It essentially provides all the data needed for a profile of strengths and weaknesses (PSW) comparison, which is relevant to SLD diagnoses.

Profile Reports provide scales of SS and PR continua for each cluster and test, and greys in the 68% CI for each. The problem is that specific SS and PR scores are not provided, just a visual grey rectangle that represents the 68% CI. Hence, this form is not useful. The Parent Report prints each cluster that was scored and places an "X" in the box under a proficiency classification. PRs are also reported, but again these pertain only to clusters and not the individual tests. Finally, there is a Data Record that prints out all of the raw scores that were entered into the program. Note that nowhere are the PRs listed for the specific tests and PRs for clusters are only available on the Parent Report. Therefore, the examiner can use the standard score to percentile rank conversion guide in Appendix A to reference approximate PRs for the various SSs.

Interpretation

Forms 8.7 and 8.8 are two versions for reporting and interpreting selected WJ IV ACH clusters, tests, and various types of data within a psychological assessment report. The principal difference lies in which data drives the reported classifications. Specifically, Form 8.7 focuses on the SSs and their associated WJ IV classifications, which emphasizes the degree of functionality. In mental health testing, this is the traditional approach because measured symptoms are considered genuine psychopathology when they cause or are associated with a sufficient degree of dysfunction. As an alternative, Form 8.8 affords a principal focus on the RPIs because they determine the proficiency classification rather than the SSs. Both continue to utilize the DSM–5 criteria of a SS of 78 or below (i.e., PR ≤ 7), thus indicating SLD symptoms. However, the chief difference between the two is which type of data drive the enumerated classifications. If the clinician wishes to emphasize functionality, then Form 8.7 is a more felicitous selection. In contrast, if the clinician wishes to emphasize proficiency levels, then Form 8.8 is more suitable.

Before proceeding with these forms, some terminology is important to briefly clarify. First, a WJ IV cluster is equivalent to a composite score or level 2 broad domain as employed in the WIAT–III. Second, a test in the WJ IV is equivalent to a subtest or narrowly defined skill (i.e., subskill) in the WIAT–III. The diagnostic significance is that a cluster with a SS of 78 or less is sufficiently low and broadly defined to indicate a SLD in that academic domain or academic area. The same *SS* for a test, however, indicates an impairment in a specific skill (i.e., subskills) and, of itself, falls short of a complete SLD diagnosis. At the same time, they are important in that they show which subskills should be listed as impaired with a valid diagnosis to assist in targeting instructional intervention. Note that this same diagnostic approach was used with the WIAT–III, hence showing consistency between both tests.

As stated previously, the DSM–5 now incorporates all learning disorders together, then subtypes them according one of three academic curricula or domains (i.e., reading, written language, and mathematics), each differentiated by their own diagnostic code. Furthermore, all subskills that are found to be impaired are also to be listed. Therefore, the data tables are apportioned so as to match this nosological organization and sequence of presentation. Also, because SLDs are diagnosed at the cluster broad domain level, the data tables proceed from the more broad-level clusters to the more specifically defined test-level skills (or subskills). It should be noted that because both Forms 8.7 and 8.8 are virtually identical, with the single exception of which scores drive the reported classification scheme, they are discussed together with differences mentioned only when necessary.

Before proceeding, it is prudent that Figure 8.4 be reviewed briefly, which is available on Routledge's e-resources website, along with the organization of the ensuing sections of the chapter that vary somewhat from that of this figure. Specifically, the interpretive process outlined in the Figure 8.4 flowchart (see e-resources) proceeds within each academic area as follows: (a) reading achievement; (b) written expression achievement; and (c) mathematics achievement. This mirrors the nosological organization of SLDs in the DSM–5. Within each academic area, the analysis proceeds from the broad domain clusters to the more specific tests, and finally, an ipsative analysis in order to detect the relative pattern of strengths and weaknesses (PSW) within an academic area at both the cluster and test levels. Although the flowchart proceeds within each academic area in such manner, the ensuing sections discuss the process according to analysis at the cluster level across the achievement domains (viz., Curricular Area Analysis in Figure 8.4), followed by analysis at the test level (viz., Academic Area Analysis in Figure 8.4), and finally, analysis at the ipsative level (viz., Intra-Achievement Variations PSW Analysis in Figure 8.4). This organization makes more pedagogical sense compared to the actual test reporting process delineated in Figure 8.4. This should be considered throughout the subsequent discussion.

CURRICULAR AREA ANALYSIS

As just stated, the WJ IV ACH data are chiefly apportioned by academic area, which mirrors the DSM–5 diagnostic scheme. Hence, Figure 8.4 presents three levels portrayed in large arrow-like figures, each representing a separate area

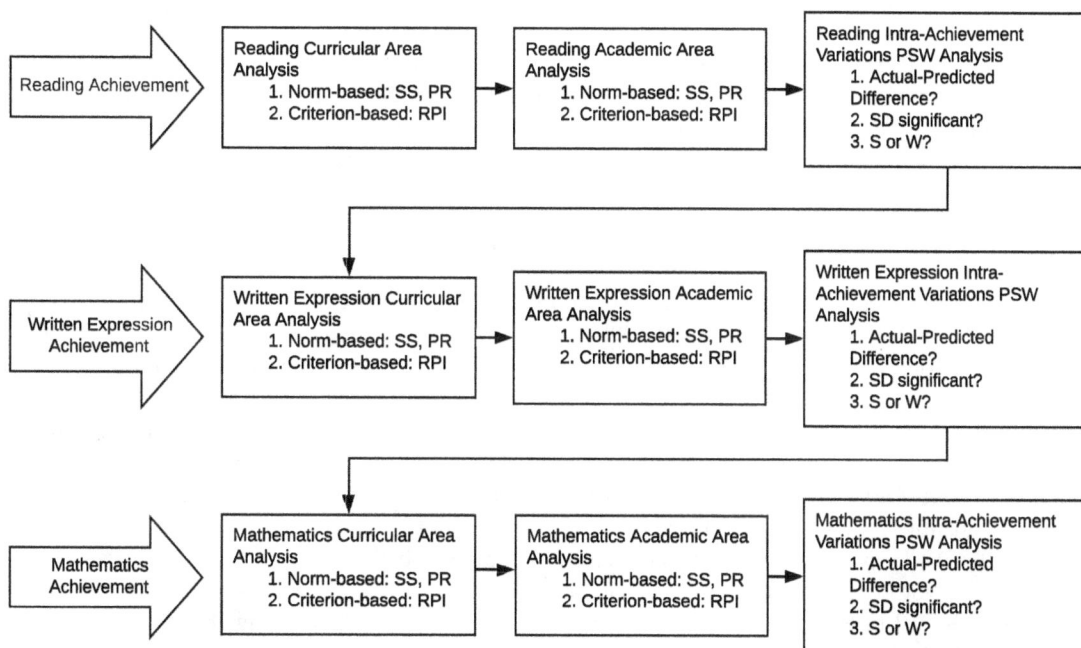

Note. Curricular area = broad academic domain (Stratum level II). Academic area = narrowly defined specific skills (i.e., subskills; Stratum I). Norm-based = comparison with standardization sample performance. Criterion-based = comparison with a preselected standard; here, 90% mastery of an academic curricular area at an examinee's grade level. SS = standard score (mean = 100, standard deviation = 15, range = 54–146). PR = percentile rank. RPI = relative proficiency index. SD = standard deviation. S = strength; W = weakness.

Figure 8.4. Woodcock Johnson, Fourth Edition, Tests of Achievement (WJ IV ACH) Interpretive Process

of achievement as follows: (a) Reading Ac^hievement (1st row); (b) Written Expression Ac^hievement (2nd row); and (c) Mathematics Ac^hievement (3rd row). The first box following each achievement arrow represents the "Cluster Level Analysis," which represent broad domains analogous to composites in the WIAT–III and Stratum II factors when referring to the structure of intelligence (see Chapter 7). Therefore, this represents the first line analysis for each achievement area.

Tables 1, 4, and 7 are constructed to report the cluster level analyses for reading, written expression, and mathematics, respectively (see Forms 8.7 and 8.8). Specifically, these tables consist of seven columns as follows: (a) cluster name; (b) standard score (*SS*); (c) 95% CI of the *SS*; (d) percentile rank (PR); (e) relative proficiency index (RPI); (f) WI IV classification (i.e., Form 8.7) or proficiency classification (i.e., Form 8.8), and (g) measured skills. As portrayed in Figure 8.4 (e-resources), the *SS* and PR norm-based comparisons drive this beginning analysis. In particular, the *SS* appends an asterisk if it is equal to or less than the DSM–5 criteria for a SLD, which is defined in the general table notes. Next, the criterion-based RPI should be interpreted in order to predict the percent mastery the examinee is expected to manifest within the classroom. Note that pre-drafted interpretive statements follow Tables 1, 4, and 7, which are intended to facilitate this analysis for each achievement area. Of course, they may be modified as needed depending upon the data pattern.

ACADEMIC AREA ANALYSIS

Tables 1, 4, and 7 are principally designed to determine if there is sufficient evidence for the presence of a SLD with impairment in reading (i.e., F81.0), written expression (i.e., F81.81), and mathematics (i.e., F81.2), respectively. Therefore, it makes logical sense to follow these data with scores at the test-level, proceeding from broad to more specific levels of analysis for each of the achievement areas. In Figure 8.4, the test level boxes are titled, "Academic Area Analysis," with the achievement area name immediately preceding this title. Note that each are positioned immediately to the right of their respective cluster level analyses. In Forms 8.7 and 8.8, Tables 2, 5, and 8 are designed to report and interpret the test level results for each achievement area. The principal purpose here is to identify which specific skills (or subskills) are impaired in order to list them with the SLD diagnosis and direct the instructional intervention plan.

Therefore, if the cluster level results are negative, it is discretionary whether or not the test level results need to be reported. This can save time and focus the report effectively on only the key results. In the presence of negative cluster data, it is advised that the test-level data be reported when either of the following two conditions apply: (a) there is value in communicating that the examinee possesses some isolated difficulties in specific skills or subskills that falls short of a full diagnosis; and/or (b) there is value in reporting the examinee's degree of proficiency in various specific skills in the classroom. Tables 2, 5, and 8 are designed in the same manner as their companion Tables 1, 4, and 7, although the interpretation is modified to be at the specific skill test level. The same interpretive pattern is followed, beginning with the norm-based comparisons and ensued by the criterion-based RPI proficiency scores. However, note that SLDs are not diagnosed here but are supplemented by reporting which subskills within those achievement areas are showing levels of impairment and requiring intervention.

INTRA-ACHIEVEMENT VARIATIONS PSW ANALYSIS

One factor that may be considered in facilitating a diagnosis of one or more SLDs is a student's relative *pattern of strengths and weaknesses* (*PSW*; IDEA 2004, §300.309[a][2][ii]) (U.S. Department of Education, 2006). PSW analyses are essentially ipsative or relative comparisons that are recognized by law as contributing to a diagnosis of SLDs. This means that significant within-subject variability in test scores represents an acceptable approach to diagnosing SLDs. In the mental health system, such analysis would be supplementary to the *SS* criterion of 78 and below, and contribute to identifying which skill sets are especially impaired. The statistical process, however, is somewhat different than done in the WIAT–III wherein pairwise comparisons are done among the composite scores and selected subtest scores. Here, the quantitative approach is more comparable to an ability achievement discrepancy (AAD) analysis.

In particular, the WJ IV procedure compares the cluster or test *SS* obtained by the examinee to that expected or predicted by an averaging of the *SS*s from other pertinent achievement areas. To perform such analyses, at minimum the first six tests of the WJ IV ACH must be administered (i.e., the core tests). Essentially, the predicted score for each of the core tests is derived by averaging the *SS*s on the other five core tests. Hence, for instance, the predicted score for Test 1–Letter-Number Sequencing is computed by an averaging of the *SS*s on Tests 2 through 6, and so on for the remaining 5 core tests. When additional tests are administered (e.g., Test 7–Word Attack and Test 12–Reading Recall from the extended battery), then both they and their resulting cluster (e.g., Basic Reading Skills) are both compared to the same predicted *SS* as was computed for Test 1. In the online computer generated Score Report, auxiliary intra-achievement comparisons are enumerated under the heading, "Intra-Achievement [Extended] Variations."

In Figure 8.4 (see e-resources), these analyses are portrayed in the third and final box in the sequence of three for each achievement area titled, "Intra-Achievement Variations PSW Analysis," with the name of the achievement area immediately preceding this label. In Forms 8.7 and 8.8, these data are reported in Tables 3, 6, and 9. Each of these tables is organized as follows: (a) cluster or test name (clusters listed first); (b) obtained or actual *SS*; (c) predicted *SS* (i.e., an averaging of the SSs on the other pertinent core and added tests); (d) difference score; (e) PR of the difference score obtained in the norm reference sample; (f) standard deviation (*SD*) of the difference score; and (g) interpretation of the difference score. The interpretation result is either "Weakness," "Strength," or neither, which is based upon the absolute value and direction of the *SD*. Specifically, any *SD* that is equal to or exceeds 1.50 is statistically significant. If the sign is negative, the interpretation is a weakness, whereas a plus sign denotes a strength. The more weaknesses that are detected within an examinee's PSW profile, the more this supports a SLD diagnosis. It also illustrates that the examinee's skill sets are showing remarkable degrees of variability, a pattern consistent with one or more SLDs. As alluded to prior, the PSW analysis has a good deal of pragmatic value in that it effectively directs where intervention should be targeted.

WOODCOCK–JOHNSON ACHIEVEMENT INTERPRETIVE PROCESS

Now that the substantive types of analyses have been reviewed, this section reviews the recommended process of interpreting the WJ IV ACH data yield. Although there are a number of cross-domain clusters available on this measure, they have been eliminated from this analysis because they are peripheral to detecting SLDs. That is, SLD diagnoses are made within and not between or across areas of achievement, at least by DSM–5 standards.[5] Therefore, although they may be interesting, they are superfluous to the objective of SLD diagnosis. For example, Broad Achievement is based upon an averaging of nine tests within the standard battery. Although extremely reliable and valid due to the amount of data upon which it relies, it is diagnostically much too general or broad to be of diagnostic use. It is much more pragmatic to begin analysis immediately at the cluster level with a particular area of achievement, followed by test-level and intra-achievement comparisons.

Therefore, Figure 8.4 (e-resources) begins the analysis with reading achievement, principally because reading disorder is the most common of the three achievement areas, estimated at a prevalence rate of 7% in the population of children, including mostly males (Peterson & Pennington, 2015; Rutter et al., 2004). The sequence begins with the reading-related clusters, followed by test-level and intra-achievement comparisons. The chief reason why preference is afforded to all relevant analyses within an achievement area is that the test-level and intra-achievement comparisons may either not be necessary at all, or may be significantly curtailed due to negative results. For example, of all reading-related clusters are clearly above threshold for diagnosing a SLD, the ensuing test-level and intra-achievement comparisons may be deleted entirely, hence saving both time and space. If only some of the clusters are significant for a SLD, then follow-up analyses may be reported and interpreted although in reduced number.

The written expression achievement area immediately follows reading because the skills are related, both requiring the use of language. Finally, the mathematics achievement area is done last, although in the same cluster, test, and intra-achievement sequence as for the reading and written language areas. This made the most sense considering that mathematics is not as similar in terms of content as are the reading and written expressions areas. Its prevalence rate is also much lower, estimated at only 1% in the population of children (Tannock, 2005).

POSITION VERSUS PROFICIENCY

This final section concerns the issue of whether norm-based data or proficiency measures are more useful in the context of achievement testing. In academic achievement evaluations, the relative proficiency index (RPI) makes an important contribution that cannot be derived from norm-based peer-comparison scores. For example, if a child's *SS* in a cognitive skill is not significantly low (e.g., a *SS* of 85, low average), the examiner may not consider this as a genuine weakness. However, the weakness may become more obvious when the RPI is considered. As has been apparent in prior examples, the low average *SS* appeared significantly higher than an examinee's accompanying RPI that is derived much differently. Many psychologists have had the experience of telling a teacher that a student scored in the average or low average range on a test, only to have the teacher respond with disbelief because the score did not reflect the child's struggles in daily class work (see, e.g., Jaffe, 2009). Because of the divergence between the information provided by peer-comparison scores and that provided by the RPI, the results of an evaluation might be misinterpreted if RPI scores are not considered. Woodcock (1999) illustrated the importance of recognizing the dissimilarity between position in a distribution and level of competence by explaining that people with sensory limitations are classified as disabled based upon weaknesses in the quality of their performance, not because they fall below some point on a norm-referenced scale (p. 109). For this reason, (a) the WJ IV ACH has been included as part of the test battery in achievement, (b) the RPI has been added to the data tables for this measure, and (c) a second alternative form (viz., Form 8.8) has been designed that emphasizes proficiency in classification labels that are driven by the RPI.

Recapitulation

This chapter defined achievement as the degree of learning and accomplishment in various areas of instruction, then focused upon major areas of achievement wherein SLDs are diagnosed, including reading, written expression, mathematics, and oral communication or language. Thereafter, two individually administer tests of achievement were discussed in detail, including (a) the WIAT–III, and (b) the WJ IV ACH. The WIAT–II was discussed first because it is somewhat more conducive to testing in the mental health field for a number of reasons, and it is selected for use when an AAD analysis is required or desired. Hence, the WIAT–III was first discussed in terms of its data yield for PK and for individuals from K though grade 12 and adulthood. Next, AAD analyses were reviewed, including the data tables that facilitated such analysis and the statistical procedures contained therein. Thereafter, the WJ IV ACH was presented in detail, with special emphasis on components that make this test unique from that of the WIAT–III and why this test was added to the book's inventory. In particular, the WJ IV ACH yields both norm-based and criterion-based data, the latter including a measure of predicted proficiency in the classroom. However, this test must be computer scored on the online program and tests of oral language are not included among the achievement tests; that is, they must be purchased separately, hence adding to the costs of using this test if oral language skills need to be measured. Looking ahead, the ensuing Chapter 9 is the third and final chapter wherein cognitive abilities are measured. However, the focus shifts to the measurement of brain-behavior relationships and functioning; that is, the diagnosis of neurocognitive disorders (previously known as dementias and delirium).

Key Terms

- ability achievement discrepancy (AAD)
- ability memory discrepancy (AMD)
- accountability
- accuracy disability
- achievement
- achievement batteries
- adaptive testing
- age-equivalent (AE)
- brisk administration
- chronological age (CA)
- communication disorders
- confidence intervals (CIs)
- co-norming
- criterion-based approach
- criterion-based test
- cross-validation
- crystalized intelligence
- Diagnostic and Statistical Manual of Mental Disorders, Fifth Edition (DSM–5)
- Diagnostic and Statistical Manual of Mental Disorders, Fourth Edition, Text Revision
- discontinue rules
- dyslexia
- Dyslexia Index
- exact administration
- experimentwise error rate
- extended battery
- extended percentile ranks
- familywise error rate
- fluid intelligence
- Gf-Gc model of intelligence
- grade equivalents (GEs)
- grade scores

- grade-equivalent (GE)
- growth scale values (GSVs)
- Individuals with Disabilities Education Improvement Act of 2004
- inferential norming
- instructional zone
- intelligence
- Iowa Assessments (Iowa Test of Basic Skills)
- item sets
- language disorder
- learning disabilities
- math fluency
- Memory for Sound Patterns (UM)
- moments
- normal curve equivalent (NCE)
- norm-based test
- orthographic mapping
- orthographic skills
- parallel tests
- percentile rank (PR)
- Percentile ranks (PRs)
- percentiles
- phoneme–grapheme correspondence
- phonic decoding
- phonological abilities
- phonological awareness
- phonological disorder
- phonological processing
- phonological recoding
- phonological-orthographic relationships
- preauthorization (PA)
- predicted difference discrepancy analyses
- proficiency
- pseudowords
- rate disability
- reference W
- relative proficiency index (RPI)
- relative proficiency index (RPI)
- reliability
- reverse rules
- semantics
- short-term working memory (Gwm)
- simple difference discrepancy analyses
- specific learning disorders (SLDs)
- speech sound disorder
- Speed of lexical analysis (LA)
- standard battery
- standard error of measurement (SEM)
- standard score (*SS*)
- standards-based education
- stanines
- start points
- stop points
- syntax
- teratogens
- three stratum hierarchical model of intelligence
- trait

- utility
- validity
- *W* ability
- *W* difference (W DIFF)
- *W* difficulty
- *W* score
- Wechsler Individual Achievement Test (WIAT)
- Wechsler Individual Achievement Test, Second Edition (WIAT–4)
- Wechsler Individual Achievement Test, Second Edition (WIAT–II)
- Wechsler Individual Achievement Test, Third Edition (WIAT–III)
- Woodcock–Johnson Psycho-Educational Battery (WJ)
- Woodcock–Johnson Psycho-Educational Battery–Revised (WJ R)
- Woodcock–Johnson, Fourth Edition, Tests of Achievement (WJ IV ACH)
- Woodcock–Johnson, Third Edition (WJ III)
- word retrieval

Notes

1. The terms learning disability and specific learning disorders (SLDs) will here be used interchangeably, although the former is usually more commonly utilized in the educational system and more generally whereas the latter is particular to the DSM–5 nosology.
2. Inferential norming will be broached again with other standardized test that measure personality. Hence, this statistical procedure is not limited to norming cognitive-type tests.
3. However, the Woodcock–Johnson achievement test battery also uses the SS for both its tests, which are comparable to the WIAT–III subtests, and for its clusters, which are comparable to the WIAT–III composites.
4. This is the exact strategy employed with the Woodcock–Johnson as it speeds the interpretation process considerably. Although the overall and cross-domain achievement scores may be of interest, they are too broad for effective psychodiagnosis and thus can be omitted.
5. Recall that the ICD–10 has F81.3 Specific Learning Disorder, Mixed disorder of scholastic skills, as a listed diagnosis that could be used for a disorder that crosses academic areas. Examples of cluster scores on the WJ IV ACH that consists of several academic curricula include Academic Fluency (viz., Sentence Reading Fluency, Math Facts Fluency, and Sentence Writing Fluency) and Academic Applications (viz., Applied Problems, Passage Comprehension, and Writing Samples). Both of these scales measure a type of skill set (e.g., degree of fluency, ability to apply knowledge) versus mastery of a content area. In mental health, the disorders are classified principally by content area, hence, this is what is emphasized in the data tables. The same information can be communicated, although within each academic area rather than across these areas. However, the clinician who wishes to add these cross-domain clusters can do so easily.

References

Adams, M. (1990). *Beginning to read: Thinking and learning about print*. Cambridge, MA: MIT Press.

Alfonso, V. C., Flanagan, D. P., & Radwan, S. (2005). The impact of Cattell-Horn-Carroll theory on test development and the interpretation of cognitive abilities. In D. P. Flanagan & P. L. Harrison (Eds.), *Contemporary intellectual assessment: Theories, f*ts and issues* (2nd ed.; pp. 185–202). New York, NY: Guilford Press.

American Psychiatric Association. (2000). *Diagnostic and statistical manual of m*tal disorders* (4th ed., text rev.; DSM–IV–TR). Washington, DC: Author.

American Psychiatric Association. (2013). *Diagnostic and statistical manual of m*tal disorders* (5th ed.; DSM–5). Arlington, VA: Author.

Bailet, L. L. (2001). Development and disorders of spelling in the beginning school years. In A. M. Bain, L. L. Bailet, & L. C. Moats (Eds.), *Written language disorders: Theor* into practice* (2nd ed., pp. 1–41). Austin, TX: Pro-Ed.

Beitchman, J., & Brownlie, E. B. (2014). *Language disorders in children and adolescents*. Cambridge, MA: Hogrefe & Huber.

Benasich, A. A., Curtiss, S., & Tallal, P. (1993). Language, learning, and behavioral disturbances in childhood: A longitudinal perspective. *Journal of the American Academy of Child & Adolescent Psychiatry, 32*, 585–594.

Berninger, V. (1998). *Process assessment of the learner. Guides for intervention: Reading and writing*. San Antonio, TX: Pearson.

Berninger, V., Cartwright, A., Yates, C., Swanson, H., & Abbott, R. (1994). Developmental skills related to writing and reading acquisition in the intermediate grades: Shared and unique variance. *Reading and Writing: An Interdisciplinary Journal, 6*, 161–196.

Berninger, V., Yates, C., Cartwright, A., Rutberg, J., Remy, E., & Abbott, R. (1992). Lower-level developmental skills in beginning writing. *Reading and Writing: An Interdisciplinary Journal, 4*, 257–280.

Bradley, L., & Bryant, P. E. (1978). Difficulties in auditory organisation as a possible cause of reading backwardness. *Nature, 271*, 746–747.

Braze, D., Tabor, W., Shankweiler, D., & Mencl, W. E. (2007). Speaking up for vocabulary: Reading skill differences in young adults. *Journal of Learning Disabilities, 40*, 226–243.

Breaux, K. C. (2020a). *Wechsler individual achievement test, fourth edition (WIAT–4): Administration manual*. Bloomington, MN: NCS Pearson.

Breaux, K. C. (2020b). *Wechsler individual achievement test, fourth edition (WIAT–4): Scoring manual.* Bloomington, MN: NCS Pearson.

Breaux, K. C. (2020c). *Wechsler individual achievement test, fourth edition (WIAT–4): Technical and interpretive manual.* Bloomington, MN: NCS Pearson.

Bryant, D. P., Bryant, B. R., & Hammill, D. D. (2000). Characteristic behaviors of students with LD who have teacher-identified math weaknesses. *Journal of Learning Disabilities, 33,* 168–177.

Bull, R., & Scerif, G. (2001). Executive functioning as a predictor of children's mathematics ability: Inhibition, task switching, and working memory. *Developmental Neuropsychology, 19,* 273–293.

Calhoon, M. B., Emerson, R. W., Flores, M., & Houchins, D. E. (2007). Computational fluency performance profile of high school students with mathematics disabilities. *Remedial and Special Education, 28,* 292–303.

Carlisle, J. (1991). Language comprehension and text structure. In J. F. Kavanagh (Ed.), *The language continuum: From infancy to literacy* (pp. 115–145). Parkton, MD: York Press.

Carroll, J. B. (1993). *Human cognitive abilities: A survey of factor analytic studies.* Cambridge, England: Cambridge University Press.

Catts, H. W., Gillispie, M., Leonard, L. B., Kail, R. V., & Miller, C. A. (2002). The role of speed of processing, rapid naming, and phonological awareness in reading achievement. *Journal of Learning Disabilities, 35,* 510–525.

Cizek, G. J. (Ed.). (2001). *Setting performance standards: Concepts, methods, and perspectives.* Mahwah, NJ: Lawrence Erlbaum Associates.

Cummins, J. (1984). Language proficiency and academic achievement revisited: A response. In *Note 100p.; Selected papers of the Language Proficiency Assessment Symposium* (Warrenton, VA, March 14–18, Vol. 400, p. 90).

de Jong, D. E. (1998). Working memory deficits of reading disabled children. *Journal of Experimental Child Psychology, 170,* 75–76.

DuBois, P. H. (1966). A test-dominated society: China 1115 B.C.E–1905 A.D. In A. Anastasi (Ed.), *Testing problems in perspective* (pp. 29–36). Washington, DC: American Council on Education.

DuBois, P. H. (1970). *A history of psychological testing.* Boston: Allyn & Bacon.

Flanagan, D. P., & Dixon, S. G. (2013). The Cattell-Horn-Carroll theory of cognitive abilities. In C. R. Reynolds, K. J. Vannest, & E. Fletcher-Janzen (Eds.), *Encyclopedia of special education* (pp. 368–382). Hoboken, NJ: John Wiley & Sons.

Gathercole, S. E. (2004). Working memory and learning during the school years. *Proceedings of the British Academy, 125,* 365–380.

Gathercole, S. E., & Baddeley, A. D. (1989). Evaluation of the role of phonological memory and vocabulary in children: A longitudinal study. *Journal of Memory and Language, 28,* 200–213.

Gathercole, S. E., Lamont, E., & Alloway, T. P. (2006). Working memory in the classroom. In S. J. Pickering (Ed.), *Working memory and education* (pp. 220–241). Burlington, MA: Elsevier Press.

Gathercole, S. E., Willis, C., Emslie, H., & Baddeley, A. D. (1992). Phonological memory and vocabulary development during the early school years: A longitudinal study. *Developmental Psychology, 28,* 887–898.

Gathercole, S. E., Willis, C., Emslie, H., & Baddeley, A. D. (1994). The Children's Test of Nonword Repetition: A test of phonological working memory. *Memory, 2,* 103–127.

Geary, D. C. (2004). Mathematics and learning disabilities. *Journal of Learning Disabilities, 37,* 4–15.

Goldman-Rakic, P. S. (1992). Working memory and the mind. *Scientific American, 267,* 110–117.

Gough, P. B., & Tunmer, W. E. (1986). Decoding, reading, and reading disability. *Remedial and Special Education, 7,* 6–10.

Gregg, N., & Hafer, T. (2001). Disorders of written expression. In A. M. Bain, L. L. Bailet, & L. C. Moats (Eds.), *Written language disorders: Theory into practice* (2nd ed., pp. 103–136). Austin, TX: Pro-Ed.

Gregg, N., & Mather, N. (2002). School is fun at recess: Informal analyses of written language for students with learning disabilities. *Journal of Learning Disabilities, 35,* 7–22.

Gregg, N., Coleman, C., Davis, M., & Chalk, J. C. (2007). Timed essay writing: Implications for high-stakes tests. *Journal of Learning Disabilities, 40,* 306–318.

Gregory, R. J. (2011). *Psychological testing: History, principles, applications.* Boston, MA: Pearson Education.

Groth-Marnat, G. (2003). *Handbook of psychological assessment* (4th ed.). New York, NY: John Wiley & Sons.

Holmes, D. R., & McKeever, W. F. (1979). Material specific serial memory deficit in adolescent dyslexics. *Cortex, 15,* 51–62.

Hoover, H. D., Dunbar, S. B., Frisbie, D. A., Oberley, K. R., Bray, G. B., Naylor, R. J., . . . Qualls, A. L. (2007). *Iowa tests of basic skills: Norms and score conversions.* Itasca, IL: Riverside Publishing.

Horn, J. L. (1991). Measurement of intellectual capabilities: A review of theory. In K. S., McGrew, J. K. Werder, & R. W. Woodcock (Eds.), *WJ–R technical manual* (pp. 197–232). Chicago, IL: Riverside Publishing.

Houck, C. K., & Billingsley, B. S. (1989). Written expression of students with and without learning disabilities: Differences across the grades. *Journal of Learning Disabilities, 22,* 561–572.

Individuals with Disabilities Education Improvement Act of 2004, Pub. L. 108–446, 118 Stat. 328 (2004).

Jaffe, L. E. (2009). *Development, interpretation, and application of the W score and the relative proficiency index* (Woodcock-Johnson III Assessment Service Bulletin No. 11). Rolling Meadows, IL: Riverside Publishing. Explanation of the W score and RPI score metrics).

Johnson, D. J. (1982). Programming for dyslexia: The need for interaction analyses. *Annals of Dyslexia, 32,* 61–70. Baltimore, MD: The Orton Dyslexia Society.

Johnson, D. J., & Myklebust, H. R. (1967). *Learning disabilities: Educational principles and practices.* New York, NY: Grune & Stratton.

Jorm, A. F. (1979). The cognitive and neurological basis of developmental dyslexia: A theoretical framework and review. *Cognition, 7,* 19–33.

Jorm, A. F. (1983). Specific reading retardation and working memory: A review. *British Journal of Psychology, 74,* 311–342.

Kaplan, D. S., Damphous, K. R., & Kaplan, H. B. (1994). Mental health implications of not graduating from high school. *Journal of Experimental Education, 62,* 105–123.

Katzir, T., Kim, Y., Wolf, M., Morris, R., & Lovett, M. W. (2008). The varieties of pathways to dysfluent reading: Comparing subtypes of children with dyslexia at letter, word, and connected text levels of reading. *Journal of Learning Disabilities, 41*, 47–66.

Kaufman, A. S., & Lichtenberger, E. O. (1999). *Essential of the WAIS–III assessment.* New York, NY: John Wiley & Sons.

Kaufman, S. B., Reynolds, M. R., Lin, X., Kaufman, A. S., & McGrew, K. (2012). Are cognitive *g* one and the same *g*? An exploration on the Woodcock–Johnson and Kaufman tests. *Intelligence, 40*, 123–138.

Kavale, K. A., & Forness, S. R. (1995). *The nature of learning disabilities: Critical elements of diagnosis and classification.* Mahwah, NJ: Erlbaum.

Kavale, K. A., & Forness, S. R. (1996). Social skill deficits and learning disabilities: A meta-analysis. *Journal of Learning Disabilities, 29*, 226–237.

Kavale, K. A., Holdnack, J. A., & Mostert, M. P. (2005). Responsiveness to intervention and the identification of learning disability: A critique and alternative proposal. *Learning Disability Quarterly, 28*, 2–16.

Kavanagh, J. F. (1991). Preface. In J. F. Kavanagh (Ed.), *The language continuum: From infancy to literacy* (pp. vii–1). Parkton, MD: York Press.

Kim, Y. S. G., & Wagner, R. K. (2015). Text (oral) reading fluency as a construct in reading development: An investigation of its mediating role for children from grades 1 to 4. *Scientific Studies of Reading, 19*, 224–242.

LaBerge, D., & Samuals, S. J. (1974). Toward a theory of automatic information processing in reading. *Cognitive Psychology, 6*, 293–323.

Lane, S. E., & Lewandowski, L. (1994). Oral and written compositions of students with and without learning disabilities. *Journal of Psychoeducational Assessment, 12*, 142–153.

Larsen, R. J., & Buss, D. M. (2021). *Personality psychology: Domains of knowledge about human nature* (7th ed.). New York, NY: McGraw Hill.

Lennon, J. E., & Slesinski, C. (1999). Early intervention in reading: Results of a screening and intervention program for kindergarten students. *School Psychology Review, 28*, 353–364.

Lewandowski, L. J., & Lovett, B. J. (2014). Learning disabilities. In E. J. Mash & R. A. Barkley (Eds.), *Child psychopathology* (pp. 625–669). The Guilford Press.

Linacre, J. M. (2005). *WINSTEPS Rasch measurement computer program.* Chicago: Winsteps.com.

Lovett, M. (1987). A developmental approach to reading disability: Accuracy and speed criteria of normal and deficient reading skill. *Child Development, 58*, 234–260.

Lyon, G. R., Shaywitz, S. E., & Shaywitz, B. A. (2003). Defining dyslexia, comorbidity, teachers' knowledge of language and reading: A definition of dyslexia. *Annals of Dyslexia, 53*, 1–14.

Mann, V. A., Cowin, E., & Schoenheimer, J. (1989). Phonological processing, language comprehension, and reading ability. *Journal of Learning Disabilities, 22*, 76–89.

Mann, V. A., Liberman, I. Y., & Shankweiler, D. (1980). Children's memory for sentences and word strings in relation to reading ability. *Memory and Cognition, 8*, 329–335.

Matarazzo, J. D., & Herman, D. O. (1985). Clinical uses or WAIS–R: Base rates of differences between VOQ and PIQ in the WAIS–R standardization sample. In B. B. Wolman (Ed.), *Handbook of intelligence: Theories, measurement, and applications* (pp. 899–932). New York, NY: John Wiley & Sons.

Mather, N., & Wendling, B. J. (2014). *Woodcock–Johnson, fourth edition, tests of achievement (WJ IV ACH): Examiner's manual.* Rolling Meadows, IL: Riverside Publishing.

Mayes, S. D., Calhoun, S. L., & Lane, S. E. (2005). Diagnosing children's writing disabilities: Different tests give different results. *Perceptual and Motor Skills, 101*, 72–78.

Mayringer, H., & Wimmer, H. (2000). Pseudoname learning by German-speaking children with dyslexia: Evidence for a phonological learning deficit. *Journal of Experimental Child Psychology, 75*, 116–133.

McCrae, R. R., & Costa, P. T., Jr. (2010). *NEO inventories for the NEO personality inventory, third edition (NEO–PI–3), NEO five factor inventory, third edition (NEO–FFI–3), NEO personality inventory, revised (NEO PI–R): Professional manual.* Lutz, FL: Psychological Assessment Services (PAR).

McCutchen, D., Abbott, R. D., Green, L. B., Beretvas, S. N., Cox, S., Potter, N. S., et al. (2002). Beginning literacy: Links among teacher knowledge, teacher practice, and student learning. *Journal of Learning Disabilities, 35*, 69–86.

McGrew, K. S. (1986). *Clinical interpretation of the Woodcock–Johnson test of cognitive ability.* Boston, MA: Allyn & Bacon.

McGrew, K. S. (1994). *Clinical interpretation of the Woodcock–Johnson test of cognitive ability–revised.* Boston, MA: Allyn & Bacon.

McGrew, K. S. (2005). The Cattell-Horn-Carroll (CHC) theory of cognitive abilities: Past, present, and future. In D. P. Flanagan, & P. L. Harrison (Eds.), *Contemporary intellectual assessment: Theories, tests, and issues* (2nd ed., pp. 136–202). New York, NY: Guilford Press.

McGrew, K. S. (2008). *The Australian standardization of the Woodcock Johnson III cognitive and achievement battery.* Paper presented at the Conference of the Australian Psychological Society, Hobart, Tasmania, Australia.

McGrew, K. S., & Woodcock, R. W. (1989). *Woodcock–Johnson psycho-educational battery–revised: Technical manual.* Rolling Meadows, IL: Riverside Publishing.

McGrew, K. S., & Woodcock, R. W. (2001). *Woodcock–Johnson, third edition (WJ III): Technical manual.* Rolling Meadows, IL: Riverside Publishing.

McGrew, K. S., LaForte, E. M., & Schrank, F. A. (2014). *Woodcock–Johnson, fourth edition (WJ IV): Technical manual.* Rolling Meadows, IL: Riverside Publishing.

MedFriendly. (2020). *Standard score to percentile conversion.* Retrieved June 26, 2020, from www.medfriendly.com/standardscoretopercentileconversion.html

Mertler, C. A. (2002). *Using standardized test data to guide instruction and intervention.* College Park, MD: ERIC Clearinghouse on Assessment and Evaluation. (ERIC Document Reproduction Service. Retrieved from www.eric.ed.gov/ (No. ED470589)

Miller, G. A., Galanter, E. & Pribram, K. H. (1960). *Plans and the structure of behavior.* New York, NY: Holt, Rinehart, & Winston.

Miller, L. A., McIntire, S. A., & Lovler, R. L. (2011). *Foundations of psychological testing* (3rd ed.). Thousand Oaks, CA: SAGE Publications.

Moats, L. C. (2001). Spelling disability in adolescents and adults. In A. M. Bain, L. L. Bailet, & L. C. Moats (Eds.), *Written language disorders: Theory into practice* (2nd ed., pp. 43–75). Austin, TX: Pro-Ed.

Mok, P. L. H., Pickles, A., Durkin, K., & Conti-Ramsden, G. (2014). Longitudinal trajectories of peer relations in children with specific language impairment. *Journal of Child Psychology and Psychiatry, 55*, 516–527.

Moran, M. R. (1981). Performance of learning disabled and low achieving secondary students on formal features of a paragraph-writing task. *Learning Disability Quarterly, 4*, 271–280.

Myklebust, H. R. (1973). *Development and disorders of written language: Studies of normal and exceptional children* (Vol. 2). New York, NY: Grune & Stratton.

National Center for Education Statistics. (2001). *The condition of education 2001.* Washington, DC: U.S. Department of Education. (For web copy on pdf. file, go to nces.ed.gov).

National Council of Teachers of Mathematics. (2000). *Principles and standards for school mathematics.* Reston, VA: Author.

National Institute of Child Health and Human Development. (2000). *Report of the national reading panel. Teaching children to read: An evidence-based assessment of the scientific research literature on reading and its implications for reading instruction* (NIH Publication No. 00–4769). Washington, DC: U.S. Government Printing Office.

NCS Pearson. (2020). *Wechsler individual achievement test, fourth edition (WIAT–4).* Bloomington, MN: Author.

Neely, J. H. (1977). Semantic priming and retrieval from Lexical memory: Roles of inhibitionless spreading activation and limited capacity attention. *Journal of Experimental Psychology: General, 106*, 226–254.

Pearson. (2005). *Wechsler individual achievement test, second edition (WIAT–II): Update 2005.* San Antonio, TX: Author.

Pearson. (2009a). *Wechsler individual achievement test, third edition (WIAT–III): Examiner's manual.* San Antonio, TX: Author.

Pearson. (2009b). *Wechsler individual achievement test, third edition (WIAT–III): Technical manual (on CD-ROM).* San Antonio, TX: Author.

Pearson. (2009c). *WIAT–III Scoring Assistant* [CD-ROM]. San Antonio, TX: Author.

Pearson. (2010). *Wechsler individual achievement test, third edition (WIAT–III): WIAT–III adult standardization, norms development, and norms tables.* San Antonio, TX: Author.

Pearson. (2021). *Q–global: Better insights. Anytime. Anywhere.* [Internet Web-Based Computer Scoring]. Retrieved from https://qglobal.pearsonclinical.com/qg/login.seam.

Perfettie, C. A. (1985). *Reading ability.* New York, NY: Oxford University Press.

Peterson, R. L., & Pennington, B. F. (2015). Developmental dyslexia. *Annual Review of Clinical Psychology, 11*, 283–307.

Poplin, M. S., Gray, R., Larsen, S., Banikowski, A., & Mehring, T. (1980). A comparison of components of written expression abilities in learning disabled and non-learning disabled students at three grade levels. *Learning Disability Quarterly, 3*, 46–53.

Poteet, J. A. (1978). *Characteristics of written expression of learning disabled and non-learning disabled elementary school students* (ERIC Document ED159–830). Muncie, IN: Ball State University.

Psychological Corporation (PsychCorp). (1992). *Wechsler individual achievement test (WIAT).* San Antonio, TX: Author.

Puolakanaho, A., Ahonen, T., Aro, M., Eklund, K., Leppänen, P. H. T., Poikkeus, A., et al. (2008). Developmental links of very early phonological and language skills to second grade reading outcomes: Strong to accuracy but only minor to fluency. *Journal of Learning Disabilities, 41*, 353–370.

Rayner, K., Foorman, B. R., Perfetti, C. A., Pesetsky, D., & Seidenberg, M. S. (2001). How psychological science informs the teaching of reading. *Psychological Science in the Public Interest, 2*, 31–74.

Riverside Score™. (2021). *Internet-based scoring platform.* Retrieved from https://riversidescore.com/.

Roth, P. L., Bevier, C. A., Switzer, F. S., & Schippmann, J. S. (1996). Meta-analyzing the relationship between grades and job performance. *Journal of Applied Psychology, 81*, 548–556.

Rutter, M., Caspi, A., Fergusson, D., Horwood, L. J., Goodman, R., Maughan, B., . . . Carroll, J. (2004). Sex differences in developmental reading disability: New findings from 4 epidemiological studies. *Journal of the American Medical Association, 291*, 2007–2012.

Sattler, J. M. (2001). *Assessment of children: Cognitive functions* (4th ed.). San Diego, CA: Author.

Sattler, J. M. (2014). *Foundations of behavioral, social, and clinical assessment of children* (6th ed.). LaMesa, CA: Jerome M. Sattler Publisher.

Sattler, J. M., & Ryan, J. J. (2009). *Assessment with the WAIS–IV.* San Diego, CA: Jerome M. Sattler Publisher.

Schneider, W. J., & McGrew, K. (2012). The Cattell-Horn-Carroll model of intelligence. In D. P. Flanagan & P. L. Harrison (Eds.), *Contemporary intellectual assessment: Theories, tests, and issues* (3rd ed., pp. 99–144). New York, NY: Guilford.

Schrank, F. A., & Dailey, D. (2014). *Woodcock–Johnson, online scoring and reporting* [Online format]. Rolling Meadows, IL: Riverside Publishing.

Schrank, F. A., Mather, N., & McGrew, K. S. (2014a). *Woodcock–Johnson, fourth edition, tests of achievement (WJ IV ACH).* Rolling Meadows, IL: Riverside Publishing.

Schrank, F. A., Mather, N., & McGrew, K. S. (2014b). *Woodcock–Johnson, fourth edition, tests of oral language (WJ IV ORL).* Rolling Meadows, IL: Riverside Publishing.

Schrank, F. A., McGrew, K. S., & Mather, N. (2014a). *Woodcock–Johnson, fourth edition (WJ IV).* Rolling Meadows, IL: Riverside Publishing.

Schrank, F. A., McGrew, K. S., & Mather, N. (2014b). *Woodcock–Johnson, fourth edition, tests of cognitive abilities (WJ IV COG).* Rolling Meadows, IL: Riverside Publishing.

Siegel, L. S., & Ryan, E. B. (1989). The development of working memory in normally achieving and subtypes of learning disabled children. *Child Development, 60*, 973–980.

Silverstein, A. B. (1981). Reliability and abnormality of test score differences. *Journal of Clinical Psychology, 37*, 392–394.

Spores, J. M. (2012). *Clinician's guide to psychological assessment and testing: With forms and templates for effective practice.* New York, NY: Springer Publishing.

Stevens, S. S. (1946). On the theory of scales of measurement, *Science,* 1103, 677–680.

Swanson, H. L. (1994). Short-term memory and working memory: Do both contribute to our understanding of academic achievement in children and adults with learning disabilities? *Journal of Learning Disabilities, 27*, 34–50.

Swanson, H. L., Ashbaker, H. J., & Lee, C. (1996). Learning disabled readers' working memory as a function of processing demands. *Journal of Experimental Child Psychology, 61*, 242–275.

Tallmadge, G. K., & Wood, C. T. (1978). *User's guide: ESEA Title I evaluation and reporting system.* Mountain View, CA: RMC Research Corporation.

Tannock, R. (2005). Mathematics disorder. In B. J. Sadock & V. A. Sadock (Eds.), *Kaplan & Sadock's comprehensive textbook of psychiatry* (pp. 3116–3123). Philadelphia: Lippincott Williams & Wilkins.

Thomas, C. C., Englert, C. S., & Gregg, S. (1987). An analysis of errors and strategies in the expository writing of learning disabled students. *Remedial and Special Education, 8*(1), 21–30.

Thurlow, M. L., & Ysseldyke, J. E. (2001). Standard setting challenges for special populations. In G. J. Cizek (Ed.), *Setting performance standards: Concepts, methods, and perspectives* (pp. 387–409). Mahwah, NJ: Lawrence Erlbaum.

Traweek, D., & Berninger, V. (1997). Comparison of beginning literacy programs: Alternative paths to the same learning outcome. *Learning Disability Quarterly, 20*, 160–168.

U. S. Department of Education. (2006, August 14). Assistance to states for the education of children with disabilities and preschool grants for children with disabilities; Final rule. Part II: 34 CFR Parts 300 and 301. *Federal Register, 71*(156).

U.S. Bureau of the Census. (2005). *Current population survey, October 2005: School enrollment supplement file* [CD-ROM]. Washington, DC: Author.

U.S. Bureau of the Census. (2010). *Current population survey, October 2010: School enrollment supplement file* [CD-ROM]. Washington, DC: Author.

van der Leij, A., & van Daal, V. H. P. (1999). Automatization aspects of dyslexia: Speed limitations in word identification, sensitivity to increasing task demands, and orthographic compensation. *Journal of Learning Disabilities, 32*, 417–428.

Vars, G. F. (2001). Can curriculum integration survive in an era of high-stakes testing? *Middle School Journal, 33*(2), 7–17. doi:10.1080/00940771.2001.11494658

Wechsler, D. (1939). *The measurement of adult intelligence.* Williams & Wilkins.

Wechsler, D. (2008a). *Wechsler Adult Intelligence Scale, Fourth Edition (WAIS–IV): Administration and scoring manual.* San Antonio, TX: The Psychological Corporation (PsychCorp)-Pearson.

Wechsler, D. (2008b). *Wechsler Adult Intelligence Scale–Fourth Edition (WAIS–IV): Technical and interpretive manual.* San Antonio, TX: The Psychological Corporation (PsychCorp)-Pearson.

Wechsler, D. (2012a). *Wechsler Preschool and Primary Scale of Intelligence, Fourth Edition (WPPSI–IV): Administration and scoring manual.* Bloomington, MN: The Psychological Corporation (PsychCorp)-Pearson.

Wechsler, D. (2012b). *Wechsler Preschool and Primary Scale of Intelligence, Fourth Edition (WPPSI–IV): Technical and interpretive manual.* Bloomington, MN: The Psychological Corporation (PsychCorp)-Pearson.

Wechsler, D. (2014a). *Wechsler Intelligence Scale for Children, Fifth Edition (WISC–V): Administration and scoring manual.* Bloomington, MN: The Psychological Corporation (PsychCorp)-Pearson.

Wechsler, D. (2014b). *Wechsler Intelligence Scale for Children, Fifth Edition (WISC–V): Technical and interpretive manual.* Bloomington, MN: The Psychological Corporation (PsychCorp)-Pearson.

Whitaker, D., Berninger, V., Johnston, J., & Swanson, H. L. (1994). Intraindividual differences in levels of language in intermediate grade writers: Implications for the translating process. *Learning and Individual Differences, 6*, 107–130.

Wikipedia Contributors. (2020, February 13). Richard Woodcock. In *Wikipedia, the free encyclopedia.* Retrieved 02:24, September 22, 2020, from https://en.wikipedia.org/w/index.php?title=Richard_Woodcock&oldid=940541768

Wilkins, C., Rolfhus, E., Weiss, L., & Zhu, J. (2005, April). *A new method for calibrating translated tests with small sample sizes.* Paper presented at the 2005 annual meeting of the American Educational Research Association, Montreal, Canada.

Woodcock, R. W. (1978). *Development and standardization of the Woodcock–Johnson psycho-educational battery.* Rolling Meadows, IL: Riverside Publishing.

Woodcock, R. W. (1984). A response to some questions raised about the Woodcock–Johnson II: Efficacy of the aptitude clusters. *School Psychology Review, 13*, 355–362.

Woodcock, R. W. (1987). *Woodcock reading mastery tests–Revised.* Circle Pines, MN: American Guidance Service.

Woodcock, R. W. (1998). *Woodcock reading mastery tests–Revised/Normative Update.* Circle Pines, MN: American Guidance Service.

Woodcock, R. W. (1999). What can Rasch-based scores convey about a person's test performance? In S. E. Embretson & S. L. Hershberger (Eds.), *The new rules of measurement: What every psychologist and educator should know* (pp. 105–127). Mahwah, NJ: Erlbaum.

Woodcock, R. W., & Dahl, M. N. (1971). *A common scale for the measurement of person ability and test item difficulty* (AGS Paper No. 10). San Antonio, TX: Pearson.

Woodcock, R. W., & Johnson, M. B. (1977). *Woodcock–Johnson psycho-educational battery.* Rolling Meadows, IL: Riverside Publishing.

Woodcock, R. W., McGrew, K. S., & Mather, N. (2001). *Woodcock–Johnson, third edition (WJ III).* Rolling Meadows, IL: Riverside Publishing.

See Routledge's e-resources website for forms. (www.routledge.com/9780367346058)

9 Neuropsychological Tests

Overview

Neuropsychology constitutes the study of brain–behavior relationships (Gregory, 2011), or, more specifically, how the brain functions to produce human thought and behavior (Andrewes, 2016). The focus of study is typically on higher mental functions that consist of cognition (i.e., thought), emotion, and movement (Andrewes, 2016). As such, the construct of *neuropsychological testing* (also known as *neurocognitive testing*) may be defined as performance on mental and behavioral tasks which are direct indicators of underlying neurological or organic brain integrity (Barlow, Durand, & Hofmann, 2018; Gregory, 2011).

Neuropsychological test batteries and individual subtests are designed to measure varying aspects of brain functioning. In so doing, it is important that this chapter first provide an overview of the brain and its major areas such that the reader has an opportunity to gain a working knowledge of what these tests tap into in terms of neuropsychological function and dysfunction. Therefore, prior to presenting the neuropsychological tests in the book's inventory (see Chapter 1), a review of the brain, its major areas, and their functions is provided. This is followed by a macro-model (i.e., general model) of brain functioning, which also integrates concepts from the *DSM–5*. The latter is especially designed to facilitate diagnosis when employing neuropsychological test batteries.

When the actual tests are reviewed, they are presented in order of increasing chronological age and from general test batteries to more narrowly designed independent tests. It should be noted here that any of the intelligence tests discussed in Chapter 7 can be incorporated into a neuropsychological test battery, especially if diagnostic issues concern higher level cortical functioning, or in the event an ability memory discrepancy (AMD) analysis is desired (discussed subsequently). Now, onto a succinct review of the human brain and its major areas of functioning.

The Human Brain

This section reviews the major areas of the human brain, beginning with the outermost cortical areas and moving inward toward subcortical structures. This discussion espouses a *localization of function approach*, meaning that areas of the brain are defined in terms of (a) where they are and (b) what they essentially do in terms of function. Admittedly, this is an oversimplification, as damage to any area can reflect (a) impairment in that location, (b) dysfunction between related areas, (c) hindrance along a sequence of interconnected areas, and/or (d) imbalance in neurotransmitter levels. In addition, the ensuing discussion is based upon a generic or typical individual. That is, the organization of any individual's brain can vary.

To begin, the human brain has the largest proportional mass relative to body size when compared to other species. This is an important fact considering that such a characteristic is related in a general way to increased sophistication in abilities and culture. It is estimated that the brain is contains 86 billion *neurons* (i.e., nerve cells), including *glial cells* for support and protection, and an enormous assembly of interconnections (Azevedo et al., 2009).[1]

An overall and vital tenet of the human brain is that its structures permit us to adapt extraordinarily well, especially referring to our abilities to communicate and remember. Keep them in mind because when they are hindered by injury or disease, this frequently leads to requests for neuropsychological testing.

In examining the brain, the *cerebral cortex* (hereafter *cortex*) is the outermost covering and is most highly developed when compared to other species (Stephan & Andy, 1969). Figure 9.1 displays the cortex where *convolutions* or folds can be seen. The creases or valleys are referred to as *sulci* (singular form *sulcus*), and the protuberances are called *gyri* (singular form *gyrus*). The folds produce a corrugated-like surface designed to efficiently permit a larger number of cells to exist within a circumscribed space. The cortex is colored gray because it consists of dense neural cell bodies (i.e., gray matter), while white-colored axons proceed to lower brain areas analogous to telephone lines that transmit signals (see also Chapter 2 on the neuron). Approximately 2–4 millimeters (0.08–0.16 inches) thick, it represents the

DOI: 10.4324/9780429326820-11

largest site of neural integration and generally controls the most complex functioning, including attention, perception, thought, memory, language, and consciousness (i.e., functions that make us distinctly human).

In general, the cortex is apportioned into two *hemispheres* (i.e., halves), with four lobes in each hemisphere. Figure 9.1 shows the left and right hemispheres of the brain, which are specialized for different functions. This is referred to as *lateralization (of function)*. In most people, the *left hemisphere* controls language, sequential processing, logical reasoning (e.g., mathematics and science), and the right side of the body, while the *right hemisphere* controls visual spatial and holistic processing, interpretation of emotion and implied meaning (i.e., connotation), and the left side of the body. The *corpus callosum* (not pictured in Figure 9.1) is a subcortical band of fibers that permits the two hemispheres to communicate, hence accounting for people being generally unaware of technically possessing two brains.

Next, each hemisphere comprises four *lobes*, which are naturally divided by large sulci called *fissures*. The two fissures, or large sulci, of interest here include the *central sulcus*, which is the dark line running vertically down between the frontal lobe and the parietal lobe in Figure 9.2, and the *lateral sulcus* (also known as the *Sylvian fissure*), which is the dark line running horizontally between the frontal and parietal lobes (above) and the temporal lobe (below). The frontal lobe has the largest relative size and complexity relative to other species and includes complex problem-solving ability, preparation for motor movements, attention, planning, self-monitoring, and other executive-type functions that give our behavior organization, direction, purpose, adaptability, and ingenuity; essentially, the human personality. The *parietal lobe* lies at the top of the brain behind the frontal lobe and controls sensation perception (i.e., temperature, taste, touch, and movement) and higher-level sensory integration. Visual information processing and mapping is primarily done in the *occipital lobe*, which is located at the back of the brain and is why people see

Cerebral Hemispheres

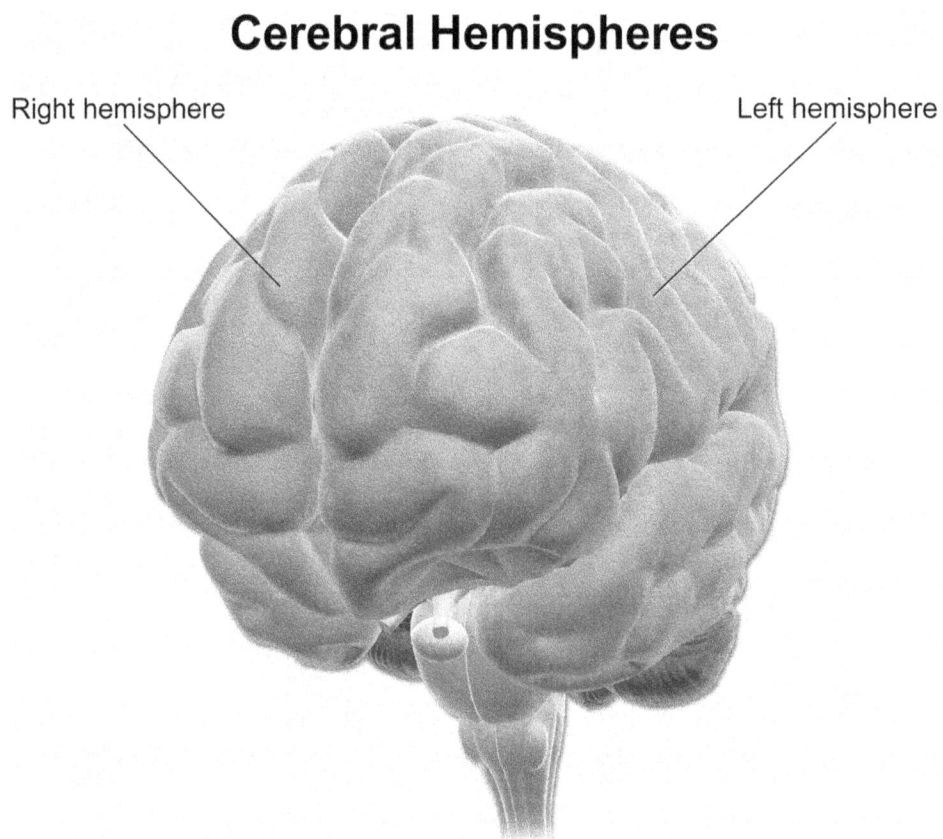

Right hemisphere   Left hemisphere

Figure 9.1 The Cerebral Hemispheres of the Human Brain

Note. The cerebral cortex, which controls the most complex higher-order functions, is divided into two hemispheres by the longitudinal fissure. The hemispheres are independent and control different functions, although they communicate through a strand of fibers called the *corpus callosum* (not shown). The *left hemisphere* controls language, sequential reasoning, logic, and the right side of the human body. The *right hemisphere* controls holistic reasoning, attention, visual-spatial processing, emotions and implied meaning, and the left side of the human body.

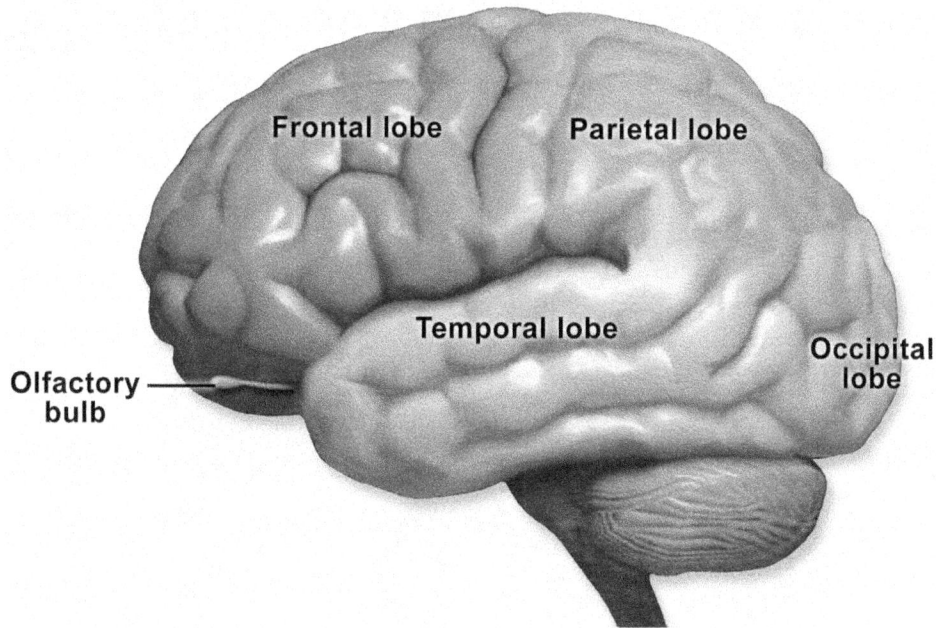

Figure 9.2 The Four Lobes of the Human Brain

Source. Downloaded November 28, 2020, by Blausen.com staff (2014). "Medical gallery of Blausen Medical 2014." *WikiJournal of Medicine* 1 (2). DOI:10.15347/wjm/2014.010. ISSN 2002–4436., CC BY 3.0 <https://creativecommons.org/licenses/by/3.0>, via Wikimedia Commons, with no changes made, *https://commons.wikimedia.org/wiki/File:Blausen_0111_BrainLobes.png*

Note. The cortex or outermost covering of the brain is divided into four lobes, each controlling different major functions. The *frontal lobe* controls high-level executive functioning, including planning, organizing, initiating behavior, self-monitoring, and goal-directed behavior (i.e., personality functioning). The *parietal lobe* controls sensation perception (i.e., temperature, taste, touch, and movement) and higher-level sensory integration. The *occipital lobe* controls visual processing and mapping. Finally, the *temporal lobe* controls auditory processing, including speech reception, visual memory, language comprehension, pain, and recalling emotion. Of note, the olfactory bulb located just above the sinus cavity (not shown) controls the sensation and perception of smell. Also note that the cortex is folded, called *convolutions*, so as to compact more neural material into this area of the brain. The cortex is what makes people distinctly human, as it controls the highest levels of neurocognition.

"stars" after striking the back of their heads on a hard surface (see Figure 9.2). Finally, the *temporal lobe* is located on the sides next to each ear, and controls auditory processing, including speech reception, visual memory, language comprehension, pain, and the recollection of emotion.

Figure 9.3 shows the outer portion of the left hemisphere, which highlights sensorimotor, language, and related areas of the cortex. First, the sensory and motor functions are located in long strips or major convolutions that form gyri. The sensory strip, called the primary sensory cortex (see Figure 9.3), has connections to various bodily locations (e.g., fingers, lips, arms) and registers tactile and *haptic senses*, including *proprioception*, which is an awareness of body position and movement. It is located at the front of the parietal lobe and immediately subsequent to the central sulcus, hence it is also termed the *postcentral gyrus* (see Figure 9.3). The motor strip, called the *primary motor cortex* (see Figure 9.3), has parallel connections to various bodily locations and controls intentional movement. It is located at the back of the frontal lobe and just prior to the central sulcus, hence it is also referred to as the *precentral gyrus*. Any damage or injury to these areas will hinder sensory and motor functioning in the locations of the body controlled by those portions of the sensory or motor strip. Of note, the axons of each strip cross over in the lower sections of the brain to control the opposite (i.e., *contralateral*) side of the body. Hence, damage to the right motor strip will cause *apraxia* (i.e., impairment of movement) on the contralateral left side of the body and vice-versa. This crossing over is referred to as *decussation*, which is pertinent to diagnosis.

Figure 9.3 also displays the language centers, both of which lie in the left hemisphere in the majority of people. Damage in these areas will generally result in *aphasia* (Tobias, 1995), which refers to any language dysfunction that can be attributed to brain damage. First, *Wernicke's area* traverses the temporal and parietal lobes and controls speech reception or receptive language (see Figure 9.3). It makes anatomical sense that it is proximate to the *auditory cortex*, which is responsible for decoding hearing signals and the ear. Damage here will interfere with speech comprehension, although speech production remains intact. Second, *Broca's area* is located in the frontal lobe in proximity to the motor strip and is specialized for speech production. Damage here will interfere with expressive language.

Motor and Sensory Regions of the Cerebral Cortex

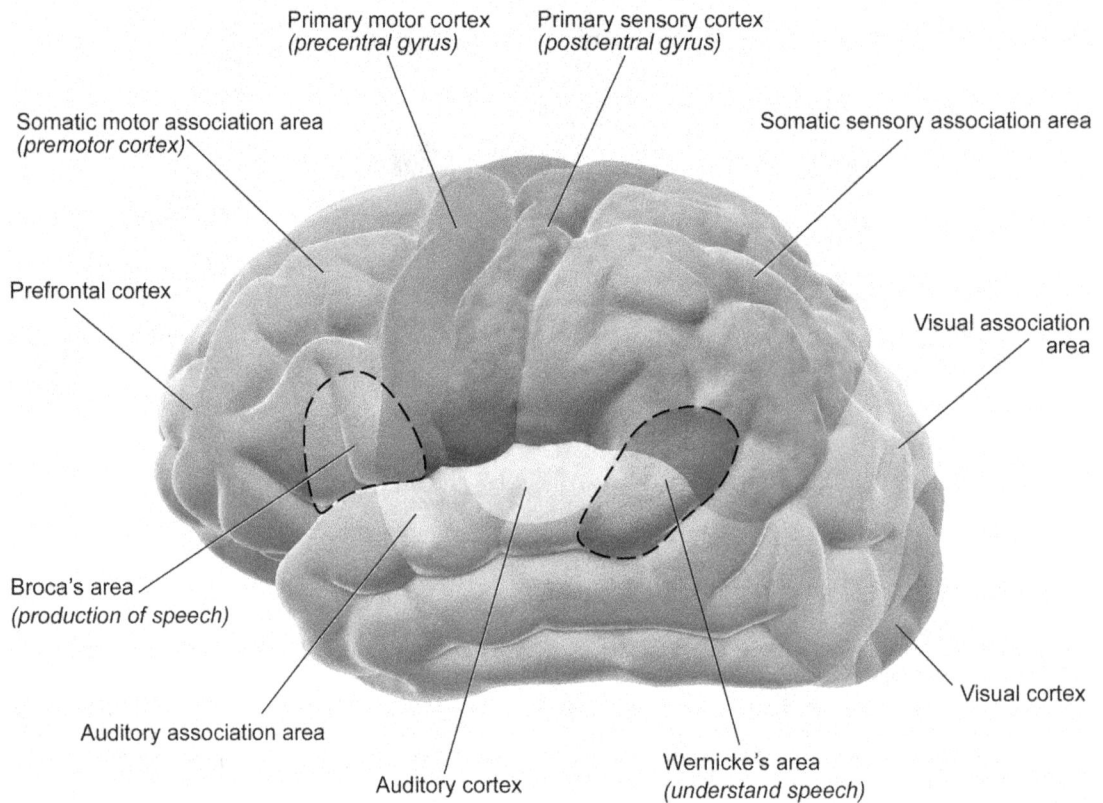

Figure 9.3 Sensorimotor, Language, and Related Areas of the Human Brain

Source. Downloaded November 28, 2020, by Blausen.com staff (2014). "Medical gallery of Blausen Medical 2014." *WikiJournal of Medicine* 1 (2). DOI:10.15347/wjm/2014.010. ISSN 2002–4436., CC BY 3.0 <https://creativecommons.org/licenses/by/3.0>, via Wikimedia Commons, with no changes made, *https://commons.wikimedia.org/wiki/File:Blausen_0102_Brain_Motor%26Sensory.png*

Note. The diagram shows the sensorimotor and language-center areas of the human brain, along with some related areas. They include the following: (a) *prefrontal cortex* controlling higher executive functions and personality; (b) *primary motor cortex* controlling movement (opposite side of the body); (c) *primary sensory cortex* controlling sensation (i.e., touch); (d) *visual cortex* controlling visual perception; and (e) *auditory cortex* controlling auditory perception. *Association areas* are devoted to long-term memory storage for a particular sensory modality. Finally, the language centers (typically the left hemisphere, as shown) are as follows: (a) *Wernicke's area* for speech reception (near the auditory cortex) and (b) *Broca's area* for speech production (near the motor strip).

Another vital facet of Figure 9.3 is the insertion of several association areas, including visual, somatic sensory, somatic motor, and auditory locations. Specifically, *association areas* permit the combined analysis or integration of all sensory information (i.e., cross-modal sensory-perception), in effect functioning as large amodal areas separate and independent from any particular sensory system. In fact, the human brain has more area compared to other species that is not attributed to any specific sensory system such that more complex processing can be accomplished, including the storage of long-term memories (see Figure 9.3). For instance, when one views an object visually, 60–90% of all energy utilized by the brain occurs in regions unrelated to the external event (Raichle, 2010). Additionally, long-term memory (LTM) is integrated into various association areas of the cortex via the hippocampus (Binder, Desai, Graves, & Conant, 2009; Goldman-Rakic, 1998; Rao, Rainer, & Miller, 1997; Weis, Klaver, Reul, Elger, & Fernandez, 2004; see also later in this chapter) and maintained by stable neural connections, sometimes referred to as physical *memory traces*. Further, recent evidence shows that memory *consolidation* is the consequence of numerous physical changes in the brain at the cellular level, including dendritic changes in neurons (Alkon, 1989; Kandel & Schwartz, 1982; Squire & Kandel, 1999), synaptic plasticity (Kandel, 2012), and neuron structure (Deger, Helias, Rotter, & Diesmann 2012; Fioriti et al., 2015; Griggs, Young, Rumbaugh, & Miller, 2013; Hill, Vasireddi, Wang, Bruno, & Frost, 2015; Krüttner et al., 2012). Physical blows to the head can disrupt consolidation and cause *retrograde* (i.e., information prior to the injury) and *anterograde* (i.e., information subsequent to the injury) *amnesia* (see

Hodges, 1994; Squire, Slater, & Chace, 1975). The latter is frequently observed in cases of *major neurocognitive disorder* (previously known as *senile dementia*).

The diagram in Figure 9.4 shows the brain sectioned down its length along the *longitudinal fissure* (refer back to Figure 9.1). This illustrates a network of structures beneath the cortex that is not seen from the outside, together referred to as the *limbic system*, which generally controls emotion, motivation, learning, and memory in humans. More specifically, the *amygdala* (see amygdaloid body in Figure 9.4) controls motivational behaviors, such as response to reward, aversion, fear conditioning, anger, emotional memories, and appetite. It is especially involved in the emotional system that assists people in judging emotional faces. The *hypothalamus*, which controls basic kinds of motivation (e.g., hunger, thirst, sleep), activates the *sympathetic nervous system* (i.e., the fight-or-flight response) in coping with stress. The *hippocampus* is a horseshoe-shaped structure that is vital for the formation and storage of new memories, along with learning and emotions. Hippocampal damage can hinder an individual's ability to form new memories and cause profound *amnesia* (i.e., memory loss). Finally, the *thalamus* is located just above the hypothalamus and is specialized for relaying all senses (except smell) to the proper cortex for further processing. The structures in the limbic system are significantly more advanced when compared to other species and permits us to learn, remember, and adapt (Stephan et al., 1988; Semendeferi & Damasio, 2000). Diseases and injury that deleteriously affects this system (e.g., Alzheimer's disease) are clearly devastating, which is why it is reviewed in this chapter on neuropsychological testing. The *cerebellum* is part of the *hindbrain*, which among other functions integrates incoming sensations with motor movements to help regulate balance (see bottom-right circular structure in Figure 9.4). Damage to this area can cause problems with body balance and coordination, as in chronic alcoholism.

This completes the succinct review of the human brain and it major features. The purpose was to provide neurological context to the behaviors measured by neuropsychological tests to be later reviewed in this chapter. In particular, the various behaviors and constructs measured by these tests (e.g., memory, learning, and attention) can now be related to various functions and thus likely brain locations. This will afford increased relevance and purpose

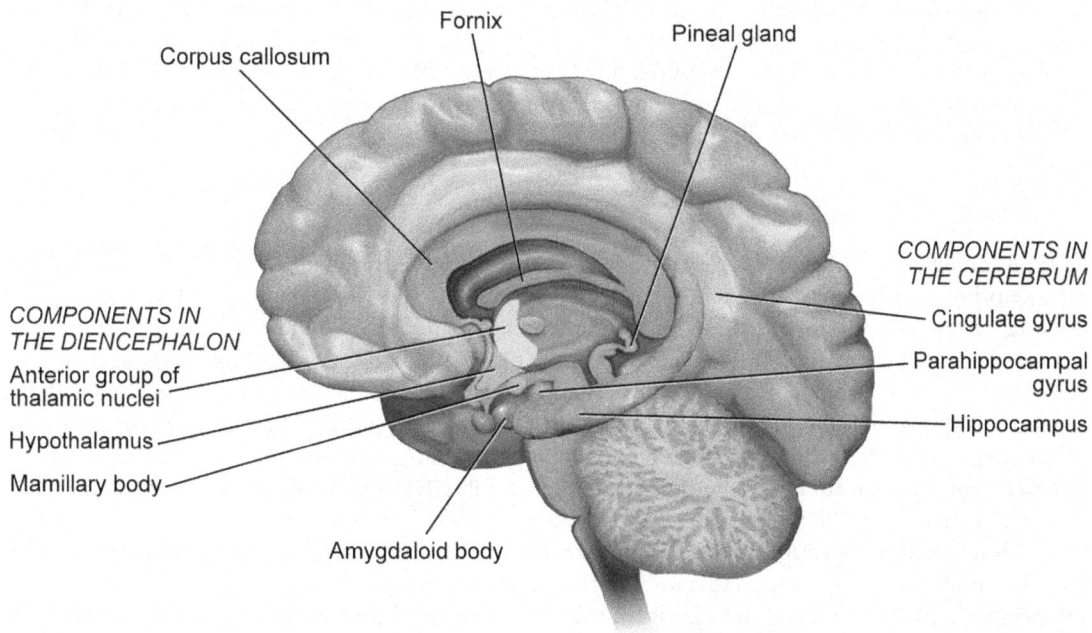

Figure 9.4 The Subcortical Areas of the Human Brain

Note. The *limbic system* consists of a set of structures beneath the cortex that regulates motivation, emotion, learning, and memory in humans. It includes the *hippocampus*, which controls the learning of new memories, the *amygdala* (see *amygdaloid body* in the diagram), which controls emotional and motivational behavior, the *hypothalamus*, which controls the fight-or-flight stress response, and the *thalamus* (see *thalamic nuclei* in the diagram) through which most senses are sent to the appropriate cortex for further processing. The cerebellum (lower-right circular structure) is part of the hindbrain, which integrates incoming sensations with outgoing motor movements.

when these tests are discussed. Next, a general model of brain functioning will be presented, which is intended to add theoretical context to neuropsychological testing.

A Level-of-Processing Categorical Model of Brain Functioning

It is important that an examiner utilize a theoretical model of brain–behavior relationships when conducting neuropsychological testing in order to organize and interpret the garnered data effectively. Although the previous section actually did imply a model, that is, a *localization of function approach*, such a model is too simplistic in that vital interrelationships among the various areas and how they interact is not addressed. Sometimes referred to as the "father of neuropsychology," Alexander Luria proposed an early functional systems model (Luria, 1973), which continues to be influential and from which other models have evolved to some degree. Because it is conceptually consistent with the model that is utilized in interpreting neuropsychological test data, his theorizing will first be briefly reviewed and thereafter succeeded by a presentation of Bennet's more contemporary model with *DSM–5* integration. Of note, the models reviewed subsequently are referred to as macro-models in that they attempt to account for general brain functioning. Micro-models are more circumscribed in explaining only a limited neurocognitive activity (e.g., speech production, short-term memory) and thus will not be addressed.

Luria's Functional Systems Model of Brain Functioning

In Luria's macro-model, *functional systems* consist of a complex interaction of brain regions, with each contributing a specialized role (i.e., a sub-role). Hence, he proposes different functional systems for perception, memory, and language, although each is contingent upon an integration of several brain regions working in concert. In total, he postulates the presence of three units that overlap to provide a functional system.

First, there is a unit for regulating tone and mental states, which is necessary for optimal levels of nervous system arousal. This includes a *reticular activating system* that traverses the brain stem (i.e., the lowest brain area that regulates survival functions) and through the thalamus, located within the limbic system (see Figure 9.4). Second, there is a unit for areas that analyze and store information, which refer to regions within the various lobes, including occipital for visual information, temporal for auditory information, and parietal for tactile or haptic information. Third, and finally, there is a unit for programming, regulating, and verifying activity. Not surprisingly, the frontal lobe regions are referenced here for directing and controlling all other brain tasks and activities, where actions are prepared, planned, and finally executed. The principal concept running through Luria's ideas regards functional units or regions of the brain that work in coordinated fashion.

Bennet's Model of Brain Functioning

Bennet's (1988) model of brain–behavior relationships is consistent with Luria's ideas regarding functional systems or specific areas working in tandem to effectuate a particular action (e.g., speech production). More specifically, Bennet proposes a total of seven categories of neurocognitive activities that are ordered in terms of degrees or levels of information processing (see Figure 9.5). The initial levels consist of more simplistic kinds of processing, with succeeding levels becoming increasingly complex. These actions are coordinated to produce meaningful behavior, although they can be analyzed and measured by neuropsychological tests to determine (a) the type of impairment and (b) what regions of the brain are most likely implicated. These include the neuropsychological tests and test batteries appearing in the test inventory put forth by this book (see Chapter 1, Table 1.1) and presented in detail later in this chapter.

Bennet actually built upon the model proposed by Reitan and Wolfson (1985, 1986), by separating out attention and memory from the other six categories, and effectively organizes the major categories of abilities into increasingly deeper levels of processing. In successive order of brain processing, they include: (a) sensory input, (b) attention and concentration, (c) learning and memory, (d) language and sequential processing (i.e., left hemisphere functions) occurring contemporaneously with spatial processing and manipulatory ability (i.e., right hemisphere functions), (e) executive functioning (i.e., logical analysis, concept formation, reasoning, planning, and flexibility of thinking), and (f) motor output (Bennet, 1988). In addition to Bennet's levels, the more recent *DSM–5* categories of abilities are integrated and addressed when diagnostic issues arise. Note that each successive category reflects a deeper, more complex, and increasingly sophisticated level of processing.

More specifically, Level 1 represents initial sensory input, which can be in the form of external stimulation (e.g., tactile form recognition while blindfolded) or internal stimulation (e.g., one's own thoughts and images). Once senses are registered, the information moves to Level 2, which includes attention and concentration. An individual can register a significant amount of sensory information; however, attention and concentration are required for further

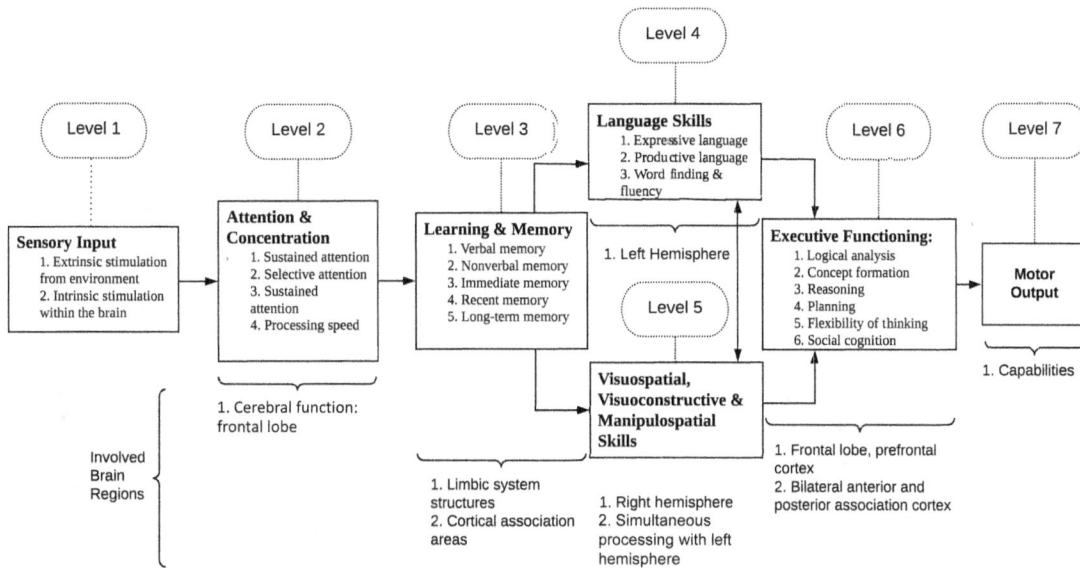

Figure 9.5 Model of Brain Functioning

Note. Level 1 = initial registration of stimuli by the senses or intrinsically within the brain (e.g., imagery); Level 2 = initial information processing that permits encoding and additional processing; Level 3 = determining the significance of the stimulation and storing information for later reference; Level 4 = left hemisphere bidirectional flow of language processing; Level 5 = right hemisphere bidirectional flow of visual-spatial processing; Levels 4 and 5 processing occurs simultaneously; Level 6 = highest and most complex degree of abstract processing and reasoning; Level 7 = motor output contingent upon personal capabilities.

processing to take place. In Bennet's model, *attention* can be defined as the ability to focus on specific activities and suppress irrelevant stimuli. However, this level would also comprise complex attention as employed in the *DSM–5*. *Complex attention* is multifaceted, including *sustained attention* (i.e., maintaining attention over time), *selective attention* (i.e., maintaining attention in the presence of competing or distracting stimuli), and *divided attention* (i.e., paying attention to two tasks simultaneously). All these are measured by current neuropsychological tests (e.g., continuous performance tests discussed later) and subtests (e.g., digit span tasks) and are largely controlled by frontal lobe functioning. This is because complex attention requires the assistance of executive system control (see subsequently).

Learning and memory occurs at Level 3. Once an individual has successfully paid attention to selected stimuli, it can then be learned and transferred into memory for later retrieval. *Learning* includes the ability to acquire new information. *Memory* involves the process of retaining and retrieving information. Therefore, *learning* and *memory* work together and include the ability to acquire, retain, and access new information. The latter includes *working memory*, which involves holding immediate memory traces while executing cognitive tasks. Indeed, because learning and memory may be considered as on the same continuum, the *DSM–5* classifies them together. The *DSM–5* also differentiates memory by content (i.e., semantic, visual-spatial, autobiographical), type of task (i.e., recognition, cued recall, and free recall), and duration (i.e., immediate, recent, long term). As discussed in the prior section, learning and memory are controlled by many structures in the limbic system. Also, long-term memory would be stored in the cortical association areas. These can be seen in all the tests to follow.

Level 4 language skills and Level 5 visual-spatial skills occur simultaneously in the left and right hemispheres, respectively. *Language* is the ability to express and understand verbal communication. This consists of (a) receptive speech involving the comprehension and decoding of speech, and (b) expressive speech or language production. The *DSM–5* apportions verbal abilities into *expressive language* (i.e., confrontational naming of objects or pictures, fluency, and phonemics), grammar and syntax (e.g., sentence structure, word omissions), and *receptive language* (i.e., reading comprehension, following verbal commands). All of these are typically measured by neuropsychological test batteries. Impairments indicate the presence of aphasia and left hemisphere dysfunction within the language centers. *Visuospatial processing* is the capacity to understand the orientation of visual information in two- and three-dimensional space. The *DSM–5* combines the category of visual processing with motor functioning, hence referring to the combination as perceptual-motor abilities. Such is further apportioned into *visual perception* (i.e., visuospatial processing as defined prior), *visuoconstruction* (i.e., creating items requiring eye-hand coordination, such as drawing a figure), *perceptual-motor* (i.e., integrating perception with intentional movement), *praxis* (i.e., integrity of learned movements), and *gnosis* (i.e., perceptual integrity of awareness and recognition, for example, of faces). Note that Levels 4 and 5 reflect cortical function in the two hemispheres as shown in Figure 9.1, although the processing is simultaneous and shared via the nerve bundles that make up the corpus callosum (see Figure 9.4). The information managed at this level can be relayed to the deepest and most sophisticated processing reflected at Level 7, which occurs within the frontal lobe (see Figure 9.2), especially the *prefrontal cortex* located in the anterior portion of this lobe (see Figure 9.3).

The frontal lobe specializes in *executive functioning*, which involves the ability to (a) engage in activities necessary for achieving objectives and (b) regulate one's actions based on environmental feedback. The prefrontal cortex is implicated in planning complex behavior, decision-making, and moderating one's own behavior, which amounts to the expression of personality. The *DSM–5* divides executive functioning into six subcategories, including *planning* (e.g., thinking done to achieve an end objective, such as finding one's way out of a maze), *decision-making* (i.e., choosing the correct action in the face of several alternatives), *working memory* (i.e., holding information until it can be manipulated in some way, such as digits backward), *error utilization* (i.e., the ability to benefit from feedback), *overriding habits/inhibition* (i.e., ability to select a more complex solution, such as naming the color of a word's font and not the word), and *mental flexibility* (i.e., the ability to shift to different rules, such as naming the correct arrow direction followed by naming the opposite direction). Again, measures of these aspects of executive functioning will become apparent among the neuropsychological tests to follow. Because this category represents the highest level of neurocognitive functioning, impairment here implicates dysfunction in the frontal lobe and prefrontal cortex.

The *DSM–5* has appropriately added social cognition and perception to the neurocognitive abilities that should be appraised when attempting to detect a disorder in this class of psychological disorders. *Social cognition* refers to two components, including recognition of emotions and *theory of mind*. The former examines whether the individual can accurately interpret various facial expressions as representing various negative and positive emotions, especially happiness, anger, fear, disgust, surprise, and sadness (Ekman, 1973; Ekman & Friesen, 1969, 1971). *Theory of mind* is the ability to consider another individual's mental state (e.g., motives, thoughts, desires, feelings) or experience and act accordingly (e.g., understanding why a person might be angry). This would most obviously fall under the category of executive functioning, which represents the deepest level of neurocognition (see Figure 9.5). Impairment in this skill accounts for the changes in personality observed in cases of major neurocognitive disorder (e.g., dementia of the Alzheimer's type).

Summary

To conclude this section, Bennet's macro-model of brain functioning covers seven categories of neurocognitive activities that are ordered in terms of levels of processing, progressing from simple and superficial types of activities (e.g., sensory input) to deep and complex activities (e.g., executive functioning). The model is presented visually in Figure 9.5 and explicated in the narrative portion of this chapter. It provides useful context for the ensuing review of the various neuropsychological tests listed in the overall inventory in Chapter 1 and may be referenced when discussing the measurement of various brain functions. The next section discusses the circumstances under which neuropsychological tests should be included in an assessment battery in mental health practice. Thereafter, the central portion of the chapter reviews the actual tests, including the data tables designed for reporting and interpreting their results within a final neuropsychological or psychological assessment report.

Diagnostic Reasons for Inclusion within a Test Battery

Neuropsychological testing is principally ordered to rule out, establish *baseline functioning*, or measure the progression of major or minor *neurocognitive disorders* (previously known as *dementias*). Irrespective of etiology, neurocognitive disorders involve the essential symptom of a cognitive decline from a previous level of functioning, as reflected by any one or more of the following symptoms: (a) impaired complex attention, (b) language dysfunction (i.e., *aphasia*), (c) perceptual-motor disability (e.g., *apraxia* or an inability to perform specific purposive acts; *agnosia* or the failure to interpret objects accurately despite normal sensory function), and (d) impaired executive functioning (American Psychiatric Association, 2013). Testing should be based upon the stated concerns of the patient or those who are intimately knowledgeable of the patient's *premorbid level of functioning* relative to current functioning. These facts should be clearly documented among the presenting symptoms, in addition to a referral source who may have also documented the observed decline. Having a knowledgeable collateral is sometimes vital because the prospective examinee may be in denial or otherwise unaware of the decline paradoxically caused by the actual deterioration, namely, *anosognosia*. Having a medical referral, especially from a neurologist, is extremely useful in establishing *medical necessity* for this type of testing. For some of the more stringent insurers, documentation of neuroimaging that detects the neuropathology is required.

By listing these kinds of pathology under the rubric *neurocognitive disorders*, the *DSM–5* continues to acknowledge that neuropsychological dysfunction is associated with many previously conceptualized *nonorganic mental disorders* (e.g., schizophrenia; American Psychiatric Association, 1987). As a consequence, neuropsychological tests can and should be used when attempting to detect psychopathology that is not technically classified under the neurocognitive disorders. In particular, two previously conceptualized non-organic disorders now necessitate neuropsychological testing as part of an effective battery. They include: (a) *attention-deficit/hyperactivity disorder* (*ADHD*), and (b) *autism spectrum disorder* (*ASD*). First, with respect to ADHD, research using neuroimaging techniques convincingly shows evidence of neurocognitive dysfunction in brain regions responsible for regulating executive functions, attention, and inhibitory control, particularly within the prefrontal cortex (Peterson et al., 2009; Shaw et al., 2009).

Second, ASDs have been linked to the malfunctioning of *mirror neuron systems*, thus accounting for deficits in theory of mind, social perception, empathy, and language (Oberman & Ramachandran, 2007). Succinctly, mirror neurons permit the comprehension of others' thoughts and feelings by reacting to them as if they were one's own (Mcintosh, Reichmann-Decker, Winkielman, & Wilbarger, 2006). Theory of mind is the ability to understand that people possess internal mental states, including feelings, desires, beliefs, and intentions, which direct and explain their behavior (Sigelman & Rider, 2018). Therefore, measured deficits in theory of mind in particular, and in social perception generally, are diagnostic of both neuron dysfunction and the presence of ASD. Neuropsychological subtests that measure social perception and theory of mind in children and adolescents are available (see NEPSY–II) and increase the accuracy and veracity of ASD diagnoses, along with indicating valuable targets for treatment intervention.

Neuropsychological tests are also useful for addressing a referring clinician's more general question as to whether there exists neurocognitive dysfunction in a particular case, which may be considered a distinct comorbid disorder, thus complicating treatment intervention. In these cases, an age-appropriate neuropsychological test battery is ordered to rule out an *other specified neurodevelopmental disorder* or *unspecified neurocognitive disorder* (insurance permitting), and more particularly attempt to (a) identify the various functional deficits, (b) quantify their severity (i.e., mild, moderate, severe), (c) identify likely areas of brain impairment, and (d) render neurocognitive diagnoses, ultimately to assist in treatment planning or rehabilitation.

Additionally, neuropsychological testing is indicated when there exists a need to rule out a *mental disorder due to another medical condition* (e.g., psychotic, bipolar, depressive, anxiety) that can potentially affect brain functioning, most especially *traumatic brain injury* (*TBI*). Another applicable disorder would be personality change due to TBI. Finally, all neurocognitive disorders may be supplemented by a specifier *with or without behavioral disturbance*, which includes symptoms of psychosis, mood disorder, agitation, apathy, and any other hindering behavioral problems, such as anger outbursts. For these cases, a symptom-relevant personality test (see Chapters 11 and 12) or adaptive behavior measure (see Chapter 10) may accompany the neuropsychological tests.[2] The neuropsychological tests within the assessment battery measure whether and to what extent head trauma has resulted in significant brain damage, while the personality and adaptive behavior tests assist in measuring the presence of the maladaptive traits, clinical symptoms, and/or behavioral impairment.

Occasionally, referring clinicians will directly request a standardized measurement of a particular neurocognitive ability (see Bennet's 1988 model). The most frequently requested specific ability includes memory and its facilitator, learning. Lastly, selected neuropsychological language subtests are useful in screening for a possible reading disorder or *dyslexia*, and one of the following communication disorders: (a) *speech sound (phonological) disorder* and (b) language disorder. Admittedly, this overlaps with achievement testing, as noted in Chapter 8. However, in some cases, requesting neuropsychological testing for such disorders may be more likely to receive preauthorization (PA) by insurance companies considering that such is more consistent with a mental health versus a psychoeducational issue.

It is also consistent with research that has identified various forms of subtle brain dysfunction and genetics as being responsible for learning disabilities. A number of genes have been linked to reading problems, especially word recognition (Cope et al., 2012; Siegel & Mazabell, 2013; Zou et al., 2012). In addition, both reading difficulties and mathematics disorder have been linked to dysfunction in several areas located in the left hemisphere (Ashkenazi, Black, Abrams, Hoeft, & Menon, 2013; Peterson & Pennington, 2012). The principal point here is that specific neuropsychological tests and subtests can be legitimately requested to assist in detecting the presence of an SLD, both from a research and pragmatic perspective.

Finally, the most likely referral sources for neuropsychological testing purposes include (a) physicians (i.e., psychiatrists, neurologists, pediatricians, family practitioners), (b) non-medical mental health professionals, and (c) attorneys (e.g., *tort law*, probate law, disability). Referrals from family members are possible when there exists a history of dementia diagnoses in immediate or extended family relatives, and they are sufficiently sophisticated regarding the usefulness of neuropsychological testing in such instances.

The Neuropsychological Tests

This section represents the core of this chapter. It begins with two complete neuropsychological test batteries, the first for child and adolescents and the second for adults, hence following chronological order. Together, these two batteries effectively cover this specialized type of testing from ages 4–97, thus virtually the entire life span in which such testing is relevant. Prior to age four, developmental testing is a more felicitous choice because a failure to obtain expected milestones is the major concern here, whereas for older ages, declines in previously obtained levels of functioning increasingly becomes the principal focus. Both of these batteries can be effectively utilized in whole or in part as the case facts determine and therefore possess the capability of being specially tailored rather than employed rigidly as a complete test battery, especially the younger child and adolescent test.

Following the complete batteries, the subsequent neuropsychological tests are more circumscribed in terms of the abilities measured. One covers individuals from middle adolescence through older adulthood and focuses on measuring various kinds of memory (i.e., visual, auditory, visual working, immediate, delayed), and is effective when presenting complaints are restricted to memory function in this age grouping. The remaining three are specifically designed to measure various components of executive functioning, including attention, sustained attention, impulse control, and sustained impulse control. As a genre, they are referred to as *continuous performance tests* (*CPTs*), which are designed to be tedious, ongoing, and without the affordance of breaks, and are fully automated in terms of computer administration and scoring. As will be seen, these are employed largely to determine the presence of ADHD, although they can be used more generally as part of a neuropsychological test battery. Together, these cover examinations ranging in age from four years through adulthood. The ensuing section begins with the NEPSY–II.

NEPSY–II

Synopsis

The *NEPSY–II*[3] (Korkman, Kirk, & Kemp, 2007a, 2007b) is a comprehensive neuropsychological test battery normed on children and adolescents from 3 years, 0 months through 16 years, 11 months. It is a flexible battery that principally yields subtest scores for various specific neurocognitive abilities, rather than composite or index scores. The complete battery of subtests is classified conceptually by the general neurocognitive ability or domain that they have in common, including the following: (a) attention and executive functioning, (b) language, (c) memory and learning, (d) sensorimotor, (e) social perception, and (f) visuospatial processing. This test structure is theoretically based, although it is supported empirically by expected patterns of intercorrelations among the various subtests (Korkman et al., 2007b).

There are two forms based upon age, including Ages 3–4 and Ages 5–16. Each form consists of a full battery (i.e., all the subtests for that age range), a general battery (i.e., only those subtests that have empirically proven to be the best predictors of brain dysfunction), and a specialized battery (i.e., only those subtests that address the diagnostic issues in a case). The subtests are co-normed and thus may be directly compared as part of a test profile. Overall, the NEPSY–II is a flexible battery that is considered by some to be one of its greatest assets. Next, the test structure is more closely examined, which is intended to facilitate the interpretation of its scores (discussed later).

Test Structure

The NEPSY–II test organization is designed to measure neurocognitive constructs and abilities not covered by intelligence and achievement tests (see Chapters 11 and 12, respectively). Rather, the various NEPSY–II subtests measure more basic processing difficulties underlying many neurodevelopmental, behavioral, and psychiatric disorders. For example, many children with social and interpersonal difficulties manifest impairments in affect recognition and theory of mind. Therefore, their relationship difficulties may be traced to problems in understanding how to interpret people's reactions toward them and react appropriately rather than to emotional or personality etiology. As the NEPSY–II is apportioned into different neurocognitive domains, its test structure will be discussed according to such classification. Key concepts will be defined in each neurocognitive classification or domain to clarify the abilities measures by this test battery, which supplements the review of brain–behavior relationships and model of brain functioning discussed in the opening sections of this chapter.

ATTENTION AND EXECUTIVE FUNCTIONING

Attention and executive functions concern goal-directed or objective-based activities, including forethought, planning, and behavioral regulation based upon feedback provided by environmental input (Barkley, 1997; Pennington & Ozonoff, 1996; Pineda et al., 1998). Executive functioning consists of several components, including cognitive flexibility, fluency, and planning (Miyake, Friedman, Emerson, Witzki, & Howerter, 2000; Pennington & Ozonoff, 1996; Smith & Jonides, 1999). *Cognitive flexibility* concerns the ability to modify one's behavior, problem-solving strategy, or approach to a task or social circumstance. Repeatedly engaging in the same behavior, especially making the same mistake without modification, is referred to as *perseveration* and represents a classic sign of brain dysfunction in the form of cognitive inflexibility or rigidity. As seen in Chapter 8, *fluency* regards the facility, smoothness, speed, and accuracy of completing a task. As mentioned previously, planning refers to arranging a method or scheme to reach an objective and consists of both initiation and cognitive flexibility. *Initiation* regards the ability to begin a task, the impairment of which is observed in children who appear to lack motivation but actually cannot effectively direct their own behavior. Also included in executive functioning is the ability to initiate activity and to evaluate the results of activity (Gioia & Isquith, 2004; Lezak, 1995). A final component of executive functioning worthy of mention is again working memory, which is holding information actively in the mind while cognitive tasks that are dependent on such information are being executed (i.e., multitasking).

As referenced prior, attention is a concentration of the mind on an object or thought. Two key elements of attention consist of inhibition and selective attention (Barkley, 1997; Klimkeit, Mattingley, Shappard, Lee, & Bradshaw, 2005; Nigg, 2000, 2001; Quay, 1997; Sargeant, 1996, 2000, 2005; Tsal, Shalev, & Mevorach, 2005). *Inhibitory control* refers to the ability to resist urges to engage in enticing behavior and to consciously stop automatic (i.e., overlearned or habitual) behaviors when so desired. Impairments in this neurocognitive ability are indicated by impulsive behaviors and are a principal deficit in children with ADHD (Barkley, 2003). Selective attention again represents the ability to focus effectively on a task or activity while simultaneously suppressing competing but irrelevant stimuli. As referenced previously, sustained attention is essentially selective attention that is maintained over a particular duration of time as needed in the circumstances. *Distractibility* is an impairment in sustained attention in the context of extraneous stimuli (i.e., actions, sounds). Children who evidence mind-wandering and problems listening for extended periods of time are showing symptoms of distractibility, which is commonly observed in cases of ADHD.

LANGUAGE

As seen in Chapter 8, language concerns the ability to produce and comprehend verbal kinds of communication and is an essential neurocognitive function. Language can be dichotomized into input (i.e., receptive) and output (i.e., expressive) functions. *Receptive language* refers to both comprehending and decoding speech. Children with impairments in receptive language manifest difficulties in processing words and sentences, especially sentences with longer sequences and that are syntactically more complex (Deevy & Leonard, 2004; Dick, Wulfeck, Krupa-Kwiatkowski, & Bates, 2004; Evans & MacWhinney, 1999). *Expressive language* regards speech production. Children with impairments in this skill may speak on *holophrases* (i.e., single words with accompanying gestures) or evince short and simplistic responses (Dalal & Loeb, 2005; Klee, Stokes, Wong, Fletcher, & Gavin, 2004; Marinellie, 2004).

Both receptive and expressive language abilities are based upon several more specific processes, including oromotor control, phonological processing, and naming (Bishop & McArthur, 2005; Burlingame, Sussman, Gillam, & Hay, 2005). *Oromotor control* is the ability to regulate movement-type actions that are necessary for speech production, including the proper articulation of words (e.g., replacing the *s* sound with the *t* sound in a word such as toy, tall, or tail). *Phonological processing* is the ability to decode sounds associated with words, while *naming* refers to the ability to assign verbal labels to objects, people, events, and actions. As seen in Chapter 8, both of these neurocognitive abilities are intimately involved in learning to read (Bishop & Snowling, 2004; Kail & Hall, 1994).

Two other language abilities measured by the NEPSY–II are repetition and word generation and continue to illustrate the overlap here between achievement testing and neuropsychological testing. Repetition is the capability of duplicating exactly what has been said. Repetition of nonwords is measured by the NEPSY–II because impairment here has been associated with language disorders, especially of expressive speech (Bishop & Snowling, 2004; Gray, 2003). Finally, *word generation* is the ability to produce words quickly and accurately according to themes or categories (e.g., colors, animals, foods). Problems in word generation or fluency may be indicative of a variety of underlying problems related to language and communication disorders.

LEARNING AND MEMORY

Together, the related neurocognitive functions of learning and memory concern the ability to acquire, retain, and access new information (Budson & Price, 2005; Cowan & Hulme, 1997; Gathercole, 2002; Kapur, 1994; Squire & Butters, 1984; Stringer, 1996; Temple, 1997). More specifically, learning as referenced previously represents the ability to acquire new information which, conceptually speaking, renders it a component of intelligence as previously defined in Chapter 7. Again, memory here refers to abilities more related to acquisition and retrieval. Hence, it is evident as to how these two constructs work together, which accounts for why they are similarly measured together on the NEPSY–II.

Memory possesses a number of sub-components that are tapped by the NEPSY–II subtests, which can be effectively represented by the information-processing or multi-store model of memory (Atkinson & Shiffrin, 1968) presented in Figure 3.1 (see Chapter 7). Some types of memory refer to different durations of time after exposure to information. *Immediate memory* concerns recall of information instantly after exposure and conceptually represents short-term memory (STM). *Immediate memory span* is the quantity of verbal information that can be retained after a single exposure. *Supraspan learning* is the ability to memorize new information that exceeds immediate memory span by means of repeated exposure. For example, repeating a list of 15 words that the examinee must memorize over 7 trials. The amount of effort put forth by examinees, along with the utilization of mnemonic strategies, determines performance on supraspan learning tasks. *Rote memory* is the simple verbatim recall of presented information.

In contrast, *delayed memory* is the recall of learned information 20–30 minutes subsequent to exposure, which conceptually refers to long-term memory (LTM). *Encoding* is defined as the process of transferring information into LTM storage, hence making it relatively permanent. The quality of encoding depends upon the degree to which such information is organized and associated within existing knowledge stores. As described previously in this chapter, memory traces must be consolidated to remain in LTM. *Retrieval* regards the ability to extract information from LTM when needed. This can be measured in two ways, including *free recall* (i.e., retrieving information without hints) and *cued recall* (i.e., retrieving information with hints or clues). A deficit in retrieval is measured by poor performance in such recall tasks, although especially free recall. Working memory was defined previously when discussing executive functioning due to its involvement there.

SENSORIMOTOR

The measurement of sensorimotor functioning on the NEPSY–II is restricted to fine-sensorimotor coordination and speech production. As shown earlier in this chapter, tactile (or haptic) sensation is controlled by the primary sensory cortex (i.e., sensory strip), while motor functioning is controlled by the proximate primary motor cortex (see Figure 9.3). It is a complex system with unique terminology (see, e.g., Kolb & Whishaw, 2003; Purves, Williams, Nundy, & Lotto, 2004). These include sensorimotor functioning, dyspraxia, and visuomotor functioning (Polatajko & Cantin, 2006; Sanger et al., 2006). Next, such terms are defined as they are used by the NEPSY–II sensorimotor subtests.

Sensorimotor functioning specifically refers to motor control that needs neural feedback from the senses for proper coordination, including kinesthetic, tactile, and visual signals. *Motor coordination* is defined here as muscle groups that work together to produce accurate manual output. *Dyspraxia* (also known as *apraxia*) is the inability to perform intentional actions as the result of brain dysfunction or injury. As referenced previously, *visuomotor skills* refer to vision interacting with movement to effectuate specified actions, including a variety of fine motor movements and sensorimotor functioning (as defined prior). Visuomotor accuracy depends upon the coordination of visual input or mental imagery with manual output. Finally, the NEPSY–II measures the ability to imitate fine motor positions and sequences, specifically with the hands and fingers. The purpose is to attempt to detect manual motor problems in learning a producing smooth motor sequences, which were first identified by the first edition of this test (Denckla, 1985; Korkman, Kettunen, & Autti-Rämö, 2003).

SOCIAL PERCEPTION

Social perception involves several cognitive abilities that facilitate both the effectiveness and appropriateness of one's interpersonal interactions. These abilities include the following. First, this includes the interpretation, encoding, and recognition of faces. The ability to encode, recall, and recognize faces has a significant impact on social relationships and communication. In fact, impairment in this aspect of social perception has been linked to autism (Dakin & Frith, 2005; Tanaka & Farah, 1993). Second, social perception includes the ability to recognize affect and facial emotional expression, which also has an association with autism (Ashwin, Wheelwright, & Baron-Cohen, 2006; Linder & Rosen, 2006). This makes sense since the ability to recognize and accurately detect emotional states portrayed on an individual's face (e.g., sadness, happiness, anger) facilitates effective interpersonal communication.

Finally, a third and perhaps most pertinent facet of social perception is the aforementioned theory of mind, which again refers to the ability to understand that people possess internal thoughts, beliefs, and expectations that guide their behavior and that are distinct and separate from that of the self. A robust finding is that children with autism perform poorly on theory of mind tasks (Baron-Cohen, 2001; Baron-Cohen, Leslie, & Frith, 1985; Happé, 1995; Pilowsky, Yirmiya, Arbelle, & Możes, 2000). Children with deficits in theory of mind are unlikely to understand the subtleties in social communication, including sarcasm and figures of speech. Hence, the measurement of these components of social perception are included in the NEPSY–II battery, which is consistent with the *DSM–5* recently adding deficits in social perception as a bona fide symptom of neurocognitive disorder (American Psychiatric Association, 2013).

VISUOSPATIAL PROCESSING

A final neurocognitive domain is *visuospatial processing*, which includes elements of visual perception, spatial or visuospatial perception, and visuoconstructive skills (Benton, Hamsher, Varney, & Spreen, 1983; Lezak, Howieson, & Loring, 2004; Strauss, Sherman, & Spreen, 2006). *Visual perception* is the interpretation of sensory input that is transmitted from our eyes, through the thalamus, and lastly into the occipital lobe's visual cortex. It is expressed in tasks such as the matching of pictorial patterns or pictures, or by identifying forms embedded within complex pictures. *Spatial processing* is the ability to comprehend the orientation of visual information in two- and three-dimensional space. This ability permits individuals to perceive objects in three-dimensions (i.e., from a two-dimensional retina), estimate distance, complete mental rotation tasks (i.e., perceiving the same object in different orientations), and construct objects. Finally, *visuoconstruction* refers to our ability to organize and manually manipulate spatial information to produce a design. This requires the coordination of fine motor skills with the understanding of visual-spatial relationships. Visuoconstruction is frequently tested using block construction subtests and tasks requiring the reproduction of geometric figures, including such activities as clock drawing.

SUMMARY

This section covered the six domains of neurocognitive abilities measured by the NEPSY–II. Although they are theoretical, intercorrelations among the subtests have supported this organization with empirical data (see Korkman et al., 2007b, pp. 51–130). At the same time, it must be acknowledged that many subtests do have some overlap with other domains that should be considered when interpreting the results of the NEPSY–II data yield.

Norm Reference Sample

The standardization sample consisted of 1,200 individuals in 12 age groups, ranging in age from 3 years through 16 years, inclusive. A total of 100 individuals were in each age group, which were apportioned into one-year intervals from ages 3 to 12. Ages 13–14 years and 15–16 years were combined into two-year intervals, which again comprised 100 in each group. This sample was stratified according to age, race/ethnicity, geographic region, and parent education level. Sex was apportioned equally so that 50% were males and 50% were females. The remaining categories were proportioned according to data collected by the U.S. Census Bureau in October 2003 (U.S. Bureau of the Census, 2004). Race/ethnicity included White, African American, Hispanic, or Other. Geographic region was divided into Northeast, Midwest, South, and West. Finally, parent educational level was divided into groups of 0–11 years, 12 years, 13–15 years, and 16 or more years.

Administration

There are two basic issues concerning NEPSY–II administration. The first concerns the type of battery that is to be selected, which stems directly from the fact that the NEPSY–II is intentionally designed as a flexible battery. The second issue refers to some general administration rules that are analogous to those used by the intelligence and achievement tests, namely, *adaptive testing* rules. The former is more unique to this instrument, so this is where the discussion begins.

SELECTING THE PROPER NEPSY–II BATTERY

When using the NEPSY–II, the first consideration is selecting the subtests to be administered. As illustrated by the test structure, the NEPSY–II is organized by two variables; that is, by (a) chronological age (CA) of the examinee (i.e., ages 3–4 and 5–16), and (b) by neurocognitive domain. The former is due to the fact that the array of NEPSY–II subtests apply to varying age ranges within these two larger classes. Therefore, the first choice is rather straightforward. The second is contingent upon the diagnostic issues that must be resolved according to the case facts. There are essentially four alternatives as follows: (a) administer a full battery, (b) administer a general battery, (c) administer a recommended cluster of subtests for a specified diagnostic issue, or (d) administer a specially tailored combination of subtests to address issues presented by unique case facts.

The full battery (i.e., a Full Assessment) consists of all subtests that fit the CA of the examinee (with the exception of the social perception subtests). Such is recommended for a comprehensive neuropsychological evaluation. Estimated administration time for the younger three- to four-year age group is 90 minutes, thus requiring a two-hour appointment for test administration. Estimated administration time for the older 5- to 16-year age group is three and a half hours, hence requiring the scheduling of two, two-hour appointments. A general battery (i.e., a General Assessment) consists of those subtests from each domain that have the proven capability of best detecting the presence of brain dysfunction (i.e., subtests that are most sensitive to brain impairment), which is advised for an overview of the individual's neuropsychological status (Korkman et al., 2007a, p. 1). If results are positive for brain dysfunction, the general battery will need follow-up testing for more precise differential diagnosis; that is, if such is desired. Administration time for the general battery is 45 minutes for the younger group and 60 minutes for the older group.

The third type of battery is referred to as a Diagnostic Assessment, which is a combination of subtests advised when searching for certain commonly known diagnoses or issues. In the NEPSY–II administrative manual (Korkman et al., 2007a, p. 12), there are batteries recommended for learning problems in reading, learning problems in math, attention/concentration (i.e., ADHD), behavioral management (i.e., *oppositional defiant disorder* or *ODD*), *language disorder*, perceptual/motor disorder, school readiness, and social/interpersonal issues. The fourth and final battery is referred to as a Selective Assessment, from which several permutations have evolved over years of testing practice using this instrument and is reflected in some of the uniquely designed data tables using NEPSY–II subtests.

SPECIFIC ADMINISTRATIVE RULES

In general, subtests may be administered in any order. The exception to this rule refers to the administration of immediate and delayed versions of certain subtests wherein the delayed task must be administered between 20 and 30 minutes subsequent to initial exposure for valid results (e.g., Memory for Designs and Memory for Designs–Delayed have a 15–25-minute interval). Recording the time after immediate exposure and testing has been completed helps to ensure that the delayed task is completed within the proper interval of elapsed time.

Subtest items are ordered by increasing degrees of difficulty. Adaptive testing rules are utilized to reduce testing time and help maintain motivation and rapport with the examinee. Although some subtests have single start points, most have age-appropriate start points as done in the administration of the intelligence and achievement tests. Reverse rules accompany the age-appropriate start points. Thus, in the event the examinee fails at the start point, the examiner is to reverse course until two consecutive items are passed, after which all previous items are awarded full credit under the assumption that easier items would have been passed if administered. Similarly, discontinue rules dictate the stoppage of a subtest subsequent to a predetermined number of consecutive failures. Compared to the intelligence and achievement tests for this age range, the discontinue rules are remarkably generous (e.g., discontinues after five consecutive failures on Affect Recognition). Some subtests have *stop points* that are based upon age. In fact, some subtests have both discontinue rules and stop points.

There are a number of timed tests on the NEPSY–II. Some provide a total time limit. For example, Word Generation asks examinees to report as many animals as they can within 60 seconds. Other subtests time at the level of the item, awarding more points if done correctly within a predefined time limit, and fewer points when completed in a greater amount of time (e.g., Block Construction). As a general rule, the examiner attempts to elicit maximum performance by the examinee. Therefore, providing prompts (i.e., brief statements of encouragement) and queries (i.e., questions that ask for clarification of a vague but potentially correct response) are not only permitted but are encouraged. Examples of prompts include "Just give it a try," Keep going," or "Try it one more time." Examples of queries are, "Tell me more about that" or "Explain what you mean" (see Korkman et al., 2007a, p. 27). Although these are technically phrased as statements, the question is implied as, "Can you. . .?"

Finally, the test has two record forms in which the subtests are included in alphabetical order as follows: (a) Record Form Ages 3–4 (colored purple) and (b) Record Form Ages 5–16 (colored green). The latter includes various age ranges for each subtest, along with different stop points defined by age. The principal purpose of the record form is to enter examinee responses, item scores, raw score totals, and a graph on the front where scaled scores can be entered manually for profile analysis. Although verbal instructions are provided on some subtests (e.g., Comprehension of Instructions), other subtests require the administrative manual (e.g., Oromotor Sequences).

Scoring

Forms 9.1, 9.2, 9.3, and 9.4 present the NEPSY–II subtests and their data tables used for reporting them within final psychological assessment reports in clinical practice. They are apportioned according to age grouping (viz., Ages 3–4 and Form Ages 5–16) and battery type (viz., Full Battery and General Battery). The combination of these two components renders four Forms as follows: (a) Form Ages 3–4, Full Battery (Form 9.1); (b) Form Ages 5–16, Full Battery (Form 9.2); (c) Form Ages 3–4, General Battery (Form 9.3); and (d) Form Ages 5–16, General Battery (Form 9.4). It is important to note that for the Age 5–16 Forms 9.2 and 9.4, specific table notes had to be appended to subtests that can be administered to less than the full 5–16-year age range (e.g., age 7–16 years or 5–6 years). In cases where a subtest does not apply to an examinee (e.g., the Statue subtest for an examinee who is 12 years old), double-dash lines can be inserted in that subtest row or that subtest can simply be deleted from the table.

The NEPSY–II offers two types of subtest data, including primary scores and process scores. *Primary scores* measure key clinical neurocognitive abilities, as evinced by such terms as, "Total" or "Combined," in the subtest moniker. In contrast, *process scores* measure more narrowly defined neurocognitive abilities that qualify the primary scores. An excellent example is the percentile rank (PR) metric provided for errors made interpreting certain emotions on the Affect Recognition subtest. Therefore, if an examinee scores poorly on that subtest (e.g., scaled score = 3), these data are capable of showing which emotion(s) were most difficult for the examinee to read accurately. As can be seen even by a cursory examination of Forms 9.1–9.4, the focus is clearly and consistently on primary scores. The NEPSY–II also offers contrast scores, which are designed to compare if there are differences between selected types of neurocognitive functioning. In lieu of using these, however, confidence intervals (CIs) among the primary scores can simply be compared for their degrees of overlap.

Irrespective of the score type, however, the subtests use a scaled score metric with a mean of 10, standard deviation (*SD*) of 3, and a range of 1–19, all of which are included in general table notes (see Forms 9.1–9.4). The Full Battery forms (i.e., Forms 9.1 and 9.2) organize the subtests by neurocognitive domain as presented in the section on the NEPSY–II test structure. That is, each table lists subtests that measure a single domain or general neurocognitive ability. Within each table, the subtests are enumerated according to the conceptual similarity of the ability measured. For example, Inhibition-Inhibition Combined, which measures inhibitory control, is immediately ensued by Inhibition-Switching Combined, which also measures inhibitory control but with the addition of cognitive flexibility. In contrast, the General Battery consists of subtests and their primary scores that best discriminate between individuals with and without brain dysfunction. Because this is the chief component that binds these subtests together, they are listed within a single table. The measured abilities column, however, clearly shows which domain each subtest represents. Note that in the General Battery, all domains save social perception are represented by one or more subtests.

Following the subtest name in the first column are the following: (a) scaled score, (b) 95% confidence interval (CI), (c) percentile rank (PR), (d) classification, and (e) measured abilities. The scaled score metric has already been shown. The 95% CI was determined by use of the average *standard error of measurement* (*SEM*) listed for each subtest scaled score in the clinical and interpretive manual (see Korkman et al., 2007b, Tables 4.3–4.4, pp. 58–59). Recall that the *SEM* represents the average spread of scores around an individual's true score on a particular test or subtest. *SEM*s are used to compute a confidence interval or range around an estimated true score. Where an *SEM* was not reported in the manual for a particular subtest primary score, the average *SEM* for its neurocognitive domain was used. Next, to estimate the 95% CI, the *SEM* was rounded to the nearest 0.5 points, doubled, and finally rounded to the nearest whole number for convenience. To report the 95% CI for a subtest then, the examiner merely adds and subtracts the value entered immediately under the brackets in that subtest's column. For example, imagine a 4-year-old earns a scaled score of 10 on the Statue subtest in the Full Battery. Next, in Table 1 of Form 9.1, the examiner would add and subtract 3 points to the score of 10 and compute a 95% CI of 7 to 13. Therefore, it can be stated with 95% certainty that the examinee's true Statue scaled score falls somewhere between 7 and 13. If the examiner desires more precision in such estimates, a 68% CI can be employed by adding and subtracting half the value entered below the brackets in that subtest's column (rounding up or down to the nearest whole number. In the immediate example, the examiner could add and subtract one point (i.e., half of 3, which is 1.5, rounded down to 1.0); that is, the obtained score of 10 would have a 68% CI of 9 to 11. Here, an increase in precision would be balanced with a concomitant decrease in confidence.

The PR is based upon the theoretical normal curve. As usual, it has a median of 50 and range of 1–99. Because they are areas scores, they minimize changes in the extremes of the distribution and exaggerate those occurring in the distribution center. Next, the NEPSY–II classification represents an ordinal-nominal type score that is categorical in nature, although it incorporates an approximate order of functioning. This is described in more detail in the interpretation section. Lastly, the neurocognitive abilities that are tapped by each subtest is summarized to facilitate interpretation. Lastly, note that the CI and PR are both defined in the specific tabular notes to benefit the reader, who may not be familiar with these data.

Although the NEPSY–II can be scored manually by using the many tables in the clinical and interpretation manual for transforming raw scores into scaled scores and PRs (Korkman et al., 2007b), this would not be recommended due to the significant amount of time required. Furthermore, because of its flexibility and abundant primary, process, and contrast scores, the likelihood of human error when manually scoring a full NEPSY–II battery is considerable. Rather, the *NEPSY–II Scoring Assistant and Assessment Planner* (Pearson, 2007) provides rapid and efficient computer scoring. There is also a NEPSY–II training CD available for new users (2007). However, it should be reiterated that the former is essential for utilizing this complex yet flexible test battery in an efficient and accurate manner.

Interpretation

Interpretation of the NEPSY–II data yield is intimately associated with which type of battery has been administered, irrespective of age. As such, this section will be further subdivided according to the type of battery given to the examinee, which guides the interpretative strategy. Prior to this, however, the aforementioned classification scheme will be reviewed because this is integral to test interpretation irrespective of battery or subtest combination used.

Table 9.1 presents the scaled score ranges associated with each descriptive classification relative to same age peers. The wording of each classification is in terms of performance level. Hence, for example, *at expected level* refers to performance by a child that is normal, typical, or ordinary based on chronological age (CA). Likewise, *below expected level* is performance that is atypical or abnormal based on CA. An interpretive scheme that has proven to be useful is to interpret borderline scores as showing mild impairment or dysfunction, below expected level to show moderate impairment or dysfunction, and well below expected level to show severe impairment or dysfunction as applied to the neurocognitive abilities measured by that subtest. These classifications apply notwithstanding the various types of batteries that can be applied to a case. The discussion now begins with the most comprehensive battery and moves to increasingly specialized batteries.

NEPSY–II FULL BATTERY

The *NEPSY–II Full Battery* provided the most comprehensive assessment of a child or adolescent's neurocognitive functioning among all six domains measured by this flexible instrument (see Forms 9.1 and 9.2). Because the battery consists of only primary scores that measure key clinical neurocognitive abilities, there is no hierarchical interpretive strategy to be employed as is done on the intelligence and achievement tests. Therefore, the interpretative strategy is to note the following aspects within each domain: (a) the number of subtest primary scores that are borderline or lower; (b) the degree of impairment of each low score (i.e., mild, moderate, or severe, as outlined earlier); and (c) the specific neurocognitive abilities that are most impaired.[4]

Notice that after each data table, both Forms 9.1 and 9.2 include (a) definitions of the major neurocognitive concepts representing each domain and (b) pre-drafted interpretative statements for deriving clinical meaning of the score patterns. The former ensure that the reader comprehends the principal neurocognitive abilities that define each domain. The interpretive statements invariably begin by summarizing a "normal" profile of scaled scores for that domain. This is followed by a necessarily complex set of statements that describe patterns of impaired functioning with spaces to be filled in depending upon the particular data pattern. These are intended to provide a beginning interpretation of the results and should be modified and added to as needed.

Table 9.1 NEPSY–II Classification Guide

Scaled score	Classification
13–19	Above expected level
8–12	At expected level
6–7	Borderline
4–5	Below expected level
1–3	Well below expected level

Source. Adapted from Korkman, M., Kirk, U., & Kemp, S. (2007b). *NEPSY, Second Edition (NEPSY–II): Clinical and interpretive manual.* San Antonio, TX: NCS Pearson, Table 6.2, p. 136.

Note. Scaled score mean = 10, standard deviation = 15, range 1–19.

After all domains are analyzed in this manner, they can be integrated thereafter within a "summary of results" section of the report for purposes of determining if sufficient areas are impaired, and to what degree, to meet the criteria for a minor or major neurocognitive disorder, along with indicating etiology if such has not yet been determined. Finally, the location(s) of the dysfunction can be estimated based upon what neurocognitive abilities are impaired and which brain areas are implicated according to the examiner's model of brain functioning (see prior). The Full Battery is justified when a child or adolescent has been referred to determine if a neurocognitive disorder is present; if so, what are the functional impairments and parts of the brain that are implicated, and what is the likely etiology?

NEPSY–II GENERAL BATTERY

The *NEPSY–II General Battery* can be used when a simple overview of an examinee's neurocognitive status is desired. Here, sufficient data is provided to make a general diagnosis of minor or major neurocognitive disorder, although it is less likely that such information will be sufficient to determine etiology (if unknown), the degree and type of functional impairments that the examinee will manifest in daily life and identifying the location of brain dysfunction. The General Battery, however, is sufficient as a neurocognitive screening for this age group to determine if more comprehensive follow-up neuropsychological testing or neurological referral is needed. The latter is especially important when one considers the lack of mental status screening devices available for individuals under the age of 18 years, and most especially younger than 16 years.

The General Battery consists of one or more subtests from each domain, with the exception of social perception (see Forms 9.3 and 9.4). Hence, the measured abilities final column includes added language (compared to the Full Battery forms) to ensure the clarity of the neurocognitive domain measured by each particular subtest. As stated, these subtests best discriminate between those with and without significant brain impairment in each of their respective domains. Hence, these data can indicate if neurocognitive pathology is present, although it is not sufficiently comprehensive for a more detailed diagnosis and treatment planning.

Note that an added section has been inserted immediately after the single General Battery table, termed, "neurocognitive abilities defined" (see Forms 9.3 and 9.4). As should now be apparent, neuropsychology has its own special nomenclature and jargon. This is why such terms are defined throughout the Full Battery forms after each domain data table. To provide useful definitions of these concepts to both professionals and laypeople who may read the General Battery results, these same definitions are provided in one summary paragraph prior to the interpretative statements. Next, two pre-drafted interpretive paragraphs are provided. The first represents an interpretation of a completely normal protocol, which effectively rules out neurocognitive dysfunction. In contrast, the second interprets the presence of signification dysfunction and a listing of all domains that were measured by the subtests. Those that showed impairment can simply be retained while those that were measured to be within normal limits can be deleted. Here, follow-up testing is recommended.

DIAGNOSTIC AND SELECTIVE BATTERIES

While the NEPSY–II manual discriminates between these types of batteries, the two are here conflated. Technically, Diagnostic Assessments are subtest groupings recommended by the NEPSY–II manual for various common diagnostic problems (e.g., behavioral problems). Selective Assessments are those designed by the examiner according to the distinctive case facts. In either case, they may be considered specially tailored batteries that are determined by the unique diagnostic issues and idiographic case facts. Hence, this distinction has no meaningful difference, which justifies their being combined in such manner.

When a unique combination of tests has been employed, it is most typically as follows: (a) Attention and Executive Functioning subtests for attention-deficit/hyperactivity disorder (ADHD), (b) Social Perception subtests for autism spectrum disorder (ASD) and *social pragmatic communication disorder*, and (c) Language subtests for language disorder and speech sound (phonological) disorder or *other specified communication disorder*. The former two have by far been the most common, especially when used with continuous performance tests (see later) and the *Autism Diagnostic Observation Schedule, Second Edition* (*ADOS–2*; Lord, Luyster, Gotham, & Guthrie, 2012b; Lord et al., 2012a), respectively. When using a specially devised battery, the examiner can simply select the proper subtests from Forms 9.1 and 9.2 and report them independently, in groups according to their domain or in an organization that is consistent with the objectives of the testing case, whether it be with the context of a final neuropsychological or psychological assessment report. If an examiner uses a particular subtest combination frequently, creating a permanent table that includes only those subtests for the purpose of saving time and for convenience is strongly advised.[5]

Neuropsychological Assessment Battery

Synopsis

The *Neuropsychological Assessment Battery* (*NAB*; Stern & White, 2003; White & Stern, 2003c) is a comprehensive yet efficient and flexible measure, which is comparable in many ways to the NEPSY–II in that it affords the testing psychologist with both a fixed and flexible battery approach. All the tests that comprise this instrument are co-normed on individuals aged 18 years, 0 months through 97 years, 11 months. More specifically, the full battery comprises five main modules, each of which measures a general neuropsychological ability or domain consistent with both Bennet's 1988 model and the criteria established for the *DSM–5* neurocognitive disorders (American Psychiatric Association, 2013). They may be administered in whole or in part contingent upon the diagnostic and referral questions.

In order of administration, the main modules include Attention, Language, Memory, Spatial, and Executive Functions. Note the similarity in content to the NEPSY–II. In contrast to the NEPSY–II, however, this measure provides an overall NAB Total index comparable to the Full Scale IQ score that symbolizes the *g* or general factor. Other unique and advantageous features of the NAB include the following: (a) availability of equivalent Forms A and B, (b) choice between demographically corrected norms (White & Stern, 2003a) and U.S. census-matched norms (White & Stern, 2003c), (c) optional neuropsychological test screening, and (d) inclusion of pragmatic daily living subtests within each module. Some brief comments on each of these features are in order.

Equivalent Forms A and B permit a more accurate measure of symptom progression because it reduces practice effects. Demographically corrected norms compare the examinee's performance to neurologically healthy individuals of the same age, sex, and education, and are recommended for clinical diagnostic purposes (White & Stern, 2003a, 2003b). In the alternative, if for some utilitarian reason the testing psychologist prefers comparing the examinee's performance to the U.S. population, the U.S. census-matched norms may be employed (White & Stern, 2003b, 2003c). This sample more closely represents key U.S. demographic characteristics, including geographic region by age group, education, sex, and ethnicity.

The Neuropsychological Assessment Screening Battery (NASB) is an abbreviated measure of an examinee's functioning in each of the domains or modules. This provides empirical data to determine whether follow-up testing with the respective complete modules is necessitated. The measurement of practical daily living skills enhances (a) ecological validity (White & Stern, 2003b), (b) generalizability of the results, and (c) meaningful feedback to referring clinicians, patients, and family members regarding the nature and extent of dysfunction.

Test Structure

The NAB test structure is reviewed in this section to facilitate test interpretation. First, empirical support for the NAB structure is presented. Second, this is followed by succinct reviews of each of the main modules and the screening module.

EMPIRICAL SUPPORT

The NAB test structure was empirically supported by (a) intercorrelations of internal structure, (b) exploratory factor analyses, and (c) confirmatory factor analyses. First, the Screening Domain scores had their highest correlations with their respective main module index scores. Further, intercorrelations of tests within each main module showed positive and moderate level correlations, with the exception of the language tests where the correlation magnitudes were somewhat lower. However, the latter was likely due to the restriction in range among the language tests, which all tend to be negatively skewed (i.e., many high scores) due to the large proportion of healthy nonimpaired people in the population in terms of language function. In addition, the tests had their lowest intercorrelations with those of other modules. Therefore, the patterns of intercorrelations manifested a consistent pattern of both convergent and divergent validity.

Exploratory factor analyses (EFAs) consistently showed both five-factor and six-factor solutions that accounted for 48.3% and 52.8% of the variance, respectively, and represented the best fit of the data. The former consisted of the following distinct factors: attention, language, memory, spatial skills, and executive functions. The six-factor model separated out a psychomotor speed factor from that of executive functions. This latter finding was not surprising, as it was apparent from the NAB's inception that the tests were multifactorial in nature with a good deal of overlap in skills.

Finally, confirmatory factor analyses (CFAs) were done on both the main modules and the screening module. Although the aforementioned five-factor model was generally supported for both the screening module and the five main modules, there was evidence of a number of cross-factor and shared loadings among the many test scores, including a psychomotor speed factor that was a salient component of many of tests (e.g., Design Construction and Mazes tests). Therefore, although organizing the tests within each of the modules is empirically justified, it should also be recognized that many of these neurocognitive processes are multifactorial in nature. This fact should especially be considered during test interpretation.

To summarize, the NAB tests are organized according to five main modules, each of which measure a general neurocognitive ability. These include the Attention Module, Language Module, Memory Module, Spatial Module, and the Executive Functioning Module. The five modules contribute to a NAB Total index that represents an examinee's overall level of neurocognitive functioning. There is also a NASB that consists of a screening module for each of the five general neurocognitive abilities. These also contribute to a Screening Total index that represents a gross estimate of likely neurocognitive functioning. Next, the more specific neurocognitive abilities measured by each of the principal NAB tests are presented to facilitate later test interpretation. They are organized according to module or organizational structure.

ATTENTION MODULE

The Attention Module begins with a measure of *orientation* (i.e., awareness of oneself in relation to one's environment), which is commonly impaired in a variety of brain disorders (Lezak, 1995). There are a total of 16 items that measure orientation to self, time, place, and situation. Also included is the repetition of orally presented digits, both in a forward and backward sequence. This is a common method of measuring auditory attentional capacity, although the backward sequence also includes working memory (Kaplan, Fein, Morris, & Deis, 1991; Lezak, 1995). The Dots test comprises a sequence of presenting an initial page with an array of dots, a blank interference page, and a page of the same array although with one added dot. The examinee is asked to identify the new dot. This is referred to as a *spatial delayed-recognition span paradigm*, which is a measure of working memory and visual scanning found to be sensitive to major neurocognitive disorder (Moss, Killiany, Lai, Rosene, & Herndon, 1997) and subcortical dysfunction (Partiot et al., 1996). The Numbers and Letters test consists of a variety of tasks that together measure selective, sustained, and divided attention, along with concentration and psychomotor speed.

These include using a controlled search paradigm (i.e., selecting a specific target among similar distractors during the course of a *cancellation task*). A *cancellation task* asks the examinee to search for and mark a target letter or symbol among comparable stimuli. Such a task requires selective or focused attention (Ruff & Allen, 1996) in addition to information processing and psychomotor speed (Williamson, Scott, & Adams, 1996). Recognizing that attention has many facets that are interrelated, the NAB included four different Numbers and Letters tasks that together measured sustained attention (also known as *vigilance*), psychomotor speed, selective attention, divided attention, information processing speed, impulsivity, and disinhibition. Finally, the Driving Scenes test incorporated a *useful field of view (UFOV) paradigm* (see Ball, Beard, Roenker, Miller, & Griggs, 1988; Ball & Roenker, 1998) in which examinees' scan a scene as if they were sitting behind the steering wheel of a car. After a brief exposure, the scene is changed and examinees must identify which aspects are different, new, or missing. In addition to measuring content related to everyday life (see, e.g., Robertson, Ward, Ridgeway, & Nimmo-Smith, 1994), this test taps visual scanning, working memory, attention to detail, and selective attention.

LANGUAGE MODULE

The Oral Production test is a measure of *proposition speech output*, which essentially measures language production in terms of quantified units of content (see, e.g., Goodglass et al., 2000; Yorkston & Beukelman, 1980). Hence, examinees are asked to describe all they see happening in a picture of an outdoor interpersonal scenario. Measured in this manner, oral language production has been found to be key in identifying aphasia (i.e., language impairment due to brain dysfunction) and impairment in executive functioning (Boone, 1999).

Auditory comprehension tasks involve giving the examinee commands of increasing complexity, who subsequently responds by manipulating objects as instructed (Boller & Vignolo, 1966; DeRenzi & Vignolo, 1962). Other auditory comprehension tasks include pointing and responding to dichotomous "yes-no" questions (Goodglass et al., 2000). This ability has also been found to be essential in detecting language dysfunction (see, e.g., Benton, Hamsher, & Sivan, 1994).

The Naming test requires examinees to accurately identify photos of common objects (e.g., a ruler). This test primarily taps word-finding ability, which is common to most if not all individuals who suffer from aphasia (Benson & Ardilla, 1996; Goodglass & Wingfiled, 1997). Next, the NAB Reading Comprehension test requires examinees to match single words and sentences to a photograph that represents the object or main idea expressed by the item. This exemplifies a common strategy in detecting the presence of aphasia in individuals (Benson & Ardilla, 1996). Most patients with aphasia or language dysfunction manifest difficulties in written expression or *agraphia* (Benson & Ardilla, 1996). The NAB Writing test is therefore designed to quantify several major aspects of writing ability, including legibility, syntax, spelling, and conveyance of major themes illustrated in a picture of a scene (see, e.g., Goodglass et al., 2000). Finally, Bill Payment is the daily living test in the Language Module. Generally, it represents a complex task that people are required to execute in the real world, which people with aphasia find to be very difficult in performing (see, e.g., Frattali, Thompson, Holland, Wohl, & Ferketic, 1995; Holland, 1980; Holland, Frattali, & Fromm, 1999). This test taps multiple areas of language function, including auditory comprehension, reading comprehension, writing, simple calculations, and expressive speech.

MEMORY MODULE

The NAB Memory Module consists of a number of tests that have significant empirical support. They include the following: (a) list-learning of words with repeated trials (i.e., supraspan learning seen in the NEPSY–II), word list interference, immediate free recall, delayed free recall, and delayed (yes-no) forced-choice recognition trials (viz., a List Learning test); (b) a visual shape-learning test, with immediate multiple-choice recognition, delayed multiple-choice recognition, and delayed forced-choice recognition trials (viz., a Shape Learning test); (c) short narrative story learning with two trials, verbatim and gist recall, and immediate free recall and delayed free recall trials (viz., a Story Learning test); and (d) a Daily Living Memory test, including memory for medication instructions and memory for an individual's identifying information, both involving immediate free recall, delayed free recall, and delayed multiple-choice recognition trials.[6] Next, a brief rationale for each of these types of memory tests is provided.

List-learning tests using words permit measures of a learning curve, sensitivity to interference, use of semantically based coding strategies, perseveration, and changes in central nervous system functioning (see, e.g., Curtiss, Vanderploeg, Spencer, & Salazar, 2001; Killiany et al., 2002). Shape-learning tasks commonly involve the recall of geometric shapes and figures (Meyers & Meyers, 1995; Sivan, 1992), largely to reduce the influence of previous learning (Williams, 1991). Additionally, these NAB visual memory tests are motor-free to eliminate a potential confound of graphomotor skills with visual memory (Hannay, Levin, & Grossman, 1979). The forced choice recognition trials for both the List Learning and Shape Learning tests was supported by evidence that such data could assist in detecting true memory impairments (see, e.g., Snodgrass & Corwin, 1988). Regarding the Story Learning test, the learning and recall of logically connect material has proven to be extremely sensitive to detecting early memory impairment (Locascio, Growdon, & Corkin, 1995; Morris et al., 2001; Wefel, Hoyt, & Massman, 1999). Finally, the Daily Living Memory test was included principally because the learning and recall of such material has proven to be more efficacious in predicting memory for practical information (see, e.g., Makatura, Lam, Leahy, Castillo, & Kalpakjian, 1999).

The ensuing evidence concerns comparisons between tests and the decisions regarding the selected test time intervals. First, the inclusion of both List Learning and Story Learning tests was bolstered by evidence showing that differential performance between these two tasks contributed to valuable differential diagnosis. For example, poorer performance on list-learning versus logically organized story learning was associated with deficits in executive functioning (see, e.g., Tremont, Halpert, Javorsky, & Stern, 2000). Second, length of delay intervals (e.g., immediate versus a 10–15-minute delay) was based upon research showing that relative brief delays of 2–10 minutes were significantly more efficacious in discriminating between patients with neurocognitive impairment versus normal controls, as opposed to longer 10–60-minute intervals Albert & Moss, 1992; Berry & Carpenter, 1992; Chapman, White, & Storandt, 1997; Somerville & Stern, 2001).

SPATIAL MODULE

The Spatial Module tests consist of both (a) pure visuospatial tasks and (b) visual-motor tests. First, visuospatial functioning relies principally upon visual perceptual precision. That is, in the absence of accurate visual perception, drawing, object assembly, visual organization, and all other such multifactorial skills would also be impaired. Hence, the NAB Visual Discrimination test employs a visual match-to-target paradigm (see Benton, Sivan, Hamsher, Varney, & Spreen, 1994). More specifically, the examinee must select which of four irregular geometric shapes, consisting of multiple curves and straight lines, matches the target shape at the top of the stimulus page. This measures pure visuoperception and visuospatial skills, along with attention to detail.

Next, the Design Construction test requires the assembly of two to seven geometrically shaped puzzle pieces to match two-dimensional designs of the same size printed on stimulus pages. This test measures a combination of skills, including visual perception, motor output and integration, and spatial analysis, which is distinct from a drawing task that is measured by the ensuing test (Lezak, 1995). Next, the Figure Drawing test asks the examinee to sketch a figure that includes a number of distinct components, including major vertical and horizontal bisectors, an oval, a crisscross figure, a rectangle, triangular shape, and other embedded patterns. Examinees can use these components to organize their approach to drawing the entire figure, then recreating the drawing from memory. Such drawing tasks are extremely common in neuropsychological test batteries because they are remarkably sensitive to neurological dysfunction (Kessler, 1998; Walsh & Darby, 1999). The Figure Drawing Immediate Recall simply adds an encoding and immediate retrieval element to the task.

Finally, Map Reading represents the daily living test for the Spatial Module. This task requires examinees to follow verbal directions, given both orally and in written format, and identify (a) final destinations, (b) estimated distances, and (c) required turns on a map of a hypothetical town. Like other daily-living NAB tests, this test is designed to maximize *ecological validity* (i.e., does test performance generalize to the real world?), and measures visuospatial skills, spatial/directional orientation, right-left orientation, and visual scanning.

EXECUTIVE FUNCTIONS MODULE

In general, the NAB Executive Functions Module is designed to tap planning and foresight, both of which are prime components of this more advanced neurocognitive ability (see Bennet's 1988 model; see also Stern & Prohaska, 1996). As such, these tests are frequently associated with frontal lobe dysfunction (see Figure 9.2; Milner, 1968; Porteus, 1959). The NAB Mazes test is founded upon a *maze-tracing paradigm* in which examinees must use a pen and trace their way out of a sequence of increasingly complex mazes, including multiple blind alleys, and without lifting their pen once they begin the maze. Examinees are timed and earn added points for faster completions. This test measures planning and foresight, impulse control, and psychomotor speed.

The Judgment test requires the examinee to answer questions that require practical decision-making, including aspects of independence or autonomy in daily living. In particular, the questions regard home safety, health, and medical issues people may encounter in daily living. Poor judgment is associated with impairment in the prefrontal cortex (see Figure 9.3; Parker, 1990), along with major neurocognitive disorder (Knopman et al., 2001). Next, the Categories test requires examinees to classify six individuals according to their identifying information, including physical, psychological, and personal characteristics and facts. This test measures concept formation, cognitive response set, mental flexibility, and generativity, all of which are shown to be sensitive to frontal lobe dysfunction (Berg, 1948; Delis, Kaplan, & Kramer, 2001; Heaton, Chelune, Talley, Kay, & Curtis, 1993). Finally, Word Generation asks examinees to report as many three-letter words as they can produce in 120 seconds from a list of eight letters with consonants and vowels. This was included because such tasks are sensitive indicators of neurocognitive dysfunction (see, e.g., Mutchnick, Ross, & Long, 1991; Spreen & Benton, 1977). This test measures generativity, verbal fluency, and self-monitoring. The latter is further detected by recording the number of perseverative responses.

SUMMARY

This section reviewed the overall NAB test organizational structure. It began with a succinct review of supporting evidence, including internal consistency and its factorial structure. This was followed by a delineation of each test according to its module. Here, each test was described in terms of task, specifically measured neurocognitive abilities, and empirical support for its inclusion in the NAB battery. The objective was to facilitate test interpretation, a topic which is discussed in more detail subsequently.

Norm Reference Samples

Empirical evidence indicates that performance on neuropsychological test batteries is significantly influenced by age, educational attainment, and sex, independent from that of an individual's brain functioning. In consequence, there is general agreement that demographically corrected norms are the most felicitous normative standard to employ when inferring brain–behavior relationships (Heaton et al., 1993; Heaton et al., 1991; Lezak, 1995; Mitrushina et al., 1998; Spreen & Strauss, 1998). Therefore, the NAB offers two types of norms as follows: (a) demographically corrected norms and (b) age-referenced, U.S. Census–matched norms.

Demographically corrected norms are grouped according to age, education level, and sex (White & Stern, 2003a, 2003b). Hence, a sufficient number of participants were included in each Age x Education x Sex group to achieve the objective of providing stable estimates of performance (White & Stern, 2003a, 2003b; see also Fastenau & Adams, 1996, for criticizing past neuropsychological test batteries for having insufficient numbers in demographically corrected standardization samples). The demographically corrected normative sample totaled 1,448 healthy individuals, ranging in age from 18 years, 0 months through 97 years, 11 months. This total was divided into 711 for Form 1 and 737 for Form 2 (White & Stern, 2003a, 2003b).

In contrast, the age-based, *U.S. Census–matched sample* totaled 950 individuals of comparable age range, which was stratified according to the Population survey, March 2001 (U.S. Bureau of the Census, 2002) with respect to education, sex, race/ethnicity, and geographic region (White & Stern, 2003b, 2003c). These norms may be used when the examinee's performance is to be compared to the general U.S. population. However, the authors advised that the demographically corrected norms are to be prioritized when used in clinical practice because they are adjusted or corrected for the three variables that have the greatest impact upon neuropsychological test performance (viz., age, educational attainment, and sex).

Administration

Administration of the NAB consists of two general issues. One issue regards which of three administrative approaches the examiner wishes to pursue. The second issue concerns the convenient administrative materials and rules that facilitate data collection. These issues are discussed subsequently.

APPROACH

The NAB offers options for a number of administrative approaches as follows: (a) fixed battery; (b) flexible battery; or (c) screening battery with optional follow-up administration of indicated main modules. The *fixed battery approach* consists of all five of the main modules, which permits an overall score, index scores for each module or general neurocognitive function, and scores for the primary and secondary tests that comprise each module. The main modules are to be administered according to their numerical order as Attention, Language, Memory, Spatial, and Executive Functions. Note that the NAB refers to the specific measures comprising each module as "tests," whereas the NEPSY–II refers to them as "subtests." However, notwithstanding the different names, they are identical in both function and substance. Estimated administration time for the complete fixed battery is 3 hours, or 180 minutes.

The *flexible battery approach* targets single modules and their primary and secondary tests, or even customized combinations of individual tests. The diagnostic issues and case facts would drive the selection of modules and tests. For example, the Attention Module could be selected when testing for adult ADHD (see Form 9.7 delineated subsequently). Administration times for each module range from 25 minutes for Spatial to 45 minutes each for Attention, Language, and Screening.

Finally, the *screening battery approach* initiates administration with the Screening Module. The Screening Module results would then be used to determine the need for any follow-up neuropsychological testing, either for selected main modules, external neuropsychological tests, or both. As will be seen, the Screening Module yields a set of scoring criteria that guides decisions as to whether the follow-up administration of selected main modules would provide added differential diagnostic information. Thus, the Screening Module is invariably administered first, followed by any one or more of the main modules if so indicated.

MATERIALS AND RULES

Based upon clinical experience, the NAB administrative materials have proven to be by far the most user friendly. Most NAB modules possess both Record Forms and Response Booklets. Each module is color coded for easy identification (e.g., green for Attention and orange for Language). The Record Forms consist of all the oral instructions to the examinee (including permitted queries and prompts), administrative instructions for the examiner, start points, discontinue rules, time limits, spaces for recording examinee responses, item points, and spaces for raw score point totals. As such, the examiner can administer the entire test from the Record Forms, with only occasional use of the administrative and scoring manual (Stern & White, 2003) for clarification of special scoring rules (e.g., determining whether a line-crossing should be penalized in the Mazes test). The Response Booklets are designed for garnering required written responses to items by the examinee, whether they are verbal (e.g., providing a written description of an outdoor scene) or nonverbal (e.g., drawing a figure or tracing one's way through a series of mazes). There are also stimulus books with large printing of stimuli so that examinees with visual sensory limitations are not unfairly penalized and the results so confounded by peripheral impairments. Other tests would do well to use the NAB as a model in designing their stimulus materials, including record and response booklets.

The majority of test instructions are to either administer all items to the examinee or to discontinue after a designated duration of time. Examinees routinely begin each test with item 1, and therefore there are no reversal rules.

Furthermore, there are few discontinue rules for untimed tests. These features can be attributed to several facets of this instrument as follows: (a) the overall battery is relatively brief (i.e., 3 hours); (b) the instructions are designed to maintain a consistent flow (e.g., after so many seconds without a response the examinee is asked to "Take your best guess"); and (c) the tasks frequently have designated time limits, which prevents unnecessary delays between items and tests. Administration of the Memory Module requires special practice because each independent cluster of information to be learned and recalled (e.g., word lists, shapes, narrative story facts) is examined both immediately and then again after 10–15 minutes to remain accordant with standardized administration. Forms 1 and 2 are administered in identical fashion. The only difference involves the specific item content.

Finally, this neuropsychological test is accompanied by a detailed, comprehensive, and laudable video training program that can rival most if not all others. More specifically, the NAB administrative training program is comprised of six disks, the first introducing the test and reviewing the NAB Screening Module (2004a), and the remaining disks each devoted to an entire module, including NAB Attention (2004b), NAB Language (2004c), NAB Memory (2004d), NAB Spatial (2004e), and NAB Executive Functions (2004f). The training program also demonstrates how the scores are input into the Neuropsychological Assessment Battery Software Portfolio (NAB-SP; 2008), which provides rapid and efficient computer scoring, a felicitous segue into the next section.

Scoring

The NAB full battery and screening battery data are presented in Forms 9.5 and 9.6, which represent the manner in which they are reported within the context of a final assessment report. Because they possess the same types of scores and metrics, both forms will be discussed together.

STANDARD SCORES

Table 1 of Forms 9.5 and 9.6 present the total index and domain data. Indexes refer to the NAB Total and the six modules (viz., Screening [Screening Total], Attention, Language, Memory, Spatial, and Executive Functions). Domains refer to the general neurocognitive areas (i.e., attention, language, memory, spatial, and executive functions) and their screening data. The index and domain data are typical *standard scores* (SSs) with a mean of 100, standard deviation (SD) of 15, and a range of 45 to 155. Lower scores indicate greater degrees of neurocognitive impairment or brain dysfunction. The NAB Total is based upon an aggregation of the five main modules (excluding the Screening Module). The Screening Total is similarly based upon an aggregation of the five screening domains.

Confidence intervals (CIs) can be reported in the typical 90% or 95% degree of certainty that reflects the limits within which the examinee's true score is likely to fall (again the latter is selected in an attempt to be consistent with other cognitive tests). The PR is an area transformation that is based upon the theoretical standard normal distribution, which represents the percent of the population that the examinee scores equal to or higher than. The PR has a *median* of 50 and a range of 1–99. The NAB interpretive categories represent a combined nominal-ordinal measurement scale in that each class is associated with an increasing degree of functioning (i.e., if proceeding from lower to higher score ranges). Hence, in this scheme, the lower the class, the more impaired the functioning. These will be reviewed in more detail in the interpretation section that follows. The final column summarizes the neurocognitive abilities measured by that index SS.

As alluded to prior, the Screening Module Total index SS is the abbreviated companion to the NAB Total index SS. Accordingly, it has the same metric and is the result of a combination of all the screening areas; the latter being referred to as screening domains (e.g., Screening Language domain). Because each screening domain is an abbreviated companion to its respective module, they also share the same metrics. As will become apparent, although they share the same interpretive category, the screening domains have an optional secondary classification that determines whether follow-up testing with the companion full module is indicated. This is discussed in detail in the interpretation section.

General table notes delineate the data metrics and abbreviations, while specific table notes provide definitions for key neuropsychological concepts that are likely esoteric to many potential readers of the report. For example, executive functions is a concept that is not only complex but also may vary somewhat among various tests, theories, and investigators. Therefore, it is important to clarify in a brief yet informative note how this concept is being defined and ostensibly measured. Furthermore, key facts about some of the tests that can significantly impact the score's meaning are also enumerated in specific tabular notes. For instance, recognition memory is clarified by identifying for the reader exactly how it was tested (i.e., by multiple choice or yes-no format). Note that this was also done on the NEPSY–II using the same rationale.

PRIMARY AND SECONDARY SCORES

At the most specific test level are the NAB primary and secondary scores. Of most importance, the primary scores measure the fundamental neurocognitive abilities that contribute to the NAB Module index standard scores, which in turn contribute to the NAB Total index. Hence, they are most essential for measuring performance on this battery. Primary scores are measured according to the *T*–score metric, with a mean of 50, standard deviation (*SD*) equal to 15, and a range of 19–81. In Form 9.5, the primary scores are reported for all tests appearing in Tables 2, 3, 4, 5, and 6. The tests are organized in each subsequent table according to the module in which they belong and contribute. That is, each NAB Main Module index *SS* listed in Table 1 is based upon an aggregation of the test primary scores assigned to that respective module. Therefore, the ensuing sequence of tables lists the tests and their primary scores in the same order as the Main Modules appear in Table 1. As such, the sequence is as follows: (a) Table 2 lists the attention test primary scores; (b) Table 3 lists the language test primary scores; (c) Table 4 lists the memory test primary scores; (d) Table 5 lists the spatial test primary scores, and (e) Table 6 lists the executive functions test primary scores. The purpose of the Screening Module is to garner only that data needed to determine if more testing is needed. Consequently, the reporting of specific tests in this instance has little if any diagnostic purpose, hence rendering them superfluous and deleted from further analysis. In lieu of such data, an interpretive table appears that facilitates the decision-making process for potential further testing. This is discussed in the ensuing section.

Each primary score is also supplemented by a CI, PR, interpretive category, and a succinct description of the measured abilities. The CIs are not provided by the NAB manuals (Stern & White, 2003; White & Stern, 2003a, 2003b, 2003c) or the computer software (NAB–SP, 2008). In addition, the *SEM*s are also not provided by the NAB manuals (Stern & White, 2003; White & Stern, 2003a, 2003b, 2003c). Therefore, the internal consistency alpha coefficients for the module tests reported in the psychometric manual were culled (White & Stern, 2003b, Tables 5.2–5.6, pp. 96–98), then used in the following formula to compute the *SEM* values:

$$SEM = SD\sqrt{1 - r_{xx}} \qquad\qquad \text{Equation 9.1}$$

where *SEM* is the standard error of measurement, *SD* is the standard deviation for the test, and *r* represents the internal consistency coefficient, or the test correlated with itself. To facilitate the computation of the CIs, the resulting quantities were rounded to the nearest whole number. The *SEM*s were 5 for the Attention and Memory Module tests and 6 for the remaining three Modules. They are relatively high due to the multifactorial nature of many neurocognitive tests. Therefore, the decision was made to break with the characteristic selection of 95% CIs because it would result in a remarkably imprecise estimate when measuring neurocognitive constructs and change to a more precise (although less confident) 68% CI. In such case, added and subtracting 1 *SEM* results in the desired 68% confidence limits and a much more reasonable degree of precision despite the loss of certainty. The PR and interpretive category data as applied to the primary scores are essentially the same as in Table 1 of Form 9.5.

Secondary scores contribute to test interpretation, although greater caution must be utilized due a reduced quality of psychometric features. For example, they have poorer quality reliability coefficients and significantly skewed distributions that render them conducive only to score metrics that are less statistically powerful. More specifically, secondary scores provide only nonparametric PR data and cannot be converted to linear *T*–scores. Consequently, they also do not contribute to the Main Module index scores or the Screening Module. Two secondary scores are included in the data tables in Form 9.5. They include Orientation (Table 2, Form 9.5) and Reading Comprehension (Table 3, Form 9.5). Both are negatively skewed, meaning that few examinees miss these tests. However, when they are responded to incorrectly, such results weigh heavily in terms of detecting neurocognitive dysfunction. That is, they are *pathognomonic*, which essentially means that, although rarely missed, when they are, it represents a distinctive sign of a disorder. A specific table note designates that such a test only provides a PR and interpretive category. A brief note is in order here. The NAB also includes descriptive scores, which represent the lowest level type score provided by this instrument. They are raw scores that are converted to *cumulative percentages* (i.e., the sum of percentages in a data set). These are not used because their diagnostic value is infinitesimal.

COMPUTER SCORING SOFTWARE

Finally, the NAB Software Portfolio (NAB–SP, 2008) provides computer scoring for all of its modules and tests, including either type of norms (see prior). It can be loaded on a personal computer and delivers unlimited scoring. More specifically, it can produce two general types of score reports, including the NAB Screening Module Score Report and the NAB Main Modules Score Report. The latter will score some or all of the Main Modules wherein raw scores are entered. After all, selected raw scores are entered, a score report is created in a matter of seconds and without clerical errors (assuming accurate data entry). Although manual scoring is also possible, the investment in this computer scoring software is worth the savings in time and precision.

Interpretation

NAB interpretation depends upon which administrative approach was selected. Therefore, this section is further apportioned into the full battery, partial battery, and screening battery. They are hereafter discussed in said order.

NAB FULL BATTERY

The NAB full battery includes all five Main Modules and their tests (excluding the Screening Module). As indicated in the scoring section, the NAB results and interpretation tables for the full battery are presented in Form 9.5. The boldfaced and underlined title includes "Form 1/2," thus requiring the examiner to delete the number of the form that was not used. Table 1 presents the most essential results pertinent to interpretation and diagnosis, analogous to the Wechsler intelligence test Table 1 composite score results (see Chapter 11). The NAB Total data are listed in the first row and appear in boldface to highlight the examinee's overall neuropsychological functioning. The focus should be on the NAB Total *SS*; the 95% CI to show the degree of certainty in the examinee's true overall score; the associated PR to interpret the examinee's ranking compared to the population of healthy people of analogous age, education, and sex; and perhaps most importantly, the interpretive category.

The NAB SSs and their associated categories may be quickly referenced in Table 9.2.

The SSs ranges are listed in the first column and are juxtaposed with the final two columns that show (a) a dichotomous (i.e., two-category) scheme and (b) a more traditional 10-category scheme. The former simply apportions the scores into a nonimpaired (i.e., normal functioning) or impaired (i.e., abnormal dysfunctioning) classification. However, it does not make any further distinctions; that is, it does not show varying degrees of normality or abnormality. The latter is the more preferred diagnostic or interpretive scheme because it renders greater degrees of discrepancy, while not being overly detailed so as to obfuscate the point of a diagnostic scheme (i.e., to summarize and communicate effectively). Additionally, it should be noted that the dichotomous and interpretive schemes are not in contravention, as one merely provides more information. When interpreting the NAB Total index, note whether the *SS* is on a threshold between two categories. If so, this should be noted in the interpretation. The 10-category scheme, however, with marginal thresholds incorporated into some of the categories (e.g., mildly to moderately impaired) obviates this result. Table 9.2 will be revisited when interpreting the module test scores.

After interpreting an examinee's overall neurocognitive status, analysis proceeds to the Main Module index SSs, first interpreting each module individually, then examining their relation to the overall score. It is preferable to interpret impact of the Main Modules on the NAB Total *SS*, beginning with the lowest Main Module SSs, then moving to the highest, and finishing with those that are most commensurate with the overall score. Beginning with the lowest Main Module SSs makes the most sense since the primary goal is detecting neuropathology or brain

Table 9.2 Neuropsychological Assessment Battery (NAB) Interpretive Category Guide

Standard scores	Primary T–scores	Secondary PRs	Dichotomous classification	Clinical interpretation
130–155	---	---	Nonimpaired	Very superior
				Superior
115–129	---	---	---	
107–114	55–81	75–99	---	Above average
92–106	45–54	25–50	---	Average
85–91	40–44	16–24	---	Below average
77–84	35–39	6–15	Impaired	Mildly impaired
				Mildly-to-moderately
70–76	30–34	3–5	---	impaired
62–69	25–29	2	---	Moderately impaired
55–61	20–24	1	---	Moderately to
45–54	19	< 1	---	severely impaired
				Severely impaired

Source. Adapted from Stern, R. A., & White, T. (2003b). *Neuropsychological Assessment Battery (NAB): Administrative, scoring, and interpretation manual.* Lutz, FL: Psychological Assessment Resources (PAR), Tables 6.8, 6.9, & 6.10, pp. 124, 128–129.

Note. Standard score mean = 100, standard deviation = 15, range 45–155. *T*–score mean = 50, standard deviation = 10, range = 19–81. PRs = percentile ranks; PR median = 50, range = 1–99.

dysfunction. Also, the more extreme scores having the greatest impact on the overall NAB Total, which is why they are the initial focus of interpretation. Finally, the Main Modules can be compared to each other in an ipsative (i.e., intraindividual manner) by scrutinizing the 95% CIs and their degree of overlap. Specifically, 95% CIs with little or especially no overlap should be interpreted as likely being significantly discrepant. The pre-drafted narrative excerpts following Table 1 (Form 9.5) provide language that can guide the examiner through the recommended interpretation of the data.

The interpretive manual does provide tables showing the needed degree of discrepancy for all pairwise comparisons involving the six modules and between each module and the total score, for obtaining statistical significance at the .05 and .01 levels (see White & Stern, 2003b, Table 5.27, p. 127). The manner in which this is done is relatively straightforward and is edifying, hence the manual computation will be briefly demonstrated.

To determine the point-spread needed between the scores on two scales to conclude they are significantly different (also known as a *critical value*), the following formula can be used:

$$x = z\sqrt{SEM^2 + SEM^2}$$

Equation 9.2

where X is the difference score or critical value between the two scales needed to reach statistical significance (i.e., to conclude that the scores on two scales are truthfully or actually different and not due to chance), z is the normal curve value (or z–score) associated with either the *two-tailed* .05 or .01 probability (i.e., alpha) levels, and *SEM* represents the standard error of measurement as previously defined for each of the two scales being compared. Of note, the z–score value must reflect a two-tailed probability level because the test is to determine if two scores are truthfully different (i.e., lesser or greater) when subtracted from each other (hence bi-directional).

For example, assume one wants to discern the *SS* difference between the NAB Total and Language Module index at a 5% probability level. The *SEMs* for the NAB Total and Language Module index are 3.00 and 6.87, respectively (White & Stern, 2003b, Table 5.25, p. 124). The two-tailed z–score value at a .05 probability level is 1.96. Putting these values into Equation 9.1, the following is found:

$$1.96\sqrt{3.00^2 + 6.87^2} = 14.69 = 14.7$$

Rounding to the nearest tenth as in the NAB psychometrics manual, the result is 14.7, which comports exactly as reported in said manual (White & Stern, 2003b, Table 5.27, p. 127). This means that differences between the scales of 14 points or greater in either direction means the scores are actually different and not due to chance factors. The Type I error rate would be 5% here, indicating that there is only a 5% chance that this conclusion is incorrect (remember that probabilities are being considered here). The computations are not complex, although one does need two pieces of information: (a) the *SEMs* for each of the scales that are being compared; and (b) the obtained scores on these scales, which also need to be on the same metric. However, if the scales are on different metrics, they can always be linearly transformed to be on the same scale, then inserted into Equation 9.2.

That being said, the most reliance is placed on the NAB Total and Main Modules norm-based analyses, which compare an examinee's performance with a healthy population of peers when attempting to detect brain malfunction. Secondarily, one can informally examine between-module differences using the 95% CIs. However, it is more meaningful to consider moving quickly into norm-based analyses of the tests that contributed to the Main Modules SSs if so indicated. Consequently, tables for formal comparisons of the NAB Total and the Main Modules are not included.

In deciding whether to report and interpret a Main Module's tests, the following criteria are employed: (a) the module's SS falls within the impaired range (i.e., the lower the SS, the more imperative), (b) there appears to be a high degree of variability among that Main Module's test scores upon visual inspection, and (c) at least one or more test scores fall within the impaired range. These criteria are only meant to be guidelines. Occasionally, reporting individual test scores is indicated, for example, if normal functioning in a particular area needs to be emphasized.

The Main Module test tables are listed in the order they appear in Table 1, which also reflects the order of standard administration (see prior). These tables have the same organization, with two exceptions as follows: (a) primary *T*–scores supplant the SSs, and (b) there are two secondary scores that, by definition, report only a PR and interpretive category. The interpretive categories for the primary and secondary scores are also listed in Table 9.2, including both the dichotomous and 10-category interpretive scheme. Of note, the latter applies only 8 of the 10 categories that apply to the SSs because of their more constricted range. In particular, the superior and very superior categories are not applicable to the primary and secondary scores, which does not present a problem since the focus favors identification of impairment.

Interpretation of the test scores prioritizes norm-based analyses, comparing the examinee's performance to a sample of neurologically healthy individuals who represent such populations on variables known to significantly influence performance (viz., sex, education, and age). Ipsative comparisons (i.e., within-subject or intra-individual) can be done by comparing the CIs and their degree of overlap. A caveat here is that the CIs possess only 68% certainty of including the true score (i.e., almost one-third less confidence). Therefore, a more conservative approach is warranted. Specifically, interpreting differences should be reserved for CIs with clear separation or no overlap, the greater the discrepancy, the more confident the difference. Again, tables are not provided for conducting formal analyses of score difference among the tests, although they are provided in the manual for both .05 and .01 probability levels. For example, the psychometrics manual reports the needed difference scores for statistically significant discrepancies for the Attention Module test scores in Table 5.29 (White & Stern, 2003b, p. 129). Next illustrated is the NAB flexible approach using a partial battery.

PARTIAL BATTERY

A partial battery exploits the flexible design of the NAB in that selected Main Modules can be used to measure targeted neurocognitive abilities. An excellent example is the use of the Attention Module when testing for signs of ADHD in adults. When used in conjunction with standardized rating scales and continuous performance tests (CPTs; see subsequent discussion of Conners CPT tests), these data can contribute to a more reliable and valid diagnostic outcome. In fact, the NAB attention module has been used for adult ADHD testing referrals of such frequency that it was prudent to simply create a template for reporting the Attention Module index and its accompanying tests. Form 9.7 consists of data tables for reporting such NAB data and provides an example of how to organize a partial battery involving less than the entire complement of NAB modules, hence precluding the calculation of the NAB Total index.

More specifically, the title that immediately precedes the data should be modified to reflect whether Form 1 or 2 was used. Next, Table 1 (Form 9.7) is designed to display the Attention Module index *SS*, 95% CI, PR, and interpretive category. Table notes report the *SS* metric, designate abbreviations, and define key concepts to explicate the reported data. Pre-drafted narrative statements follow Table 1, with fill-in-the-blanks to be completed as indicated by the results. These excerpts are meant to guide the examiner through the process of interpretation as delineated prior. Of course, the language in these statements may be modified as needed. For example, the continuous measurement scales of the SSs, *T*-scores, PRs, and even the interpretive categories permit estimates of degrees of severity, which is allowable and even encouraged in the *DSM–5* diagnostic scheme.

Irrespective of the results in Table 1 (Form 9.7), all the primary scores and single secondary score (i.e., Orientation) are routinely reported. This is because scores in both the nonimpaired and impaired range have an impact upon the ultimate diagnostic result. That is, the overall interpretive strategy should be analogous to that of the NEPSY–II and consider (a) the number of tests in the impaired range versus the nonimpaired range (i.e., frequency), and (b) their degree of impairment or nonimpairment (i.e., intensity). Therefore, they should be reported and interpreted to bolster the final diagnostic outcome. Hence, Table 2 is organized to report and interpret all the Attention Module tests and their *T*-scores, 68% CI, PR, category, and measured symptoms. The Orientation secondary scores are included in the latter three columns of the table. Again, table notes elucidate the metrics, test abbreviations, and concepts to completely understand the meaning of the reported data. Finally, pre-written quotes follow Table 2 (Form 9.7) and guide the examiner through the process of interpretation, which begin with norm-based comparisons and then ipsative analyses. The former is more pertinent to diagnosis as they compare the examinee to normal healthy peers that are corrected for key variables known to affect performance. Ipsative or intraindividual comparisons can be made by investigating the CIs and their degrees of overlap. Formal analyses of score differences can be done as set out prior when discussing the full battery. The continuous nature of the *T*-score metric facilitates estimates of the level of severity of any detected impairment. The final use of the NAB regards its Screening Module and its accompanying domains.

SCREENING BATTERY

The NAB screening battery employs the Screening Module and its five domains. Each domain uses a briefer version of the same tests that contribute to the complete Main Module. For example, the Mazes test is used for both the complete Executive Functioning Module and the Executive Functions Screening domain. The difference is that the Mazes test for the complete module consists of seven mazes versus three for the screening version. As indicated in the scoring section (see prior), the metrics are the same as in the complete modules; that is, the domains are measured using SSs, while the screening tests are measured using *T*-scores. The template used to report and interpret the NAB Screening Module results within an assessment report is presented in Form 9.6, as indicated previously. It consists of only two tables, the second of which has been rarely used because the objective in interpretation here diverges from that of the authors. This will become clear as Form 9.6 is reviewed in more detail.

First, Table 1 is organized in the same fashion as Table 1 for the full battery (see Form 9.5), beginning with the preceding title in which Form 1 or 2 must be designated. The Screening Total index data are in boldface to effectively highlight these results, ensued by the five domains that mirror the Main Modules. Following the scale names are the SS, 95% CIs, PRs, interpretive category, and measured abilities for interpretation purposes. The analyses here are exclusively rather than principally norm based as in the full battery. The question here is whether there may be neurocognitive dysfunction that is in need of being corroborated and more completely measured. The Total Screening Module index works in similar fashion to a full-scale IQ score or total achievement score in that it shows overall functioning. If it falls proximate to or clearly within the impaired range (see Table 9.2), then further testing is suggested or indicated, respectively, and this should be stated within the interpretation.

Next, the norm-based analyses of the Screening Domain SSs are done in the same manner as for the total score. Any SSs that fall within the impaired range show empirical evidence that further neurocognitive testing is needed at least within that area. Additional testing may also be advised to provide a more complete diagnostic picture. Pre-drafted interpretive statements follow Table 1 (Form 9.6) that guide the examiner through the aforementioned analysis. Even when less than five domains show impairment, administering the NAB full battery is advisable. The rationale is that a comprehensive assessment of brain functioning is desired to yield a complete diagnostic picture; that is, the following questions should be addressed: (a) what is impaired; (b) if impairment is discovered, what functions are deleteriously affected; (c) how severe are the deficits; (d) what functions remain intact; and (e) if nonimpairment is discovered, what functions are intact and to what degree? When assessing brain function, it is perhaps more important than in other areas of testing to provide as complete a picture as possible, as such a profile contributes to an overall more accurate diagnosis. The reason is that rehabilitation frequently involves attempting to train intact areas of the brain and their functions to adopt or compensate for those functions that are impaired or completely lost. This strategy capitalizes on a characteristic called *plasticity*, which refers to the ability of the brain to modify its structure, and thus functioning, in response to training, intervention, stimulation, and/or experience. For example, patients with amnesia for explicit memory have been trained to use their intact implicit memory as a retrieval aid (Andrewes & Gilewski, 1999; Cramon & Matthes-von Cramon, 1990; Glisky, Schacter & Tulving, 1986; Sohlberg, White, Evans, & Mateer, 1992). Notice that the preceding questions could largely be answered by norm-based comparisons with perhaps some secondary ipsative examination if needed.

The NAB authors, however, take an alternate tact (Stern & White, 2003). In particular, they provide a scheme that guides the decision as to whether testing with the complete module is needed. Table 9.3 lists the SS values and the categories that determine the necessity for further testing for each domain. Notice that they vary somewhat for each module, and thus all had to be listed for greatest precision. The categories work as follows. First, a sufficiently low score shows unequivocal impairment. Further testing is therefore not needed, as it would not provide added information. Second, a sufficiently high score also shows that no further testing is needed. That is, nonimpairment is clearly shown, and further testing likely would not change the result. Finally, moderate-level scores are interpreted as ambiguous concerning the decision of whether there exists brain dysfunction in that domain or area. In this case, administration of the full main module is advised.

I do not use this interpretive scheme for several reasons. First, it does not provide a sufficiently complete diagnostic picture. Second, and related to the first reason, this scheme is based upon the dichotomous classification scheme of nonimpairment–impairment, which is typically insufficient in terms of discriminatory power for both diagnostic and treatment objectives. However, if a dichotomous interpretive approach is for some reason sufficient for purposes

Table 9.3 Neuropsychological Assessment Battery (NAB) Screening Module Interpretive Guide

Screening domain	Impairment—no further administration	Borderline—further administration	Nonimpairment—no further administration
Attention	45–74	**75–113**	114–155
Language	45–75	**76–125**	126–155
Memory	45–75	**76–118**	119–155
Spatial	45–74	**75–119**	120–155
Executive functions	45–73	**74–114**	115–155

Source. Adapted from Stern, R. A., & White, T. (2003). *Neuropsychological Assessment Battery (NAB): Administrative, scoring, and interpretation manual.* Lutz, FL: Psychological Assessment Resources, Tables 6.3–6.7, pp. 122–124.

of addressing the referring issues, then such a screening approach is available and quite efficient. To conclude this section, the use of Table 2 is explained.

In columnar order of presentation, Table 2 (Form 9.6) provides the following: (a) screening domain name, (b) dichotomous affirmative or negative recommendation on whether to administer the respective complete NAB module, and (c) the rationale for the recommendation enumerated in column two. Regarding the latter, two standardized statements have been entered. The first reads, "Significant/No evidence of impairment; further testing unlikely to provide additional diagnostic information." If the recommendation is, "Negative," delete either the word "Significant" or the word "No," whichever alternative applies, then delete the entire second statement, indicating that further testing is needed. On the other hand, if the recommendation is, "Affirmative," the latter statement applies verbatim, "Further testing needed for differential diagnosis," while the entire former statement is now dropped as being inapplicable. In this manner, Table 2 can be completed rapidly and efficiently by the testing psychologist. A simple narrative summary of Table 2 highlighting recommendations for further testing should suffice and is provided. If a partial or full battery ensues, these data can be added within a separate supplementary report.

Summary

This completes the presentation of the NAB, which represents a comprehensive fixed or flexible neuropsychological battery for adults. This instrument mirrors that of the NEPSY–II, which is also a fixed and flexible neuropsychological battery for children and adolescents. Together, they cover the majority of the life span. When testing is needed for a 17-year-old, which is not covered by norms for either test, the same reasoning is used when deciding whether to administer an older or younger version of an IQ test to an individual whose age matches both tests. If impairment in the 17-year-old is extremely severe and a lower basal is needed, administer the NEPSY–II while noting such reasoning in the test report. In contrast, if the 17-year-old possesses estimated higher cognitive functioning and a higher ceiling is needed, administer the NAB with the same out-of-norm caveat. If the decision is ambiguous, it is advisable to begin administration with the NAB and transition to the NEPSY–II if early test results so indicate. The reason is that the NAB would produce a baseline if future retesting is requested, whereas the NEPSY–II younger norms would be obsolete for such a purpose. Next, the chapter moves into tests that are more circumscribed in terms of the constructs measured and their diagnostic objectives.

Wechsler Memory Scale, Fourth Edition

Synopsis

The *Wechsler Memory Scale, Fourth Edition* (*WMS–IV*; Wechsler, 2009a, 2009b) fundamentally measures *declarative episodic memory* (also known as *explicit memory*), which is defined as the neurocognitive ability to consciously learn and remember novel information that is bound by the testing situation. To the extent that all information must first be processed through *semantic memory* prior being encoded into episodic memory, both of which are declarative types of memories, the WMS–V may also be considered an indirect measure of the episodic memory (see Wechsler, 2009b). Briefly, *semantic memory* involves general knowledge, such as language and information learned through formal education, while *episodic memory* includes recollection for events that occur in people's lives (e.g., the meal one had during breakfast that morning; special events such as birthdays; exposure to visual figures, symbols, or grid patterns). Furthermore, the WMS–IV measures both immediate memory, which involves short-term or temporary storage (i.e., seconds), and delayed memory, which involves longer-term or more stable storage and retrieval (i.e., 20–30 minutes), consistent with empirically supported theoretical concepts (Atkinson, & Shiffrin, 1968; see also Figure 7.1).

Therefore, generally speaking, the WMS–IV provides one of the most comprehensive standardized measures of memory functioning available, beginning in middle adolescence and extending through older adulthood. In terms of Bennet's 1988 model of neuropsychological abilities (see Figure 9.5), this instrument measures in more detail than a general neuropsychological battery (e.g., NEPSY–II; NAB) the various aspects that define Level 3, Learning and Memory. Thus, this memory test has been used most frequently when a referral source, for various reasons, specifically requests a thorough, detailed, or comprehensive measure of memory functioning, or when the presenting symptoms and/or signs are circumscribed to impairments in Level 3 processing, as per Bennet's model (see Figure 9.3). Next reviewed is the WMS–IV test structure, which is ensued by an expanded diagram of the information-processing model of memory, with added short-term memory components and special emphasis on long-term memory. The objective is to introduce some relevant theory to clarify key memory concepts, along with the various kinds of memory that is measured by the WMS–IV.

Structure of the WMS–IV

The WMS–IV is the immediate successor to the *Wechsler Memory Scale, Third Edition* (*WMS–III*; Wechsler, 1997). It consists of (a) a detailed measure of declarative (i.e., semantic and episodic) memory functioning and (b) a brief evaluation of neurocognitive status introduced in Chapter 5 when discussing screening measures; namely, the *Wechsler Memory Scale, Fourth Edition, Brief Cognitive Status Exam* (*WMS–IV, BCSE*; Wechsler, 2009a, 2009b; see Form 9.9). Because the screening aspect of this instrument was previously discussed under the felicitous topic of screening measures, the focus here will be upon the more comprehensive memory portion of the WMS–IV. Also, because the WMS–IV test structure has been significantly modified from that of the WMS–III, and historical perceptive will neither be useful nor provided, hence saving space for the more pertinent ability memory discrepancy (AMD) feature of this instrument. For example, in transitioning from the WMS–III, 8 subtests were dropped in their entirety, 3 were significantly modified, and 4 completely new subtests were added to the new edition, totaling 15 fundamental changes. Such changes constitute a virtual overhaul of this memory test. Consequently, the WMS–IV psychometric properties have been significantly improved, including its utility and matching the needs of prospective examinees, especially the older adult population. This will become more apparent as the discussion delves more into the test structure.

There are actually two batteries that comprise the WMS–IV, apportioned by age as follows: (a) Adult Battery, Ages 16–69 (hereafter Adult Battery), and (b) Older Adult Battery, Ages 65–90 (hereafter Older Adult Battery); hence, together covering an age span from 16 years, 0 months through 90 years, 11 months (i.e., middle adolescence through older adulthood). As such, there is a five-year overlap in which the examiner is presented with a choice of batteries. The criteria for such selection are discussed in the administration section subsequently.

The WMS–IV Adult Battery contains six subtests, including four with immediate and delayed versions, which in various combinations contribute to five domains as follows (subtests in parentheses): (a) Auditory Memory (Logical Memory I/II; Verbal Paired Associates I/II), (b) Visual Memory (Designs I/II; Visual Reproduction I/II), (c) Visual Working Memory Spatial Addition; Symbol Span), (d) Immediate Memory (Logical Memory I; Verbal Paired Associates I; Designs I; Visual Reproduction I), and (e) Delayed Memory (Logical Memory II; Verbal Paired Associates II; Designs II; Visual Reproduction II). Notice the immediate and delayed versions of subtests that contribute to the first three domains are reshuffled to compute the latter two domains.

In comparison, the Older Adult Battery consists of four subtests, including three with immediate and delayed versions, which in various combinations contribute to four domains as follows (subtests in parentheses): (a) Auditory Memory (Logical Memory I/II; Verbal Paired Associates I/II), (b) Visual Memory (Visual Reproduction I/II), (c) Immediate Memory, and (d) Delayed Memory. The Symbol Span subtest is also included, although it does not contribute to a domain index because it is not accompanied by a second subtest. Therefore, the Older Adult Battery contains two less subtests (viz., Designs I/II; Spatial Addition) and one less domain, namely, Visual Working Memory. Further, the Immediate and Delayed domains do not have the two versions of the Designs subtest contributing to them.

As alluded to prior, each domain yields an index score, which is contributed to by all the assigned subtests. This will be explained in more detail within the scoring section subsequently. Next, the domains and their subtests will be delineated in terms of the constructs they measure. Where there are differences between the two WMS–IV batteries, these will be mentioned explicitly.

AUDITORY MEMORY DOMAIN

The Auditory Memory domain consists of both Logical Memory and Verbal Paired Associates subtests, including both immediate and delayed versions; the delay being presented after a 20–30-minute hiatus with interference (i.e., other tests are being administered to hinder *maintenance rehearsal*). Logical Memory comprises short stories with a coherent fact pattern and social context. The examinee must retell the story both immediately and after delay under free recall (i.e., without hints) conditions. The latter taps working memory and LTM due to interference and the time delay. A yes-no delayed recognition task follows the second free recall task. The Verbal Paired Associates subtest presents four trials of the same 10–14 word pairs in different orders that the examinee must memorize and recall immediately after each list and then after delay; that is, a cued recall task (i.e., hints are given). Subsequently, a list of word pairs is read to the examinee who must identify whether that pair was in the prior lists (i.e., a cued recognition task). Note how both subtests are presented orally and processed through the auditory (i.e., hearing) sensory-perceptual system. Therefore, it can be concluded that the Auditory Memory domain and its index score measures the examinee's ability to recall orally presented information.

VISUAL MEMORY DOMAIN

The Visual Memory domain is comprised of the Designs and Visual Reproduction subtests, both of which have immediate and delayed (i.e., a 20–30-minute interval) versions. The Designs subtest presents a grid with 4–8 designs on a page for 10 seconds, after which the examinee must select the proper designs from a set of cards and place them in the correct grid locations. This subtest measures spatial memory for novel visual material using free recall. This is ensued by a visual-spatial recognition task in which the examinee must select two designs on a page that are the correct shapes and in the same grid location. The Visual Production subtest presents 5 nonverbal designs each for 10 seconds, after which the examinee is asked to draw the figure(s) from immediate memory as accurately as possible. The designs have either one or two figures. In the delayed condition, the examinee is asked to reproduce the designs in any order, although the figures that were paired must be reproduced together. Subsequently, the examinee must recognize which two of six figures matches one seen previously. Of note, the Designs subtest is not included in the Older Adult Battery and thus does not contribute to the Visual Memory index score in this case. Also, note how this information is presented in a visual-spatial modality and requires motor output; hence visual sensorimotor abilities. Therefore, it can be concluded that the Visual Memory domain and its index score measures the examinee's ability to remember visually presented information.

VISUAL WORKING MEMORY DOMAIN

The Visual Working Memory domain includes both Spatial Addition and Symbol Span subtests, which appears only on the Adult Battery. The Spatial Addition subtest presents a series of two-grid page sequences with blue and red circles placed in selected locations. The task is to place a blue circle where a blue circle was placed in a location on only one of the pages, and a white circle where a blue circle was placed in the same location on both pages, all this while simultaneously ignoring any red circle (the latter representing distractors). Because STM here engaged in alternative tasks, WM must be initiated by the executive system to perform such a task; hence, visual working memory. Analogously, Symbol Span shows a series of novel abstract symbols on a page for several seconds, and the examinee must select the correct symbols from a larger array in the same order previously presented. Because the examinee must report both the correct symbols and their order, STM is taxed, hence requiring WM controlled by the executive system. Therefore, it can be concluded that the Visual Working Memory domain and its index score measures the examinee's ability to remember and manipulate visually presented information in STM. Finally, as indicated, Spatial Addition is not included in the Older Adult Battery. Consequently, a Visual Working Memory index is not computed for older adults.

IMMEDIATE AND DELAYED MEMORY DOMAINS

The Immediate and Delayed Memory domains are discussed together because they involve the same subtests, although are grouped by duration. That is, both domains consist of Logical Memory, Verbal Paired Associates, Visual Reproduction, and Designs (Adult Battery only), with the immediate versions contributing to the Immediate Memory Domain and the delayed versions (i.e., 20–30-minute intervals) contributing to the Delayed Domain. In addition, the Immediate and Delayed index scores on the Adult and Older Adult batteries differ in terms of subtest contribution. Specifically, notice that the Immediate and Delayed Memory domain index scores on the Older Adult Battery do not include the Designs subtest.

These minor differences notwithstanding, it can be concluded that the Immediate Memory domain and its index score measures the examinee's ability to recall both visually and orally presented information instantly after exposure. Analogously, it can be established that the Delayed Memory domain and its index score measures the examinee's ability to recall both visually and orally presented information subsequent to a 20–30-minute interval with interference of recall. *Interference* occurs under two conditions as follows: (a) when maintenance rehearsal of the information is hindered in any way and (b) when information to be held in STM exceeds its capacity. Briefly, *maintenance rehearsal* occurs when an individual continues to pay attention to the information so it does not fade or decay, which is portrayed in Figure 9.6 by the rectangular shape with rounded edges and labeled "Attention," occurring between sensory memory and STM. It has been shown that information will only remain in STM for 12–20 seconds in the absence of rehearsal (Atkinson & Shiffrin, 1968; Brown, 1958; Peterson & Peterson, 1959), after which the information disappears rapidly. Of further relevance, the capacity of STM has been shown to be limited to seven, plus or minus two unrelated pieces of information (i.e., from five to nine bits of unrelated information; Miller, 1956), although it can be as low as four or five items, according to more recent research (Baddeley & Lieberman, 1980; Cowan, 2001; Cowan et al., 2005; Palva, Monto, Kulashekhar, & Palva, 2010).

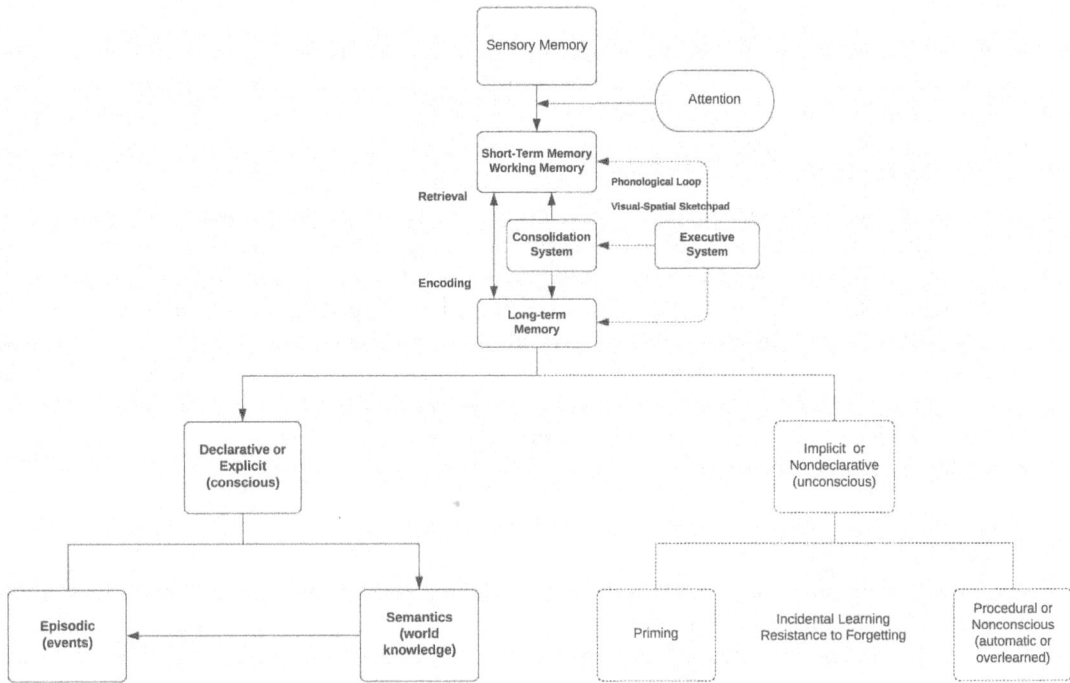

Figure 9.6 Structure of Human Memory with Emphasis on Long-Term Memory Organization

Note. Bold typeface and solid lines are essential for declarative long-term memory, which is directly measured by the WMS–IV. Normal typeface and broken lines are part of the long-term memory system, although not directly tapped by the WMS–IV test. The arrow direction shows the direction in which information becomes encoded into long-term memory through the sensory store, short-term store, and finally, into declarative long-term memory, first processed through semantic memory (using words and factual knowledge to organize the information), and then to episodic memory where the events and experiences of a person's life are stored. Episodic memories are based on personal experience and may or may not be shared with others depending on the volition and ability of the individual to recall the events. Encoding is the transfer of information from STM into LTM. Retrieval is the transfer of LTM back into STM; if modified, the process is referred to as working memory. Consolidation is the neurobiological process of strengthening a physical memory trace or engram via an intentional processing into one of the many cortical association areas of the brain. The consolidation system is responsible for maintaining and strengthening longer-term memories. The executive system is required when short-term memory needs to upgrade to a working memory, hence permitting the retention of information before it fades in the face of interference. Incidental learning is the acquisition of knowledge without intention. The phonological loop stores auditory verbal information while the visual-spatial sketchpad stores visual-spatial information, both as part of working memory controlled by the executive system.

SUMMARY

This section summarized the organizational structure of the WMS–IV by reviewing the various domains of memory measured by this instrument. It also described the subtests that contributed to the index scores of each domain to better delineate the constructs measured. Next, the structure of human memory is presented in more detail than done in the review of brain functioning presented at the beginning of this topic to better appreciate what is known about memory function.

The Structure of Human Memory

Memory has been referred to as the *final common pathway* because it represents the culmination of perception, attention, and executive functioning (Andrewes, 2016). This is illustrated by the observation that memory tests have been capable of detecting dysfunction where measures of perception, attention, and executive functions appear normal due to the brain's ability to compensate for damage or injury. This is one reason why a detailed and comprehensive test of human memory that covers mid-adolescence through adulthood represents a vital component of a psychologist's test inventory.

The structure of human memory is presented in Figure 9.6. It builds upon the *information processing* or *multistore model* proposed by Atkinson and Shiffrin (1968) and shown in Figure 3.1 (see Chapter 3). To begin the process, the receptors for each sense are the first line of neurons specialized for reacting to various types of physical energy (e.g., cones and rods in the eye retina fire when stimulated by electromagnetic waves located in the visual spectrum). At that juncture, the physical energy transforms into electrochemical signals, which is the language of the brain; a process called *transduction*. Thereafter, the neural signals are relayed, largely through the thalamus (except for *olfaction*, or smell) to the proper areas of the cortex for higher-order processing and interpretation. This sequence of events is referred to as *sensation–perception*, a process of encoding sensory information and interpreting it to give it meaning.

The neurocognitive process of attention, which again is the ability to focus on specific activities and suppress irrelevant stimuli, is required for sensory information to be transferred into STM. Here, limited information will remain for about 30 seconds unless processed further (e.g., maintenance rehearsal). The STM is upgraded by the executive system into *working memory (WM)* when the capacity to remember is challenged; for example, when multiple alternative tasks are simultaneously required, which stresses the STM system (see Baddeley, 2000; Gathercole, 2008; Gathercole & Alloway, 2008). This is denoted by the two-way arrow interposed between STM and LTM (see Figure 9.6).

WM is critical for transient storage and the manipulation of information, which facilitates language comprehension, learning ability, and the ability to reason (Baddeley, 2000). A model of WM that controls information storage and processing consists of three specific components as follows: (a) a phonological loop, (b) a visual-spatial sketchpad, and (c) an executive system (Baddeley, 2000; Baddeley & Hitch, 1974). The *phonological loop* retains information by means of maintenance rehearsal based upon acoustic and phonemic elements that utilizes speech-planning motor circuits (Gathercole, 2008). The phonological loop is vital for the acquisition, processing, and development of language (Gathercole, 2008). The *visual-spatial sketchpad* works in identical fashion except that it stores and processes visual-spatial information, especially for single complex images (Gathercole, 2008). Both the phonological loop and visual-spatial sketchpad are WM elements. Finally, WM is regulated by the *executive system* that provides supervisory actions, including information flow, selective and sustained attention, and engagement of the LTM system. Essentially, the executive system (also known as the *central executive system*) is invoked when more complex processing is needed and accounts for the correlation between WM and *fluid reasoning* abilities (Haavisto & Lehto, 2004; see also Figure 9.6 and Chapter 11).

More specifically, the double-sided arrow proceeding from STM to LTM symbolizes the process of encoding and retrieval. In particular, encoding is the transfer of information into LTM that occurs when information is sufficiently or deeply processed. One can make the case that this is where learning occurs. The related concepts of learning and memory have a close association because the latter can be understood as the natural outcome of the former. As stated by Squire (1987), "*Learning* is a process of acquiring new information, while *memory* refers to the persistence of learning in a state that can be revealed at a later time" (p. 3). This is why the NEPSY–II authors link these concepts together when labeling this domain of neurocognition. Once in LTM, the memory will remain indefinitely depending on a number of factors, including how it is incorporated (i.e., the level of processing or novelty of the information), how often it is used (i.e., repetition and any degree of decay), and if there exists any competing information (i.e., degree of interference).

There is also newly emerging evidence that as time elapses, new memories are capable of being reorganized to be reintegrated into previously established long-term memories and to accommodate new learning. This process is termed *binding*, which essentially represents a method of assimilating new information into previously learned information. The degree of difficulty of such a task is contingent upon the novelty of the new information; that is, the more novel, the more difficult it is to assimilate it into previously established memories. The reason there is a broken line in Figure 9.6 between the executive system and both STM and LTM is that such a system is not needed when there is no alternative task involved. In such case, STM is capable of holding information in mind without the need for executive system facilitation. If sufficiently processed in STM, such information can be transferred into LTM.

Consolidation refers to the neurobiological process that solidifies information into LTM stores, hence accounts for its retention within the many association areas of the brain (Squire & Butters, 1992). The *consolidation system* includes many structures, although the two principal ones are the *hippocampus* and *thalamus*, both of which are interconnected (see Figures 9.6 and 9.7). This system is crucial for creating and maintaining new memories into LTM. An infamous patient, HM, underwent a surgical procedure involving bilateral (i.e., both sides) excision and resection of the majority of the hippocampus among other temporal lobe structures. The purpose was to reduce severely impairing temporal lobe seizure activity due to *refractory epilepsy* (i.e., seizure disorder that is resistant to drug therapy). Subsequent to the procedure, HM could no longer create new long-term memories, although his early memories remained normal and intact (Annese et al., 2014; Scoville & Milner, 1957). As a follow-up, it has been confirmed that bilateral removal of temporal lobe cortical areas and hippocampus result in pervasive anterograde amnesia (i.e., loss of memory for future events), although it leaves long-term early memories both vivid and intact (Rempel-Clower, Zola, Squire, & Amaral, 1996; Zola-Morgan et al., 1993).

At the cellular level, a memory trace, or *engram*, is represented in the cortex by what Hebb (1949) referred to as a *cell assembly*, which is a hypothetical cluster of neurons that represent a memory. This cluster of neurons habitually fires in a specific sequence, which essentially is the beginnings of an LTM trace. Thereafter, Hebb believed repeated

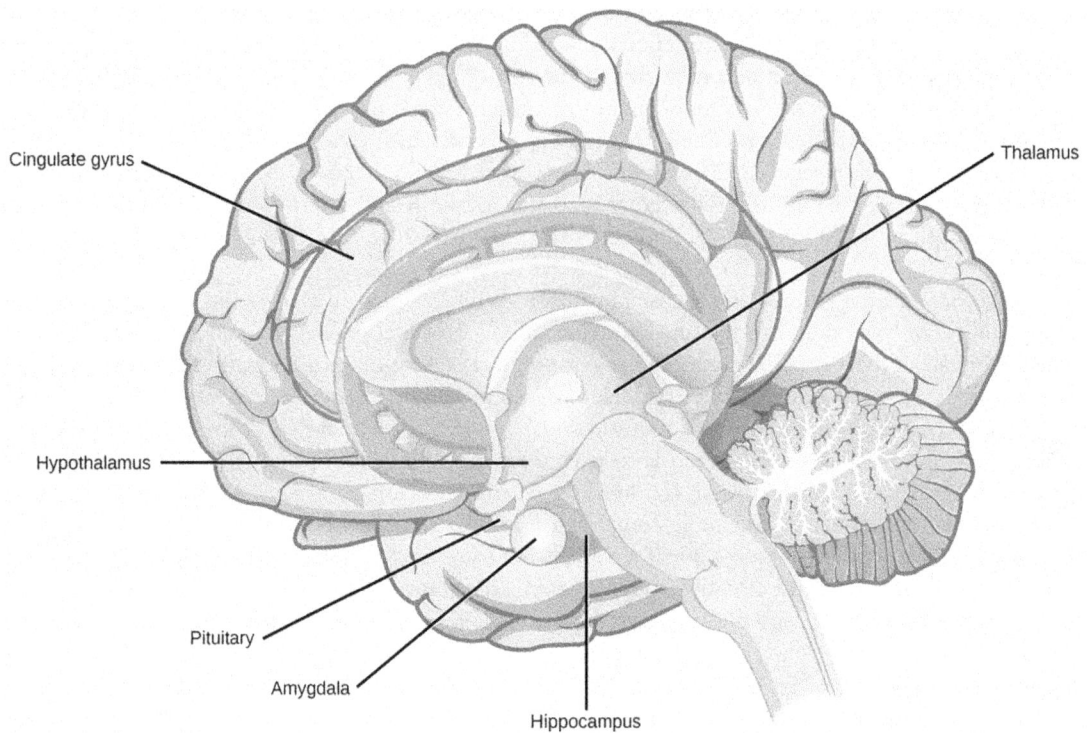

Figure 9.7 Neurobiological Memory Model: The Consolidation System

Source. Downloaded July 16, 2021, by CNX OpenStax, CC BY 4.0 <https://creativecommons.org/licenses/by/4.0>, via Wikimedia Commons, with no changes made, *https://commons.wikimedia.org/wiki/File:Figure_35_03_06.jpg*

Note. The hippocampus is located within the medial (i.e., middle) portions of the temporal lobe and adjacent to the cortical areas (see the convolutions or folds). The thalamus is connected to the hippocampus as part of the *memory consolidation system* and is vital for assisting in the storage of new memories into the LTM store. The consolidation system also is crucial in retrieving memories, especially those that have been stored in more recent years. The executive system, which is largely located in the prefrontal cortex of the frontal lobe (front-left of the diagram), upgrades STM to WM when needed and assists in locating and retrieving needed information when needed.

and intense firing of this neuronal sequence in a reliable pattern caused structural inter-neuronal changes so that eventually they became enduringly linked, hence permitting these cell connections to fire with increasing facility and resulting in a relatively enduring circuit; that is, a long-term memory. *Long-term potentiation* refers to the enduring modifications in electrical potential between neurons that make up this lasting circuit or relatively permanent memory (Bliss & Lomo, 1973). This theory is an attractive explanation for how new memories are created in the cortex. Of course, the area of the cortex where the memory is formed and maintained is contingent upon the type of memory formed (e.g., episodic; semantic). The discussion has now progressed fully into the LTM system, which is the principal focus when testing individuals with the WMS–IV. As can be seen in Figure 9.6, LTM can be dichotomized into *declarative* or *explicit memory* and *nondeclarative* or *implicit memory*. This discussion prioritizes the former because, as previously stated, the WMS–IV is designed to measure that class of LTM.

Succinctly, declarative memory consists of the conscious recollection of facts or events. These memories can be evoked by one's volition and include vocabulary and facts, such as one's name and date of birth, who won the championship game last week, and what one wore to work the day prior. Further, declarative memory can be apportioned into semantic and episodic types (Tulving, 1983; see also Figure 9.6). *Semantic memory* consists of ideas, facts, and concepts that are part of our ever-expanding knowledge base and are acquired by formal learning over time. Examples of semantic memories include vocabulary, historical facts, academic knowledge (e.g., physics, statistics), and personal information. In contrast, *episodic memory* involves the recollection of specific events, situations, and personal experiences. Examples include remembering one's first date, graduation, or one's last vacation. These are personal experiences that people can choose to keep private.

The fact that semantic and episodic memories represent separate systems in LTM was first supported by patients who manifested relatively isolated dysfunction in semantic memory in the absence of other confounding impairments (Snowden, Goulding, & Near, 1989; Hodges, Patterson, Oxbury, Funnell, 1992). That is, such patients were able to easily recall daily events (i.e., episodic memory) while failing tests of vocabulary, general information, and picture naming (i.e., tests of sematic memory). These patients were thereafter diagnosed as having *semantic dementia*. Further investigations have shown that sematic LTM is distributed throughout the cortex adjacent to areas with the functional mechanism they represent (Binder et al., 2009). For example, concepts of artifacts (e.g., hammer, saw) are stored in areas in proximity to movement or skills areas represented by cell assemblies that are activated when such tools are manipulated in their proper way (Binder et al., 2009).

The main point here is that the WMS–IV measures declarative episodic memory that has been initially processed by means of semantic memory. Furthermore, this is done both immediately while in STM and then again after 20–30 minutes subsequent to encoding into LTM (see Figure 9.6). There is now robust evidence that the hippocampus and the proximate perirhinal cortex control the creation of episodic and semantic memory functions, respectively (Figure 9.7; Nyberg, 2008). Additionally, the frontal lobe (Figure 9.2) controls the efficiency of the encoding and retrieval strategies (i.e., the executive system in Figure 9.6) so that an individual is not susceptible to interference effects from competing memories (Malloy & Richardson, 1994; Stuss, Alexander et al., 1994; Stuss, Eskes, & Foster, 1994; Stuss & Knight, 2002). In similar fashion, the occipital cortex controls visual memory while the parietal cortex is associated with spatial memories. During recognition tasks (versus recall or cued recall tasks), the frontal and parietal cortices are activated (Stern & Hasselmo, 2008). To provide more complete context without being overly pedantic, the rest of LTM will be reviewed, which includes an interesting type that is unusually resistant to forgetting referred to as *implicit* or *nondeclarative memory* (see Figure 9.6).

Implicit memory uses past experiences for remembering in the absence of conscious awareness. The more commonly known of these is *procedural* or *nonconscious memory*, which consists of automatic or overlearned motor tasks that people engage in without cognizance. Much of implicit memory is formed by *incidental learning*, which is the gaining of knowledge without intention (also known as *automatic learning*). A good example is a classically conditioned fear of dogs after such an animal has been paired with being injured or attacked (also known as *conditioned emotional responses*; see, e.g., Rescorla, 1968, 1988). Here, information is stored so that an individual remains knowledgeable about how to perform certain skills or procedures or react to certain stimuli without having to utilize cognitive resources, hence keeping them in reserve to perform other tasks simultaneously. These include walking, riding a bicycle, driving a car, and even inhibiting behavior so that people do not roll off the bed at night while sleeping. These are usually tasks that people have done repeatedly (hence overlearned) and in a mechanical automatic fashion. An interesting phenomenon about this kind of memory is its resistance to forgetting. For example, people can recall how to ride a bicycle or play checkers even after not playing for years.

Finally, *priming* is a phenomenon wherein the introduction of a prior stimulus prepares an individual to respond in a particular way to a subsequent stimulus. This is a viable process because an association is created in memory just prior to another stimulus being presented. Another way to view this is that exposure to a prior stimulus can alter future behaviors or thoughts. For example, when a child sees a certain cereal on television, she might begin to recall that cereal next time she watches television. In therapy, relaxation is associated with a feared stimulus (e.g., a snake), hence priming a relaxation response to that stimulus (i.e., a counterconditioning technique).

Priming was at the core of a debate about *subliminal perception* (meaning registering a stimulus below the threshold of awareness) where stimuli were presented in a movie just under the threshold of consciousness (e.g., popcorn) in an attempt to prime the eating of popcorn in moviegoers. It was eventually shown that subliminal perception did not influence direct voluntary behavior, such as eating popcorn (Bargh, Chen, & Burrows, 1996; Broyles, 2006; Moore, 1988; Pratkanis & Greenwald, 1988; Trappey, 1996; Vokey & Read, 1985), although it did influence automatic reactions, such as thinking about popcorn or related concepts (Babiloni et al., 2010; Bernat, Shevrin, & Snodgrass, 2001; Fazel-Rezai & Peters, 2005; Sabatini et al., 2009). In any case, such findings demonstrate the presence of a semantic network model of memory wherein concepts that are related in meaning are stored in physical proximity in the cortex versus concepts that are unrelated (Collins & Loftus, 1975; Collins & Quillian, 1969). The more cues associated with a concept, the greater the retrieval or recollection of that concept. Furthermore, people are frequently unaware of all the cues that trigger a memory for a concept, which explains why priming is classified under implicit LTM. Finally, this evidence shows how, in reality, these various LTMs work together in the brain to produce memories. The divisions made here in the narrative, and as visually presented in Figure 9.6, are made for pedagogical purposes. It must be recognized that the various brain areas are integrated in complex ways.

To summarize, Figure 9.6 builds upon the information-processing model of memory by expanding LTM and apportioning it into its various classes. This was done to delineate what kinds of immediate and longer-term memories the WMS–IV targets and measures while providing a comprehensive view of the entire memory system for context. Next, the WMS–IV is described further, as the Wechsler intelligence measures are in Chapter 11, primarily due to their similar organizational structures, although also due to the fact that a special AMD analysis is possible, as was done for AAD investigations.

Norm Reference Sample

The WMS–IV standardization sample consisted of 1,400 individuals ranging in age from 16 years, 0 months through 90 years, 11 months. This total sample was apportioned into 900 who completed the Adult Battery and 500 who completed the Older Adult Battery. The total sample was divided into 13 cohorts (in years) as follows: 16–17, 18–19, 20–24, 25–29, 30–34, 35–44, 45–54, 55–64, 65–69, 70–74, 75–79, 80–84, and 85–90. Therefore, the age bans became larger with increasing age. The 65–69 group was bifurcated into two subgroups, one who completed the Adult Battery and the other who completed the Older Adult Battery. Further, there was an equivalent quantity of males and females in all age groups between 16 and 64 years. Age groups of 65 years and older consisted of more women than men in concert with the 2005 census data (U.S. Bureau of the Census, 2005). Race/Ethnicity included White, African American, Hispanic, Asian, and Other. Education levels consisted of 0–8 years, 9–11 years, 12 years, 13–15 years, and 16 or more years. Finally, geographic region was apportioned into West, Midwest, Northeast, and South. The latter three categories again comprised proportions according to the 2005 census (U.S. Bureau of the Census, 2005).

Administration

The WMS–IV has separate Adult Battery and Older Adult Battery Record Forms, along with a Response Booklet, two stimulus books, and Memory Grids with cards. The Record Forms contain many of the instructions to examinees, spaces to record responses, item raw scores and totals, and places for raw score conversions, graphic profiles, and tables to compute contrast scores and AMD analyses. The Response Booklet is principally for both the immediate and delayed versions of the Visual Reproduction subtest wherein the examinee draws the figures previously presented on printed pages of the stimulus book.

Administration times for the WMS–IV depend upon a variety of factors. However, the overall range for total administration times concerning the norm reference sample are 82–116 minutes. These times are in accord with clinical experience in using this test as administration time has rarely ever exceeded 120 minutes, especially for the shorter Older Adult Battery. These times are based upon the assumption that the subtests are administered in the order that they appear in the Record Forms, which is required in order to comport with test standardization. There also must be a 20–30-minute hiatus between the immediate and delayed versions of Logical Memory, Verbal Paired Associates, Designs, and Visual Reproduction subtests.

Fortunately, clinical experience demonstrates that administering the subtests within the standardized order, with a continuous, smooth, and uninterrupted pace, typically results in administering the delayed versions within the designated time intervals. Occasionally, the delayed subtest versions may be reached somewhat sooner than the minimum 20-minute interval because the examinee has reached discontinuation criteria in an unusually rapid manner and/or recollection is extremely poor in amount reported (e.g., reporting few story facts in Logical Memory). In such case, the examinee can be given a respite until the proper time has elapsed. A circumstance in which the time interval was in jeopardy of exceeding the 30-minute interval has yet to occur. However, these must be taken seriously to help ensure valid results. In addition, once started, this test should be completed within one two-hour session. The many immediate and delayed subtest versions precludes standardized administration in two separate sessions.

The WMS–IV incorporates adaptive testing in comparable manner to previously discussed cognitive tests (see Chapters 7 and 8). However, with one exception (viz., Spatial Addition), all subtests begin at Item 1. On Spatial Addition, the start point depends on the chronological age (CA) of the individual, which is computed in the same manner as done for the Wechsler IQ (see Chapter 7) and achievement (see Chapter 8) tests. Therefore, Spatial Addition is also the only subtest that requires a *reverse rule*, which is designed to extend the floor by reverting to easier items until either a specified number of consecutive correct responses are recorded or Item 1 is reached. Finally, discontinue rules direct the termination of a subtest after a consecutive number of items are responded to incorrectly. However, the majority of subtests do not have discontinue rules (i.e., only Spatial Addition and Symbol Span utilize such rules). Taken together, the objective of these administrative instructions is to shorten test time, which in turn maximizes motivation and minimizes fatigue.

Finally, prompts and repetitions are provided at select times to maintain a consistent pace and encourage responses. First, *prompts* are brief verbal inducements to respond and are employed to either (a) remind the examinee how to perform the task or (b) afford cues to elicit a response. An example includes, "Please try it again." *Repetitions* consist of reiterations of items or their attendant instructions, the purpose of which is to redirect the examinee's attention or ensure understanding of the task. However, some subtests have restrictions on the latter.

Scoring

As is typical of Wechsler tests, the WMS–IV data yield is considerable. Thus, for purposes of clinical practice, it is prudent to be remarkably selective concerning the scores to report and interpret. Therefore, this section begins with those scores found to be most clinically useful, followed by those which are available but culled from the WMS–IV data tables used for report generation. Of course, the principal focus is on the former.

SCORES USED IN TEST REPORTING

Forms 9.8, 9.9, 9.10, and 9.11 include all the data used in reporting and interpreting the WMS–IV results in neuropsychological and psychological test reports. The first two cover data for reporting only WMS–IV scores for the Adult and Older Adult batteries. The latter two are specially designed for AMD analyses, which includes the following: (a) WAIS–IV General Ability Index (GAI) data; (b) WMS–IV data; and (c) the AMD analysis using data from the predicted-difference method. The latter features analogous statistical analyses and logic used in the ability achievement discrepancy (AAD) analysis employed in Chapter 12 using the age-appropriate Wechsler IQ test and the Wechsler Individual Achievement Test, Third Edition (WIAT–III; PsychCorp-Pearson, 2009a, 2009b). Thus, the discussion will begin with the fundamental WMS–IV scores, making references to Forms 9.8 and 9.9, then move to the more technical AMD data, referring to Forms 9.10 and 9.11.

Subtest total raw scores are converted into primary subtest scaled scores (hereafter scaled scores), with a mean of 10 and standard deviation (*SD*) of 3 (range 1–19). These may be seen in Forms 9.8 and 9.9, Tables 3, 4, and 5, which represent the fundamental data for the WMS–IV subtests. These scores were developed using the statistical procedure of *inferential norming* (Gorsuch, 2003; Roid, 2003; Wilkins, Rolfhus, Weiss, & Zhu, 2005), which has been seen in prior tests and will appear again with the personality tests subsequently. That is, specified moments (i.e., mean, *SD*, skewness) of each score were computed across the age bands reported in the norm reference sample section prior. Regression techniques were then employed as a fit to the moment data. Subsequently, for each subtest, the computed functions were used to derive estimates of the population moments, after which theoretical distributions were created for each of the age groups. Finally, percentiles for each raw score were derived and converted to scaled scores with the aforesaid mean, *SD*, and range. Succinctly, population distributions are estimated by means of regression analyses using sample moments for each age band in the norm reference sample.

The confidence intervals are set at 95%, which means the examinee's true scaled scores have a 95% likelihood of falling within such interval. The WMS–IV scoring and technical manuals (Wechsler, 2009a, 2009b) do not provide these intervals, although the average standard errors of measurement (*SEM*s) for each subtest can be found in Table 3.3 of the technical manual (Wechsler, 2009b, p. 49). These *SEM*s ranged from 0.55 to 1.55, with virtually all, save one, being under 1.5. Therefore, using the grand average and rounding to the nearest *SEM*, the result is an even 1. To easily estimate the 95% CI, the examiner may simply add and subtract 2 *SEM*s to the examinee's obtained score. This is entered as a specific table note in the respective tables. The percentile rank (PR) indicates the percentage of standardization sample, which is corrected for both age and education, that the examinee scores equal to or better than. These were derived as delineated prior.

The next score type is a qualitative description (see Table 9.4), which are technically a combined nominal-ordinal measurement scale; that is, these are classes that are ordered or ranked from least to most effective neurocognitive

Table 9.4 Wechsler Memory Scale, Fourth Edition (WMS–IV) Qualitative Description Guide

Index standard scores	Scaled scores	Standard deviations from the mean	Qualitative description
130 to 160	16 to 19	+2 to +4	Very superior (extremely high)
120 to 129	14 to 15	+1⅓ to +1⅔	Superior (very high)
110 to 119	12 to 13	+ ⅔ to +1	High average
90 to 109	8 to 11	−⅔ to +⅓	Average
80 to 89	6 to 7	−1⅓ to −1	Low average
70 to 79	4 to 5	−2 to −1⅔	Borderline (very low)
40 to 69	1 to 3	−4 to −2⅓	Extremely low

Source. Adapted from Wechsler, D. (2009b). *Wechsler Memory Scale, Fourth Edition (WMS–IV): Technical and interpretive manual.* Bloomington, MN: NCS Pearson, Table 5.1.

Note. Updated Wechsler balanced qualitative descriptive labels are in parentheses when divergent from the scheme used for prior editions of cognitive tests, including the WMS–IV.

functioning (or in the contrary direction, from least to most impairment). The descriptions follow the previous (not outdated) scheme used for the prior IQ test editions. If an examiner wishes to follow the balanced updated scheme, simply supplant *borderline* with *very low*, superior with *very high*, and very superior with *extremely high*. These are set out in parentheses in Table 9.4. Use of the more contemporary scheme is preferred simply because it is well balanced, logically speaking, and introduces consistency into test interpretation.

As denoted, index scores are assigned for each domain of memory. Such scores are derived by aggregating the scaled scores for the subtests that load on each domain. As indicated by the test structure section, there is some redundancy in that the immediate and delayed versions of four subtests also contribute to an Immediate and Delayed Memory domain index score. Index scores have a mean of 100, *SD* of 15, and a large range from 40 to 160, which is equivalent to 4 *SD*s toward both the low and high end, the objective being to minimize floor (i.e., not going sufficiently low) and ceiling (i.e., not going sufficiently high) effects. The index scores are presented in the first table that is numbered, namely, Table 1 (see Forms 9.8 and 9.9). The index score metric is listed in a general table note, as was done for the scaled scores in the concatenation of ensuing tables. The only discrepancy between Table 1, Form 9.8, and Table 1, Form 9.9, is the lack of a Visual Working Memory domain in the latter. As indicated, the purpose was to reduce the administration time for older examinees.

As also introduced previously, examinees who fit within the age range of 65–69 years can be given either the Adult Battery or the Older Adult Battery. The decision rule relates to the degree of impairment such examinees demonstrate upon initial examination; if significant dysfunction and frailty is noted, the Older Adult Battery is a more felicitous choice because it is briefer and less cognitively demanding. In borderline cases, it is prudent to begin with the Adult Battery, and if the examinee is palpably laboring, then switching to the Older Battery is viable, especially because they both begin with Visual Reproduction (or the optional Brief Cognitive Status Exam or BCSE). As a practice note, administering the BCSE during the initial assessment when anticipating later use of the WSM–IV may be worth the extra time because such data can be used to (a) bolster the case for the medical necessity of follow-up testing, (b) assist in determining which WMS–IV battery to administer, and (c) supplement the more comprehensive WMS–IV data interpretation. Finally, the index scores are associated with the same CIs (i.e., 90% or 95%), PRs, and qualitative descriptions, as done for the scaled scores.

Both Forms 9.8 and 9.9 actually begin with a non-numbered table that includes columns for the Brief Cognitive Status Exam (BCSE). The reason is that the BCSE is optional. More specifically, it may (a) be given to initiate administration of the WMS–IV, (b) be omitted altogether, or as suggested previously, (c) have been already administered during the initial assessment as a screening for follow-up neuropsychological testing. In the latter case, it would be redundant to report such results again with the rest of the WMS–IV scores. In contrast to reporting detailed item raw scores, as done when using the BCSE as a screening device (see Chapter 5), Forms 9.8 and 9.9 provide a summary table, listing CA in years and months, years of education (especially considering that the scores are adjusted for both CA and level of formal academic training), aggregated raw score, base rate (i.e., the percentage of the standardization sample that manifested the examinee's raw score), and classification level.

The BCSE provides two kinds of diagnostic data: (a) base rate; and (b) classification level. Both are empirically determined. First, the base rate is an effect size datum, which informs the examiner of the degree of typicality associated with the total raw score. The same diagnostic scheme as was used for all previous base rate analyses is used here (see Sattler, 2001, 2014; Sattler & Ryan, 2009). Second, the classification level is determined by a table that is provided on the inside page of the Record Form, which is organized by age, years of education, and BCSE total raw score, and with the following classes in increasing order of functioning: Very Low, Low, Borderline, Low Average, and Average.

Table 2 of both Forms 9.8 and 9.8 present formal pairwise comparisons between a select number of domain index scores, including Auditory Memory versus Visual Memory, Visual Working Memory versus Visual Memory (Adult Battery only), and Immediate Memory versus Delayed Memory. These comparisons are done using a unique method. More specifically, the difference between the two domains index scores is converted into a scaled score, again with a mean of 10, *SD* of 3, and range of 1–19. Scaled scores of 8–12 (i.e., average range) indicate that the two index scores are statistically equivalent. Extreme lower scaled scores (viz., 1–7) indicate that the first listed domain index score is significantly higher than the second listed domain index score; the lower the more divergent in that direction. Conversely, extreme scaled scores in the higher direction (viz., 13–19) show that the first listed domain index score is lower, with increasingly large scaled scores denoting growing discrepancies. Admittedly, interpreting these contrast scale scores can easily obfuscate the analysis, and it may be more direct and clear to simply examine the degree of overlap among the domain index score CIs and drop the contrast scaled score analysis altogether.

This completes review of the fundamental scores employed in the WMS–IV data yield, both for the Adult Battery and Older Adult Battery. The ensuing scores form the basis of the AMD analysis. Before delving into these special scores, the rationale behind the need to upgrade to a more complex analysis should be explicated, which immediately follows.

The AMD analysis necessarily begins with the reporting of the ability score that represents the individual's overall intellectual competency. The WMS–IV was co-normed with the WAIS–IV, hence this intellectual measure would be the IQ test of choice, covering the same age range from 16 through 90 years. Within this IQ measure, the WMS–IV provides a selection of the General Ability Index (GAI), Verbal Comprehension Index (VCI), and Perceptual Reasoning Index (PRI). The GAI provides a measure of an examinee's overall intelligence that includes the latter two indexes (i.e., verbal and perceptual abilities), excluding working memory and processing speed indexes. Because the latter two abilities are considered an integral part of human memory, especially the former, excluding these effectively controls for their confounding effects on the AMD analysis. That is, without removing these two index scores from the overall IQ score, the ability and memory data would be artificially correlated because they would be measuring similar constructs. In turn, this would mask any true differences between ability and memory, hence risking Type II errors (i.e., missing true differences or concluding that there are no differences when in fact they exist). The end result of this unfortunate concatenation of events is an increased risk of false negative results, which means missing a true diagnosis of neurocognitive dysfunction.

Additionally, it has never become necessary or proper to use either the VCI or PRI as representative of an individual's overall intellectual ability, even in cases where there is a significant discrepancy between the two indexes. The reason is that it would be too limiting a measure for overall intelligence, especially when considering that these abilities represent hemispheric specialization; that is, VCI or verbal abilities within the left hemisphere and visual-spatial or perceptual abilities in the right hemisphere (see Figure 9.1). Why would an examiner use an overall intellectual ability score that effectively ignores an entire hemisphere or brain functioning? Actually, the only instance in which the PRI or VCI should be used is when an examinee cannot complete one or the other index, although in such a case, it is also most likely that neither would the examinee be able to complete the WMS–IV. However, if an examiner does find it appropriate to use the PRI or VCI, it can be done by simple electronic cutting and pasting or using the previous data tables provided in the first edition (Spores, 2012). They are not included any longer because they muddle or obfuscate the analysis in the absence of a rational reason for retaining them.

Table 1 in both Forms 9.10 and 9.11 list the relevant ability scores, including the GAI, 95% CI, PR, and qualitative descriptor, which possesses the exact metrics, as does the WMS–IV domain index scores. The GAI is explicated in the specific table notes, although it is interpreted in the pre-drafted narrative statements as representing an examinee's overall intelligence, as did the full-scale IQ score, the latter including both the working memory index and the processing speed index (see Chapter 7). Following this initial ability table are the WMS–IV memory scores as presented in Forms 9.8 and 9.9, beginning with the domain index scores (again without the Visual Working Memory domain index in the Older Adult Battery in Form 9.11), the domain index level contrast scaled scores, and the subtest scaled scores organized by the Auditory Memory, Visual Memory, and Visual Working Memory domains.

The AMD begins in earnest just prior to Table 7 with the bold font and underlined title *Ability Memory Discrepancy (AMD) Analysis*. Only the predicted-difference method is used for the same reasons delineated in Chapter 8 when discussing the ability achievement discrepancy (AAD) analysis. Essentially, the GAI is used to predict an examinee's performance on the WMS–IV domain index scores. The *predicted-difference method* is based upon the correlation between ability and memory, with the ability score being employed in a regression equation as the *predictor* and the memory score as the *criterion*. Statistically significant differences are calculated at both the .05 and .01 probability levels (i.e., two-tailed). Because only the .01 level is used to minimize the cumulative effect of repeated hypothesis tests (viz., *the familywise error rate*), that formula will be illustrated (Shepard, 1980) only for said probability level as follows:

$$SE_{resid(.01)} = 2.58\, SD\sqrt{1 - r_{xy}^2}\,\sqrt{1 - r_{resid}} \qquad\qquad \text{Equation 9.3}$$

which would determine the critical value needed to show whether the difference between the GAI and selected domain index score is beyond chance expectations. Compared to Equation 9.2, this formula utilizes the degree of correlation between the scores being analyzed as opposed to the *SEM*s (see Equation 9.2). Therefore, in Table 7 of both Forms 9.10 and 9.11, the WMS–IV domain name is listed in the first column, the domain index score obtained (i.e., earned) by the examinee is listed in the second column, and in the third column is the domain index score predicted by the GAI score (i.e., using a regression equation based upon the correlation between the GAI and domain index score). The computed difference is enumerated in the fourth column, followed immediately by the critical value computed by Equation 9.3. If the difference score *equals or exceeds the critical value in the negative direction*, the discrepancy is considered to be true or real. That is, the examinee's obtained score is significantly lower than that predicted by the ability score. The analysis then proceeds to the base rate column to determine the degree to which the result is unusual or atypical (i.e., an effect size measure). In contrast, if the difference is less than the critical value, *or is significantly different in the positive direction*, the analysis stops and a double dash line is entered into the final column.

Lastly, the base rate measures the proportion of the standardization sample, which represents the population of normal healthy individuals adjusted for both age and education, that obtained the examinee's difference score. The same interpretative scheme is used here as employed by previous tests in this book that report base rate data (see Sattler, 2001, 2014; Sattler & Ryan, 2009). This information is listed in the specific table notes to Table 7 to assist the examiner in such analysis. Instances in which AMD analyses are useful are discussed in the interpretation section (see subsequently). Next, additional WMS–IV scores not incorporated in Forms 9.8 through 9.11 are briefly presented.

SCORES NOT USED IN TEST REPORTING

The ensuing data are not used in the forms that have been created for reporting the WMS–IV results within a final test report in clinical practice. Some of them can be recognized as partially used, for example, as applied to index scores but not to subtest scores. In other instances, they are entirely excluded.

First, process scores are subtest scaled scores that can provide some added insight regarding an examinee's memory skills and deficits, although they do not contribute to the index scores. They are computed on the same metric as the primary scaled scores or as cumulative percentages (i.e., base rates). For example, imagine an examinee scores the following: (a) Designs II Recognition I = 0–16%; and (b) Verbal Paired Associates II Recognition ≤ 2%. This result indicates that, although both tend to be atypical, the examinee's recognition of word pairs is profoundly abnormal as compared in an ipsative manner with recognition of visual-spatial material, hence implicating greater left hemisphere dysfunction. These are not used, as they provide data that are (a) redundant with the index and primary subtest scaled scores and (b) more unreliable (see Wechsler, 2009b).

Subtest-level comparisons within each domain are also available. Essentially, the average of all subtest primary scaled scores within a domain (e.g., Auditory Memory) is first computed. Subsequently, this average is subtracted from each subtest primary scaled score to determine if it is significantly higher or lower at either the .15 or .05 probability level, after which a base rate is reported as an effect size. In such manner, an examinee's relative strengths and weaknesses within each domain can be computed and analyzed for diagnostic and treatment-planning purposes. These are not used because the norm-based comparisons are sufficient for diagnosing brain dysfunction (i.e., compared to healthy peers with age and education corrections).

Contrast scaled scores are also used to determine if there are significant relative (i.e., ipsative) differences among selected primary and process subtest scaled scores. Suffice it to say that the reticence to report such scores for index comparisons generalizes to analyzing relative differences among subtests. Although having an opportunity for formal relative comparisons of selected domain indexes is borderline justifiable, such is not the case when referring to the less reliable subtests. Simply put, the contrast scaled score approach is too confusing to justify using it with subtest scores.

Finally, contrast scaled scores can be used when conducting an AMD analysis. Here, the domain index score is subtracted from either the GAI, PRI, or VCI, whichever the examiner chooses as the IQ representative. This difference score is then converted into a scaled score with a mean of 10 and *SD* of 3. As applied to domain index score comparisons, scaled scores in the average range (i.e., 8–12) indicate that the two scores are equivalent, whereas more extreme scores in either direction show evidence that the scores are significantly different as delineated previously. Obviously, the predicted-difference method discussed previously is preferred and set out in Forms 9.10 and 9.11. Finally, the simple-difference method performs the AMD by subtracting the domain index score directly from the ability score. Some examiners prefer this method because it is easier to explain to referral sources, examinees, and family members. However, this method assumes a perfect correlation between the ability and memory scores and measurement error is essentially ignored. Therefore, greater accuracy is preferred over that of simplicity.

COMPUTER SCORING

At the time this memory test was published, a *WMS–IV Scoring Assistant* (Pearson, 2009a) was available that provided unlimited scoring and data analysis consistent with the Wechsler intelligence and achievement tests. This software included all possible AMD analyses between the WAIS–IV composite scores, including the GAI and all the WMS–IV index scores at both the .05 and .01 levels. However, this is no longer available. Currently, the WMS–IV can be computer scored only on the Q-global (Pearson, 2021) website in the same manner as the other Wechsler cognitive. However, there is also a training CD available that can assist new examiners in learning to administer and score this measure effectively (Pearson, 2009b).

Interpretation

WMS–IV interpretation is somewhat more straightforward than the Wechsler intelligence and achievement tests because it consists of only a two-level hierarchy of scores, namely, domain index scores (i.e., standard scores) and primary subtest scaled scores. Analogous to the NEPSY–II, there is no higher-order complex memory factor akin to the complex general *g* intelligence factor. Perhaps the many forms of memory do not converge naturally upon such a unitary complex factor. Hence, an interpretive flowchart is not needed in this instance. Additionally, the norm-based comparisons predominate the interpretative process because brain functioning is best compared to healthy peers of comparable age and educational level.

Hence, the ensuing discussion begins with the optional BCSE, although it quickly moves to the norm-based domain index score and primary subtest scaled score interpretative approach. Note that each table includes a final column that summarizes the measured memory abilities and pre-drafted excerpts that guide the examiner through a norm-based interpretive process. Ipsative analyses are secondary and limited to treatment-planning strategies. This section ends with discussion upon when and why an AMD analysis should be done.

BCSE ANALYSIS

The BCSE appears in Forms 9.8 and 9.9 as an unnumbered table denoting its optional status. The variables CA and years of education are reported because they are accounted for in the interpretation. Here, the raw score is interpreted in terms of base rate and classification level. Regarding the latter, low and very low classifications are interpreted as clinically significant; that is, the result is interpreted as positive for neurocognitive dysfunction. One asterisk is appended to a *low* classification, which is associated with a 2–4% base rate, while two asterisks are attached to a *very low* level, which is related to a base rate of less than 2% (see also Chapter 9). Typically, these data will not need to be reported or interpreted because they are most useful as screening data. However, this table was inserted in the event that their interpretation would be useful (e.g., for ordering a more comprehensive neuropsychological test battery, such as the NAB). If not, this table should be deleted.

DOMAIN INDEX ANALYSIS

The domain index data should principally be compared to those of the standardization sample, noting especially those that fall within the very low to extremely low range. Prior to the narrative statements, there appears a listing of key memory concepts and their definitions as set out by this measure. Thereafter, narrative statements guide the examiner through the interpretive process. The focus is on the domain index score, its qualitative description, and PR. If the index falls near the threshold of two classes, these should both be mentioned, as shown in the pre-drafted statements with blanks wherein the classifications should be entered. The index scores should be diligently interpreted individually, starting with the lowest score that falls within the impaired range and working up to those that fall within normal limits. If there are palpable discrepancies between indexes, especially if CIs have no overlap at a 95% level of certainty, these can be mentioned secondarily as relative strengths and weaknesses.

The indexes that show impairment should be followed up by reporting and interpreting their primary subtest scaled scores that contributed them, especially if there exists large variability among those scaled scores. If a domain index score is normal, along with all its subtest scaled scores, then reporting them is optional; for example, when a comprehensive reporting of all memory scores is desired.

PRIMARY SUBTEST SCALED SCORES

Reporting and interpreting the primary subtest scaled scores is most imperative when (a) the associated domain index score falls within the impaired range and (b) when there are salient discrepancies among the primary scaled scores that contributed to that domain index score. Occasionally, it is imperative to show that normalcy is present, in which case all the subtest scores should be interpreted using a norm-based strategy. Additionally, all scaled scores should be reported if a referring clinician is asking for a baseline measure of the examinee's memory functioning. Forms 9.8 and 9.9 report only the fundamental WMS–IV data, which present the subtest scores organized according to their associated domain index (except the immediate and delayed indexes due to redundancy) in Tables 3–5. These same tables are presented in the AMD Forms 9.10 and 9.11 in Tables 4–6. Each table is followed by interpretive statements, beginning with a short interpretation of completely normal results, followed by a second that describes impairments among the measured abilities and a suggestion of an unnamed disorder to be completed by the examiner if applicable. Note that there are no interpretive statements addressing ipsative analyses, as they are second-ary to the norm-based interpretations, although they can be added by borrowing from the IQ subtest interpretive statements (see Chapter 7). If done, the analysis should focus on the relative positions of the CIs.

INDEX-LEVEL CONTRAST SCALED SCORE ANALYSIS

Interpretation here determines whether there exist significant differences among some selected domain index scores. For the Adult Battery, there are three such comparisons; Auditory versus Visual, Visual Working versus Visual, and Immediate versus Delayed. The Older Adult Battery does not include the Visual Working versus Visual comparison because the former is not computed. To attempt to clarify this analysis, the interpretive scheme is listed in a specific tabular note. Note that interpretation focuses on the contrast scaled score. Essentially, scores of 8–12 signify no dif-ference, 1–7 indicate the first score is higher, and 13–19 denote that the second listed score is higher. The interpre-tive scheme set out in the table uses language that concentrates on the position of the first score, although that can be changed to the language used here, which focuses on which score is considered the higher when a discrepancy is indicated. Both versions begin with the clearest interpretation of no difference within the average range because it commences at the center of the distribution and logically works toward both extremes and their meanings. It is listed third in this section because this approach is least preferred in interpreting score differences. In particular, readers (and even examiners) can become easily nonplussed when the comparison of two index scores on a much larger metric is abruptly reduced to a single scaled score that purportedly denotes their degree of discrepancy, not to mention correctly interpreting the direction of a significant difference.

ABILITY MEMORY DISCREPANCY ANALYSIS

This final interpretive section refers only to Forms 9.10 and 9.11, which are specially designed for ability memory dis-crepancy (AMD) analysis determinations. The principal question here is, "Under what circumstances should upgrad-ing the complexity of memory testing to an AMD analysis be done?" The answer is, "When there is convincing evidence upon initial examination that an examinee falls at either extreme of the intelligence spectrum." Operation-ally defined, extreme may be defined as being in excess of one *SD* from the mean, either in the positive or negative direction (i.e., outside the range of about 80–120; refer back to Table 7.2). When this is the case, the risk is that such examinees may score significantly low or high on the WMS–IV due to their deficit or superior intelligence, which risks a false positive or false negative result, respectively. In either case, there is a risk of rendering an incorrect deci-sion, resulting in needless or delayed treatment. The most efficacious way to avoid such result is to interpret such examinees' memory performance in the context of their intellectual exceptionalism; in effect, controlling for intellec-tual ability. Another way to look at this circumstance is to ask, "To whom should I compare this examinee's memory performance, a sample of healthy peers corrected for age and education, or the individual him or herself, who has the same age, education, and IQ level?" The latter is fundamentally a within-subject design, in which individuals serve as their own control (more specifically, a single subject nonexperimental design; see Shaughnessy, Zechmeister, & Zech-meister, 2015). Considering that the standardization sample contains individuals with an IQ distribution comparable to that of a normal curve, it is likely more accurate to use such examinees as their own comparison or control group.[7]

Therefore, Forms 9.10 and 9.11 begin with interpreting the examinee's GAI, followed by the fundamental WMS–IV scores as construed prior, and culminating in the AMD analysis organized by the rows and columns of Table 7. In the event the examinee does not score 120 or above or 79 or below on the IQ measure, the intelligence test score can be reported and interpreted in Table 1, although the examiner need not proceed with the AMD. In such case, an expla-nation as to why the AMD is no longer indicated would be advised. However, if the examinee scores as predicted on the GAI, then such a score should be listed prior to Table 7, hence proceeding with the analysis. Pre-drafted interpretative statements follow Table 7, beginning with a brief description of consistent negative discrepancies. This is followed by language intended to list all difference scores that are statically significant, followed by any needed base rate interpretations. Statistically significant differences are denoted by an appended asterisk, while atypical base rates have affixed crosses. A greater number of crosses designates increasing abnormality or effect size. Finally, a base rate should not be reported for statistically nonsignificant differences. In their stead should be a double dash, which is defined for the reader in a general table note. AMD analyses are not available for primary subtest scores.

Summary

The WMS–IV is a standardized test that provides a detailed analysis of memory functioning from middle adolescence through adulthood. This type of test is extremely useful in clinical practice to resolve differential diagnostic questions concerning memory issues. That is, are a person's memory difficulties due to a psychiatric clinical syndrome, such as depression or anxiety, or do they reflect a bona fide neurocognitive disorder? It can also be used to determine if more comprehensive follow-up neuropsychological testing is needed, to measure any progression from baseline (i.e., using Equation 9.3), or to determine if a particular treatment for memory functioning is showing symptom remission.

At this juncture of the chapter, two comprehensive neuropsychological test batteries have been presented, which together cover the majority of the life span, along with a detailed test of memory that is considered to be one of the most important neurocognitive abilities from the standpoint of functioning in the real world. Imagine for a moment attempting to function without the ability to store and retrieve memories learned from day to day. The final genre of neuropsychological tests to be covered next have even greater specificity in that they focus on the measurement of attention and inhibitory control, which are key components of executive functioning (see Figure 9.6; the executive system as supervising STM–LTM integration and reciprocity). Together, they are referred to as *continuous performance tests* and are unique in that they are fully automated in terms of both administration and scoring. They are also ideal as performance-based measures for detecting the presence of attention deficit/hyperactivity disorder (ADHD). It is to these tests the discussion turns to next, which will conclude this vital chapter on neuropsychological testing and brain functioning.

Conners Continuous Performance Tests

Synopsis

There are three Conners *continuous performance tests* (*CPTs*) in this book's inventory. They include the following: (a) the *Conners Kiddie Continuous Performance Test, Second Edition* (*Conners K–CPT 2*; Conners, 2015); (b) the *Conners Continuous Performance Test, Third Edition* (*Conners CPT–3*; Conners, 2014); and (c) *Conners Continuous Auditory Test of Attention* (*Conners CATA*; Conners, 2014). They are all designed, organized, administered, scored and interpreted in like manner, such that they will be presented simultaneously as a group. Similar to the combination of the NEPSY–II and NAB, these cover the majority of the life span; that is, from ages 4 years, 0 months through 89 years, 11 months.

Essentially, examinees are to continuously respond, or not respond, by computer mouse click (or keyboard space bar press) to random presentations of target and nontarget stimuli, respectively. The procedure is intentionally tedious and without the provision of any breaks or respites. The principal clinical use of a CPT test is in determining the likelihood that an individual manifests a disorder of attention and impulse control (Conners, 2001, 2004). Hence, these CPT tests are used exclusively for ADHD evaluations, although they may be easily incorporated into a more comprehensive neuropsychological test battery. Prior to presenting these three CPT tests in terms of standardization samples, administration, scoring, and interpretation, a brief history of this genre of tests will provide interesting context as to how these tests were initially designed for research purposes, then later for clinical practice, as used currently.

History of CPT Tests

The first CPT test was introduced in a study including patients with some form of brain injury (Rosvold, Mirsky, Sarason, Bransome, & Beck, 1956). The objective was to design a test that incorporated two components as follows: (a) random responding and (b) uninterrupted attention over a considerable period of elapsed time. There were two task paradigms. The first simply required a key press upon presentation of a target letter (viz., the *X paradigm*), while the more difficult paradigm required a response to a target letter only when preceded by a designated prior letter (viz., the *AX paradigm*). The former represented a pure measure of selective sustained attention while the more difficult latter task required the use of working memory, as set out previously (see Smid, de Witt, Homminga, & van den Bosch, 2006; see also Figure 9.6, the working memory system). Thus, CPT tests began as they are today as neuropsychological tests, although within the context of scientific research.

Thereafter, various modifications to CPT tests were instituted, including the use of multiple modalities, such as auditory stimuli (Loeb & Binford, 1968), numbers versus letters (Anderson, Siegel, Fisch, & Wirt, 1969), the employment of signal detection statistical methods (Broadbent, 1971), and finally, the use of *image degradation techniques* (Nuechterlein, Parasuraman, & Jiang, 1983). Image degradation techniques present the stimuli according to graded levels of blurring to determine if this has a differential impact upon sustained and selective attention. During the 1990s, CPT techniques were adopted as clinical tests, especially in concert with standardized rating scales to detect ADHD and other types of psychopathology that included attention problems as a principal part of the symptom cluster (Riccio, Reynolds, & Lowe, 2001).

More specifically, CPT tests have shown sensitivity to a number of neurological impairments, including mild traumatic brain injuries (TBIs; Allen, Leany, Thaker, & Cross, 2010), *Alzheimer's disease* (Sherod et al., 2009), epilepsy (Borgatti et al., 2004), mild concussion (Nauheim, Mattero, & Fucetola, 2008), major neurocognitive disorders (Sanchez-Castaneda et a., 2009), *Parkinson's disease* (Ibarretxe-Bilbao et al., 2009), and brain tumors (White & Levin, 2004). However, the greatest impact of CPT tests has been on measuring and understanding attention deficits, including differences in developmental trajectories (Miller & Hineshaw, 2010; Miller, Ho, & Hinshaw, 2012; Vaughn et al., 2011), sex differences (Balint et al., 2009; Rucklidge, 2006; Wodka et al., 2008), and different ADHD presentations (Bauermeister et al., 2005; Egeland, Johansen, & Ueland, 2009; Pasini, Paloscia, Alessandrelli, Porifirio, & Curatolo, 2007; Riccio, Homack, Jarratt, & Wolfe, 2006; Wodka et al., 2008). This scientific research is accordant with the manner in which the CPT tests are used here in clinical practice.

Norm Reference Samples

The norm reference samples for each of the three Conners CPT tests will be presented separately in increasing order of age. Comparisons and contrasts will be made where indicated.

CONNERS K–CPT 2 NORMS

The Conners K–CPT 2 standardization sample included 320 children ranging in age from 4 years, 0 months through 7 years, 11 months, with equal proportions of males and females. The sample demographics were based on the 2010 Census Bureau data (U.S. Bureau of the Census, 2010) and stratified according to race/ethnicity, geographic region, and parental education level. The latter was apportioned according to the following four categories: no high school diploma, high school diploma or equivalent, some college, and four or more years of college.

CONNERS CPT–3 **NORMS**

The Conners CPT–3 norms were based on a total sample size of 1,400 individuals, including 800 minors ranging in age from 8 years, 0 months through 17 years, 11 months, and 600 adults, ranging in age from 18 years, 0 months through 89 years, 11 months; hence 8 years through 89 years. The age range was selected to be compatible with the Conners K–CPT 2 age norms. The Conners CPT–3 standardization sample contained equal proportions of males and females and was also matched according to the 2010 Census Bureau data (U.S. Bureau of the Census, 2010) using race/ethnicity, geographic region, and parental education level as stratification variables. The latter matched the categories used for the Conners K–CPT 2.

CONNERS CATA NORMS

The Conners CATA standardization sample included a total of 1,080 individuals, further broken down into a subgroup of 600 minors with an age range from 8 years, 0 months through 17 years, 11 months, along with an adult subgroup of 480 participants between the ages of 18 years, 0 months through 83 years, 11 months. The sample contained an even proportion of males and females and was garnered using a stratification strategy based on the same 2010 Census Bureau data (U.S. Bureau of the Census, 2010). The stratification variables were the same as employed for both the Conners CPT–3 and Conners K–CPT 2.

SUMMARY

As can be seen, the Conners K–CPT 2, Conners CPT–3, and Conners CATA norms were all collected in proximity and are compatible in terms of age ranges. That is, together, they cover from ages 4 through 89. Furthermore, the age range 8–83 offers standardized CPT tests via two modalities, namely, auditory and visual (see subsequently). Finally, the samples are all well matched to the 2010 Census Bureau using the same equality of gender and stratification variables that are known to impact CPT performance. Next, CPT administration will be reviewed as done here.

Administration

As previously stated, administration for all three CPT tests is fully automated, which augments objectivity, along with both test reliability and validity. Each uses succinct instructions to examinees, a brief practice administration (with added practices as needed), and the actual test. Because the various CPT tests differ in terms of test stimuli, length, and other specifics, each administration will be briefly described in the same sequence as was their norms.

CONNERS K–CPT 2 PROCEDURE

The program begins with written instructions to the examinee to respond as quickly and accurately as possible to all pictures except for the ball (i.e., a soccer ball). The pictures are distinctive drawings of objects familiar to young children (e.g., a house, horse, a fish). The written directions are best supplemented by oral instructions provided by the examiner that clarify any words the child shows difficulty understanding. Having children in this four- to seven-year age range repeat back the instructions to ensure their comprehension is an effective strategy. Responses are made by either space bar or mouse button press, which is programmed by the examiner using the computer software settings (I prefer the left-mouse button option). In technical *signal-detection theory* terms, the ball is referred to as a *non-target stimulus* because a response to its presence is to be inhibited. Any alternate picture is referred to as a *target stimulus* because a rapid response to its presence is required.

The program flashes solid black pictures on a white screen (i.e., to reduce glare) randomly with an overall average 4:1 ratio of targets to non-targets. This higher proportion of targets to non-targets has been found to be most sensitive to detecting attention problems (Conners, 2000), which is the principal function of this test. Furthermore, the higher target probability produces a responding mode in the examinee, which also renders response inhibition to the lower likelihood non-targets more challenging. Another key feature of this CPT test regards the time interval between stimuli, referred to as an *interstimulus interval* (*ISI*). Shorter ISIs require the examinee to respond more quickly, although one-second ISIs were deemed to be too fast for this younger age group. Hence, the program alternates between 1.5- and 3.0-second ISIs. Display time is also a key feature, which is essentially the length of time the stimulus appears on the screen. The Conners K–CPT 2 stimulus display time is 500 milliseconds, hence twice the time (i.e., slower) than for older examinees (i.e., 250 milliseconds). Lastly, the duration of the test is reduced to 7.5 minutes versus 14 minutes for older individuals.

The practice administration runs for one minute. In the event the child manifests greater than 25% *omission errors* (i.e., not responding to targets), then a warning message appears with a recommendation for the child to, "Practice Again," with the "Start" button deactivated. The "Start" button can be activated manually, although with this type of performance, it is most likely that the child has misunderstood the instructions. However, a child can pass the test and still show evidence of not comprehending the instructions, in which case the child can practice again despite the "Start" button being activated.

It is recommended that the examiner administer the test individually and be present for the entire test. Although examiners may not coach the child during actual administration, they are permitted to encourage the child on a one-time basis to continue responding if they become disengaged from the task (i.e., no longer responding). A second disengagement results in a termination of the test, otherwise the program will record an excessive number of omissions and still require the examinee to retake the test without it being scored.

The 7.5-minute test is apportioned into 5 blocks or sets of trials. In turn, each block contains 2 sub-blocks that are comprised of 20 trials. Each sub-block has either all 1.5-second ISIs or all 3-second ISIs. Therefore, the entire test presents 200 trials (i.e., 10 sub-blocks with 20 trials each). These are used to compute all the standard scores for the test (see subsequent). The program will automatically end when the 7.5 mark has been reached.

CONNERS CPT–3 PROCEDURE

The CPT–3 procedure is much like that of the Conners K–CPT 2, hence only those differences between the two CPT tests will be reviewed here. That is, if a feature is not mentioned in this section, it should be assumed that it is exactly as described in the prior Conners K–CPT 2.

First, the stimuli represent capital block letters of the alphabet, which again are dark on a white background for the purpose of minimizing glare. The instructions are to respond as quickly as possible to all letters except the "X." Hence, in this case the "X" is the nontarget, whereas the remaining letters, or non-Xs, are targets. The practice test works in the same fashion as for the Conners K–CPT 2. However, the actual test is 14 minutes in duration and consists of 3 ISIs; that is, 1-second, 2-second, and 4-second intervals that are presented randomly. There are 6 time blocks or trial sets, including 60 trials in each set for a total of 360 trials. The first letter to initiate the actual test is omitted from scoring due to an unusually high error rate to such stimulus. All remaining key features are equivalent to that of the Conners K–CPT 2.

CONNERS CATA PROCEDURE

The Conners CATA procedure is quite different than either of the two previous CPT tests because it requires use of the auditory versus visual sensory-perceptual modality. Although it also has both a practice administration and an actual test, the instructions are more complicated. Based on clinical experience, younger children closer to age eight tend to have more difficulty understanding the commands. Although the same input device is used (viz., space bar or mouse click), a pair of headphones are placed on the examinee for auditory reception. Essentially, examinees are asked to respond to low-tone/high-tone pairings and not to low tones that are not paired with high tones. The low/high-tone pairings are set about two seconds apart, and examinees are instructed to respond as soon as the high tone is played. Hence, low/high-tone pairs represent the targets, while singular low tones are nontargets.

The practice administration is also about one minute, although there are two criteria used to elicit a warning to practice again. First, as in the prior two CPT tests, more than 25% omissions errors (i.e., not responding to low/high-tone pairs) will trigger a recommendation to practice again. Second, an excess of 50% commission errors (i.e., responding to a single high tone without the preceding warning stimulus) will result in the same "practice again" warning. If examinees are confused, it is typically concerning which tone the examinee is to respond to. A small number of examinees do not grasp the instruction even after several attempts, including a direct demonstration done by the examiner with the examinee observing. In such instance, the Conners CATA can be supplanted by comparable attention tests as part of the NEPSY–II or NAB.

The actual test runs 14 minutes and includes 200 trials. There are two types of trials: warned and unwarned. A warned trial consists of the low/high-tone pairing, with the low tone being the warning stimulus, followed by a two-second ISI, and them the high-tone target (viz., the target; viz., the AX paradigm). The unwarned trials have no preceding low tone, a four-second ISI, then a high tone (viz., nontargets). Other ISIs are as follows: (a) 1,000 milliseconds between the warning (low) tone and target (high) tone; (b) 2,000 milliseconds between the target tone and the next warning tone; and (c) 4,000 milliseconds to the high tone in unwarned trials. There are no ISI modifications from those just delineated.

Scoring

Although administration among the three CPT tests are sufficiently different to justify separate sections, scoring is extremely similar and completely automated by the same computer software that administered the test. Therefore, all three CPT measures and their scores will be described in one section to preserve space. Areas of divergence will be delineated as needed. This section will be subdivided into validity checks and actual scores. Scores that are available although not used are briefly mentioned. Forms 9.12, 9.13, and 9.14 present the tables used for reporting and interpreting the Conners K–CPT 2, Conners CPT–3, and Conners CATA test results in a final clinical assessment report, respectively.

VALIDITY CHECKS

There are three validity checks that are not actual scores, although they indicate whether the overall results may or may not reflect the examinee's true abilities. First, the run time of the test is checked to ensure it was the proper duration. This is essentially a computer issue. For example, an outdated computer may not be able to administer the test within the programmed time due to limitations in memory or processing speed, hence exceeding the standardized duration. This summarily invalidates the results. Second, the program checks if scoring some of the specific measures was precluded due to insufficient responding on the part of the examinee (e.g., a lack of responding to targets or insufficient hits), referred to as "computable scores." Third, an excessive number of omission errors (i.e., not responding to targets) may invalidate the results if excessive, hence similar to that used during the practice administration. This is similar to the prior validity check on computable scores, although focuses only on the omission error issue rather than on potential deleterious effects of upon several non-computable specific measures. In the case of the latter two checks, the computer typically scores the actual test, in which case the examiner must decide whether the results truly reflect the individual's ability or are due to extraneous variables (e.g., oppositional behavior).

Table 1 in each of the aforementioned forms contains these three validity checks. There are four columns, including the validity check names, issue, dichotomous yes or no result, and an interpretation (see subsequently). The "issue" column describes succinctly what is being securitized to ensure that the test was run properly and that the results can be relied upon. Most typically, in cases where the examinee has passed the practice test, all three checks will result in an affirmative conclusion.

Briefly, the program also provides a *response style analysis*, which is a signal detection theory concept. This is analogous to an examinee's approach to completing a self-report inventory and, in the extreme, can affect test scores. In *signal detection theory* (Swets, 1964; Tanner & Swets, 1954), the decision a person renders as to whether a physical stimulus was present depends on the following two variables: (a) the person's ability to detect the stimulus and (b) the degree to which the person is mentally prepared to state that it was present or not. The latter reflects more of a personality style, proclivity, or approach versus an ability variable. The interaction of these two variables results in four potential outcomes, two correct and two incorrect, as follows: (a) the person states that the stimulus was present when it actually was present (viz., a correct hit); (b) the person responds that the stimulus was not present when it actually was not present (viz., a correct rejection); (c) the person responds that the stimulus was not present when it was actually present (viz., an incorrect a miss); and (d) the person responds that the stimulus was present when it actually was not present (viz., an incorrect false alarm).[8]

As applied to the CPT test, when individuals are uncertain, some will tend toward stating that the stimulus was present, hence increasing the odds of hits, although accompanied by a concomitant escalation in the likelihood of false alarms. This is referred to as a *liberal response style* and will tend to exaggerate commission errors while minimizing omission errors. In complementary fashion, a *conservative response style* is a tendency to conclude that the stimulus was not present when uncertain, which will tend toward increasing omission errors and decreasing commission errors. The Conners CPT tests provide an analysis of such response style, classifying the individual into one of the following: (a) *Conservative or Very Conservative*; (b) *Balanced*; or (c) *Liberal or Very Liberal*. This response style score is not used as even very conservative and liberal styles will tend to cancel each other out when analyzing all the specific measures. Hence, it does not justify the time to report and interpret this kind of data. Furthermore, anecdotally there has not been any observed association between examinee response style and overall outcome.

Examinees' raw scores are all transformed into standardized *T*–scores, with a mean of 50, *SD* of 10, and range from 0 to 90. The highest score is capped at 90 to prevent over-interpretation or the excessive influence of one extreme score or outlier on interpretation. The specific measures are listed in Table 2 of Forms 9.12–9.14. The only variation among these forms is that the Conners CATA possesses two fewer specific measures as compared to the Conners K–CPT 2 and Conners CPT–3, both of which pertain to the fact that there are no changes in ISIs in the Conners CATA administration.

Scrutinizing the specific measures not included in the Conners CATA is instructive. First, the *HRT ISI Change* measures the degree to which examinees remain consistent with longer ISIs versus impulsively responding prior to stimulus presentation. Second, *Variability* examines an individual's response speed variability to differing ISIs relative to his or her own average. Because the Conners CATA is the only one of the three CPT tests that does not vary its ISIs in a random manner, the inclusion of these measures is precluded. Other than these two exceptions, the three CPT tests yield the same specific measures. For example, in addition to omission errors and commission errors reviewed previously when discussing the practice administration, *Detectability (d')* measures the ability of the examinee to discriminate targets from nontargets, thus basically comparing the accuracy in responding to each.

All the specific measure names are listed in the first column of Table 2 (see Forms 9.12–9.14). This is ensued by the *T*–score, 90% CI, PR, interpretive classification (see below), and a succinct description of the specific measure. The CI and PR have the same meaning as for the previous three neuropsychological tests presented in this chapter. The definition of each measure can be scrutinized in Forms 9.12, 9.13, and 9.14 and will not be repeated here.

Interpretation

The interpretive strategy is the same for all three Conners CPT tests and thus will be discussed together. The discussion will be divided into validity interpretation and actual test interpretation.

First, using Table 1 the examiner must ensure that the validity issues have all been satisfied, that is, answered in the affirmative. There are three potential interpretations as follows: (a) valid; (b) qualified valid; and (c) invalid. When all three issues are answered in the affirmative, which is the vast majority of cases, the decision is valid. Following Table 1 are pre-drafted excerpts for the most common conclusions. Here, the valid option should be retained while deleting the rest. Second, if either the Computable Scores or Typical Response Patterns results are no or negative, and the program provides a scored profile, the interpretation should either be a qualified valid or qualified invalid. Qualified valid results usually manifest when the examinee has passed a practice administration and was observed to be responding as instructed throughout the vast majority of the actual test. In this instance, the profile should be interpreted as being valid, and the aberrant scores (usually including outliers and/or some non-scored specific measures) are the results of significantly impaired attention and impulse control. Hence, the qualified valid interpretive option should be retained and the others deleted. Finally, if the examinee did not pass a practice administration, or several practice administrations were needed to reach a passing result, and there are one or two validity issues with negative results, then the invalid option should be selected. In such cases, examinees may respond more favorably to a more traditional individually administered table test that incorporates more interpersonal interaction between examiner and examinee. Viable alternatives include the NEPSY–II attention and executive function subtests and the NAB Attention Module (see Form 9.7).

There is one additional option for the Conners CATA. Occasionally, there will be an individual who has a hearing handicap in one ear. In such cases, desktop computer audio speakers or computer laptop speakers can be used. Because this modifies administration instructions, this should be noted by selecting the "non-standardized administration" excerpt that follows Table 1 (Form 9.14). The only feature that will be missing from the standardized administration is differential performance between left ear–right ear (i.e., alternating) versus same-ear (i.e., non-alternating) tone presentations, which is not really imperative, at least when testing for the presence or absence ADHD.

ACTUAL TEST INTERPRETATION

Briefly, the two predecessors of the current tests (viz., *Conners CPT-II* and *Conners K-CPT*; Conners, 2001, 2004, respectively) utilized a *discriminant analysis* (*DA*) to predict whether an examinee's T–score profile was more correlated with non-clinical profile norms or clinical profile norms (Conners, 2001, 2004). Briefly, DA predicts group membership on a Y outcome variable (i.e., nonclinical and clinical) from a combination of numerical scores on several X predictor variables (e.g., CPT–specific measure T–scores; Warner, 2021a, 2021b). However, this was dropped from these editions as excessively unreliable.

The current approach mirrors that of the NEPSY–II. That is, diagnosis of significant impairment rests on two criteria: (a) the number of specific measures that have T–scores falling within the clinical range, and (b) the extremity of individual T–scores. Regarding the latter, all the specific measures except one are unidirectional (i.e., higher scores indicate more impairment). More specifically, the unidirectional scores are interpreted as follows: (a) 0–59 is considered nonclinical or normal responding; (b) 60–69 represents a clinical elevation; and (c) 70– 90 is a high clinical elevation. The single bidirectional specific measure is *Hit Reaction Time* (*HRT*), which quantifies the examinee's mean or average reaction time to stimuli. Extremely high scores reflect consistently slow reaction time, hence an indicator of inattention. More specifically, 60–69 is a high elevation, while 70–90 is a markedly high elevation. In contrast, extremely low scores show excessively rapid average reaction time, thus an indicator of impulsivity. Here, 40–44 is a low elevation, while 0–39 is a markedly low elevation. The middle-most scores, 45–59, are interpreted to be within normal limits on the bidirectional measure. Overall, these CPT test address the following abilities or signs: (a) general attention, (b) sustained attention (i.e., vigilance),[9] (c) impulsivity, and sustained impulsivity (the latter not measured by the Conners CATA).

Therefore, if a specific measure shows a nonclinical elevation, the interpretive term "normal" can be inserted. If there is a clinical elevation or high clinical elevation, the sign that is manifested is entered as attention, sustained attention, impulsivity, or sustained impulsivity. Not only does this show the presence of impairment but also what *kind* of impairment that is so integral to accurate differential diagnosis; here considering the presence of ADHD. The degree of extremity is shown by the number of asterisks affixed to the T–score (i.e., zero, one, or two). The interpretive scheme for both unidirectional and bidirectional specific measures is incorporated into the specific notes to Table 2 (Forms 9.12–9.14). Although the computer software employs alternate terms, these have been found to be more effective for clinical practice.

Finally, several pre-drafted interpretations of potential test results follow Table 2 data. In general, they describe the following outcomes: (a) positive for neurocognitive impairment, including ADHD; (b) negative for neurocognitive impairment, including ADHD; or (c) borderline results that are either insufficiently negative or mildly positive. In addition, there is an excerpt for (a) integrating the CPT results with other test results (i.e., show consistency or inconsistency), (b) describing a false positive result (i.e., an elevated profile that is an anomaly when compared to all other negative data), and (c) explaining a false negative outcome (i.e., a normal profile juxtaposed with clear and consistent evidence of impairment among other tests in the battery).

Summary

The CPT tests are relatively rapid, automated, and specific in terms of the neurocognitive abilities measured: principally, attention and secondarily impulse control. Of all the neuropsychological tests presented in this chapter, the CPT tests should probably be accompanied by other tests to help ensure their validity. For example, several children who are otherwise severely hyperactive and impulsive have passed computerized CPT tests by using their imagination, such as pretending the CPT was a game or simply having a proclivity for performing well on computer tasks. Also, CPT tests are administered individually and in an artificially quiet environment, which should also be considered; hence referring to the issue of ecological validity (i.e., do the results generalize to the real-world environment). With these caveats, CPT tests are convenient, largely automated, and usually accurate.

Recapitulation

This concludes a sequence of three chapters covering standardized tests that measure some aspect of cognitive functioning. These included the complex constructs of intelligence, achievement, and lastly, neuropsychological testing; the latter being the topic of the current chapter. Neuropsychological testing was defined as measuring brain–behavior relationships, principally for detecting the presence of neurocognitive disorders. As such, a model of brain functioning was presented with diagrams to provide a contextual understanding of what neuropsychological tests tap into, especially focusing on cortical areas, although with some examination of key subcortical structures. There was also some brief discussion of when neuropsychological tests should be ordered in clinical practice as part of an assessment battery. However, the key portion of the chapter focused on two comprehensive neuropsychological test batteries, the NEPSY–II and the NAB, including their structure, data yield, and how their scores can be reported and interpreted as part of an assessment report. Next, the WMS–IV memory test was presented, including its organizational structure, data yield, and tables for reporting and interpreting results. Here, an expanded model of human memory was presented, with special focus on declarative semantic and episodic LTM, which is the focus of the WMS–IV. Finally, three Conners CPT tests were presented, which measure the more specific neurocognitive abilities of attention and impulse control. The next chapter covers a variety of standardized rating scales, some of which are multidimensional (i.e., measuring a variety of symptoms and disorders), along with others that provide a detailed analysis of a particular type of psychopathology (e.g., trauma-related disorder).

Key Terms

- ability memory discrepancy
- adaptive testing
- agnosia
- agraphia
- Alzheimer's disease
- amnesia
- amygdala
- anosognosia
- anterograde amnesia
- aphasia
- apraxia
- association areas
- attention
- attention-deficit/hyperactivity disorder (ADHD)
- Autism Diagnostic Observation Schedule, Second Edition (ADOS–2).
- autism spectrum disorder (ASD)
- baseline functioning
- binding
- Broca's area
- cancellation task
- cell assembly
- central sulcus
- cerebellum
- cerebral cortex
- cognitive flexibility
- complex attention
- conditioned emotional responses
- Conners Continuous Auditory Test of Attention (Conners CATA)
- Conners Continuous Performance Test, Third Edition (Conners CPT–3)
- Conners CPT–II
- Conners K–CPT
- Conners Kiddie Continuous Performance Test, Second Edition (Conners K–CPT 2)

- conservative response style
- consolidation
- consolidation system
- continuous performance tests (CPTs)
- contralateral
- convolutions
- corpus callosum
- criterion
- critical value
- cued recall
- cumulative percentages
- decision–making
- declarative episodic memory (explicit memory)
- decussation
- delayed memory
- dementia/s
- demographically corrected norms
- Detectability (d')
- discriminant analysis (DA)
- distractibility
- divided attention
- dyslexia
- dyspraxia (apraxia)
- ecological validity
- encoding
- engram
- episodic memory
- error utilization
- executive functioning
- executive system (central executive system)
- expressive language
- final common pathway
- fissure/s
- fixed battery approach
- flexible battery approach
- fluency
- fluid reasoning
- functional systems model
- glial cells
- gnosis
- gyri (gyrus, singular form)
- haptic
- hemispheres
- hindbrain
- hippocampus
- Hit Reaction Time (HRT)
- holophrases
- HRT ISI Change
- hypothalamus
- image degradation techniques
- immediate memory
- incidental learning (automatic learning)
- inferential norming
- information processing (multistore model)
- inhibitory control
- initiation

- interference
- interstimulus interval (ISI)
- language
- language disorder
- lateral sulcus (Sylvian fissure)
- lateralization (of function)
- learning
- learning and memory
- left hemisphere
- liberal response style
- limbic system
- lobes
- localization of function approach
- longitudinal fissure
- long-term memory (LTM)
- long-term potentiation
- maintenance rehearsal
- major neurocognitive disorder
- maze-tracing paradigm
- medical necessity
- memory
- memory trace/s (engram)
- mental disorder due to another medical condition
- mental flexibility
- mirror neuron systems
- motor coordination
- naming
- NEPSY–II
- NEPSY–II Full Battery
- NEPSY–II General Battery
- neurocognitive disorder/s
- neuron/s
- Neuropsychological Assessment Battery (NAB)
- neuropsychological (neurocognitive) testing
- neuropsychology
- nonorganic mental disorders
- nontarget stimulus
- olfaction
- omission errors
- oppositional defiant disorder (ODD)
- orientation
- oromotor control
- other specified communication disorder
- other specified neurodevelopmental disorder
- overriding habits/inhibition
- parietal lobe
- Parkinson's disease
- pathognomonic
- perceptual-motor
- perseveration
- phonological loop
- phonological processing
- planning
- plasticity
- postcentral gyrus
- praxis

- precentral gyrus
- predicted-difference method
- predictor
- prefrontal cortex
- premorbid level of functioning
- primary motor cortex
- primary scores
- primary sensory cortex
- priming
- procedural (nonconscious) memory
- process scores
- prompts
- proposition speech output
- proprioception
- receptive language
- refractory epilepsy
- repetitions
- response style analysis
- reticular activating system
- retrieval
- retrograde amnesia
- reverse rule
- right hemisphere
- rote memory
- screening battery approach
- selective attention
- semantic dementia
- semantic memory
- senile dementia
- sensorimotor functioning
- short-term memory
- signal-detection theory
- social cognition
- social perception
- social pragmatic communication disorder
- spatial delayed-recognition span paradigm
- spatial processing
- speech sound (phonological) disorder
- standard error of measurement (*SEM*)
- standard scores (*SS*s)
- stop point/s
- sulci (sulcus, singular form)
- supraspan learning
- sustained attention
- sympathetic nervous system
- target stimulus
- temporal lobe
- thalamus
- theory of mind
- tort law
- transduction
- traumatic brain injury (TBI)
- unspecified neurocognitive disorder
- U.S. Census-matched sample
- useful field of view (UFOV) paradigm
- variability

- vigilance
- visual perception
- visual-spatial sketchpad
- visuoconstruction
- visuospatial processing
- Wechsler Memory Scale, Fourth Edition (WMS–IV)
- Wechsler Memory Scale, Fourth Edition, Brief Cognitive Status Exam (WMS–IV, BCSE)
- Wechsler Memory Scale, Third Edition (WMS–III)
- Wernicke's area
- with or without behavioral disturbance
- WMS–IV Scoring Assistant
- word generation
- working memory (WM)
- X paradigm
- XA paradigm

Notes

1. Neurons and interneural connections will not be discussed here, as this information is available in numerous other titles. Therefore, the reader is referred to external sources for such information in the interests of preserving space.
2. Recall that all tests used for the purposes of assessing neurocognitive disorder should be billed as neuropsychological testing, even if they are principally classified as personality or developmental tests (refer back to Chapter 3 on billing codes for psychological services; see also Figure 3.2). The manner in which a test is being employed within a test battery is the controlling factor when determining the proper billing code, not the test's individual classification.
3. NEPSY is an abbreviation for neuropsychological rather than an acronym.
4. Because NEPSY-II interpretation is more straightforward as compared to a test with multiple levels of analysis (e.g., intelligence tests), an interpretative flowchart is not needed for any of the NEPSY-II batteries.
5. I have created selective forms for ADHD testing and autism testing because of the frequency with which such batteries are used. The reader is welcome to them by simply contacting the author and requesting them. They are not included in this book to save space and due to the fact that they are redundant with the Full Battery Forms.
6. Note that these memory tests include both learning and memory tasks as in the NEPSY-II, although here the authors have chosen for some reason not to use the term "Learning and Memory." This is pointed out simply to show how similar these two neuropsychological test batteries are in terms of the constructs they measure and their comparability to the model of brain functioning presented in Figure 9.5.
7. This line of reasoning palpably demonstrates the virtues of a scientist–practitioner model of training in psychology, wherein clinical practice and research are reciprocal skills that enhance each other.
8. In actuality, there is a third situational variable that affects the outcome, which is the consequence of a miss that must be balanced against that of a false alarm. This variable is not a consideration in this instance, although it should be acknowledged in the interest of being complete and accurate.
9. Vigilance used within the context of CPT neurocognitive testing refers to sustained attention, an ability trait. Vigilance will be revisited when discussing personality testing, here associated with trauma-related psychopathology (i.e., hypervigilance or extreme sensitivity to potential danger) or a sign of personality disorder (i.e., paranoia). This is one of those constructs in psychology that can change significantly in meaning depending upon context.

References

Albert, M. S., & Moss, M. B. (1992). The assessment of memory disorders in patients with Alzheimer's disease. In L. R. Squire & N. Butters (Eds.), *Neuropsychology of memory* (2nd ed., pp. 211–219). New York, NY: Guilford Press.

Alkon, D. (1989). Memory storage and neural systems. *Scientific American, 261*, 42–50.

Allen, D. N., Leany, B. D., Thaker, N. S., & Cross, C. (2010). Memory and attention profiles in pediatric traumatic brain injury. *Archives of Clinical Neuropsychology, 25*, 618–633.

American Psychiatric Association. (1987). *Diagnostic and statistical manual of mental disorders* (3rd ed., rev., DSM–III–R). Washington, DC: Author.

American Psychiatric Association. (2013). *Diagnostic and statistical manual of mental disorders* (5th ed., DSM–5). Arlington, VA: Author.

Anderson, V. E., Siegel, F. S., Fisch, R. O., & Wirt, R. D. (1969). Responses of Phenylketonuric children on a continuous performance test. *Journal of Abnormal Psychology, 74*, 358–362.

Andrewes, D. G. (2016). *Neuropsychology: From theory to practice* (2nd ed.). New York, NY: Routledge.

Andrewes, D. G., & Gilewski, E. (1999). Rehabilitation back to work of an amnesic patient. *Neuropsychological Rehabilitation, 9*, 70–99.

Annese, J., Schenker-Ahmed, N., Bartch, H., Maechler, P., Sheh, C., Thomas, N., . . . Corkin, S. (2014). Post-mortem examination of patient HM's brain based on histological sectioning and digital reconstruction. *Nature Communications, 5*, 3122.

Ashkenazi, S., Black, J. M., Abrams, D. A., Hoeft, F., & Menon, V. (2013). Neurobiological underpinnings of math and reading learning disabilities. *Journal of Learning Disabilities, 46*, 549–569.

Ashwin, C., Wheelwright, S., & Baron-Cohen, S. (2006). Finding a face in the crowd: Testing the anger superiority effect in Asperger syndrome. *Brain and Cognition, 61,* 78–95.

Atkinson, R. C., & Shiffrin, R. M. (1968). Human memory: A proposed system and its control processes. In K. W. Spence & J. T. Spence (Eds.). *The psychology of learning and motivation* (Vol. 2, pp. 89–105). New York, NY: Academic Press.

Azevedo, F. A. C., Carvalho, L. R. B., Grinberg, L. T., Farfel, J. M., Ferretti, R. E. L., Renata, E. P., . . . Herculano-Houzel, S. (2009). Equal numbers of neuronal and nonneuronal cells make the human brain an isometrically scaled-up primate brain. *Journal of Comparative Neurology, 513,* 532–541.

Babiloni, C., Vecchio, F., Buffo, P., Buttiglione, M., Cibelli, G., & Rossini, P. M. (2010). Cortical responses to consciousness of schematic emotional facial expressions: A high-resolution EEG study. *Human Brain Mapping, 8,* 8.

Baddeley, A. D. (2000). The episodic buffer: A new component of working memory? *Trends in Cognitive Sciences, 4,* 417–423.

Baddeley, A. D., & Hitch, G. J. (1974). Working memory. In G. A. Bower (Ed.), *The psychology of learning and motivation* (Vol. 8, pp. 47–90). New York, NY: Academic Press.

Baddeley, A. D., & Lieberman, K. (1980). Spatial working memory. In R. Nickerson (Ed.), *Attention and performance* (Vol. VIII, pp. 521–539). Hillsdale, NJ: Lawrence Erlbaum Associates.

Balint, S., Czobor, P., Komlosi, S., Meszaros, A., et al. (2009). Attention-deficit/hyperactivity disorder (ADHD): Gender- and age-related differences in neurocognition. *Psychological Medicine, 39,* 1337–1345.

Ball, K. K., & Roenker, D. L. (1998). *Useful field of view.* San Antonio, TX: The Psychological Corporation.

Ball, K. K., Beard, B. L., Roenker, D. L., Miller, R. L., & Griggs, D. S. (1988). Age and visual search: Expanding the useful field of view. *Journal of Optical Society of America, 5,* 2210–2219.

Bargh, J. A., Chen, M., & Burrows, C. (1996). Automaticity of social behavior: Direct effects of trait construct and stereotype activation on action. *Journal of Personality & Social Psychology, 71,* 230–244.

Barkley, R. A. (1997). Behavioral inhibition, sustained attention, and executive functions: Constructing a unified theory of ADHD. *Psychological Bulletin, 121,* 65–94.

Barkley, R. A. (2003). Issues in the diagnosis of attention-deficit/hyperactivity disorder in children. *Brain & Development, 25,* 77–83.

Barlow, D. H., Durand, M. V., & Hofmann, S. G. (2018). *Abnormal psychology: An integrative approach* (8th ed.). Boston, MA: Cengage Learning.

Baron-Cohen, S. (2001). Theory of mind and autism: A review. *International Review of Research in Mental Retardation, 23,* 169–184.

Baron-Cohen, S., Leslie, A. M., & Frith, U. (1985). Does the autistic child have a "theory of mind"? *Cognition, 21,* 37–46.

Bauermeister, J. J., Matos, M., Reina, G., Salas, C. C., et al. (2005). Comparison of the DSM–IV combined and inattentive types of ADHD in school-based sample of Latin\Hispanic children. *Journal of Child Psychology and Psychiatry, 46,* 166–179.

Bennet, T. (1988). Use of the Halstead–Reitan neuropsychological test battery in the assessment of head injury. *Cognitive Rehabilitation, 6,* 18–25.

Benson, D. F., & Ardilla, A. (1996). *Aphasia: A clinical perspective.* New York, NY: Oxford University Press.

Benton, A. L., Hamsher, K. deS., & Sivan, A. B. (1994). *Multilingual aphasia examination* (3rd ed.). Iowa City, IA: AJA Associates.

Benton, A. L., Hamsher, K. deS., Varney, N. R., & Spreen, O. (1983). *Contributions to neuropsychological assessment: A clinical manual.* New York, NY: Oxford University Press.

Benton, A. L., Sivan, A. B., Hamsher, K. deS., Varney, N. R., & Spreen, O. (1994). *Multilingual aphasia examination* (3rd ed.). Iowa City, IA: AJA Associates.

Berg, E. A. (1948). A simple objective technique for measuring flexibility of thinking. *Journal of General Psychology, 39,* 15–22.

Bernat, E., Shevrin, H., & Snodgrass, M. (2001). Subliminal visual oddball stimuli evoke a P300 component. *Clinical Neurophysiology, 112,* 159–171.

Berry, D. T. R., & Carpenter, G. S. (1992). Effect of four different delay periods on recall of the Rey-Osterrieth complex figure by older persons. *The Clinical Neuropsychologist, 6,* 80–84.

Binder, J. R., Desai, R. H., Graves, W. W., & Conant, L. I. (2009). Where is the semantic system? A critical review and meta-analysis of 120 functional neuroimaging studies. *Cerebral Cortex, 19*(12), 2767–2796.

Bishop, D. V. M., & McArthur, G. M. (2005). Individual differences in auditory processing in specific language impairment: A follow-up study using event-related potentials and behavioural thresholds. *Cortex, 41,* 327–341.

Bishop, D. V. M., & Snowling, M. J. (2004). Developmental dyslexia and specific language impairment: Same or different? *Psychological Bulletin, 130,* 858–886.

Bliss, T. V., & Lomo, T. (1973). Long-lasting potentiation of synaptic transmission in the dentate area of the anaesthetized rabbit following stimulation of the perforant path. *The Journal of Physiology, 232,* 331–356.

Boller F., & Vignolo, L. (1966). Latent sensory aphasia in hemisphere-damaged patients: An experimental study with the token test. *Brain, 89,* 815–831.

Boone, K. B. (1999). Neuropsychological assessment of executive functions. In B. L. Miller & J. L. Cummings (Eds.), *The human frontal lobes: Functions and disorders* (pp. 247–260). New York, NY: Guilford Press.

Borgatti, R., Pccinelli, P., Montirosso, R., Donati, G., et al. (2004). Study of attentional processes in children with idiopathic epilepsy by conners' continuous performance test. *Journal of Child Neurology, 19,* 509–515.

Broadbent, D. E. (1971). *Decision and stress.* Oxford, UK: Academic Press.

Brown, J. (1958). Some tests of the decay theory of immediate memory. *Quarterly Journal of Experimental Psychology, 10,* 12–21.

Broyles, S. (2006). Subliminal advertising and the perpetual popularity of playing to people's paranoia. *Journal of Consumer Affairs, 40,* 392–406.

Budson, A. E., & Price, B. H. (2005). Memory dysfunction. *New England Journal of Medicine, 352,* 692–699.

Burlingame, E., Sussman, H. M., Gillam, R. B., & Hay, J. F. (2005). An investigation of speech perception in children with specific language impairment on a continuum of format transition duration. *Journal of Speech, Language, and Hearing Research, 48,* 805–816.

Chapman, L. L., White, D. A., & Storandt, M. (1997). Prose recall in dementia: A comparison of delay intervals. *Archives of Neurology, 54,* 1501–1504.

Collins, A. M., & Loftus, E. F. (1975). A spreading activation theory of semantic processing. *Psychological Review, 82,* 407–428.

Collins, A. M., & Quillian, M. R. (1969). Retrieval time from semantic memory. *Journal of Verbal Learning and Verbal Behaviour, 8,* 240–247.

Conners, C. K. (2000). *Conners' continuous performance test II: Computer program for windows technical guide and software manual.* Toronto, Canada: Multi-Health Systems.

Conners, C. K. (2001). *Conners' kiddie continuous performance, version 5 for windows (K–CPT): Technical guide and software manual.* North Tonawanda, NY: Multi-Health Systems.

Conners, C. K. (2004). *Conners' continuous performance test II, version 5 for windows (CPT–II): Technical guide and software manual.* North Tonawanda, NY: Multi-Health Systems.

Conners, C. K. (2014). *Conners continuous performance test, third edition (conners CPT–3) and conners continuous auditory test of attention (Conners CATA): Technical manual.* North Towanda, NY: Multi-Health Systems (MHS).

Conners, C. K. (2015). *Conners Kiddie continuous performance test, second edition K–CPT 2): Technical manual.* North Towanda, NY: Multi-Health Systems (MHS).

Cope, N., Eicher, J. D., Meng, H., Gibson, C. J., Hager, K., Lacadie, C., & Gruen, J. R. (2012). Variants in the DYX2 locus are associated with altered brain activation in reading-related brain regions in subjects with reading disability. *NeuroImage, 63,* 148–156.

Cowan, N. (2001). The magical number 4 in short-term memory: A reconsideration of mental storage capacity. *Behavioral and Brain Sciences, 24,* 97–185.

Cowan, N., & Hulme, C. (1997). *The development of memory in childhood.* East Sussex, UK: Psychology Press.

Cowan, N., Elliott, E. M., Saults, J. S., Morey, C. C., Mattox, S., Hismjatullina, A., & Conway, A. R. A. (2005). On the capacity of attention: Its estimation and its role in working memory and cognitive aptitudes. *Cognitive Psychology, 51,* 42–100.

Cramon, D. Y. von, & Matthes-von Cramon, G. (1990). Frontal lobe dysfunctions in patients—therapeutical approaches. In R. L. Wood & I. Fussey (Eds.), *Cognitive rehabilitation in perspective* (pp. 164–179). London, UK: Taylor & Francis.

Curtiss, G., Vanderploeg, R. D., Spencer, J., & Salazar, A. M. (2001). Patterns of verbal learning and memory in traumatic brain injury. *Journal of the International Neuropsychological Society, 7,* 574–585.

Dakin, S., & Frith, U. (2005). Vagaries of visual perception in autism. *Neuron, 48,* 497–507.

Dalal, R. H., & Loeb, D. F. (2005). Imitative production of regular-past tense—*ed* by English-speaking children with specific language impairment. *International Journal of Language and Communication Disorders, 40,* 67–82.

Deevy, P., & Leonard, L. B. (2004). The comprehension of *Wh-* questions in children with specific language impairment. *Journal of Speech, Language, and Hearing Research, 47,* 802–815.

Deger, M., Helias, M., Rotter, S., & Diesmann, M. (2012). Spike-timing dependence of structural plasticity explains cooperative synapse formation in the neocortex. *PLoS Computational Biology, 8,* e1002689.

Delis, D. C., Kaplan, E., & Kramer, J. H. (2001). *Delis-Kaplan executive functioning system.* San Antonio, TX: The Psychological Corporation.

Denckla, M. B. (1985). Motor coordination in dyslexic children: Theoretical and clinical implications. In F. H. Duffy & N. Geschwind (Eds.), *Dyslexia: A neuroscientific approach to clinical evaluation* (pp. 187–195). Boston, MA: Little, Brown.

DeRenzi, E., & Vignolo, L. (1962). The Token Test: A sensitive test to detect receptive disturbances in aphasics. *Brain, 85,* 665–678.

Dick, F., Wulfeck, B., Krupa-Kwiatkowski, M., & Bates, E. (2004). The development of complex sentence interpretation in typically developing children compared with children with specific language impairments or early unilateral focal lesions. *Developmental Science, 7,* 360–377.

Egeland, J., Johansen, S. N., & Ueland, T. (2009). Differentiating between ADHD sub-types on CPT measures of sustained attention and vigilance. *Scandinavian Journal of psychology, 50,* 347–354.

Ekman, P. (1973). Darwin and cross-cultural studies of facial expression. In P. Ekman (Ed.), *Darwin and facial expression: A century of research in review.* New York: Academic Press.

Ekman, P., & Friesen, W. (1969). The repertoire of nonverbal behavior: Categories, origins, usage, and coding. *Semiotica, 1,* 49–98.

Ekman, P., & Friesen, W. (1971). Constants across cultures in the face and emotion. *Journal of Personality and Social Psychology, 17,* 124–129.

Evans, J. L., & MacWhinney, B. (1999). Sentence processing strategies in children with expressive-receptive specific language impairments. *International Journal of Language & Communication Disorders, 34,* 117–134.

Fastenau, P. S., & Adams, K. M. (1996). Heaton, Grant, and Matthews' comprehensive norms: An overzealous attempt. *Journal of Clinical and Experimental Neuropsychology, 18,* 444–448.

Fazel-Rezai, R., & Peters, J. F. (2005). *P300 wave feature extraction: Preliminary results.* Proceedings of the 18th Annual Canadian Conference on Electrical and Computer Engineering (CCECE'05, pp. 390–393). Saskatoon, Saskatchewan, Canada.

Fioriti, L., Myers, C., Huang, Y. Y., Li, X., Stephan, J. S., Trifilieff, P., . . . Kandel, E. R. (2015). The persistence of hippocampal-based memory requires protein synthesis mediated by the prion-like protein cpeb3. *Neuron, 86,* 1433–1448.

Frattali, C. M., Thompson, C. K., Holland, A. L., Wohl, C. B., & Ferketic, M. M. (1995). *American speech-language-hearing association functional assessment of communication skills for adults.* Rockville, MD: American Speech-Language-Hearing Association.

Gathercole, S. (2002). *Short-term and working memory*. University of Durham, UK: Psychology Press.

Gathercole, S. E. (2008). Working memory. In J. H. Byrne & H. L. Roediger (Eds.), *Learning and memory: A comprehensive reference: Cognitive psychology of memory* (Vol. 2, pp. 33–48). San Diego, CA: Elsevier Science.

Gathercole, S. E., & Alloway, T. P. (2008). *Working memory and learning: A practical guide for teachers*. London, UK: Paul Chapman.

Gioia, G. A., & Isquith, P. K. (2004). Ecological assessment of executive function in traumatic brain injury. *Developmental Neuropsychology, 25*, 135–158.

Glisky, E. L., Schacter, D. L., & Tulving, E. (1986). Learning and retention of vocabulary words in amnesic patients: Method of vanishing cues. *Journal of Clinical and Experimental Neuropsychology, 8*, 292–312.

Goldman-Rakic, P. S. (1998). The prefrontal landscape: Implications of functional architecture for understanding human mentation and the central executive. In A. C. Roberts, T. W. Robbins, & L. Weiskrantz (Eds.), *The prefrontal cortex: Executive and cognitive functions* (pp. 87–102). Oxford, UK: Oxford University Press.

Goodglass, H., & Wingfield, A. (Eds.). (1997). *Anomia: Neuroanatomical and cognitive correlates*. New York, NY: Academic Press.

Goodglass, H., Kaplan, E., & Barresi, B. (2000). *Boston Diagnostic Aphasia Examination* (3rd ed.). Philadelphia: Lippincott, Williams & Wilkins.

Gorsuch, R. L. (2003, August). *Update on continuous norming*. Paper presented at the annual meeting of the American Psychological Association, Toronto, Canada.

Gray, S. (2003). Diagnostic accuracy and test-retest reliability of nonword repetition and digit span tasks administered to preschool children with specific language impairment. *Journal of Communication Disorders, 36*, 129–151.

Gregory, R. J. (2011). *Psychological testing: History, principles, applications*. Boston, MA: Pearson Education.

Griggs, E. M., Young, E. J., Rumbaugh, G., & Miller, C. A. (2013). MicroRNA-182 regulates amygdala-dependent memory formation. *Journal of Neuroscience, 33*, 1734.

Haavisto, M. L., & Lehto, J. E. (2004). Fluid/spatial and crystalized intelligence in relation to domain-specific working memory: A latent-variable approach. *Learning and Individual Differences, 15*, 1–21.

Hannay, H. J., Levin, H. S., & Grossman, R. G. (1979). Impaired recognition memory after head injury. *Cortex, 15*, 269–283.

Happé, F. G. E. (1995). The role of age and verbal ability in the theory of mind task performance of subjects with autism. *Child Development, 66*, 843–855.

Heaton, R. K., Chelune, G. J., Talley, J. L., Kay, G. G., & Curtis, G. (1993). *Wisconsin Card Sorting manual: Revised and expanded*. Odessa, FL: Psychological Assessment Resources (PAR).

Heaton, R. K., Grant, I., & Matthews, C. G. (1991). *Comprehensive norms for an expanded Halstead-Reitan Battery: Demographic corrections, research findings, and clinical applications*. Odessa, FL: Psychological Assessment Resources.

Hebb, D. O. (1949). *Organization of behaviour*. New York, NY: John Wiley & Sons.

Hill, E. S., Vasireddi, S. K., Wang, J., Bruno, A. M., & Frost, W. N. (2015). Memory formation in tritonia via recruitment of variably committed neurons. *Current Biology, 25*(22), 2879–2888.

Hodges, J. R. (1994). Retrograde amnesia. In A. Baddeley, B. A. Wilson, & F. Watts (Eds.), *Handbook of memory disorders* (pp. 81–107). New York, NY: John Wiley & Sons.

Hodges, J. R., Patterson, K., Oxbury, S., & Funnell, E. (1992). Semantic dementia. *Brain, 115*, 1783–1806.

Holland, A. (1980). *Communicative activities of daily living*. Austin, TX: Pro-Ed.

Holland, A., Frattali, C. M., & Fromm, D. (1999). *Communicative activities of daily living* (2nd ed.). Austin, TX: Pro-Ed.

Ibarretxe-Bilbao, N., Junque, C., Tolosa, E., Marti, M. J., Valldeoriola, F., Bargallo, N., & Zarei, M. (2009). Neuroanatomical correlates of impaired decision-making and facial emotion recognition in early Parkinson's disease. *European Journal of Neuroscience, 30*, 1162–1171.

Kail, R., & Hall, L. K. (1994). Processing speed, naming speed, and reading. *Developmental Psychology, 30*, 949–954.

Kandel, E. R. (2012). The molecular biology of memory: cAMP, PKA, CRE, CREB-1, CREB-2, and CPEB. *Molecular Brain, 5*(14).

Kandel, E. R., & Schwartz, J. H. (1982). Molecular biology of learning: Modulation of transmitter release. *Science, 218*, 433–443.

Kaplan, E., Fein, D., Morris, R., & Deis, D. (1991). *WAIS–R as a neuropsychological instrument*. San Antonio, TX: The Psychological Corporation (PAR).

Kapur, N. (1994). *Memory disorder sin clinical practice*. Hove, UK: Lawrence Erlbaum Associates.

Kessler, H. R. (1998). The bedside neuropsychological examination. In P. J. Nussbaum (Eds.), *Clinical neuropsychology: A pocket handbook for assessment* (pp. 54–75). Washington DC: American Psychological Association.

Killiany, R. J., Hyman, B. T., Gomez-Isla, T., Moss, M. B., Kikinis, R., Jolesz, F., et al. (2002). MRI measures of entorhinal cortex versus hippocampus in preclinical AD. *Neurology, 58*, 1188–1196.

Klee, T., Stokes, S. F., Wong, A. M. Y., Fletcher, P. & Gavin, W. J. (2004). Utterance length and lexical diversity in Cantonese-speaking children with and without specific language impairment. *Journal of Speech, Language, and Hearing Research, 47*, 1396–1410.

Klimkeit, E. L., Mattingley, J. B., Shappard, D. M., Lee, P., & Bradshaw, J. L. (2005). Motor preparation, motor execution, attention, and executive functions in attention deficit/hyperactivity disorder (ADHD). *Child Neuropsychology, 11*, 153–173.

Knopman, D. S., DeKosky, S. T., Cummings, J. L., Chui, H., Corey-Bloom, J., Relkin, N., et al. (2001). Practice parameter: Diagnosis of dementia (evidence-based review): Report of the quality standards subcommittee of the American academy of neurology. *Neurology, 56*, 1143–1153.

Kolb, B., & Whishaw, I. Q. (2003). *Fundamentals of human neuropsychology*. New York, NY: W. H. Freeman.

Korkman, M., Kettunen, S., & Autti-Rämö, I. (2003). Neurocognitive impairment in early adolescence following prenatal alcohol exposure of varying duration. *Child Neuropsychology, 9*, 117–128.

Korkman, M., Kirk, U., Kemp, S. (2007a). *NEPSY–II: Administrative manual*. San Antonio, TX: The Psychological Corporation-Pearson.

Korkman, M., Kirk, U., & Kemp, S. (2007b). *NEPSY–II: Clinical and interpretative manual.* San Antonio, TX: The Psychological Corporation-Pearson.

Krüttner, S., Stepien, B., Noordermeer, J. N., Mommaas, M. A., Mechtler, K., Dickson, B. J., & Keleman, K. (2012). Drosophila CPEB Orb2A mediates memory independent of its RNA-binding domain. *Neuron, 76,* 383.

Lezak, M. D. (1995). *Neuropsychological assessment* (3rd ed.). New York, NY: Oxford University Press.

Lezak, M. D., Howieson, D. B., & Loring, D. W. (2004). *Neuropsychological assessment* (4th ed.). New York, NY: Oxford University Press.

Linder, J. L., & Rosén, L. A. (2006). Decoding of emotion through facial expression, prosody, and verbal content in children and adolescents with Asperger's syndrome. *Journal of Autism & Developmental Disorders, 36,* 769–777.

Locascio, J. J., Growdon, J. H., & Corkin, S. (1995). Cognitive test performance in detecting, staging, and tracking Alzheimer's disease. *Archives of Neurology, 52,* 1087–1099.

Loeb, M., & Binford, J. R. (1968). Variation in performance on auditory and visual monitoring tasks as a function of signal and stimulus frequencies. *Perception and Psychophysics, 4,* 361–367.

Lord, C., Rutter, M., Dilavore, P. C., Risi, S., Gotham, K., & Bishop, S. L. (2012a). *Autism Diagnostic Observation Schedule, Second Edition (ADOS–2) [Manual: Modules 1–4].* Torrance, CA: Western Psychological Services (WPS).

Lord, C., Rutter, M., Dilavore, P. C., Risi, S., Gotham, K., & Bishop, S. L. (2012b). *Autism diagnostic observation schedule, second edition (ADOS–2) [Manual: Modules 1–4].* Torrance, CA: Western Psychological Services (WPS).

Luria, A. R. (1973). *The working brain.* Harmondsworth: Penguin.

Makatura, T. J., Lam, C. S., Leahy, B. J., Castillo, M. T., & Kalpakjian, C. Z. (1999). Standardized memory tests and the appraisal of everyday memory. *Brain Injury, 13,* 355–367.

Malloy, P. F., & Richardson, E. D. (1994). Assessment of frontal lobe functions. Special issue: The frontal lobes and neuropsychiatric illness. *The Journal of Neuropsychiatry and Clinical Neurosciences, 6,* 399–410.

Marinellie, S. A. (2004). Complex syntax used by school-age children with specific language impairment (SLI) in child-adult conversation. *Journal of Communication Disorders, 37,* 517–533.

Mcintosh, D. N., Reichmann-Decker, A., Winkielman, P., & Wilbarger, J. L. (2006). When the social mirror breaks: Deficits in automatic, but not voluntary, mimicry of emotional facial expressions in autism. *Developmental Science, 9,* 295–302.

Meyers, J. E., & Meyers, K. R. (1995). *Rey complex figure test and recognition trial: Professional manual.* Odessa, FL: Psychological Assessment Resources (PAR).

Miller, G. A. (1956). The magical number seven, plus or minus two: Some limits on our capacity for processing information. *Psychological Review, 63,* 81–97.

Miller, M., & Hineshaw, S. P. (2010). Does childhood executive function predict adolescent functional outcomes in girls with ADHD? *Journal of Abnormal Child Psychology, 38,* 315–326.

Miller, M., Ho, J., & Hinshaw, S. P. (2012). Executive function in girls with ADHD followed prospectively into young adulthood. *Neuropsychology, 26,* 278–287.

Milner, B. (1968). Visual recognition and recall after right temporal-lobe excision in man. *Neuropsychologia, 6,* 191–209.

Mitrushina, M. N., Boone, K. B., & D'Elia, L. F. (1998). *Handbook of normative data for neuropsychological assessment.* New York, NY: Oxford University Press.

Miyake, A., Friedman, N. P., Emerson, M. J., Witzki, A. H., & Howerter, A. (2000). The unity and their contributions to complex "frontal lobe" tasks: A latent variable analysis. *Cognitive Psychology, 41,* 49–100.

Moore, T. E. (1988). The case against subliminal manipulation. *Psychology and Marketing, 5,* 297–316.

Morris, J. C., Storandt, M., Miller, P., McKeel, D. W., Proce, J. L., Rubin, E. H., et al. (2001). Mild cognitive impairment represents early-stage Alzheimer's disease. *Archives of Neurology, 58,* 397–405.

Moss, M. B., Killiany, R. J., Lai, Z. C., Rosene, D. L., & Herndon, J. G. (1997). Recognition memory span in rhesus monkeys of advanced age. *Neurobiology of Aging, 18,* 13–19.

Mutchnick, M. G., Ross, L. K., & Long, C. J. (1991). Decision strategies for cerebral dysfunction IV: Determination of cerebral dysfunction. *Archives of Clinical Neuropsychology, 6,* 259–270.

Nauheim, R. S., Mattero, D., & Fucetola, R. (2008). Assessment of patients with mild concussion in the emergency department. *Journal of Head Trauma Rehabilitation, 23,* 116–122.

Nigg, J. T. (2000). On inhibition/disinhibition in developmental psychology: Views from cognitive and personality psychology and working inhibition taxonomy. *Psychological Bulletin, 126,* 220–246.

Nigg, J. T. (2001). Is ADHD a disinhibitory disorder? *Psychological Bulletin, 127,* 571–598.

Nuechterlein, K. H., Parasuraman, R., & Jiang, Q. (1983). Visual sustained attention: Image degradation produces rapid sensitivity decrement over time. *Science, 220,* 327–329.

Nyberg, L. (2008). Structural basis of episodic memory. In J. H. Byrne & H. Eichenbaum (Eds.), *Learning and memory: A comprehensive reference: Memory systems* (Vol. 3, pp. 99–109). San Diego, CA: Elsevier.

Oberman, L. M., & Ramachandran, V. S. (2007). The simulating social mind: The role of the mirror neuron system and simulation in the social and communicative deficits of autism spectrum disorders. *Psychological Bulletin, 133,* 310–327.

Palva, J. M., Monto, S., Kulashekhar, S., & Palva, S. (2010). Neuronal synchrony reveals working memory networks and predicts individual memory capacity. *Proceedings of the National Academy of Sciences, USA, 107,* 7580–7585.

Parker, R. S. (1990). *Traumatic brain injury and neuropsychological impairment: Sensorimotor, cognitive, emotional, and adaptive problems of children and adults.* New York, NY: Spinger-Verlag.

Partiot, A., Verin, M., Pillon, B., Teixeira-Ferreira, C., Agid, Y., & Dubois, B. (1996). Delayed response tasks in basal ganglia lesions in man: Further evidence for a striato-frontal cooperation in behavioral adaptation. *Neuropsychologia, 34*, 709–721.

Pasini, A., Paloscia, C., Alessandrelli, R., Porifirio, M. C., & Curatolo, P. (2007). Attention and executive functions profile in drug naïve ADHD subtypes. *Brain Development, 29*, 400–408.

Pearson. (2007). *NEPSY–II scoring assistant and assessment planner.* [CD-ROM Computer software]. San Antonio, TX: Author.

Pearson. (2007). *NEPSY–II training CD version 1.0.* [CD-ROM Computer software]. San Antonio, TX: Author.

Pearson. (2009a). *WMS–IV scoring assistant.* [CD-ROM Computer software]. San Antonio, TX: PsychCorp Center-II, Author.

Pearson. (2009b). *WMS–IV training CD Version 1.0* [CD-ROM Computer software]. San Antonio, TX: Author.

Pearson. (2021). *Q-global: Better insights. Anytime. Anywhere.* [Internet Web-Based Computer Scoring]. Retrieved from https://qglobal.pearsonclinical.com/qg/login.seam.

Pennington, B. F., & Ozonoff, S. (1996). Executive functions and developmental psychopathology. *Journal of Child Psychology and Psychiatry, 37*, 51–87.

Peterson, B. S., Potenza, M. N., Wang, Z., Zhu, H., Martin, A., Marsh, R., & Yu, S. (2009). An fMRI study of the effects of psychostimulants on default-mode processing during Stroop task performance in youths with ADHD. *American Journal of Psychiatry, 166*, 1286–1294.

Peterson, L. R., & Peterson, M. J. (1959). Short-term retention of individual items. *Journal of Experimental Psychology, 58*, 193–198.

Peterson, R. L., & Pennington, B. F. (2012). Developmental dyslexia. *The Lancet, 379*(9830), 1997–2007.

Pilowsky, T., Yirmiya, N., Arbelle, S., & Mozes, T. (2000). Theory of mind abilities in children with schizophrenia, children with autism, and normally developing children. *Schizophrenia Research, 42*, 145–155.

Pineda, D., Ardila, A., Rosselli, M., Cadavid, C., Mancheno, S., & Mejia, S. (1998). Executive dysfunctions in children with attention-deficit/hyperactivity disorder. *International Journal of Neuroscience, 96*, 177–196.

Polatajko, H. J., & Cantin, N. (2006). Developmental coordination disorder (dyspraxia): An overview of the state of the art. *Seminars in Pediatric Neurology, 12*, 250–258.

Porteus, S. D. (1959). *The Maze Test and clinical psychology.* Palo Alto, CA: Pacific Books.

Pratkanis, A. R., & Greenwald, A. G. (1988). Recent perspectives on unconscious processing: Still no marketing applications. *Psychology and Marketing, 5*, 337–353.

Psychological Assessment Resources (PAR). (2004a). *NAB screening module: Training disk 1.* [DVD computer software]. Lutz, FL: Author.

Psychological Assessment Resources (PAR). (2004b). *NAB screening module: Training disk 2.* [DVD computer software]. Lutz, FL: Author.

Psychological Assessment Resources (PAR). (2004c). *NAB screening module: Training disk 3.* [DVD computer software]. Lutz, FL: Author.

Psychological Assessment Resources (PAR). (2004d). *NAB screening module: Training disk 4.* [DVD computer software]. Lutz, FL: Author.

Psychological Assessment Resources (PAR). (2004e). *NAB screening module: Training disk 5.* [DVD computer software]. Lutz, FL: Author.

Psychological Assessment Resources (PAR). (2004f). *NAB screening module: Training disk 6.* [DVD computer software]. Lutz, FL: Author.

Psychological Assessment Resources (PAR). (2008). *Neuropsychological assessment battery software portfolio (NAB-SP).* [CD-ROM computer software]. Lutz, FL: Author.

Purves, D., Williams, M. S., Nundy, S., & Lotto, B. R. (2004). Perceiving the intensity of light. *Psychological Review, 111*, 142–158.

Quay, H. C. (1997). Inhibition and attention deficit hyperactivity disorder. *Journal of Abnormal Child Psychology, 25*, 7–13.

Raichle, M. E. (2010, March). The brain's dark energy. *Scientific American*, 44–48.

Rao, S. C., Rainer, G., & Miller, E. K. (1997). Integration of what and where in the primate prefrontal cortex. *Science, 276*, 821–824.

Reitan, R. M., & Wolfson, D. (1985). *The Halstead–Reitan Neuropsychological Test Battery: Theory and clinical interpretation.* Tucson, AZ: Neuropsychology Press.

Reitan, R. M., & Wolfson, D. (1986). *Traumatic brain injury, Volume 1: Pathophysiology and neuropsychological evaluation.* Tucson, AZ: Neuropsychology Press.

Rempel-Clower, N. L., Zola, S. M., Squire, L. R., & Amaral, D. G. (1996). Three cases of enduring memory impairment after bilateral damage limited to the hippocampal formation. *The Journal of Neuroscience, 16*, 5233–5255.

Rescorla, R. A. (1968). Probability of shock in the presence and absence of CS in fear conditioning. *Journal of Comparative and Physiological Psychology, 66*, 1–5.

Rescorla, R. A. (1988). Pavlovian conditioning—It's not what you think. *American Psychologist, 43*, 151–160.

Riccio, C. A., Homack, S., Jarratt, K. P., & Wolfe, M. E. (2006). Differences in academic and executive function domains among children with ADHD predominantly inattentive and combined types. *Archives of Clinical Neuropsychology, 21*, 657–667.

Riccio, C. A., Reynolds, C. R., & Lowe, P. A. (2001). *Clinical applications of continuous performance tests.* Toronto, Canada: John Wiley & Sons.

Robertson, I. H., Ward, T., Ridgeway, V., & Nimmo-Smith, I. (1994). *Test of everyday attention.* Bury St. Edmunds, England: Thames Valley.

Roid, G. H. (2003, August). *Continuous norming of tests and research scales: Twenty year update.* Paper presented at the annual meeting of the American Psychological Association, Toronto, Canada.

Rosvold, H. E., Mirsky, A. F., Sarason, I., Bransome, E. D., & Beck, L. H. (1956). A continuous performance test of brain damage. *Journal of Consulting Psychology, 20*, 343–350.

Rucklidge, J. J. (2006). Gender differences in neuropsychological functioning of New Zealand adolescents with and without attention-deficit/hyperactivity disorder. *International Journal of Disability, Development and Education, 53*, 47–66.

Ruff, R. M., & Allen, C. C. (1996). *Ruff 2&7 selective attention test*. Odessa, FL: Psychological Assessment Resources (PAR).

Sabatini, E., Della Penna, S., Franciotti, R., Ferretti, A., Zoccolotti, P., Rossini, P. M., . . . Gainotti, G. (2009). Brain structures activated by overt and covert emotional visual stimuli. *Brain Research Bulletin, 79*, 258–264.

Sanchez-Castaneda, C., Rene, R., Ramirez-Rutz, B., Campdelacreu, J., et al. (2009). Correlations between gray matter reductions and cognitive deficits in dementia with Lewy Bodies and Parkinson's disease with dementia. *Movement Disorders, 24*, 1740–1746.

Sanger, T. D., Daofen, C., Delgado, M. R., Gaebler-Spira, D., Hallet, M., & Mink, J. W. (2006). Definition and classification of negative motor signs in childhood. *Pediatrics, 118*, 2159–2167.

Sargeant, J. (1996). A theory of attention: An information processing perspective. In G. R. Lyon & N. A. Krasnegor (Eds.), *Attention, memory, and executive function* (pp. 57–69). Baltimore: Brookes.

Sargeant, J. (2000). The cognitive-energetic model: An empirical approach to attention-deficit hyperactivity disorder. *Neuroscience and Biobehavioral Reviews, 24*, 7–12.

Sargeant, J. (2005). Modeling attention-deficit/hyperactivity disorder: A critical appraisal of the cognitive-energetic model. *Biological Psychiatry, 57*, 1248–1255.

Sattler, J. M. (2001). *Assessment of children: Cognitive applications* (4th ed.). San Diego, CA: Jerome M. Sattler Publisher.

Sattler, J. M. (2014). *Foundations of behavioral, social, and clinical assessment of children* (6th ed.). LaMesa, CA: Jerome M. Sattler Publisher.

Sattler, J. M., & Ryan, J. J. (2009). *Assessment with the WAIS–IV*. San Diego, CA: Jerome M. Sattler Publisher.

Scoville, W. B., & Milner, B. (1957). Loss of recent memory after bilateral hippocampal lesions. *Journal of Neurology, Neurosurgery & Psychiatry, 20*, 11–21.

Semendeferi, K., & Damasio, H. (2000). The brain and its main anatomical subdivisions in living hominids using MRI. *Journal of Human Evolution, 38*, 317–332.

Shaughnessy, J. J., Zechmeister, E. B., & Zechmeister, J. S. (2015). *Research methods in psychology* (10th ed.). New York, NY: McGraw Hill Education.

Shaw, P., Lalonde, F., Lepage, C., Rabin, C., Eckstrand, K., Sharp, W., Greenstein, D., & Rapoport, J. (2009). Development of cortical asymmetry in typically developing children and its disruption in attention-deficit/hyperactivity disorder. *Archives of General Psychiatry, 66*, 888–896.

Shepard, L. (1980). An evaluation of the regression discrepancy method for identifying children with learning disabilities. *Journal of Special Education, 14*, 79–91.

Sherod, M. G., Griffith, H. R., Copeland, J., Belue, K., et al. (2009). Neurocognitive predictors of financial capacity across the dementia spectrum: Normal aging, mild cognitive impairment, and Alzheimer's disease. *Journal of the International Neuropsychological Society, 15*, 258–267.

Siegel, L. S., & Mazabell, S. (2013). Basic cognitive processes and reading disabilities. In H. L. Swanson, K. R. Harris, & S. Graham (Eds.), *Handbook of learning disabilities* (2nd ed., pp. 186–213). New York, NY: Guilford.

Sigelman, C. K., & Rider, E. A. (2018). *Life-span human development* (9th ed.). Boston, MA: Cengage Learning.

Sivan, A. B. (1992). *Benton visual retention test* (5th ed.). San Antonio, TX: The Psychological Corporation.

Smid, H. G., de Witt, M. R., Homminga, I., & van den Bosch, R. (2006). Sustained and transient attention in the continuous performance tasks. *Journal of Clinical and Experimental Neuropsychology, 28*, 859–883.

Smith, E., & Jonides, J. (1999). Storage and executive processes in frontal lobes. *Science, 283*, 1657–1661.

Snodgrass, J. G., & Corwin, J. (1988). Pragmatics and recognition memory: Applications to dementia and amnesia. *Journal of Experimental Psychology: General, 117*, 34–50.

Snowden, J. S., Goulding, P. J., & Neary, D. (1989). Semantic dementia: A form of circumscribed cerebral atrophy. *Behavioural Neurology, 2*, 167–182.

Sohlberg, M. M., White, O., Evans, E., & Mateer, C. (1992). Background and initial case studies into the effects of prospective memory training. *Brain Injury, 6*, 129–138.

Somerville, J. A., & Stern, R. A. (2001). Effects of length of delay on Rey-Osterrieth Complex Figure Recall [Abstract]. *Journal of the International Neuropsychological Society, 7*, 132.

Spores, J. M. (2012). *Clinician's guide to psychological assessment and testing: With forms and templates for effective practice*. New York, NY: Springer Publishing Company.

Spreen, O., & Benton, A. L. (1977). *Neurosensory Center Comprehensive Examination for Aphasia*. Victoria, BC, Canada: University of Victoria Neuropsychological Laboratory.

Spreen, O., & Strauss, E. (1998). *A compendium of neuropsychological tests: Administration, norms, and commentary* (2nd ed.). New York, NY: Oxford University Press.

Squire, L. R. (1987). *Memory and brain*. New York, NY: Oxford University Press.

Squire, L. R., & Butters, N. (1984). *Neuropsychology of memory*. New York, NY: Guilford Press.

Squire, L. R., & Butters, N. (Eds.). (1992). *Neuropsychology of memory* (2nd ed.). New York, NY: The Guilford Press.

Squire, L. R., & Kandel, E. (1999). *Memory: From mind to molecule*. New York: Scientific American Library.

Squire, L. R., Slater, P. C., & Chace, P. M. (1975). Retrograde amnesia: Temporal gradient in very long-term memory following electroconvulsive therapy. *Science, 187*, 77–79.

Stephan, H., & Andy, O. J. (1969). Quantitative comparative neuroanatomy of primates: An attempt at phylogenic interpretation. *Annals of the New York Academy of Science, 167*, 370–387.

Stephan, H., Baron, G., & Frahm, H. D. (1988). Comparative size of brains and brain structures. In H. Steklis & J. Erwin (Eds.), *Comparative primate biology* (pp. 1–38). New York, NY: Liss.

Stern, C. E., & Hasselmo, M. E. (2008). The neurobiological basis of recognition memory. In J. H. Byrne & H. Eichenbaum (Eds.), *Learning and memory: A comprehensive reference: Memory systems* (Vol. 3, pp. 131–141). San Diego, CA: Elsevier Science.

Stern, R. A., & Prohaska, M. L. (1996). Neuropsychological evaluation of executive functioning. In L. J. Dickenstein, M. B. Riba, & J. M. Oldman (Eds.), *American psychiatric press review of psychiatry* (Vol. 15, pp. 243–266). Washington, DC: American Psychiatric Press.

Stern, R. A., & White, T. (2003). *Neuropsychological Assessment Battery (NAB): Administrative, scoring, and interpretation manual*. Lutz, FL: Psychological Assessment Resources (PAR).

Strauss, E., Sherman, E., & Spreen, O. (2006). *A compendium of neuropsychological tests: Administration, norms, and commentary* (3rd ed.). New York, NY: Oxford University Press.

Stringer, A. Y. (1996). *A guide to neuropsychological diagnosis*. Philadelphia, PA: F. A. Davis.

Stuss, D. T., & Knight, D. F. (Eds.). (2002). *Principles of frontal lobe function*. Oxford, UK Oxford University Press.

Stuss, D. T., Alexander, M. P., Palumbo, C. L., Buckle, L., Sayer, L., & Pogue, J. (1994). Organizational strategies of patients with unilateral or bilateral frontal lobe injury in word list learning tasks. *Neuropsychology, 8*, 355–373.

Stuss, D. T., Eskes, G. A., & Foster, J. K. (1994). Experimental neuropsychological studies of the frontal lobe functions. In F. Boller & J. Grafman (Eds.), *Handbook of neuropsychology* (Vol. 9, pp. 149–185). Amsterdam: Elsevier.

Swets, J. A. (1964). *Signal detection and recognition by human observers*. New York, NY: John Wiley & Sons.

Tanaka, J. W., & Farah, M. J. (1993). Parts and wholes in face recognition. *The Quarterly Journal of Experimental Psychology A: Human Experimental Psychology, 46*, 225–245.

Tanner, W. P., Jr., & Swets, J. A. (1954). A decision-making theory of visual detection. *Psychological Review, 61*(6), 401–409.

Temple, C. M. (1997). Cognitive neuropsychology and its application to children. *Journal of Child Psychology and Psychiatry, 38*, 27–52.

Tobias, P. V. (1995). The brain of the first hominids. In J. P. Changeux & J. Chavaillon (Eds.), *Origins of the human brain*. Oxford: Clarendon Press.

Trappey, C. (1996). A meta-analysis of consumer choice and subliminal advertising. *Psychology and Marketing, 13*, 517–530.

Tremont, G., Halpert, S., Javorsky, D. J., & Stern, R. A. (2000). Differential impact of executive function on verbal list learning and story recall. *The Clinical Neuropsychologist, 14*, 295–302.

Tsal, Y., Shalev, L., & Mevorach, C. (2005). The diversity of attention deficits in ADHD: The prevalence of four cognitive factors in ADHD versus controls. *Journal of Learning Disabilities, 38*, 142–157.

Tulving, E. (1983). *Elements of episodic memory*. Oxford, UK: Clarendon Press.

U.S. Bureau of the Census. (2002). *Statistical abstract of the United States census: 2001*. Washington, DC: Government Printing Office.

U.S. Bureau of the Census. (2004). *Current population survey, October 2003: School enrollment and computer use supplement (Machine-readable data file)*. Washington, DC: Author.

U.S. Bureau of the Census. (2005). *Statistical abstract of the United States: 2004–2005 census*. Washington, DC: Government Printing Office.

U.S. Bureau of the Census. (2010). *United States American community survey 2010*. Washington, DC: Government Printing Office.

Vaughn, A., Epstein, J. N., Rausch, J., Altaye, M., et al. (2011). Relation between outcomes on a continuous performance test and DHD symptoms over time. *Journal of Abnormal Child Psychology, 39*, 853–864.

Vokey, J. R., & Read, J. D. (1985). Subliminal messages: Between the devil and the media. *American Psychologist, 40*, 1231–1239.

Walsh, K. W., & Darby, D. (1999). *Neuropsychology: A clinical approach* (4th ed.). Edinburgh, Scotland: Churchill-Livingston.

Warner, R. M. (2021a). *Applied statistics I: Basic bivariate techniques* (3rd ed.). Thousand Oaks, CA: Sage.

Warner, R. M. (2021b). *Applied statistics II: Multivariable and multivariate techniques* (3rd ed.). Thousand Oaks, CA: Sage.

Wechsler, D. (1997). *Wechsler memory scale, third edition (WMS–III)*. San Antonio, TX: The Psychological Corporation.

Wechsler, D. (2009a). *Wechsler memory scale, fourth edition (WMS–IV): Administration and scoring manual*. San Antonio, TX: The Psychological Corporation-Pearson.

Wechsler, D. (2009b). *Wechsler memory scale, fourth edition (WMS–IV): Technical and interpretative manual*. San Antonio, TX: The Psychological Corporation-Pearson.

Wefel, J. S., Hoyt, B. D., & Massman, P. J. (1999). Neuropsychological functioning in depressed versus nondepressed participants with Alzheimer's disease. *The Clinical Neuropsychologist, 13*, 249–257.

Weis, S., Klaver, P., Reul, J., Elger, C. E., & Fernandez, G. (2004). Temporal and cerebellar brain regions that support both declarative memory formation and retrieval. *Cerebral Cortex, 14*, 256–267.

White, H. K., & Levin, E. D. (2004). Chronic transdermal nicotine patch treatment effects on cognitive performance in age-associated memory impairment. *Psychopharmacology, 171*, 465–471.

White, T., & Stern, R. A. (2003a). *NAB demographically corrected norms manual*. Lutz, FL: Psychological Assessment Resources (PAR).

White, T., & Stern, R. A. (2003b). *NAB psychometric and technical manual*. Lutz, FL: Psychological Assessment Resources (PAR).

White, T., & Stern, R. A. (2003c). *NAB U.S. census-matched norms manual*. Lutz, FL: Psychological Assessment Resources (PAR).

Wilkins, C., Rolfhus, E., Weiss, L., & Zhu, J. (2005, April). *A simulation study comparing inferential and traditional norming with small sample sizes*. Paper presented at the 2005 annual meeting of the American Educational Research association, Montreal, Canada.

Williams, J. M. (1991). *Memory assessment scales*. Odessa, FL: Psychological Assessment Resources (PAR).

Williamson, D. J. G., Scott, J. G., & Adams, R. L. (1996). Traumatic brain injury. In R. L. Adams, O. A. Parsons, J. L. Culbertson, & S. L. Nixon (Eds.), *Neuropsychology for clinical practice: Etiology, assessment, and treatment of common neurological disorders* (pp. 9–64). Washington, DC: American Psychological Association.

Wodka, E. L., Mostofsky, S. H., Prahme, C., Gidley Larson, J. C., et al. (2008). Process examination of executive function in ADHD: Sex and subtype effects. *The Clinical Neuropsychologist, 22*, 826–841.

Yorkston, K. M., & Beukelman, D. R. (1980). An analysis of connected speech samples of aphasic and normal speakers. *Journal of Speech and Hearing Disorders, 45,* 27–36.

Zola-Morgan, S., Squire, L. R., Clower, R. P., & Rempel, N. L. (1993). Damage to the perirhinal cortex exacerbates memory impairment following lesions to the hippocampal formation. *The Journal of Neuroscience, 13,* 251–265.

Zou, L., Chen, W., Shao, S., Sun, Z., Zhong, R., Shi, J., & Song, R. (2012). Genetic variant in KIAA0319, but not in DYX1C1, is associated with risk of dyslexia: An integrated meta- analysis. *American Journal of Medical Genetics Part B: Neuropsychiatric Genetics, 159B,* 970–976.

See Routledge's e-resources website for forms (www.routledge.com/9780367346058).

10 Rating Scales Tests

Overview

This chapter consists of a variety of tests designed to help diagnose *clinical syndromes* or *disorders*. Succinctly, these disorders refer to clusters of intercorrelated symptoms with an identifiable onset, course, and remittance, and which tend to respond to intervention. Although this type of psychopathology is delineated in more detail subsequently, let it suffice to state at this juncture that they were explicitly recognized by the *Diagnostic and Statistical Manual of Mental Disorders, Fourth Edition, Text Revision* (*DMS–IV–TR*; American Psychiatric Association, 2000), which was the last of such editions to employ the *multiaxial system* of diagnosis. This system specifically examined each case according to five dimensions considered to be useful in rendering a comprehensive diagnosis, the first two representing clinical disorders (Axis I) and personality disorders (Axis II). Although such a system was not impeccable, it was believed by many to be pragmatic in terms of conceptualizing psychopathology.

Hence, this organization is reflected at several points within the organization of this book. The first was back in Chapter 3, Section 2, when delineating the diagnostic scheme located in the "Initial Psychological Assessment Report" (see Forms 3.3–3.6). Note the title, "Mental Health, Developmental, and Personality Disorders," just prior to diagnosis wherein personality psychopathology was intentionally culled out. The former two broad labels (i.e., mental health and developmental) represent clinical syndromes, including the latter identifying the frequent disorders seen that manifest early in life and thus implicate neurodevelopmental factors (e.g., *attention-deficit/hyperactivity disorder* or *ADHD*). The second point in the book where the clinical versus personality disorders groupings are readily apparent is here; that is separating rating scales, which have an exclusive focus on detecting clinical syndromes, from personality inventories (Chapter 11) and performance personality tests (Chapter 12). Although the latter do assist in identifying clinical disorders, they are sufficiently comprehensive such that they also detect maladaptive personality traits. In fact, it is arguable that personality psychopathology is their principal focus, which predispose one to various clinical syndromes (see, e.g., McWilliams & Shedler, 2017; Millon, Tringone, Grossman, & Millon, 2020).

With this introduction, what follows is a discussion of what constitutes (a) a clinical disorder and (b) a rating scale. The reason for this is that there are different varieties of each. What constitutes a clinical disorder will be addressed first because the various rating scales are designed to measure different numbers and kinds of such psychopathology. This discussion is ensued by a section devoted to delineating the circumstances under which rating scales should be employed as part of a test battery. Lastly, special insurance coverage issues are discussed, along with suggestions of how they can be managed. Subsequent to these prelusory issues, the rating scales appearing in the book's inventory are presented (see Table 1.1), which represents the core portion of this chapter. As in previous chapters, data tables designed for presenting their scores and interpreting them within a psychological assessment report are also provided.

The Construct of Clinical Disorder

A *clinical disorder* or *clinical syndrome* (hereafter *clinical disorder*) is a clustering or covariance of psychological symptoms which cause dysfunction and typically exhibit the following characteristics: (a) identifiable onset, (b) acute presentation, (c) precipitant for seeking professional therapeutic intervention, and (d) amenability to treatment (American Psychiatric Association, 2000). As it is currently designed, the *DSM–5* classifies disorders according to a categorical system which adopts a *prototypical approach*, although it is increasingly incorporating dimensional aspects into the overall nosology (Barlow, Durand, & Hofman, 2018). That is, each disorder is defined by essential symptoms, which are accompanied by nonessential variations. Furthermore, dimensional facets are progressively being integrated into the diagnostic scheme to improve precision and comprehensiveness (e.g., degree of severity). To meet the criteria for a particular disorder, an individual must manifest the essential symptoms, in addition to a minimum number of nonessential variations. For select disorders, essential criteria include age of onset and symptom duration. Furthermore, certain disorders contain particular characteristics that are deemed relevant to prognosis and treatment planning, including symptom course and degree of severity (e.g., mild, moderate, severe). These are referred to as *specifiers* and is where dimensional facets of diagnosis can be frequently found.

The clinical disorders include all psychological disorders enumerated in each of the initial assessment forms (see Forms 3.3–3.6), with the single exception of *personality disorders*. Personality disorders consist of maladaptive traits or relative consistencies in behavior over time and, to some extent, across different situations. Because many traits are interpersonal in nature, personality disorders are also regarded as lifestyle problems (Widiger, 1997). In either case, their onset is insidious or extremely gradual, usually initiated by both biological and environmental factors that occur during childhood (Nigg & Goldsmith, 1994). Some of these etiological variables include the following: disturbed emotional attachments (Kernberg, 1975, 1984; Nigg & Goldsmith, 1994); exposure to abuse, maltreatment, and early pathogenic care (Guzder, Paris, Zelkowitz, & Marchessault, 1996; Pollock et al., 1990; Westen, 1990); chaotic home environments that included the impulsive behaviors of adults (Millon, 2000); and genetic factors (Lykken, 1995; Nigg & Goldsmith, 1994). The maladaptive traits become increasingly ingrained over time and are usually fully developed by young adulthood (American Psychiatric Association, 2013). Because their onset, course, and nature are considerably different from that of clinical disorders, it is preferable to retain the distinction between the two. This dichotomy is logically consistent with this chapter on rating scales, which focus on the detection of clinical disorders and do not address personality psychopathology per se.

As a final note, because the clinical disorders are still principally categorical in nature as defined and recognized in the *DSM–5*, there continues to exist a considerable amount of symptom overlap. For example, impaired attention and concentration may be associated with ADHD, persistent depressive disorder, bipolar disorder, and generalized anxiety disorder (GAD). Thus, comorbidity is not uncommon, which renders precise differential diagnosis a complicated and arduous task (Krueger & Markon, 2006). The rating scales included in the selected inventory (see Table 1.1 and subsequently) contain many features that render them remarkably useful in making accurate differential diagnoses among the many clinical disorders, including the detection of *comorbidity* (i.e., the presence of co-occurring disorders). Next, the various components of such rating scales are presented, including cautions regarding their use in clinical practice.

Types of Rating Scales Tests

As stated prior, the *rating scales* tests presented in this chapter are used in outpatient mental health and other clinical settings to assist in diagnosing a variety of common clinical disorders, many of them recognized by the *Diagnostic and Statistical Manual of Mental Disorders, Fifth Edition*, (*DSM–5*; American Psychiatric Association, 2013). The various rating scales have formats, domains of coverage, and concerns for response sets as they attempt to enhance their *reliability* (i.e., consistency or accuracy of a test; Cohen & Swerdlik, 2018; Hogan, 2019; Shum, O'Gorman, Creed, Myors, 2017) and *validity* (i.e., precision or truthfulness of a test; Cohen & Swerdlik, 2018; Hogan, 2019; Shum et al, 2017). This section is intended to provide a review of these general issues such that they are readily understood when presented within the core section of this chapter subsequently.

Formats

Rating scale formats concern the (a) type of respondent and the (b) type of item. The respondent refers to the individual who is asked to complete the test and provide its data. The item type regards the manner in which statements or questions are presented to the respondent and the means by which the informant's responses are converted into quantities or scores. These will be discussed next in this order.

Type of Respondent

Rating scales can be classified as *multi-score systems* or *single-score systems* (Hogan, 2019). *Multi-score systems* are a collection of related instruments that act as parallel forms, although they are completed by different respondents who may be in different settings (e.g., parent, teacher, self, other). The forms that comprise multi-score systems contain virtually the same item content and domain(s), although they are worded to match the type of respondent and his or her particular context (i.e., home, school, community). The reader will see a number of rating scales subsequently that are multi-score systems, which provides an opportunity for the examiner to obtain standardized scores concerning an examinee's symptoms from various informants in different environments (e.g., self, parent, teacher).

Data provided by oneself (i.e., a self-report form) is referred to felicitously as self-report data or *S-data* (Larson & Buss, 2021). Because rating scales present items to all respondents using the same content and order, such S-data are tightly controlled and regulated, analogous to a structured interview format (see Chapter 2). Most multi-score systems incorporate self-report forms as one component of the entire measure, usually with a minimum age of about eight years to ensure that sufficient cognitive development has occurred. S-data possesses several advantages, the most obvious being that the individual has access to a wide array of information not available to others (recall episodic long-term memory from Chapter 13; see also Vazire, 2010; Larson & Buss, 2021). However, some caveats associated with S-data are the need for cooperation on the part of the individual, along with the ability to introspect. Thus, if the individual manifests *alexithymia* (i.e., an inability to recognize one's feelings, emotions, and beliefs), or more problematically, *anosognosia* (i.e., an inability to perceive the severity of one's condition due to severe mental distur-bance and/or brain dysfunction), the opportunity to collect S-data would be precluded. This brings us to a viable complementary type of data termed observer data.

Examinees typically have developed meaningful relationships with others who develop impressions of them in various situations or contexts. Therefore, these individuals become potential sources of information regarding the examinee's symptoms and/or functioning. When such individuals complete rating scales from a multi-score system, this is referred to as observer-report data or *O-data* (Larson & Buss, 2021). A key advantage of O-data is that such informants may have access to facts about the examinee not obtainable from other sources, including the individual him- or herself (see, e.g., Fetchenhauer, Groothuis, & Pradel, 2010). Furthermore, in this instance, multiple observ-ers can be employed (e.g., parents, various teachers), which is obviously not possible with S-data (Connelly & Ones, 2010; Paunonen & O'Neill, 2010).

Multi-score systems are invaluable principally from the fact that they permit the accumulation of comparable data from a variety of sources or informants. Comparing the degree of consistency across such ratings affords the oppor-tunity to examine two vital components of psychological testing and measurement: (a) interrater reliability and (b) convergent validity.

First, *interrater reliability* concerns the degree to which individuals who provide separate ratings of an examinee are consistent with each other, hence indicating the degree of consistency or accuracy of the ratings. *Convergent validity* simply asks, "To what degree do different tests provide the same results with respect to a particular construct (e.g., the presence of bipolar disorder)?" Thus, if both the teacher and parent ratings are in the clinical range for symptoms of ADHD, the examiner has both interrater reliability and convergent validity evidence for such diagnosis. Further-more, obtaining data showing the presence of the same disorder (e.g., ADHD) using a different test format (e.g., a performance-based continuous performance test or CPT) would add further convergent validity for that diagnosis, which represents a scientific approach to psychodiagnosis espoused by this book. Attempting to accumulate both interrater reliability and convergent validity for diagnoses using test data accounts for the employment of multi-score systems that are presented in this chapter's major section.

Type of Item

Rating scales most typically present items in the form of brief statements describing mental health symptoms and behavioral problems, along with a variety of formats designed to transform a response into a quantity or score (i.e., the practice of measurement). Examples of statements include, "I feel sad," "I have trouble sleeping," or "I feel worthless." Examples of different response formats include the following: (a) *True–False*; (b) *Yes–No*; or (c) *Disagree Strongly* (score = 1), *Disagree Somewhat* (score = 2), *Neutral* (score = 3), *Agree Somewhat* (score = 4), and *Agree Strongly* (score = 5). The last format represents a *Likert-type scale* (Likert, 1932), which requires respondents to rate the extent to which they disagree or agree with a statement (i.e., a stem). Traditionally, Likert scales present an odd number of response choices to create a middle neutral score, as in the last example. The original Likert scale included 5 choices, although there may be 3, 7, 9, or as many as 11 alternatives, which depends on the degree of discrimination needed or desired when measuring a construct. If there is a preference for essentially forcing respondents toward a direction on the scale (viz., in the *disagree* or *agree* direction), there can be an even number of alternatives, hence having no middlemost alternative.

In most cases, responses to items on a particular scale are added together for a total raw score, hence creating a *sum-mative scale*, which is analogous to adding the number of items answered correctly on a neuropsychological subtest to be later converted into a standard score. Thus, a *summative scale* is one in which responses are added across all its items to create an aggregate or total raw score. Subsequently, total raw scores are usually transformed into a standard score that shows the examinee's exact position in a distribution of peers. The majority of the rating scales presented in this chapter possess one or more summative scales that measure an examinee's degree of symptoms on a specific clinical disorder.

As a final comment regarding item format, the rating scales that are presented subsequently ask respondents to estimate the presence of specified mood, cognitive, affective, or behavioral symptoms during a specified duration (e.g., the past month or six months). They accomplish this in somewhat different ways, although a common approach is to ask about symptom frequency (e.g., ranging from "not at all" to "very often"). Another approach is to ask informants to rate the truthfulness of a statement as applied to the examinee (e.g., ranging from "not true at all" to "very true"). Lastly, some rating scales combine two dimensions (e.g., to rate both the frequency and the degree of truth represented by a particular statement). Taken together, these rating scales represent structured interviews that provide standardized data concerning an examinee for which accurate diagnosis is being sought. Specifically, their ability to quantify a variety of symptoms and disorders in such an efficient manner renders them an invaluable tool in the process of psychological testing in mental health practice. However, there are a number of cautions concerning the use of rating scales that need to be recognized such that they are used appropriately and with due diligence on the part of the examiner. These are addressed when discussing response sets, which threaten the reliability and validity of rating scale diagnostic data.

Domains of Coverage: Multidimensional versus Unidimensional Tests

This section concerns the number and type of clinical disorders that are measured by the rating scales delineated subsequently. A *domain* essentially represents a clinical disorder or general type of clinical disorder (e.g., ADHD, trauma-related disorders). The core section of the chapter begins with presenting *multidimensional tests* (here, rating scales), which means they measure a wide array of clinical disorders or problems. These tests provide scores for multiple scales, each of which measure a different clinical disorder or problems. They are designed to cover different age ranges. The instrument covering the youngest ages do not include self-report forms, although they do provide developmental scales designed to detect potential delays in various skill areas (e.g., play, motor skills).

The *unidimensional tests* focus on one clinical disorder or area of psychopathology and provide detailed data regarding its symptom pattern. This includes such facets as degree, the presence of qualifiers or specifiers (e.g., with or without dissociation), and/or range of effects or *sequelae* (e.g., deficits in one's sense of self, character pathology). An area of psychopathology may refer to its *etiology* (i.e., cause or origin) or general pattern of symptoms (e.g., anxiety disorder, depressive disorder). A good example are measures of trauma-related psychopathology or autism spectrum symptoms (see subsequently). Typically, these tests delve into a single type of psychopathology in such a degree of detail not available on more broad-based multidimensional measures. These are invaluable in cases where the examiner is reasonably certain an examinee manifests a specific type of psychopathology but desires a more detailed profile of unique symptoms along with their severity. For example, an examiner may have convincing evidence that a trauma-related disorder is present but needs an in-depth examination of the symptom profile (e.g., is there dissociation or damage to the examinee's sense of self?). Provision of such detail would be vital in treatment planning or even providing direction for any needed follow-up testing (e.g., personality testing).

It will become apparent that the rating scales to be covered consist of a balanced combination of both multidimensional and unidimensional tests. The former is best used when an examiner is searching for co-occurring disorders or needs to render a refined differential diagnosis among disorders that share similar symptoms yet are fundamentally different (e.g., higher-functioning autism versus social anxiety disorder). The latter are best when the examiner has confidence that a particular class of psychopathology is present and wishes a detailed description of symptoms for well-matched or targeted treatment interventions. Furthermore, many of these are multi-score systems that provide the opportunity to gather data from various sources. The next and final section discusses caveats regarding the use of rating scales. Some of these cautions have been well researched and are accompanied by guidelines for managing them. Others are based on clinical experience. Although anecdotal, they are legitimate concerns to be considered.

Response Sets

As has been stated, rating scales assume a distinctive questionnaire format, essentially representing a structured clinical interview that has been reduced to writing. The assumption here is that there are measurable individual differences in symptom presentation. One of the most efficient ways to measure the quantity and degree of symptoms examinees manifest is to simply ask them or someone who knows them well. However, this assumes that the individual and collaterals are both willing and able to accurately report such symptoms and behavior. Hence, when using rating scales, examiners must be concerned with variables that may impede the accuracy of their answers to items. This section is devoted to examining what are referred to as *response sets*, which are approaches or styles respondents may have to answering rating-scale items that have nothing to do with their content. Because such answers are not based on item content, such response sets are deleterious to both the reliability and validity of the results. Therefore, they must be recognized when they occur in clinical practice. As will be seen, some of the rating scales incorporate attempts to identify one or more of these response sets. All the examples set out in this chapter assume the respondent has sufficient cognitive and reading abilities. Furthermore, some response sets are intentional and done by volition, while others are done without premeditation or conscious awareness.

Careless and Inconsistent Responding

Careless responding occurs when a respondent is unmotivated to complete the rating scale and consequently answers the items rapidly and in a haphazard or random manner. A frequently used stratagem for detecting careless responding is to include items that the vast majority of people will respond to in a particular manner (e.g., "The sun rises in the morning," *True* or *False*). Answers made recurrently in the incorrect direction on a summative scale indicates careless responding, which is commonly referred to as an *infrequency scale* (see, e.g., Jackson & Messick, 1967).

A cousin to careless responding is *inconsistent responding*. In this instance, the respondent is answering similar items in contradictory ways. An example of such responding on a *True–False* rating scale is as follows: "I feel sad most of the time," *True*; "I have felt down about things," *False*. Inconsistent responding can be attributed to several potential reasons, including lack of motivation, being indecisive, or lack of attention and concentration.

Faking

In general, *faking* is a deliberate attempt to distort the presence of symptoms. Faking can manifest in two directions: exaggerating or minimizing symptoms. Exaggerating (also known as faking bad) occurs when the respondent over-reports, embellishes, or amplifies the examinee's symptoms. This could be due to a number of reasons, including *malingering*, which is faking bad for an identifiable reward or desired outcome (see Chapter 17). The underlying reason notwithstanding, exaggerating subverts the accuracy of the results and should be seriously questioned. Some of the instruments in this chapter have scales designed to detect possible faking, although they tend to miss such response sets. Scales designed to detect faking shall be revisited in Chapter 11 on personality inventory tests, which are more effective at detecting such response sets.

Acquiescence

Acquiescence (also known as *yea saying*) represents a proclivity for the respondent to simply agree with the item content irrespective of what is states. Counteracting acquiescence is most effectively done by *reverse scoring* some of the items on a summative scale. Reverse scoring is done by wording two items in opposite directions, then adjusting the scores such that their valence is consistent (e.g., higher scores on both mean more of the construct). For example, on a *depression scale*, an item may read, "I am sad," to which the respondent must answer *True* (score = 1) or *False* (score = 0), followed by an oppositely worded item, "I am happy," to which the respondent again must answer *True* (score = 0) or *False* (score = 1). Notice the reverse in scoring such that higher numbers denote increased depression, which is the construct being measured in this case. Such rewording helps counterbalance an acquiescent response set and also encourages the person to read items more carefully.

Extreme and Middle Responding

Extreme responding reflects a response set in which an individual tends to answer toward either far end of a Likert scale (e.g., *Disagree Strongly* or *Agree Strongly*), hence avoiding the center of the scale. Of course, there may be some individuals who represent the antithesis of extreme responding and prefer *middle responding* (usually the neutral or moderate) portion of the scale. A dichotomous response format (e.g., True–False) may offset either tendency, while an even-numbered set of alternatives helps correct a neutral response tendency by eliminating a centermost score.

Social Desirability

Social desirability represents a tendency to answer items such that the individual appears to be interpersonally accepted, likeable, and attractive. Such respondents tend to deny the presence of any flaws or negative attitudes that may cause others to judge them negatively. This particular response set applies more exclusively to self-report forms and is the most investigated by personality psychologists (see, e.g., Larsen & Buss, 2021). There are two opposing approaches to dealing with social desirability, including (a) viewing it as a distortion to be neutralized or (b) viewing it as a valid personality trait to be measured. Of note, most of those who consider social desirability as a distortion do not also argue that it is done consciously or intentionally. In any case, it should be considered as a potential influence on any self-report forms.

The most effective way to counter this response set is via a *forced-choice* response format wherein examinees must choose which of two or more alternatives of equivalent social desirability best describes their behaviors, attitudes, or symptoms. Of note, none of the rating scales presented subsequently adopt a forced-choice format.

Halo Effect

The *halo effect* occurs when a prior global impression created in one area influences succeeding impressions in other areas (Rosenzweig, 2007; Lachman & Bass, 2010). This preceding broad-based impression can be either positive, producing what has been referred to as a "good guy bias," or negative, hence generating a "bad guy bias" (Hare, 2003, p. 20). In either instance, this represents an error in reasoning. The term "halo" has been applied to this effect as it represents an analogy to the religious concept of a glowing circle surrounding the heads of saints, which signifies that the individual must be an entirely good, moral, and utmost worthy individual.

There are actions a respondent can take to minimize this effect. First, each item should be rated independently. That is, later ratings should not be influenced at all by scores on prior ratings. Second, the rater should review evidence for and against higher or lower ratings and make written notes justifying the final rating. Third, the rater should avoid resolving uncertain scores in the same direction. Thus, if one rating is estimated to be questionably higher, then the next ambiguous rating should be resolved in the lower direction with the overall objective of evenly balancing the tentative ratings. Fourth, and finally, informing each rater that there will be a second informant who provides ratings will augment the motivation of all informants to be more precise in their scoring decisions, which also provides an opportunity for interrater reliability analyses. This concludes a general description of rating scales used in clinical practice. The ensuing section discusses the circumstances under which rating scales should be considered as part of a test battery.

Reasons for Inclusion within a Test Battery

There are three principal uses of rating scales in mental health testing practice. First and foremost, they assist the examiner in detecting the presence of one or more clinical disorders as defined prior. Second, they provide succor in obtaining the medical necessity required by health insurance companies for *preauthorization* (*PA*) of requested testing units. In this role, they essentially act as screening tests. Third, they can be employed to measure the effectiveness of a treatment intervention. These issues will be expounded upon next in such order.

Corroborating the Presence of Clinical Disorders

This section is apportioned into the general supporting role of rating-scale data in diagnosing clinical disorders, the manner in which such data can specifically provide both reliability and validity for a diagnosis (both theoretically and pragmatically), and finally, the more specific and controversial issue of diagnosing bipolar disorder in children. The latter issue is broached by the fact that rating scales yield data that purport to measure unstable mood or mood cycling, which ultimately may lead to a bipolar diagnosis and the prescription of invasive mood stabilizing medication with potentially dangerous side effects (e.g., lithium carbonate). This issue is discussed here because it seemed to be the most felicitous point in the book.

Providing Supplementary Data for Psychodiagnosis

Especially concerning multi-score systems, rating scales can be used to provide corroborating evidence of the presence of clinical disorders that have been evinced by tests with enhanced reliability and validity. Recall that rating scales act as structured interviews that are administered in written format. Thus, their accuracy is contingent upon the opinions of laypeople who typically possess little or no training in psychology or the behavioral sciences. Although the rating scales presented in this book are all standardized and use norms, they typically are not subject to the extensive research afforded both the personality inventories and performance personality tests. Therefore, rating scales should always play a supporting role and never determine a diagnosis independently and without corroboration from either a performance-based cognitive, neuropsychological, or personality test, or by a well-researched personality inventory.

Working within a subsidiary role, multisystem rating scales can yield interrater reliability checks, convergent validity evidence, and/or add increased detail to a diagnosis that have treatment implications, such as degree (e.g., mild, moderate, severe) or subtype of a particular disorder (e.g., ADHD, predominantly inattentive presentation). Single systems of unidimensional rating scales can confirm a strongly suspected diagnosis while adding a significant amount of detail to the diagnosis, especially regarding nonessential symptom variations (e.g., PTSD with or without dissociation).

Interrater Reliability and Convergent Validity in Psychological Testing

The approach to psychological testing espoused in this book borrows from the *Multitrait-Multimethod Matrix* (*MTMM*) logic proposed by Campbell and Fiske (1959), which was developed to provide a research methodology for the theoretically based notion of the *nomological network* (Cronbach & Meehl, 1955). Briefly, the nomological network was a lawful organization of psychological constructs and their observable manifestations, which together provided evidence that a psychological test was actually measuring the trait it claimed to measure (i.e., *construct validity*). The problem with this proposal was that it was entirely theoretical and did not provide guidance as to how to put this into practice. The MTMM method did just that, claiming that validity could be empirically shown in two ways; convergent validity and discriminant validity. In particular, *convergent validity* was demonstrated when tests that measured similar constructs were significantly correlated (e.g., narcissism and psychopathy), while *discriminant validity* was shown when tests that measured different constructs were not significantly correlated (e.g., IQ and show size).

The MTMM method put these two kinds of validity into action by comparing tests of the same and dissimilar traits and the same and dissimilar methods. Of special significance were high correlations between tests of the same trait but of different methods (e.g., a rating scale versus a performance-based personality test both measuring the presence of clinical levels of depression), also known monotrait–heteromethod comparisons that showed the strongest evidence of validity. Additionally, monomethod–monotrait correlations are also expected to be significant and perhaps the largest correlations because they shared the most characteristics and are taken as evidence for test reliability.

So how are these seminal ideas applied to psychological testing cases? It is most prudent for a testing psychologist to order tests of different informants and formats because when they provide similar outcomes, they provide the most convincing evidence for the construct validity of a particular diagnosis. Technically, two different informants using the same rating scale would be considered a monomethod–monotrait strategy, hence providing interrater reliability for a diagnosis. Further, a test of a different format (e.g., a performance-based personality test; see Chapter 16), and in this example, a different informant (i.e., the examinee), which provides evidence consistent with a rating scale, would represent a heteromethod–monotrait comparison and hence the strongest evidence for the validity of a diagnosis.

What is being advised here is that the testing psychologist merely utilize the MTMM logic in the practice of psychological testing. Within the context of a report, the concurrence between raters is framed as providing interrater agreement or reliability for a diagnosis, and an agreement between tests of different methods or formats as evidence for the convergent validity of a diagnosis, the latter of which is also correct considering that the American Psychological Association (2007) defines all types of validity as contributing to construct validity, with the latter superseding all types of validity. Convergent validity is simply when two tests agree on the same trait or construct and such evidence is considered to contribute to overall construct validity.

The Issue of Diagnosing Bipolar Disorder in Childhood

Diagnosing bipolar psychopathology in children is controversial among many clinicians. Furthermore, rating-scale data may play at least a partial role in rendering that diagnosis because such measures contain scales that purport to measure such symptomatology. Therefore, this issue is briefly addressed with both research data and the author's opining prior to moving on to subsequent topics.

Empirical findings indicate that children and young adolescents can and do develop bipolar disorder, although usually with a somewhat different symptom presentation as compared to older adolescents and adults (Geller & Luby, 1997). In particular, symptoms more commonly manifest as a mixed episode including depression, irritability, and outbursts of temper (versus euphoria), and cycling is significantly more rapid and ongoing, thus rendering differential diagnosis from that of ADHD and *oppositional defiant disorder* (*ODD*) extremely challenging (National Institute of Mental Health, 2001; Weller, Weller, & Fristad, 1995).

Furthermore, early detection is crucial considering the accumulating evidence that such early onset may indicate a more virulent variety of bipolar disorder, compared to the more typical onset in older adolescence and young adulthood (Carlson & Kashani, 1988; Geller & Luby, 1997). Also relevant, 2003 survey data revealed that as many as 1% of children and adolescents were diagnosed with bipolar disorder, which represents an increase of 40% over the previous ten years (Holden, 2008). Such a remarkable increase, at least in part, may be attributed to our enhanced ability to measure and diagnose bona fide cases of this disorder using such symptom rating scales as the Conners EC. Finally, it is anticipated that future editions of the *DSM* will amend the diagnostic criteria for bipolar psychopathology as applied to children such that it becomes more correspondent with evidence of its idiosyncratic symptom presentation (Nevid, Rathus & Green, 2011).

Obtaining Preauthorization for Supplemental Testing

Another valid use of a rating scale is for scanning the data for any disorders that may have to this point gone undetected but now show a distinct potential to be present for a comprehensive accounting of the presenting symptoms. However, this use pertains to multidimensional-type rating scales, which by design provide standard scores for a variety of disorders. For example, a six-year-old child was once referred for testing with a directive to rule out *obsessive-compulsive disorder* (*OCD*). In this case, the presenting symptoms included repetitive behaviors, such as lining up toys for hours in a particular order, along with a fascination about washing machines and how they operated. Although the personality and rating-scale data were only subthreshold regarding OCD, the parent and teacher ratings were both positive for *autism spectrum disorder* (*ASD*); in fact, both manifested near maximum scores. Consequently, such rating-scale data were sufficient for (a) detecting the potential presence of a previously unsuspected disorder and (b) obtaining PA to formally test for such psychopathology using the *Autism Diagnostic Observation Schedule, Second Edition* (*ADOS–2*; Lord, Luyster, Gotham, & Guthrie, 2012; Lord, Rutter, Dilavore, Risi, Gotham, & Bishop, 2012; see Chapter 9); *NEPSY–II* Social Perception subtests (reference; see Chapter 13); and *Gilliam Autism Rating Scale, Third Edition* (*GARS–3*; Gilliam, 2014a; see later in this chapter). In this sense, the rating-scale measure is assuming the unintended role of a screening device. As such, rating scales can also be employed as a screening device in the event PA for testing has been denied.

For example, the state of Indiana offers families with low income levels a health insurance program termed Healthy Plan Indiana (HIP), with remarkably stringent criteria for determining the medical necessity for psychological testing. In part, this program does not recognize rating scales as psychological tests for purposes of PA, irrespective of whether measure is standardized and includes a representative sample of peers. However, rating scales can be used to supplement clinical interview data to demonstrate the medical necessity for testing even when dealing with insurance carriers such as HIP.

For example, a nine-year-old female was referred to determine if she had ADHD. Subsequent to clinical interview, a multi-score system rating scale was ordered, including parent and teacher forms, along with two CPT tests. Because this family had HIP for health insurance, the requested testing units for the rating scales were summarily denied, although so were the units requested for the CPT tests. The lack of medical necessity was ostensibly due to the fact that the presenting symptoms were sufficiently clear and consistent to provide such diagnosis. Consultation with the parents was done regarding the denial, and the parents were advised to complete the rating scales irrespective of said denial. After scoring the parent and teacher forms, there was an unequivocal discrepancy between the data, with the former being negative for ADHD and the latter providing scores that were clearly elevated within the clinical range. These data were added to the initial assessment report, which was resubmitted with a request for a peer consultation with a representative from HIP. Because there was now conflicting evidence regarding ADHD, all units for the two CPT tests were afforded PA. To complete this case, the girl scored consistently in the normal range on both CPT tests, hence being negative for ADHD. She was ultimately diagnosed with a stress-related adjustment disorder with anxiety, associated with conflict occurring between her parents, which accounted for her difficulty paying attention at school and the presenting symptoms. To conclude, rating-scale data in this case were instrumental in obtaining PA for ADHD testing, which assisted in avoiding the prescription of psychostimulants to a nine-year-old who did not have ADHD (i.e., a false positive result leading to unnecessary treatment). Furthermore, this was accomplished with an insurance program that does not even recognize rating scales as bona fide psychological tests.

Measuring the Effectiveness of Treatment Intervention

Finally, rating scales can be employed to measure the effectiveness of particular types of treatment intervention, whether they be biomedical, psychotherapeutic, or behavioral. This can be done in two contexts: (a) as part of a psychological testing case and (b) during a therapy session. In the former case, this occurs when a patient is being treated for a working diagnosis, and testing is focused on detecting other co-occurring disorders. For instance, a patient may have a working diagnosis of ADHD and is being referred to rule out a mood or anxiety disorder. In such cases, if a multisystem, multidimensional rating scale has been ordered as part of the test battery, it behooves the examiner to report and interpret any data relevant to that working diagnosis. The principal rationale for doing this is to ensure that the current treatment regimen is being efficacious in remitting the symptoms of the incoming working diagnosis. For example, in a number of child cases, an examinee's ADHD symptoms remained elevated well within the clinical range on both parent and teacher forms, despite being medicated for the disorder, and thus the examinee was either acting out in frustration or was actually developing a mood or anxiety disorder due to their failure to control such symptoms.

The other treatment-related use of rating scales is to administer and score them at various points during therapy sessions. In fact, many of the instruments presented subsequently possess computer scoring capable of comparing multiple administrations across time and to graph the results. A visual presentation of symptom type and degree over time can be extremely therapeutic and can be employed to determine whether termination is indicated. Because this use of rating scales is not relevant to testing per se, it is beyond the scope of this book and is not discussed further. Suffice it to state that many rating scales have this capability, principally due to their efficiency.

Summary

To reiterate, this section delineated three ways rating scales can be employed in mental health practice, two of which pertain to psychological testing. They included corroborating the presence of disorders, helping to establish the medical necessity for testing, and measuring the effectiveness of treatment intervention for certain disorders. The various rating scales are presented in the ensuing section, which represents the principal part of this chapter. The section will begin with multi-score, multidimensional rating scales, presenting them in chronological order, followed by unidimensional rating scales that provide a detailed analysis of a particular disorder, type, area, or genre of psychopathology.

The Rating Scales Tests

This section presents each of the rating scales enumerated within this book's test inventory (see Table 1.1, Chapter 1). As such, it represents the central portion of this chapter. It begins with two multisystem, multidimensional measures, which are presented in chronological order (i.e., according to the age range of their standardization samples). These are the most frequently used in clinical practice, largely attributed to their comprehensiveness and multi-score features that permit interrater reliability and convergent validity analyses so crucial to measuring children's symptoms and behaviors.

Conners Early Childhood

The Conners Early Childhood begins presentation of the rating-scale instruments because it covers the youngest age cohort. This is also evinced by its inclusion of both behavior problem scales and developmental milestones scales. The latter is a special feature not found in other rating scales, especially those that are applicable to older age groups.

Synopsis

The *Conners Early Childhood* (*Conners EC*; Conners, 2009) is a multi-informant (i.e., multi-score) rating-scale instrument, which is normed on young children aged 2 years, 0 months to 6 years, 11 months. It includes five forms based on the type of (a) observer respondent and (b) type of data desired. The two kinds of informants are parents or parent surrogates (e.g., foster parents, guardians), and teacher/childcare workers. As alluded to previously, this age range precludes self-report ratings due to insufficiently developed cognitive abilities and psychological mindedness (see, e.g., Wellman, 1990, 2014). Additionally, for each informant, there are the following versions: (a) full-length forms that provide data on clinical and behavioral symptoms, global problem areas, and developmental milestones; (b) short forms that yield the same data as the former, although including only a partial set of scale items more conducive for screening purposes (see Chapter 5); (c) behavior forms that cover only the clinical and behavioral symptom scales; (d) global index forms that are circumscribed to measuring general problem areas (see subsequent); and (e) developmental forms that focus only on the measurement of various milestones as observed by the informant (i.e., these are not performance-based scales). The principal focus in this section will be on the full-length forms because they provide all the scores used by the data tables designed for reporting and interpreting the Conners EC results within a psychological assessment report.

The Conners EC consists of a number of features that make this rating scale extremely useful in the assessment of very young children, especially those transitioning from infancy and toddlerhood to the preschool and early elementary grades (i.e., K–1). With such a young population, testing must rely on performance-based developmental and cognitive tests and on observer-based ratings. The special features of the Conners EC include the following: (a) assessment of precursors to major clinical syndromes, (b) detection of developmental delays, (c) the use of multiple informants, (d) validity scales, (e) computer scoring, and (f) English and Spanish versions.

Norm Reference Sample

Standardization consisted of 3,281 assessments, both from the general population (from which norms were produced) and a clinical sample. Hence, the focus here is on delineating the characteristics of the sample drawn from the general population. The general population sample was apportioned into 1,315 assessments using the Parent Form and 1,252 assessments using the Teacher/Childcare Form. Of these, 800 assessments were extracts from each to represent the norm reference sample for that particular form. The remaining assessments were utilized for other analyses, such as for *construct validity*.

Data collection was done from September 2006 through October 2008. The samples for both the Parent and Teach/Childcare Forms consisted of 40 males and 40 females in each of 10 6-month age groupings ranging from 2 to 6 years; hence, 400 boys and 400 girls. The samples were stratified according to race/ethnicity, parent education level, and geographic region according to proportions reported in the 2000 U.S. census (U.S. Bureau of the Census, 2000). Parent education level was defined as (a) high school diploma or lower; (b) two-year college, vocational training, or apprenticeship; and (c) four-year college or higher.

Administration

The beginning administrative issue is determining which of the various Conners EC forms to employ. Because this instrument is being considered as part of a formal test battery, the choices are focused on the two full-length forms for parent and teacher/childcare provider. If the child is enrolled in daycare, preschool, a combined daycare–preschool program, or formal schooling (i.e., kindergarten or first grade), both parent and teacher/childcare forms should be given. If a child is just beginning such a program, a minimum of one month of observation of the child (see subsequently) is needed prior to rendering such ratings. If two parents want to provide ratings, they are usually asked to complete the items in consultation with each other and to resolve any discrepancies between themselves. This tends to result in more reliable and valid results compared with two separate forms wherein discrepancies can be measured although not resolved. The rationale is that the child's behavior is being observed in comparable home environments where discrepancies in ratings can be attributable mostly to the informants and not so much the environment. This stratagem is especially appropriate if a teacher or childcare provider is available to afford ratings in a completely different environment. If the teacher/childcare ratings are not available, obtaining ratings from two separate individuals in parenting roles is a more viable strategy.

These forms provide the maximum data yield without placing inordinate demands on the respondent that may threaten the reliability and validity of the ratings. More specifically, the full-length forms can be completed in approximately 25 minutes. This provides data on all validity scales, behavior scales, the global impairment scales, and developmental milestones scales. A sixth-grade reading level is required to sufficiently comprehend the items, which should cover the vast majority of selected respondents. The informants are asked to rate the child according to their observed behavior over the past month. This implies that the informant be familiar with the child's behavior for a minimum of 30 days, especially when considering teachers and childcare workers.

There are generally two types of items, one for behavior items and one for developmental milestone items. The former asks the respondent to rate the child's behavior according to either the degree of truth or the degree of frequency as follows: (a) 0 = *Not true at all* (*Never, Seldom*); (b) 1 = *Just a little true* (*Occasionally*); (c) 2 = *Pretty much true* (*Often, Quite a bit*); and (d) *Very much true* (*Very often, Very frequently*). The latter items ask the respondent to rate how frequently the child demonstrates each skill without assistance as follows: (a) 0 = *No* (*Never or rarely*), (b) 1 = *Sometimes*, and (c) *Yes* (*Always or almost always*). Of note, the developmental milestones scales are reverse scored to make them consistent with the behavior scales (viz., higher scores indicate greater indications of delays or problems). Informants are asked to provide a single rating for each item, to consider whether the examinee's behavior is more or less typical than for a child of the same age, and to make their best estimate even if uncertain.

Administration can be done by the rater online or by pencil-and-paper hard copy. The latter is preferable because frequently there is a request to obtain both parent and teacher/childcare ratings, which is easier to obtain by hard copy forms. They also become part of the testing file for easier reference. Lastly, omitted items are those which are (a) not marked or are (b) improperly marked (e.g., double-marked, marked in-between two alternatives). The Conners EC manual (Conners, 2009) provides a table that indicates the maximum number of omissions permitted before certain scales become invalid (Table 3.2, p. 24), along with a computational scheme to use for prorating final raw score totals if the total number of omissions does not exceed the aforesaid maximum.

Scoring

Scoring the full-length forms can be accomplished online for a fee per score report and by computer scoring software. The Conners EC Scoring Software (Multi-Health Systems, 2009) provides unlimited scoring for a single fee and is loaded onto a computer via thumb drive. The analyses include optional test–retest statistical comparisons to measure changes in symptom course and response to treatment, along with interrater comparisons. If this instrument is to be used frequently, including the *Conners Early Childhood, Behavior, Short Version, Parent Form* (*Conners EC-BEH-SP*; Conners, 2009) for screening purposes, then the latter is advised because the unlimited scoring USB key will pay for itself in time. This is a consistent rule to follow for the majority of psychological testing instruments that provide an unlimited computer-scoring option.

The computer scoring will deliver all the following data: (a) standardized *T*–scores with a *mean* of 50 and *standard deviation* (*SD*) of 10, which are *linear transformations* of the total raw scores for each scale; (b) *percentiles* (P) and *percentile ranks* (*PR*), which are empirically based upon the distribution of raw scores in the norm reference sample and not the theoretical standard normal distribution; and (c) a *standard error of measurement* (*SEM*) for each scale. The latter two types of data are optional, although are vital to report for a more comprehensible and complete interpretation of the diagnostic results. All of these scores are based upon gender-specific norms; that is, the child is compared only to their biologically assigned sex, which is the most common considering that this variable has a significant impact on behavior (e.g., males are more aggressive than females [see, e.g., Archer, 2009]). However, a combined gender-norms option is available in the event the examiner desires an age-corrected comparison without controlling for the effects of sex.

Recall that PRs show the percentage of the norm reference sample (which represents the population of same-aged peers) that the examinee scores equal to or higher than, a datum that is much easier for laypeople to understand. Also recall that the *SEM* represents the potential error in estimating the examinees' true scores from their observed scores, which is especially noteworthy when using non-experts in providing test data for purposes of psychodiagnosis. When two *SEM*s are added to and subtracted from the obtained score, an estimated 95% confidence interval is obtained; that is, it can be stated that the examinee's true score falls in such interval with 95% certainty, which is a high degree of confidence. In any case, all these data are needed when using the data tables that have been prepared for reporting the Conners EC results within a psychological testing report, which is presented next.

I have prepared two data tables for reporting the Conners EC results within a psychological assessment report. The first is the Conners Early Childhood, Parent Form (Conners EC-P) when reporting only parent ratings (see Form 10.1). This form is to be used when the child is not currently enrolled in either daycare or an academic program and will not be for the foreseeable future. The second includes entries for both the Conners Early Childhood, Parent Form and Teacher/Childcare Form (Conners EC-P and Conners EC-T/C), which is to be employed when both types of informants are available, hence exploiting the multi-score feature of this instrument (see Form 10.2). Having access to only the teacher/childcare ratings without the parent ratings has been so rare that such a form has not been devised for such a scenario. If such occurs, the data tables for parent ratings only (Form 10.1) can be easily transformed into a teacher/childcare provider form by simply supplanting the titles, or the parent and teacher/childcare provider form (Form 10.2) can be used by simply inserting double-dashed marks in all of the parent rows, each of which denote an absence of score reporting due to excessive item omissions on the part of the informant and/or improper administration.

Because both forms present virtually identical data for one (Form 10.1) and two different informants simultaneously (Form 10.2), both are described at the same time while apportioning the subsequent sections into the different types of scales. Where the two forms diverge in terms of substance, these discrepancies will be delineated in more detail. In order of appearance, three tables report the following core data: (a) validity scales; (b) behavioral scales or BEH (which include global index scales); and (c) developmental milestones scales, or DM. These tables shall be discussed in said sequence.

VALIDITY SCALES

The validity scales are reported directly in raw score units. Note that the parent ratings and teacher/childcare ratings are juxtaposed to facilitate interrater comparisons, in addition to maximizing the efficiency of data presentation. Data within Table 1 (Forms 10.1 and 10.2) identify test-taking response sets (see prior discussion on response sets) that may compromise the veracity of the subsequent ratings. Thus, Table 1 should always be included first in the analysis. There are three such response sets, including (a) overly favorable ratings, (b) overly harsh ratings, and (c) contradictory ratings. The top row of Form 10.2 apportions the table equally into parent ratings (denoted by "P") and teacher/caregiver ratings (denoted by T/C). This order prioritizes the parent ratings when both informants are available because such ratings are based on a greater sampling of behavior across both time and situations. As regarding both Forms 10.1 and 10.2, Table 1 enumerates first the validity scale name, followed by the ensuing order for each respondent: (a) raw score and (b) dichotomous interpretation (i.e., either the scale showed or did not show the stipulated invalid response set). The language used to describe the scale interpretations was based on the more elaborate narrative descriptions provided in the accompanying manual (Conners, 2009, pp. 37–38). The raw scores should be inserted first and the corresponding results so indicated.

General tabular notes define the directional meaning of higher raw scores and the "--" symbol for identifying non-scorable scales. For convenience, three of the most frequently occurring narrative interpretations of Table 1 results have been drafted. Fortunately, both parent and teacher/childcare ratings typically show valid results. Hence, this is the first available narrative interpretation for both Forms 10.1 and 10.2. However, occasionally the parent ratings alone or one of the two raters' manifests evidence of invalidity. In practice, negative impressions have been found to be most common, followed by inconsistency.

Hence, as applied to the parent ratings alone, two versions of invalidity have been drafted; that is, questionably valid and completely invalid. The former shows an invalid tendency that renders the subsequent ratings reasonably accurate, although in need of some supporting evidence. The latter shows an exaggerated response set that virtually invalidates the remaining ratings and precludes reporting them to avoid giving a distorted interpretation of the child's functioning. Diagnostic terms can be misleading even when reported within a context of extreme caution. Hence, the better practice in such instances is to simply not report the results.

As regarding Form 10.2, narrative interpretations must address instances wherein one rater shows consistent validity while the second evinces invalid response tendencies. These interpretations argue that the latter's subsequent scores should be deemed as accurate only when consistent with the valid ratings and/or other test data or diagnostic information deemed reliable and valid. That is, sufficient corroboration is required before validity is attributed to such results. Interpretations have been drafted to cover either scenario. Finally, there are two pre-drafted excerpts that cover both parent and teacher/childcare ratings being either questionably valid or consummately invalid. These are comparable to those drafted for the parent ratings that interpret questionable and clearly invalid results. The latter precludes reporting the subsequent ratings, as was done for the parent ratings alone.

BEHAVIORAL SCALES

Table 2 in both Forms 10.1 and 10.2 provides the standard *T*–scores for selected Conners EC behavioral scales. Those listed in the table are those found to be most useful in rendering *DSM–5* differential diagnoses within this young age group. They have been enumerated within the table based on two criteria: (a) their measuring the same or similar *DSM–5* disorders and (b) the frequency with which that particular disorder is tested for in clinical practice among this cohort. Therefore, those that measure the most frequently suspected disorders appear first or toward the top of the listing.

Prior to reviewing the specific organization of Table 2, behavior scale names and *DSM–5* disorders most germane to those scales will be listed. This is necessary because there is not as direct a correspondence between the two as there is for the older-age *Conners Comprehensive Behavior Rating Scales* (*Conners CBRS*; Conners, 2008) discussed in the succeeding section.

Using the same row sequence as presented in Table 2, the behavior scales and their respective *DSM–5* disorders are as follows: (a) Inattention-Hyperactivity—ADHD; (b) Restless-Impulsive—ADHD; (c) Defiance-Temper—ODD; (d) Aggression—*conduct disorder (CD)*; (e) Social Functioning—*social pragmatic communication disorder (SPCD)*; (f) Atypical Behaviors—*ASD*; (g) anxiety—*generalized anxiety disorder (GAD)*; (h) Mood and Affect—*persistent depressive disorder* (also known as *dysthymic disorder*); and (i) Emotional Lability—*disruptive mood dysregulation disorder (DMDD)*, *cyclothymic disorder*, or pediatric bipolar disorder.

In Form 10.2, Table 2 maintains the juxtaposition of parent and teacher/childcare ratings for purposes of interrater comparisons, hence exploiting the multi-informant facet of this instrument. This is reflected in columns two, three, and four as parent (all denoted "P") and columns four, five, and six as teacher/childcare ratings (all denoted "T/C"). In columnar order of presentation, the body of Table 2, Form 10.1 includes the following: (a) behavior scale name; (b) parent standardized *T*–scores, including potential asterisk denoting statistical significance; (c) 68% CI; (d) empirically measured PR (i.e., the distribution of raw scores in the norm reference sample); and (e) the symptoms measured by each scale. Note that the CI that is used increases precision, although with a concomitant loss in confidence. Hence, the examiner merely adds and subtracts one *SEM*, which is provided by the computer-scoring software (see subsequent). This is in contrast to the cognitive measures (i.e., Chapters 7, 8, and 9), which tend to produce greater reliability or precision in measuring its intended constructs. This practice will be apparent throughout this and the ensuing two chapters, which target clinical and personality-type constructs that are less precisely measured. The only exception applies to the *sensory processing (integration)* measures presented later in this chapter, which manifest the greatest degree of measurement precision. Hence, a reduction in confidence to achieve more reasonable precision was not necessary in this instance. Perhaps the reason lies in the fact that sensory perception most resembles a cognitive versus behavioral construct. Form 10.2 retains the same order of data for each rater, beginning with the parent ratings, followed by the teacher/childcare provider ratings, and ending with the measured symptoms of each scale. The latter are based upon the behavior scale and global index descriptions available in the manual (Conners, 2009, Tables 4.4 and 4.6, pp. 40–41). The symptom descriptions are emended to enhance test interpretation and reader comprehension while maintaining accuracy. Also emphasized are certain symptom descriptors that had considerable evidence of validity (Conners, 2009, pp. 137–142).

General tabular notes denote the following: (a) *T*–score mean and *SD*, (b) directional meaning of higher scores, (c) import of the statistical significance asterisk(s), and (d) "--" the meaning of the not-reported symbol. Specific tabular notes define the meaning of the various *T*–score elevations, which are delineated in the interpretation section to follow, and the meaning of various table abbreviations (e.g., defining the meaning of PR, *SEM*, and CI). For purposes of brevity, it is advisable to delete the behavior scales that are either (a) not relevant to a particular case's differential diagnostic issues or (b) fail to detect previously unsuspected disorders that may actually be present and account for the presenting symptoms. The reason is that rating-scale data play an auxiliary role in test interpretation. As such, only those data relevant to the principal analysis should be reported, otherwise the main points may be obfuscated by excessive amounts of supplementary scores.

DEVELOPMENTAL MILESTONES SCALES

Lastly, Table 3 provides the developmental milestones (DM) scale data. In contrast to Tables 1 and 2, which are typically requisite to the analysis, Table 3 is discretionary and most pertinent in cases containing suspected neurodevelopmental delays. These involve testing for ADS, *intellectual disability (ID)*, early screening for a potential *specific learning disorder (SLD)*, and *neurocognitive disorder*, which, although rare, can manifest in early childhood (Anderson, Northam, Hendy, & Wrennall, 2001).

Table 3 is designed as was Table 2, although here the focus is on potential developmental delays in key skill sets. The measured skills were culled from Table 4.7 in the manual (Conners, 2009, Table 4.7, p. 42). The same *T*–score ranges are employed in interpreting abnormal elevations (Conners, 2009, p. 34), which is further delineated in the ensuing section. Once again, this permits the same discretionary application of the statistical significance asterisk(s) in Table 3 as in Table 2. Lastly, general table notes are analogous to those of Table 2.

Interpretation

Assuming the validity data show accurate and truthful responding, interpretation of the Conners EC data focuses on the *T*–score elevations and, as regarding the multi-informant Form 10.2, the analysis of interrater agreement or reliability. According to the manual (Conners, 2009, Table 4.1, p. 34), the *T*–score ranges are apportioned into five categories, with the lowest three essentially representing within–normal limits symptom levels. In particular, 30–39 is a low score, 40–59 is an average score, and 60–64 is a high average score, which leaves the highest two ranges as atypically elevated (i.e., 65–69) and very elevated (i.e., 70–90). Because testing in clinical practice focuses on the identification of pathological functioning, the interpretive scheme can be curtailed into a more efficient three-category system, which effectively integrates the lowest three ranges into a larger within–normal limits category. That is, in clinical practice, there is no need to make discriminations between different levels of normal functioning, although differentiating normal versus select levels of abnormal functioning is more efficient and thus a more prudent decision.

Therefore, the behavioral scales employ a trichotomous interpretation scheme based on the standardized scores as follows: (a) *T*–score 30–64 is *within normal limits*, (b) *T*–score 65–69 is *elevated* (one asterisk is amended to the numerical score), and (c) *T*–score 70–90 is *very elevated* (two asterisks are amended to the numerical score). This interpretation scheme is conveniently placed within a specific note to Table 2 to assist the examiner in data analysis and the reader of the report in comprehending the data output. In Form 10.1, the examiner should search for scores that corroborate other test results based on more reliable and valid measures. In Form 10.2, the examiner should engage in the added analysis of interrater reliability. Hence, not only is the examiner to search for corroboration of other test data but he or she is also to attempt to determine if and to what extent the raters agree on their observations of the child's behavior and symptom presentation.

To assist in the interpretative process, inserted pre-drafted excerpts of varying test-result scenarios have been inserted. They are organized in terms of clinical syndrome or disorder, which can be identified by a diagnostic acronym or summary label. Regarding the parent ratings only (Form 10.1), there are most commonly two excerpts per clinical disorder as follows: (a) two scales measuring clinically similar disorders (e.g., ODD and CD as *externalizing behavior disorders*) are either both normal or both clinically elevated (i.e., an elevated or very elevated score) or both consistent with each other, or (b) only one of the two scales measuring similar but diagnostically divergent disorders is clinically elevated. In the latter case, there is likely a crucial differential diagnosis between two very similar disorders that needs to be corroborated (e.g., inattentive versus hyperactive-impulsive ADHD types). Ipsative analysis of the relative positions of the scale CIs can assist in determining significant differences among the scales. Occasionally, a scale does not have a companion of similar symptoms (e.g., the anxiety behavioral scale) in which only one excerpt is needed (i.e., either it is or it is not clinically elevated), or there are more than two potential diagnoses (e.g., emotional lability may indicate three different mood disorders, including depressive disorder, pediatric bipolar disorder, and disruptive mood dysregulation disorder for those six years of age). In such cases, the excerpt is modified to adjust for the different possible scenarios. Finally, Form 10.2 consists of one additional excerpt per clinical disorder, which describes a scenario in which the two raters are providing significantly conflicting results, which could mean symptoms are atypical or manifesting in different environments (i.e., they are situation specific, which suggests a stress-induced disorder). In any case, the advice is to search for additional data that can help resolve the discrepant ratings.

Lastly, Table 3 DM data are interpreted using the same trichotomous scheme based on *T*–score elevations. Here, high scores show increasing evidence of delay, which seems paradoxical in the sense that performance-based cognitive or adaptive behavior scores are usually interpreted in the opposite direction (i.e., higher scores mean more adequate functioning or ability). However, it must be recalled that these items are reverse scored to be consistent with the behavior scales (viz., higher scores mean more problems). Therefore, the psychologist must be cautious here to correctly interpret higher scores as evidence of increasing delay. Pre-drafted excerpts follow Table 3 for both Forms 10.1 and 10.2. Once again, note the added language that addresses interrater agreement among the DM scales in Form 10.2, with discrepancy among the ratings most likely indicating variable development among the DM skill sets. In such cases, the examiner should consider which rater may be most accurate in estimating the particular skills in question. For example, the teacher may be in a more opportune position to estimate the child's pre-academic skills, whereas the parent may be more accurate in estimating the child's overall adaptive skills. In general, the pre-drafted excerpts are offered to expedite the interpretive process and may be employed in whole or in part as deemed necessary and useful by the examiner.

Conners Comprehensive Behavior Rating Scales

This ensuing instrument can be accurately conceived of as an older companion to the Conners EC. Although it does not feature developmental milestones scales because it covers an older age cohort, it provides some added facets to its data to enhance reliability and validity analyses.

Synopsis

The *Conners Comprehensive Behavior Rating Scales* (*Conners CBRS*; Conners, 2008, 2014) is also a multi-score, multi-informant system that comprises three respondent forms, including a parent form, a teacher form, and a self-report form. The first two observer respondent forms are based on norm reference samples ranging in age from 6 years, 0 months to 18 years, 11 months and afford identical data, while the self-report form is normed on individuals aged 8 years, 0 months to 18 years, 11 months, which affords comparable, although not identical, data.

In general, the CBRS data are more *DSM* driven, with a cluster of scales that are designed to measure many of the major *DSM* clinical disorders. These are referred to as the *DSM* symptom scales. When this measure was initially published, the *Diagnostic and Statistical Manual of Mental Disorders, Fourth Edition, Text Revision* (*DSM–IV–TR*; American Psychiatric Association, 2000) was still being used. Therefore, the items on these scales were designed to detect clinical disorders as defined by the criteria in that edition. However, subsequent to the publication of the *DSM–5* in 2013, a supplement to the Conners CBRS was published (see Conners, 2014) to make the proper adjustments in symptom counts such that the forms were accordant with the new criteria.

More specifically, adjustments were made to the following *DSM–5* symptom scales: attention deficit hyperactivity disorder, oppositional defiant disorder, major depressive episode, manic episode, mixed episode, social anxiety disorder (social phobia), obsessive-compulsive disorder, and especially autism spectrum disorder. For example, the Asperger's disorder scale was subsumed into the autistic disorder scales, and the symptoms were thereafter adjusted to be in harmony with the modified criteria. Although the updated computer-scoring software now scores the forms using the *DSM–5* criteria, the option to use the prior *DSM–IV–TR* criteria continues to be available.

The CBRS also provides content scales, which measure constructs and subject matter that have been useful based on clinical experience and practice. Although there is some perhaps unavoidable degree of redundancy between the *DSM* and content scales, there are also some unique scales that can be extremely useful in psychodiagnosis (e.g., the violence potential content scale). These are listed in a separate table because they offer only a dimensional *T*–score metric, whereas the *DSM–5* symptom scales yield two types of scores, including a categorical symptom counts metric and a dimensional *T*–score metric. The only data that are lacking when compared to the younger Conners EC forms are the *DSM* scales, which is understandable since the Conners CBRS forms begin at age six.

Lastly, it may already be apparent that the Conners EC and Conners CBRS overlap at six years of age. As such, the examiner has the option of using either form depending on the needs of the case. Succinctly, if the case consists of issues concerning developmental delay (e.g., ID, ASD, communication disorder), then the Conners EC tends to be most useful because it includes the *DSM* scales. In contrast, if the case is focusing more on *DSM* disorders without a developmental delay component (e.g., ADHD, CD, ODD), and especially if such disorders tend to have a later onset (e.g., bipolar disorder), then the older Conners CBRS instrument is more useful.

Norm Reference Samples

Standardization consisted of an extremely large 6,702 assessments, both from the general population (from which norms were produced) and a clinical sample. Thus, the general population sample was further apportioned into a norm reference sample, which consisted of 1,200 assessments using the parent form, 1,200 assessments using the teacher form, and 1,000 assessments using the self-report form, with the remainder employed to examine construct validity.

Data collection was done from March 2006 through August 2008. The samples for both the parent and teacher forms consisted of 600 males and 600 females distributed equally within each of 12 1-year age groups ranging from 6 to 18 years (the 17- and 18-year-old groups being combined); hence, 100 males and 100 females in each age cohort. Analogously, the self-report form comprised 500 males and 500 females divided equally in each of 10 1-year age cohorts ranging from 8 to 18 years (once again, the 17- and 18-year-old groups were combined); thus, 100 males and 100 females in each age group. The samples were stratified according to race/ethnicity, parent education level, and geographic region according to proportions reported in the 2000 U.S. census (U.S. Bureau of the Census, 2000). Parent education level was defined as (a) no high school diploma; (b) high school diploma; (c) two-year college, vocational training, or apprenticeship; and (d) four-year college or higher.

Administration

There are two general topics concerning Conners CBRS administration. They include (a) which forms to utilize and (b) outlining the general administrative rules.

SELECTION OF CONNERS CBRS FORMS

As for the companion Conners EC forms, the prevailing administrative issue here concerns which informants are to be used in any particular case. Most typically, ordering the parent and teacher Forms for this age range best exploits the multi-score feature of the Conners CBRS. More specifically, this age range effectively covers the compulsory school years and extends further through high school graduation. As such, obtaining standardized clinical data from two independent observers, further assuming that the examinee will be providing his or her own test data with greater reliability and validity characteristics, takes most advantage of these rating scales. Having three sources provide clinical data in the same case makes possible more advanced analyses of interrater reliability (i.e., do independent informants agree when using similar data?) and convergent validity (i.e., do tests of different formats and informants indicate the presence of the same disorders or type of psychopathology?).

However, examinees who are matriculating through middle school and high school most likely have multiple teachers, which is due to their more diverse subject matter and schedule. In such instances, it is prudent to investigate whether there exists a teacher who has observed the examinee in environments that are not highly structured. For example, if a homeroom teacher or study hall teacher is asked to provide ratings, they are most likely to be spuriously negative, hence making a false negative result more likely. This is because behavior is always a function of both personality characteristics (including relatively consistent clinical symptoms or characteristics) interacting with situational forces or as follows:

$$B = f(P \times S)$$

Equation 10.1

where *B* symbolizes overt or observable behavior, *f* symbolizes the term function, *P* denotes relatively consistent symptoms or personality characteristics, and *S* designates the presence of situational forces (see Funder, 2006; Moskowitz &Fournier, 2015). If situational effects are formidable, they will tend to suppress the individual's characteristic patterns of behavior and symptoms, hence rendering it more likely that they will be erroneously missed. The ideal environments for such behavior ratings are those in which the situation is relatively weak in terms of influence and control (e.g., gym class), or if the respondent has opportunities to observe the examinee in various environments over time.

My point here is that, if there is no such teacher, it may be more effective to obtain self-report-type ratings; the older the examinee, the more the self-report form should be considered in lieu of the teacher ratings. Irrespective of the fact that the examinee will be providing the bulk of the data, this practice is acceptable, especially if the examinees show themselves to be both motivated and able to report their symptoms. The structure of the items should also assist the examinee, along with the fact that the parent ratings can be used for interrater reliability analyses.

Finally, occasionally obtaining only parent or self-report data alone is appropriate. The former can be chosen if teacher ratings are not available (e.g., the assessment is being done during the academic summer recess from school) and overwhelming the examinee with tests is to be avoided so as to avert deleteriously affecting the examinee's motivation to complete tests that possess greater degrees of reliability and validity.

To summarize this initial section of Conners CBRS administration, the examiner has a number of alternative combinations of informants to select from when using this multi-score system. For each of the most common combinations that have been employed in clinical testing practice, data tables have been created that are designed to report the results of such ratings within the context of a psychological assessment report. These include the following, with the designated form in parentheticals: (a) parent ratings alone (Form 10.3), (b) parent and teacher ratings together (Form 10.4), (c) self-report ratings alone (Form 10.5), and (d) parent and self-report ratings together (Form 10.6). The teacher form has never been used by itself, hence there is not a form created for presenting these data in isolation. However, by virtue of the Conners CBRS Parent Form and Teacher Form yielding the exact same data, all that needs to be done is supplanting the word "Parent" with the word "Teacher" using the *Replace* function in Microsoft Word and the form is immediately ready for such reporting. The ensuing section discusses general rules that govern the administration of this multi-score system.

GENERAL CONNERS CBRS RULES

After selecting the Conners CBRS forms to be employed in a testing case, the informants are directed to provide a scorable response to each item. Administration time is estimated at 25 minutes, although respondents usually provide valid protocols in less time. The parent and teacher forms require a sixth-grade reading level for adequate comprehension, while the self-report form requires approximately a fourth-grade reading level (Conners, 2008, p. 22). Observer-respondents should have witnessed the examinee's behavior for a minimum of one month since this is the time frame of symptoms used in the instructions. If possible, the informants are asked to complete the forms the same day and immediately after the initial interview, which by definition applies to the parent and self-report forms. It is usually at these times that such respondents are most motivated to provide data, along with the content of the interview being recent in their memory systems. Furthermore, obtaining such data sooner rather than later renders it possible to use these data to bolster the case for the medical necessity of testing if so needed. The single drawback is that the forms will in essence be wasted in cases where formal testing is ultimately not pursued (e.g., the examinee moves or otherwise decides not to follow through with testing or PA is summarily denied). However, this is usually worth the risk because a drawback of waiting for a later submission of the forms is that they are lost, destroyed, or forgotten. In the case of the teacher form, this must be completed and submitted latter, either by giving the form back to the parent or via the U.S. postal service.

In general, the item instructions ask the respondent to rate the examinee's behavior according to either the degree of truth or the degree of frequency as follows: (a) 0 = *Not true at all* (*Never, Seldom*); (b) 1 = *Just a little true* (*Occasionally*); (c) 2 = *Pretty much true* (*Often, Quite a bit*); and (d) *Very much true* (*Very often, Very frequently*). These response choices are the same as for the Conners EC behavior scales. The forms must be completed independently and especially without consultation of the second informant, who is also asked to complete a Conners CBRS form. This avoids correlating the data from different forms, which would otherwise subvert an accurate measure of interrater reliability; that is, it would artificially inflate the correlation between raters.

Administration can be done by the rater online or by hard copy. Again, there is a preference for the hard copy forms, as they can easily become part of the testing file for later reference. Lastly, omitted items are those which are improperly marked or not marked at all. The Conners CBRS manual (Conners, 2008) provides a table that indicates the maximum number of omissions permitted before certain scales become invalid (Table 4.1, p. 28), along with a computational scheme to use for prorating final raw score totals if the total number of omissions does not exceed the aforesaid maximums (p. 27).

Scoring

In general, scoring can be done online for a fee per score report or by computer software. The Conners CBRS Scoring Software (Multi-Health Systems, 2008) provides unlimited computer scoring for a one-time fee. The same optional test–retest and interrater statistical comparisons are available as on the Conners EC computer software. Once again, if the examiner anticipates using this multi-score system fairly frequently, the unlimited scoring software is the most prudent selection. It can be loaded onto the psychologist's computer by means of a thumb drive and thereafter activated when inserted into the computer during scoring. It essentially works in the same manner as the Conners EC computer software.

In terms of data, there are three categories of scales on the Conners CBRS forms. They are as follows: (a) validity scales; (b) *DSM–5* symptom scales; and (c) content scales. Each grouping has different content and purpose. Hence, the three clusters are presented in as many parts and in such order. Because all the data tables designed for reporting the Conners CBRS scores with varying informants yield essentially the same data, they will be discussed simultaneously. Where there are substantive differences, they will be made explicit.

VALIDITY SCALES

The Conners CBRS contains the same three validity scales as the Conners EC, although as will become apparent shortly, there is an additional datum on the inconsistency index. Note that the data table that includes two informants (i.e., Forms 10.4 and 10.6) juxtapose the scores to facilitate interrater comparisons, in addition to maximizing the efficiency of data presentation. Data within Table 1 (Forms 10.3–10.6) identify test-taking response sets (see prior discussion on response sets) that may compromise the veracity of the subsequent ratings. Thus, Table 1 should always be included first in the analysis. There are three such response sets, including (a) overly favorable ratings, (b) overly harsh ratings, and (c) contradictory ratings. The latter scale is somewhat more elaborate than seen in the Conners EC, as it includes the following two metrics: (a) raw score (i.e., sum of the discrepancies in ratings on comparable items) and an added (b) *differentials* (i.e., absolute frequency of occurrence of discrepant ratings on similar items of two or more points). Therefore, the differentials column is only pertinent to the inconsistency index scale; that is, the "--" symbol should invariably be retained in the differentials column for the positive and negative impression scales as being inapplicable.

Note that the top row of Forms 10.4 and 10.6 apportions the table equally into parent ratings (denoted by "P"), and either teacher ratings (denoted by T) or self-report ratings (designated by SR). This order prioritizes the parent ratings when both informants are available because such ratings are either based on (a) a greater sampling of behavior across both time and situations (i.e., compared to teacher ratings) or (b) a unique third-person perspective that is not available among other data in the report (i.e., compared to self-report ratings).

As regarding all Conners CBRS data tables (Forms 10.3–10.6), Table 1 enumerates first the validity scale name, followed by the ensuing order for each respondent: (a) raw score and (b) dichotomous interpretation (i.e., either the scale showed or did not show the stipulated invalid response set). The language used to describe the scale interpretations are based on the more elaborate narrative descriptions provided in the accompanying manual (Conners, 2008, pp. 44–46). The raw scores should be inserted first and the corresponding results so indicated.

General tabular notes define the directional meaning of higher raw scores and the "--" symbol for identifying non-scorable scales. For convenience, three of the most frequently occurring narrative interpretations of Table 1 results have been drafted. Fortunately, these ratings typically show valid results for all types of informants. Hence, this is the first available narrative interpretation for Forms 10.3–10.6. However, occasionally one of the respondents alone or one of the two raters' manifests evidence of invalidity. Hence, as applied to the parent and self-report ratings alone, two versions of invalidity have been drafted; that is, questionable validity and completely invalid. The former shows an invalid tendency that renders the subsequent ratings reasonably accurate, although in need of some supporting evidence. The latter shows an exaggerated response set that virtually invalidates the remaining ratings and precludes reporting them to avoid offering a distorted impression of the examinee's overall functioning.

As regarding Forms 10.4 and 10.6, narrative interpretations must address instances wherein one rater shows consistent validity while the second evinces invalid response tendencies. These interpretations argue that the latter's subsequent scores should be deemed accurate only when consistent with the valid ratings and/or other test data or diagnostic information deemed reliable and valid. Interpretations have been drafted to cover either scenario. Finally, there are two pre-drafted excerpts that cover both ratings being either questionably valid or per se invalid. These are comparable to those drafted for the single informant ratings that interpret questionable and clearly invalid results. Again, the latter precludes reporting the subsequent ratings as was done for the parent ratings alone.

DSM–5 SYMPTOM SCALES

The Conners CBRS *DSM* symptom scales are enumerated in Table 2 (Forms 10.3–10.6) and vary somewhat in design as compared to the Conners EC behavior scales. First, consistent with their name, they have direct correspondence to the following *DSM–5* clinical syndromes or disorders: (a) ADHD (including all types of presentations), (b) ODD, (c) CD, (d) *major depressive episode (MDE)*, (e) *manic episode*, (f) GAD, (g) *separation anxiety disorder*, (h) *social anxiety disorder* (previously *social phobia*), (i) OCD, and (j) ASD. The reader is referred to Chapter 4 of this book for a more detailed presentation of these clinical disorders. Second, these disorders are measured by both the dimensional *T*–score metric (mean = 50, *SD* = 10; range = 30–90), and by the *DSM–5* categorical metric referred to as *DSM symptom counts* (hereafter and in the data tables, *DSM count*). Recall that these symptom counts were adjusted since initial publication to be consistent with the *DSM–5* modifications (Conners 2014).

The *DSM* count is unique to the Conners CBRS and augments test reliability and validity regarding *DSM–5* differential diagnoses, including most especially the detection of comorbidity. Briefly, selected Conners CBRS items correspond directly to *DSM–5* criteria for the previously listed disorders. When a respondent rates an item on the aforesaid Likert-type scale sufficiently high to be classified as either *indicated* or *may be indicated*, which varies somewhat from item to item, it is, in effect, marked as a *DSM* count. If ample essential and nonessential *DSM–5* symptom items are so classified, that diagnosis is identified as a dichotomous *Probably Met* (versus *Probably Not Met*), hence consistent with a categorical approach to psychodiagnosis.

Specific guidelines are provided for interpreting the integration of *T*–score and *DSM* count results (Conners, 2008, p. 50). Briefly, a *T*–score at or above 65 coexisting with a positive *DSM* count (i.e., *Met*) indicates the presence of a *DSM–5* diagnosis, whereas a lower *T*–score and negative *DSM* count indicates that such diagnosis is not supported. Guidelines are also provided in resolving discrepancies between these two measures (Conners, 2008, p. 49). Supplemental guidelines have been drafted consistent with the design of Table 2, which have been found to be reliable in practice (discussed subsequent).

CONTENT SCALES

The Conners CBRS content scales provide data that measure the presence of problems, issues, and symptoms that have been observed and managed in psychological testing and psychotherapeutic practice. Although they are in some respects redundant with the *DSM* scales, they also serve as extremely useful supplements, including the identification of problematic personality issues, such as perfectionism and low self-confidence, along with the identification of vital issues, such as danger to self and others, and screening for learning disabilities. These content scales are listed in Table 3 of Forms 10.3–10.6. Their listing in a separate table was determined by their role as effective supplements to the *DSM* scores and the fact that they only yield dimensional *T*–scores.

Interpretation

Once again, the ensuing interpretive guidelines apply assuming the validity scales did not detect extreme response sets that would be deleterious to the reporting and interpreting of the clinically related data. First, the analysis will typically begin with the *DSM–5* symptom scales, considering that the majority of testing referrals concern *DSM–5* differential diagnoses and related issues. Here, the dimensional *T*–score elevations must be interpreted by integrating them with the *DSM* count categorical or dichotomous metric, hence employing a combination of both approaches to psychodiagnosis. According to the manual (Conners, 2008, Table 6.1, p. 41), the *T*–score ranges are apportioned into four categories, with the lowest two essentially representing within–normal limits symptom levels. In particular, 30–39 is a low score, and 40–59 is an average score, which leaves the highest two ranges as atypically elevated (i.e., 60–69) and very elevated (i.e., 70–90). As for the Conners EC, because testing in clinical practice trends toward the identification of abnormality, the interpretive scheme can be abridged to a more efficient three-category system, which effectively integrates the lowest two ranges into a somewhat larger within–normal limits category.

Therefore, the *DSM* symptom scales employ a trichotomous dimensional (i.e., ordinal) interpretation scheme based on the standardized scores as follows: (a) *T*–score 30–59 is *within normal limits*; (b) *T*–score 60–69 is *elevated* (one asterisk is amended to the score); and (c) *T*–score 70–90 is *very elevated* (two asterisks are amended to the score). This interpretation scheme is conveniently placed within a specific note to Table 2 (Forms 10.3–10.6) to assist the examiner in data analysis and the reader of the report. Next, the *DSM* count dichotomous result (*Met* or *Not Met*) is considered. Hence, in the event the T–score is elevated and the associated *DSM* count is met, there is clear evidence of the presence of that psychopathology. The degree of T–score elevation is then used as an estimate of the symptom level (i.e., mild, moderate, or severe), although the actual symptom counts can also be of use. The specific symptom counts are not included in the table because this would produce clutter. However, such data can be entered into the narrative if it would assist in interpretation. Another reason the symptom counts are not reported is that they are similar to item responses, which are lacking in reliability. Mixed results can occur with elevated T–scores and negative *DSM* counts or within–normal limits T–scores and positive *DSM* counts. In either case, the data are to be interpreted as equivocal and in need of further support in either the positive or negative direction. Obviously, within–normal limits T–scores and negative *DSM* counts are unequivocally negative results for that type of psychopathology.

To facilitate test interpretation, Table 2 (Forms 10.3–10.6) lists the scale name, T–score, CI, and PR for each rater, and concludes with a summary of the measured symptoms. Thus, for the double-informant forms, the T–score, CI, PR sequence is repeated twice, once for each rater. One asterisk is appended to denote elevated T–scores, while two asterisks are appended for very elevated T–scores. This is to provide a visual marker for clinical elevations among the data. The first row of the table designates the rater to which the data belong (i.e., "P" for parent ratings, "T" for teacher ratings, and "SR" for self-report ratings). Table notes summarize the metrics, the meaning of higher scores, the T–score interpretive scheme, and definitions for various abbreviations. The single difference in informants is that the self-report ratings do not include the autism spectrum disorder scale. This is because if an examinee has this disorder, a lack of theory of mind (which is an integral component of this disorder) would preclude the provision of accurate self-ratings.

Following Table 2, excerpts that guide the interpretation of the data have been inserted. The language can be adjusted to report clearly negative, positive, or ambiguous results. Further, there usually appear statements that additional test data is needed to corroborate the rating-scales findings, consistent with the tenet that this type of data is to be considered supplemental in nature. These interpretive statements cover the single informant forms (viz., Forms 10.3 and 10.5). However, the double-informant data tables add the dimension of interrater reliability. Hence, an added interpretative statement is inserted into these forms that address whether interrater agreement with the reported results is obtained. The examiner has the discretion to elaborate upon this statement, thus qualifying the ambiguous results; for example, affording more validity to the parent ratings due to observing the examinee in more types of situations and across a greater length of time. Also note that the pre-drafted excerpts are organized by type of clinical disorder, which approximates the order in which the scales appear in the table. This makes locating the proper interpretive summary both easier and faster.

The data tables end with a listing of the Conners CBRS content scales, which are organized according to various issues in Table 3. For example, the first two scales are pertinent to ADHD, while the second pair of scales addresses violence and aggression. These content scales are extremely pragmatic supplements to the *DSM* symptom scales. For example, in the event an adolescent manifests symptoms of CD, then the violence potential and aggressive behaviors content scales can assist in estimating the risk of danger to others or risk for violence. The academic-related scales can be used as screening data for the presence of a specific learning disorder, which can be used to bolster the medical necessity for follow-up achievement testing. Finally, there are some scales that suggest the presence of problematic personality issues, including perfectionism and poor social skills, that can be the target of psychotherapy.

While the content scales represent issues that may be the objective of future therapy or testing, they do not represent clinical syndromes per se. Hence, they are measured exclusively by the dimensional T–score metric with the same interpretative scheme as employed for the *DSM* symptom scales. As in Table 2, Table 3 reports the content scale name, T–score, CI, PR, and a summary of the measured symptoms. Asterisks are appended to the T–score to visually denote clinical elevations, as is done for Table 2. Tabular notes immediately follow Table 3, which again clarify all the data and abbreviations reported within the tabular rows and columns. Finally, pre-drafted excerpts have been incorporated that guide the interpretation of the various content scales. Once again, they are listed in the approximate order in which they appear in the table.

Summary

This section was devoted to presenting the multi–score Conners CBRS system, its essential features, and how its data can be reported and interpreted effectively within a formal psychological assessment report. To render its use most efficiently, the examiner is advised to report only those scales that are pertinent to the diagnostic issues in a particular case or that flag a particular disorder that previously had gone unsuspected. Otherwise, the reporting of data can become overwhelming to the reader, in which case the scores will detract from, rather than provide increased focus on, the most important test results. Furthermore, the use of two raters has the advantage of adding an interrater reliability check to the analysis, which can lead to more precise diagnostic conclusions. Next, the discussion moves to rating-scales tests that are more unidimensional in nature (i.e., focused on one clinical disorder or type of psychopathology), although they provide a much more detailed profile of symptoms that can represent specific targets for intervention. Although the multidimensional instruments previously described cover a broad array of clinical disorders, they do not provide the depth and detail of the ensuing measures. Hence, the latter provide much more guidance in terms of what specific symptoms are present and need to be goals of intervention. However, the examiner must be reasonably certain that the examinee manifests that particular type of psychopathology, otherwise such a test will manifest negative results and miss the opportunity to detect other disorders that may be present due to its overly narrow focus.

Autism-Related Measures

There are two autism-related rating scales in this book's test inventory (see Table 1.1). They include the *Gilliam Autism Rating Scale, Third Edition* (GARS–3; Gilliam, 2014a) and the *Gilliam Asperger's Disorder Scale* (*GADS*; Gilliam, 2001). The latter measure continues to be employed when such symptom pattern is present, although it never renders an ASD diagnosis based entirely or even principally upon such data. Recall the principle that rating-scale data should be supplemental only and never used solely or primarily in determining ultimate diagnoses.

More specifically, both are especially vulnerable to a negative impression or overreporting response set (see prior section on response sets). This may be related to the fact that children with such diagnoses may be eligible for special services through the *Individuals with Disabilities Education Improvement Act of 2004* (*IDEA*, 2004) or other vital programs, such as the *Affordable Care Act*, which requires health insurance companies to cover treatment for preexisting conditions, including treatments for diagnosed cases of autism (Autism Speaks, 2015). The fact that each of these rating scales includes the disorder's label in its title, hence being explicit about what is being measured, may also be suggestive that such a disorder is present and skew results in the positive direction. In either case, because of this vulnerability, the examiner must use these rating scales judiciously and advise prospective respondents to be conservative as to how they rate each item (e.g., interpreting a child's desire to go to sleep at the same time every night as constituting a rigid and repetitive behavior versus a normal and expected habit pattern). With these caveats in mind, both measures will be briefly presented in the aforementioned sequence, with an ultimate focus on the data tables that have been prepared for purposes of presenting their results within a psychological assessment report.

Gilliam Autism Rating Scale, Third Edition

The Gilliam Autism Rating Scale, Third Edition (GARS–3; Gilliam, 2014a) is presented first because it is patterned directly after this disorder as currently defined by the *DSM–5*. The examiner's manual (Gilliam, 2014a) is accompanied by a resource guide (Gilliam, 2014b), which contains instructional objectives and goals for teaching individuals who have ASD. The objectives are patterned after the GARS–3 scores at the item level, which is at the most detailed level of analysis. In that sense, it explains why the GARS–3 data trend toward overreporting. That is, it is more important to error on the side of reporting a symptom that may not be present because then the child will at least be provided some type of potentially useful intervention. On the other hand, in the event there was an overreporting of the measured symptom, this would become apparent quickly during the course of intervention and then adjustments could be made quite rapidly. In such case, there would be minimal harm to the child. However, missing an opportunity for intervention, especially when considering the impairing effects of autism, would be considered a more deleterious error in measurement.

The concern that is manifest regarding false positive results or an overestimation of symptoms when using the GARS–3 to assist in diagnosis should be clear if the objective is to maximize measurement accuracy. The first step in adjusting for this tendency is to acknowledge its presence and reasons, which has now been done. The second step is to actually incorporate a stratagem for making the needed adjustments in quantifying and interpreting the GARS–3 data, which will be done as the current presentation unfolds. Succinctly, the GARS–3 can be a very useful measure in diagnosing autism, as long as the proper modifications are enacted.

SYNOPSIS

The GARS–3 is designed as a measuring device that assists in the identification of ASD in an individual aged 3 years, 0 months through 22 years, 11 months. It comprises 58 items that are apportioned into six subscales. Each item is worded in such a manner that the target behaviors are specific, observable, and quantifiable. Together, the six subscales contribute to an overall autism index score.

The instrument consists of three components. First, the examiner's manual (Gilliam, 2014a) possesses all the information required to administer, score, and interpret the measure, along with technical data concerning its characteristics, such as reliability and validity. Second, the summary/response form provides space to document examinees' demographics, rater responses, raw scores and totals, subsequent data transformations, and other information relevant to making an autism determination. Finally, there is an instructional objective resource guide that assists in developing a detailed intervention program based directly on the GARS–3 results. Therefore, this instrument is designed to assist in the detection of ASD, although it incorporates significant treatment-related information to evaluate the effectiveness of intervention and for use in empirical research. Therefore, the guiding principle of using rating-scale data as strictly supplementary for purposes of psychodiagnosis is emphasized to an even greater extent when applying the GARS–3 to testing practice.

NORM REFERENCE SAMPLE

The GARS–3 was standardized on 1,859 individuals who had valid diagnoses of ASD, were 3–22 years of age, and who were citizens of the United States. Of these, 1,139, or 61.3%, had no co-occurring mental health disorders. The remaining individuals had one or more comorbid disabilities. The latter were retained in the final sample due to the fact that comorbidity is a common occurrence in ASD diagnoses. Stratification variables included geographic region, gender, race, and parental education. Analysis of the normative sample showed that the aforesaid stratification variables conformed to an acceptable degree with the 2010 census (U.S. Census Bureau, 2010). Of note, the gender ratio of ASD in the population is 5:1 males-to-females, which was approximated in the normative sample. The subsample sizes per year of age ranges from 157 for 5-year-olds to 25 for 21-year-olds. Finally, autism is found in all states, cultures, and geographic regions, the diversity of which was matched by that standardization sample (e.g., individuals in the sample were garnered from 48 U.S. states).

ADMINISTRATION

Raters are to be given a copy of the summary/response form and instructed to enter (a) the examinee's identifying information and (b) their own information, including the number of years or months they have known the individual to be rated. Informants are to be encouraged to read each item twice before responding to maximize comprehension, although they should make themselves available in the event they need assistance in deciphering the intent of each behavior to be rated. Thus, the implication is that respondents should complete the form during or after an initial interview or during a testing session where the respondent has access to the examiner if needed. Administration time is a very brief five to ten minutes.

More specifically, the respondent is to use the ensuing guidelines in answering each item: (a) 0 = *Not at all like the individual* (i.e., you have never seen the person behave in this manner); (b) 1 = *Not much like the individual* (i.e., the person seldom behaves in this manner; perhaps one to two times per six-hour period); (c) 2 = *Somewhat like the individual* (i.e., the person sometimes behaves in this manner; perhaps three to four times per six-hour period); or (d) 3 = *Very much like the individual* (i.e., the person frequently behaves in this manner; at least five to six times per six-hour period). Of note, respondents must not consider the individual's age when making their ratings, as this variable is accounted for in the norm reference data (see prior). That is, their responses must be contingent upon how well the items describe the examinee's behavior. The time frame for making the ratings is two weeks. Therefore, if a respondent is just beginning to work with the examinee (e.g., teacher, foster parent), they should observe the individual for a two-week period prior to completing the form. To help guard against overreporting, the prospective informants are asked to be conservative in making their ratings; that is, if in doubt, rating an item as being less (versus more) descriptive of the person's behavior, keeping in mind that autism is both a severe and pervasive disorder by definition.

SCORING

Scoring is done manually on the summary/response form with the assistance of data tables in the examiner's manual that permit the conversion of total raw scores into PRs and scaled scores (mean = 10; SD = 3; range = 1–20), and subsequently, total scaled scores into an autism index (mean = 100; SD = 15; range = 43–140). Briefly, items target behavioral symptoms according to the *DSM–5* criteria (American Psychiatric Association, 2013). Such items are apportioned into subscales as follows: (a) restricted/repetitive behaviors (RB); (b) social interaction (SI); (c) social communication (SC); (d) emotional responses (ER); (e) cognitive style (CS); and (f) maladaptive speech (MS). Item raw scores in each of the six subscales are summed and converted into as many scaled scores and PRs (Gilliam, 2014a, Appendix A, pp. 49–50).

However, there is an alternate circumscribed version for examinees who are nonverbal. Note that the latter two subscales assume that the examinee has verbal abilities. If these were to be scored for such individuals, the results would be artificially low (viz., zero) because such a result would be due to an absence of the ability to use words and not on true symptoms of ASD. Therefore, the nonverbal version deletes the latter two subscales from the analysis by instructing the informant not to provide ratings for such items if the examinee is indeed nonverbal. In consequence, item raw scores in each of the first four subscales are aggregated and converted into as many scaled scores and PRs (Gilliam, 2014a, Appendix A, pp. 49–50).

Next, the scaled scores are summed for either verbal (i.e., all six subscales) or nonverbal (i.e., four of six subscales) examinees, and converted into a composite autism index score and PR. Conversions are provided for both the six summed subscales and the four summed subscales (Gilliam, 2014a, Appendix B, pp. 51–53). The scaled score and index data together form what is referred to on the summary/response form as the composite performance (Section 3 of the form). The *SEM*s for the index and scaled scores are 4 and 1, respectively. Both are conveniently listed directly on the summary/response form in different sections. The only other data to be inserted in the composite performance are the probability of ASD and the severity level, both of which are enumerated in the interpretive guide (Section 4) of the summary/response form. At this juncture, scoring on the GARS–3 form is complete. The remainder of the scoring process regards inputting these scores into the data tables that have been designed for reporting the GARS–3 results within a psychological assessment report.

In particular, Forms 10.7 and 10.8 provide a sequence of two data tables for reporting the verbal and nonverbal GARS–3 results, respectively. Table 1 focuses on the composite autism index, a 95% CI, PR likelihood of autism, severity level, and descriptor. All of these are listed on the summary/response form. The latter three columns are actually linked. Therefore, to assist the examiner, the autism index score ranges are listed in a specific table note and associated with the indicated sequence of probability of autism, severity level, and descriptor. For example, if an examinee's autism index is 112, the 68% CI would be 108–116 (i.e., ± 4 points), PR would be 79, and the remaining three columns would together read: *Very likely-profound*, *Level 3*, and *Requiring very substantial support*. Although they are linked in the specific table note "e," they can be easily selected for each independent column by simply deleting the language that does not apply. Also note that Forms 10.7 and 10.8 are identical, with the exception of Table 1 note "a," which delineates for the reader which subscales contributed to the autism index results. In all other quantitative respects, however, the data are identical.

Table 2 data, however, do diverge between Forms 10.7 and 10.8. More specifically, Form 10.7 includes all six subscales, whereas Form 10.8 includes only the first four subscales. The remaining components are the same. The first column shows the subscale label, scaled score, 68% CI, PR symptoms severity, and measured symptoms. Hence, the design is similar to Table 1, although it is based on a smaller metric and different symptom severity descriptor. Because the GARS–3 does not provide such a descriptor, one is created that is useful in gauging degree or level and is accordant with *DSM–5* standards. That is, *DSM–5* asks for a separate severity rating for social communication and behavioral impairment, whereas the GARS–3 provides only a single severity descriptor. Hence, an examiner can scrutinize various scaled scores and 95% CIs and estimate a severity rating for the two areas of functioning, social and behavioral. In particular, the subscales restricted/repetitive behaviors (RB) and perhaps emotional responses (ER) can be analyzed in terms of behavioral impairment, the latter contributing to behavioral outbursts and lack of behavioral control. The remaining subscales can be analyzed in terms of the overall social area of functioning.

Admittedly, the following scaled scores ranges and severity descriptors have been selected somewhat arbitrarily, although an attempt was made to incorporate some of the language used by this instrument in the examiner's manual and the summary/response form. They are listed in specific table note "d" and are as follows: (a) *Absent* is an *SS* of 1–4, (b) *Mild* is an *SS* of 5–7, (c) *Moderate* is an *SS* of 8–12, (d) *Severe* is an *SS* of 13–16, and (e) *Profound* is an *SS* of 17–20. Of course, these may be modified and interpreted in different ways and as appropriate to the case facts. These are intended as scoring guidelines that have shown to be viable in clinical practice and may be modified at the examiner's discretion.

INTERPRETATION

It may have already been apparent that the GARS–3 does not provide validity scales designed to detect response sets that threaten the accuracy of the results. This means the examiner must be vigilant to any evidence that may show one of the aforesaid response sets, or including in the battery an instrument that does provide such validity scales. For example, the examiner can ask the respondent to complete both the Conners CBRS and the GARS–3 for a

12-year-old examinee. Hence, the validity scale results on the Conners CBRS can be extrapolated to his or her test-taking approach on the GARS–3 and the latter interpreted accordingly.

In any case, for Table 1 GARS–3 data (Forms 10.7 and 10.8), several pre-drafted excerpts have been inserted that cover several of the most common interpretive outcomes. These can be used to expedite and guide interpretation. They include three versions for results that are consistent with other data, two versions that are inconsistent with other data, and one for results that are hopelessly mixed (i.e., a testing psychologist's worst nightmare). The three consistent versions are for positive results, subthreshold results, and negative results. The two inconsistent results explain the presence of a false positive and false negative interpretation. Of note, the false positive version has been used fairly frequently. The overall equivocal result provides an open-ended statement leaving room for the examiner to attempt to account for such complete ambiguity, which is usually considered an obligation of the test interpreter.

If the outcome is a consistent negative, not reporting any of the subscales is advised. The autism index is by far the most reliable score this measure has to offer (Gilliam, 2014a, Table 5.1, p. 28). Hence, when results are so consistently negative, the GARS–3 has done its job. It does not add anything substantive to the analysis to report the subscales. Hence, such language is included in the consistent negative outcome. Similarly, reporting the subscales is unnecessary when the GARS–3 has produced false positive and negative results. In such an instance, reporting them would be confounding to the reader. That is, why report a detailed profile if they afford a false impression? In consequence, language to that effect has been inserted into these versions. However, the opposite is not true; that is, consistent positive results require an analysis of the subscale data to estimate degree of severity of both social communication and behavioral functioning, along with providing information relevant to treatment intervention.

Therefore, interpretive language has been inserted immediately following Table 2 that is designed to provide an ipsative analysis of the various subscales. Because the autism index is showing positive results that are bolstered by additional test data, it implies that there exist positive results among the contributing subscales that need to be explicated. The examiner simply needs to report the most to least severely prominent subscales, which will ultimately contribute to an estimate of severity levels for the social and behavioral domains as prompted by *DSM–5* standards.

SUMMARY

This concludes a brief presentation of the GARS–3, which is a unidimensional rating scale that can effectively supplement performance-based data showing evidence of autism. Although this measure tends to result in overreported symptoms to some degree, it can also provide a more detailed profile of an individual's specific symptoms in the real world. Next, a unidimensional rating scale designed to measure symptoms previously associated with Asperger's disorder is succinctly presented. Although this disorder has been technically removed from the *DSM–5*, the symptoms measured can still assist in detecting signs of autism, especially higher-functioning cases with intact intellectual and language functioning.

Gilliam Asperger's Disorder Scale

The Gilliam Asperger's Disorder Scale (GADS; Gilliam, 2001) was designed to measure what was previously conceptualized as one of several related but distinct versions or *pervasive developmental disorder* (PPD; American Psychiatric Association, 2000; World Health Organization, 1992/2010). PDDs were severe and generalized disorders that manifested impairments in several major developmental domains, including reciprocal social interaction skills; communication; and the presence of stereotyped behaviors, activities, and interests (American Psychiatric Association, 2000, p. 69). Because this measure is continually used to assist in detecting some symptoms of autism as currently defined by *DSM–5*, it is prudent that the symptoms measured by the GADS is succinctly reviewed; this after a synopsis.

SYNOPSIS

The GADS is a rating scale that focuses on helping to detect Asperger's syndrome–type symptoms in individuals aged 3–22. The items presented in the response form were founded upon the criteria set out for this type of psychopathology as defined by both the *DSM–IV–TR* and ICD–10 (International Classification of Diseases, Tenth Revision). There is also a parent interview portion of this instrument designed to rule out symptoms more indicative of autism, including significant delays in language, cognitive, and adaptive behavior skills, along with ensuring adequate curiosity about the environment. The purpose was make an effective differential diagnosis between Asperger's syndrome, which did not include these delays, and autism, in which such delays were expected (American Psychiatric Association, 2000). Finally, the GADS was normed on 371 individuals who had documented diagnoses of Asperger's syndrome within the aforementioned age range from 46 U.S. states, the District of Columbia, Canada, the U.K., Mexico, Australia, and several other countries around the world.

ASPERGER'S SYMPTOMS

The GADS yields information concerning four categories of behavior, including social interaction, restricted patterns of behavior, cognitive patterns, and pragmatic skills. Irrespective of an individual's ultimate diagnosis, these areas of functioning provide useful information regarding differential diagnosis. *Social interaction* items target the inability to engage in reciprocal interpersonal interaction (e.g., cooperating with others), lack of cognizance of social conventions or rules (e.g., engaging in casual conversation, such as "How are you?"), inability to empathize with others' feelings, misunderstanding implied meanings in conversation, and problems regulating affect effectively. *Restricted patterns* of behavior include not reacting appropriately to compliments from others, showing eccentric forms of behavior, lack of coordination in motor skills, being insensitive to others' needs, and requiring a significant amount of directions from others.

Cognitive patterns target intensive interest in single and/or esoteric subjects (e.g., washing machines); using overly precise or pedantic speech as if lecturing (i.e., didactic speech); interpreting speech or comments literally or concretely; demonstrating obsessive interest in certain intellectual subjects; and showing unusually excellent memory ability, especially for certain facts. Finally, *pragmatic skills* generally measure one's ability to use and understand pragmatic, everyday speech. This includes an inability to understand sarcasm or slang, difficulty comprehending when one is being teased or rejected by others, problems predicting the consequences of engaging in certain behaviors (e.g., being inappropriately honest with someone without proper censuring), and lack of being able to pretend or use fantasy.

Taken together, items in these four areas help detect classic symptoms of *Asperger's disorder* or *syndrome*. Furthermore, the parent interview assists in ensuring that particular lines of development proceeded normally, including language, intelligence, and adaptive behavior, which effectively discriminates Asperger's syndrome from autistic disorder as defined in *DSM–IV–TR*. The latter is, in large part, responsible for considering Asperger's syndrome a higher-functioning form of autism (see, e.g., Bishop, 1989; see also Klin & Volkmar, 1995; Rutter 1985; Wing, 1991; regarding the controversial nature of Asperger's being a separate and distinct form of PPD, Gilliam, 2001). In conclusion, interpretation of the GADS data (see later in this section) is consistent with the conceptualization of Asperger's symptoms as a higher-functioning form of ASD as currently listed in the *DSM–5*. While some clinicians may disagree with such utilization of the GADS, it has been found to be pragmatically useful in some referrals to rule out ASD, especially when one suspects the presence of a subtler, higher-functioning form of this disorder.

NORM REFERENCE SAMPLE

The GADS was standardized on a sample of 371 individuals between the ages of 3 years, 0 months through 22 years, 11 months with documented diagnoses of Asperger's disorder as defined by *DSM–IV–TR* or ICD–10. The relatively small standardization sample was attributed to the rarity of the Asperger's diagnosis, including an estimated prevalence rate of 0.26% in the general population. Furthermore, this low prevalence rate resulted in little knowledge concerning the demographic characteristics of individuals with Asperger's syndrome. Other than the small sample size, the other major concern was that the norm reference sample statistics did not fit those in the population for race and ethnicity. For example, 76% of the sample was White, 2% Black, and 22% Other.

However, the one most consistently reported demographic characteristic of those with Asperger's disorder is a gender ratio of 4:1 favoring males over females (Bauer, 1996; Ehlers & Gillberg, 1993; Klin, Volkmar, Sparrow, Ciccetti, & Rourke, 1995). Consistent with this, the norm reference sample was 85% male versus 15% female. Furthermore, the sample was culled from the four major regions in the U.S. and other countries as follows: 18% Northeast; 21% Midwest; 25% South; 28% West; and 8% International. Hence, the proportions were approximately equal when scrutinizing U.S. regions and including some international individuals. As there were no data to doubt that those with Asperger's disorder would manifest such diversity in a geographic region, these data were considered a reasonable representation of this special population of individuals. Ultimately, it was concluded that the GADS, "for the most part, appears representative of the Asperger's disorder population" (Gilliam, 2001, p. 22). For the interested reader, the demographic characteristics of the sample are reported in Table 4.1 (Gilliam, 2001, p. 22).

ADMINISTRATION

In many ways, GADS administration parallels that of the GARS–3, which is not surprising when one considers that (a) the same author designed both instruments that (b) measure related constructs. The required time frame of observation is once again a minimum of two weeks. Administration time for the response form section that includes the aforementioned four subscales is also five to ten minutes, although this does not include the parent interview form section of the summary/response booklet.

There are a total of 32 items across the 4 subscales that use objective frequency-based ratings. More specifically, the respondent is to use the ensuing guidelines in answering each item: (a) 0 = *Never Observed* (i.e., you have never seen the person behave in this manner); (b) 1 = *Seldom Observed* (i.e., the person seldom behaves in this manner; perhaps one to two times per six-hour period); (c) 2 = *Sometimes Observed* (i.e., the person sometimes behaves in this manner; perhaps three to four times per six-hour period); or (d) 3 = *Frequently Observed* (i.e., the person frequently behaves in this manner; at least five times per six-hour period). The informant is encouraged to rate every item and to make additional observations if uncertain as to how to respond. The principal divergence between the GARS–3 and the GADS is in the requirement of the parent interview form as a key part of the latter.

The parent interview form of the summary/response booklet is to be answered by those with direct and continued contact with the examinee during the first three years of life. The examiner is responsible for recording yes or no responses to the questions posed to the informant. As stated, these questions are designed to rule out developmental delays that are not indicative of Asperger's syndrome. That is, if such delays are present, this argues against a diagnosis of Asperger's syndrome and suggests the presence of a more severe form of PDD; most likely, a more virulent degree and quality of autism as currently conceptualized by *DSM–5*.

SCORING

In the event there are no developmental delays that tend to rule out Asperger's symptoms, the response form portion of the summary/response booklet can be scored. Again, although there are no other validity checks on the GADS, the examiner can administer any other available rating-scale device that measures threatening response sets and generalize the findings to the GADS. The other option is to rely on other test data considered to be more reliable and valid in rendering an ASD diagnosis and use the GADS only in a supplementary role, which is invariably recommended, considering this measure provides rating-scale data completed by laypeople.

The scoring is done manually and very similarly to that of the GARS–3. In particular, the items within each of the subscales are aggregated and converted to scaled scores with a mean of 10, SD of 3, and range of 1–20, along with PRs (Gilliam, 2001, Appendix A, pp. 41–42). The SEMs for the subscales are all 1, hence adding and subtracting this quantity from the obtained score will provide an estimated 68% CI. Next, the subscale scaled scores are summed and converted to an Asperger's disorder quotient, with a mean of 100, SD of 15, and range of 40–132, along with PRs (Gilliam, 2001, Appendix B, pp. 43–44). The SEM for the Asperger's quotient is 4, hence an estimated 68% CI would add and subtract four points from the obtained score to provide an eight-point interval with this degree of certainty of including the true score. Of note, a 95% degree of confidence would require an unreasonably imprecise 16-point interval, which exceeds the range of some of the descriptive categories; hence, the use of a 68% CI.

Form 10.9 includes a sequence of two data tables designed for reporting the GADS results within a psychological assessment report. Table 1 is organized for reporting the overall results, including the Asperger's disorder quotient score, 68% CI, PR, and finally the odds that such a syndrome is present, organized into three ordinal ranges (see interpretation). General table notes defined the Asperger's disorder quotient metrics, the meaning of higher scores, and the definition of table abbreviations. Specific tabular notes define the different columns and interpretative scheme.

Table 2 in Form 10.9 is designed for reporting the Asperger's disorder subscales as defined earlier. Columns are provided for the subscale label, scaled score, 68% CI, PR, and succinct description of the measured symptoms. General table notes define the metrics and abbreviations, while specific notes define the meaning of the various derivatives of the scaled scores, along with the interpretive scheme.

INTERPRETATION

The interpretive process mirrors that of the GARS–3, moving from general to specific. The interpretive scheme is provided in the manual as follows: (a) *Low* is a quotient of 40–69, (b) *Borderline* is a quotient of 70–79, and (c) *High* is a quotient of 80–132. To both facilitate and expedite the interpretive process, excerpts have been inserted that describe the most frequent outcomes. These consist of three versions for results that show consistency with other test results, including positive, negative, and subthreshold findings. There are also two versions for inconsistent findings, including one false positive and one false negative outcome. The final version addresses continuing findings of mixed or ambiguous results, with an open-ended partial statement prompting the examiner to provide an attempt at explanation. Of note, the consistent negative and false positive and negative results suggest that the subsequent reporting of Table 2 is unnecessary. That is, consistent negative results need no further explanation, while false results should not be reported, as they are by definition misrepresentative, misleading, and obfuscating in effect.

In contrast, consistently positive and subthreshold results do need an elaboration using subscale data. In both instances, the issue to examine is what made the overall result either positive or near positive. In the former case, this will work to solidify the diagnosis and profile the specific symptoms that are providing the greatest degree of hindrance to functioning. The subthreshold case may be indicating the presence of another disorder that shares elements with Asperger's or autism psychopathologies, even if it does not fit the pattern for formal diagnosis. For example, the individual could alternatively meet the criteria for a social (pragmatic) communication disorder if the social interaction, cognitive patterns, and pragmatic skills subscales show significant impairment in the absence of restricted patterns of behavior. As another possibility, the individual could be suffering from a stereotypic movement disorder if there are severe degrees of restricted patterns of behavior in the absence of social and interpersonal problems.

As was done for the GARS–3, this author developed his own interpretive scheme for the symptom severity column since the GADS manual does not provide such information. They are the same scaled score ranges and labels as were used for the GARS–3 and are presented in Table 2 specific note "d." Hence, they will not be repeated here in the narrative. The measured symptoms for each subscale are summarized in the final column of Table 2 to assist both the examiner and reader in terms of interpretation. Finally, a pre-drafted excerpt has been inserted to guide interpretation of Table 2 data. Because it is assumed that Table 2 data are being reported if there are positive or subthreshold results manifested in Table 1, the interpretive language trends toward accounting for degrees of symptom presence, with a final statement identifying if there are any absent symptom clusters.

SUMMARY

This concludes presentation of the GADS, which is a unidimensional rating scale that can be useful in detecting cases of autism that are higher functioning or separate disorders that share some symptoms of autism. Again, these data should always be employed in a supplementary role because they are most frequently based on the observation of laypeople who may have known the individual for only two weeks. The ensuing instrument is also unidimensional and designed to detect adult cases of ADHD, including type of presentation and level of symptoms.

Adult ADHD

A diagnosis of ADHD in adulthood has a history of being controversial (Smith, Waschbusch, Willoughby, & Evans, 2000). However, there is currently convincing evidence that such a disorder exists within this age group (see, e.g., Biederman, 2005). In particular, it has been found that approximately 50% of adults aged 30–40 years who were diagnosed with ADHD in childhood continued to manifest clinically significant symptoms associated with dysfunction (Biederman & Faraone, 2005). These data show that ADHD symptoms have an early onset and an ensuing chronic course. As such, testing referrals for adult ADHD are both valid and medically justified. Pursuant to *DSM–5* criteria, however, it is crucial during the initial diagnostic assessment to document the suspected presence of at least some of these symptoms prior to the age of 12 (American Psychiatric Association, 2013). If such onset criterion is met, then the administration of rating-scale data can be extremely useful in detecting the presence, type, and degree of symptoms.

Conners' Adult ADHD Rating Scales, Long Version

The rating scale instrument that is employed for helping to diagnose ADHD in adults is the *Conners' Adult ADHD Rating Scales, Long Version* (*CAARS–L*; Conners, Erhart, & Sparrow, 1999). This measure is presented subsequently, including data tables designed to report its data yield within a psychological assessment report.

SYNOPSIS

There are actually three CAARS versions, including long, short, and screening (Conners, Erhardt, & Sparrow, 1999). The *long version* is utilized in helping to detect adult ADHD for several reasons. First, it possesses approximately twice the number of items (i.e., 9 and 12) on pertinent *DSM* subscales compared to the short form (i.e., 5). Second, because of the greater item coverage, the long version contains two subscales that measure both ADHD symptom cluster criteria as defined by the *DSM–IV* (American Psychiatric Association, 1994), whereas the short form lacks such subscale discrimination due to item brevity. The CAARS–L is also a multi-score instrument, consisting of self-report and observer report forms. Therefore, this measure provides the option of including an interrater reliability component to diagnosing adult ADHD.

Unfortunately, this measure has not yet been updated to be completely accordant with the *DSM–5* standards. However, this is not a fatal flaw because rating-scale data are here being employed solely within a supplementary role. That is, these data should never be used in isolation to render a diagnosis of adult ADHD. In particular, clinical interview information should attempt to determine symptom onset, development, and course over time, and performance-based continuous performance tests should represent the primary data used to determine if symptoms of inattention and impulse control difficulties are manifest. The *DSM–IV* and *DSM–IV–TR* ADHD symptom criteria are identical (cf. American Psychiatric Association, 1994, 2000), hence the content validity of the long version remains intact, at least when using those prior criteria.

In addition to detecting symptoms of adult ADHD, the long version possesses some supplementary subscales that are useful in screening for possible mood problems (i.e., impulsivity/emotional lability) and self-confidence personality issues (i.e., problems with self-concept). Scrutinizing these data have been useful in several past cases in which adult ADHD was suspected, although alternate mood and/or personality issues were found to be responsible for the presenting symptoms. In such cases, these findings are reported in the narrative because they occur infrequently and are considered screening measures in need of follow-up formal testing.

NORM REFERENCE SAMPLE

The norm reference sample for the CAARS–L self-report and observer forms (including long, short, and screening versions) ranged in age from 18 to 80 and 18 to 72, respectively. The self-report forms sample totaled 1,026 individuals, which included 466 males and 560 females. The self-report form mean age for men was 38.99 years (*SD* = 12.54), and the mean age for women was 38.84 years (*SD* = 12.32). The observer forms sample totaled 943 assessments, including 433 males and 510 females. For both samples, the norms were apportioned by gender and mostly 10-year age groups, including 18–29 years, 30–39 years, 40–49 years, and 50 and older. The observer forms mean age for men was 38.04 years (*SD* = 13.21), and the mean age for women was 39.40 years (*SD* = 12.68). These were nonclinical adults who were garnered from the various U.S. states and Canada from 1996 through 1998.

Looking ahead to the CAARS–L data yield, the form does not provide the data for directly computing the CIs. Hence, the reported *SEM*s for both forms were important to reference. The manual does list *SEM*s for the total self-report forms sample, further broken down by gender (Conners, 1999, Table 6.11, p. 63), along with the total observer forms sample, again further apportioned by gender (Conners, 1999, Table 6.13, p. 64). In addition, this was done for all three ADHD scales employed in the data tables, including *DSM*–Inattentive Symptoms, and *DSM*–Hyperactive/Impulsive Symptoms, *DSM*–Symptoms Total, and ADHD Index. These *SEM*s were computed by using internal consistency reliability estimates. The largest *SEM* was 2.53 versus the smallest at 1.73, which means the largest variability is only about 1.5 times the smallest variability. Accordingly, homogeneity of variance is satisfied (Howell, 2014), which justifies taking the average of all the *SEM*s (i.e., pooling the variance). The average *SEM* is 2.13, hence 2 when rounding to the nearest whole number. Therefore, to compute the 68% CI when reporting the CAARS–L data, simply adding and subtracting two points will provide a reasonable estimate of the 68% CI or degree of certainty of including the examinee's true score.

ADMINISTRATION

Informants are instructed to complete all items and to use their "best" answer if uncertain. Also, it is important that informants (a) realize there is both a front and back page, as it is not uncommon for the latter to be inadvertently missed, and (b) use a ballpoint pen on a hard surface because responses must be recorded through a response sheet to a scoring sheet. Average time to complete the long form is 25 minutes and requires a fourth-grade reading level. There are 66 items in total. Response alternatives are as follows: (a) 0 = *Not at all, never*; (b) 1 = *Just a little, once in a while*; (c) 2 = *Pretty much, often*; and (d) 3 = *Very much, very frequently*. Interestingly, the form does not provide a specific time frame for rendering answers to the items. The form simply states how frequently each item describes the individual "recently." Therefore, the advice provided by the CBRS forms is followed, which instructs the informant to base the ratings on the individual's behavior during the past month, or 30 days. This instruction is vital because ADHD symptoms are by definition chronic (i.e., enduring over time) and should manifest in more than one environment, hence distinguishing such symptoms from situational variables and a state (versus trait).

SCORING

Scoring is done manually and consumes between five and ten minutes for each form. The scoring sheet is located between the front and back response sheets. Responses are transferred automatically to the scoring sheet by having the informant press hard on the response sheets. Missing scores for two or more items on a particular scale renders it invalid. If five or more items are omitted, the entire form is considered invalid. Also, there is one validity scale that measures the consistency of ratings by comparing raw scores on similarly worded items. There are eight pairs of items on this scale that are entered at the bottom of the score form and subtracted from each other. The scores differences are summed for a total raw inconsistency score. A raw score total of eight or greater invalidates the protocol on the basis of excessive inconsistency among the ratings.

The scales that have proven to be most useful in reporting are as follows: (a) *DSM–IV* Inattentive Symptoms; (b) *DSM–IV* Hyperactive-Impulsive Symptoms; (c) *DSM–IV* ADHD Symptoms Total; and (d) ADHD Index. The raw scores for each of these scales are aggregated and then entered into norms that are gender and age specific; that is, male or female, and age groupings 18–29 years, 30–39 years, 40–49 years, and 50 years and older. The latter age cohorts were based on statistical analyses done on the standardization sample (see prior), which showed a gender by age interaction effect according to the aforesaid age groupings.

Raw scores are converted to dimensional *T*–scores by graphing them on the profile sheets that are part of the response sheet packet. Confidence intervals (CIs) can be rapidly computed by using the average of the *SEMs* reported in the technical manual (see prior), here estimated as two points. Hence, to create an interval that contains the examinee's true score with 68% certainty, the examiner would simply add and subtract two points. The PRs for these *T*–scores would be assigned according to the standard normal distribution (see Appendix A of this book).

Forms 10.10 and 10.11 provide a sequence of two data tables for reporting the results of the CAARS–L self-report rating-scale data alone or accompanied by the observer ratings, respectively. The latter juxtaposes the data for the two informants to facilitate interrater reliability analyses. Table 1 is reported first because it pertains to whether the subsequent data can be trusted or relied upon. Again, the inconsistency index represents a summation of the differences between eight pairs of similarly worded items. A difference score of eight or more invalidates the profile, with increasingly greater scores demonstrating more inconsistency.

Table 2 (Forms 10.10 and 10.11) presents the actual standardized data for the self-report alone or accompanied by observer ratings. The juxtaposition of the data maximizes the effectiveness of the interrater-reliability analysis. For each informant, the data are listed as follows: (a) *T*–score (mean = 50; *SD* = 10, range = 26–90); (b) 95% CI; and (c) PRs (median = 50; range = 1–99). Table notes define metrics, abbreviations, descriptive statistics, and the interpretative scheme (see next section).

INTERPRETATION

Deriving meaning from the CAARS–L data is relatively straightforward. First, the validity scales must be checked. Several pre-drafted outcomes have been prepared for both forms 10.10 and 10.11. The self-report ratings in Form 10.10 are initially apportioned into valid and invalid results. The latter describe either (a) cautionary valid results or (b) completely invalid results. The former represents invalid results that are just above the threshold, hence permitting a cautious interpretation of the clinical data, which must be checked against other scores that are deemed to be of greater reliability and validity. The latter represents an extraordinary degree of inconsistency that precludes any further reporting of data to avoid presenting misleading results. Interpreting the self-report and observer data is more intricate due to an increased number of potential outcomes. Here, there are four potential scenarios, including both being valid, one being valid and the other invalid (i.e., two possible combinations), and both being invalid. The mixed result places more credence on the valid ratings and other data, while both being invalid seeks other data to corroborate any results shown among the clinical data. Although rating scale data are always conceptualized as supplementary, potentially invalid ratings require extended degrees of corroboration. This outcome can also lead to a recommendation not to report the rating scale clinical data due to the risk of presenting misleading scores. Of course, this decision is left to the examiner, who is in the best position to render such a decision.

Table 2 presents the ADHD-related clinical data. Note that the scale labels in the first column are abbreviated such that the *DSM* edition is not entered. This is because the items were based on *DSM–IV* criteria (American Psychiatric Association, 1994) and are being applied to current *DSM–5* standards. However, this is again justified by using the rating scales data solely within a supplementary or supporting role. The initial clinical interview data, together with the performance-based *continuous performance test* (*CPT*) results and rating-scales scores, should provide a reliable and valid final diagnosis regarding the presence of adult ADHD. The scales that have been selected are also empirically on point. Scrutinizing both their labels and measured symptoms, the scales cover the inattentive cluster separately, the hyperactive-impulsive cluster separately, the combined cluster, and a scale that includes items that best discriminate between adults with a documented diagnosis of ADHD and a nonclinical sample (viz., the ADHD Index). The latter is similar to empirical criterion keying used by many of the best quality personality inventories. Briefly, *empirical criterion keying* is a statistical strategy that seeks to find items that best discriminate between a sample who has a particular disorder and a nonclinical sample, irrespective of the item content. This is discussed further in Chapter 15 and thus will not be elaborated further in this part of the book. Suffice it to state that the ADHD Index can be considered a useful scale due to its ability to discriminate individuals with and without such a disorder, especially when used in a supplementary role and bolstered by other data measuring the same construct by different means.

The interpretive scheme is founded upon the *T*–score elevation as follows: (a) 26–65 is within normal limits; (b) 66–70 is elevated; and (c) 71–90 is very elevated. Asterisks are appended to the score when statistically significant, including one for an elevated score and two for a very elevated score. To facilitate interpretation, this scheme is listed within a specific table note, followed by pre-drafted excerpts of the most common outcomes immediately following Table 2. For the single self-report case, there are three scenarios, including clear and consistent results for the presence of any of the three types of ADHD or absence of any such disorder. There are also excerpts that cover false negative and false positive ratings, which also must be accounted for if they occur.

For the self-report and observer case, an interrater-reliability analysis must be incorporated. Thus, there is a scenario describing interrater agreement, both raters being either positive or negative for this diagnostic outcome, and a scenario that covers interrater disagreement. The latter instance ends with a recommendation to seek other data in an attempt to resolve the inconsistency. However, the examiner may also want to add an explanation as to why the disagreement occurred; for example, inferring that the observer's negative results may have been due to observing the examinee in environments that were structured and regimented, hence situational forces engulfed the field and masked any symptoms. In any case, the data are sequenced such that the scores for each rater can be easily compared across each row of the table, ending in a succinct description of the measured symptoms.

Two final notes are in order here prior to moving on to the next instrument. First, the self-report ratings are listed first to afford them greater priority. This is because, all other things being equal, an individual sees him- or herself in many more circumstances and longitudinally across linear time. Second, there is no form for an observer-only situation. Because such a situation has never been encountered, such was not needed. If an examiner may repeatedly use only observer ratings, either Form 10.11 can be used by entering the double-dashed no score symbol within all the self-report columns, or Form 10.10 can be converted into an observer-only form by simply supplanting the self-report label with the observer label.

Sensory Processing Measures

What are sensory processing disorders, and why should a psychologist possess tests that measure such problems? Until about ten years ago, sensory processing disorders were not considered when taking developmental histories of children and adolescents during an initial clinical interview. This class of disorder was not covered in prominent abnormal psychology texts, including several this author had adopted for use in advanced undergraduate courses on this subject (viz., Barlow et al., 2018; Nolen-Hoeksema, 2020), including, for example, abnormal child psychology (viz., Mash & Wolfe, 2019). Gradually, this author became increasingly aware of an association between a premorbid history of sensory processing difficulties and testing for the subsequent onset of various neurodevelopmental (e.g., ADHD), behavioral (e.g., ODD), and mood (e.g., disruptive mood dysregulation disorder, or DMDD) disorders. Furthermore, sensory processing impairments were more recently added to the diagnostic criteria for ASD. More specifically, Criterion B.4 of the *DSM–5* description of autism states, "Hyper- or hyporeactivity to sensory input" (American Psychiatric Association, 2013, p. 50).

Next, this author was assigned to provide psychological testing services within a medical pediatric clinic where referrals to rule out a sensory processing disorder became common practice. In researching this disorder, the *Diagnostic Classification of Mental Health and Developmental Disorders of Infancy and Early Childhood* (*DC:0–5*; Zero to Three, 2016) listed a general class of *sensory processing disorders*. Succinctly, these are defined as abnormalities in regulating sensory input, which cause significant distress or impairment in a young child's daily activities. Although the *DSM–5* considers sensory processing symptoms as part of ASD, the DC:0–5 indicates that there is sufficient evidence to consider these problems as separate and independent from other types of neurodevelopmental and psychopathological syndromes and as stable throughout the first five years of life.

Within this general class of early childhood disorder, there are three more specific manifestations. Specifically, sensory processing problems can manifest as *over-responsivity* (i.e., an abnormally low sensory threshold to environmental stimuli), *under-responsivity* (i.e., an abnormally high threshold to environmental stimuli), or atypical responses to sensory input (i.e., extended sensory exploration to environmental stimuli). These three different reactions to environmental stimuli are general referred to as (a) *sensory over-responsivity disorder*, (b) *sensory under-responsivity disorder*, and (c) *other sensory processing disorder*. These disorders are linked to *DSM–5* as an *other specified neurodevelopmental disorder* (code F88) and in the ICD–10 as *other disorders of psychological development* (code F88).

Finally, the *Psychodynamic Diagnostic Manual, Second Edition* (*PDM–2*; Lingiardi & McWilliams, 2017) also recognized sensory processing disorders as "constitutionally based maladaptive responses to sensory stimuli that may lead to difficult behaviors and complicate a child's interactions with the environment" (Speranza & Mayes, 2017, p. 674). Hence, the *PDM–2* went further and actually proposed an etiological or causal link between different sensory processing disorders and problematic behavioral patterns. For example, the *PDM–2* proposes a *hypersensitive disorder* that is linked with either a fearful–anxious pattern, a negative–stubborn pattern, or a self-absorbed pattern (i.e., difficult to engage). The point here is that sensory processing problems are increasingly recognized as representing a bona fide independent class of early onset neurodevelopmental psychopathology that cause distress and dysfunction and that predispose an individual to other kinds of behavioral problems. This means that a testing psychologist, especially one who works with individuals in early childhood, should have tests that measure the construct of sensory processing disorder and associated behavioral problems. Next, the sensory processing measures that have been selected for use in mental health testing practice are presented, beginning with the one that is designed for the younger preschool population, then moving in chronological order to the measure that is normed on older children largely of elementary school age through middle school or preadolescence. Sensory processing measures are available for adolescents and adults, although a demand for such testing in these older populations has not been found, at least not in mental health practice.

Sensory Processing Measure–Preschool

This first of two sensory processing measures is generally designed for the preschool-age population. Thus, it will be presented first to maintain this book's preference in presenting measures of similar kinds of psychopathology in chronological order (i.e., from younger to older populations).

SYNOPSIS

The *Sensory Processing Measure–Preschool* (*SPM–P*; Ecker, Parham, Kuhaneck, Henry, & Glennon, 2010) consists of observer-based rating scales that measure preschool children's real-world processing across a number of sensory modalities, including the visual, auditory, tactile, *proprioceptive* (i.e., body position awareness), and vestibular (i.e., balance and motion) systems, along with *praxis* (i.e., the ability to plan and organize movement) and social participation, the last two representing higher-level integrative functions that are frequently affected by a child's sensory processing abilities (Miller, Anzalone, Lane, Cermack, & Osten, 2007). Covering ages 3–5, this instrument is intended to be a younger companion to the *Sensory Processing Measure* (*SPM*; Parham, Ecker, Kuhaneck, Henry, & Glennon, 2007), which virtually provides the same data on children ages 5–12. Together, these instruments provide continuity in measuring the same sensory processing constructs from ages 2–12 (i.e., toddlerhood through childhood and preadolescence). The one-year overlap at age five was by design in that if an examinee of that age happens to be enrolled in Grade K (i.e., formal schooling), the older version is to be administered, otherwise the preschool version is to be used in its stead. Not surprisingly, the SPM–P consists of two forms: the home form and school form, covering home and preschool environments, respectively. Technically, the home form also implicates sensory processing functioning within the community, considering that such is typically completed by a parental figure who frequently observes the child in many different environments in addition to that of the home. However, for brevity's sake, this will be hereafter inferred from use of the single term "home."

The SPM–P is based on the same sensory integration theory proposed by Ayers (1972, 1979, 2005) as was the companion SPM. Succinctly, *sensory integration* (also known and hereafter referred to as *sensory processing*) is defined by Ayers as the "organization of sensation for use" (1979, p. 184). Hence, he proposes that such ability directly impacts both learning and adaptive behavioral functioning, including the higher-level integrative functions mentioned previously. Early detection of sensory problems is thus critical in this young population, which justifies the clinical use of this measure and its older companion in mental health testing practice.

NORM REFERENCE SAMPLE

The SPM–P standardization sample consisted of 651 typically (i.e., normally) developing children recruited from mainstream education preschools, hence including an expected proportion of children in the population with mild pre-academic or behavioral difficulties. None of the five-year-olds were enrolled in kindergarten. The sample was stratified in terms of age, gender, ethnicity, and SES (socioeconomic status), the latest defined by the parents' education level, and corresponded to the 2006/2007 U.S. census (U.S. Census Bureau, 2006, 2007a, 2007b, 2007c). Any discrepancies that were considered potential moderating variables were analyzed in terms of effect size. All except *age* yielded small effects and hence were considered clinically meaningless. Regarding age, medium-to-large effect sizes were consistently observed between the two-year-olds and the two- to five-year-olds, with significantly higher raw scores being associated with the youngest age group. Therefore, the SPM–P provides separate norms for these two groups, as reflected by a doubled-sided profile form with raw to *T*–score conversions for ages three to five on the front side and those for age two on the back side.

ADMINISTRATION

The home form is to be completed by the child's primary caregiver (typically a parent or parent surrogate) and contains 75 items, while the school form is to be completed by the child's primary preschool teacher or day care provider and also contains 75 items. Both take about 15–20 minutes of administration time. They are color coded for easier reference; that is, orange for the home form and blue for the school form. These forms consist of parallel items worded somewhat differently to match their particular environments.

More specifically, items are rated in terms of behavioral *frequency* or the child's most *typical* behavior on a four-point Likert-type scale, including the following: (a) N = *Never* (i.e., the behavior *never* or *almost never* happens); (b) O = *Occasionally* (i.e., the behavior happens *some of the time*); (c) F = *Frequently* (i.e., the behavior happens *much of the time*); and (d) A = *Always* (i.e., the behavior *always* or *almost always* happens). With one exception, items have a negative valence, meaning higher ratings indicate more problems. For social participation, items have a positive valence and thus are reversed scored such that higher raw scores consistently indicate greater pathology.

For the most consistent and accurate ratings, the authors recommend a minimum of one-month daily observation of the child; especially applicable to the school-based abilities (Ecker et al., 2010, p. 5). This time frame is consistent with that advised for the Conners EC and Conners CBRS, both of which are multidimensional scales that cover comparable age ranges (see prior). Finally, informants are encouraged to answer all items to the best of their ability. Because several items ask informants to rate the child's degree of manifested "distress," this term is concretely defined in terms of both verbal expressions (e.g., whining, crying, yelling) and nonverbal expressions (e.g., withdrawing, gesturing, pushing, running away, wincing, and striking out aggressively).

SCORING

The home form and school form are scored manually within an estimated time of five to ten minutes (Ecker et al., 2010, p. 3). The respondent's ratings are recorded by means of carbon paper onto a scoring worksheet. For each of the eight scales, including total sensory systems, raw scores are totaled and transformed into standardized *T*–scores (mean = 50, standard deviation = 15, range = 40–80) and associated percentile ranks (PRs) using a profile sheet with such tabled information. As alluded to previously, this measure is quantified such that higher scores indicate the presence of more problems. This profile sheet is to be removed by the clinician just prior to administration and is doubled-sided with norms for ages three to five on the front and those for age two on the back. These scales and their measured abilities appear in Forms 10.12 and 10.13, where the former includes columns for the home form only and the latter includes juxtaposed columns for reporting both the home form and school form data together. On the home form, there is also a DIF (differential item functioning) calculation available at the bottom of the profile summary sheet in which the total sensory systems scores for home and school are subtracted in said order. This feature is only available on Form 10.13, upon which data from both forms are input. This permits comparison of overall sensory functioning between the two environments.

When looking at Table 1 on both Forms 10.12 and 10.13, there are a number of scoring components to highlight. First, note that the total sensory systems score is computed by a summation of the five scale raw scores that measure functioning within a sensory modality (viz., vision, hearing, touch, body awareness, and balance and motion), along with raw scores from four free-standing items addressing *taste* and *smell* that do not contribute to an independent scale. This information is available in specific table notes "e" and "g." Hence, from an interpretation perspective, the total sensory systems score does not include the two higher-level integrative functioning scales social participation and planning and ideas (i.e., praxis), a fact that is addressed further in the interpretation section. Second, in Form 10.13 only, the school-based data are juxtaposed with the home-based data to facilitate comparison of functioning between the two environments. Third, a 95% CI column has been incorporated after the dimensional *T*–score, which can be easily computed based on the *SEM* for each form and scale. This information is available in Table 13 of the manual (Ecker et al., 2010, p. 46).

The particular values chosen were those provided by the test–retest coefficients (versus the internal consistency reliability coefficients) because sensory processing stability across time appeared to be the more central feature upon which to base such an estimated interval of certainty, as compared to within-test consistency, especially regarding children whose behavior is more vulnerable to fluctuation across both situations and time. The clinician merely adds and subtracts the value appearing within the table to the obtained score to compute the interval. Specifically, the listed number reflects the addition of two *SEM* units, which were already rounded to the nearest whole number for computational simplicity, for purposes of computing an estimated 95% CI. That listed value can then be deleted from the final psychological assessment report as no longer necessary to the interpretation. For instance, if the vision clinical scale on the home form (see both Forms 10.12 and 10.13) obtained *T*–score of 70, the 95% CI would be 66–74 (70 ± 4). As can be seen, the *SEM* values are sufficiently low so that the 95% CIs are generally eight- to ten-point intervals, which is a reasonable range when applied to *T*–scores. Therefore, a high degree of confidence can be used here, as was done for the cognitive constructs. Next, the intended interpretive sequence for these data is described.

INTERPRETATION

As there are no validity scales, test interpretation begins immediately with the clinical scale data, which are included on the one and only table for this measure (see both Forms 10.12 and 10.13). The table is configured to guide interpretation, which proceeds in the following order for both Forms 10.12 and 10.13 unless otherwise noted: (a) overall sensory system processing; (b) quantitative (i.e., environmental difference or DIF calculation) and qualitative (i.e., DIF interpretation as No [0–9 points], Probable [10–14 points], or Definite [≥ 15 points] difference) comparison of overall sensory processing ability in the home versus school environments, with positive differences indicating more home problems, whereas negative scores indicate more school problems (Form 10.13 only); (c) analysis of functioning within and across the specific sensory systems and environments (Form 10.13 only) by examining the *T*–score elevations; (d) investigation of higher-level integrative functioning and its relationship (if any) to sensory system processing ability within and across both environments (as proposed by Ayers' sensory integration theory); (e) item analysis to explore any underlying evidence of sensory integration vulnerabilities (contingent upon any prior evidence of sensory processing impairment); (f) rendering of an opinion of whether the overall evidence supports a sensory processing regulation disorder; and (g) offering of an opinion as to whether the data support a current, or risk of a future, *DSM* disorder, especially within the neurodevelopmental class of syndromes.

The *T*–score interpretive scheme is as follows: (a) *T*–score of 40–59 is the *typical* range (i.e., no problems); (b) *T*–score of 60–69 is the *some problems* range; and (c) *T*–score 70–80 is the *definite dysfunction* range. This scheme is reported in a specific table note for ease of interpretation. To further facilitate interpretation, pre-drafted excerpts follow Table 1 in both Form 10.12 and 10.13. The statements are ordered so as to easily identify the steps. Note that the Form 10.13 interpretive sequence contains five steps versus four in Form 10.12 because of the added differential analysis between home and school environments. Furthermore, the between-environment comparison of the child's sensory processing functioning also renders each step more intricate because of garnering data from two raters and in different environments.

More specifically, even prior to proceeding with the interpretive sequence, note that two points are made concerning the sensory processing construct. First, the fact that sensory processing and sensory integration are defined as synonymous terms is necessary because they are frequently used interchangeably in the literature, although if left undefined, they carry the risk of being confused as representing different constructs. Second, the association between sensory processing functioning and other mental health disorders is made explicit to further justify its measurement. Hence, the reader will immediately be informed of both (a) the meaning of sensory processing and (b) its relevance to mental health diagnosis. Following this prologue, the initial step is designed to investigate the overall sensory functioning of the child. For Form 10.13 only, the next step focuses on the differential between the two environments. Next, the *T*–score scale elevations are scrutinized to determine the particular profile, largely using norm-based comparisons. Here, scale names are listed at each of the three interpretive levels (i.e., typical, some problems, and definite dysfunction). The subsequent level of interpretation examines the profile of higher-level integrative functions. If there are clear problems here, an attempt to discern any relationship to previously identified sensory impairments should be done. This comparison investigates if there is evidence that any sensory processing dysfunction is causing higher-level behavioral or neurodevelopmental issues.

Perhaps the most vital portion of the interpretive process for diagnostic purposes is item analysis. Clusters of items are associated with different sensory processing vulnerabilities. Hence, it is critical to identify any patterns of elevated items, namely, those that are rated either *F* for *Frequently* or especially *A* for *Always*. Items that are associated with different sensory vulnerabilities are enumerated in the interpretation narratives of different sensory vulnerabilities and color coded for ease of detection; that is, red font for the home form items and blue font for the school form items (Form 10.13 only). For example, if items 16, 17, 18, 20, 21, 23, 24, 26, 27, 28, 29, 30, 31, 32, 33, 35, 37, 38, 39, 40, 41, 45, and 46 showed *F* or *A* ratings, then a sensory over-responsivity disorder would be diagnosed. Such information can be obtained from the interpretive manual, which lists the principal sensory integration vulnerability associated with each item in tabular form (Ecker et al., 2010, Tables 2 and 3, pp. 15–20). It is listed in the interpretative summary for convenience and may be deleted after the interpretation is made. Lastly, as suggested in the aforementioned example, the interpretation should conclude with an opinion regarding the presence or absence of a sensory processing disorder. If such is indicated, then further addressing the risk or presence of a related *DSM–5* disorder should also be done prior to concluding interpretation.

Sensory Processing Measure

This second and final sensory processing measure is designed in the same manner as was the prior instrument. Thus, it is presented in like fashion, with special attention to the differences in the norm reference sample, along with some differences in item content. As a result, the data forms created for this measure are strikingly similar to those of the preschool version.

SYNOPSIS

The *Sensory Processing Measure* (*SPM*; Parham et al., 2007) consists of observer-based rating scales that measure children's real-world processing across a number of sensory modalities, including the visual, auditory, tactile, proprioceptive (i.e., body position awareness), and vestibular (i.e., balance and motion) systems, along with *praxis* (i.e., the ability to plan and organize movement) and social participation, the last two representing higher-level integrative functions that are frequently affected by a child's sensory processing abilities (Parham et al., 2007). From a diagnostic perspective, the two most useful rating scales included in this instrument are the home form (Parham & Ecker, 2007), which measures a child's functioning in the home and community environments, and the main classroom form, which measures a child's functioning in the principal classroom.[1] The SPM covers an age range of 5 years, 0 months through 12 years, 11 months (i.e., K–6th grade). Hereafter, it will be implicitly understood that the home form also represents the child's functioning in the community, although this will no longer be stated explicitly for purposes of pithiness, including in the upcoming data tables.

Similar to its younger version, the SPM is based on the sensory integration theory proposed by Ayers (1972, 1979, 2005), which defines the construct of *sensory integration* (or *sensory processing*, as used principally here) as the "organization of sensation for use" (Ayers, 1979, p. 184). In essence, the theory proposes that sensory processing and integration is a neurodevelopmental ability that directly impacts adaptation.[2] Specifically, it is argued that impairments in sensory processing in turn deleteriously affects learning and adaptive behavioral functioning, the latter including the aforementioned higher-level integrative functions that are measured as part of this instrument. Consistent with this proposition, the research indicates an association between sensory processing problems and *DSM* disorders, including ASD (see e.g., Lai, Parham, & Ecker, 1999) and ADHD (see e.g., Miller, 2006), both appropriately classified as *DSM–5* neurodevelopmental disorders.

NORM REFERENCE SAMPLE

The SPM home form and main classroom form are normed on a representative sample of 1,051 typically (i.e., normally) developing children in Grades K through 6 (i.e., ages 5–12). Included were children with mild sensory problems, which were considered to be a natural component of the typical population of children in this age group. The sample was stratified in terms of age, gender, ethnicity, and SES, the last defined by the parents' education level, and which corresponded to the 2001 U.S. census (U.S. Census Bureau, 2001a, 2001b). Any discrepancies that were considered potential moderating variables were analyzed in terms of effect size. All yielded small effects and hence were deemed to be not clinically meaningful, including especially age (Parham et al., 2007, p. 47). The latter was critical in that it justified the use of a single set of norms for the entire age group.

ADMINISTRATION

The home form is to be completed by the child's primary caregiver and contains 75 items, while the main classroom form is to be completed by the child's primary teacher and contains 62 items. Both take about 15–20 minutes of administration time. These two principal forms consist of parallel items worded somewhat differently for their particular environment. Items are rated in terms of behavioral *frequency* on a four-point Likert-type scale, including the following: (a) *N = Never* (i.e., the behavior *never* or *almost never* happens), (b) *O = Occasionally* (i.e., the behavior happens *some of the time*), (c) *F = Frequently* (the behavior happens *much of the time*), and (d) *A = Always* (the behavior *always* or *almost always* happens).

With the exception of the social participation clinical scale, items have a negative valence (i.e., higher ratings indicate greater pathology of dysfunction). Therefore, for all scales to be scored in that same direction, the social participation items are reverse scored. For the most reliable ratings, the authors recommend a minimum of one month of daily observation and to focus on the child's *typical behavior*, especially applicable to the school-based data (Parham et al., 2007, p. 5). Hence, the item instructions focus the rater on the examinee's average tendencies over time, consistent with the definition of sensory processing ability. It is interesting that the home form and main classroom form are not color coded for easier detection; that is, both are printed in black ink with a white background. All the remaining administration procedures are exactly the same as for the SPM–P and thus will not be repeated here for space-saving purposes.

SCORING

The home form and main classroom form are scored manually within an estimated time of five to ten minutes (Parham et al., 2007, p. 3). The respondent's ratings are recorded by means of carbon paper onto a scoring worksheet. For each of the eight scales, including total sensory systems, raw scores are totaled and transformed into standardized *T*–scores (mean = 50, standard deviation =15, range = 40–80) and associated PRs using a profile summary sheet with such tabled information wherein higher scores indicate more problems; this profile sheet is to be removed by the clinician just prior to administration for later scoring and optional graphing. These scales and their measured abilities appear in Forms 10.14 and 10.15, which have been designed for reporting the SPM results within a final psychological assessment report.

As done for the preschool SPM, Form 10.14 is created for entering only the home form data; hence, in cases where the main classroom ratings are not available (e.g., when done during the summer recess from school). On Form 10.15, the home form and main classroom form data are juxtaposed to facilitate interrater (and between environment) comparisons. As on Form 10.13, discrepancies between the home and main classroom ratings can be due to genuine differences in sensory processing between environments and/or interrater inconsistency. Examiner discretion must be employed in making such a determination, which is made more difficult due to the absence of validity scales. In the event both the home form and main classroom forms were employed, the former contains a DIF calculation at the bottom of the profile summary sheet in which the total sensory systems scores for home and school can be subtracted from each other in this order. This permits an empirical comparison of overall sensory functioning between the environments, which is in the form of a difference score and can be reported in the interpretation portion of Form 10.15 (see the subsequent interpretation section).

When looking at Table 1 in both Forms 10.14 and 10.15, there are a number of points to highlight. These points apply to both Forms 10.14 and 10.15 unless otherwise noted. First, note that the total sensory systems score is computed by a summation of the five scale raw scores that measure functioning within a sensory modality (viz., vision, hearing, touch, body awareness, and balance and motion), along with raw scores from four free-standing items addressing *taste* and *smell* that do not contribute to an independent scale. This information is available in specific table notes "e" and "g." Hence, from an interpretation perspective, the total sensory systems score does not include the two higher-level integrative function scales social participation and planning and ideas (i.e., praxis). Second, the school-based data immediately follow the home-based data in the same row to facilitate comparison of functioning between the environments. Third, the *T*–score elevations determine the overall and specific levels of dysfunction among the scales to which has been appended a 95% CI column. The latter can be easily computed based on the standard error of measurement (*SEM*) reported for each form and scale.

As was done for the SPM–P, this information is available in Table 18 of the manual (Parham et al., 2007, p. 57), where the quantities are listed to add and subtract to the obtained score so as to estimate the interval. The values chosen were those provided by the test–retest coefficients (versus the internal consistency reliability coefficients) because ensuring stability across time is most central to measuring sensory processing ability as defined earlier. The clinician merely adds and subtracts the confidence value appearing within the table to the obtained score to compute the interval; that is, it already reflects the addition of two SEM units rounded to the nearest whole number. The values used for creating the CIs can then be deleted, as they are no longer necessary to interpretation. For instance, if the home form vision clinical scale had a *T*–score of 60, the 95% CI would be 57–63 (i.e., 60 ± 3). Next, the SPM interpretive steps are delineated, which mirror those for the SPM–P.

INTERPRETATION

Table 1 in both Forms 10.14 and 10.15 is configured to guide interpretation, which proceeds in the following order: (a) overall sensory system processing ability; (b) quantitative (i.e., environmental difference or DIF calculation) and qualitative (i.e., DIF interpretation as No [0–9 points], Probable [10–14 points], or Definite [≥ 15 points] Difference) comparison of overall sensory processing ability in the home versus school environments, wherein positive differences indicate more home problems and negative scores indicate more school problems (Form 10.15 only); (c) analysis of functioning within and across the specific sensory systems and environments (the latter pertaining to Form 10.15 only); (d) investigation of higher-level integrative functioning and its relationship (if any) to sensory system processing ability within and across both environments (the latter pertaining to Form 10.15 only); (e) item analysis to explore any underlying evidence of sensory integration vulnerabilities (contingent upon any prior evidence of sensory processing impairment); (f) render an opinion of whether or not the overall evidence supports a sensory processing disorder (and if so what type as indicated by item analyses); and (g) offer an opinion of whether or not the data either support a current, or risk of a future, DSM disorder, especially within the neurodevelopmental class of syndromes.

The interpretive scheme is based on the *T*–score range as follows: (a) 40–59 is the *typical* range (i.e., no problems); (b) 60–69 is the *some problems* range (denoted by appending one asterisk); and (c) 70–80 is the *definite dysfunction* range (denoted by appending two asterisks). These ranges mirror those used for the SPM-P. The interpretive steps for both Forms 10.14 and 10.15 also parallel those for Form 10.12 and Form 10.13, beginning with defining the sensory processing construct and its synonym and associating it with mental health disorder. This is followed by a general to specific sequence of interpretation, starting with overall sensory functioning and moving to the sensory clinical scales and higher-order functioning scales, any available environment discrepancies, items analyses, a determination of sensory processing disorder diagnosis, and finally, whether there is a *DSM–5* disorder present or a risk thereof. Pre-drafted narrative templates have also been inserted here, as was done for the preschool versions that guide the examiner through the interpretive steps. Because these steps were already reviewed in sufficient detail, they will not be repeated here. The only difference regards some variation among the item clusters that are associated with somewhat different sensory processing vulnerabilities. Once again, they are color coded for easy reference; that is, red font for home ratings and blue font for school ratings. Once again, the item numbers should be deleted after the interpretation is complete.

SUMMARY

This ends the presentation of the two sensory processing rating scales that measure disorders of said construct as manifested in the real world. Note that these data are based on observations of a child's typical behavior in the home setting and various environments in the community, along with a school setting, rather than on performance-based data obtained in an artificial clinical office where sensory issues likely do not manifest in similar fashion. This maximizes what has been referred to as *ecological validity*, which is the ability to generalize psychological test results to the real-world environment. It is also assumed that dysfunction in this ability represents independent pathology that also contributes to comorbid mental health disorders, especially in the neurodevelopmental category. Next, the last of the unidimensional rating scales are presented, here focused on disorders that are caused by trauma and their *sequelae* (i.e., supplemental conditions of a prior disorder or injury).

Trauma-Related Measures

The ensuing trilogy of rating scales are unidimensional in design in that they focus on measuring trauma-related disorders and associated conditions. This consists of primary disorders resulting therefrom, along with collateral symptoms, problems, issues, and sequelae. *Sequelae* are common consequences of a prior disorder, disease, or injury (*sequela* as singular). The three instruments presented next can be conceptualized as companion measures for several related reasons. First, they are published by the same author and company. Second, they are remarkably similar in design, organization, and format. Third, as a triad, they cover the vast majority of the life span. The last two reasons shall become apparent when the various tests are considered. As a final introductory note, these instruments are most useful when examinees have suspected or confirmed trauma in their history and are showing psychological symptoms that are interfering with functioning. This is a direct consequence of these measures' unidimensional quality. Because of this, a review of (a) what constitutes trauma and (b) its consequential symptoms will first be provided. This will be ensued by a presentation of these three measures following chronological age, as has been done for all prior test sequences. The ensuing two sections present the following in such order: (a) what constitutes a trauma according to the *DSM–5* and empirical research, and (b) what types of disorders, symptoms, symptom clusters, and sequelae are commonly exhibited subsequent to a bona fide trauma or series of traumas?

What Is Trauma? A Review

To begin, the *DSM–5* defines *trauma* as exposure to death or endangerment, grave injury, or profound violence, whether it be a direct insult to the self, direct witnessing of such an event, learning that such an event has happened to one who represents a close emotional attachment, or repeated exposure to such traumatic experiences or details. Therefore, for an event to be potentially considered as constituting a trauma, it must at minimum fit the aforesaid conceptualization. In addition, there is an expectation that trauma has the capability of precipitating the onset of subsequent psychopathology (see the next section). This definition also clearly differentiates trauma from the more ordinary stressors people experience on a daily basis, which have been referred to as hassles. Briefly, *hassles* are small frustrations, annoyances, aggravations, or minor disagreements that occur on a daily basis or fairly frequently and can cause some degree of irritation or distress (Lazarus, 1993; Lazarus & Folkman, 1984). In contrast, traumas must rise to the level of being catastrophic or at least near catastrophic. These aversive events can also be somewhat less intense but repetitive such that there is an accumulating effect. So much for a working definition. What does the research tell us?

First examined are events that have caused PTSD (post-traumatic stress disorder) and other trauma-related syndromes in children and adolescents. Not surprisingly, earthquakes (Scott, Knot, Beltran-Quines, & Gomez, 2003), hurricanes (Russoniello et al., 2002), and natural disasters in general have proven capable of leading to PTSD (Green et al., 1991). Events caused by negligence are also relevant, including motor vehicle collisions (Briere, 2005; Ehlers, Mayou, & Bryant, 2003; Saigh, Yasik, Oberfield, Halamandaris, & McHugh, 2002) and residential fires (Jones, Ribbe, Cunningham, Weddle, & Langley, 2002). The experience of terrorist attacks (Pfefferbaum et al., 2002; Stuber et al., 2002) and war-related events (Peltzer, 1999; Smith, Perrin, Dyregrov, & Yule, 2003) are clearly occurrences commonly associated with trauma-associated psychopathology.

Unfortunately, perhaps the largest number and variety of traumatic events causing subsequent psychopathology are associated with family, and especially involving parents or primary caretakers. Specifically, they include parental suicides (Clements & Burgess, 2002); parental alcoholism (Briere, 2005); domestic violence in the presence of children (Jaffe, Wolfe, & Wilson, 1990; Kashani, Daniel, Dandoy, & Holcomb, 1992), including the murder of a parent (Malmquist, 1986); severe illness of a family member (Briere, 2005); physical and sexual abuse perpetrated by primary caretakers (Briere, 1992; Brier & Elliot, 2003; Browne & Finkelhor, 1986; Finkelhor, Hotaling, Lewis, & Smith, 1990; Graziano & Namaste, 1990; Kiser, Heston, Millsap, & Pruit, 1991; Kolko, Moser, & Weldy, 1988; Lanktree, Briere, & Zaidi, 1991); and even marital dissolution between children's parents (Evans, Briere, Boggiano, & Barret, 1994).

Being a victim of crime also represents a class of events shown to cause trauma-related disorders. These comprise interpersonal victimization (Brownstein, Haltry, Altschuler, & Blair, 1989; Schubiner, Scott, & Tzelepis, 1993), including sexual battery, being shot or shot at, and being attacked or stabbed with a knife (Singer, Anglin, Song, & Lunghofer, 1995; Tjaden & Thoennes, 2000); physical and sexual batteries perpetrated by peers (Boney-McCoy & Finkelhor, 1995; Freeman, Mokros, & Poznanski, 1993; Singer et al., 1995); and finally, school violence (Ruchkin, Scwab-Stone, Koposov, Vermeiren, & Steiner, 2002). Further, being incarcerated at juvenile detention can also induce a trauma-related disorder via exposure to intimidation, bullying, threats, and violence (Crimmins, Cleary, Brownstein, Spunt, & Warley, 2000; Kroll et al., 2002; Rcuhkin et al., 2002).

Regarding adults, experiences such as rape, combat, and torture are causes of trauma-related psychopathology (Breslau, Davis, & Andreski, & Peterson, 1991; Kessler, Sonnega, Bromet, Hughes, & Nelson, 1995; Marshall, Schell, Elliot, Berthold, & Chun, 2005; Ramchand et al., 2010; Steel et al., 2009). In addition, working in certain professions predisposes adults to PTSD and trauma-related symptoms. For instance, a meta-analysis of police, firefighters, and emergency medical technicians (EMTs) found that 10% met the criteria for PTSD (Berger et al., 2012). Furthermore, soldiers have been found to experience trauma-related syndromes 10–20 years following their combat experience (Elder & Clipp, 1989; Sutker, Allain, & Johnson, 1993; Sutker, Allain, & Winstead, 1993).

Of the factors that exacerbate trauma symptoms, severity, duration, and proximity to the event were the three most prominent (Cardozo, Vergara, Agani, & Gotway, 2000; Ehlers et al., 1998; Hoge et al., 2004; Kessler et al., 1995). For instance, soldiers who were involved in more intense combat, and for a longer period of time on the front lines, had the highest probability of later manifesting PTSD (Iversen et al., 2008). As another example, women who experienced rape that was both violent and repeated over time were most likely to develop PTSD (Epstein, Saunders, & Kilpatrick, 1997; Zinzow et al., 2012).

At this juncture, a definition of trauma has been offered, along with empirical data as to what kinds of experiences are ensued by psychopathology. Next scrutinized are the kinds of disorders that typically result from exposure to trauma; a topic that is directly relevant to its accurate measurement.

Trauma-Related Disorders and Symptoms

Before presenting the three trauma-related rating scales, this section will briefly cover some of the disorders and symptoms that eventuate after trauma exposure. Not surprisingly, one of the most common clinical disorders resulting from trauma is PTSD, which principally includes dysphoria, chronic arousal, hypervigilance, emotional numbing, partial amnesia, avoidance of reminders of the event(s), flashbacks, nightmares, reliving of the event(s), self-blame, excessive guilt, acting out the trauma in play (as applied particularly to children), anger outbursts, irritability, and dissociative symptoms (i.e., alterations in conscious awareness). Not surprisingly, PTSD is one of the most prevalent disorders listed under the new general category of trauma-related disorders in the *DSM–5* (American Psychiatric Association, 2013). For instance, the lifetime prevalence of PTSD in the general population is estimated at 8% (Breslau et al., 1991; Kessler et al., 1995; Marshall et al., 2005; Ramchand et al., 2010; Steel et al., 2009), which rivals an estimated 7% 12-month prevalence for major depressive disorder and 0.6% for bipolar I disorder (American Psychiatric Association, 2013). Additionally, PTSD with dissociative symptoms has also been found in young children who have experienced trauma (Boney-McCoy & Finkelhor, 1995; Breslau et al., 1991; Green et al., 1991; Singer et al., 1995; Wolfe, Gentile, & Wolfe, 1989). However, PTSD is certainly not the only clinical disorder or symptom cluster that can result from trauma.

As concerning children, trauma has been linked to the following mental health disorders and symptoms: (a) anxiety and depression (Fergusson, Horwood, & Lynskey, 1996; Freeman et al., 1993; Hurt, Malmud, Brodky, & Giannetta, 2001; Lanktree, Briere, & Zaidi, 1991; Martinez & Richters, 1993; McDermott & Palmer, 2002; Pynoos et al., 1993); (b) sexual symptoms and age-inappropriate sexual behavior (Friedrich 1994; Friedrich et al., 2001; Hall, Mathews, & Pearce, 2002); (c) ODD and CD (Ford, 2002; Guterman, Cameron, & Hahm, 2003); (d) anger and aggression (Flannery, Singer, & Wester, 2001; Kolbo, Blakely, & Engleman, 1996; Singer et al., 1995); (e) somatization symptoms (Abdalla & Elklit, 2001; Darves-Bornoz, Choquet, Ledoux, Gasquet, & Manfredi, 1998); (f) self-injurious and suicidal behavior (Finzi et al., 2001; Johnson et al., 2002); and (g) low self-esteem and other cognitive distortions from a cognitive-behavioral perspective (Hurt, Malmud, Brodky, & Giannetta, 2001; Ryan, Kilmer, Cauce, Watanabe, & Hoyt, 2000).

Regarding adults, research on trauma has similarly shown that it has extensive effects on victims, resulting in an array of non-PTSD-specific symptoms. Some of these include (a) anxiety and depressive disorders (Gilboa-Schechtman & Foa, 2001; Heim & Nemeroff, 2001); (b) somatization disorders (Dietrich, 2003; Walker, Katon, Roy-Byrne, Jemelka, & Russo, 1993); (c) impaired identity formation (Briere & Richards, 2007; Cole & Putnam, 1992); (d) disorders involving severe emotion dysregulation (van der Kolk et al., 1996; Zlotnick, Donaldson, Spirito, & Pearlstein, 1997); (e) attachment disorders (Cloitre, Stovall-McClough, Zorbas, & Charuvastra, 2008; Harari, Bakermans-Kranenburg, & Van IJzendoorn, 2007); (f) maladaptive personality traits associated with interpersonal problems (Elliott, 1994; Pietrzak, Goldstein, Malley, Johnson, & Southwick, 2009); (g) dissociative psychopathology (Briere, Scott, & Weathers, 2005; Chu, Frey, Ganzel, & Matthews, 1999); (h) substance use disorders (Ouimette & Brown, 2003; Najavits, 2002); (i) suicidal ideation, gestures, and attempts, and more generally risk of self-harm (Panagioti, Gooding, & Tarrier, 2009); and (j) externalizing or acting-out behavioral symptoms and more generally risk of harm to others (Briere & Gill, 1998; Zlotnick et al., 1997).

Because trauma experiences can lead to such variegated patterns of psychopathology, any particular case that meets the criteria for a diagnosis of PTSD can also present with multiple cotemporaneous problems and disorders. This is especially the case when an individual's traumas consist of early, repetitive, and profound violations of interpersonal trust, which are exacerbated by subsequent traumas (van der Kolk, Roth, Pelcovitz, Sunday, & Spinazzola, 2005). For such cases, the construct of *complex PTSD* (*c-PTSD*) has been proposed (Briere & Spinazzola, 2005; Cloitre et al., 2009; Ford, 1999; Herman, 1992; van der Kolk et al, 2005). Alternative challenging cases present with more ingrained-type symptoms, including frequent and intense episodes of emotional dysregulation, acting-out behaviors (including aggression), and severe and chronic interpersonal conflict, from which the presence of personality psychopathology can be inferred, including disturbed attachment patterns.

Trauma Symptom Checklist for Young Children

The *Trauma Symptom Checklist for Young Children* (*TSCYC*; Briere, 2005) will be presented first as it applies to the youngest of the three age cohorts covered by the ensuing three measures. Specifically, the TSCYC covers an age range from 3 years, 0 months through 12 years, 11 months.

SYNOPSIS

The TSCYC is an observer-based rating scale instrument designed to detect post-traumatic stress symptom clusters and some nonessential sequelae in individuals from early childhood through preadolescence. It does not have a self-report version because (a) it begins at an early age wherein examinees do not have sufficient cognitive development to accurately report their symptoms (i.e., ages 3–7 that largely cover the preoperational stage of cognitive development in Piaget's influential theory where logical reasoning is not yet developed; Piaget, 1952, 1962, 1983), and (b) it continues into the middle-to-older childhood age range (i.e., 8–12 years) where there exists large individual differences in metacognitive ability, including the ability to introspect (see Flavell, Green, & Flavell, 1995a, 1995b).

Therefore, if an examinee from ages 8 to 12 shows evidence of the ability to introspect, the older self-report trauma instrument should be selected (see subsequent). In contrast, if the examinee is poor at describing their internal feelings and mental state, then this observer-report younger version is the measure of choice. Of note, it should be increasingly apparent these instruments are to be considered components of the same multi-score, multi-informant system. If the examiner is unsure as to which form to use when the examinee fits within the overlapping age range, however, there is nothing prohibiting the use of both measures so as to best detect the particular profile of potential symptoms present in a case. This practice is especially acceptable as applied to trauma-related disorders due to the multitude of possible symptoms that may manifest, which is why some time was devoted to reviewing the host of symptoms that have been found in consequence to experienced trauma.

NORM REFERENCE SAMPLE

The standardization group was obtained via Internet-based sampling wherein 41,446 emails were sent out with screening questions. These questions inquired as to ethnicity, parental educational level, geographic region, and age of children living in the residence. About 95% of those meeting the desired demographic criteria completed the TSCYC. The overall sample was stratified to match the 2002 U.S. census data (U.S. Census Bureau, 2002) according to geographic region, parent education level, race, child age, and child gender. The final normative sample totaled 750 who completed the TSCYC online.

In terms of the final sample demographics, 50% were males and 50% were females, and age was approximately evenly apportioned for each year beginning at age 3 through age 12 (i.e., each year comprised about 10% of the sample). About 62% were White, 17% Hispanic, 16% Black, and 6% Asian or Other. Of the caretaker informants, 39% were male and 61% were female. Regarding geographic region, the South had the largest proportion at 37%, whereas the remaining three regions each contained about 20%. Education level of the rater was apportioned into (a) less than 12 years (i.e., 17%), (b) 12 years (i.e., 31%), (c) 13–15 years (i.e., 28%), and (d) greater than 15 years (i.e., 24%). A series of multivariate analyses with post-hoc analyses of variance resulted in six normative subgroups for the TSCYC, including gender (viz., male, female) by age cohort (viz., 3–4 years, 5–9 years, and 10–12 years).

ADMINISTRATION

The intended informant is a parent or an adult who is in a primary caretaker role for the child. In complementary fashion, the intended examinees are 3–12 years of age and have experienced a traumatic event. Although there is nothing prohibiting this measure from being employed with children who do not have trauma histories, perhaps other ratings scales that cover a wider array of symptoms are a more felicitous selection for the non-traumatized population. The TSCYC consists of three component parts as follows: (a) a reusable "item booklet" that includes written instructions on the front page, along with an enumeration of 90 items printed on the two middle pages and back page (including a reprinting of the Likert scale at the top of each item page); (b) an "answer sheet" upon which the respondent records all identifying information, demographics of both examinee and informant, and item answers; and (c) a "profile form" upon which the examiner creates a profile by transforming the raw scores to dimensional *T*–scores (see scoring section). The profile form is not needed when the TSCYC scoring software (Briere & PAR Staff, 2008b) is obtained for such use, as it creates such a graphic representation of standard scores.

The item booklet instructs the informant to rate the frequency with which the child's described behaviors, feelings, and experiences have occurred within the past month, hence indicating a time frame of 30 days. The response alternatives are as follows: (a) 1 = *Not At All*; (b) 2 = *Sometimes*; (c) 3 = *Often*; and (d) 4 = *Very Often*. Administration time is estimated at 15–20 minutes, and the required reading level is seventh grade. Informants are asked to respond to every item and to be as honest as possible. Three or more missing items precludes scoring on any one scale. However, if there are only one or two missing items, these can be scored as 1 without hindering test results. Because this measure can be administered in under 20 minutes, the parent or caretaker is typically asked to complete this measure immediately after the initial assessment interview; that is, if the identified informant is present and available for immediate administration. The rationale is the same as provided when discussing the Conners multidimensional rating scales and thus will not be repeated here.

The answer sheet is divided into two major sections. The smaller upper section is further subdivided into three subsections as follows: (a) examinee's identifying information, (b) informant's identifying information, and (c) information that measures the degree of familiarity of the informant with the child. The last consists of information indicating whether the child lives with the respondent, and if so for how long, along with the number of hours each day the informant and examinee spend together. These data are used as one of several validity scales. The larger bottom section of the answer sheet contains five columns of item numbers and response alternatives 1, 2, 3, or 4 juxtaposed, one of which is to be circled based on the informant's opinion concerning the examinee's behavior as set out previously.

SCORING

Scoring the TSCYC can be done manually or preferably by the unlimited-use computer software scoring program (Briere & PAR Staff, 2008b). If done manually, the respondent's entered information and item answers are recorded automatically to a carbonless scoring sheet located immediately underneath the answer sheet. After separating the two sheets, the item scores from the scoring sheet are entered into a TSCYC worksheet, which is located on the back of the answer sheet. Missing responses are defined as those that are either omitted, double-scored, or improperly scored. As stated in the administration section, if there are two or fewer missing responses, they can be each counted as a score of 1. Three or more missing responses invalidates that scale.

Each row of item scores is summed and represents a validity scale or a clinical scale total raw score. There are two exceptions to this aggregating rule as follows: (a) the response level (RL) validity scale involves summing up the number of 1 scores; and (b) the post-traumatic stress–total represents the sum total raw score for all three PTSD-related scales. Other than these two exceptions, raw scores for each scale are added for a total raw score. All scale total raw scores are then converted to standardized *T*–scores (mean = 50, standard deviation = 10, range = 35–110) by means of plotting them on the proper norms profile form, each of which is apportioned according to gender and age grouping, as shown in the norms section. After circling the total raw scores for each scale in the graph, the examiner then reads across the profile form to the far left or right where a listing of *T*–scores is located. After finding the associated *T*–score, each is entered at the bottom of the form under each scale name. The total raw scores in the graph can be connected by straight lines to create a visual profile that facilitates interpretation. In general, higher scores are an indication of a greater degree of the measured test-taking response set on the validity scales and greater symptoms as described on each of the clinical scales. Fortunately, the computer scoring software provides all the aforementioned data after entering in the item raw scores, including the profile (Briere & PAR Staff, 2008b).

Form 10.16 is designed for reporting all the key TSCYC data within a final psychological assessment report. Prior to Table 1, optional information about the rater and his or her relationship to the child being evaluated is listed. Although such information does not determine test validity, it can be used to bolster or qualify the subsequent results if such is indicated. Following this introductory information, there are two validity scales. The first quantifies the degree of familiarity between the informant and the examinee, *operationally defined* by the average number of waking hours spent between the two individuals. Anything less than an average six hours per week invalidates the remaining data. Thus, it is good practice to ask a potential rater this question prior to administration. In this manner, the Table 1 result will invariably produce a valid outcome and bolster the rater's credibility. Pre-drafted excerpts have been inserted after Table 1 to facilitate interpretation, with both valid and invalid versions. Note that, contrary to the ensuing tables, the percentile rank data is based on that found in the norm reference sample and thus does not assume a normal curve. Also, the term "cumulative" preceding percentile rank has the same meaning as percentile rank defined in the succeeding tables; that is, they all represent the proportion of individuals the individual scores equal to or higher than.

Table 2 of Form 10.16 reports two validity scales, both with dimensional *T*–scores, 95% CIs, and PRs, as done for the subsequent clinical scales. Each scale's validity is determined by the *T*–score, although using somewhat different interpretative schemes. In particular, the RL validity scale measures an underreporting response set, with *T*–scores of 35–64 being valid, 65–69 being cautiously valid, and 70–110 being invalid. The atypical response (ATR) validity scale measures an overreporting tendency, although with a dichotomous interpretive scheme of *T*–scores 35–89 being valid and 90–110 being invalid. Once again, pre-drafted excerpts have been inserted after Table 2 with descriptions for valid outcomes, cautiously valid underreporting, and two invalid versions covering both under-reporting and overreporting. Note that part of the cautious interpretation makes use of the CIs in that, when an informant underreports symptoms, it is logical to assume the child's true scores fall somewhere toward the higher end of such intervals. Also note that the overreporting set does not need a cautious interpretation because of its dichotomous nature. The manner in which the 95% CIs can be used to augment test interpretation will be provided when discussing the clinical scales subsequently. The PRs can be referenced in the Appendix A, Table A.1, Standard Score to Percentile Rank conversion guide.

Finally, Table 3 of Form 10.16 reports the clinical scales or diagnostic data. The tabular organization follows that of all prior rating scales for a single informant, including five columns as follows: (a) scale name; (b) dimensional *T*–score; (c) 95% CI, (d) PR, and (e) a succinct description of the measured symptoms. Concerning the clinical scales, there are eight as follows (in the order they appear in the professional manual; Briere, 2005): (a) anxiety, (b) depression, (c) anger/aggression, (d) post-traumatic stress–intrusion, (e) post-traumatic stress–avoidance, (f) post-traumatic stress–arousal; (g) dissociation; (h) sexual concerns, and (i) post-traumatic stress–total (viz., a general PTSD scale). Regarding the CIs, the professional manual (Briere, 2005) does not provide the *SEM*s for the individual clinical scales. Hence, they must be computed from the available psychometric data.

More specifically, reliability coefficients are reported for all clinical scales but not for the complete set of validity scales (see Briere, 2005, Table 5.2, p. 29). However, Cronbach's coefficient alpha internal reliability coefficients are provided for the complete set of validity and clinical scales (see Briere, 2005, Table 5.1, p. 28), hence the average (i.e., median due to wide variability among the coefficients) of those are used to compute the estimated *SEM* for the 95% CIs. It is also consistent with that done with the companion Trauma Symptom Checklist for Children (TSCC; Briere, 1996), which is delineated in the next section. The median Cronbach's coefficient alpha turned out to be 0.85. Therefore, using the formula

$$SEM = SD\sqrt{1-\alpha}$$

Equation 10.2

where *SD* = 10 (for *T*–scores), and α = 0.85 (Chronbach's alpha), one has $SEM = 10\sqrt{1-.85} = 3.87 = 4$. Therefore, the CI is based on an estimated *SEM* of 4 (rounded to the nearest whole number). All of this is reported in specific table notes to both Table 2 for the prior validity scales and Table 3 for the clinical scales. Again, the PR values are derived from the theoretical standard normal distribution, which can be referenced in Appendix A of this book. It is now appropriate to discuss the interpretive strategy for Table 3. The ensuing interpretation assumes the validity scales all showed truthful and accurate outcomes.

INTERPRETATION

The focus here is on providing meaning to the data input into Table 3 of Form 10.16, again because it is assumed the data have been declared either valid, or at minimum, qualified or cautionary valid. The first feature to note is the revised order of the clinical scales. In particular, the clinical scales have been sequenced according to two criteria, including (a) from general to more specific, and (b) from most to least pertinent to PTSD diagnoses as listed in the *DSM–5*. As a consequence, the order in Table 3 is as follows: (a) post-traumatic stress–total (PTS–TOT) in bold font to highlight its predominance; (b) clinical scales contributing directly to the PTS–TOT to delineate the symptom clusters and degree of severity of each if present; (c) the dissociation clinical scales to inform as to whether such a specifier applies; (d) anxiety as either an integral component of the syndrome or as an independent disorder; (e) depression as either an integral component of the syndrome or as an independent disorder, along with any potential suicidal risk; (f) anger and potential aggression as either an integral component of the syndrome or as an independent problem; and (g) any evidence of a potential sexual preoccupation that suggests direct or indirect exposure to sexual molestation.

For all clinical scales, the standard score interpretive ranges are as follows: (a) *T*–score of 35–64 is *within normal limits*, (b) *T*–score of 65–69 is *elevated*, and (c) *T*–score of 70–110 is *very elevated*. This scheme is reported within a specific table note, with one and two asterisks appended to highlight clinically elevated and very elevated scores, respectively. A series of pre-drafted excerpts follow Table 3, which are intended to guide the examiner through the interpretive process by covering the three most common scenarios. They are as follows.

The first statement applies to the PTS–TOT score results, including normal, elevated, and very elevated outcomes. Thereafter, the interpretation first addresses positive results, either elevated or very elevated, assuming that these will be the most common outcomes, consistent with the rule of using this measure only in cases of a suspected or confirmed trauma history and likely consequential symptoms. The very elevated initial language is more unequivocal in interpreting the presence of PTSD and the need to scrutinize a symptom profile, whereas the elevated overall result is somewhat more tentative, although it also advises further investigation. The interpretive analysis addresses the clinical scales that directly contributed to the overall results, as they show the essential PTSD symptom clusters and provide information regarding severity level. Next, the dissociation (DIS) clinical scale is addressed, as this informs whether the PTSD single specifier should be added to such a diagnosis.

The following three scales cover symptoms that may be interpreted as either an integral part of the PTSD diagnosis (i.e., related but nonessential symptoms) or, if sufficiently severe with corroborating test data, an independent comorbid clinical disorder or disorders (e.g., generalized anxiety disorder) or personality issue or disorder (e.g., anger management difficulties, borderline traits or full disorder). The final scale addresses symptoms suggesting that sexual abuse or exposure was a component of the experienced trauma, which should be subject to further investigation. Notice that the same potential language is used for both very elevated and elevated overall results, as they differ only in degree. Separate conclusions have been drafted for these two positive outcomes, one concluding the presence of PTSD and the other an atypical symptoms pattern.

Thereafter, a separate series of interpretive steps have been pre-drafted for negative results. Depending on the needs of the case, more or fewer details may be needed in reporting and interpreting negative outcomes. For example, if the case is not controversial and the results are both consistent with other data and clear, a simple interpretive statement indicating that the overall results are negative for PTSD and any associated trauma-related psychopathology may be sufficient. In contrast, if the case is controversial, includes ambiguous or mixed results, and/or some individuals involved in the case would benefit from a more comprehensive and detailed interpretation of the negative findings, the sequence guides the examiner through the process of delineating such outcomes. The steps mirror those for the positive findings, the only exception being the negative versus positive wording. Thus, the PTSD-related clinical scales are addressed first, ensued by the DIS clinical scale, and finally, the nonessential variation scales and symptoms. The final statement integrates all the negative results and offers a conclusion that a diagnosis of PTSD is not supported. The discussion now moves to the second trauma measure in the trilogy.

Trauma Symptom Checklist for Children

The *Trauma Symptom Checklist for Children* (*TSCC*; Briere, 1996) is the second of three measures designed to detect trauma-related psychopathology for older children and continuing through most of adolescence. In contrast with its younger counterpart, it is a self-report form. If examinees fall within the age range of 8–12 and there are serious questions about whether the examinee can or is willing to provide accurate and honest ratings, the preceding TSCYC should be selected in its stead, along with an implicit personality measure that has the capability of detecting trauma and related symptoms (see Chapter 16). Another pertinent consideration is that the mere presence of certain PTSD symptoms has the capability of interfering, at least to some extent, with examinees' ability to effectively report them. These include amnesia, emotional numbing, and avoiding reminders of the trauma. Again, in such instances, alternate measures should be considered. With these caveats in mind, the TSCC will be presented as was the TSCYC.

SYNOPSIS

The TSCC is a self-report measure of post-traumatic stress and related symptoms in reaction to unspecified traumatic events. The target population consists of children and young-to-middle adolescents ages 8–16 who have experienced traumatic events (e.g., physical abuse, sexual molestation, physical and/or sexual assault perpetrated by peers, losses of primary attachment figures, the witnessing of severe violent events, and natural disasters; see also the prior review). Symptoms are queried in terms of the frequency with which selected feelings, thoughts, and behaviors occur.

There is a full and reduced version of the TSCC. The full version contains 54 items, while the reduced version excludes items with sexual content in an attempt to minimize any chances of inducing distress. The latter is to be considered in cases where the trauma involved extraordinarily invasive, disturbing, or violent sexual maltreatment and/or a remarkably vulnerable examinee who is showing signs of profound emotional disturbance (e.g., a psychotic process or borderline personality pathology).

Lastly, the TSCC comprises two validity scales (viz., underresponse and hyperresponse), along with six clinical scales as follows: (a) anxiety; (b) depression; (c) anger; (d) post-traumatic stress; (e) dissociation; and (f) sexual concerns. This brief introduction should illustrate the high degree of resemblance between the TSCC and TSCYC.

NORM REFERENCE SAMPLE

The standardization sample consisted of 3,008 children and adolescents that were combined from three smaller nonclinical subsamples. These included 2,399 schoolchildren who were involved in a study regarding the impact of neighborhood violence on functioning (Singer et al., 1995), 387 schoolchildren in a study regarding the effects of stressful events on functioning (Evans et al., 1994), and 222 children undergoing physical examinations at the Mayo Clinic (Friedrich, 1994). The total sample consisted of 47% males and 53% females, and race was composed of 44%

White, 27% Black, 22% Hispanic, 2% Asian, and 4% Other. Age cohorts were as follows: 8–10 ($n = 111$); 11–12 ($n = 400$); 13–14 ($n = 462$); and 15–16 ($n = 2,035$).

Based on a series of multivariate and univariate follow-up analyses of variance done on the aforementioned demographic variables and TSCC scores provided by the standardization sample, four subgroupings of norms were formed according to as many age by sex combinations. They were as follows: (a) male, ages 8–12; (b) female, ages 8–12; (c) male, ages 13–16; and (d) female, ages 13–16.

ADMINISTRATION

This instrument is administered by giving examinees the TSCC booklet, a ballpoint pen, and a hard surface to record their responses. The instructions are written on the front page, which can be opened vertically, thus exposing the two middle pages of items. The instructions indicate that the items describe things that children think, feel, and do and that they are to report how often these happen to them as follows: (a) 0 = It *never* happens; (b) 1 = It happens *sometimes*; (c) 2 = It happens *lots of times*; or (d) 3 = It happens *almost all the time*. The examinees are also asked to respond to every item and to makes their best guess if uncertain. Curiously, the reading level of the TSCC is not reported. Hence, the examiner should feel free to clarify any word the examinee is uncertain about by providing a denotative definition.

The full version includes 54 items and an estimated 15–20 minutes of administration time. The items contributing to the clinical scales were derived from a review of the literature on symptoms resulting from various childhood traumas. Content validation was afforded by child psychologist experts specializing in traumas occurring in this population, with subsequent inter-scale correlations, and correlations with other tests, which provided evidence of their internal reliability and convergent, discriminant, and construct validities.

As stated, there is also an alternate or reduced version (viz., TSCC–A) that excludes the ten items that contribute to the sexual concerns clinical scale. Of note, this version is not used because of the vital diagnostic information that may be missed. Also, eliminating these items risks communicating that such topics are not to be discussed, which is antithetical to the child's therapeutic interests and may inadvertently embolden any pathological family secrets that keep any abuse from being revealed and reported. In the event the examinee is truly vulnerable to an exacerbation of symptoms if such items are asked, then the administration instructions permit them to be read to the examinee in whole or pertinent part. In such instance, the examinee can be provided with emotional support and empathy if distressed, and the pace of questioning can be adjusted to facilitate accurate responses. Again, if the examinee is within the age range of the TSCYC, this measure can supplant the TSCC, as indicated previously. The point here is that the TSCC–A is not necessary and therefore is not part of the test inventory or book.

Omissions are items that are not answered, have multiple marks, or have ambiguous markings, as was defined in the TSCYC. However, they should not occur because the scale is sufficiently brief and can be easily corrected by the examiner (a) giving a cursory examination of the completed form when submitted to ensure all the items have been properly answered and, if necessary, (b) asking the examinee to correct any errors or missed items. However, the rules regarding item omissions are as follows. Six or more omitted items invalidates the TSCC. Three or more items omitted on a scale invalidates that scale. Subscales (see later) should not be scored if any items are missing. Lastly, omissions of less frequency may be scored as 0.

SCORING

Analogous to the TSCYC, scoring can be done manually or by TSCC scoring software (Briere & PAR Staff, 2008a). If hand scoring, the perforated strip at the top of the open TSCC booklet should be torn off, thus exposing the bottom scoring sheet. The respondent's answers are automatically copied onto the scoring sheet via a carbonless form. Item raw scores are transferred to columns for each scale, which are then summed at the bottom of the score sheet. The raw score totals are next transferred onto the proper profile form for the correct age group and sex of the examinee, as was done for the TSCYC. The *T*–scores are found on the far right or left of the profile form and recorded at the bottom under the graph.

Form 10.17 is organized for purposes of reporting the TSCC data within the context of a final psychological assessment report. It resembles Form 10.16 that was created for the TSCYC because of the similarity of the resulting scores. It includes three tables: two that address various response sets that can potentially affect test validity and the accuracy of the final clinical data. This section will discuss the validity scales first, followed by the clinical scales and the data yield.

Regarding Table 1 (Form 10.17), the manual advises that children are to be specifically instructed by the psychologist to answer every item in as much time as they need (Briere, 1996, p. 6). If they miss one to five items, it may affect the provision of scores for particular scales and subscales, although it will not invalidate the entire test. If the child misses six or more items, the entire test is deemed invalid. Table 1 is designed to report this result. The scale is in raw score units, one point for each missing item. Following Table 1 are two pre-drafted excerpts, one for a valid interpretation and one for an invalid outcome. The former continues the validity analysis to the issue of response sets, while the latter ends the TSCC score report for want of data.

Table 2 (Form 10.17) contains two validity scales, as did the second table in Form 10.16, including underreporting and overreporting response sets. There are five columns going across each of the two rows, including scale name, *T*–score, 68% CIs, PRs, and succinct definition of the response set. Each has an alternative interpretation, which includes the use of denial and feelings of being overwhelmed, respectively. Therefore, both interpretations are listed as possibilities in the succinct definition of the particular response sets in Table 2. The 68% CI is based on an *SEM* of 4, the computation of which is explained in a specific table note and in more detail later in this section when delineating the 68% CIs for the clinical scales. The interpretive schemes for each validity scale each use three ranges, although they are measured using slightly different intervals. Hence, they are defined in separate specific table notes to facilitate their interpretation. Note that the invalid result for the underresponse (UND) validity scale represents the top 2% of the normal distribution, whereas the hyperresponse (HYP) validity scale represents an even more extreme top 1%. The HYP has a higher threshold score for invalidity because (a) some children attempt to answer truthfully but score in this range because they are genuinely overwhelmed by trauma, and (b) there is an empirically supported tendency for children being evaluated in mental health clinics to score in this range on such measures for bona fide reasons. The higher threshold adjusts for these proclivities.

Following Table 2 are pre-drafted excerpts that describe valid, cautiously valid, and invalid outcomes. The interpretative language remains as objective as possible by focusing simply on whether the ratings are accurate or tend to over- or underestimate symptoms. That is, no reference is made to denial or feelings of being overwhelmed in these interpretive excerpts because such statements require additional evidence and inference. Therefore, the default interpretation is the most objective, whereas the alternate interpretations can be inserted if supported by clinical judgment.

Table 3 begins the diagnostically relevant TSCC data. The table organization is the same, including columns for scale (and subscale) labels, 68% CIs, PRs, and a succinct description of measured symptoms. The *T*–score metric is the same as prior, including a mean of 50, *SD* of 10, and range from 35 to 111. The CI is based on an estimated *SEM* of 4, which again is estimated by Equation 10.2, $SEM = SD\sqrt{1-\alpha}$, where *SD* is 10 (as defined by a *T*–score) and α is the median of the internal reliability Cronbach's alpha coefficients for the TSCC variables reported in the professional manual. In the professional manual (Briere, 1996, Table 7, pp. 28–29), the median is 0.82, which results in a *SEM* of 4.24, or 4 when rounded to the nearest whole number. Hence, the examiner merely adds and subtracts 4 points to and from the obtained score to estimate the 68% CI. This is all listed in a specific note to Table 3. The PR is based on the standard normal distribution, which can be referenced in Appendix A, Table A.1 in this book.

INTERPRETATION

This final section assumes the TSCC validity scales are all valid or at least cautiously valid; thus, interpretation focuses on Table 3 data. First, the order of the clinical scales is designed to expedite test interpretation, beginning from most to least pertinent to a PTSD diagnosis as listed in the *DSM–5*. Hence, the sequence is as follows: (a) PTSD scale (i.e., PTS); (b) dissociation scale with its two subscales; (c) negative symptomatic mood-related scales (i.e., anxiety, depression, anger, or irritability); and (d) sexual concern scale and its two subscales most relevant to detecting sexual elements to the reported trauma. The two scales that possess accompanying subscales are dissociation (DIS) and sexual concerns (SC). Specific table notes identify these scale–subscale sequences, which have different interpretive schemes and are also identified by table notes.

Following Table 3 are pre-drafted excerpts whose order, organization, and language are very similar to that found in Form 10.16 in interpreting the TSCYC. The interpretation is initiated by the PTS scale result, which is either normal, elevated, or very elevated. Either of the latter two results are considered positive, with the very elevated result being associated with a more definitive statement of PTSD being present, whereas the elevated result being associated with a more qualified "may be present" interpretation. Thereafter, both follow similar steps, the choices of which depend on the particular data profile. These steps first address potential dissociative symptoms (and subsystems); nonessential clusters of mood-related symptoms (i.e., anxiety, depression, and irritability); and finally, sexual concerns, preoccupations, and behavioral symptoms. As in the TSCYC interpretation, the SC scale and subscales suggest the reported or suspected trauma included sexual aspects, which require further inquiry. The two positive results culminate in either (a) a diagnosis of PTSD with added symptoms or comorbidity or (b) an atypical symptom profile.

Lastly, the negative result has its own language, although it follows similar steps. How much detail to provide when reporting negative results is contingent upon the case facts and objectives. As stated for the TSCYC, the more controversial and ambiguous the data, the more detail should be provided in the report. The greater the ambiguity and controversy, the greater the need for factual detail to clarify matters and to communicate that the conclusions are based on as much objectivity as possible. This leads us to the third and final trauma-related measure, this being designed for individuals in adulthood.

Trauma Symptom Inventory, Second Edition

The *Trauma Symptom Inventory, Second Edition* (*TSI–2*; Briere, 2011) is again a self-report measure of post-traumatic stress and trauma-related symptoms for individuals aged 18–90. It is the last of the trilogy designed to measure trauma-related disorders and sequelae across the majority of the life span. Although the 17-year-old age group is not captured by these three measures, either the TSCC or TSI–2 can be used as long as this fact is mentioned during test interpretation and other valid data are employed to corroborate the ultimate results. In general, if the 17-year-old appears more immature in terms of personality development and autonomy, then the TSCC is likely to be a more felicitous fit. However, if the individual is more mature and independent based on the initial assessment data, the TSI–2 can be used with the same caveats. In terms of format, they both are self-report, hence this is not a factor in the decision. Finally, if the individual's personality development does not assist in the decision of which measure to use, scrutiny of the different clinical scales and the data yield should be considered, the question here being which is a better fit to the case issues and facts.

SYNOPSIS

The TSI–2 succeeds the Trauma Symptom Inventory (TSI; Briere, 1995) and includes updated norms and revised and added factors, scales, and subscales, including 87 new items. The validity scales in particular possess new and improved items that permit the assessment of both (a) general overreporting test-taking response patterns and (b) the misrepresentation of post-traumatic stress symptoms in particular. In addition to measuring PTSD, the related symptoms include various types of dissociation, disturbed attachment patterns, disruption in the sense of self, depression, and anxiety, along with symptoms addressing danger to self and/or others. It also evaluates both acute and chronic symptom patterns resulting from sexual and physical abuse, intimate partner violence, combat, torture, automobile collisions, and mass casualty incidents (including the witnessing of such events), traumatic loss, and the sequelae associated with early child maltreatment.

In all, the TSI–2 contains 136 items, 2 validity scales, 4 general factor scales, 12 clinical scales, and 12 subscales. It is considered a *broadband measure* of PTSD because it measures both PTSD-specific and non-specific associated symptoms, the latter providing useful context for a complete PTSD diagnosis that better informs treatment intervention. The prior review of trauma and the many types of psychopathology to which it can lead attests to the importance of designing the TSI–2 in such a manner.

TEST STRUCTURE

As shown previously, trauma-related disorders are complex and consist of a multitude of symptom patterns and clusters. As a consequence, the TSI–2 test structure is also complex, and its qualities deserve a quick review. First, test reliability was measured by means of internal consistency coefficients (viz., coefficient alpha), average inter-item correlations, and test–retest coefficients (viz., stability coefficients). *Coefficient alpha* evaluates the extent to which items measure the same psychological construct (Cronbach, 1951). The TSI–2's factors, clinical scales, and clinical subscales ranged from 0.72 to 0.94, hence within acceptable limits. Similarly, inter-item correlations ranged from 0.61 to 0.84. Lastly, all stability coefficients were statistically significant save one; namely, the suicidality–behavior clinical subscale. The latter was an understandable result considering the variability in that symptom over time.

Second, validity was evaluated using convergent and discriminant validity, factorial validity, and criterion validity. First, TSI–2 factors, clinical scales, and clinical subscales were strongly correlated with their TSI counterparts, especially defensive avoidance ($r = 0.98$), intrusive experiences ($r = 0.96$), anger ($r = 0.94$), and impaired self-reference ($r = 0.94$) (see Briere, 2011, p. 41, Table 5.5). *Confirmatory factor analysis* (*CFA*) of the norm reference sample showed that the most parsimonious model consisted of the three predicted latent factors self-disturbance (SELF), post-traumatic stress (TRAUMA), and externalization (EXT), along with a fourth factor, somatization (SOMA). Further, this model was also an acceptable fit to two other samples completing the TSI–2 (see Godbout, Hodges, Briere, & Runtz, 2010a, 2010b). Regarding criterion validity, the TSI–2 was shown to be significantly associated with actual trauma exposure (Briere & Jordan, 2009), experience in combat, being a victim of domestic violence, and borderline personality diagnosis (Briere, 2011, pp. 46–47, Tables 5.9 and 5.10).

The TSI–2 standardization sample was selected to be representative of the U.S. population of adults, ages 18 years, 0 months through 90 years, 11 months. It was designed to match data reported by the 2007 U.S. Census Bureau (U.S. Bureau of the Census, 2007d) and stratified for age, gender, race/ethnicity, education, and geographic region of the country. Exclusionary criteria included those who were incarcerated, hospitalized, diagnosed with a psychotic disorder, visual or hearing impairment, and those who lacked reading comprehension abilities at the third-grade level and below.

The sample totaled 637 individuals. About 54% were female and 46% were male, with an average age of 53.4 years. In terms of race/ethnicity, the breakdowns were 73% White, 11% Black, 9% Hispanic, and 7% Other. Regarding education, 32% earned a high school diploma, 15% had less than a 12th-grade education, 27% completed some college, and 26% were college graduates and beyond. Regarding relationship status, 19% were single, 55% were married or cohabitating, 13% were divorced, and 13% were widowed. Finally, 32% reported that they had experienced a trauma and 8% had seen a therapist.

Multivariate analysis of variance (MANOVA) was done to determine if different norms were needed for various subgroups. Succinctly, there were main effects for gender (male versus female), age group (younger versus older), along with a gender by age group interaction. Follow-up relationship-based effect sizes were done. Results showed that gender accounted for 28.1% of the variance in TSI–2 scores, while age accounted for 17.4% of such variance. In the end, the authors determined that different norms were justified for the following four groups: (a) males, ages18–54; (b) males, ages55–90; (c) females, ages18–54; and (d) females, ages55–90.

The TSI–2 actually consists of two versions. The TSI–2 complete version comprises all 136 items, factors, scales, and subscales referenced previously and takes approximately 20–30 minutes to complete. The TSI–2–A is the alternative form, hence the appended letter A to the acronym, which includes 126 items and, in particular, excludes all data referencing sexual symptoms. As a result, the following are not available on this form: (a) sexual disturbance scale (SXD); (b) sexual concerns subscale (SXD–SC); and (c) dysfunctional sexual behavior subscale (SXD–DSB). However, it seems most prudent to include such data in all trauma assessments, considering that the literature shows such wide-ranging deleterious effects of trauma experiences.

In cases where an examinee is quite disturbed and vulnerable to a severe or psychotic breakdown in functioning if asked about such matters, testing should most often be deferred until a later time when such data can be more accurately garnered. Accurate results supersede rapid results in such cases. If results are needed more rapidly, an alternative is to administer an implicit personality test with the capability of measuring trauma and related symptoms (see Chapter 16). Additionally, the structure of the self-report administration format, along with the support and guidance that can be afforded by the testing psychologist, should be sufficient to obtain valuable information. Lastly, as discussed previously, it is prudent and even therapeutic to give the examinee permission to talk about such intimate matters and to avoid inadvertently reinforcing their *suppression* (i.e., conscious avoidance) or *repression* (i.e., unconscious avoidance). As such, the focus of the ensuing discussion will pertain only to the TSI–2, including the scoring and interpretation tables. If the TSI–2–A is given for some reason, the testing psychologist can simply omit the sexual concerns scores from the TSI–2 tables and analyses (see Form 10.18).

The TSI–2 is designed to be administered within an individual or group setting. Concerning psychological testing, the administration format would be individual and face to face. Instructions to be read to the examinee are printed on page six of the manual (Briere, 2011).

Essential points incorporated into such instructions include (a) identifying the item booklet and the answer sheet, (b) completing the demographic information accurately on the answer sheet, (c) replying to each item in terms of how often it has happened within the last six months (hence the time frame of this measure), (d) reviewing and clarifying the meaning of each alternative selection (viz., 0 = *never*; 1 = *only rarely*; 2 = *sometimes*; 3 = *often*), (e) answering all items, and (f) answering as honestly as possible. Written instructions on the front of the item booklet are also provided in sufficient detail to guide the examinee through the booklet if necessary. The administration should be done in one session, although short breaks are permitted for examinees who are especially distressed and distractible. Lastly, the completed answer sheet is to be given a cursory examination to ensure all items have been answered with one selection and, if not, to assist in correcting improperly answered items to avoid excessive omissions that will invalidate many of the scales, subscales, and factors.

The TSI–2 uses standardized *T*–scores as its principal metric, with a mean of 50, *SD* of 10, and range of approximately 30–100 (i.e., ≤ 30 and ≥ 100, as reported on the TSI–2 profile form). Percentile ranks (PRs) are also provided, although they are computed based on the empirical distribution of raw scores for each scale. Because the raw score distributions for each scale differ, most of which have varying degrees of negative skew, the association between *T*–scores and PRs will differ somewhat across the scales (cf. to inferential *T*–scores discussed elsewhere throughout this book). Hence, interpretation should focus mostly on *T*–scores versus their PRs. In general, higher *T*–scores indicate more of the measured symptoms.

Although CIs are not provided, the standard *SEM*s are given for each factor, scale, and subscale across the four standardization subgroupings with different norms (viz., male, 18–54; male, 55–90; female, 18–54; female, 55–90; Briere, 2011, pp. 32–35, Tables 4.6–4.9).[3] The four *SEM*s for each factor and scale were then averaged and rounded to the nearest whole number. For example, the average *SEM* for the post-traumatic stress factor is 3.58. Rounding to the nearest whole unit is 4. Therefore, the 68% CI for this factor score is estimated by adding or subtracting four points to/from the obtained *T*–score. As can be seen, a ±4 appears under the CI brackets to inform the testing psychologist the number to add and subtract from the obtained score, and which is intended to be deleted after the interval is computed and inserted into this cell. Such *SEM* values were subsequently rounded to the nearest whole number and inserted into the 68% CI column of the scoring and interpretation tables (i.e., the obtained *T*–score ± 1 *SEM*). Using this scheme, the 68% CIs are reasonably precise 6–10-point intervals rather than 12–20-point intervals if 95% CIs are desired. Therefore, the testing psychologist can efficiently report estimated 68% CIs for all scales, further supplemented by a PR area transformation score. As discussed for prior tests in this book, the CIs are vital to analyses of likely *ipsative* (i.e., intra-individual) differences across the scales, which facilitates differential diagnosis by identifying unique symptom clusters that are relatively more and less prominent in a particular case. It also communicates the important fact that such scores are not completely accurate and are accompanied by some degree of error, as does any quantity that is measured. Of course, the examiner may change the CIs to any degree of confidence desired for a particular case. Although PRs are *area transformations* and can distort interpretation, they are easier for the non-expert to comprehend and are thus inserted into the data tables.

Scoring can be done manually or by the TSI–2 scoring software (Briere & PAR Staff, 2011). If done by hand, the answer sheet is torn off, revealing the scoring sheet in which the circled answers are automatically recorded. In general, each row of items and their answers represent a clinical scale or validity scale, which are summed across from left to right (with some slight modifications for special scales). The four factors are determined by summing selected scale raw score totals. The raw score totals are then transformed into *T*–scores and PRs by entering them on the TSI–2 summary sheet and using the proper appendices in the manual to find the two raw score conversions for the pertinent norm group (Briere, 2011, Appendices A and B, pp. 71–93). Lastly, a profile form is available upon which an examinee's raw scores, *T*–scores, and PRs can be entered again, and the *T*–scores can be entered onto a graph and connected by lines to provide a visual presentation of standard scores.

Compared to manual scoring, the computer software is much faster, efficient, and accurate, and it is worth the financial investment, as it provides unlimited scoring (Briere & PAR Staff, 2011). Client demographics are entered, including name, sex, age, date of birth, and test date, followed by entering the item raw scores. The rest is provided by the software, including all the aforementioned scores (except the CIs and *SEM*s) for all factors, scales, and subscales, in both tabular and profile graphic format, along with a summary description of each question, the provided answer, answer key, and finally, a critical item summary and the examinees responses.

Some special scoring rules apply to item omissions. Omissions are answers that are skipped entirely or improperly marked. In particular, if any scale has two or fewer omissions, or a subscale has one omission, those omissions are given a score of 0. This is referred to as a *zero-substitution* method and is considered a conservative approach to prorating because it can result in a minor underestimation of true psychopathology. This is typically not a problem in trauma cases because it has been shown that those with extensive child maltreatment histories are more likely to endorse extensive symptomatology (Briere & Elliot, 1997; Klotz Flitter, Elhai, & Gold, 2003). If there are three or more omissions, scoring those scales or subscales is prohibited, including any subsequent scale or factor in which a subscale or scale score is required for computation. There are no validity criteria that involve total item omissions and possible invalidation of the entire test, although the test can be invalidated by certain response sets to which the discussion now turns.

Validity considerations are dealt with prior to data interpretation. Hence, these issues are discussed here in the scoring section, as were the item omissions. Form 10.18 includes all the data tables for reporting the TSI–2 scores, beginning with the validity scales in Table 1. First, the response level (RL) scale consists of eight items designed to detect if an examinee is either (a) responding indiscriminately or (b) denying feelings, thoughts, and behaviors that most others would typically report. It accomplishes this by adding the number of zero ratings (viz., 0 = *never*) an examinee provided on items rarely answered in such manner by the standardization sample (e.g., answering "never" to an item such as "Making a mistake"). In the standardization sample, a T–score above 75 on this validity scale is at or above the 96th percentile. Therefore, this criterion was selected as indicating an invalid TSI–2 protocol, specifically due to indiscriminant zero responding. Alternative interpretations for such results are responding with excessive denial, defensiveness, avoidance, or opposition. Note that these are all listed as possible interpretations in the final column in Table 1 that describes in the measured response set, which leaves it to the discretion of the examiner as to which alternative to consider as being most applicable. Hence, a T–score below 75 on this validity scale is considered valid.

In contrast, the atypical response (ATR) validity scale assesses an overreporting test-taking response pattern. More specifically, higher scores reflect any of the following: (a) overreporting all types of symptoms, (b) overreporting specific PTSD symptoms, (c) indiscriminant responding that happens to result in endorsement of rarely reported symptoms, and/or (d) genuinely high levels of distress produced by repeated traumas or catastrophic experiences. The last element was alluded to in the prior review when discussing a noted trend for individuals exposed to early and repeated maltreatment to report symptoms as being more intense and frequent versus the general population as a "cry for help" and urgently needing assistance (Briere, 2004; Briere & Elliot, 1997; Klotz Flitter et al., 2003). In clinical and forensic contexts, a raw score of 15 or greater indicates that the TSI–2 is invalid due to any of the aforementioned possibilities. Because the ATR validity interpretation is based on a raw score versus T–score value, the association of which can vary across the different age-by-gender norms, a raw score sub-cell is provided in Table 1 for this validity scale, along with the standard score columns for continuity. Although the author advises that if an examinee has a reasonable explanation for endorsing a particular ATR item, the average of all the ATR items should supplant the score on that item, this seems too costly in terms of time. It also does not result in much of an adjustment. Therefore, a more efficient solution is to examine the assessment information to determine if early and prolonged maltreatment, or a catastrophic exposure, would otherwise justify a high ATR score. In the alternative, the testing psychologist can proceed with a cautious interpretation and search for corroborating evidence (see the subsequent discussion).

Immediately following Table 1, alternative narrative excerpts are offered for rapid validity interpretation. They include versions for (a) valid, (b) invalid underreporting, (c) cautiously valid overreporting, and (d) invalid overreporting. Version (c) in this listing is offered for cases in which there is assessment evidence of early and prolonged maltreatment or catastrophic and extreme experiences such that the resulting data may be usefully diagnostic. The selection between the last two versions should be based on clinical judgment. However, in either case, the diagnostic data true scores should be interpreted as falling toward the lower end of the reported CIs, which is one reason why such data are included in all data tables incorporated into formal psychological assessment reports.

INTERPRETATION

Assuming Table 1 validity scales show truthful and accurate responding in the absence of invalidating response sets, the interpretative procedures can begin in earnest. Continuing with the rule of proceeding from general to specific, the most general factors represent the first set of diagnostic scores to report. Table 2 lists the four available TSI–2 factors, although beginning with the most construct relevant post-traumatic stress (TRAUMA) factor rather than the order listed in the manual- and computer-scoring printout. In contrast to the clinical scales and clinical subscales, these factors were found by confirmatory factor analysis (*CFA*), as discussed in the preceding test structure section. The test manual conveniently provides a table showing which subclinical scales and clinical scales contribute to each factor within a three-tiered hierarchical organization (Briere, 2011, p. 19, Table 3.1). For virtually all factors, clinical scales, and clinical subscales, the T–score range interpretative scheme is as follows: (a) 30–59 is *normal*; (b) 60–64 is *problematic* (i.e., above-average symptom endorsement with probable clinical implications); and (c) 65–100 is *clinically elevated* (i.e., endorsement of symptoms of sufficient degree that it represents a significant clinical concern). These T–score ranges and qualitative descriptions are presented in specific table notes.

Test interpretation should invariably begin with Table 3, which lists all the most general TSI–2 factors. Assuming PTSD is a major rule-out diagnosis when using this test, the post-traumatic stress (TRAUMA) factor is listed first. In the likely event that personality issues also form an additional diagnostic focus, especially in the case of early, severe, and repetitive trauma, the self-disturbance (SELF) factor is listed next. The externalizing (EXT) factor is vital in cases where danger to self and others is a concern or a diagnostic question. Lastly, Table 2 lists the somatization (SOM) factor, which may be relevant especially if conversion or somatic symptoms are manifest. Note that the clinical scales and subscales contributing to each of these factors are enumerated in independent tables and in the same sequence as the factors in Table 2. Therefore, the TRAUMA clinical scales and subscales follow first in Table 3, followed by SELF (Table 4), EXT (Table 5), and SOM (Table 6) clinical scales and subscales.

In addition to enhancing the organization of the test data, the intent here is to provide an option for the examiner to omit the reporting of any clinical scales and subscales in which the associated factor was negative. So, for example, if the TRAUMA and SELF factors are elevated and hence showing symptoms, and the remaining factors are negative, the examiner can interpret clinical scales and subscales only for the former two factors, hence (a) focusing the interpretation on pertinent positive results and (b) curtailing the report to accentuate the positive findings. As such, the report will focus only on the data most relevant to delineating the examinee's symptoms for purposes of customizing the treatment plan. In most cases, there is no need to inundate the report and reader with detailed negative findings and thus risk obfuscating matters. In addition, if all factor data are negative, and most if not all clinical scales and clinical subscales are negative or near negative, the analysis may terminate at the factor level in an efficient manner, with a practitioner's note that the clinical scales and subscales are similarly negative and not reported for purposes of brevity.

To facilitate interpretation of the factor data in Table 3 (Form 10.18), pre-drafted excerpts follow Table 2, beginning with the likely most pertinent TRAUMA factor, and followed by the remaining factors in the order they appear in the table. Each factor has its own paragraph appropriately labeled with italics (e.g., *PTSD* for the TRAUMA factor). The interpretive language is diligent in first indicating the degree to which those symptoms are present, followed by CI and PR interpretation, and concluding with a statement regarding the need for any follow-up analysis of the clinical scales and subscales.

Assuming factor data are positive, the clinical scale and subscales should also be interpreted to describe the unique symptom profile. Because PTSD would most likely represent a core rule-out diagnosis, it would be prudent to begin analysis of the TRAUMA scales (see Table 3, Form 10.18). This table essentially consists of scales for symptoms of anxiety, hypervigilance, and the most fascinating dissociative symptoms as a potential *DSM–5* specifier. The inclusion of a host of anxiety symptoms explains why PTSD was first classified as an anxiety disorder in the *DSM* nosology. That is, it includes symptoms resulting from excessive sympathetic nervous system (SNS) arousal, especially *hypervigilance*, which maintains the sufferer in a state of high alertness for any form of threat or attack, although gradually drains the individual of energy and quality of life. Intrusive and avoidance symptoms are also measured here, both of which assist in diagnosis. Lastly, *dissociation* is defined as the unconscious, defensive alteration of awareness, developed as an avoidance response to overwhelming psychological distress; here, trauma-related memories. Such a symptom has been proposed as an adaptive means of coping in circumstances where physical escape was precluded (e.g., child sexual abuse perpetrated by a parent), hence leaving psychological escape as the only remaining means of adjustment without succumbing to shock or a psychotic break. It is measured here in the clinical scale aptly named dissociation (DIS) and is key to determining if the PTSD *DSM* specifier applies; that is, "with dissociative symptoms." Once analyses of these scales are done, the remaining analysis determines the broader picture of whether other trauma-related disorders are comorbid, especially personality- and attachment-type relational disorders.

The self-disturbance clinical data are listed immediately after the PTSD scales, with or without dissociation, have been addressed. These data focus on potential co-occurring personality disorders and emotional attachment problems. Although the table begins with a measure of depression, the remaining clinical scales and subscales assess the examinee's attachment pattern and sense of self. As indicated in the test manual, disturbed relationships and sense of self is strongly predictive of classic depressive symptoms, including internal emptiness, hopelessness, and suicidal symptoms, which accounts for depression leading off this set of trauma-related data. The insecure attachment clinical scale first detects such disturbance, followed by its two clinical subscales, which apportions insecure attachment into (a) the use of avoiding intimacy as a defense mechanism, and (b) identification of an underlying fear of rejection and abandonment. The next scale directs attention to a lack of a sense of self and personal identity, which breaks down into two subscales: (a) identity diffusion and (b) excessive dependency upon others. The latter predictably renders an individual at risk for remaining in an abusive relationship. Further, taken together, because these data measure key aspects of personality (i.e., self and attachment to others), they inform as to the possible presence of personality psychopathology, including especially borderline, avoidant, and dependent types.

Externalizing (EXT) clinical scales and clinical subscales (see Table 5, Form 10.18) address severe impairments in affective regulation, including acts that are potentially destructive to self and others. Internal and external aspects of anger are addressed by the anger clinical scale, including the likelihood of anger outbursts that are clearly in excess of situational circumstances. Next, the sexual disturbance clinical scale warns of impairments in this area of functioning, with two clinical subscales measuring (a) potential sexual dysfunction and (b) the presence of sexual acting-out behaviors that are potentially self-destructive (e.g., risk-taking). The suicidality clinical scale comes next, including two subscales addressing (a) thoughts and (b) actual behavior. Both suicidality subscales identify a measurable risk of a danger to self, especially the clinical subscale addressing actual behavior. The final clinical scale is unique in the sense that it measures the presence of self-destructive and self-injurious behaviors as a means for coping; that is, as a means for reducing internal tension. This last scale would be of special interest in trauma cases involving self-injurious behavior (e.g., cutting, burning). High scores on such clinical scales help appraise such things as the risk, frequency, and intensity of such behavior.

Finally, the somatization (SOM) clinical scale and clinical subscales would be of least relevance due to its peripheral symptom content, along with its redundancy. In cases where conversion disorder or somatization disorder are rule-out diagnoses, these data would be relevant. However, somatization rule-outs typically do not accompany PTSD or trauma rule-out diagnoses. Of note, the single somatic preoccupations clinical scale is exactly the same as the somatization (SOMA) factor. Hence, such data is entirely redundant, and care should be taken not to interpret these symptoms as indicative of greater severity, chronicity, or intensity. Especially in cases where the SOMA factor is negative, this table can be justifiably eliminated from the analysis due to its redundancy. Lastly, in cases where these data are clinically elevated, this table can still be deleted unless it adds an important facet to the diagnostic workup.

Summary

This concludes the trilogy of related instruments designed to detect psychopathology resulting from trauma as defined previously. They include an observer-report format for the youngest age cohort, covering early to late childhood, and a self-report format for each of the two older measures, covering middle childhood through adolescence and adulthood. These rating scales are sufficiently similar to be considered a multi-score, multi-informant system, all of which may be either hand scored or computer scored. This also completes the rating scales included in the test inventory introduced in Chapter 1. Thus, a chapter summary ensues, which provides a succinct description of the chapter and where the discussion is headed next.

Recapitulation

This chapter was devoted to defining clinical disorders and how various standardized rating scales can be used to assist in their diagnosis. First, clinical disorders were defined and differentiated from other types of psychopathology, especially personality disorders. Second, rating scales were defined and compared and contrasted with other types of tests, especially personality inventories with whom they are most similar. This discussion consisted of reviewing different formats (i.e., various respondents and items), domains (i.e., multidimensional versus unidimensional), and response sets that may deleteriously affect the validity of the data yield. Next, reasons for including rating scales within a test battery were reviewed. The remainder of the chapter focused on presenting the various rating scales in the book's test inventory, beginning with the multidimensional, multi-informant, multi-score systems, followed by the unidimensional measures that focused on one disorder (e.g., adult ADHD) or domains of psychopathology (e.g., trauma-related disorders). In each case, the psychopathology being measured was diligently delineated, followed by presenting the rating scales designed to detect its major symptoms. For each measure, data tables were presented to illustrate how the results could be most effectively reported and interpreted within a formal psychological assessment report.

Key Terms

- acquiescence (yea saying)
- Affordable Care Act
- alexithymia
- anosognosia
- area transformations
- Asperger's disorder or syndrome
- Autism Diagnostic Observation Schedule, Second Edition (ADOS–2)
- autism spectrum disorder (ASD)
- broadband measure
- careless responding
- clinical disorders (syndromes)

- Coefficient alpha
- comorbidity
- complex PTSD (c-PTSD)
- conduct disorder (CD)
- confirmatory factor analysis (CFA)
- Conners' Adult ADHD Rating Scales, Long Version (CAARS–L)
- Conners Comprehensive Behavior Rating Scales (Conners CBRS)
- Conners Early Childhood (Conners EC)
- Conners Early Childhood, Behavior, Short Version, Parent Form (Conners EC–BEH–SP)
- construct validity
- continuous performance test (CPT)
- convergent validity
- cyclothymic disorder
- *Diagnostic and Statistical Manual of Mental Disorders, Fourth Edition, Text Revision (DMS–IV–TR)*
- Diagnostic Classification of Mental Health and Developmental Disorders of Infancy and Early Childhood (DC:0–5)
- differentials
- disruptive mood dysregulation disorder (DMDD)
- dissociation
- domain
- *DSM* symptom counts (*DSM* count)
- ecological validity
- empirical criterion keying
- etiology
- externalizing behavior disorders
- extreme responding
- faking
- forced choice
- generalized anxiety disorder (GAD)
- Gilliam Asperger's Disorder Scale (GADS)
- Gilliam Autism Rating Scale, Third Edition (GARS–3)
- halo effect
- hassles
- hypervigilance
- inconsistent responding
- Individuals with Disabilities Education Improvement Act of 2004 (IDEA)
- intellectual disability (ID)
- interrater reliability
- ipsative
- Likert-type scale
- linear transformations
- major depressive episode (MDE)
- mean
- middle responding
- multiaxial system
- multidimensional tests
- multi-score systems
- Multitrait-Multimethod Matrix (MTMM)
- neurocognitive disorder
- nomological network
- obsessive-compulsive disorder (OCD)
- O-data
- oppositional defiant disorder (ODD)
- other disorders of psychological development
- other sensory processing disorders

- other specified neurodevelopmental disorders
- over-responsivity
- percentile rank (PR)
- percentiles (P)
- persistent depressive disorder (dysthymic disorder)
- pervasive developmental disorder (PPD)
- praxis
- preauthorization (PA)
- proprioceptive
- prototypical approach
- rating scale/s
- reliability
- repression
- response sets
- reverse scoring
- S-data
- sensory integration
- sensory over-responsivity disorder
- sensory processing (integration)
- Sensory Processing Measure (SPM)
- Sensory Processing Measure–Preschool (SPM–P)
- sensory under-responsivity disorder
- separation anxiety disorder
- sequelae (singular, sequela)
- single-score systems
- social anxiety disorder (social phobia)
- social desirability
- social pragmatic communication disorder (SPCD)
- specific learning disorder (SLD)
- specifiers
- standard deviation (*SD*)
- standard error of measurement (*SEM*)
- summative scale
- suppression
- trauma
- Trauma Symptom Checklist for Children (TSCC)
- Trauma Symptom Checklist for Young Children (TSCYC)
- Trauma Symptom Inventory, Second Edition (TSI–2)
- under-responsivity
- validity
- zero-substitution

Notes

1. This measure also has a school environments form (Miller Kuhaneck, Henry, & Glennon, T. J., 2007), which consist of 6 very brief 10–15-item rating sheets for as many school environments, including special classes, recess, bus, and cafeteria. These provide a single total score and are only to be used with the main classroom form. These are not typically used in clinical outpatient practice. In particular, they do not provide enough additional diagnostically useful information over and above that provided by the home form and main classroom form, to justify the added time and expense of administration (which involves the addition of several observers), scoring, and interpretation. Furthermore, the respondents associated with these school environments will likely be less familiar and adept at completing such forms and will be relatively less familiar with the child's typical behavior.
2. As stated previously in this chapter and bearing reiteration, the terms *sensory processing* and *sensory integration* have typically been employed as synonyms, referring to the neurocognitive organization of incoming sensory information both within and across the major sensory modalities or systems (Ayers, 1972, 2005). Hence, they are continually used in similar fashion, with a preference for sensory processing to be consistent with the DC:0–5 use of the label in the abnormal sense.
3. The *SEM*s themselves were computed in the test manual by using the formula , where *SD* was the *T*–score standard deviation of 10, and *r* was the internal consistency reliability coefficient for each scale (Briere, 2011, p. 32).

References

Abdalla, K., & Elklit, A. (2001). A nation-wide screening survey of refugee children from Kosovo, *Torture, 11*, 45–49.

American Psychiatric Association. (1994). *Diagnostic and statistical manual of mental disorders* (4th ed.; DSM—IV). Washington, DC: Author.

American Psychiatric Association. (2000). *Diagnostic and statistical manual of mental disorders* (4th ed., text rev.; DSM—IV—TR). Washington, DC: Author.

American Psychiatric Association. (2013). *Diagnostic and statistical manual of mental disorders* (5th ed.; DSM—5). Arlington, VA: Author.

American Psychological Association. (2007). *APA dictionary of psychology* (2nd ed.). Washington, DC: Author.

Anderson, V., Northam, E., Hendy, J., & Wrennall, J. (2001). *Developmental neuropsychology: A clinical approach*. Philadelphia: Psychology Press.

Archer, J. (2009). Does sexual selection explain human sex differences in aggression? *Behavioral and Brain Sciences, 32*, 249–311.

Autism Speaks. (2015). *The affordable care act and autism*. Retrieved June 1, 2016, from http://autismspeaks.org.

Ayers, A. J. (1972). *Sensory integration and learning disorders*. Los Angeles: Western Psychological Services (WPS).

Ayers, A. J. (1979). *Sensory integration and the child*. Los Angeles: Western Psychological Services (WPS).

Ayers, A. J. (2005). *Sensory integration and the child, 25th anniversary edition*. Los Angeles: Western Psychological Services (WPS).

Barlow, D. H., Durand, M. V., & Hofmann, S. G. (2018). *Abnormal psychology: An integrative approach* (8th ed.). Boston, MA: Cengage Learning.

Bauer, S. (1996). *Asperger's syndrome*. Internet article from asperger syndrome coalition of the United States. Retrieved from www.asperger.org.

Berger, W., Coutinho, E. S. F., Figueira, I., Marques-Portella, C., Luz, M. P., Neylan, T. C., . . . & Mendlowicz, M. V. (2012). Rescuers at risk: A systematic review and meta-regression analysis of the worldwide current prevalence and correlates of PTSD in rescue workers. *Social Psychiatry and Psychiatric Epidemiology, 47*, 1001–1011.

Biederman, J. (2005). Attention-deficit/hyperactivity disorder: A selective overview. *Biological Psychiatry, 57*, 1215–1220.

Biederman, J., & Faraone, S. V. (2005). Attention-deficit/hyperactivity disorder. *The Lancet, 366*, 237–248.

Bishop, D. V. M. (1989). Autism Asperger's syndrome and semantic-pragmatic disorder: Where are the boundaries? *British Journal of Disorder of Communication, 24*, 107–121.

Boney-McCoy, S., & Finkelhor, D. (1995). Psychosocial sequelae of violent victimization in a national youth sample. *Journal of Consulting and Clinical Psychology, 63*, 726–736.

Breslau, N., Davis, G. C., Andreski, P., & Peterson, E. (1991). Traumatic events and posttraumatic stress disorder in an urban population of young adults. *Archives of General Psychiatry, 48*, 216–222.

Briere, J., & Elliot, D. M. (2003). Prevalence and psychological sequelae of self-reported childhood physical and sexual abuse in a general population sample of men and women. *Child Abuse and Neglect, 27*, 1205–1222.

Briere, J. (1992). *Child abuse trauma: Theory and treatment of the lasting effects*. Newbury Park, CA: Sage.

Briere, J. (1995). *Trauma symptom inventory (TSI)*. Odessa, FL: Psychological Assessment Resources (PAR).

Briere, J. (1996). *Trauma symptom checklist for children (TSCC): Professional manual*. Lutz, FL: Psychological Assessment Resources (PAR).

Briere, J. (2004). *Psychological assessment of adult posttraumatic states: Phenomenology, diagnosis, and measurement* (2nd ed.). Washington, DC: American Psychological Association.

Briere, J. (2005). *Trauma symptom checklist for young children (TSCYC): Professional manual*. Lutz, FL: Psychological Assessment Resources (PAR).

Briere, J. (2011). *Trauma symptom inventory* (2nd ed.; TSI—2): Professional manual. Lutz, FL: Psychological Assessment Resources (PAR).

Briere, J., & Elliot, D. M. (1997). Psychological assessment of interpersonal victimization effects in adults and children. *Psychotherapy: Theory, Research & Practice, 34*, 353–364.

Briere, J., & Gill, E. (1998). Self-mutilation in clinical and general population samples: Prevalence, correlates, and functions. *American Journal of Orthopsychiatry, 68*, 609–620.

Briere, J., & Jordan, C. (2009). Childhood maltreatment, intervening variables, and adult psychological difficulties in women: An overview. *Trauma, Violence & Abuse, 10*, 375–388.

Briere, J., & PAR Staff. (2008a). *Trauma symptom checklist for children (TSCC): Scoring software*. [CD-ROM]. Lutz, FL: Psychological Assessment Resources (PAR).

Briere, J., & PAR Staff. (2008b). *Trauma symptom checklist for young children (TSCYC): Scoring software*. [CD-ROM]. Lutz, FL: Psychological Assessment Resources (PAR).

Briere, J., & PAR Staff. (2011). *Trauma symptom inventory, second edition (TSI—2): Scoring software*. [CD-ROM]. Lutz, FL: Psychological Assessment Resources (PAR).

Briere, J., & Richards, S. (2007). Self-awareness, affect regulation, and relatedness: Differential sequels of childhood versus adult victimization experiences. *Journal of Nervous and Mental Disease, 195*, 497–503.

Briere, J., & Spinazzola, J. (2005). Phenomenology and psychological assessment of complex posttraumatic states. *Journal of Traumatic Stress, 18*, 401–412.

Briere, J., Scott, C., & Weathers, F. W. (2005). Peri-traumatic and persistent dissociation in the presumed etiology of PTSD. *American Journal of Psychiatry, 162*, 2295–2301.

Browne, A., & Finkelhor, D. (1986). Impact of child sexual abuse: A review of the research. *Psychological Bulletin, 99*, 66–77.

Brownstein, J., Haltry, H. P., Altschuler, D. M., & Blair, L. H. (1989). *Patterns of substance use and delinquency among inner-city adolescents: Report to the national institute of justice.* Washington, DC: The Urban Institute.

Campbell, D. T., & Fiske, D. W. (1959). Convergent and discriminant validation by the multitrait-multimethod matrix. *Psychological Bulletin, 56*, 81–105.

Cardozo, B. L., Vergara, A., Agani, F., & Gotway, C. A. (2000). Mental health, social functioning, and attitudes of Kosovar Albanians following the war in Kosovo. *Journal of the American Medical Association, 284*, 569–577.

Carlson, G. A., & Kashani, J. H. (1988). Phenomenology of major depression from childhood through adulthood: Analysis of three studies. *American Journal of Psychiatry, 145*, 1222–1225.

Chu, J. A., Frey, L. M., Ganzel, B. L., & Matthews, J. A. (1999). Memories of childhood abuse: Dissociation, amnesia, and corroboration. *The American Journal of Psychiatry, 156*, 749–755.

Clements, P. T., & Burgess, A. W. (2002). Children's response to family member homicide. *Family and Community Health, 25*, 32–42.

Cloitre, M., Stolbach, B. C., Herman, J. L., van der Kolk, B., Pynoss, R., Wang, J., & Petkova, E. (2009). Developmental approach to complex PTSD: Childhood and adult cumulative trauma as predictors of symptom complexity. *Journal of Traumatic Stress, 22*, 399–408.

Cloitre, M., Stovall-McClough, C., Zorbas, P., & Charuvastra, A. (2008). Attachment organization, emotion regulation, and expectations of support in a clinical sample of women with childhood abuse histories. *Journal of Traumatic Stress, 21*, 282–289.

Cohen, R. J., & Swerdlik, M. E. (2018). *Psychological testing: An introduction to tests and measurement* (9th ed.). New York, NY: McGraw-Hill Education.

Cole, P. M., & Putnam, F. W. (1992). Effect of incest on self and social functioning: A developmental perspective. *Journal of Consulting and Clinical Psychology, 60*, 174–184.

Connelly, B. S., & Ones, D. S. (2010). Another perspective on personality: Meta-analytic integration of observers' accuracy and predicative validity. *Psychological Bulletin, 136*, 1092–1122.

Conners, C. K. (2008). *Conners comprehensive behavior rating scales (Conners CBRS): Manual and interpretive update.* North Tonawanda, NY: Multi-Health Systems (MHS).

Conners, C. K. (2009). *Conners Early Childhood manual (Conners EC).* North Towanda, NY: Multi-Health Systems (MHS).

Conners, C. K. (2014). *Conners comprehensive behavior rating scales: DSM—5 update.* Canada: Multi-Health Systems (MHS).

Conners, C. K., Erhardt, D., & Sparrow, E. (1999). *Conners' adult ADHD rating scales (CAARS): Technical manual.* North Tonawanda, NY: Multi-Health Systems (MHS).

Crimmins, S. M., Cleary, S. D., Brownstein, H. H., Spunt, B. J., & Warley, R. M. (2000). Trauma, drugs and violence among juvenile offenders. *Journal of Psychoactive Drugs, 32*, 43–54.

Cronbach, L. J. (1951). Coefficient alpha and the internal structure of tests. *Psychometrika, 16*, 297–334.

Cronbach, L. J., & Meehl, P. E. (1955). Construct validity in psychological tests. *Psychological Bulletin, 52*, 281–302.

Darves-Bornoz, J. M., Choquet, M., Ledoux, S., Gasquet, I., & Manfredi, R. (1998). Gender differences in symptoms of adolescents reporting sexual assault. *Social Psychiatry and Psychiatric Epidemiology, 33*, 111–117.

Dietrich, A. (2003). Characteristics of child maltreatment, psychological dissociation, and somatoform dissociation of Canadian inmates. *Journal of Trauma and Dissociation, 4*, 81–100.

Ecker, C., Parham, L. D., Kuhaneck, H. M., Henry, D. A., & Glennon, T. J. (2010). *Sensory processing measure—preschool (SPM—P): Manual.* Los Angeles, CA: Western Psychological Services (WPS).

Ehlers, A., Clark, D. M., Dunmore, E., Jaycox, L., Meadows, E., & Foa, E. (1998). Predicating response to exposure treatment in PTSD: The role of mental defeat and alienation. *Journal of Traumatic Stress, 11*, 457–471.

Ehlers, A., Mayou, R., & Bryant, B. (2003). Cognitive predictors of posttraumatic stress disorder in children: Results of a prospective longitudinal study. *Behaviour Research and Therapy, 41*, 1–10.

Ehlers, S., & Gillberg, C. (1993). The epidemiology of Asperger syndrome: A total population study. *The Journal of Child Psychology and Allied Disciplines, 34*, 1327–1350.

Elder, G. H., Jr., & Clipp, E. C. (1989). Combat experience and emotional health: Impairment and resilience in later life. *Journal of Personality, 57*, 311–341.

Elliott, D. M. (1994). Impaired object relationships in professional women molested as children. *Psychotherapy, 31*, 79–86.

Epstein, J., Saunders, B. E., & Kilpatrick, D. G. (1997). Predicting PTSD in women with a history of childhood rape. *Journal of Traumatic Stress, 10*, 573–588.

Evans, J. J., Briere, J., Boggiano, A. K., & Barret, M. (1994, January). *Reliability and validity of the Trauma Symptom Checklist for Children in a normal sample.* Paper presented at the San Diego Conference on Responding to Child Maltreatment, San Diego, CA.

Fergusson, D. M., Horwood, L. J., & Lynskey, M. T. (1996). Childhood sexual abuse and psychiatric disorder in young adulthood: II. Psychiatric outcomes of childhood sexual abuse. *Journal of the American Academy of Child and Adolescent Psychiatry, 35*, 1365–1374.

Fetchenhauer, D., Groothuis, T., & Pradel, J. (2010). Not only states but traits—Humans can identify permanent altruistic dispositions in 20's. *Evolution and Human Behavior, 31*, 80–86.

Finkelhor, D., Hotaling, G., Lewis, I. A., & Smith, C. (1990). Sexual abuse in a national survey of adult men and women: Prevalence, characteristics, and risk factors. *Child Abuse and Neglect, 14*, 19–28.

Finzi, R., Ram, A., Shnit, D., Har-Even, D., Tyano, S., & Weizman, A. (2001). Depressive symptoms and suicidality in physically abused children. *American Journal of Orthopsychiatry, 71*, 98–107.

Flannery, D. J., Singer, M. I., & Wester, K. (2001). Violence exposure, psychological trauma, and suicide risk in a community sample of dangerously violent adolescents. *Journal of the American Academy of Child and Adolescent Psychiatry, 40*, 435–442.

Flavell, J. H., Green, F. L., & Flavell, E. R. (1995a). The development of children's knowledge about attentional focus. *Developmental Psychology, 31*, 706–712.

Flavell, J. H., Green, F. L., & Flavell, E. R. (1995b). Young children's knowledge about thinking. *Monographs of the Society for Research in Child Development, 60*, 1–96. doi:10.2307/1166124

Ford, J. D. (1999). Disorders of extreme stress following war-zone military trauma: Associated features of posttraumatic stress disorder or comorbid but distinct syndromes? *Journal of Consulting and Clinical Psychology, 67*, 3–12.

Ford, J. D. (2002). Traumatic victimization in childhood and persistent problems with oppositional defiance. *Journal of Aggression, Maltreatment and Trauma, 6*, 25–28.

Freeman, L. N., Mokros, H., & Poznanski, E. O. (1993). Violent events reported by normal urban school-aged children: Characteristics and depression correlates. *Journal of the American Academy of Child and Adolescent Psychiatry, 32*, 419–423.

Friedrich, W. N. (1994). Assessing children for the effects of sexual victimization. In J. Briere (Ed.), *Assessing and Treating Victims of Violence* (pp. 17–27). San Francisco, CA: Jossey-Bass.

Friedrich, W. N., Fisher, J. L., Dittner, C. A., Acton, R., Berliner, L., Butler, J., et al. (2001). Child sexual behavior inventory: Normative, psychiatric, and sexual abuse comparisons. *Child Maltreatment, 6*, 37–49.

Funder, D. C. (2006). Towards a resolution of the personality triad: Persons, situations, and behaviors. *Journal of Research in Personality, 40*, 21–34.

Geller, B., & Luby, J. (1997). Child and adolescent bipolar disorder: A review of the past 10 years. *Journal of the American Academy of Child and Adolescent Psychiatry, 36*, 1168–1176.

Gilboa-Schechtman, E., & Foa, E. B. (2001). Patterns of recovery from trauma: The use of intraindividual analysis. *Journal of the Abnormal Psychology, 110*, 392–400.

Gilliam, J. E. (2001). *Gilliam Asperger's disorder scale (GADS) examiner's manual.* Austin, TX: Pro—Ed.

Gilliam, J. E. (2014a). *The Gilliam Autism rating scale, third edition (GARS—3), examiner's manual.* Austin, TX: Pro-Ed.

Gilliam, J. E. (2014b). *Instructional objectives for individuals who have autism.* Austin, TX: Pro-Ed.

Godbout, N., Hodges, M., Briere, J., & Runtz, M. G. (2010a). *TSI-2 Structural Analyses on three samples: The dimensions of trauma symptoms—A measurement study.* Unpublished manuscript.

Godbout, N., Hodges, M., Briere, J., & Runtz, M. G. (2010b). *Confirmatory Factor Analysis of the Trauma Symptom Inventory-2: A four factor model.* Poster presented at the annual meeting of the International Society for Traumatic Stress Studies. Montreal, Quebec, Canada.

Graziano, A. M., & Namaste, K. A. (1990). Parental use of physical force in child discipline: A survey of 679 college students. *Journal of Interpersonal Violence, 5*, 449–463.

Green, B. L., Korol, M., Grace, M. C., Vary, M. G., Leonard, A. C., Gleser, G. C., & Smitson-Cohen, S. (1991). Children and disaster: Age, gender, and parental effects on PTSD symptoms. *Journal of the American Academy of Child and Adolescent Psychiatry, 30*, 945–951.

Guterman, N. B., Cameron, M., & Hahm, H. C. (2003). Community violence exposure and associated behavior problems among children and adolescents in residential treatment. *Journal of Aggression, Maltreatment, and Trauma, 6*, 111–135.

Guzder, J., Paris, J., Zelkowitz, P., & Marchessault, K. (1996). Risk factors for borderline personality in children. *Journal of the American Academy of Child and Adolescent Psychiatry, 35*, 26–33.

Hall, D. K., Mathews, F., & Pearce, J. (2002). Sexual behavior problems in sexually abused children: A preliminary typology. *Child Abuse and Neglect, 26*, 289–312.

Harari, D., Bakermans-Kranenburg, M. J., & Van IJzendoorn, M. H. (2007). Attachment, disorganization, and dissociation. In E. Vermetten, M. J. Dorahy, & D. Spiegel (Eds.), *Traumatic dissociation: Neurobiology and treatment* (pp. 31–54). Washington, DC: American Psychiatric Publishing.

Hare, R. D. (2003). *The hare psychopathy checklist—Revised* (2nd ed.). Toronto, ON: Multi-Health Systems.

Heim, C., & Nemeroff, C. B. (2001). The role of childhood trauma in the neurobiology of mood and anxiety disorders: Preclinical and clinical studies. *Biological Psychiatry, 49*, 1023–1039.

Herman, J. L. (1992). Complex PTSD: A syndrome in survivors of prolonged and repeated trauma. *Journal of Traumatic Stress, 5*, 377–391.

Hogan, T. P. (2019). *Psychological testing: A practical introduction* (4th ed.). Hoboken, NJ: John Wiley & Sons.

Hoge, C. W., Castro, C. A., Messer, S. C., McGurk, D., Cotting, D. I., & Koffman, R. L. (2004). Combat duty in Iraq and Afghanistan, mental health problems, and barriers to care. *New England Journal of Medicine, 351*, 13–22.

Holden, C. (2008). Bipolar disorder: Poles apart. *Science, 321*, 193–195.

Hurt, H., Malmud, E., Brodky, N. L., & Giannetta, J. (2001). Exposure to violence: Psychological and academic correlates in child witnesses. *Archives of Pediatrics and Adolescent Medicine, 155*, 1351–1356.

Individuals with Disabilities Education Improvement Act of 2004, Pub. L. 108–446, 118 Stat. 328 (2004).

Iversen, A. C., Fear, N. T., Ehlers, A., Hacker Hughes, J., Hull, L., Earnshaw, M., . . . Hotopf, M. (2008). Risk factors for posttraumatic stress disorder among UK Armed Forces personnel. *Psychological Medicine, 38*, 511–522.

Jackson, D. N., & Messick, S. (1967). *Problems in human assessment.* New York, NY: McGraw-Hill.

Jaffe, P. G., Wolfe, D. A., & Wilson, S. K. (1990). *Children of battered women.* Newbury Park, CA: Sage.

Johnson, J. G., Cohen, P., Gould, M. S., Kasen S., Brown, J., & Brook, J. S. (2002). Childhood adversities, interpersonal difficulties, and risk for suicide attempts during late adolescence and early adulthood. *Archives of General Psychiatry, 59*, 741–749.

Jones, R. T., Ribbe, D., Cunningham, P., Weddle, J., & Langley, A. K. (2002). Psychological impact of fire disaster on children and their parents. *Behavior Modification, 26*, 163–186.

Kashani, J. H., Daniel, A. E., Dandoy, A. C., & Holcomb, W. R. (1992). Family violence: Impact on the child. *Journal of the American Academy of Child and Adolescent Psychiatry, 31*, 181–189.

Kernberg, O. (1975). *Borderline conditions and pathological narcissism*. New York: Jason Aronson.

Kernberg, O. F. (1984). *Severe personality disorders*. New Haven, CT: Yale University Press.

Kessler, R. C., Sonnega, A., Bromet, E., Hughes, M., & Nelson, C. B. (1995). Posttraumatic stress disorder in the national comorbidity survey. *Archives of General Psychiatry, 52*, 1048–1060.

Kiser, L. J., Heston, J., Millsap, P. A., & Pruit, D. (1991). Physical and sexual abuse in childhood: Relationship with post-traumatic stress disorder. *Journal of the American Academy of Child and Adolescent Psychiatry, 30*, 776–783.

Klin, A., & Volkmar, F. R. (1995). *Asperger's syndrome: Guidelines for assessment and diagnosis*. New Haven, CT: Yale Child Study Center.

Klin, A., Volkmar, F. R., Sparrow, S. S., Ciccetti, D. V., & Rourke, B. P. (1995). Validity and neurological characterization of Asperger syndrome: Convergence with nonverbal learning disabilities syndrome. *The Journal of Child Psychology and Allied Disciplines, 36*, 1127–1140.

Klotz Flitter, J. M., Elhai, J. D., & Gold, S. N. (2003). MMPI—2 *F* scale elevations in adult victims of child sexual abuse. *Journal of Traumatic Stress, 16*, 269–274.

Kolbo, J. R., Blakely, E. H., & Engelman, D. (1996). Children who witness domestic violence: A review of empirical literature. *Journal of Interpersonal Violence, 11*, 281–293.

Kolko, D. J., Moser, J. T., & Weldy, S. R. (1988). Behavioral/emotional indications of sexual abuse in child psychiatric inpatients: A controlled comparison with physical abuse. *Child Abuse & Neglect, 12*, 529–542.

Kroll, L., Rothwell, J., Bradely, D., Shah, P., Bailey, S., & Harrington, R. (2002). Mental health needs of boys in secure care for serious or persistent offending: A prospective, longitudinal study. *Lancet, 359*, 1975–1979.

Krueger, R. F., & Markon, K. E. (2006). Reinterpreting comorbidity: A model-based approach to understanding and classifying psychopathology. *Annual Review of Clinical Psychology, 2*, 111–133.

Lachman, S. J., & Bass, A. R. (2010). A direst study of the halo effect. *The Journal of Psychology, 119*, 535–540.

Lai, J. S., Parham, L. D., & Ecker, C. (1999). Sensory dormancy and sensory defensiveness: Two sides of the same coin? *Sensory Integration Special Interest Section Quarterly, 22*, 1–4.

Lanktree, C. B., Briere, J., & Zaidi, L. Y. (1991). Incidence and impacts of sexual abuse in a child outpatient sample: The role of direct inquiry. *Child Abuse & Neglect, 15*, 447–453.

Larsen, R. J., & Buss, D. M. (2021). *Personality psychology: Domains of knowledge about human nature* (7th ed.). New York, NY: McGraw-Hill.

Lazarus, R. S. (1993). From psychological stress to the emotions: A history of changing outlooks. *Annual Review of Psychology, 44*, 1–22.

Lazarus, R. S., & Folkman, S. (1984). *Stress, appraisal and coping*. New York: Springer.

Likert, R. (1932). A technique for the measurement of attitudes. *Archives of Psychology, 22 140*, 55.

Lingiardi, V., & McWilliams, N. (Eds.). (2017). *Psychodynamic diagnostic manual, second edition* (PDM—2). New York, NY: The Guilford Press.

Lord, C., Luyster, R. J., Gotham, K., & Guthrie, W. (2012). *Autism diagnostic observation schedule, second edition (ADOS—2)* [Manual: Toddler Module]. Torrance, CA: Western Psychological Services (WPS).

Lord, C., Rutter, M., Dilavore, P. C., Risi, S., Gotham, K., & Bishop, S. L. (2012). *Autism diagnostic observation schedule, second edition (ADOS—2)* [Manual: Modules 1–4]. Torrance, CA: Western Psychological Services (WPS).

Lykken, D. T. (1995). *The antisocial personalities*. Hillsdale, NJ: Erlbaum.

Malmquist, C. P. (1986). Children who witness parental murder: Post-traumatic aspects. *Journal of the American Academy of Child and Adolescent Psychiatry, 25*, 320–325.

Marshall, G. N., Schell, T. L., Elliot, M. N., Berthold, S. M., & Chun, C. (2005). Mental health of Cambodian refugees 2 decades after resettlement in the United States. *Journal of the American Medical Association, 294*, 571–579.

Martinez, P., & Richters, J. E. (1993). The NIMH community violence project, II: Children's distress symptoms associated with violence exposure. *Psychiatry, 56*, 22–35.

Mash, E. J., & Wolfe, D. A. (2019). *Abnormal child psychology* (7th ed.). Boston, MA: Cengage Learning.

McDermott, B. M., & Palmer, L. J. (2002). Postdisaster emotional distress, depression and event-related variables: Findings across child and adolescent developmental stages. *Australian and New Zealand Journal of Psychiatry, 36*, 754–761.

McWilliams, N., & Shedler, J. (2017). Personality syndromes: P Axis. In V. Lingiardi & N. McWilliams (Eds.), *Psychodynamic diagnostic manual* (2nd ed., PDM—2; pp. 15–74). New York, NY: The Guilford Press.

Miller, L. J. (2006). *Sensational kids: Hope and help for children with sensory processing disorder (SPD)*. New York, NY: G. P. Putnam's Sons.

Miller, L. J., Anzalone, M. E., Lane, S. J., Cermack, S. A., & Osten, E. (2007). Special issue: Cenceptualizing and identifying sensory processing issues. *American Journal of Occupational Therapy, 61*, 135–259.

Millon, T. (2000). Sociocultural conceptions of the borderline personality. *Psychiatric Clinics of North America Special Issue: Borderline Personality Disorder, 23*, 123–136.

Millon, T., Tringone, R., Grossman, S., & Millon, C. (2020). *Millon adolescent clinical inventory* (2nd ed.; *MACI—II*): Manual. Bloomington, MN: Dicandrien.

Moskowtiz, D. S., & Fournier, M. A. (2015). The interplay of persons and situations: Retrospect and prospect. In L. Cooper & R. J. Larsen (Eds.), *Handbook of personality and social psychology: Personality processes and individual differences*. Washington, DC: American Psychological Association.

Multi-Health Systems (MHS). (2008). *Conners CBRS scoring software*. [USB Key Computer software]. North Tonawanda, NY: Author.

Multi-Health Systems (MHS). (2009). *Conners EC scoring software*. [USB Key Computer software]. North Tonawanda, NY: Author.

Najavits, L. M. (2002). *Seeking safety: A treatment manual for PTSD and substance abuse*. New York, NY: Guilford.

National Institute of Mental Health. (2001). *Bipolar disorder*. Author. Retrieved from www.nimh.nih.gov./publicat/bipolar.cfm

Nevid, J. S., Rathus, S. A., & Greene, B. (2011). *Abnormal psychology in a changing world* (8th ed.). Upper Saddle River, NJ: Prentice Hall.

Nigg, J. T., & Goldsmith, H. H. (1994). Genetics of personality disorders: Perspectives from personality and psychopathology research. *Pathological Bulletin, 115,* 346–380.

Nolen-Hoeksema, S. (2020). *Abnormal psychology* (8th ed.). New York, NY: McGraw Hill Education.

Ouimette, P., & Brown, P. J. (2003). *Trauma and substance abuse: Causes, consequences, and treatment of comorbid disorders.* Washington, DC: American Psychological Association.

Panagioti, M., Gooding, P., & Tarrier, N. (2009). Posttraumatic stress disorder and suicidal behavior: A narrative review. *Clinical Psychology Review, 29,* 471–482.

Parham, L. D., & Ecker, C. (2007). *Sensory Processing Measure (SPM) home form.* Los Angeles, CA: Western Psychological Services.

Parham, L. D., Ecker, C., Kuhaneck, H. M., Henry, D. A., & Glennon, T. J. (2007). *Sensory processing measure (SPM): Manual.* Los Angeles, CA: Western Psychological Services (WPS).

Paunonen, S. V., & O'Neil, T. A. (2010). Self-reports, peer ratings, and construct validity. *European Journal of Personality, 24,* 189–206.

Peltzer, K. (1999). Trauma and mental health problems of Sudanese refugees in Uganda. *Central African Journal of Medicine, 45,* 110–113.

Pfefferbaum, B. D., Doughty, D. E., Reddy, C., Patel, N., Gurwitch, R., Nixon, S., & Tivis, R. (2002). Exposure and peri-traumatic response as predictors of posttraumatic stress in children following the 1995 Oklahoma City bombing. *Journal of Urban Health, 79,* 354–363.

Piaget, J. (1952). *The origins of intelligence in children.* New York: W. W. Norton.

Piaget, J. (1962). *Play, dreams and imitation in childhood.* New York: W. W. Norton.

Piaget, J. (1983). Piaget's theory. In W. Kessen (Ed.), *Handbook of child psychology: Volume 1. Theoretical models of human development* (pp. 103–128). New York: Wiley.

Pietrzak, R. H., Goldstein, M. B., Malley, J. C., Johnson, D. C., & Southwick, S. M. (2009). Subsyndromal posttraumatic stress disorder is associated with health and psychosocial difficulties in veterans of operations enduring freedom and Iraqi freedom. *Depression and Anxiety, 26,* 739–744.

Pollock, V. E., Briere, J., Schneider, L., Knop, J., Mednick, S., & Goodwin, D. W. (1990). Childhood antecedents of antisocial behavior: Parental alcoholism and physical abusiveness. *American Journal of Psychiatry, 147,* 1290–1293.

Pynoos, R. S., Goenjian, A., Tashjian, M., Karakashian, M., Manjikian, R., Manoukian, G., . . . Fairbanks, L. (1993). Posttraumatic stress reactions in children after the 1988 Armenian Earthquake. *British Journal of Psychiatry, 163,* 239–247.

Ramchand, R., Schell, T. L., Karney, B. R., Osilla, K. C., Burns, R. M., & Caldarone, L. B. (2010). Disparate prevalence estimates of PTSD among service members who served in Iraq and Afganistan: Possible explanations. *Journal of Traumatic Stress, 23,* 59–68.

Rosenzweig, P. (2007). *The halo effect: . . . and the eight other business delusions that deceive managers.* New York, NY: The Free Press.

Ruchkin, V. V., Schwab-Stone, M., Koposov, R., Vermeiren, R., & Steiner, H. (2002). Violence exposure, posttraumatic stress, and personality in juvenile delinquents. *Journal of the American Academy of Child and Adolescent Psychiatry, 41,* 322–329.

Russoniello, C. V., Skalko, T. K., Thomas, A., O'Brien, K. F., McGhee, S. A., Bingham-Alexander, D. B., & Beatley, J. (2002). Childhood post-traumatic stress disorder and efforts to cope after Hurricane Floyd. *Behavioral Medicine, 28,* 61–71.

Rutter, M. (1985). Infantile autism and other pervasive developmental disorders. In M. Rutter & L. Hersov (Eds.), *Child and adolescent psychiatry: Modern approaches* (2nd ed., pp. 545–566). Oxford: Blackwell.

Ryan, K. D., Kilmer, R. P., Cauce, A. M., Watanabe, H., & Hoyt, D. R. (2000). Psychological consequences of child maltreatment in homeless adolescents: Untangling he unique effects of maltreatment and family environment. *Child Abuse and Neglect, 24,* 333–352.

Saigh, P. A., Yasik, A. E., Oberfield, R. O., Halamandaris, P., & McHugh, M. (2002). An analysis of the internalizing and externalizing behaviors of traumatized urban youth with and without PTSD. *Journal of Abnormal Psychology, 111,* 462–470.

Schubiner, H., Scott, R., & Tzelepis, A. (1993). Exposure to violence among inner-city youth. *Journal of Adolescent Health, 14,* 214–219.

Scott, R., Knoth, R., Beltran-Quines, M., & Gomez, N. (2003). Assessment of psychological functioning in adolescent earthquake victims in Colombia using the MMPI–A. *Journal of Traumatic Stress, 16,* 49–57.

Shum, D., O'Gorman, J., Creed, P., & Myors, B. (2017). *Psychological testing and assessment* (3rd ed.). Sydney, NSW: Oxford University Press.

Singer, M. I., Anglin, T. M., Song, L. Y., & Lunghofer, L. (1995). Adolescents' exposure to violence and associated symptoms of psychological trauma. *Journal of the American Medical Association, 273,* 477–482.

Smith, B. H., Waschbusch, D. A., Willoughby, M. T., & Evans, S. (2000). The efficacy, safety, and practicality of treatments for adolescents with attention-deficit/hyperactivity disorder (ADHD). *Clinical Child and Family Psychology Review, 3,* 243–267.

Smith, P., Perrin, S., Dyregrov, A., & Yule, W. (2003). Principal components analysis of the impact of event scale with children in war. *Personality and Individual Differences, 34,* 315–322.

Speranza, A. M., & Mayes, L. (2017). Personality syndromes: P Axis. In V. Lingiardi & N. McWilliams (Eds.), *Psychodynamic diagnostic manual* (2nd ed., PDM—2; p. 674). New York, NY: The Guilford Press.

Steel, Z., Chey, T., Silove, D. M., Marnane, C., Bryant, R. A., & Van Ommeren, M. H. (2009). Association of torture and other potentially traumatic events with mental health outcomes among populations exposed to mass conflict and displacement: A systematic review and meta-analysis. *Journal of the American Medical Association, 302,* 537–549.

Stuber, J., Fairbrother, G., Galea, S., Pfefferbaum, B., Wilson-Genderson, M., & Vlahov, D. (2002). Determinants of counseling for children in Manhattan after the September 11 attacks. *Psychiatric Services, 53,* 815–822.

Sutker, P. B., Allain, A. N., & Winstead, D. K. (1993). Psychopathology and psychiatric diagnoses of World War II Pacific theater prisoners of war and combat veterans. *American Journal of Psychiatry, 150,* 240–245.

Sutker, P. B., Allain, A. N., Jr., & Johnson, J. L. (1993). Clinical assessment of long-term cognitive and emotional sequelae to World War II prisoner-of-war confinement: Comparison of pilot twins. *Psychological Assessment, 5,* 3–10.

Tjaden, P., & Thoennes, N. (2000). Prevalence and consequences of male-to-female and female-to-male intimate partner violence as measured by the national violence against women survey. *Violence Against Women, 6*, 142–161.

U.S. Bureau of the Census. (2000). *Population data for 2000*. Retrieved from www.census.gov/popest/statesasrh/files/SC-EST2000-AGESEX-RES.csv

U.S. Census Bureau. (2001a). *Census 2000 summary file 1 (SF1)*. [Data file]. Retrieved from www.census.gov/main/www/cen2000.html

U.S. Census Bureau. (2001b). *Census 2000 summary file 3 (SF3)*. [Data file]. Retrieved from www.census.gov/main/www/cen2000.html

U.S. Census Bureau. (2002). *Current population survey, March 2002*. Washington, DC: U.S. Census Bureau, Population Division.

U.S. Census Bureau. (2006). *Annual estimates of the population by five-year age groups and sex for the United states: April 1, 2000 to July 1, 2006* [Table 1]. Retrieved from www.census.gov/popest/national/asrh/NC-EST2006/NC-EST2006-01.xls

U.S. Census Bureau. (2007a). *Monthly post census resident population, by single year of age, sex, race, and Hispanic origin* (Data file). Retrieved from www.census.gov/popest/national/asrh/2007-nat-res.htm

U.S. Census Bureau. (2007b). *Educational attainment of the population 18 years and over, by age, sex, race, and Hispanic origin* [Table 1]. Retrieved from www.census.gov./population/socdemo/education/cps2007/Table1-01.csv

U.S. Census Bureau. (2007c). *Annual estimates of the resident population for the United States, regions, states, and Puerto Rico: April 1, 2000 to July 1, 2008* [Data file]. Retrieved from www.census.gov.popest/states/NST-ann-est.html

U.S. Census Bureau. (2007d). *Current population survey, March 2007* (Data file). Washington, DC: U.S. Department of Commerce.

U.S. Census Bureau. (2010). *Statistical abstract of the United States: 2010*. Washington, DC: Author.

van der Kolk, B. A., Pelcovitz, D., Roth, S., Mandel, F. S., McFarlane, A., & Herman, J. (1996). Dissociation, somatization, and affect dysregulation: The complexity of adaptation to trauma. *American Journal of Psychiatry, 153*, 83–93.

van der Kolk, B. A., Roth, S. H., Pelcovitz, D., Sunday, S., & Spinazzola, J. (2005). Disorders of extreme stress: The empirical foundation of a complex adaptation to trauma. *Journal of Traumatic Stress, 18*, 389–399.

Vazire, S. (2010). Who knows what about a person? The self-other knowledge asymmetry (SOKA) model. *Journal of Personality and Social Psychology, 98*, 281–300.

Walker, E. A., Katon, W. J., Roy-Byrne, P. P., Jemelka, R. P., & Russo, J. (1993). Histories of sexual victimization in patients with irritable bowel syndrome or inflammatory bowel disease. *The American Journal of Psychiatry, 150*, 1502–1506.

Weller, E., Weller, R., & Fristad, M. (1995). Bipolar diagnosis in children: Misdiagnosis, underdiagnosis, and future directions. *Journal of the American Academy of Child and Adolescent Psychiatry, 34*, 709–714.

Wellman, H. M. (1990). *The child's theory of mind*. Cambridge, MA: MIT Press.

Wellman, H. M. (2014). *Making minds: How theory of mind develops*. New York, NY: Oxford University Press.

Westen, D. (1990). Psychoanalytic approaches to personality. In L. A. Pervin (Ed.), *Handbook of personality: Theory and research* (pp. 21–65). New York, NY: The Guilford Press.

Widiger, T. A. (1997). Personality disorders as maladaptive variants of common personality traits: Implications for treatment. *Journal of Contemporary Psychotherapy Special Issue: Personality Disorders, 27*, 265–282.

Wing, L. (1991). The relationship between Asperger's syndrome and Kanner's autism. In U. Frith (Ed.), *Autism and Asperger syndrome* (pp. 93–121). Cambridge: Cambridge University Press.

Wolfe, V. V., Gentile, C., & Wolfe, D. A. (1989). The impact of sexual abuse on children: A PTSD formulation. *Behavior Therapy, 20*, 215–228.

World Health Organization (WHO). (1992/2010). *The ICD–10: Version 2010 classification of mental and behavioural disorders: Clinical descriptions and diagnostic guidelines*. Geneva: Author.

Zero to Three. (2016). *Diagnostic classification of mental health and developmental disorder of infancy and early childhood (DC:0–5)*. Washington, DC: Author.

Zinzow, H. M., Resnick, H. S., McCauley, J. L., Amstadter, A. B., Ruggiero, K. J., & Kilpatrick, D. G. (2012). Prevalence and risk of psychiatric disorders as a function of variant rape histories: Results from a national survey of women. *Social Psychiatry and Psychiatric Epidemiology, 47*, 893–902.

Zlotnick, C., Donaldson, D., Spirito, A., & Pearlstein, T. (1997). Affect regulation and suicide attempts in adolescent inpatients. *Journal of the Academy of Child & Adolescent Psychiatry, 36*, 793–798.

See Routledge's e-resources website for forms. (www.routledge.com/9780367346058).

11 Personality Inventory Tests

Overview

The genre of measures presented in this chapter are referred to as *personality inventory tests* (or simply *personality inventories*). Because these tests measure a fundamental construct that heretofore has not been addressed in earnest in this book, a few introductory comments regarding their format structure and organization is in order. First, these are tests that present the informant with a rather extensive listing of standard statements describing behaviors, thoughts, feelings, and/or symptoms, along with a forced-choice response format (e.g., *True* or *False*; the extent of agreement), which use summative scales to measure the extent to which the examinee possesses a variety of maladaptive traits and, secondarily, the presence of clinical disorders or syndromes as defined in Chapter 10. Regarding the latter, whether the personality inventory measures the presence of clinical disorders varies in degree among the specific tests presented here as part of this book's test inventory. That is, some afford clinical disorders a nearly equivalent emphasis, while others conceptualize personality psychopathology primarily as predisposing factors for clinical disorders, and still others focus exclusively on measuring personality traits and dispositions.

Second, while most of the personality inventories here focus on measuring psychopathology or abnormal traits, one began as a measure of "normal" traits that were presumed to be a universal part of the human condition. Only more recently has the latter test mentioned been applied to measuring maladaptive or problematic traits as the *DSM–5* progresses toward a dimensional approach to diagnosing personality disorders. Third, these measures are remarkably sophisticated in both design and empirical support. For example, some were developed by empirical criterion keying, some by factor analysis, and some were guided by theory and thereafter supported by statistical methods. Their degree of sophistication, empirical or scientific support, and focus on personality with perhaps secondary attention to clinical disorders renders these measures superior to rating scales that were covered in Chapter 10. So, while they will seem very similar to many of the rating scales, they are fundamentally different and should be considered superior measures. If these are used along with rating scales in the same test battery, the personality inventories should routinely be reported first and afforded more diagnostic weight in terms of test interpretation.

Fourth, and finally, the vast majority of these personality inventories are self-report or S-data in format. Hence, it will become immediately apparent that the majority also employ the use of multiple validity scales in an attempt to detect *response sets* (see Chapter 10). In fact, several personality inventories not only detect response sets but proceed further in an attempt to statistically adjust the diagnostic scales to counteract their potential deleterious effects on test validity. There is only one exception to this rule in which there is available both a self-report form (i.e., *S-data*) and observer-report form (i.e., *O-data*). This inventory also possesses validity scales that are more direct and straightforward in the way they function (e.g., asking respondents directly if they are answering the items in an honest and accurate manner).

To reiterate, personality inventories are principally designed to measure just that, personality, typically maladaptive forms within the domain of clinical psychology and mental health testing practice. Hence, as this chapter proceeds, four introductory issues will be presented as follows. First, a brief history of personality inventories will be provided to afford context to the contemporary versions of these tests. Second, the construct of personality disorder deserves a more refined definition and elaboration. This will be accomplished by comparing and contrasting the construct of personality disorder with that of clinical disorder in an extended fashion due to the fact that the latter is also implicated when discussing the various personality inventories.

Third, the *DSM–5* continues to employ a categorical approach to diagnosing personality disorders, although it is introducing an alternative dimensional model in its appendix section. Because one of the personality inventories presented in this chapter is being used to diagnose disorders as defined by this new model, the issue of whether these disorders are best conceptualized as one of type or degree is addressed. The former assumes that an individual either has the disorder and is "abnormal" or does not have the disorder and is, hence, "normal." The latter assumes

DOI: 10.4324/9780429326820-13

all individuals possess such traits to some degree, although those with a personality disorder manifest certain traits to greater or lesser degrees. Therefore, this issue is delineated in more detail such that it is more readily understood when it arises during the presentation of the designated personality inventories.

Fourth, diagnosing people with mental health disorders can be controversial due to potential negative connotations (Hinshaw & Stier, 2008; Martinez, Piff, Mendoza-Denton, & Hinshaw, 2011; Parcesepe & Cabassa, 2013). Of further import, diagnosing people with a disorder of personality can additionally communicate that there is something disturbed about their very character or being. Hence, personality disorder diagnoses in particular have the potential of being extraordinarily controversial due to the greater likelihood of stigma that accompanies such a label, even greater than that for clinical disorder. Now contemplate giving such a diagnosis to a young individual, for instance a 16-year-old. The issues here are exactly when and under what set of facts can or should psychologists diagnose personality disorders in people. This will be addressed using facts, logic, and a consideration of current *DSM–5* standards.

Fifth, and finally, the reasons for including and excluding a personality inventory within a test battery in mental health practice will be reviewed. The latter refers to the issue of selecting the proper personality test for a particular case. More specifically, there are two principal types of personality tests, namely, the *personality inventory test* and the *performance personality test*. Each have advantages and disadvantages. Here, it will be addressed how to exploit what the personality inventory test has to offer, along with assets of this instrument and circumstances in which its use is contraindicated. After processing these three key introductory issues, the chapter presents the personality inventories in the test inventory, along with data tables that are designed for presenting their results within a formal psychological assessment report. As in Chapter 10, this will represent the core of the current subject matter.

Personality Inventory Tests: A Brief History

A major demand for personality testing was afforded by World War I, wherein a large number of recruits needed to be screened to assess their degree of psychological adjustment for duty. In response, the *Woodworth Personality Data Sheet* (Woodworth, 1920) was developed as a 116-item self-report rating scale. Items were put into question form (e.g., "Do you feel depressed?"), to which the forced-choice response options were a dichotomous *Yes* or *No*. Items were drafted based on clinical experience and logic and not on theory or empirical methods. That is, items were selected because the authors, Woodworth and Poffenberger, believed they were associated with psychological instability.

It was discovered that nonclinical individuals would, on average, provide ten psychopathological responses. Therefore, those that scored 20 or more responses in the pathological range were referred for follow-up psychiatric assessment. Some items were deemed to be *pathognomonic*, meaning that if they were responded to in the keyed abnormal direction, they were immediately referred for psychiatric assessment irrespective of the total score.

The next test that was highly influential was the *Bernreuter Personality Inventory* (Bernreuter, 1933), which essentially measured self-sufficiency, introversion, dominance, and neuroticism. The chief advancement was the inclusion of multiple scales or personality dimensions. Similar to the Woodworth Personality Data Sheet, its format was self-report, the items were in question form and based upon logical reasoning rather than empirical methods, and the response choices were also a dichotomous *Yes* or *No*. Hence, items were phrased so that they were logically consistent with the ostensibly measured trait or construct. For example, an item that measured neuroticism might be phrased, "Are you frequently anxious?" This aspect of the test turned out to represent its most glaring weakness as research discovered that people frequently did not respond as expected. For example, it was found that 90% of people with schizophrenia (i.e., a psychotic disorder) scored above the 90th percentile on a neurotic scale (Landis & Katz; 1934; see also, Super, 1942). The cardinal lesson here was that the exclusive use of logical reasoning in test development was inappropriate and would lead to inaccurate results. In consequence, formal validation methods were now considered to be a critical phase in test construction.

The final test worthy of mention, which led to the introduction of the MMPI (Minnesota Multiphasic Personality Inventory) inventories presented later, was the Humm and Wadsworth (1935) *Temperament Scale*. This scale was founded upon Rosanoff's theory of personality (Rosanoff, 1927) and was designed to detect temperament constructs that purportedly assessed an individual's likely adjustment within a work environment. This theory was very similar to many contemporary personality inventories in that abnormality was measured in terms of degree and not of kind. In other words, it was assumed that all individuals could be measured on the same temperament traits. Those displaying psychopathology simply had more of these traits than others, hence manifesting uncontrolled versions of them.

From this theory, seven elements of temperament were evinced. These included normal (i.e., balance and equilibrium), antisocial (i.e., self-preservation), cycloid (i.e., bipolar depressed or manic), schizoid (i.e., autistic or paranoid), and *epileptoid* (i.e., achievement oriented and meticulous). The initial set of items were composed once again according to logical and clinical experience. However, Humm and Wadsworth quickly discovered what was also apparent in the Bernreuter Personality Inventory test development; that is, examinees frequently failed to answer the items according to logical reasoning. For example, they discovered that only 25% of the questions were responded to in the expected direction. Once again, the lesson learned was how vital it was to validate the manner in which people respond to test items versus simply relying upon logic and experience.

To remediate the situation, Humm and Wadsworth assigned scores to each item according to its ordinal position in the distribution of scores on that temperament scale. In particular, an item was assigned a score of 1, 2, 3, 4, or 5 depending on its rank order on that scale divided into intervals of 20%; that is, if an item fell in the bottom 20%, it was given a score of 1, whereas if it fell in the top 20%, it was given a score of 5. The total score for examinees on each scale was the summation of these ordinal score values. Total scores were then classified as strong (0.5 standard deviations above the average category), weak (0.5 standard deviations below the average category), or average (mid-range between the strong and weak categories) on each temperament dimension. The temperament with the highest score represented the examinee's personality diagnosis. The total number of items on the final scale was 318. Hence, this represented one of the first attempts at empirical validation for a personality inventory.

Finally, Humm and Wadsworth were also concerned about the examinee's approach to the self-report task. That is, was the individual providing answers that were truthful, honest, and accurate? Until this point, it was simply assumed that examinees were responding in a valid manner, as evidenced by the notable absence of validity scales on the previously cited personality inventories. In contrast, the temperament scale was one of the first such measures that incorporated validity scales. Here, there were two such scales as follows: (a) the total number of *No* responses and (b) the total number of missed items. In terms of the former, there were three categories. First, if 145–193 of 318 total items were answered *No*, this was acceptable. Second, 132–144 and 194–214 *No* responses were classified as doubtful. Third, fewer than 132 or more than 214 *No* responses were deemed unacceptable. Regarding missed items, greater than 25 omissions invalidated the test.

Although the highest component indicated the person's diagnosis, it was rare that only one scale elevated significantly. More frequently, one scale was predominant with accompanying secondary elevations, therefore leading to a unique profile pattern that described mixed traits of varying degrees. This result is important to highlight because contemporary personality inventories also typically yield a unique personality profile showing several significant elevations of varying degrees, which together describe an individual's dominant and secondary traits.

The temperament scale received continued support through the 1940s, although by the 1950s its ascendancy and use dissipated. However, this test provided some notable advances, including items that distinguished between known groups, a multidimensional test structure, summative scales, quantitative scales of similar metrics that could be compared, and the use of profile interpretation. At this point, test construction moved toward the use of more reliable and sophisticated empirical methods and continued to build upon the innovations afforded by the temperament scale, which included the introduction of the first MMPI. This completes the brief history of personality inventories. Additional historical information is provided subsequently, when each of the ensuing series of tests are presented independently in sequence. Next, the constructs of personality disorder and clinical disorder are examined.

Comparing and Contrasting the Personality Disorder and the Clinical Disorder

The *clinical disorder* (or *clinical syndrome*) was previously defined as a cluster of essential symptoms and nonessential variations that cause dysfunction and/or distress and that has an identifiable onset, being capable of precipitating a request for professional intervention, and tending to be responsive to treatment (refer also to Chapter 10). To reiterate, clinical disorders are classified by major nomological systems (see, e.g., *DSM–5*; ICD–10) by employing a categorical system that assumes a prototypical approach. The prototype aspect refers to the *essential symptoms* that define a clinical disorder (e.g., depressed mood or lost pleasure for at least two weeks for a major depressive episode; American Psychiatric Association, 2013, p. 160), without which the disorder is considered absent. The *nonessential variations* are largely responsible for rendering the symptoms of two individuals with the exact same diagnosis as appearing very different. For example, one individual with *major depressive disorder* (*MDD*) may appear extremely sad, having no interests, and sleeping excessively (viz., *hypersomnia*), whereas another individual with MDD may appear irritable, angry, agitated, and having difficulty getting to sleep (viz., *insomnia*).

In contrast, the *personality disorder* is defined as a continuing pattern of aberrant thinking, feeling, and behavior, which is inflexible and pervasive and which causes dysfunction and/or distress (American Psychiatric Association, 2013, p. 647). The terms continuing, inflexible, and pervasive imply that the symptoms should manifest temporal consistency and, to some degree, situational consistency depending on the strength of the environmental demands. In essence, it represents a chronic, enduring lifestyle problem due to its deleterious effects chiefly impacting interpersonal relationships. Thus, personality disorder is different in quality or nature as contrasted with a clinical disorder.

In fact, the two main features these disorders have in common are their dysfunctional effects and, at least currently, their categorical nature. The latter is further elaborated on later and is subject to change in the years to come.

In addition, evidence indicates that the onset of personality psychopathology typically begins in childhood by a host of deleterious factors. These include the following: (a) disturbed attachments with parental figures (Benjamin, 1996; Kernberg, 1975, 1984; Livesley, 1995; Nigg & Goldsmith, 1994); (b) childhood sexual abuse (Westen, 1990); (c) general abuse, victimization, and maltreatment during childhood (Pollock et al., 1990); and (d) early deficient learning caused by excessive punishment (Newman, 1987). There is also evidence for predisposing genetic influences on the development of personality disorder (see, e.g., Kendler et al., 2006; Lykken, 1995; Reichborn-Kjennerud, 2008; Reichborn-Kjennerud et al., 2007; Torgersen et al., 2008), including neurobiological variables, such as deficiencies in processing rewards and reacting to punishment (Arnett, Smith, & Newman, 1997; Blair et al., 1995; Glenn, Raine, Mednick, & Venables, 2007; Patrick, Drislane, & Strickland, 2012; Seara-Cardoso & Viding, 2015). Once the incipient behavioral problems begin to manifest during child development, they gradually escalate and become increasingly ingrained on an insidious course through adolescence, typically coalescing in full form during young adulthood (Widiger, 2012). In fact, there is evidence that early pathogenic care can lead to neurobiological changes that, in turn, contribute to later personality pathology, including abnormal functioning in the hypothalamus and pituitary gland (i.e., the master endocrine gland; e.g., Mason et al., 1994). Taken together, this evidence demonstrates that personality psychopathology begins in childhood, develops gradually over years of development, and manifests an *insidious onset* that typically culminates in early adulthood. For purposes of psychological assessment, testing, and psychodiagnosis, these features are used to differentiate personality disorder from that of clinical disorder.

From this standpoint, personality functioning comprises the complete matrix of the individual human, which is anchored to multiple areas of both structure and functioning, including behavioral, phenomenological, intrapsychic, cognitive, and biophysical (Millon & Millon, 2008, p. 58). As such, clinical disorders are most accurately conceptualized as being nested within the context of personality psychopathology. The analogy would be an art painting embedded with a beautiful frame. The artwork represents the clinical disorder, while the framework affords the influential surrounding context without which the painting is deprived of its essential meaning. This discussion would not be complete without examining an elemental aspect of both personality disorder and clinical disorder that both (at least currently) share.

At present, the *DSM–5* principal approach to diagnosing a personality disorder is the same as for clinical disorder, namely, a categorical system that employs a prototypical approach as defined previously. Thus, a personality disorder also comprises essential symptoms, without which the disorder would not be present, along with nonessential variations. Of course, in this case, the "symptoms" would represent problematic *traits*, which are defined as average tendencies in a person's behavior that are relatively consistent over time and, to some extent, across situations depending on the strength of environmental forces; recall behavior is a function of personality traits and the strength of situational forces as follows:

$$B = f\left(P \times S\right)$$

Equation 11.1

where B symbolizes overt or observable behavior, f symbolizes the term function, P denotes relatively consistent patterns or personality traits, and S designates the presence of situational forces (see Funder, 2006; Moskowtiz & Fournier, 2015). In the case of maladaptive traits, however, one would expect such to supersede situational factors to a much greater extent by virtue of their rigidity, inflexibility, and temporal stability, hence causing dysfunction and distress to a concomitant degree. The reason this current commonality between personality disorder and clinical disorder is emphasized is to broach the topic of a newly proposed alternative model of diagnosing personality psychopathology using a *dimensional approach* (see American Psychiatric Association, 2013, pp. 761–779). Here will be explicated arguments in favor of the current categorical model that the *DSM–5* continues to espouse as its principal diagnostic scheme. Later, the discussion will revisit the dimensional model of diagnosing personality disorder when presenting the final test in this chapter that is used in this manner.

Personality Disorder: Type or Degree?

There continues to be an enduring and arduous debate as to whether the personality disorder represents a disturbance in type or degree (Widiger & Trull, 2007). Those who advocate the latter position espouse a dimensional versus categorical nosology of diagnosis (Shedler & Westen, 2004). The remarkably high rate of comorbidity, even exceeding that for clinical disorders, bolsters the argument for a dimensional approach (Zimmerman, Rothschild, & Chelminski, 2005). However, current dimensional diagnostic frameworks are more complex and therefore more cumbersome to employ in clinical practice, thus hindering consensus regarding the most useful standardized system (see Larsen & Buss, 2021). This will be illustrated later in this chapter when presenting the personality inventory that is currently being used for deriving dimensional personality diagnoses.

These issues notwithstanding, the current categorical system endures by offering clinicians a pragmatic balance between diagnostic accuracy and utility in mental health practice. Furthermore, assessing personality by typology dates back to Hippocrates (460–370 B.C.) and Galen (130–200 A.D.) and has continued as an influential approach in personality psychology or the study of individual differences (see, e.g., Block, 1971, 1977; Friedman & Rosenman, 1974; Myers, 1998; Myers, McCaulley, Quenk, & Hammer, 1998).

However, some have cogently argued that the categorical (i.e., nominal) and dimensional (i.e., ordinal/interval/ratio) distinction is a false dichotomy and represents an artificial outcome of varying statistical assessment methods (see, e.g., Chamorro-Premuzic, 2011). This shall become most evident when the unique *base rate* (*BR*) standard scores of some of the subsequent personality inventories are introduced, which are a unique combination of nominal and ordinal data. These will be contrasted with the traditional standardized *T*–scores most typically considered to be interval data (see, e.g., Warner, 2021a, 2021b) and hence singularly dimensional in nature.[1] Whichever position one supports, the *DSM–5* and all major diagnostic systems continue to employ the categorical approach. Thus, with one exception, the subsequent personality inventories will be discussed in terms of how their results can be reported and interpreted in ways that provide a personality disorder diagnosis according to the dominant categorical approach. The final measure to be covered within the NEO inventories, however, is presented using a dimensional approach; more specifically, as applied to the new *alternative DSM–5 model for personality disorders*. As a result, readers of this book will be informed of the most contemporary developments in the field of conceptualizing and diagnosing personality disorders. The ensuing section addresses the issue of diagnosing personality disorders in individuals who have not yet reached adulthood.

At What Age and Circumstances Should a Personality Disorder be First Diagnosed?

The issue to be presented in this section regards when and under what circumstances a personality disorder should be diagnosed in young individuals. This issue is analogous to the one previously presented wherein the question concerned the bipolar diagnosis in children (see Chapter 10). There, the controversy centered upon the potentially deleterious effects of such diagnosis, most especially the prescription of mood stabilizers to young individuals so diagnosed. In this instance, however, the diagnosis of a personality disorder in childhood and adolescence pertains more to (a) the degree to which it is empirically justified in individuals who are still developing both psychologically and physically and (b) the potential negative connotations and effects of such a label (Hinshaw & Stier, 2008).

First, as indicated previously, there is substantial evidence that personality disturbance originates in childhood, has an insidious onset, and continues on a chronic and gradually escalating course, culminating at some point during early adulthood, when it becomes fully established (see, e.g., Widiger, 2012; Yasgur, 2017). However, this information renders onset difficult to discern, which does not assist in answering the question regarding the age at which these disorders can first be diagnosed. Thus, a vital issue to clarify is the particular point in development at which a personality disorder can or should be diagnosed?

The *DSM–5* advises that personality disorders "may be applied with children or adolescents in those relatively unusual instances in which the individual's particular personality traits appear to be pervasive, persistent, and unlikely to be limited to a developmental stage or another mental disorder" (American Psychiatric Association, 2013, p. 647). A pertinent *DSM–IV–TR* qualifier is that a childhood-onset personality disorder "will often not persist unchanged into adult life" (American Psychiatric Association, 2000, p. 687). Thus, the minimum duration of symptoms is one year, and it is recognized that the particular manifestation may change over time because of the recognized malleability of the young and developing personality. This means the maladaptive traits may diminish, exacerbate, and/or manifest differently with age after diagnosis and is consonant with evidence of the malleability of child and adolescent personality (Caspi & Roberts, 2001; McCrae & Costa, 2003).

Interestingly, it is also accordant with the concept of *personality coherence* in which rank order stability in a trait is maintained longitudinally, although the particular behavioral expressions change predictably with chronological age (Larsen & Buss, 2021). For example, explosive temper tantrums in childhood were shown to be reliable predictors of poor occupational performance and marital dissolution 30 years later (Caspi, Elder, & Bem, 1987). Other experts believe that even the most disturbed varieties of personality disorder (e.g., borderline; Yasgur, 2017) begin in childhood and progressively exacerbate thereafter.

The single exception to permitting child and adolescent personality diagnoses is the *antisocial personality disorder* (*APD*), which is precluded for individuals younger than 18 years of age (American Psychiatric Association, 2013, p. 659).

Therefore, with the exception of APD, it appears that personality disorders can be legitimately diagnosed from the point of early adolescence; perhaps 13 or 14 years of age. Logically, the younger the individual, the more the identified traits should be shown to be pervasive, rigid, and maladaptive, while ruling out other plausible explanations, most especially developmental factors, situational issues, or clinical syndromes (e.g., mood or anxiety disorders). Prior to age 13 or 14, if there is clear test evidence for personality psychopathology, this fact should first be noted, then qualified by appending either one of the following terms: (a) "risk" of developing a personality disorder with such traits or (b) "emerging" personality disorder. For example, if an 11-year-old was showing evidence of borderline pathology, the following could be listed: (a) "*Noted:* Emerging borderline personality disorder"; or (b) "*Noted:* Risk of developing borderline personality disorder."

Reasons for Including a Personality Inventory Within a Test Battery

This section discusses when and under what circumstances a personality inventory should be used as part of a test battery, although it is apportioned into three more specific issues. The first concerns the type of referral questions that are most conducive to using personality inventories. The second is related to insurance coverage issues; that is, for what issues do insurance companies consider the use of personality inventories as most medically necessary? Third, and finally, if a personality test is indicated, what kind should be used? The ensuing discussion proceeds in such order.

Referral Issues Conducive to Personality Inventories

Concerning individuals from adolescence through adulthood, especially the latter, mental health testing referrals frequently present differential diagnostic questions involving a clinical disorder as opposed to a personality disorder, which is why this chapter was diligent in discriminating between the two kinds of psychopathology. A frequent example is a referral to rule out bipolar disorder versus borderline personality disorder, as both involve mood swings or unstable mood. The potential borderline psychopathology may present intense affective instability and transient psychotic symptoms (Kernberg, 1967; McWilliams, 2011) or extremely severe dissociative symptoms (American Psychiatric Association, 2013) suggestive of bipolar disorder with psychotic features. In the absence of objective standardized clinical and personality testing, even the most sagacious mental health clinician would be taxed to render such precise differential diagnostic decisions based only on a clinical interview.

Considering that the *DSM–5* adopts the position that personality disorders can most accurately be diagnosed over time and across multiple sessions by means of clinical interviewing, standardized psychological testing can be employed to significantly expedite such determination. Hence, even if it is assumed that clinical interviewing can be as accurate as standardized testing in pursuit of a personality disorder diagnosis, which is a tenuous position based on empirical data (Aegisdottir et al., 2006), the latter method can provide such diagnostic results much more rapidly. In such cases, without the assistance of standardized psychological testing, excessive comorbid diagnoses, along with imprecise, poorly designed, and protracted trial-and-error treatment interventions, are extremely likely and done at the expense of the patient who is seeking effective treatment.

Differential diagnoses between clinical and personality disorders are also becoming remarkably more common concerning adolescents (i.e., ages 13–17). For preadolescents (i.e., ages 9–12), it is more likely that testing issues will focus more exclusively on differential diagnosis involving exclusively clinical disorders, although there may be more specific questions concerning self-esteem, emotion regulation, social skills, social perception, and other personality-related issues. However, it is not infrequent that an assessment of emerging maladaptive personality traits and risk for later development of a particular personality disorder is indicated in preadolescent referrals. Therefore, it is judicious testing practice concerning this younger age group to measure whether a personality disorder is either in its incipient stages so as to identify risk, or in the alternative, sufficiently pervasive, rigid, and maladaptive pursuant to *DSM–5* guidelines for legitimate diagnosis (discussed earlier).

Insurance Coverage Issues

Regarding insurance coverage issues, because effective psychiatric and psychotherapeutic intervention is contingent upon accurate *DSM–5* diagnoses as defined by the American Psychiatric Association (2013), substantiating medical necessity for such testing is routinely feasible. This is especially the case for testing requests to rule out one or more personality disorders, as such diagnoses are readily recognized as being more difficult to make based solely on the clinical method (see American Psychiatric Association, 2013, p. 647; Aegisdottir et al., 2006). Many insurance companies are cognizant of the cost effectiveness of standardized personality testing for personality disorder differential diagnosis, although evidence of a long course of treatment ineffectiveness for a clinical disorder bolsters the case that there may be a heretofore undiagnosed personality disorder that has been masked by the more acute clinical symptoms.

Which Type of Personality Test to Use

Finally, if testing for a personality disorder is apparent, the question remains as to what type of personality test is indicated; that is, self-report (i.e., S-data), observer-report (i.e., O-data), or performance personality testing (i.e., test data or *T-data*). As will become apparent subsequently, self-report personality inventories provide the greatest degree of selection. As such, these are the most likely to be selected of the personality inventories. The self-report format is susceptible to all the vulnerabilities discussed in Chapter 10 as applied to self-report rating scales, including all the response sets that can distort the findings, along with the sometimes tenuous assumption that the informant possesses the ability to introspect and report one's feelings, behaviors, and thoughts accurately. In cases where there is likely to be intentional distortion or lack of ability to introspect, then either the observer-report format is a more felicitous choice (i.e., assuming it provides the personality data needed to address the referral issues), or in the alternative, selecting performance personality testing. Here, a brief discussion regarding explicit versus implicit personality tests is relevant.

An *explicit personality test* presents stimuli to the respondent that clearly reveal the kind of traits and symptoms being measured. Usually, these are in the form of a personality inventory test wherein the listing of standardized statements openly describes what behaviors, thoughts, and feelings the informant is responding to in terms of degree of truth or agreement. In contrast, an *implicit personality test* is much more discreet regarding the traits it is measuring. For example, answering the question "What might this be?" in response to an inkblot largely disguises what traits are being measured. These tend to be the performance personality tests discussed in Chapter 12, which also require more testing time and are more indirect regarding personality disorder diagnosis. Therefore, in the event the examinee is assessed as having the requisite ability to introspect and has no apparent reason to intentionally distort the findings, a self-report personality inventory is the most felicitous selection. That is, such a measure is more efficient and more direct and requires less time and expense. If the individual does not meet these criteria, and there is a collateral who is sufficiently familiar with the examinee, then an observer-based personality inventory is a second-best selection, but only if the test provides the requisite data needed to resolve the differential diagnostic issues in the case. Lastly, if neither of these options are viable, then a performance personality test should be selected.

The Personality Inventory Tests

The personality inventory tests reviewed next represent the core section of this chapter and are represented by three different systems. They include (a) the Millon inventory tests, (b) the MMPI inventory tests, and (c) the NEO inventory tests. The Millon inventory tests are presented first for three reasons. First, these instruments are based on both theory and research. Second, their test structure is most effectively accordant with rendering differential diagnoses both within and among personality psychopathology and clinical disorders. Third, the scales bear a remarkable resemblance to the *DSM–5* nosology despite the fact that they are based on theory, whereas the *DSM–5* is purportedly atheoretical. The MMPI inventory tests are discussed next due to their long history and significant research backing. They also address personality and clinical differential diagnoses, although afford somewhat greater emphasis to the latter. The NEO inventory tests are discussed last because they began as measures of universal normal traits and only more recently are being applied to the diagnosis of personality psychopathology according to the new dimensional model proposed by the *DSM–5* (American Psychiatric Association, 2013). The latter were included because they provide an opportunity to review the five-factor model, which has been very influential in personality psychology and more recently to clinical psychology. They also provide an opportunity to illustrate the manner in which personality inventories designed to measure this model are being used by the *DSM–5* in diagnosing personality disorders according to the newly proposed dimensional model.

The Millon Personality Inventory Tests

The Millon inventory tests number three in total and together cover an age range from 9 to 85 years. They are all founded upon Millon's personality theory, which, as will become apparent, utilizes concepts from evolutionary psychology. Therefore, before introducing the three tests, a review of Millon's personality theory is indicated and is presented.

Millon's Biosocial Learning Evolutionary Personality Theory

Millon's biosocial learning evolutionary theory of personality (Millon, 2011; Millon & Grossman, 2005) posits that human personality comprises learned strategies to (a) secure reinforcement and (b) minimize punishment (Millon, 1990; Millon & Davis, 1996). This is accomplished through the following three polarities: (a) self–other (i.e., independent–ambivalent–dependent); (b) active–passive (i.e., initiate–accommodate); and (c) pleasure–pain (i.e., positive–negative reaction from others). Various types of personality disorders represent differing qualitative combinations of rigid, inflexible, and maladaptive positions on these polarities. This representing the gist of his theory, let us now scrutinize the concepts in more detail.

There are four areas in which evolutionary principles are illustrated, including existence, adaptation, replication, and abstraction. The initial three domains are manifested in polarities, which are employed to assemble his nosology of personality disorders that are reflected within the Millon personality inventory tests. Imbalances on these dimensions, or in some instances being conflicted regarding them, is believed to lead to personality psychopathology and predispose the individual to a variety of clinical disorders. Each polarity is next examined in such order.

First, *existence* refers to an individual's state of being versus nonbeing, which is conveyed on a pleasure versus pain dimension; that is, survival versus inevitable death. Further, this continuum concerns behaviors that improve the quality of life and that reduce the risk of harm. At its greatest level of abstraction, this polarity forms a pleasure versus pain continuum. An individual who is imbalanced on this dimension is considered to manifest personality disturbance.

Adaptation comprises a homeostatic mechanism that maintains an individual's survival and is expressed on a dimension of active versus passive. Assuming the individual indeed exists, this continuum concerns the manner in which one can endure. A passive orientation is evinced when the individual is able to accommodate to environmental demands, whereas the active orientation is manifested when the individual attempts to modify the environment to fit one's needs. This polarity is not intended to be completely unidimensional, as some personalities may simply be conflicted on this continuum and not express either extreme.

Replication regards nurturance both internally and externally and is manifested on a dimension of self versus other. Because death is inevitable, the principal way individuals attempt to circumvent this problem is to reproduce biologically, which will succeed in continuing their genetic make-up into future generations. Here, the two extremes are to nurture oneself and, on the other hand, to nurture others. Once again, some individuals can be conflicted on this continuum, hence rendering it completely unidimensional in nature.

Therefore, let us look more closely at what separates the normal versus pathological personality from this perspective. Adaptive personalities are those that show a reasonable balance between, at minimum, one of these polarities. In addition, if there is a tendency toward an extreme on another polarity, then they need to demonstrate at least some degree of flexibility to adjust to environmental demands. In other words, balance and flexibility are personality aspects that promote good adjustment, as explicated by this theory.

Together, Millon's personality theory proposes 15 personality patterns or styles, each of which can range across three levels of functioning from healthy to moderately disturbed to extremely disordered. As one moves toward the healthy end, there is a preference across the three polarities, along with exhibiting reasonable flexibility in response to environmental demands. At the moderate level of disturbance, the individual will predictably manifest symptoms in response to psychosocial stressors, which are associated with deficits in flexibility and adaptability according to their personality pattern's vulnerabilities. At the most disturbed and disordered level, individuals predictably manifest chronically impaired traits and manifest continuous episodes of various clinical disorders and psychopathology that are self-perpetuated according to their personality pattern's vulnerabilities. The three more severe personality patterns refer to more advanced stages of personality psychopathology, including breakdowns in psychological structure, especially the manifestation of psychotic episodes and severe deficits in social competence.

Together, these personality patterns are measured by each of the Millon inventory tests. Therefore, they need not be listed and explained here. However, it should be noted that the theory, along with the Millon personality inventories, affords precedence to the personality disorders and conceptualizes clinical disorders as being nested within personality psychopathology. Planned treatment intervention based on Millon's theory and measures makes the same assumptions, hence primarily targeting the personality issue. In other words, it is assumed that genuine ongoing progress in treatment will not be achieved if intervention is limited to the patient's clinical disorder. Either the clinical symptoms will predictably return or another clinical disorder will emerge. This is analogous to the psychoanalytic concept of symptom substitution in which it is believed that clinical symptoms will return if the underlying unconscious conflict is not fully resolved. This explains why each of the Millon personality inventories reports the personality data first, followed by the clinical syndrome-type scales. Also represented within the personality inventories are the three levels of personality functioning, including healthy, moderately disturbed, and severely disturbed, along with the personality patterns and severe personality psychopathology dichotomy. However, the data yield is not required to be interpreted according to Millon's personality theory, although obviously this is advised by all three manuals.

Next, the Millon personality inventory tests are introduced. As done for other tests of similar systems, the specific measures will be presented in order of increasing chronological age (CA), hence beginning with the test for the youngest age group and finishing with the adult version. Because these are principally personality tests, the youngest age group begins in preadolescence.

Millon Pre–Adolescent Clinical Inventory

The Millon test designed for the youngest cohort begins in preadolescence. This is because the construct of focus here is personality, which is not sufficiently developed for purposes of measuring personality disorder prior to this developmental stage.

SYNOPSIS

The *Millon Pre–Adolescent Clinical Inventory (M–PACI*; Millon, Tringone, Millon, & Grossman, 2005) is a personality inventory test for individuals ranging in age from 9 years, 0 months to 12 years, 11 months. It is designed as a self-report inventory, hence it relies on S-data. It is based on Millon's biosocial learning evolutionary theory and comprises emerging personality scales, clinical scales, and a listing of noteworthy responses in said order. Hence, consistent with the theory upon which it is based, personality pathology trumps the measurement of clinical disorders and takes precedence in both reporting and interpretation. The noteworthy responses are helpful in flagging urgent issues, such as indications of self-harm.

NORM REFERENCE SAMPLE

A total of 271 preadolescents comprised the standardization sample. It consisted of 191 males and 88 females, along with 11 that had missing data. There were four age groups, ranging from 9 to 12 years. The numbers in each year of age were as follows: (a) 9 years ($n = 55$); (b) 10 years ($n = 55$); (c) 11 years ($n = 67$), and (d) 12 years ($n = 104$). In terms of race/ethnicity, 81% were White, 21% African American, 5% American Indian, 2% Asian American, 4% Other, and 11% missing. Finally, 12% had been seen once by a mental health professional, whereas in excess of 50% had been seen five or more times. These data were collected from July 2002 through May 2003. This sample was then apportioned by random assignment into either a development subsample ($n = 171$) or a *cross-validation sample* ($n = 100$), the latter being used to measure the degree to which findings generalize to a sample different from that which initially standardized the test. The M–PACI uses combined gender norms in transforming raw scores to standard scores.

ADMINISTRATION

As stated, the M–PACI is administered by means of self-report. Administration time is estimated to be a relatively brief 20 minutes, which works well with this younger population. A minimum third-grade reading level is required for adequate comprehension of the items. Although this inventory can be administered via hard copy booklet and Scantron answer sheet, computer administration through the *Q-global* (Pearson, 2021) online scoring and reporting platform is most convenient and minimizes the likelihood of human error in recording responses.

Test instructions are either printed in the hard copy booklet or provided on screen by the computer. Examinees are advised that the statements they will be reading describe how people their age may feel and act and to decide if it is *True* or *False* as applied to themselves. Missing response are those in which the item is skipped, double answered, or improperly marked. Of note, the last two are precluded by computer administration. The completed inventory should be perused and any missing items completed by means of encouragement. This is because five or more missing responses invalidate the protocol.

SCORING

Scoring is also done on the Q-global (Pearson, 2021) web platform and is required if such was used to administer this test. It can also be scored by mailing the Scantron answer sheet to Pearson, although obviously the previous option affords immediate results. There are two report options for computer administration and scoring: (a) the profile report, which yields all the raw and standard scale scores, along with a brief excerpt regarding validity scale interpretation; and (b) the interpretive report, which provides all the data shown in the score report plus interpretive statements based on the diagnostic data. The latter are programmed into the computer based on the score profile, although they are not effectively qualified according to clinical judgment and should not be uncritically reported verbatim. Such practice contravenes ethical standards promulgated by the American Educational Research Association, American Psychological Association, National Council on Measurement in Education (NCME), and the Standards for Educational and Psychological Testing (1974). Utilizing the data tables that have been prepared for reporting the results of this personality test (see Form 11.1) will effectively guide an examiner through the reporting and interpretation process. Hence, using Form 11.1, discussed subsequently, negates the need for ordering the more expensive interpretive report.

The score report computer printout provides data in several sections as follows: (a) interpretive considerations (i.e., client demographics); (b) response validity; (c) emerging personality patterns (i.e., incipient personality disorder); (d) current clinical signs (i.e., clinical disorder); (e) noteworthy responses (i.e., a listing of responses that deserve immediate scrutiny); and (f) the response *True* or *False* (i.e., 1 or 2, respectively).

Regarding the actual data, the M–PACI yields *base rate* or *BR–scores* that fundamentally differ from the more familiar linearly transformed *T–scores* in terms of both measurement scale and meaning. Thus, the *BR–score* will be reviewed here in detail because (a) it is being introduced for the first time in this book and (b) all Millon personality tests employ this metric. First, the *BR–scores* account for the estimated prevalence of various personality and clinical disorders (Craig, 1999). As such, they are considered to be nonparametric nominal/ordinal data in terms of measurement scale (Stevens, 1946), with a range from 0 to 100 (Kamp & Tringone, 2008; McCann, 1999, 2008; Strack, 2002). An explanation of the way *BR–scores* are derived will clarify this definition.

First, the M–PACI norm reference sample completed the preadolescent Millon inventory to obtain raw scores for all the personality scales. Second, expert clinicians rated each individual in the sample in terms of which single diagnostic scale represented (a) the *best fit* diagnosis and (b) the *second-best fit* diagnosis. These ratings were then used as a basis for the Millon raw score to *BR–score* transformations for all diagnostic scales according to the following steps. One, the percentage of the normative sample who were first-most prominent and second-most prominent were computed for each personality patterns and clinical syndromes scales. For example, for the unstable personality scale, 17% were first-most prominent and 20% second-most prominent. Thus, *BR–score* transformations were designed such that 17% and 20% of the standardization sample would score as first- and second-most prominent on the unstable personality scale. In such manner, the estimated prevalence rates of the various personality and clinical disorders measured by the M–PACI are reflected by the raw score to *BR–score* transformations. Subsequent examinees being evaluated by this test in effect have their resulting scores adjusted for the estimated prevalence rates of all the measured psychopathology in their age group. It will be seen that the Millon personality inventories for older individuals utilize a very similar strategy and effectively provide adjustments for the estimated prevalence rates for the various disorders, whereas linear *T–scores* do not make such adjustments.

Form 11.1 provides three data tables for reporting the results of an M–PACI test. Table 1 is first because it evaluates the validity of the entire profile in terms of omissions, honesty and accuracy, and tendencies to minimize or magnify one's degree of psychopathology. The table lists the scale name, raw score, percentile rank (PR), result, and the assessed test-taking response set. First, the omissions scale is dichotomous wherein five or more missed or improperly marked items invalidates the profile. Second, the four items comprising the invalidity scale directly query whether the examinee is answering truthfully. A raw score of 1 renders the profile of questionable validity and more than this invalidates the test for want of honesty, accuracy, and motivation to answer. Hence, the first two scales are interpreted according to raw score metrics. Response negativity is a bipolar scale that hinges upon the degree of rarity of a response set. Therefore, although both a raw score and PR is reported, only the latter is interpreted for purposes of determining validity on this scale. The greater the PR, the more the examinee is producing a negative impression by endorsing an increasing number of problems and vice versa. At the extremes, a PR of 0–10 indicates significant underreporting, while a PR of 90 and greater shows significant overreporting. Either extreme invalidates the profile, whereas all other PR ranges leaves test validity intact.

To expedite interpretation of the validity scales and render a determination of whether the remaining diagnostic scales are appropriate to report and interpret, narrative excerpts immediately follow Table 1. The first describes a valid profile, the second a questionably valid profile, and the third an invalid profile. Both the questionable and invalid excerpts list all potential reasons that validity is being questioned. Hence, the examiner merely deletes those that do not apply. The questionable alternative advises the need for corroboration because of the tenuousness of M–PACI data. Finally, the invalid interpretation argues that the M–PACI diagnostic data should not be reported because of its misleading nature. Next, M–PACI interpretation is discussed, which assumes that the validity data were acceptably valid or, at minimum, questionably valid.

INTERPRETATION

Figure 11.1 is available for download on Routledge's e-resources website. It depicts an interpretive strategy for all the Millon personality inventories, which is made feasible by virtue of the fact that they are all based on the same personality theory and possess comparable test structures. In all cases, the personality patterns scales are afforded priority in the interpretive process, which is supplemented by the facets scales available on the adolescent and adult measures for a more detailed analysis of the present problematic traits. This is invariably followed by analysis of the clinical syndromes scales, which are designed to detect the presence of any clinical disorders that have been produced by the aforementioned personality disturbance. Finally, the adolescent version yields data regarding unresolved concerns that may be considered aggravating factors. The chief point here is that the three Millon personality inventories are sufficiently similar such that a single flowchart is capable of guiding the interpretive process irrespective of which age group is being discussed. The primary modification is the availability of some supplemental scales on the adolescent version, which will be discussed subsequently. Hence, Figure 11.1 (see e-resources) will be referenced when delineating the interpretive strategy that can be employed for all Millon personality inventories.

After analyzing the validity data, M–PACI interpretation necessarily begins with the personality patterns scales (Figure 11.1, second box titled "Personality Patterns"), consistent with Millon's theory that maladjustment in this domain predisposes an individual to a variety of clinical disorders. Thus, in the event there is no evidence of personality psychopathology, any subsequent clinical syndrome should be interpreted as situationally induced and thus transient. This is illustrated in Figure 11.1, box titled "Clinical Syndromes," which addresses positive clinical disorder findings (i.e., clinically significant data) in the absence of personality pathology. The most felicitous *DSM–5* disorders would fall under the *adjustment disorders*, which by definition are triggered by environmental stressors and are assumed to dissipate within six months of stressor resolution. Also, the *emerging* language employed as part of the label used for these scales is meaningful in that the personality disturbance is presumed to be in the process of forming or in its incipient stage. This is due to the young age of the standardization sample of 9–12 years. Therefore, unless there is clear and convincing evidence that the traits are sufficiently rigid, pervasive, and severe from this and other data, the interpretive language must reflect a conservative approach regarding personality disorder diagnosis.

In Form 11.1, Table 2 is organized to present the personality data across three columns, including the scale name, *BR*–score, and a succinct description of the emerging psychopathology to facilitate diagnostic interpretation. Note that each scale name includes the *DSM–5* equivalent or link, once again to assist in interpretation. General table notes define abbreviations and the directional meaning of *BR*–scores. Of perhaps greatest importance, a specific table note defines the diagnostic meaning of *BR*–score ranges, which are interpreted as follows: (a) 0–59 reflects normal or adaptive personality development; (b) 60–74 signifies a personality *feature*, which is a style that is generally considered to be healthy and adaptive, although occasionally can lead to some problems; (c) 75–84 designates the presence of *clinically significant personality traits*, which are discernable patterns of behavior that most likely are causing dysfunction; and (d) 85–100 shows an emerging or potentially fully developed *personality type*, which reflects a pervasive cluster of rigid, inflexible, and maladaptive traits that definitively cause dysfunction and that may constitute a genuine personality disorder. Considering this young age cohort, the more conservative emerging personality disorder should represent the default selection unless the fully established version is warranted by extremely high scores and other assessment information.

Of note, these designations are not found in the M–PACI manual (Millon, Tringone et al., 2005). In fact, the manual assumes the rather ambiguous position that higher elevations simply reflect more of a particular disposition, and the ultimate diagnostic decision is left to the discretion of the examiner. Therefore, this diagnostic scheme was employed for the purpose of applying it consistently to all three Millon personality inventories. This approach provides reliability of interpretation across all Millon personality measures and renders it much easier to apply from the perspective of the examiner. In testing practice, such consistency can increase both efficiency and objectivity. In any case, examiners may modify this specific interpretive scheme to better match the populations with which they test and work in their respective practices.

Once the datum is classified within one of these score ranges (i.e., a nominal measurement scale), the elevation within that category represents its degree of severity, with higher scores indicating greater severity (i.e., an ordinal scale). This reveals a nominal/ordinal integrated approach to test interpretation employed by the Millon unique *BR*–score metric. For instance, an individual may have *BR*–scores of 90 for unstable and 85 for unruly. This dual-score profile may be interpreted as an individual with an emerging borderline personality as his type, with secondary narcissism. Although both personality patterns fall within the personality type range, the unstable or borderline personality constellation of traits would be considered principal due to its being five *BR*–score points higher, and the unruly conduct-disordered type would be secondary. If both these scales were higher within the type range, this may also be interpreted as comorbid personality disorders if also substantiated by other data. Furthermore, in the event the unruly *BR*–score was 76, the conduct-disordered traits could still be listed, although here as subthreshold clinically significant traits. Hence, the Millon interpretive scheme may be seen as a quantitative guide, which leaves some degree of flexibility and discretion to the examiner. Figure 11.1 (e-resources) generally illustrates the various categories and degrees of the different types of psychopathology available on the Millon personality inventories.

To facilitate test interpretation, three narrative excerpts were drafted following Table 2 (Form 11.1). The first describes results in which the data are all negative. That is, there are absolutely no statistical elevations above a *BR*–score of 59. Considering that behavior is always a function of personality interacting with situational factors (see Equation 11.1), and assuming that other personality pathology has not gone undetected, any evidence of statistical elevations among the clinical syndromes scales must be caused by environmental stressors. This translates most probably into a diagnosis of adjustment disorder with the clinical symptoms shown among the clinical syndromes scales; for example, *adjustment disorder with anxiety* (see also Figure 11.1).

The three other narrative excerpts deal with increasing degrees of evidence for personality disturbance, one for mild level (i.e., *BR*–scores 60–74), one for moderate level (i.e., *BR*–scores 75–84), and one for severe level (i.e., *BR*–scores 85–100). All acknowledge the currently measured personality disturbance, with added language referencing a risk of the later development of a full personality disorder. Furthermore, there are statements referencing the implications that the personality findings have for the clinical data that is yet to be viewed. Finally, in the event the clinical data are not pertinent to the case (e.g., the diagnostic issues regarding personality functioning only), the Table 3 clinical syndromes scales can be disregarding as irrelevant and deleted.

More commonly, when the M–PACI has been selected as part of the test battery, the final Table 3 (Form 11.1) clinical syndromes data yield will need to be reported and interpreted. It has the same structure as Table 2 for consistency. The scales are listed in approximate order of decreasing severity and similarity in terms of classification. Therefore, the scales begin with psychotic symptoms (viz., reality distortions), while the last three scales have previously been classified together as *disruptive behavior disorders*. The *BR*–score ranges are as follows: (a) 0–74 indicates an *absence* of a clinical disorder; (b) 75–84 signifies a *presence* of a clinical disorder; and (c) 85–100 designates the *prominence* of a clinical disorder. Again, this interpretive scheme represents a guide that possesses some degree of diagnostic flexibility in the same manner as for the personality data. For instance, an examinee who manifests a *BR*–score of 95 on depressed moods, along with a *BR*–score of 80 on reality distortions, can be diagnosed with a major depressive disorder with psychotic features. Interpretively, however, this clinical diagnosis would be secondary to, and embedded within, any personality disturbance shown among the personality pattern scales, this being consistent with the personality theory upon which these measures are founded.

To be consistent with this interpretive scheme, three narrative excerpts were drafted that are reasonably parallel to those composed for the personality data. The first addresses consistent negative results, while the second and third deal with moderate-level and severe-level positive findings of clinical pathology. The negative version offers descriptions for consistent (i.e., both negative findings) and inconsistent (i.e., clinical data negative, personality data positive) results across the clinical and personality disorders and their implications. Both positive clinical findings also describe data patterns that are consistent with the personality data (i.e., positive personality pathology) and inconsistent with such data (i.e., negative personality pathology). All these potential combinations are portrayed in Figure 11.1 (e-resources), which will be referenced once again when the adolescent and adult Millon personality inventories are presented.

SUMMARY

This completes the presentation of the M–PACI. The principal focus was on providing a description of this measure that yielded sufficient information to appreciate the theory upon which it was established, its unique data and test structure, and how the results can be most effectively reported and interpreted within a psychological assessment report (see Form 11.1 and Figure 11.1). Next, the Millon personality inventory for adolescents is presented.

Millon Adolescent Clinical Inventory, Second Edition

The *Millon Adolescent Clinical Inventory, Second Edition* (*MACI–II*; Millon, Tringone, Grossman, & Millon, 2020) is a self-report personality inventory for adolescents. It mirrors the design of the preadolescent version discussed previously, although with some added features, such as personality *facet scales* and scales measuring some concerns related to personality and interpersonal relationships.

The MACI–II consists of 24 clinical scales that are presented in three sections as follows: (a) personality patterns (i.e., stable patterns of characteristics); (b) clinical syndromes (i.e., acute and transient clinical disorders); and (c) expressed concerns (i.e., distress in self-oriented and interpersonally based areas). In addition, the personality patterns scales are supplemented by facet scales, which provide a more detailed profile of maladaptive proclivities present among the most dominant personality patterns. This edition evolved from its immediate predecessor, the *Millon Adolescent Personality Inventory* (*MACI*; Millon, Millon, & Davis, 1993), which was updated in 2006 to incorporate the Grossman facet scales (Millon, Millon, Davis, & Grossman, 2006a). Items have been updated to better reflect the prototype of each personality pattern (e.g., borderline tendency) and to be more consistent with the *DSM–5* as concerning major clinical disorders (viz., adding scales for *disruptive mood dysregulation disorder*, *post-traumatic stress disorder*, and *psychotic disorder*). Finally, validity scales are designed to detect both underreporting and overreporting, along with non-content-based responding.

NORM REFERENCE SAMPLE

The standardization sample included 1,143 cases from various regions of the United States. Data collection was done from April 2017 through February 2019. Inclusionary criteria included (a) chronological age between 13 years, 0 months and 18 years, 11 months and (b) the completed test was considered to be valid. The norm reference sample data was garnered such that it represented the population of adolescents requesting mental health treatment. Thus, as all the Millon inventories, this version is intended for clinical populations. The sample was stratified according to age, education, race/ethnicity, gender, and setting.

The total sample was apportioned into two subgroups, ages 13–15 (*n* = 645) and 16–18 years (*n* = 498), inclusive. Different norms were established for these two age bands. All the demographic percentages reported in the manual (Millon et al., 2020, Table 4.1, p. 24) pertained to each subgroup. Therefore, the general figures that follow were estimated from averaging the subgroup statistics. First, there were approximately equal percentages of males and females. In terms of race/ethnicity, there was approximately 60% White, 16% Black, 12% Hispanic, 4% Asian, and 6% Other. In terms of education level, the general breakdowns were as follows: 7th grade (15%), 8th grade (15%), 9th grade (17%), 10th grade (16%), 11th grade (20%), and 12th grade (16%). Finally, treatment setting figures were as follows: clinical/group practice (39%), private/solo practice (39%), school/university (4%), juvenile corrections (10%), residential (5%), hospital (2%), and other (1%).

ADMINISTRATION

Administration can be accomplished by paper test booklet and answer sheets or by computer in both English and Spanish. Computer administration is done on the Q-global (Pearson, 2021) online scoring and reporting platform, which are advisable to use. Administration time is estimated to be 25 minutes or less and includes 160 items in total (Millon et al., 2020, p. 7). Examinees with reading problems can be given the MACI–II via audio administration on the Q-global (Pearson, 2021) platform or via an audio USB. Because Q-global (Pearson, 2021) administration is used by the author and other examiners are advised to do the same, the ensuing directions will be described according to this procedure.

After entering in the examinee's demographics, the program first asks which language, English or Spanish, is preferred, along with some optional additional information. The directions inform examinees that the test includes lists of statements that describe how people in this cohort feel, think, and behave and that they are to respond *True* if they agree or *False* if they disagree as the statement applies to them. In the event they cannot decide, they are instructed to select the *False* alternative. This latter instruction diverts from most dichotomous *True–False* inventories, which encourage the respondent to somehow break the tie in one direction and be assured that the vast number of items will effectively counterbalance any errors in measurement. They are also encouraged to be as "honest and serious" as possible and to provide an answer to all items. Furthermore, at this juncture they may also enable the audio option at the top of the screen so that the inventory is read to them, although responses must still be by a computer mouse click. They may revert to standard administration at any time during test administration should they be more comfortable in reading the items. Finally, examinees are encouraged to answer all items because five or more omissions preclude the test from being scored. Although omissions technically include both unmarked and double-marked items, the latter is not possible on the Q-global procedure, which is another reason for using it.

The focus of this section is on the derivation of the *BR*–scores, which drive test interpretation as was seen in the M–PACI. Scoring can be done manually by the examiner or by the Q-global (Pearson, 2021) platform that also administers the test. There are two types of reports provided by the Q-global (Pearson, 2021); a profile report and an interpretive report. The former provides all the validity and diagnostic scale scores, along with validity interpretation and an enumeration of *noteworthy responses*. The latter consist of items of urgency (e.g., indicating potential self-harm) that were endorsed in an affirmative manner and require follow-up inquiry. The interpretive report affords all the data provided in the profile report, along with detailed interpretations of the diagnostic scores. The latter is remarkably costly, and the interpretive statements lack discretion, consistency, and context, and thus can be extremely misleading. The profile report is preferred, which supplies everything needed for the data tables (see Form 11.2). Next are the validity scales, which determine whether the ensuing test data are useful to diagnosis and assessment. Finally, the various scales and their presentation, along with supplemental scores, are relevant to this section. The following discussion will proceed in this order.

SCORING

BR–score Derivation   First, *BR*–score transformations were done separately for the two normative subgroups, ages 13–15 and16–18. Second, base rate estimates were provided by clinician ratings of 636 individuals in the standardization sample. Specifically, they ranked each adolescent's three most prominent personality patterns and clinical syndromes and two most prominent expressed concerns. Third, the percentage of adolescents who were judged *most prominent* on each of the scales was used as an estimate of the prevalence of that personality pattern, clinical syndrome, and expressed concern in the population as being a *prominent* characteristic. Similarly, the percentage of the sample on each of the scales rated *second-most prominent* was done as an estimate of the prevalence of that characteristic as being *present* (although not prominent).

Fourth, to determine the key raw score to *BR*–score transformations, *BR* anchor points were selected using a somewhat modified procedure from that of the M–PACI. Specifically, a *BR*–score of 75 was selected as a cutting score to represent the estimated *presence* (i.e., the second-most prominent disorder) of particular scale. The raw score equivalent that measured the estimated *presence* of a disorder on a scale was then transformed into a *BR*–score of 75. Next, the raw score equivalent was determined that measured the estimated prominence of a disorder on a particular scale, which was transformed arbitrarily into an anchor *BR*–score of 85. Therefore, a *BR*–score of 85 represented the cutting score that began the prominent category for each scale. Finally, for each scale, three other anchor points were determined to complete the scale range and diagnostic cut points as follows: (a) a *BR*–score of 0 was logically assigned to a raw score equivalent of 0 (hence, representing a base rate of 0); (b) a *BR*–score of 60 was assigned to the median raw score for each scale (hence, representing a PR of 50 or the 50th percentile); and (c) a *BR*–score of 115 was assigned to the maximum raw score for each scale (hence, representing a PR of 99, which is the maximum percentile score because one cannot score higher than oneself). The PR equivalents will become relevant subsequently when the diagnostic scales are reviewed. The remaining *BR*–scores were assigned to raw scores by linear interpolation. For example, assume on any particular scale a *BR*–score of 60 (i.e., 50th percentile) represented a raw score equivalent of 10, and a *BR*–score of 0 a raw score equivalent of 0. Then, a raw score equivalent of 5, which is halfway between raw scores of 0 and 10, would transform into a *BR*–score of 30, which is halfway between a *BR*–scores of 0 and 60. In this manner, PR scores were also derived, and they will be addressed subsequently.

This is why the diagnostic scheme seen in the data tables for the Millon personality tests apportion the personality patterns categories generally as follows: (a) 0–59 is normal or adaptive; (b) 60–74 is a feature that is considered generally adaptive but with possible problems; (c) 75–84 represents clinically significant personality traits that likely cause dysfunction; and (d) 85–115 is a personality type or disorder that is considered to be a cluster of maladaptive traits with definitive dysfunction. It will become apparent that the adult version espouses the same theme. Furthermore, although the M–PACI was derived somewhat differently, it is sufficiently similar to adopt the same interpretive scheme for purposes of consistency and objectively.

Although this delineation of *BR*–score derivation may be somewhat simplistic, it is sufficiently accurate to illustrate why this metric is being conceptualized as a combined nominal–ordinal measurement scale. First, the base rate range has a minimum (i.e., 0), maximum (i.e., 115), and average or median (i.e., 60), which has cutting scores that apportion the scale into categories that indicate diagnosis (i.e., nominal classes) as normal, features, traits, and types. Furthermore, once analysis proceeds with a class, the quantity of the *BR*–score determines amount or degree. However, each *BR*–score point is not assumed to be equivalent to another, hence equal intervals are not assumed, rendering this an ordinal scale at this level of analysis. Finally, this analysis of *BR*–scores also demonstrates how each scale adjusts for the estimated prevalence of the disorder in the population. Thus, if there is a higher prevalence in the population, an individual would have to earn a much higher raw score to reach the highest *BR*–scores that designate the presence of psychopathology. In contrast, an individual would require a much lower raw score to reach the pathological cut points for a disorder that was rare in the population. As a final note, the clinical syndromes and expressed concerns scales employ a modified *BR*–score interpretive scheme that is more conducive for interpreting these kinds of problems. This will be discussed in the interpretation section subsequently.

Validity Scales   Examining Form 11.2, there are five tables, each of which lists a different group of scales as follows: (a) validity; (b) personality patterns; (c) personality facets; (d) clinical syndromes; and (e) expressed concerns. The first analysis examines whether the data can be trusted in terms of accuracy, while the ensuing two scale types provide the crux of the analysis, that is, personality psychopathology. This section reviews the former.

Table 1 (Form 11.2) consists of four validity scales. Omissions measures the number of items unmarked or improperly double marked. As stated, five or more omissions invalidates the test using a dichotomous scheme; that is, it is either valid or not valid. Hence, the raw score here is determinative. The invalidity scale directly asks examinees if they are responding in a truthful manner. Three scores in the untruthful direction invalidates the test, whereas two such responses render the subsequent data questionable. Again, the raw score determines validity. The inconsistency scale lists pairs of items that present similar content. Each time the respondent answers a pair in a discrepant manner, a point is added. Hence, the higher the score, the more contradictory of examinee has been. Raw scores of 8 or more invalidate the test, 7 renders it questionable, and 0–6 results in a valid outcome. Therefore, the first three validity scales are based upon raw scores even though PR scores are reported. The interpretation scheme for each is listed in specific table notes to facilitate interpretation.

The final validity scale measures the degree to which examinees report their symptoms. Because interpretation is based on a PR metric, the range is 0–99 with a median of 50. The two 10% extremes invalidate the test in antithetical ways. That is, a PR of 0–10 means examinees reported their symptoms at a rate equal to or higher than 0–10% of the norm reference sample, namely, serious underreporting. Assuming individuals have been referred to a mental health professional for some rational reason, reporting symptoms at such an infrequent rate would be unexpected. In contrast, reporting symptoms equal to or greater than 90–99% of the standardization sample would be considered excessive. This interpretation scheme is enumerated in a specific tabular note (Table 1, Form 11.2).

Immediately following the validity scales table are a series of interpretive excerpts that summarize the most common outcomes; namely, valid, questionably valid, and invalid. In the latter case, no further reporting of data is needed. Notice that the language used simply describes the measured response set in the most objective manner; for example, using words such as *sufficient, accurate, maximized* or *minimized* symptoms. Explanatory interpretations are avoided, such as a "cry for help" or achieving "secondary gain" of symptoms. The latter are further from the data, require greater inference, and hence must rely on added clinical information at the discretion of the examiner, who is privy to such evidence. Questionably valid results permit the diagnostic data to be reported and interpreted, although require corroboration from other test data and/or the clinical interview and should not stand by themselves. Assuming the data have been declared either valid or questionably valid, the next step is to report the personality, clinical, and concerns scales.

Diagnostic Scales   Although the personality patterns, personality facets, clinical syndromes, and expressed concerns scales form a hierarchy from most to least important, they can all be classified under the rubric of diagnostic scales because that is indeed their function. The diagnostic data necessarily begins with the personality patterns scales, which are enumerated in Table 2 of Form 11.2. There are four columns going across the tables, including name, *BR*–score, PR, and the measured personality psychopathology. Whereas the *BR*–scores are adjusted for the estimated prominence (i.e., 85–115) and presence (i.e., 75–84) of a disorder, the PR metric represents the ordinal position of the raw score equivalent in the norm reference sample.

The personality facets scales follow in Table 3 (Form 11.2). There are three facet scales for each personality pattern scale, which accounts for their abundance. Their vast number should not be intimidating, as the only personality facets that should be reported are those contributing to highest one to three personality pattern scales. The facet scales use the term *personality* in the title to ensure the reader understands their relevance and to what they pertain. Table 3 contains only three columns because it employs the single metric of a PR, which again ranges from 0 to 99, with a median of 50. This being an ordinal scale, the scores denote *greater or lesser* than type information and not how much more or less.

Table 4 (Form 11.2) begins the clinical syndromes data. These scales utilize the same metrics, as does the personality patterns scales, beginning with the *BR*–score, which adjusts for prevalence and determines interpretation and PR, which is supplementary although much easier to understand for laypeople. Finally, Table 5 (Form 11.2) enumerates the expressed concerns scales. These scales also employ the *BR*–score and PR, although they are unique in the sense that they deal with personal and interpersonal apprehensions that, if present, are likely aggravating factors. Next, the MACI–II interpretive scheme will be examined, which mirrors that of the M–PACI. Hence, Figure 11.1 (e-resources) will once again become relevant to this discussion.

INTERPRETATION

Proceeding under the assumption that validity was established, the interpretive scheme begins with the personality patterns scales enumerated in Table 2 (Form 11.2) and, if needed, the Table 3 personality facets scales. Thereafter, the clinical syndromes and expressed concerns scales are addressed. This section will examine these diagnostic scales in said order.

Personality Findings   These scales are sequenced in the order they are printed on the aforementioned profile report and are also consistent with both the facet scale order in the computer report and Table 3 of Form 11.2. More specifically, Table 3 lists the triad of facet scales that contributed to its personality patterns scale such that they bear the same sequence. For example, the first three facet scales—expressively impassive, temperamentally apathetic, and interpersonally unengaged—all contributed to the first personality patterns scale, introversive (schizoid). Note that the *DSM* analogue label is in parentheses. This provides the conceptual link between the Millon adolescent personality patterns and the *DSM–5* personality disorder. Three Millon adolescent personality patterns do not have *DSM–5* counterparts, although were incorporated in previous *DSM* editions. These include forceful (sadistic), discontented (negativistic or passive-aggressive), and aggrieved (masochistic). Once again, the *DSM* link is in parentheses. A general note informs the reader of the meaning of the parenthetical label in Table 2. Likewise, a second general Table 2 note designates that the previous *DSM* labels would now be diagnosed in *DSM–5* as an *other specified personality disorder* if it was present.

As depicted in Figure 11.1, in the "Personality Patterns" box, the results can either be negative or positive for personality disturbance. If negative, reporting and interpreting the personality facets is unnecessary, and any evidence of clinical disorders is likely to be situationally induced or reactive (e.g., an adjustment disorder or a reactive depression). Using *DSM–5* nosology, this data pattern is most indicative of an adjustment disorder with the measured symptoms (e.g., adjustment disorder with anxiety). If positive, the question is to what degree? The options are personality features, traits, or types, or some combination thereof. These degrees are denoted by appending one, two, and three asterisks, respectively. The interpretative scheme follows the *BR*–score ranges and categories discussed previously and are listed in a specific Table 2 note to facilitate interpretation (see Form 11.2). Thus, it will not be repeated here.

To further facilitate test interpretation, four drafted excerpts immediately follow Table 2. They describe the most commonly encountered outcomes, including a single negative and three positive findings of increasing degrees of severity (i.e., features, traits, types). The negative excerpt takes the position that if there are significant clinical symptoms in the subsequent data, they are most likely externally caused. The features version refers to mild or potential occasional problems that may be addressed by discretionary therapeutic intervention. The clinically significant traits version references the need for additional analysis of facets and likely current dysfunction, along with aggravating concerns or a significant risk thereof. The personality types outcome interprets the presence of an emerging or fully developed personality disorder, with a leaning toward the former considering that the focus is on adolescent psychopathology. However, it should be evident that this version employs more definitive language regarding the presence of personality psychopathology, the need for investigating the pertinent personality facets, and the expected presence of both clinical disorders and expressed concerns. The latter is consistent with the Millon personality theory upon which these scales are based.

The highest one, two, or, at the most, three personality patterns scales determine the principal personality profile and require reporting and interpreting the contributing personality facets for a more detailed personality analysis description (see Figure 11.1, the broken arrow pointing from the "Personality Patterns" box to the "Personality Facets" box). The computer-scored profile report prints both (a) the facet scales for the highest three personality patterns scales (i.e., three facets for each personality pattern, hence nine in total), and (b) all facets listed in order under their personality pattern. Only those facets associated with the most prominent personality patterns from Table 2 need to be reported, while all the remaining facets can be deleted. Furthermore, of those personality facets remaining, only those with a PR of 75–100 need to be interpreted. Therefore, although the personality facets appear to be voluminous, only three to nine would typically be reported, and from this grouping, an even smaller subset would likely exceed a PR of 75 and thus need interpretation. For these reasons, a single narrative excerpt is drafted in a manner that permits the testing psychologist to list the pertinent facets that are present and complicating the symptom picture. Next, the clinical and expressed concerns data are interpreted as being embedded within the personality findings.

Clinical Syndromes and Concerns Findings   Following the Figure 11.1 flowchart (e-resources), the clinical syndromes scales are next interpreted. This would follow either directly from the personality patterns evidence, in the event of negative findings or the presence of a few relatively non-problematic features, or from the personality facets evidence, in the event clinically significant traits or types were discovered. The clinical syndromes data are interpreted according to three versus four categories of BR–score ranges as follows: (a) BR–score 0–74 indicates an absence of a syndrome, (b) BR–score 75–84 indicates the presence of a syndrome, and (c) BR–score 85–115 indicates the prominence of a syndrome. Therefore, clinical syndrome scales falling within the highest category are considered to be present in a major or severe form, whereas those within the 75–84 range are present, although either more mild-to-moderate versions, or subthreshold if proximate to the 75 threshold. The latter also implies the nominal-to-ordinal interpretation process, as was done using the more complex personality psychopathology interpretive scheme. That is, once the category of a scale score has been determined, the ordinal position of the score becomes relevant. For instance, assume depressive affect manifests a BR–score of 105 and an anxious feelings BR–score of 100. Both would constitute prominent clinical disorders, hence severe versions, thus leading to a comorbid diagnosis of *major depressive disorder, severe* as the principal disorder, followed by *generalized anxiety disorder (GAD)*. In contrast, if the anxious feelings BR–score was only 78, then a *major depressive disorder, severe, with anxious distress, moderate* would be more appropriate.

A series of interpretive excerpts also follow Table 3 (Form 11.2). They address the most frequent combinatory outcomes, integrating the possible clinical disorders results with those of the personality data. This can be most easily discerned in Figure 11.1 (e-resources), the "Clinical Syndromes" box, where the clinical findings can be either negative or positive and either consistent or inconsistent with the personality data, comparable to the interpretation scheme used for the M–PACI. Rather than discuss all the potential permutations, suffice it to say that the narrations cover negative, moderate, and severe clinical symptoms and integrate them with various personality findings. The statements assist in guiding the examiner through the interpretive process and deleting the versions that do not match the data pattern.

Finally, for the MACI–II only (see Figure 11.1, the "Expressed Concerns" box), there are supplemental scales that measure unresolved issues with which the adolescent may be struggling, which may represent either cause or effect as regarding the detected personality and clinical problems. Two of the scales address unresolved personal issues and two refer to interpersonal difficulties. In terms of measurement, these scales employ the same BR–score interpretive scheme as used for the clinical syndrome scales. Hence, such issues may be prominent, present, or absent. Again, these are supplemental scales that may or may not be pertinent to the case at hand and can be reported and interpreted at the discretion of the examiner.

SUMMARY

This concludes the second of three Millon inventories that deals with adolescent personality functioning, along with clinical disorders and expressed concerns. Next, the last of the Millon inventories measures adult personality and clinical symptoms in a manner nearly identical to that of the MACI–II, except that expressed concerns scales are not available.

Millon Clinical Multiaxial Inventory, Fourth Edition

Presentation of the adult Millon personality inventory is done in this section. It follows the same organization as the previous tests, including synopsis, norm reference sample, administration, scoring, and interpretation.

SYNOPSIS

The *Millon Clinical Multiaxial Inventory, Fourth Edition* (*MCMI–IV*; Millon, Grossman, & Millon, 2015) is a self-report personality inventory for individuals of 18 years, 0 months to 85 years, 11 months, designed to principally identify the presence of predominant personality patterns, their more specific facets, any secondary co-occurring clinical symptoms or syndromes, and finally, a listing of noteworthy concerns. Therefore, once again, assessment of personality traits and functioning is the central concern of this measure and, secondarily, the manner in which such variables affect and modulate an individual's clinical symptoms and core concerns.

The MCMI–IV supplants its immediate predecessor the *Millon Clinical Multiaxial Inventory, Third Edition* (*MCMI–III*; Millon, 2006b), which now includes the following two essential additions: (a) a *turbulent personality pattern* that actually dates back to early psychoanalytic theorizing (Boudry, 1983; Carlson & Maniacci, 2012; Kraeplin, 1921) and (b) a more refined continuum of measured functioning, including mild, moderate, and severe degrees of psychopathology, each respectively denoted as a feature (or style), clinically significant traits, and type (or disorder). This was seen in the most recently published MACI–II, presented in the previous section, and applied to the M–PACI due to lack of specified interpretive scheme and for consistency across the three Millon personality inventories. Development of the MCMI–IV follows the historical trend of this instrument as remaining accordant with the current major diagnostic system (viz., the *DSM–5*; American Psychiatric Association, 2013) and societal changes (e.g., the new standard for a combined gender–norm reference sample and growing concerns regarding violence potential). As will be elaborated upon subsequently, the continuing close correspondence between the MCMI–IV and the contemporary principal diagnostic system, the *DSM–5*, which in turn has an increasing affinity with the *International Classification of Diseases, Tenth Edition* (*ICD–10*; World Health Organization [WHO], 1992), is this instrument's greatest asset as concerning psychological testing practice. Lastly, the MCMI–IV is theoretically derived, as are the versions for younger examinees, which is a credible asset in its continuing development as it effectively guides test construction. Scrutiny of the theory also renders these Millon personality instruments in accord with the biopsychosocial approach to assessment espoused in this book (see Forms 3.3–3.6).

NORM REFERENCE SAMPLE

The MCMI–IV was normed on a reference sample consisting of 1,547 adults (i.e., aged 18 and older) who were seeking mental health intervention in both the United States and Canada (Millon, Grossman, & Millon, 2015). Exclusionary criteria included the following: (a) not in mental health treatment; (b) the submitted MCMI–IV test was deemed to be invalid; and (c) age was less than 18 years. Hence, as in both the M–PACI and MACI–II, the MCMI–IV is intended for a population of adults who are in mental health treatment; that is, clinical populations. Hence, it is not intended as a measure of normal personality traits. The implication is that all three Millon personality measures should not be administered to nonclinical individuals, as this may result in overestimating an individual's personality disturbance.

The sample was apportioned into three age cohorts due to the more expansive age range of this measure, including 18–25 (22.4%), 26–49 (56.0%), and 50–85 (21.7%). Thus, the middle-range age group consisted of the largest percentage of the standardization sample. Gender was 54.7% female and 45.3% male. In terms of education, 8.1% had 0–12 years without a diploma, 24.6% had a high school diploma or equivalent, 29.9% had some college or associate's degree, and 37.3% had a bachelor's degree or greater. Race/ethnicity was 72.4% White, 11.1% Hispanic, 8.0% Black, 5.4% Other, and 3.2% Asian.

In terms of treatment setting, 90.1% were outpatient and 9.9% inpatient. Region of the country again showed some degree of skewness, including 38.5% from the South, 26.8% from the West, 19.7% from the Midwest, and only 15.0% from the Northeast. Lastly, relationship status consisted of 34.5% never married, 19.3% first marriage, 13.8% divorced, 10.5% remarried, 5.0% separated, 3.1% cohabiting, 2.4% widowed, and 1.5% other. To summarize these figures, it may be concluded that the norm reference sample for the MCMI–IV is skewed toward individuals who are white, with higher degrees of education and nearly two-thirds from the South and West regions of the United States, which should be taken under consideration if the prospective examinee does not fall within these demographics.

ADMINISTRATION

The MCMI–IV consists of 195 *True* or *False* forced-choice items, requires a minimum fifth-grade reading level, and takes an average 30–40 minutes to complete. The examiner is permitted to provide assistance by answering any questions the examinee may have. As for the MACI–II, an audio version is available in cases where the examinee manifests reading comprehension difficulties. The test is explicit in terms of items being symptom or trait focused and is self-administered. Hence, it relies on examinees' motivation to be accurate and honest, and upon their ability to introspect.

As for the previous Millon personality tests, computer administration via the Q-global (Pearson, 2021) web-based platform. As stated, this program permits on-screen computer administration and immediate scoring (see the next section). Prior to the first item, the computer administration guides the examinee through the test instructions, if desired. The administration then proceeds by showing a single item on the screen at a time, with ongoing progress shown on the upper left-hand portion of the screen (e.g., 30/195 indicating item 30 out of a total 195). Lastly, because the examinee is instructed to answer each item, the computer will present a final prompt giving the option to proceed to any items skipped. Further, double-marked items (i.e., both *True* and *False*), which do not provide a scorable response, are not possible during computer administration and therefore are not a concern. This test can also be administered manually by test booklet, although this format is more laborious and vulnerable to human error. Because the remaining aspects of test administration mirror those of the M–PACI and MACI–II, no more comments will be offered here in the interest of brevity.

SCORING

Form 11.3 presents all the tables needed for reporting the MCMI–IV data yield. As stated, computer scoring on the Q-global (Pearson, 2021) platform is immediate and available in two report options that can be printed in hard copy: (a) a profile report that includes all the scale standard scores, an enumeration of noteworthy responses (such as endorsement of suicidal intentions), and a pithy narrative of significant findings;[2] and (b) an interpretive report providing all scores as in the profile report, along with a lengthy and detailed narrative interpretation of personality traits, symptoms, and treatment recommendations based on Millon's biosocial evolutionary theory. The latter requires much greater remuneration and is not required when using the data tables presented in Form 11.3. The remainder of this section is divided into one that delineates the scores available on the MCMI–IV, including categories of score ranges, ensued by an extended discussion of the validity scales, which are greater in number and more complex than in the previous versions for younger populations.

Standard Scores Three types of scores are provided by the MCMI–IV, including (a) raw scores, (b) *BR*–scores, and (c) percentile rank (PR) scores. First, raw scores are pertinent only for validity purposes, as was true in the MACI–II and M–PACI. Therefore, these are discussed first. Next, as in the MACI–II, *BR*–score transformations on the raw scores provided by the norm reference sample were used to adjust for the estimated prevalence rate of each personality construct and clinical disorder in the population; that is, as an alternative to linear *T*–scores that assume each construct forms a normal distribution in the population (cf., uniform *T*–scores discussed subsequently). This was done by having clinicians rate the percentage of each personality disorder and clinical syndrome, both mild and more severe manifestations, in the norm reference sample. These percentages were then used as estimates for base rates in the population of adults and subsequently converted into PRs that were anchored into various *BR*–scores.

More specifically, and consistent with the MACI–II, the percentage of severe cases in the sample was anchored at a *BR*–score of 85, whereas the percentage of more mild versions was anchored at a *BR*–score of 75, with 0 and 115 representing minimum and maximum raw scores for each scale, and the median raw score anchored at a *BR* of 60. For example, if severe narcissistic personality disorder manifested a 5% rate in the sample, as the top 5% it would have a percentile rank of 95 (100–5 = 95). Hence, a raw score on the narcissistic personality scale obtained from the norm reference sample that fell at the 95th percentile, for example, a raw score of 15, would be transformed into a *BR* of 85. Similarly, if more mild narcissistic personality manifested an additional 10% rate in the sample, cumulatively it would have a percentile rank of 85 (100–5–10 = 85). Then, hypothetically, if a raw score of 10 on that scale provided by the norm group fell at a percentile rank of 85, it would be transformed into a *BR* of 75. The remaining raw score to *BR*–score transformations were again accomplished by linear *interpolation*, that is, finding intermediate unknown values based on the more extreme known values. Here, the known raw score to *BR*–score conversions 0, 60, 75, 85, and 115, would be used to estimate the intermediate raw score to *BR*–score transformations. In this manner, the *BR*–scores account for the estimated prevalence rates of each measured MCMI–IV personality pattern and clinical syndrome construct in the population, rather than assuming these disorders form a normal distribution in the population as does the standardized linear *T*–score distribution.

Different *BR* transformation criteria were employed for three scales designed to detect test-taking response tendencies, which are classified as *modifying indices*. These are unique to the MCMI–IV and include disclosure, desirability, and debasement (see the next section). For all three, the *BR*–score range was reduced, ranging from 0 to 100. The disclosure scale *BR*–scores of 35, 75, and 85 represent the raw score percentiles of 15, 75, and 90, respectively. The desirability and debasement scale *BR*–scores of 85, 75, and 35 represent raw score percentiles of 95, 85, and 15, respectively. Again, linear interpolation was done on the intermediate raw scores to transform them into *BR*–score values.[3]

Lastly, PR scores indicate how many individuals in the norm reference sample, and by generalization, how many individuals in the population, the examinee scores equal to or higher than (see Warner, 2021a, 2021b). Although there is some expected redundancy between PR and BR–scores that were anchored at 75 and 85 based on percentages, the majority of PR scores add significant information in terms of ranking. Next, a succinct description of how the facets were developed is offered, which can be generalized to the previous MACI–II. They are discussed here because personality development is considered largely complete in this age group (although far from intractable).

First, items from each personality patterns scales were isolated. Those items that best matched the three domains of the theory for that personality pattern, including existence, adaptation, and replication, were selected to represent facets for that primary scale. That is why there are three facets for each personality pattern. Second, item-to-facet scale assignments were essentially factor analyzed to determine each item's overall fit. Those with the best fit were retained, although this resulted in some scales having very few items, thus causing them to be highly unstable (i.e., unreliable). Therefore, items from other personality patterns scales were similarly factor analyzed to determine which manifested sufficiently high item-to-scale correlations with the objective of stabilizing each of the brief facet scales. This resulted in the 45 personality facet scales listed in Table 4 (Form 11.3). The personality facets in Table 3 of Form 11.2 for the MACI–II were done in similar fashion. As will be seen in the interpretation section, the facet scales are empirically tied to the *BR*–scores anchor points 75 and 85, where the PRs will be at or at least proximate to these quantities. In consequence, if none or very few personality patterns scales do not reach these diagnostic thresholds, there will be concomitantly low PRs among the facets; that is, they will also largely yield PRs lower than 75. Hence, facet PRs lower than 75 possess diminutive diagnostic meaning. This is relevant to how the facet scales are to be interpreted (see subsequently). Next, the scales that measure validity on the MCMI–IV will be delineated.

Validity Scales   The initial consideration regards the following two validity questions, the second being a two-part inquiry: (a) can the MCMI–IV be scored and interpreted, or is the test invalid; (b) are there test-taking response tendencies that require caution in interpretation and/or *BR*-standard score adjustments in the personality patterns and clinical syndromes scales to enhance validity (see Figure 11.1, the "Validity" box; Form 11.3, Tables 1 and 2). These questions will be addressed in the order presented, proceeding from the validity scales (Form 11.3, Table 1) to the modifying indices (Form 11.3, Table 2, leading up to the diagnostic scales consisting of the personality patterns, personality facets, and clinical syndromes scales.

With one exception, the validity scales (Table 1, Form 11.3) address the initial question above using raw scores. First, the MCMI–IV cannot be scored if 14 or more responses are omitted. Therefore, placed in Table 1 is an omissions scale (see Form 11.3), with a specific table note regarding the two pertinent ranges of valid (i.e., 0–13) and invalid (i.e., 14–195) non-responses. Next, the invalidity scale consists of three items that have an extremely high likelihood of not being answered as *True*; for instance, "I was elected president of the United States." A raw score of 0 is valid, 1 questionably valid, and 2–3 invalid. Possible reasons for invalid responding here include poor motivation, reading comprehension problems, and vacillating attention, although the test is essentially failed irrespective of the underlying reason. Third, the inconsistency scale includes 25 two-item pairs that are related by both (a) semantics or word-meaning and (b) statistical correlation. These pairs are presented at various points in the 195-item sequence and prompt examinees to answer similar questions about themselves in a consistent manner. The ranges for valid (i.e., 0–8), questionably valid (i.e., 9–19), and invalid results (i.e., 20–25) are presented in a specific table note for this scale.

Lastly, if none of the personality pattern scales exceed a *BR*–score of 60, the test is invalid. Logically, this response style represents a rather profound denial of even minor personality flaws, especially unexpected considering the person is receiving mental health services. General table notes define the *BR* abbreviation and provide a *BR*–score range, including 60 as the median or average willingness to acknowledge personality problems. From this information, the reader can better comprehend what such consistent low scoring actually means in quantitative terms. The number of such scales equal to or below a *BR*–score of 60 was chosen because (a) it is a raw score and (b) higher numbers indicate invalidity, both of which are consistent with the other validity scales in Table 1.

To facilitate interpretation of this first round of validity results, narrative excerpts have been drafted for the three most common outcomes. These include valid, questionably valid, and invalid and are drafted in similar fashion to that done for the MACI–II and M–PACI. The invalid result concludes that subsequent data are not reported to avoid misleading inferences. Questionably valid results are reported, although they require corroboration, which is stated in this version.

Assuming adequate rapport and rationale for testing has been established, the majority of examinees provide valid scores on this initial table. These validity scales are most effectual in initiating the MCMI–IV interpretation because invalid results immediately and efficiently preclude any further analysis. Next are scales employing *BR*–scores that together (a) examine an individual's test-taking response pattern and (b) assist in determining if adjustments to the final diagnostic *BR*–scores are needed.

The *modifying indices* have been aptly referred to as impression management scales (Grossman & Amendolace, 2017) and, as reflected in the scale labels, include the constructs of disclosure, debasement, and desirability (see Table 2, Form 11.3). More specifically, the disclosure index measures the degree to which the examinee is honest, self-disclosing, and therefore accurate in reporting symptoms, as opposed to being defensive and secretive. The desirability index measures the degree to which the examinee's responses were influenced by an inclination to appear socially attractive, moral, and emotionally stable. It is most akin to denying the presence of personality flaws or dysfunction. Finally, the debasement index is virtually the antithesis of desirability. That is, this index indicates an attempt to appear more symptomatic, abnormal, or psychopathological than is actually the case, although if faced with extreme stress or trauma, high scores here may represent a genuine "cry for help" in which the examinee is desperate for assistance and an alleviation of symptoms. The statistical adjustment here involves a pattern indicating underreporting or overreporting and is principally aided by the disclosure index. Briefly, the other adjustment is determined more by markedly high scores, indicating acute anxiety and depression, although this is aided more by the clinical syndrome data (reviewed later).

Interpretation of the modifying indices is intricate because different score types are used to determine validity and influence interpretation. First, the disclosure index relies on raw scores and forms a continuum from lower (i.e., more underreporting), to moderate (i.e., typical reporting), to higher (i.e., more overreporting) raw scores. Therefore, a column has been created for raw score reporting for this index, including a specific table note that provides the specific ranges for validity results, ranging from invalid to questionably valid to valid, along with the reporting tendency in parentheses (see Table 2, Form 11.3). Further, the overall measured pattern is described in the final column. Second, the desirability and debasement indexes rely on *BR*–scores and, although they do not invalidate the results, they render them questionable when scores fall within the very low and high ranges. Hence, a second score column and an additional specific table note for these *BR*–score ranges have been created. Regarding how the specific ranges were created, it has become apparent that the most logical approach is to use the increasingly high *BR*–score anchors to denote a step-wise ordinal increase in the measured test-taking response pattern, succinct descriptions of which are again conveniently available in the final column of Table 2 (Form 11.3). Recall the earlier discussion that all modifying index *BR*–scores were anchored to raw score PRs as follows (by increasing *BR*–PR sequence): (a) *BR* 0 = PR 0; (b) *BR* 35 = PR 15; (c) *BR* 75 = PR 75 or 80; (d) *BR* 85 = PR 90 or 95; and (e) *BR* 100 = PR 100.[4] These principal *BR* anchors were simply utilized to form ranges with the authors' validity recommendations (i.e., questionably valid when in the high or low extremes, with logically assigned qualitative descriptions in parentheses borrowed from those of the NEPSY–II (Korkman, Kirk, & Kemp, 2007a, 2007b). Why the NEPSY–II language? Rather than using rather trite wording such as low, average, and high, the terms involving expected levels seemed to be more felicitous when describing these approach tendencies. That is, examiners *expect* people to be honest in their approach to the test versus possessing average honesty in completing the test.

General table notes include the *BR* abbreviation being defined, along with the necessary double-dash (--) symbol denoting that the particular score was not reported because it was not relevant to validity interpretation. This is for efficiency and to ensure that the reader is well aware of which type of score is being used in the interpretation. Finally, three narratives have been composed after Table 2 that can be used to move quickly, but meaningfully, through to the most important diagnostic scales. The language used in the various interpretative versions are flexible in that they permit the examiner to remain objective or go further and provide inferences as to what may have contributed to the atypical response set.

Three other factors affect validity, one a dichotomous valid–invalid determination, the other two involving statistical adjustments. Regarding the former, if *BR*–scores on all personality scales fall below 60, save the three deemed by the test as representing severe personality pathology, the MCMI–IV is rendered invalid. How that is denoted in Table 3 will be discussed shortly. Additionally, there exist two types of statistical adjustments that computer scoring automatically invokes in arriving at the final *BR*–scores on the diagnostic scales. First, markedly low or high scores on the disclosure index aides in respective upward or downward adjustments among selected diagnostic scales to increase measurement accuracy of the examinee's current level of functioning. This is aptly termed the *disclosure adjustment*. If such adjustment was needed and done, the language of the second *questionably valid* narrative to Table 2 is to be used. Second, a response pattern that shows the presence of acute anxiety and depression invokes what is termed the *anxiety/major depression adjustment*. Here, *BR*–scores on personality and clinical scales that incorporate an intrapsychic turmoil component are affected and thus adjusted, including avoidant, melancholic, masochistic, schizotypal, and borderline. Next, the discussion moves to an interpretive approach to the MCMI–IV personality and clinical diagnostic scales. Here, it is assumed that the validity results are sufficient for diagnostic score reporting and interpretation.

INTERPRETATION

As for all three Millon inventories, personality affords the contextual framework surrounding the presence of any one or more clinical disorders. This is depicted in Figure 11.1 (see Routledge' e-resources website) in which the first and principal analysis focuses on any degree and mixture of pathology among the personality patterns and facets, ensued by the clinical syndromes data. This interpretive inquiry is accordant with the previously used multiaxial system of diagnosis in which *axis I clinical disorders* represented the acute and time-limited symptoms that typically brought the individual in for mental health assessment and treatment, whereas *axis II personality psychopathology* consisted of insidiously developing and enduring patterns of difficulties, most especially problematic personality trait clusters, that contributed to and rendered the clinical symptoms more recalcitrant. Further, biologically based clinicians, such as contemporary psychiatrists, also tend to conceptualize cases using this dichotomy, here focusing intervention on the clinical disorder(s) while secondarily considering any underlying personality issues of the patient that may hinder progress (e.g., borderline personality). As such, this section begins interpretation with the personality data and then proceeds to the clinical scores (see Figure 11.1, "Personality Patterns" box).

Personality Patterns and Facets Scales   In actuality, there are three types of personality scales on the MCMI–IV, including the personality patterns, severe personality psychopathology, and the facets. The severe personality psychopathology scales include three types that either contain transient though actual psychotic episodes (i.e., borderline), or are as near psychotic as a disorder can become without actually being so disturbed (viz., schizotypal and paranoid). For purposes of test reporting, the distinction between the former two classes is not sufficiently useful to justify cluttering the data table. Therefore, all the main personality data are listed in Table 2 (Form 11.3) under the heading of personality patterns. It is also consistent with the prior two preadolescent and adolescent Millon personality tests.

The table consists of four columns, beginning with the scale names. They are ordered according to the manner in which they are reported in the Q-global profile report so that (a) inputting the scores is easier and less prone to human error and (b) are consistent with the order that their facet scales are reported in both the Q-global profile report and in Table 3 (Form 11.3). Following the name column are the *BR*–scores, PRs, and summary description of the cluster of maladaptive traits that define each personality pattern. Interpretation of the *BR*–score ranges involve four intervals (versus three for the clinical syndromes); that is, interpretation is more refined and discriminating as one would expect considering this represents the principal analysis. Specifically, the *BR*–scores once again reflect a continuum of functioning, ranging from adaptive (lower scores) to increasingly maladaptive (higher scores), although here with the greatest number of anchor points relative to all other MCMI–IV scales. Specifically, these include *BR*–scores of 0 (*PR* = 0), 60 (*PR* = 50 or median), 75 (*PR* = the prevalence of the second to most severe manifestation of the disorder or construct in the norm group), 85 (*PR* = the prevalence of the most severe manifestation of the disorder or construct in the norm group), and 115 (*PR* = 100). Therefore, interpretation proceeds from lowest to highest as follows: (a) *BR*–scores 0–59 is normal (i.e., adaptive functioning); (b) *BR*–scores 60–74 is a *personality style* (i.e., overall adaptive functioning although with some prominent traits that occasionally create problems); (c) *BR*–scores 75–84 is a constellation of clinical significant *personality traits* (i.e., a noticeable cluster of characteristics that are predictably problematic), and (d) *BR*–scores 85–115 is a *personality type* (i.e., a paramount cluster of rigid, inflexible, and pervasive traits that clearly cause dysfunction). The latter justifies a *DSM–5* personality disorder diagnosis utilizing the as yet predominant categorical/prototypical system. These ranges are enumerated within a specific note to Table 3, with increasing asterisks appended to the *BR*–score as it rises to higher levels of psychopathology. This is ensued by a similar note that defines the general meaning of PRs.

While the vast majority of personality patterns are recognized as *DSM–5* personality disorders, four are unique to Millon's theory. They include masochistic, negativistic, sadistic, and turbulent. The latter is the newest addition to the Millon theory and very much resembles a cyclothymic mood disorder, except that it is conceptually a personality construct. In any case, if any of these are listed in the final diagnoses, *other specified personality disorder*, should be listed first with the particular disorder label that was detected in the data appended. A cross ([†]) has been attached to each of these non-*DSM–5* personality patterns to denote that they would require the *other specified* diagnostic version. Also of relevance, any single personality scale will not be scored if five or more of its items are omitted. Therefore, a double-dash (--) symbol is defined in another general table note as denoting a non-scorable scale due to more than five item omissions. In the event that occurs, the examiner merely places this symbol in any personality scale that has no final *BR*–score and PR available.

To facilitate interpretation of Table 2 data, four excerpts have been drafted. The first describes completely negative findings in which none of the scales was elevated, even into the features range. Each of the remaining three narrative interpretations describe the detection of features, traits, and types, respectively. The features version contains language that is largely positive, with advice for discretionary counseling and an ending statement indicating that scrutiny of the relevant personality facets will be done. The latter ends each excerpt so that it is discretionary as to whether the examiner believes such detailed analysis is needed. If not, this statement can be easily deleted. The final two versions address the presence of traits and types, respectively. Time permitting, the pertinent facets should be reported when pathology is measured at these levels.

In general, the analysis of the *BR*–scores mirrors that of the MACI–II and M–PACI in that, first, the category is identified, followed by an ordinal examination to measure the degree manifested within that category. For example, if borderline was a *BR*–score of 100 and histrionic was 89, then depending upon assessment information and other test data, these could be interpreted as a borderline personality disorder with secondary histrionic traits or comorbid borderline and histrionic personality disorders. In contrast, assume the same facts but histrionic is now 78. Here, the former diagnosis would clearly appear to be most accurate. Admittedly, Table 3 (Form 11.3) is of unusual length. This is because there are (a) 15 personality patterns that (b) required a lengthier descriptive summary to facilitate accurate interpretation of personality. Hence, it is advised that only those personality patterns that are being considered in the testing case facts should be reported, along with any unexpected positive findings and thereafter deleting the remaining patterns. Finally, after interpreting the reported patterns, a statement can be made that the remaining personality scales are negative and thus not reported for purposes of test brevity. A final interpretive statement is drafted to that effect just prior to Table 4, personality facets, to which the discussion now turns.

Because the personality patterns provide an extended summary description in the fourth and final column of Table 3, reporting and interpreting the personality facets scales are somewhat less vital. In other words, their omission would not be fatal to the report as Table 3 data are designed to stand on their own. However, the more severe the personality disturbance, whether in the form of greater degrees (e.g., a personality type versus feature), quality (e.g., avoidant personality versus borderline personality), or complexity (e.g., narcissistic personality versus narcissistic personality with mixed borderline traits and histrionic features), the greater the need to report the personality facets that are prime contributors to the examinee's personality organization. In large part, this is due to the fact that few, if any, of the facets will be meaningfully elevated if the personality patterns scales do not reach the *BR*–score anchor points of 75 and 85. However, if there are significant elevations among the personality patterns scales, reporting the more fine-grained facets greatly assists in treatment planning because it informs the treating clinician a more precise profile description of the problematic tendencies. For example, if the diagnosis is borderline personality disorder, the facets would inform the relative severity of unstable moods, sense of identity, and dissociative/psychotic tendencies.

Table 4 (Form 11.3) lists all the personality facets. They are enumerated in the same order as their associated personality patterns scales in Table 3. In Figure 11.1 (e-resources), this analysis is depicted by the broken arrow proceeding from the "Personality Patterns" box to the "Personality Facets" box. Whereas interpretation of the former hinged upon the *BR*–score elevation, the facets rely exclusively on PRs. Anything below a PR of 75 is simply not interpretable. Once a PR reaches 75, the facet is interpreted as a meaningful contributor to its assigned personality pattern scale, with higher PRs indicating more ingrained and problematic facets. Hence, interpretation here, once again, is initially nominal (i.e., below 75 is not applicable, 75 and above is applicable), and secondarily ordinal (i.e., higher PRs mean increasing degrees of such pathology). Only the personality facets that contribute to the highest personality patterns scales are to be reported and interpreted, with the remaining being deleted as irrelevant. Thus, although the personality facets are threefold the quantity of the personality patterns, this should not be a problem because of this interpretive rule.

The "Personality Facets" box in Figure 11.1 (e-resources) illustrates this interpretive scheme. To expedite the interpretive process, a single excerpt is inserted immediately after Table 4 (Form 11.3). This narrative simply informs that the analysis is circumscribed to those facets pertinent to the measured personality psychopathology noted in Table 3, ensued by a listing to be filled in as per test results. Only those facets above a PR of 74 should be listed in order from most to least severe (i.e., successively decreasing PRs to that of 75 and not to go lower). It is therefore implied that the remaining facets measured by the MCMI–IV are negative and not meaningful.

Clinical Scales Analysis of the MCMI–IV clinical syndromes scales will almost invariably be required, whether to resolve diagnostic issues presented in the referral for testing and/or to proceed according to the dictates of Millon's theory. This is especially the case if significant personality disturbance is found because, at minimum, this increases the risk of one or more secondary clinical disorders. Figure 11.1 (e-resources) portrays this requirement by inserting solid arrows extending from either the "Personality Patterns" box or "Personality Facets" box, whichever was last to be reported and interpreted.

Table 5 in Form 11.3 sequences the various clinical syndromes measured by the MCMI–IV according to the order in which they are reported in the Pearson assessments Q-global profile report to facilitate inputting the scores rapidly and without error. Of note, the Q-global profile report classifies the clinical disorders data as "Psychopathology" and further dichotomizes the scales as "Clinical Syndromes" and "Severe Clinical Syndromes." Once again, this distinction is not sufficiently useful to justify incorporating such subgroupings into the table and rendering it more detailed and cumbersome to digest. Rather, it is preferable to simply list the clinical syndromes, labeling them as such, and addressing degree of pathology within the narrative interpretation.

Interpretation of the clinical syndrome scales focuses on the two *BR*–score anchor points 75 and 85, ranging from 0 to 115 into three categorical (i.e., nominal) ranges. Proceeding from lowest to highest, *BR*–scores from 0 to 74 represent normal functioning (i.e., a virtual absence of symptoms). Next, a *BR*–score range from 75 to 84 shows the *presence of a disorder*. The word *present* denotes that there is a statistically significant probability that the specified clinical disorder is befalling the examinee. Lastly, *BR*–scores from 85 to 115 demonstrate the *prominence of a disorder*. Here, the word prominent denotes a stronger or more confident interpretation that the disorder is easily observable and thus conspicuous (i.e., a markedly high likelihood that the disorder has emerged into a clearly definable symptom pattern). These score ranges and the interpretative wording are listed within a specific note to Table 5. The PR standard score is also defined in table notes, although it is clearly auxiliary to the analysis.

Interpretation of the clinical syndromes score profile proceeds in similar fashion to that of the personality patterns data, with the single exception of incorporating only three and not four diagnostic categories. That is, the *BR*–score must (a) first be fitted into one of these three categories (i.e., a nominal measurement scale) then (b) interpreted in terms of degree within that category (i.e., an ordinal measurement scale). Priority is afforded the highest two or three scales, consistent with a profile analysis approach to test interpretation. Therefore, clinical syndromes with *BR*–scores of 85 and above constitute fully developed clinical disorders, those between *BR*–scores of 75 and 84 are either secondary co-occurring clinical disorders or subthreshold symptoms falling short of a formal diagnosis. The latter also may be interpreted as the presence of a *DSM–5 diagnostic specifier* if one is available.

For example, consider the following data pattern: major depression (*BR*–score = 105); and delusional (*BR*–score = 79). One likely interpretation would be a major depressive disorder, severe, with psychotic features +(i.e., delusions). The term "likely" is being used here with intent to emphasize that the final diagnosis must be corroborated by the assessment information (viz., clinical interview historical facts and mental status examination results), along with other test data that measure similar constructs, both of which provide vital contextual information. Of vital importance, however, is to integrate the clinical syndromes findings with that of the personality findings.

The integration of clinical with personality data is depicted in the "Clinical Syndromes" box of Figure 11.1 (e-resources). Scrutiny of this box shows the various broad-based permutations, first addressing negative versus

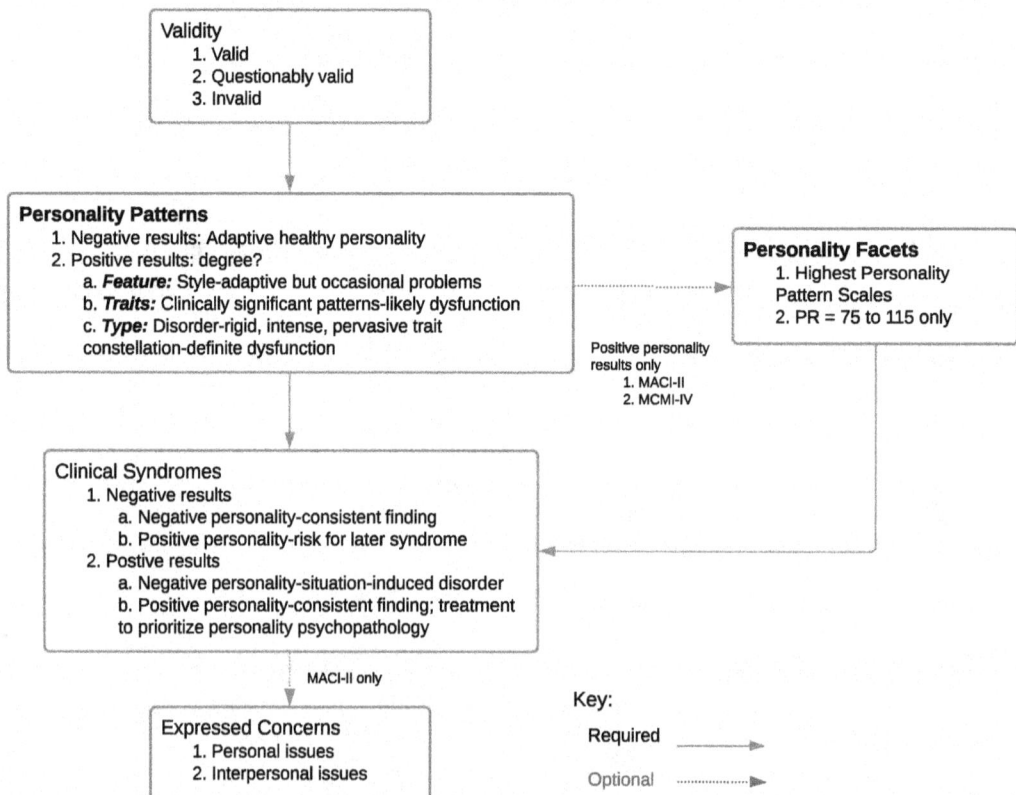

Figure 11.1 Millon Personality Inventories Interpretive Steps

positive clinical findings, followed by assimilating them into the positive or negative personality findings. For instance, if the clinical results showed the presence of depression and all the personality findings are negative, then the most likely diagnosis is an *adjustment disorder with depression*, namely, an environmentally or stress-induced clinical disorder. In contrast, if the clinical findings show the presence of depression in the context of *avoidant personality disorder*, it is likely that a persistent depressive disorder has been triggered by a lack of an adequate social support network due to the personality issues. The former has a much more favorable prognosis because (a) the clinical disorder is likely to be less severe and (b) personality functioning is adaptive and healthy. Again, all these inferences must be supported by the clinical interview information and other relevant data. Space limitations here prevent the examination of more scenarios, although this description delineated the general interpretive strategy.

Lastly, to expedite interpretation of the clinical data, excerpts immediately follow Table 5. They are apportioned according to the various permutations outlined in Figure 11.1, in the "Clinical Syndromes" box. Most generally, they are apportioned according to three potential outcomes, namely, negative findings, moderate positive findings, and severe positive findings. Within each excerpt, there is language that integrates the clinical findings with those of the personality results, namely, consistently positive or negative and inconstant in the form of one being positive and the other negative. The testing psychologist merely selects the excerpt that best fits the clinical and personality results and makes more specific modifications as indicated by the more detailed data pattern. Other narrative interpretations can be created by means of clinical experience.

SUMMARY

This completes description and use of the MCMI–IV in testing practice. It also brings to a conclusion the presentation of the Millon personality inventories, beginning from preadolescence through adulthood. Together, these personality inventories provide the testing psychologist with instruments that are ideal in rendering differential diagnostic determinations between personality disorders and clinical syndromes, along with incorporating personality disorders that are not recognized by the *DSM–5*, although they may be useful in case conceptualization and psychodiagnosis. Another strength of these measures is that they are all founded upon both theory and empiricism. That is, theory has guided the development of these measures, which have been further bolstered by empirical data.

Finally, these instruments are directly applicable to *DSM–5* nosology, which makes diagnostic inferences much easier and more straightforward. Although they are all self-report, they do offer validity scales that attempt to detect response sets that may hinder interpretative accuracy. In fact, the MCMI–IV is the most sophisticated in this sense because it not only detects over- and underreporting, but it also attempts to make statistical adjustments to specified scales to increase measurement accuracy. Finally, it should be emphasized that the interpretation of personality disorder in the forms for reporting the Millon test results (viz., Forms 11.1–11.3) assumes a conservative stance as applied to younger individuals, which is as it should be based on available theory and data on personality development. Next, a specialized Millon inventory is presented, which is designed for prospective patients who are planning to undergo bariatric weight loss surgery and require clearance by means of psychological assessment and testing.

Millon Behavioral Medicine Diagnostic

There has been an escalating obesity epidemic in both adults and children (Wadden, Brownwell, & Foster, 2002). Employing standard medical criteria, nearly 30% of the adult population qualify as candidates for bariatric weight loss surgery (Millon, Antoni, Millon, Minor, & Grossman, 2007). *Bariatric surgery* is actually a term applied to a group of related surgical procedures done for purposes of weight loss. These include a gastric bypass, sleeve gastrectomy, and duodenal switch, each of which works by modifying the anatomy or position of the stomach and small intestines. It is most appropriate for individuals who can be classified as having *obesity*, defined as a body mass index (BMI) of 30 to 39.9, or *morbid obesity* (also known as *Class 3 Obesity*), defined as a BMI of 40 and greater (Centers for Disease Control and Prevention, 2021a, 2021b), and also (a) have comorbid medical conditions that are exacerbated by the aforesaid weight condition and (b) are not responding to behavioral or biomedical drug therapies. Indeed, bariatric surgery has shown overall effectiveness as evidenced by patients manifesting an average of 60% weight loss post-surgery, with associated improvements in obesity-related conditions, including diabetes mellitus, hypertension, and heart disease (Buchwald et al., 2004), along with marked increases in the quality of life (Kral, Sjostrom, & Sullivan, 1992).

This Millon inventory was specifically designed to assist in (a) determining the appropriateness of prospective patients for such procedures in terms of their psychological functioning and (b) developing a treatment plan uniquely designed to match each patient's personality (including both assets and potential barriers to treatment progress). Furthermore, many health insurance companies require a psychological assessment prior to preauthorizing such an invasive (and expensive) medical intervention to ensure individuals' psychological functioning is such that they can follow and maintain the required post-surgical medical regimen and instructions. Although anecdotal, between 12 and 20 such referrals are received by this author annually while working within a community-based mental health center in which no advertising is done for such cases. Hence, it is worth the investment for clinicians practicing psychological testing to have at least a small inventory of this Millon or similar measure on hand for such referrals. This measure is presented next using a similar organization as for the Millon personality inventories.

SYNOPSIS

The *Millon Behavioral Medicine Diagnostic* (*MBMD*; Millon, Antoni, Millon, Minor, & Grossman, 2006) is a 165-item, *True–False*, self-report inventory for individuals aged 18 years, 0 months to 85 years, 11 months, designed to principally assess psychological factors that can potentially influence the course of treatment for medical patients. It is organized into 3 response patterns scales, 6 negative health habits scales, 5 psychiatric indications scales, 11 coping styles scales, 6 stress moderators scales, 5 treatment prognostics scales, and 2 management guides scales. In addition to general medical norms, it provides specialized targeted norms for two patient populations, including (a) those being evaluated for bariatric surgery (*Millon Behavioral Medicine Diagnostic, Bariatric Norms [MBMD, Bariatric]*; Millon et al., 2007) and (b) chronic pain patients (*Millon Behavioral Medicine Diagnostic, Pain Norms [MBMD, Pain]*; Millon, Antoni, Millon, Minor, & Grossman, 2010). As indicated, this presentation focuses on the former because it is used fairly frequently in contemporary mental health testing.

The *Millon Behavioral Health Inventory* (*MBHI*; Millon, Green, & Meagher, 1979) was the immediate predecessor to the MBMD, which was developed from 1974 through 1983 and used frequently over the approximate 20 years of its existence. As its contemporary replacement, the MBMD was essentially designed to (a) bolster its psychometric properties, (b) update and broaden its norms, and (c) modify its items and scale organization to render it more accordant with developments in the related fields of health psychology and behavioral medicine. Due to the unique design of this inventory, a description of the norm reference samples used and test development will be discussed together.

NORM REFERENCE SAMPLES AND TEST DEVELOPMENT

The MBMD was developed in three stages: (a) theoretical-substantive (i.e., the degree to which items are based upon a theoretical framework), (b) internal-structural (i.e., the degree to which item and scale inter-correlations empirically match the aforementioned theoretical framework), and (c) external-structural (i.e., the degree to which MBMD data match conceptually related constructs and standards). The theory guiding MBMD test development is based on the principle that understanding the whole patient, not simply the disease, is vital to medical intervention and outcome. As applied to bariatric populations, the objective is to identify those candidates who will most fully benefit from bariatric weight loss surgery. In fact, the MBMD has been found to be useful in determining (a) if a patient is appropriate for bariatric surgery, (b) the likely reactions of a patient after surgery, and (c) the methods of intervention that will maximize the probability of success (i.e., achieving and maintaining significant weight loss). The MBMD used two standardization samples, one for general medical populations and a specialized sample for bariatric populations. They are discussed next in said order.

General Medical Norms   Regarding the general medical norms, data were collected in two phases. The first phase included 225 general medical patients who responded to an initial set of 299 items developed according to both theory and clinical experience. Of these, 165 were retained in a revised form. These items yielded the greatest degree of internal consistency and most effectively defined each of the scales. Phase 2 consisted of 525 general medical patients who completed the revised form. Thirty patients from both samples were dropped due to incomplete data. Hence, the final norm reference sample for general medical patients was 720.

Demographic characteristics of the final general medical sample are reported based on age, gender, race, marital status, educational level, and major disease groups (Millon et al., 2006, pp. 24–25, Tables 3.1–3.5). Age ranges from one individual in the sample who was younger than 20 years old to 85 years, including the majority falling within the 30–59 range. Regarding race, the majority were White ($n = 439$), followed by Hispanic ($n = 135$), and African American ($n = 114$). Nearly half the sample was married ($n = 354$), followed by single ($n = 164$), and divorced

(n = 107). Concerning education, the majority were high school graduates (n = 273) and those who earned bachelor's degrees (n = 122). Many of these trends were affected by the fact that the bulk of MBMD data were garnered from university medical centers. Lastly, major disease groups represented in the final sample included cancer, cardiovascular disease, diabetes, HIV, neurologic disorders, pain, and other.

Bariatric Surgery Norms　To enhance specificity of the MBMD for bariatric populations, a norm reference bariatric surgery sample was employed (Millon et al., 2007). In particular, an original sample of 798 preoperative bariatric surgery candidates, representing six geographic areas, completed the MBMD from August 2004 through May 2005. However, 87 were excluded due to invalid data, hence resulting in a final sample of 711. Demographic characteristics of the bariatric sample were remarkably similar in terms of both type and proportion to those of the general medical sample (see Millon et al., 2007, pp. 22–23, Tables 2.1–2.5), including age, gender, race, marital status, education, and disease group, with one major exception; namely, about 80% of the bariatric sample were female compared to a more balanced gender proportion in the general medical sample. However, this is consistent with data showing that the vast majority of bariatric patients are indeed female (Santry, Gillen, & Lauderdale, 2005).

ADMINISTRATION

The MBMD consists of 165 forced-choice *True–False* items, requires a minimum fifth-grade reading level, and takes an average 30–40 minutes to complete. Once again, the computer-administered format is most effective and efficient because it directs the examinee through the instructions in a logical and distraction-limited order. Examinees should be informed that assuming an open and honest attitude is best and that it will assist their doctor in understanding their strengths and challenges. The examiner is permitted to provide assistance by answering any questions the examinee may have regarding the items and their wording.

The test is explicit in terms of items being symptom- or trait-focused and is self-administered. Hence, it relies on examinees' motivation to be accurate and honest and on their ability to introspect. As such, the rationale in giving the test should be comprehensible and convincing as being in the examinee's best interests. It is recommended that the test be given most conveniently using the Q-global (Pearson, 2021) web-based platform and selecting the option to administer the test to the examinee online. Such software permits on-screen computer administration and immediate scoring (see the next section).

Prior to the first item, the computer administration guides the examinee through the test instructions if desired. The administration then proceeds by showing a single item on the screen for a mouse-click response, with ongoing progress shown to examinees in the upper left-hand portion (e.g., 30/165 indicating item 30 out of a total 165). Lastly, because the examinee is instructed to answer each item, the computer will present a final prompt giving the option to proceed to any items skipped. Further, double-marked items (i.e., answered both *True* and *False*), which do not result in a scored response, are not possible during computer administration and therefore are not a concern.

SCORING

As stated, computer scoring on the Q-global (Pearson, 2021) digital web-based platform is immediate and available in two report options that can be printed in hard copy: (a) a profile report that includes all the scale standard scores, an enumeration of noteworthy responses (such as endorsement of suicidal intentions), and a pithy narrative of significant findings; and (b) an interpretive report providing all scores as in the profile report, along with a lengthy and detailed narrative interpretation of personality description, symptoms, and treatment recommendations based on Millon's theory (see prior). The latter is more expensive and can be easily and effectively supplanted by the MBMD data tables (Form 11.4), which appropriately requires logical inference and discretion on the part of the examiner in lieu of a listing of nonintegrated interpretive statements that do not consider contextual assessment information. This section is apportioned into subsections discussing the data metrics, the test structure (i.e., the clusters of provided scales), and how to use the validity scales. This will lead to the final section on test interpretation.

Prevalence Scores and Raw Scores　After the examinee completes the inventory, the clinician is presented options as to which norm reference sample to use in transforming the raw scores into standard scores, namely, general medical norms or the bariatric norms (delineated earlier). Here, the bariatric norms should be selected. If no norms are selected, the default general medical norms will be used. The MBMD, bariatric norms present both (a) raw scores and (b) *prevalence scores* (PS). The latter adjust for the estimated frequency of a characteristic in the population as opposed to linear *T*–scores that assume a normal distribution. The rationale for *PS*–scores is that medically related variables often do not form a normal frequency distribution, where a *T*–score of 50 is associated with the 50th percentile, and a *T*–score of 60 associated with the 84th percentile. To make such adjustments, clinicians were asked to rate the percentage of their patients exhibiting a problematic construct on the MBMD. They were then asked to make a differentiation between the percent of patients in whom the characteristic was moderately serious (i.e., *present*) versus clinically serious (i.e., *prominent*). For each MBMD scale, the raw score to *PS*–score transformation table was made in two steps. First, three initial transformations were anchored to as many *PS*–score ranges as follows: (a) 85–115 designated a serious or *prominent* liability; (b) 75–84 represented a moderate or *present* liability; and (c) 34 and lower was considered an asset (i.e., 0–34). This left the score interval of 35–74 to denote an absence of a liability. Hence, let us assume that for depression, 10% was the estimated prevalence of being *prominent* and 20% was the estimated prevalence of being *present*. Thus, the bariatric norm reference raw score that began the threshold of the top 10% scores (i.e., the raw score at the 90th percentile) was assigned a *PS*–score of 85. Similarly, the raw score that was located at the 70th percentile (100%–10%–20% = 70%), was assigned a *PS*–score of 75. The remaining raw to *PS*–score transformations were done by linear interpolation (i.e., estimating intermediate values from known more extreme values). This procedure is essentially identical to the raw score to *BR*–score transformations done for each of the Millon personality inventories, the only difference being the name (i.e., *PS* versus *BR*).

Test Structure: The MBMD Scales   Although *PS*–scores are comparable to the *BR*–scores used in the Millon personality tests, the MBMD test structure and diagnostic scales are remarkably different. This is due to dissimilarities in this test's core constructs and measurement objectives and the fact that a medical population of individuals is being assessed who are likely suffering from obesity and related medical conditions. Considering that this measure also incorporates a self-report format, validity scales are used (Tables 1 and 2, Form 11.4) to assess the extent to which instructions were followed and any response sets that may skew results. These validity scales use raw scores and nominal categories, which will be reviewed in more detail later in this section.

The ensuing scales (see Form 11.4) measure the following: (a) negative health habits that hinder treatment progress if present (Table 3); (b) psychiatric conditions that largely represent common clinical syndromes and symptoms that interfere with treatment, although one is more accurately conceptualized as a personality issue involving mistrust and defensiveness (Table 4); (c) coping styles that can either obstruct or facilitate treatment progress (Table 5); (d) stress moderators that influence the relationship between bariatric surgery and post-surgical progress (Table 6); (e) treatment prognostics that involve variables that influence treatment outcome (Table 7); and (f) management guides that concern factors that affect long-term treatment progress (Table 8). This overview shows the difference in measurement objectives between this behavioral medicine inventory and the Millon personality inventories. All these diagnostic scales yield *PS*–scores and raw scores, with the focus being on the former, as delineated prior. Next, the validity scales are reviewed, which then will lead to the interpretation section.

Validity Scales   Tables 1 and 2 (Form 11.4) address test validity and measure any response sets that may potentially distort the subsequent results. Table 1 is most basic and the logical starting point, as the entire test may be invalidated at this early point. That is, the test is invalidated if (a) there exist more than ten omissions (see Omissions Scale, Form 11.4) and (b) the examinee responds affirmatively to two absurd items (see Validity, Scale V). Providing only one absurd response questions test validity, although it does not preclude interpretation since it may have occurred inadvertently or by simple oversight. Narrative excerpts follow Table 1 and describe the three potential outcomes, namely, valid, questionably valid, and invalid. These have been inserted to expedite interpretation.

The Table 2 (Form 11.4) response patterns scales are more sophisticated in that they are designed to detect atypical approaches to completing the inventory that may distort the results, commonly referred to as *test-taking response sets* (see Chapter 10). These scales primarily determine if statistical score adjustments are needed as opposed to invalidating the entire test. Such patterns may represent an intentional attempt at impression management, usually associated with the testing context (here whether clearance for bariatric surgery will be obtained), or it may result from less than completely conscious internal propensities (e.g., an *acquiescence* response set). Specifically, these scales are scored in terms of nominal–ordinal categories as follows: (a) unlikely problem area, (b) possible problem area, and (c) likely problem area. For disclosure, those who score in the upper 10% using the bariatric norms are likely to be overreporting symptoms. The desirability scale classifies those scoring in the highest 15% of the norm group as attempting to appear well adjusted. Finally, the debasement scale identifies the top 15% scorers using bariatric norms as having an inclination to overreport symptoms and problems.

Thus, all who score in these extreme ranges on one or more of these scales are categorized as manifesting that response set as a likely problem area, which automatically triggers the aforesaid statistical adjustments. If examinees' scores approach these extreme ranges on any of these response patterns scales, they are classified as having a possible problem area. In such case, statistical adjustments are made, although they are slighter in degree. For example, an examinee who is classified as overreporting symptoms as a likely problem area, diagnostic scales such as depression will be adjusted downward in an attempt to reduce *error variance* imposed by the atypical response set. If such was a possible problem area, a smaller adjustment would be made. Because these statistical adjustments are computed by using a variety of intricate algorithms depending on the type and degree of the response set detected, it is much too cumbersome to report exactly which and how the *PS*–scale scores were adjusted. Rather, simply interpreting the examinee's test-taking approach qualitatively and generally indicating that statistical score adjustments were made in an attempt to increase accuracy is more than sufficient. Note that a similar approach was espoused in reporting the MCMI–IV modifying indices scales, which function in like fashion to the MBMD response patterns scales.

INTERPRETATION

On all diagnostic scales, examinee raw scores are transformed into *PS*–scores using gender-specific norms. The first round of MBMD, bariatric norms (hereafter referred to simply as MBMD) diagnostic results measure the presence and degree of certain lifestyle habits that may exacerbate or complicate treatment (Table 3, Form 11.4). Many of these address substance use, including alcohol, drugs, nicotine, and caffeine, although two are related to extremes in daily habits, namely, overeating and a sedentary lifestyle. Results are presented in the same nominal-ordinal measurement scale as the response patterns in Table 2, namely, unlikely, possible, or likely problem area. Therefore, the table is organized as Table 2, consisting of three columns as follows: (a) scale names, (b) result (i.e., nominal category), and (c) a succinct description of the measured habit. A table note defines what constitutes negative health habits to improve comprehension of the results.

Interpreting the data in Table 3 is the immediate next step. There are three excerpts that summarize interpretations for the most common outcomes. They parallel the categorical interpretive scheme. Hence, the first addresses consistently negative results, while the second and third delineate potential and unequivocal problems, respectively. The latter two are designed to list the negative habits that need addressing for maximal treatment response, with the strongest language employed in the third and last excerpt. Finally, the last excerpt includes a statement to also include habits that may be problems in the event there is a mixture of positive results at both the possible and likely levels.

The bona fide clinical scales follow these preliminary habit results and respectively include psychiatric indications, coping styles, stress modulators, treatment prognostics, and management guides. Together, they are variables that possess the greatest and most direct potential impact upon the effectiveness of bariatric weight-loss surgery. Data reported for all such scales include the raw score and *PS*–score, both as defined prior. For purposes of interpretation, the *PS*–scores determine the meaning of the data. The *PS*–scores range from 0 to 115 and are apportioned according to the four intervals consistent with the manner in which they were developed as follows (in order of increasing levels of liability): (a) 0–34 is an *asset*; (b) 35–74 is an *absence* of liability; (c) 75–84 is the *presence* of a liability; and (d) 85–115 is *prominence* of a liability. However, this interpretive scheme becomes cumbersome to employ because it is bipolar in the sense that the lowest *PS*–score interval is a strength, whereas the remaining three intervals are interpreted in the greater liability or weakness direction (viz., absence, presence, and prominence of liability). A brief explanation is in order.

When this scheme is applied to clinical scales that are all in the negative direction, such as all the psychiatric indications in Table 4 (Form 11.4), this makes logical sense. However, when applied to scales that are defined in the positive or mixed direction (i.e., both positive and negative), this scheme no longer is logically consistent. For instance, the coping styles respectful scale is defined in mostly positive terms with a potential liability; that is, the more respectful, the more responsible the patient, although they may also minimize problems. Such a scale would require a reversal of the interpretive scheme in that higher scores would be attributed to greater strengths or a trait with mixed strengths and liabilities. Therefore, it was found that combining the lowest two score intervals (viz. 0–34 and 35–74) into an *absence* of whatever is being measured significantly clarified the interpretive scheme and process. Therefore, the interpretive scheme for all clinical scales is as follows: (a) a *PS*–score of 0–74 means an absence of what is measured; (b) a *PS*–score of 75–84 means a *presence* of what is measured; and (c) a *PS*–score of 85–115 means a *prominence* of what is measured. Note that for all clinical scales, one and two asterisks are appended to *PS*–scores that fall within the latter two intervals, respectively. Within each category, the ordinal value of the score reflects its degree. This is essentially the same interpretive strategy employed with all three Millon personality tests that use the comparable *BR*–score metric.

So, let us begin with the psychiatric indications clinical scales. Table 4 (Form 11.4) consists of five psychiatric symptom clusters, three of which represent indications of a clinical syndrome (i.e., anxiety disorder, depressive disorder, and neurocognitive disorder), and two that suggest personality pathology (i.e., borderline and paranoid). The table contains four columns, including scale name, raw score, *PS*–score, and measured symptoms. The interpretive scheme is listed within a specific table note. Higher scores are negative because they designate an increased likelihood of diagnosable psychopathology, which calls for a recommendation for mental health consultation. That is, these scales are comparable to screening measures for psychopathology and not a definitive diagnosis. Four excerpts immediately follow the table. Each is designed to summarize results of three the most common outcomes, the first describing a completely negative profile wherein there are no measured indications of psychiatric symptoms. The second and third excerpts delineate different levels of indicated psychiatric disorders, including a recommendation for a follow-up mental health consultation. The language dealing with prominent indications is more assertive and unequivocal in its description and advice.

Table 5 regards coping styles, which are measured in terms of their degree of presence. As defined by this test, *coping styles* is a construct that involves cognitive, behavioral, and interpersonal strategies individuals employ to obtain rewards and avoid discomfort in both medical settings and in general (Millon et al., 2007, p. 11). Some coping styles are unequivocally negative. For example, the denigrated scale measures the self-defeating personality in Millon's theory in which individuals unconsciously subvert anything positive because they believe they are inherently undeserving. Clearly, the more prominent this trait, the more likely treatment will be similarly sabotaged. It behooves the testing psychologist to forewarn the medical provider of such proclivities. Other coping styles are either more favorable or somewhat mixed; that is, favorable at moderate levels although more of a liability at the higher end. For example, the confident style is generally positive, although if extremely high one can imagine this individual becoming somewhat arrogant and narcissistic, such as expecting special treatment. Because the interpretation of these coping styles is rather complex, the narrative excerpts list those that are most emergent and render recommendations to adjust the medical regimen to match the particular coping style profile.

There are three narrative interpretations following Table 5 (Form 11.4). The first describes a consistently negative outcome; that is, there are no coping styles that are present or prominent that require modifications in intervention. The next two are drafted so that the measured coping styles are listed with advice to make the needed adjustments. The third and final excerpt that describes prominent coping styles adds a statement to list secondary present coping styles. All coping styles are listed within the excerpts so that the ones not elevated can be simply deleted.

Table 6 (Form 11.4) presents *stress moderators*, which are defined as intrapsychic and *interpersonal* variables that influence the relationship between psychological status (previously measured in Tables 3 and 4) and treatment outcome (i.e., positive or negative; Millon et al., 2007, p. 14). This definition is offered in a general table note. A *moderator variable* influences the strength and direction of a relationship between two variables. Here, the stress moderators can modify the influence of the prior measured psychiatric indications and coping styles magnify their anticipated positive and negative effects on treatment outcome (see Figure 11.2). This is why it is important not to offer any predictions regarding prognosis, at least until all the MBMD data have been interpreted. This is principally due to the fact that a predisposition toward a psychiatric disorder can be mitigated, at least to some degree, by favorable results among the stress moderator scales. In fact, the test structure is organized in a manner in which data integration can be done using the immediately succeeding scales, namely, treatment prognostics. Finally, for these scales only, the lowest PS–score interval was reintroduced as showing evidence of an asset, meaning that if there are measured assets here, they can mitigate the effects of any unfavorable results among the psychiatric indicators and coping styles. This added discrimination is both felicitous and necessary because all these scales are clearly bipolar; that is, extremely low scores are logically interpreted as the antithesis of high scores, the latter of which are unequivocally negative (e.g., a PS–score of 24 on future pessimism means the examinee is actually optimistic, which represents resilience).

The stress moderators scale results are described by four excerpts that interpret as many common potential outcomes as follows: (a) findings of assets, (b) negative findings, (c) positive moderate findings, and (d) positive severe findings. The former interprets each scale in the opposing direction and thus as a strength. For example, social isolation is interpreted as possessing a robust social support network, which is a well-known buffer to stress (Carver & Antoni, 2004; Gonzalez et al., 2004; Gardner & Oswald, 2004; Haslam, Cruwys, Milne, Kan, & Haslam, 2016; Holt-Lunstad et al., 2003; Kroenke et al., 2012; Kulik & Mahler, 1989, 1993; Sutcliffe et al., 1999; Vaillant, 2002). The assets narrative is ensued by two optional statements if there are additional findings that are either negative or in the positive or liability direction. The first simply states that all other data are negative for the presence of stress modifiers. The second states that there are data in the direction of indicating liabilities (i.e., high scores), along with a transition phrase toward reviewing those results. The two positive findings described moderate elevations and severe

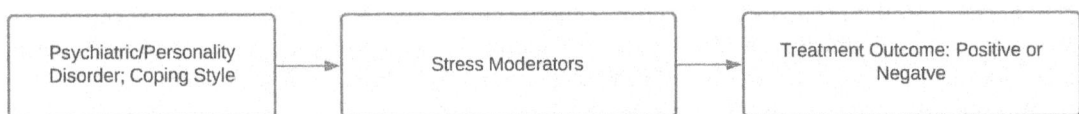

Figure 11.2 Stress Moderators on the Millon Behavioral Medicine Diagnostic (MBMD) Bariatric Norms

elevations. Both incorporate lists of the stress moderators from which the examiner can delete those scales that are not elevated. Additionally, both advise the provision of interventions designed to reduce their presence. Finally, the language used for the severe elevations are more definitive and incorporate statements describing additional moderate elevations that are interacting with the prominent stress moderators. These narrations can be extremely useful, both to guide interpretation and to vastly increase efficiency.

The treatment prognostics scales are listed in Table 7 (Form 11.4). *Treatment prognostics* are behavioral and attitudinal aspects of a patient that can complicate or subvert treatment efficacy (Millon et al., 2007, p. 17). Consistent with the stress moderators, all these scale descriptions are phrased and scored in the liability direction; that is, higher scores are in the scale name's direction, which shows greater liability. In contrast, the lowest score interval does not necessarily indicate an asset, comparable to the psychiatric indicators, but rather designates an absence of any liability that needs to be considered. Scale descriptions implicate the presence of maladaptive or dysfunctional behavioral patterns and attitudes, with higher scores representing a concomitant increase in these proclivities. Therefore, the narrative excerpts that follow Table 7 borrow much of the same interpretive language as used for the psychiatric indications scales. As such, they will not be reviewed in detail here. Suffice it to say that there are three excerpts that describe outcomes that are increasingly in the liability direction, beginning with consistently negative results, moderate positive findings, and severe positive findings. The latter also includes moderate findings at the end of the narrative in the event there are mixed moderate and severe conclusions.

Finally, Table 8 lists two management guides scales that attempt to integrate all the aforementioned findings and render conclusions as to (a) any measurable risks that psychological factors will obstruct treatment outcome and (b) the likelihood that the prospective patient will benefit from psychosocial intervention. The data are interpreted in the direction in which the scales are labeled. There are only two narrative interpretations, one for consistently negative findings and one for positive findings. The latter incorporates both the statistically significant elevations, hence being able to effectively describe mixed-level findings.

SUMMARY

This brings to an end presentation of a series of Millon inventories. The initial three measure constructs of personality patterns consistent with Millon's biosocial learning evolutionary theory, which accounts for a risk for current or future clinical syndromes. Together they cover three developmental periods, generally preadolescence, adolescence, and adulthood from 9 to 85 years. Each of these measures were normed on clinical samples and are therefore most appropriate for use with individuals who are active mental health patients. The fourth Millon inventory was normed upon two samples, the first involving a general medical sample and the second consisting of those who have completed a bariatric surgery weight-loss procedure. This book focused on the latter based on consistent referrals from medical clinics who perform the bariatric surgical procedure and require clearance from a psychological assessment for purposes of preauthorization.

Of note, the same Form 11.4 that is designed to report the Millon bariatric norms data can also be used for general medical patients (Millon et al., 2006). All that needs to be done differently is to select the general medical norms option within the Q-global (Pearson, 2021) platform rather than the bariatric norms because it uses the identical scales, which are interpreted in the same manner only as applied to general medical intervention. There is also a normative sample for chronic pain patients, although there are significantly more differences in the data yield and this author has yet to receive such a referral in mental health testing practice (Millon et al., 2010). This may be due to the fact that preauthorization for chronic pain treatment does not require psychological assessment, or perhaps what testing is done is completed in house. Next, the presentation introduces a personality inventory test series that has the longest history of use and possesses the greatest degree of empirical support compared to all contemporary personality instruments, especially among those that measure psychopathology.

The Minnesota Multiphasic Personality Inventory Tests

The *Minnesota Multiphasic Personality Inventory (MMPI)* series of tests possess the longest history of development and involvement in both research and clinical practice, beginning in 1940 and continuing to the present day. Therefore, prior to presenting the three most contemporary versions of the MMPI in this book's test inventory, the discussion should provide an informative history of their initial design and subsequent evolution. The objective here is to provide a meaningful context as to this instrument's organizational structure and contemporary usage. In pursuit of such objective, the ensuing section continues at the point where the history of personality inventories presented prior ended.

Development of the MMPI

The first edition of the MMPI was created and distributed in 1940. It consisted of eight basic clinical scales developed according to the diagnostic nosological system of the 1930s and originally published across a number of articles (Hathaway & McKinley, 1940, 1942; McKinley & Hathaway, 1940, 1942, 1944). That is, the items comprising these clinical scales were initially written to capture the core symptoms of the recognized major psychological disorders of that era (viz., the neo-Kraepelinian diagnostic system of 1921), including hypochondriasis, depression, hysteria, psychopathic deviate, paranoia, *psychasthenia*,[5] schizophrenia, and hypomania.

Subsequently, the principal approach employed for further test development was a statistical or actuarial method, which was termed *empirical criterion-keying*. This essentially meant that items retained for scale inclusion were those that best discriminated between the targeted clinical or diagnostic groups (i.e., the criterion groups) and those in the nonclinical groups (i.e., the baseline comparison groups). Hence, ongoing test development was based purely on statistical decision-making. For instance, if an apparently innocuous item such as "I like a cup of hot tea in the morning" effectively discriminated between those with and without schizophrenia, that item was retained on the schizophrenia scale. Item content was merely a logical starting point that was thereafter essentially disregarded. This method of assessment is also known as *actuarially based psychodiagnosis* versus clinical judgment. Whether or not the item content made diagnostic or theoretical sense was irrelevant to the decision of whether to retain or eliminate it. This was in contrast to many of the forerunners to the MMPI, which used logic and theory as a primary guide to developing item-scale content. The problem with this approach was that it ultimately led to extremely heterogeneous scales in terms of item content, along with a high degree of item-scale overlap.

The original MMPI standardization sample consisted of 724 non-patient adults who were representative of the Minnesota population in terms of age, sex, and marital status according to the 1930 census. The patient sample included 8 subgroups of 50, each diagnosed with only 1 of the aforementioned 8 major psychopathologies (hence, $N = 400$). A total of 504 items that effectively differentiated between patient and non-patient groups were retained for each particular scale. To help ensure these items could effectively assist in clinical diagnosis, they were cross-validated with a second group of patient and non-patient samples. Only those items that continued to show statistical discrimination between the groups were retained in the final version.

Next, two additional clinical scales were added. The masculinity–femininity scale initially consisted of items that differentiated heterosexual from homosexual males, although this was later expanded with the addition of items from the Terman and Miles I scale (1936) to discriminate traditionally masculine interests from traditionally feminine interests. As such, this scale became more of gender identity measure, with higher scores associated with the individual identifying more strongly with the opposite gender. The final social introversion scale was developed by Drake (1946) and was initially designed to discriminate females who participated in social activities from those who did not. This scale was later generalized to discriminate socially active from socially inactive individuals of both genders.

Hence, the MMPI now contained the 10 basic clinical scales and 566 items, which were later assigned numbers for code-typing purposes (see subsequent) as follows: 1–hypochondriasis (*Hs*); 2–depression (*D*); 3–hysteria (*Hy*); 4–psychopathic deviate (*Pd*); 5–masculinity–femininity (*Mf*); 6–paranoia (*Pa*), 7–psychasthenia (*Pt*); 8–schizophrenia (*Sc*); 9–hypomania (*Ma*); and 0–social introversion (*Si*). Soon thereafter, a number of validity scales were added in an attempt to measure test-taking approaches that might skew or invalidate the MMPI diagnostic scales. These included Cannot Say (?) or number of unscorable items, lie (*L*) or naïve/unsophisticated defensiveness, infrequency (*F*) or symptom exaggeration, and correction (*K*) that measured more sophisticated defensiveness. With the addition of these scales, the MMPI now had 566 items that could be answered either *True* or *False*. Raw scores were transformed into standardized linearly transformed *T*–scores with a mean of 50 and standard deviation of 10. Scores at or above 70 were considered statistically significant and indicative of psychopathology.

As the MMPI was being used as a psychodiagnostic test, it became increasingly apparent that the clinical scales did not accurately classify patients into their designated diagnostic groups as was intended (Hathaway, 1947). For example, patients who scored highest on schizophrenia (viz., Scale 8) were not ultimately diagnosed with schizophrenia. Rather, it was discovered that *patterns* of clinical scale scores, or *codetypes*, were externally correlated with various personality traits, behavioral tendencies, symptoms, and predispositions (Gilberstadt & Duker, 1965; Marks & Seeman, 1963; Marks, Seeman, & Haller, 1974). Therefore, MMPI clinical scale profile interpretation became the dominant approach in using this test. Essentially, the statistically highest clinical scales were identified in a particular case, including various one-point (i.e., single one-scale spikes), two-point, and three-point codetype patterns, which were empirically associated with specific maladaptive personality traits and symptoms using the clinical scale numbers. Using the clinical scale assigned numbers versus the original names was done to avoid diagnostic confusion. Later, content scales were added to the MMPI, which supplemented the aforementioned empirical code type (i.e., correlate type) interpretation with more direct conceptual interpretation (Wiggins, 1966). The most commonly used were the Harris Lingoes subscales, the Wiggins content scales, and some supplementary scales (Butcher, Graham, Williams, & Ben-Porath, 1990). For instance, the latter included the ego strength scale, which measured an individual's likely response to insight-oriented psychotherapy. By the 1980s, the MMPI had become one of the most frequently used tests in measuring psychopathology and personality maladjustment.

The *Minnesota Multiphasic Personality Inventory, Second Edition* (*MMPI–2*; Butcher, Dahlstrom, Graham, Tellegen, & Kaemmer, 1989) was developed to achieve the following objectives: (a) delete or modify antiquated items, (b) develop an updated and more representative norm reference sample, (c) continue the original validity scales and clinical scales (including the continuity of the codetype profile interpretive approach), and (d) develop new scales that would further advance the diagnostic use of the test. Indeed, the MMPI–2 norm reference sample was more diverse than its predecessor and included adjunctive measures of test validity and more content scales that tapped into some specific personality factors. However, there was enough resemblance between the MMPI–2 and MMPI such that valuable continuity in both research and clinical practice was observed. For instance, no more than four items were deleted from any of the original basic clinical scales, and 64 minor item revisions were found to have minimal impact on their psychometric functioning (Ben-Porath & Butcher, 1989). In addition, extensive research showed both the validity of MMPI–2 codetypes and their congruence with the codetypes of the MMPI (Ben-Porath & Tellegen, 1995; Graham, Timbrook, Ben-Porath, & Butcher, 1991).

Ultimately, the MMPI–2 was both vastly improved yet sufficiently comparable to the MMPI to facilitate its continuing popular use. Succinctly, the MMPI–2 introduced the following improvements over the preceding MMPI: (a) a standardization sample more representative of the U.S. population (see subsequent), (b) an improved method for computing standard scores (Tellegen & Ben-Porath, 1992; also see subsequent), (c) added validity scales designed to detect response inconsistency (Tellegen 1982, 1988), (d) an added infrequency validity scale toward the latter portion of the test, (e) new MMPI–2 content scales (Butcher, Graham, Williams, & Ben-Porath, 1990) supplanting the MMPI content scales (Wiggens, 1966), (f) measurement of more narrowly defined constructs by subsets of items on the clinical scales (e.g., bizarre mentation), and (g) measurement of constructs not previously addressed by the clinical scales (e.g., family problems).

Continuing major difficulties associated with the MMPI–2, however, was (a) excessive variability regarding item content within each clinical scale (i.e., intra-scale item variability), (b) a disproportionate sharing of items across the clinical scales (i.e., inter-scale item overlap), and (c) unacceptably high scale intercorrelations. These problems were largely due to Hathaway and McKinley's strategy to distinguish between non-patient and patient samples because the latter consisted of several subgroups of disorders (i.e., heterogeneous patient groups). As such, both convergent and discriminant validities were severely compromised, which precluded effective differential diagnosis. This was because when one or a few scales elevated, so did the remaining scales. Furthermore, even if a single scale elevated, there remained several diagnostic possibilities. For example, a clinical elevation on Scale 9 could be due to acute clinical hypomanic symptoms, including grandiose delusions and circumstantial speech, or characterological sensation-seeking proclivities depending on which specific items were endorsed (see, e.g., Gilberstadt & Duker, 1965). In fact, item overlap could be so extensive that reversion to the various available content scales was necessitated to accurately interpret the meaning the of clinical scale profile.

This brings us to the MMPI restructured forms which, although eliminating the codetype interpretive approach, remedied the ambiguity associated with excessive item-scale overlap by creating more item-independent diagnostic scales. This aspect is essential to effective differential diagnostic practice, which is a chief objective of using standardized psychological testing. Otherwise, testing practice offers no more accurate results than a simple clinical interview. The restructured MMPI test for adolescence will be presented first, followed by the adult version, hence being consistent with the practice of presenting these tests in chronological order. Further, the newest adult third edition will immediately follow the adult restructured version, which is comparable in structure and organization with updated norms.

Minnesota Multiphasic Personality Inventory, Adolescent Edition, Restructured Form

This is the first of two restructured MMPI tests that are part of this book's inventory. As was done for other tests, the presentation begins with a synopsis.

SYNOPSIS

The *Minnesota Multiphasic Personality Inventory, Adolescent Edition, Restructured Form* (*MMPI–A–RF;* Archer, Handel, Ben-Porath, & Tellegen, 2016) is a self-report inventory for individuals age 14 years, 0 months through 18 years, 11 months. It is principally designed to identify the presence of psychopathology in the form of both clinical disorders and maladaptive personality traits. As indicated, this design is a direct outcome of its historical evolution from the original adult MMPI. It contains a total of 241 items that are a subset of the 478 items that comprise the *Minnesota Multiphasic Personality Inventory, Adolescent Edition* (*MMPI–A*; Butcher et al., 1992). Because the MMPI–A–RF has its roots in the MMPI–A, which in turn evolved from the adult editions (reviewed subsequently), a history of the MMPI–A will also be provided for informative context.

However, the MMPI–A–RF is also modeled after the *Minnesota Multiphasic Personality Inventory, Second Edition, Restructured Form* (*MMPI–2–RF;* Ben-Porath, & Tellegen, 2011), with similar objectives, including especially reducing the degree of item overlap among the scales, hence rendering the empirical scales more construct pure. It is worth reiterating that this type of test design is essential for making difficult decisions regarding differential diagnosis, wherein there are varying degrees of symptom overlap among the many mental health and developmental disorders.

The MMPI–A–RF items ($N = 241$) consist of 48 total scales, including the following types and number: (a) validity ($n = 6$); (b) higher-order ($n = 3$); (c) Restructured Clinical ($n = 9$); (d) Specific Problems ($n = 25$); and revised PSY 5 ($n = 5$). As stated previously, because this test is in large respect a second iteration as applied to adolescents, a brief history is needed to provide context. First, development of the immediate predecessor, the MMPI–A, is provided. Second, development of the current MMPI–A–RF is discussed, which is ensued by the typical organization used in this book, namely, administration, scoring, and interpretation. Data tables for presenting this test's results within a psychological assessment report and an interpretative flowchart will accompany this discussion as pedagogical aids.

DEVELOPMENT OF THE MMPI–A

Both the adolescent and adult restructured tests began with the publication of the original MMPI (Hathaway & Mckinley, 1943), which was reviewed prior. Later, in 1967, the most frequently used adolescent norms preceding the MMPI–A were those developed by Marks and Briggs (published in Dahlstrom, Welsh, & Dahlstrom, 1972, pp. 388–399). The norm reference sample consisted of 1,800 individuals ranging in age from about 14 to 17 years and were gender specific; that is, results were reported separately for male and females. Finally, the first adolescent personality codetypes were developed in 1974 (Marks et al., 1974), which were based on 1,250 adolescents in psychotherapeutic treatment. In essence, these adolescents completed the MMPI, and their highest two or three clinical scales (i.e., codetypes) were correlated with their therapists' diagnostic descriptions. This development significantly increased the frequency with which the MMPI was employed with adolescents in both clinical and research contexts, hence providing the impetus for development of such a test whose items and scales were designed specifically for this age group.

The MMPI–A, as immediate predecessor to the MMPI–A–RF, was published in 1992 (Butcher et al., 1992). It was normed on approximately equal numbers of males and females totaling 1,620, ranging in age from 14 years, 0 months to 18 years, 11 months. It comprised 478 items, took approximately 45–60 minutes to complete, and required a minimum sixth-grade reading level. The items were responded to using a forced-choice *True–False* dichotomous format, which has been used for all MMPI tests.

Although the MMPI–A possessed many assets, there were a number of problems that impeded accurate psychodiagnosis. The most problematic was a derivative of the original empirical criterion-keying method used to initially develop this instrument and included excessive item overlap among the scales, therefore resulting in unacceptably high scale intercorrelations. A related additional problem was similarly unacceptably high correlations among the clinical scales and external constructs that were conceptually unrelated; that is, the MMPI–A scales ultimately had poor internal consistency and discriminant validity. As such, differential diagnosis was extremely hindered when using this measure, not to mention the very large item set ($N = 478$). Consequently, as one scale elevated, so would many others in concomitant fashion, not to mention the fact that such elevations were statistically related to a variety of external constructs that were not conceptually consistent. This was the principal impetus for the emergence of the MMPI–A–RF.

DEVELOPMENT OF THE MMPI–A–RF

As stated, the MMPI–A–RF was developed using the MMPI–2–RF as a model. To target the excessive item-scale overlap of the MMPI–A, along with reducing the rather extensive length of the inventory, the following steps were taken: (a) identification of a general demoralization factor (*RCd*) that pervaded all major clinical scales, hence accounting for their excessive intercorrelations; (b) empirically separating out from the broad-based demoralization factor, by means of exploratory actor analyses, the remaining principal distinctive components of the clinical scales; (c) developing diagnostically useful substantive scales (termed Specific Problems, or SP, scales) addressed by the MMPI–A item pool; (d) revising the Personality Psychopathology Five (*PSY-5*) scales that measure key dimensions of personality psychopathology (see Harkness & McNulty, 1994), here using the MMPI–A item pool; and lastly, (e) developing validity scales that measure nonresponsive, overreporting, and underreporting test-taking response sets that can deleteriously affect interpretation.

Developmental Sample The aforementioned MMPI–A–RF development was done using a sample of 15,128 adolescents, including 9,286 males and 5,842 females, with the majority being recruited from outpatient clinics, although also including inpatient, correctional, and academic settings. The age range was from 14 to 18 years inclusive, with an average of 15.61 years. To account for both gender and developmental differences, the sample was further subdivided into smaller groups as follows: (a) males 14–15 years; (b) females 14–15 years; (c) males 16–18 years; and (d) females 16–18 years. General results of the MMPI–A–RF developmental studies is presented next.

MMPI–A–RF Scale Development What follows is a succinct review of the development of the MMPI–A–RF scales. Such a review will provide a greater appreciation and understanding of scale interpretation to be discussed in detail subsequently. The discussion follows the order in which the scales were developed.

First, as expected, results for all four subsamples showed the presence of a broad (i.e., nonspecific) restructured demoralization factor (hereinafter, *RCd*). This general *RCd* factor accounted for the majority of shared variance among the more narrowly defined clinical scales and, hence, their undesired high scale intercorrelations. Once the *RCd* was statistically factored out of the remaining eight restructured clinical scales (meaning the seminal scales excluding 5 and 0 that were added later in MMPI development), the latter essentially became purer measures of their respective clinical constructs (recall that such scales were originally based on the neo-Kraepelinian nosological system). These restructured scales were aptly labeled with an *RC* to differentiate them from the original scales, followed by their assigned number 1–9 (e.g., *RC6* to designate the restructured Scale 6). Again, these excluded the clinical scales 5 and 0, which explains why they total eight restructured scales.

Second, a series of convergent and discriminant correlational analyses were done to ensure items on each of the *RC* scales had the strongest relationship to their assigned scale versus other scales. The SP scales were derived in a similar manner, although the analyses were more efficient because the parallel MMPI–2–RF scales served as starting points in the analyses (see subsequently). When completed, the SP scales possessed items that converged both conceptually and empirically on diagnostically useful problematic themes, both similar to those of the adult MMPI–2–RF discussed later, although also including problems more specific to adolescents.

The MMPI–A–RF validity scales included those measuring inconsistency, overreporting, and underreporting. The *VRIN-r* and *TRIN-r* measure variable and fixed responding, respectively. Essentially, the strongest positively correlated items (viz., *True–True, False–False*) were identified for *VRIN-r*, and the strongest negatively correlated items were targeted for *TRIN-r* (i.e., *True–False, False–True*). Therefore, answering these items in the direction opposite their correlated direction (e.g., True–False for *VRIN-r* and *True–True* for *TRIN-r*) earned a positive score on these scales. An excess of positive scores reflected that particular response set. Lastly, a combined response consistency scale (*CRIN*), which was essentially a composite of the two prior scales, was created as a more general index of response inconsistency. Overreporting was measured by infrequent responses (F-r), and consisted of items in which endorsements were found to be very low, ranging from 20% to 10% depending on the sample used. The *L-r* and *K-r* underreporting scale items were borrowed directly from the MMPI–A, although they were reduced in number based on item content.

Higher-order (*H-O*) scales were derived by conducting principal components analyses (PCAs), including the non-specific *RCd* scale and all eight more narrowly defined RC scales 1–9. However, data was limited to the most impaired inpatient sample due to the very low base rate of psychotic symptoms in adolescent samples. Results showed a three-factor higher-order structure as follows (including the *RC* scales in parentheses with the highest factor loadings): (a) emotional/internalizing dysfunction, or *EID* (*RCd, RC1, RC2*); (b) thought dysfunction, or *THD* (*RC3, RC6, RC8*); and (c) behavioral/externalizing dysfunction, or *BXD* (*RC4, RC9*). Hence, each was defined by a different array of *RC* scales that loaded most strongly on one of these broad factors. This will be pertinent when discussing test interpretation.

Included in the MMPI–A were the Personality Psychopathology Five (*PSY-5*) scales (McNulty, Harkness, Ben-Porath, & Williams, 1997), which were based on the model of personality proposed by Harkness and McNulty (1994). To develop similar scales for the new MMPI–A–RF, McNulty and Harkness chose raters with expertise for their model to review all 241 items in the test for compatibility with each of the *PSY-5* constructs, referred to as *rational item selection*. Only those with 100% interrater agreement were retained for subsequent analysis. An iterative process of internal item-scale and external item-criterion correlations were done, resulting in five non-overlapping scales (*N* = 73 items) each measuring one of the five *PSY-5* constructs as follows: (a) aggressiveness–revised (*AGGR-r*); (b) psychoticism–revised (*PSYC-r*); (c) disconstraint–revised (*DISC-r*); (d) negative emotionality/neuroticism–revised (*NEGE-r*); and (e) introversion/low positive emotionality–revised (*INTR-r*). The derivation of the *PSY-5* scales is expanded upon subsequently as it relates to their interpretation.

As can be seen, the MMPI–A–RF has a rich and informative history. Including a review of this test's origins was deemed vital to fully comprehending its current multidimensional structure, along with its many scales that measure a variety of diagnostically useful constructs. Next, the test's norm reference sample will be briefly described, including its fundamental characteristics (e.g., age, gender), to inform the extent of generalizability of its data yield (i.e., external validity).

NORM REFERENCE DATA

The MMPI–A–RF non-gendered standardization sample is a subset of that used for the MMPI–A (Butcher et al., 1992). It consists of 805 males and 805 females, totaling 1,610. The female subgroup was randomly selected from 815 females included in the MMPI–A to equalize the genders in terms of number. The age range is from 14 years, 0 months to 18 years, 11 months, with sample size per age group as follows: (a) 14 years ($n = 336$); (b) 15 years ($n = 438$); (c) 16 years ($n = 427$); (d) 17 years ($n = 292$); and (e) 18 years ($n = 87$). The overall mean age is 15.56 years ($SD = 1.18$). Grades range from 7 to 12, with a significantly smaller number in the lowest level ($n = 8$). Ethnicities are generally representative of the U.S. population, with the single exception of Hispanics, who are somewhat underrepresented. In addition, parental education tends to favor upper-level managerial and professional positions, which is associated with the modal educational level of parents being college graduates.

ADMINISTRATION

The MMPI–A–RF consists of 241 *True–False* forced-choice items, the majority of which require a fifth- to seventh-grade reading level (Dahlstrom, Archer, Hopkins, Jackson, & Dahlstrom, 1994). Average administration time varies by type of administration as follows: (a) computerized is 20–30 minutes and (b) booklet and answer sheet is 30–45 minutes. Although the test is normed on individuals 14 through 18 years, there is evidence based on the much longer MMPI–A that it is appropriate for younger individuals 13 years of age (Butcher et al., 1992; Ehrenworth & Archer, 1985; Janus, de Groot, & Toepfer, 1998; Oldenburg, 1997). Logically, then, it may be concluded that the shorter MMPI–A–RF would also be equally appropriate for 13-year-olds.

During actual administration, the examiner or assistant is encouraged to supervise the examinee, although such is not required to occur in the same room. Further, the examiner is permitted to provide dictionary definitions of any of the words if asked by the examinee, although without elaboration or "extended discussion" (Archer et al., 2016, p. 63). Computerized administration may be done on the same Q-global (Pearson, 2021) web platform that was done for all the Millon inventories and is advisable for five reasons, including (a) convenience (i.e., reading individual items on a computer screen and entering responses by computer mouse point-and-click versus reading lists of items from a booklet and entering responses via Scantron form), (b) efficiency (i.e., as much as 50% less administration time), (c) accuracy (i.e., automated step-by-step instructions and scoring), (d) optional audio administration, and (e) increased likelihood of test validity (i.e., double *True* and *False* non-scorable responses are precluded).[6] Because computer administration is the preferred modality, this will be described in lieu of manual administration.

Once on Q-global (viz., https://qglobal.pearsonclinical.com/qg/login.seam; Pearson, 2021), the examinee's demographics are entered (viz., name, case number, birth date, gender), "Assign New Assessment" is selected, and a list of all available Pearson tests appears. Once MMPI–A–RF is selected by means of radio button, the "Assign" option activates and should be clicked on. An "Assessment Details" page appears with the examinee name and demographics. There are several entries here that are considered, such as examiner's name, administrative language (i.e., English or Spanish), and, most importantly, "On-Screen Administration." Once selected, the examiner's email will appear, which notifies the examiner that the test has been completed, and a "Launch with Test Session Lock" option is also available. This option is strongly encouraged because this will lock the screen during administration such that examinees are precluded from minimizing the screen and surfing the Internet for their own purposes. The lock screen Pearson software needs only to be downloaded once to the computer, and there is no added fee. When administration is done, the screen can be unlocked by pressing Ctrl + Shift + Q. Once all these selections are made, "Start Assessment" can be clicked on. Before the screen locks, one more "Notice" appears informing test administrators that, for purposes of security, they will be logged out of Q-global (Pearson, 2021) during the administration process. Clicking upon "I Acknowledge" begins the screen-lock mode.

Once in screen-locked mode, the instructions to examinees begin with selecting the preferred language, English or Spanish. Next, a welcome screen appears, which indicates that instructions will begin. The next screen asks examinees to read each statement and decide, using their own opinion, whether it is "true as applied to you or false as applied to you." Thereafter, the instructions elaborate some, asking examinees to consider whether an item is "true" or "mostly true," or "false" or "usually not true," then answering in that direction, along with encouraging a *True* or *False* response to every item. Items appear individually on the screen, with the *True* and *False* options directly below. When completed, the administrator can unlock the screen and choose, "Generate Report," to begin the scoring process.

This section is divided into two sub-parts. The first focuses on the computerized score report, its organization, and the special *T*–score derivations used on the restructured MMPI tests. This is ensued by discussion of the validity scales in terms of how they can be reported and interpreted in determining the accuracy of the diagnostic scales.

MMPI–A–RF Score Reports and UT–scores   Proceeding with computer scoring, once the administration has been completed, "Generate Report" should be clicked on. A selection box with Report: "Please select. . . ." appears. Clicking on the down arrow in that box provides two options: (a) the MMPI–A–RF interpretative report and the (b) MMPI–A–RF score report. The latter provides the data needed for the MMPI–A–RF tables designed for reporting the results within the context of a psychological evaluation report (Form 11.5). The former also provides all the data, although it adds a multitude of automated, computer-generated statements that lack context, can be contradictory, and are not well integrated.

Within pages 2–6 of the MMPI–A–RF score report, the following is provided for each scale: (a) raw score, (b) *T*–score (also graphed), and (c) percent of items answered. Unless a specific norm reference group is selected in terms of gender and setting, the non-gendered entire sample is used to derive the standard scores as described previously. The report apportions the scales on separate pages in the following sequence: (a) validity scales; (b) H-O and RC scales; (c) somatic/cognitive and internalizing scales; (d) externalizing and interpersonal scales; and (e) *PSY-5* scales. On page 7, all scales and their *T*–scores are reported as organized by their assigned substantive domain as follows: (a) somatic/cognitive dysfunction, (b) emotional dysfunction, (c) thought dysfunction, (d) behavioral dysfunction, and (e) interpersonal functioning.

The MMPI–A–RF *T*–score metric has a mean of 50, standard deviation of 10, and range of 20–120. However, these are not linear *T*–scores, but rather *uniform T–scores* (*UT–scores*). The *UT*–score computational procedure was developed by Tellegen and Ben-Porath (1992), with the objective of creating standard scores that possessed the same percentile ranks across all substantive scales. This was deemed necessary because the raw score distributions across MMPI-type scales dating back to the original test are positively skewed to varying degrees, hence rendering *T*–scores across scales to be associated with somewhat different PR values. The *UT*–score procedure worked by first creating a composite of 16 individual raw score distributions of males and females, then essentially finding the average or composite *T*–scores corresponding to PRs 0.5 to 99.5 in increments of 0.5 on 16 selected substantive scales. Thereafter, a multiple regression procedure was used to transform the raw scores into *UT*–scores. Percentile equivalents for selected *UT*–scores are reported in the MMPI–A–RF technical manual (Archer et al., 2016). For example, a *UT*–score of 50 has a PR of 55 (versus 50 for a linear *T*–score), and a *UT*–score of 70 has a PR of 96 (versus 98 for a linear *T*–score).

Therefore, the *UT*–score procedure renders the MMPI–A–RF standard scores across scales consistent according to a positively skewed distribution that is most typical of the MMPI-type scales. Overall, percentile equivalents for *UT*–scores trend somewhat lower than for linear *T*–scores (see Archer et al., 2016, Table 5–8, p. 59). Furthermore, their discrepancies as compared to a standard normal distribution are small, especially toward the extreme values as illustrated in the previous example where there is a PR discrepancy of 5 points located at a *UT*–score of 50, compared to a difference of 2 PRs located at a *UT*–score of 70. All this being considered, Form 11.5 reports the percentile ranks for all diagnostic scales (i.e., Tables 4–9) according to the standard normal distribution because they are reasonably close to the *UT*–score percentile ranks for purposes of test score interpretation. This also provides consistency in interpreting *T*–scores when reporting other measures that employ *T*–scores. Additionally, the standard errors of measurement (*SEM*s) for all the scales are reported in the manual (Archer et al., 2016, pp. 15–17, Tables 3-2 through 3-6). For the normative sample, *SEM*s based on test–retest correlations (versus internal consistency coefficient alpha correlations) were used to make estimates of *T*–score 68% CIs (i.e., ± 1 *SEM*), largely because the temporal stability of abnormal symptoms and traits were deemed to be the most important facet and derivative to utilize. Also, the 68% CI was selected over the 95% CI because the latter resulted in excessively large (hence imprecise) intervals for purposes of ipsative (i.e., intraindividual) comparisons. The testing psychologist merely adds and subtracts the value adjacent to the "±" sign (beneath the brackets) to and from the obtained *T*–score, thus computing the 68% CI rather quickly. It also provides an idea of which scales possess more or fewer errors and can influence which data to highlight in the data analysis. The entered *SEM* value should then be deleted as being redundant information. Of note, the more common "*T*–score" label is entered into the table, in lieu of a less familiar but more technically accurate "*UT*–score," to prevent readers from becoming confused.

The reported range in the score report graphs is from 20 to 120, although this varies somewhat, with some scales having a narrower range, most typically between 30 and 100. Higher scores indicated greater degrees of either (a) aberrant test-taking response tendencies (validity scales) or (b) degrees of psychopathology according to the constructs measured by the diagnostic scales. Lastly, the score report provides a list of critical items that are endorsed in the deviant direction by examinees. Six MMPI–A–RF diagnostic scales were identified as consisting of items that, if endorsed in the keyed or pathological direction, may require immediate attention. These scales include helplessness/hopelessness (*HLP*), anxiety (*ANX*), ideas of persecution (*RC6*), aberrant experiences (*RC8*), substance abuse (*SUB*), and aggression (*AGG*). The list begins with the particular scale name and its standard score, ensued by an enumeration of the items endorsed by the examinee. Immediately after each item, the examinee's actual answer appears (viz., *True* or *False*), along with the percent of the normative sample that also answered that item in the keyed direction (i.e., the base rate). For example, an item, "I do not like myself," may appear with (True, 13.3%). This means the examinee endorsed that item in the keyed direction (i.e., *True*) and only 13.3% of the population of same-aged peers (i.e., as indicated by the norm reference sample) endorsed such an item.

Validity Scales   Consistent with generally accepted approaches in interpreting self-report inventories, presentation of the validity scales is done prior to scrutinizing the diagnostic scales. There are three classes of validity scales on the MMPI–A–RF, including non-responding (four scales), underreporting (two scales), and overreporting (one scale); hence, seven in total. Figure 11.3 is available for download on Routledge's e-resources website. It was designed as an interpretive flowchart for MMPI–A–RF interpretation using Form 11.5, which provides a method of reporting the data yield from this measure within a formal psychological assessment report. Test reporting is invariably initiated by interpreting the validity scales, as depicted in Figure 11.3 (see box "Validity Scales," located at the top of the flowchart; see e-resources). In Form 11.5, these data are reported in three different tables in the aforesaid order because (a) some rely on different metrics (i.e., raw versus *T*–scores), and especially because (b) each set has different interpretive score ranges. It is important to realize that the validity scales in Form 11.5 are ordered in the sequence in which they are to be interpreted, both within and between scales, as follows: (a) non-responding in the form of omissions, fixed responding, variable responding, and combined inconsistent responding (Table 1); (b) underreporting in the form of naïve denial or a sophisticated desire to appear well-adjusted (Table 2); and (c) overreporting (Table 3). For instance, if there are excessive item omissions at the beginning of Table 1, investigating fixed or variable responding is moot because the test at that point is immediately deemed to be invalid. Similarly, if there are either excessive item omissions or fixed responding sufficient to invalidate the profile in Table 1 data, examining additional underreporting and overreporting response sets in Tables 2 and 3 again becomes moot, and thus virtually unnecessary. In essence, excessive nonresponding invalidates all subsequent validity and substantive scales, which explains why they are interpreted first.

As indicated, Table 1 (Form 11.5) addresses non-responding. The *CNS(?)-r* Cannot Say scale relies on a raw score metric, hence notice the specific notes identifying (a) the special raw score metric and (b) the interpretative ranges of valid, qualified valid, and invalid. The qualified invalid refers to a less than 90% rule, which states that any scale with more than 10% omissions is possibly invalid. For each scale, the Q-global score report prints the

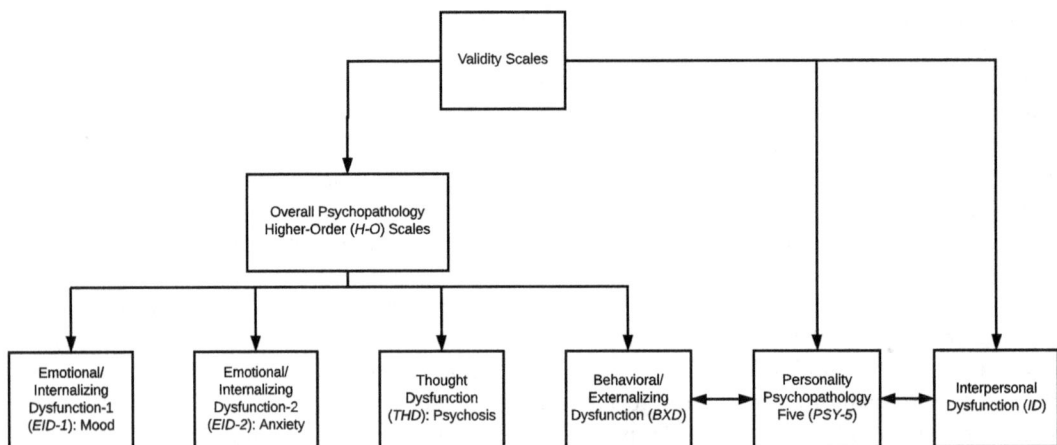

Figure 11.3 Minnesota Multiphasic Personality Inventory, Adolescent Edition, Restructured Form (MMPI-A-RF) Interpretive

raw score, *T*–score, and percent of the items answered. In this manner, the less than 90% rule for each scale can be easily examined. In addition, the MMPI–A–RF manual reports the number of items per scale (e.g., see Archer et al., 2016, Appendix B, pp. 157–169). Note that scales with fewer than five items are especially short. Those notably brief diagnostic scales used in score reporting and interpretation include the following: (a) obsession/compulsions (*OCS*); (b) anxiety (*AXY*); (c) behavior-restricting fears (*BRF*); (d) specific fears (*SPF*); (e) negative school attitudes (*NSA*); and (f) substance abuse (*SUB*). Therefore, should this validity indicator be elevated, these brief diagnostic scales should be especially scrutinized to determine if they have been deleteriously affected by item omissions.

The remaining scales measure various types of non-responding, including responding consistently *True–True* simply to agree with the items, or *False–False* simply to disagree with the items (viz., *TRIN-r*), or answering inconsistently as *True–False* or *False–True*, when the same response, *True–True* or *False–False*, would have shown consistency (viz., *VRIN-r*), or an aggregate measure of inconsistency (viz., *TRIN-r + VRIN-r = CRIN*). Because the *TRIN-r* score is computed in part by subtracting *False–False* pairs from *True–True* pairs, the directional pattern can be revealed. Therefore, for this scale only, a *T*–score with an adjacent "T" (e.g., 80T) or an adjacent "F" (e.g., 75F) indicates (a) the degree of fixed responding (i.e., the absolute *T*–score), and (b) the direction of such responding (i.e., the adjacent letter). Note that the score metric and complete scale names appear in the general table notes, along with the interpretive score ranges to facilitate interpretation for both the testing psychologist and subsequent reader of the report. In addition, three narrative excerpts follow the table: (a) valid interpretation, (b) cautiously valid interpretation, and (c) invalid interpretation with an advisement to terminate test interpretation at that point.

Next, Table 2 (Form 11.5) measures under-responding, also known as defensiveness or minimizing. The first represents a rather unsophisticated denial of any shortcomings (viz., *L-r*) while the second reflects a more sophisticated presentation of more than adequate adjustment (viz., *K-r*). Table notes identify the metric, the general meaning of high scores, scale names, and interpretive ranges. Narrative excerpts are composed for valid, cautiously valid, and invalid outcomes. The cautiously valid interpretation incorporates both mild and moderate elevations, as they are sufficiently proximate in degree such that adding a few adjectives to the excerpt can adjust for the discrepancy.

Lastly, Table 3 (Form 11.5) possesses only one scale for symptom overreporting or exaggeration. It was tempting to include this scale in the underreporting table, hence providing greater brevity. However, the interpretative ranges are quite different, not to mention the paradoxical language that would have to be input into the narrative excerpt. Regarding interpretation, a crucial difference with this overreporting scale is that a moderate elevation (i.e., *T*–score = 80–89) can indicate either moderate exaggeration or genuinely severe psychopathology, a dilemma that requires external test data and clinical judgment for proper resolution, a quandary of interpretation that reaches as far back as the original MMPI (Hathaway & Mckinley, 1943). This difference in meaning, along with the varying interpretative ranges, argued for a separate overreporting table with its own similar narrative excerpts despite the lengthier design.

If the interpretation has not yet been terminated due to one of the invalid outcomes, the validity data should then be integrated prior to initiating interpretation of the diagnostic scales. The objective here is to explicate the general approach to test interpretation that is to be followed throughout the succeeding diagnostic data. Therefore, the percentage of scored responses on each scale will be considered in the case of non-responding, and scale elevations will be interpreted as over- or underestimates of genuine psychopathology depending on the directional response set of the examinee, especially as applied to those elevations that are significantly elevated. Here, referring to the higher or lower ends of the reported CIs can be of immense assistance since the interpretation can swing toward the higher or lower ends of such intervals, therefore providing some quantitative estimates of examinees' true scores versus offering vague qualitative statements that scores are over- or underestimates of actual psychopathology. Essentially, score interpretation is being adjusted according to the measured response set of the examinee, analogous to what is done statistically in the Millon tests.

For example, if an individual's *T*–score on hypomanic activation (*RC9*) is 76, a moderately significant elevation, and the 68% CI is ±6 (*SEM* = 6), then the interval would be 70–82. In the case of moderate defensiveness, the qualified interpretation would be that the true score most likely falls toward the higher end of this interval to adjust for such defensiveness, somewhere toward 82, thus a markedly (versus moderately) significant elevation. In the case of exaggeration, the qualified interpretation would be toward the lower end of such an interval, hence somewhere near 70, and a more probable moderately significant elevation. In any case, the prevailing interpretive strategy should be clearly specified at this juncture and adhered to consistently throughout the remainder of test reporting and interpretation. Next, interpretation of the MMPI–A–RF substantive scales (i.e., diagnostic scales) is done, with references to both Figure 11.3 (see e-resources) and Form 11.5.

INTERPRETATION

The MMPI–A–RF diagnostic scales are presented in Form 11.5, Tables 4–10. They follow a pattern proceeding from the validity scales to the diagnostic-related scales, which is depicted in Figure 11.3 (e-resources). The interpretation procedure follows a logical sequence, proceeding from the three broad-based *H-O* scales, *EID* (i.e., emotion, feeling, affect), *THD* (i.e., thought process and content), and *BXD* (i.e., externalizing behavioral problems), to tables that show specific manifestations of each of the three aforesaid general types of dysfunction. The *EID* scale is apportioned into two subsets of emotion, the first showing specific symptoms or indicators of depression, including the related mood construct of hypomanic symptoms or mood cycling, and the second showing specific indicators of anxiety, including the related constructs of obsessive-compulsive symptoms (OCD), stress, trauma, and multiple fears and phobias.

In the penultimate Table 9 (Form 11.5), the *Personality Psychopathology Five (PSY-5) scales* are reported together as they were originally derived for the MMPI–2 (Butcher et al., 2001). A brief history of their development is instructive here because it informs proper interpretation. These personality constructs originated from the work of Harkness (1992), who was conducting research on using dimensional models to diagnose personality disorders using criteria listed in the *Diagnostic and Statistical Manual of Mental Disorders, Third Edition, Revised* (DSM–III–R; American Psychiatric Association, 1987). These were unique in the fact that they were derived from two non-mutually exclusive broad-based models of personality, the *clinical perspective*, which employed categorical markers to detect pathological personality, and the *normal perspective*, which utilized a dimensional model of measurement (Ben-Porath, 1994). Thus, the *PSY-5* scales began on the assumption that these two general models of personality could be effectively integrated in efforts to measure and detect personality disorders. While still in their incipient stage of development, they were refined as measures of a model of personality proposed by Harkness and McNulty (1994), at which time they assumed the felicitous title the *Personality Psychopathology Five*. More specifically, using a rational selection process, these researchers identified 5 constructs among a set of 60 descriptors representing both normal and abnormal aspects of human behavior as follows: (a) aggressiveness (*AGG*), (b) psychoticism (*PSY*), (c) constraint (*CON*), (d) negative emotionality or neuroticism (*NEN*), and (e) positive emotionality or extroversion (*PEE*).

These constructs were defined as follows. First, the *AGG* construct addressed offensive types of aggression, domination, intimidation, and the controlling of others. Second, the PSY construct regarded the cognitive ability of the individual to perceive the world in an accurate manner. Third, the *CON* construct consisted of rule-breaking and criminal conduct. Finally, the *NEN* construct assessed a general disposition to experience negative emotion, while the *PEE* measured the general disposition to experience positive emotion and enjoyment.

In 1995, Harkness, McNulty, and Ben-Porath, along with other personality researchers, compared these five personality constructs to several five-factor models of personality then in development. For example, Trull, Useda, Costa, and McCrae (1995) equated the *PSY-5* scales with the NEO Personality Inventory (Costa & McCrae, 1985; discussed subsequently), a personality test that measured the five-factor model (i.e., FFM or Big Five). Although this research concluded that the PSY-5 scales overlapped but were not identical to the FFM, they received sufficient empirical support to justify their incorporation into the MMPI–2 as described *in* the revised manual to that version of the test (see Butcher et al., 2001). In the process of integrating the *PSY-5* scales for use in the MMPI–2, two of its dimensions were reversed as follows: (a) constraint (*CON*) was transformed into disconstraint (*DISC*); and (b) positive emotionality or extroversion (*PEE*) was transformed into introversion or low positive emotions (*INTRO*). The purpose was to label and measure all the *PSY-5* scales in the abnormal or psychopathological direction, which is logical considering that they were being used to measure the presence of personality disorders (not to mention providing a more refined and tasteful acronym for the *PEE* scale). Subsequent research demonstrated that they represented useful dimensional indicators of personality psychopathology.

Thereafter, they were revised by Harkness and McNulty (2007) for use in the adult MMPI–2–RF (Tellegen & Ben-Porath, 2011; discussed subsequently). Incorporating the *PSY-5* scales for use with adolescents was first done by for the MMPI–A by Butcher, Dahlstrom, Graham, Tellegen, and Kraemer (2001, Appendix B.9). Finally, they were developed for the MMPI–A–RF with an "r" appended to the acronym so as to identify them with the restructured version of the test (Archer et al., 2016). The manner in which the *PSY-5* scales were most recently developed for both restructured MMPI tests are believed to be comparable (see Archer at al., 2016), although with the caveat that personality disorders as applied to adolescents are more prone to variations with ongoing development (see *DSM–5* and the M–PACI/MACI discussions).

To conclude this review of the *PSY-5* scales, it will be examined how they are designed to measure major issues mental health clinicians frequently confront when conducting psychological assessments on clients. These issues are as follows: (a) degree of aggressiveness and danger to others (*AGGR-r*), (b) degree of reality testing and any presence of a psychotic process (*PSYC-r*), (c) degree of impulsiveness and risk-taking or sensation-seeking (*DISC-r*), (d) degree of subjective distress and negative affect (*NEGE-r*), and (e) degree of anhedonia or lack of positive feeling or pleasure (*INTR-r*). The last two are distinct in that an individual can feel depressed although still possess the capacity to experience positive emotions. This review was provided as a rationale as to why they are reported together in Table 9 (Form 11.5), rather than as part of the broad-based O-H scales. Reporting them together as a single cluster serves three objectives. First, they are used as measuring personality psychopathology as originally intended; that is, as maladaptive traits and dispositions. Second, they assist in addressing the aforementioned assessment issues mental health clinicians commonly confront. Third, reporting them once within a single grouping avoids unnecessary redundancy among the scales contributing to the O-H scales. As will be discussed when presenting the adult versions of the restructured MMPI tests, eliminating item overlap among the MMPI clinical scales was remarkably yet not completely successful. Therefore, reducing redundancy among the scales where possible is still logically supported.

The final Table 10 contains scales that address some aspect of the respondent's functioning in relationships (viz., interpersonal dysfunction, or *ID*). The content of the constructs measured by these scales is conceptually associated with those of Tables 8 and 9. Hence, Figure 11.3 (e-resources) lists these data in proximity to the *PSY-5* scales, with options to interpret them in conjunction with either or both of these personality psychopathology data and, further, the externalizing behavioral data (*BXD*). This same interpretive strategy will be observed again when the MMPI–2–RF is reviewed, although the *PSY-5* and *ID* data are integrated into one table for the MMPI–3 for reasons that will be explicated.

The overall organization of Tables 5–10 (Form 11.5) of the diagnostic scales is consistent with (a) their contributions to their respective O-H scales in Table 4; (b) detecting the presence of *DSM–5* diagnoses (both clinical and personality disorders); and (c) answering many frequent differential diagnostic questions, such as unipolar versus bipolar psychopathology (with or without psychotic features), mood disorder with psychotic features versus schizoaffective disorder, conduct (i.e., behavior) disorder versus psychiatric disturbance, and clinical syndrome versus emergent or present personality psychopathology (see also Figure 11.3; e-resources). There is also no redundancy among the scales; that is, each scale appears only once among the diagnostic data.

That said, the MMPI–A–RF Q-global score report is organized somewhat differently according to the following sequence: (a) validity scales; (b) *H-O* scales; (c) *RC* scales; (d) Specific Problems (SP) scales (further subdivided into somatic/cognitive, internalizing, externalizing, and interpersonal scales), and (e) *PSY-5* scales. However, the two organizations are sufficiently similar such that inputting the data is a feasible task. To enhance the ease of transferring data from the computer score reports to the data tables in Form 11.5, where possible the scales are listed in a similar order, especially the validity scales, *H-O* scales, and *PSY-5* scales.

Once the overall validity and interpretive strategy of the test has been determined (discussed previously), proceeding to the diagnostic scales can occur depending on the diagnostic issues in the case. If the diagnostic issues include only clinical disorders, or both clinical disorders and (emerging) personality disorders, then the arrow proceeding from the left side of the "Validity Scales" box in Figure 11.3 to the "Higher Order (*H-O*) Scales" box should be followed. Here, interpretation is initiated with the broad *H-O* scales, analogous to hierarchical IQ test interpretation moving from general to specific (see Chapter 7). These scales, along with the focus of testing (e.g., rule out a formal thought disorder), should determine the particular interpretative approach. The question for Table 4 is "What symptom cluster, if any, is predominant in the profile, emotion, thought, or behavior?" The absolute *T*–score elevations, along with their relative differences, are both key. Do any of the scales reach or exceed marginally significant (especially in underreporting cases), moderately significant, or markedly significant thresholds? If so, what are the relative or ipsative differences in terms of CI overlap?

The more specific diagnostic scales that immediately follow, including the *RC*, SP, *PSY-5* and *ID* scales, are organized into a sequence of tables according to which of the three *H-O* scales they belong or contribute; in the language of the MMPI–A–RF manual, each of the *H-O* scales' "specific manifestations" (see Figure 11.3, Flowchart of "Higher Order (*H-O*) Scales" box and its division into tables according to their specific manifestations). The objective here is to eliminate scales that do not need to be reported, either because they are irrelevant to the diagnostic issues in the case and/or their assigned *H-O* scale is within normal limits. The reason is that a large amount of data is being reported for each scale, including its *T*–score, the meaning the of the *T*–score elevation denoted by asterisks, CI, and PR according to the standard normal distribution. This is more information than is typically reported for MMPI data, which most frequently includes only the scale *T*–scores in quantitative and graphic profile format. The strategy here is to report only the most pertinent data but do so in a comprehensive manner such that normative and ipsative comparisons can be made in more precise terms (e.g., CI overlap, PRs).

To further facilitate the interpretive process, excerpts have been drafted immediately following Table 4 (Form 11.5). The first excerpt describes what has historically been referred to as a *within-normal-limits* (*WNL*) profile, namely, all *H-O* scales are negative in terms of showing psychopathology. In such instances, no further score reporting or interpretation is necessary, unless there are isolated statistical elevations among the specific manifestations that are vital to the case at hand. This is ensued by an excerpt devoted to each *H-O* scale, analogous to IQ test interpretative language for the full scale IQ and index scores. Next, there is an excerpt for addressing ipsative comparisons among the *H-O* scales and a description of the follow-up interpretative strategy concerning any relevant specific manifestations. If there is a distinct profile pattern among the three *H-O* scales, then the highest elevation determines the set of particular clinical scales that should be prioritized. For instance, if the emotional/internalizing dysfunction (*EID*) is significantly elevated and represents the highest relative score, then Tables 5 (i.e., depression/hypomanic) and 6 (i.e., anxiety, OCD, stress, trauma) in Form 11.5 should be interpreted first. Analogously, should the highest statistically significant elevation appear on either thought dysfunction (*THD*) or behavioral/externalizing dysfunction (*BXD*), then prioritizing Table 7 (i.e., psychosis) or Table 8 (i.e., acting out) specific manifestations would be indicated. That being said, the principal diagnostic issues of the case should always take precedence. Therefore, if psychosis is the primary issue, these scales should be reported irrespective of the *THD H-O* scale elevation.

Now, note the bottom row of five boxes in Figure 11.3 (e-resources). The first two illustrate that the *EID H-O* scale specific manifestations have been dichotomized into those most relating more to mood (*EID-1*; see also Table 5, Form 11.5), including both depression and hypomanic symptoms, versus those relating more to anxiety, including OCD, stress, and trauma (*EID-2*; see also Table 6, Form 11.5). All of the latter were previously listed under the more general cluster of anxiety disorders in the DSM–IV–TR (see American Psychiatric Association, 2000). Therefore, in addition to all of them contributing to the *EID H-O* scale, they seemed to be sufficiently related conceptual constructs so as to integrate them into one table independent from mood disorders for purposes of differential psychodiagnosis.

In Figure 11.3 (e-resources), the next box to the right is "Thought Dysfunction (*THD*)," which has only two specific manifestations related to psychotic-type symptoms (see also Table 7, Form 11.5). The term "psychotic" and its derivatives are somewhat vague, and it was nearly eliminated from the *DSM* nosology, as was the fate of the term "neurosis." Hence, it should be defined here for clarification. By *psychotic*, as used in this chapter discussing explicit personality tests, it is meant that such symptoms are (a) profoundly severe, (b) involve a breakdown in reality testing or disconnection from consensual reality (also known as a *formal thought disorder*), and (c) require intensive intervention (likely including psychiatric hospitalization). The term psychotic will be addressed further when discussing implicit personality tests in the ensuing chapter.

The adjacent "Behavioral/Externalizing Dysfunction (*BXD*)" box in Figure 11.3 (e-resources) addresses the under-controlled specific manifestations that all involve some type of acting-out defenses (i.e., conduct-disordered behavior), including severe anger management problems, antisocial or major rule-breaking behavior, oppositional and defiant behavior, and substance misuse (see also Table 8, Form 11.5). Such symptoms can also be conceptualized as an emerging personality disorder with impulsive, acting-out, antisocial traits, which may be further supported among the *PSY-5* cluster in Table 9.

Subsequently, the *PSY-5* scales are reported in a table termed Personality Psychopathology Five. As discussed, these scales are interpreted consistent with their original intent as enduring maladaptive traits suggestive of an emerging or present personality disorder. For example, significant elevations on *AGGR-r* and *DISC-r* strongly suggest an emerging antisocial personality. In addition, elevations on *NEGE-r* and *INTR-r* are indicative of a borderline personality disorder. Regarding the latter, a supplemental elevation on *PSYC-r* would designate an especially disturbed borderline case that includes potential psychotic or severe dissociative episodes. Consistent with the Millon tests, these personality constructs are backed by both theory and research, the principal difference here being that personality is not assumed to supersede the presence of clinical disorders. It should be emphasized, however, that these diagnostic tables can be used in a flexible manner. For instance, the *H-O* table can be omitted, and interpretation can focus on a particular cluster of related scales based solely on the diagnostic issues in a case (e.g., testing for psychosis). Additionally, analysis can proceed immediately from the validity scales to the *PSY-5* scales, which is portrayed in Figure 11.3 by the arrow extending from the right side of the validity scales box to the "PSY-5: Personality Psychopathology" box. The double arrows between the *PSY-5* and *BXD* boxes illustrate that *PSY-5* scale interpretation can be prioritized over the clinical disorders data as done in the Millon tests.

Lastly, Form 11.5 ends with the interpersonal dysfunction (*ID*) Table 10. These scales all measure various aspects of relationship functioning (e.g., family relationships). Most are virtually indistinguishable from personality data. Hence, double arrows are placed between the *ID* variables and *PSY-5* variables, which are subsequently connected by a second set of double arrows to the behavioral scales. This final cluster of variables may be reported independently or with the other diagnostic data.

Validity Scales

Overall Psychopathology
Higher-Order (*H-O*) Scales

| Emotional/ Internalizing Dysfunction-1 (*EID-1*): Mood | Emotional/ Internalizing Dysfunction-2 (*EID-2*): Anxiety | Thought Dysfunction (*THD*): Psychosis | Behavioral/ Externalizing Dysfunction (*BXD*) | Personality Psychopathology Five (*PSY-5*) | Interpersonal Dysfunction (*ID*) | Somatic/Cognitive Dysfunction (*SCD*) |

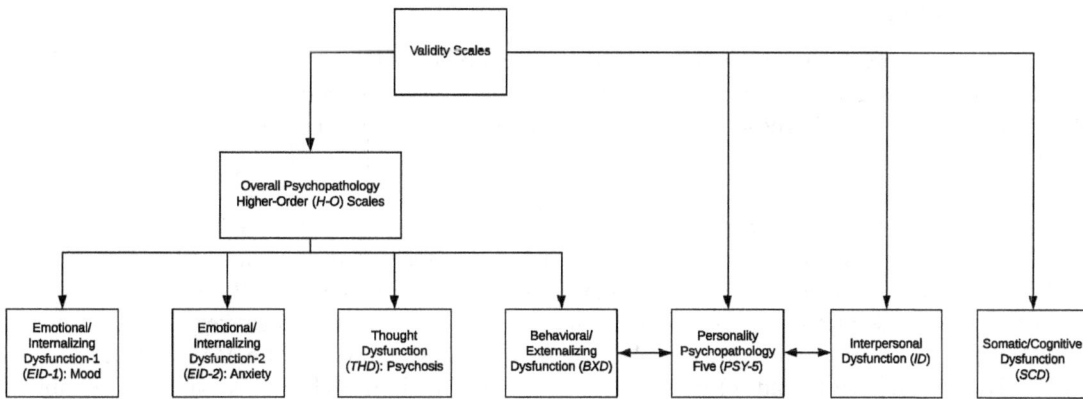

Figure 11.4 Minnesota Multiphasic Personality Inventory, Second Edition, Restructured Form (MMPI-2-RF) Interpretive Process

SUMMARY

This section was devoted to presenting the MMPI–A–RF in terms of its test structure, organization of scales, and data yield designed for reporting the results within a psychological assessment report (Form 11.5). Figure 11.3 (e-resources) provided a flowchart that visually illustrated an interpretive strategy that can be both efficient and effective when used in clinical testing practice. Special focus was made on the origin and development of the *PSY-5* scales for use with the restructured MMPI tests to explain how they are to be most effectively interpreted. Next, the adult version of the MMPI restructured form is presented. Here, special focus will be provided on how the restructured clinical scales were developed, as this procedure was first done on the adult version of the MMPI and only secondarily on the adolescent test that was just presented.

Minnesota Multiphasic Personality Inventory, Second Edition, Restructured Form

Presentation of the adult version of the MMPI restructured test will be organized in similar fashion to previous tests. This includes an introductory synopsis, a brief description of its development from the MMPI–2 predecessor, a review of the norm reference sample, an administrative section, scoring, and interpretation. The latter will be supplemented by an interpretive flowchart (Figure 11.4), which is available for download on Routledge's e-resources website for reference throughout the ensuing discussion, and data tables for score reporting and interpretation within a psychological assessment report (Form 11.6).

SYNOPSIS

The *Minnesota Multiphasic Personality Inventory, Second Edition, Restructured Form* (*MMPI–2–RF*; Ben-Porath & Tellegen, 2011; Tellegen & Ben-Porath, 2011) is a self-report inventory intended for individuals 18 years, 0 months through 85 years, 11 months. It is designed to principally identify the presence of psychopathology in the form of both clinical disorders and personality psychopathology. It contains a total of 338 items that are a subset of the 567 items that make up the *Minnesota Multiphasic Personality Inventory, Second Edition* (*MMPI–2*; Butcher et al., 1989).

Succinctly, the MMPI–2–RF is an updated multivariate factor reanalysis of MMPI-2 items using essentially the same standardization sample, namely, ages 18 years, 0 months to 89 years, 11 months (Ben-Porath & Tellegen, 2011; Tellegen & Ben-Porath, 2011; Tellegen et al., 2003). The cardinal purpose of this reanalysis was to improve both the discriminant and convergent validity of the major clinical scales by reducing scale intercorrelations, the latter being caused by remarkable item overlap characteristic of the MMPI-2 (Butcher et al., 1989). A secondary major objective was to provide a comprehensive measure of psychopathology that either assessed aspects of the clinical scales requiring independent analysis, or symptom patterns that were only indirectly or not at all assessed by the clinical scales. The 338 items consist of 51 total scales, including the following types and numbers in parentheses: (a) validity (*n* = 9); (b) higher-order (*n* = 3); (c) Restructured Clinical (*n* = 9); (d) Specific Problems (*n* = 23); (e) Interest Scales (*n* = 2); and (f) revised Personality Psychopathology Five (*PSY-5*) scales (*n* = 5). This version of the MMPI represents a third iteration as applied to adults. Therefore, a brief history of its emergence from the MMPI-2 will be instructive.

DEVELOPMENT OF THE MMPI–2–RF

This section first presents research that demonstrates the compatibility of the MMPI–2 to that of the MMPI–2–RF in terms of both item arrangement and norms. Thereafter, a discussion will ensue concerning the development of the MMPI–2–RF validity and diagnostic scales, with a special focus on the statistical methods used to create the restructured scales.

MMPI–2 and MMPI–2–RF Comparability   Because the MMPI–2 norms were garnered 20 years prior, along with using a booklet with 567 items of a different sequence, it was necessary to determine if (a) score results from the longer 567-item MMPI–2 test booklet would be comparable to those of the MMPI–2–RF, and (b) if the 1989 MMPI–2 norms would adequately represent key population demographics approximately 20 years later in 2008. To examine the first assumption, three samples were administered as follows: (a) the MMPI–2 test and retest, (b) the MMPI–2–RF test and retest, and (c) the MMPI–2 test and MMPI–2–RF test. Mean *T*–scores and standard deviations were computed and compared for all MMPI–2–RF scales, whether derived from the MMPI–2 or the MMPI–2–RF. Furthermore, inferential z test statistics were done on all mean comparisons to determine if there were any significant differences, along with test–retest correlations. This investigative strategy was borrowed from the methodology employed by Ben-Porath and Butcher (1989). Results showed very few significant differences (viz., 5 of 41 comparisons), and median test–retest correlations of 0.79 (see Tellegen & Ben-Porath, 2011, Appendix C, pp. 287–293). The latter indicates that 62% of the variance in the initial MMPI–2/MMPI–2–RF derived substantive scales can be accounted for by the second administration scores, which is a large effect (see Cohen, 1988).

To test the comparability of norms, scores obtained for the MMPI–2–RF at the time the MMPI–2 norms were garnered between 1984 and 1986, including 561 college students, were compared with the following two samples: (a) 775 adults tested with the MMPI–2 test booklet between 1992 and 1993 and (b) 229 adults tested with the MMPI–2–RF test booklet between 2007 and 2008. Once again, mean *T*–scores and standard deviations were computed and compared for all MMPI–2–RF scales (see Tellegen & Ben-Porath, 2011, Appendix C, pp. 294–312). In general, there was "substantial comparability" across different cohorts, using different MMPI booklets, and most importantly, longitudinally over time. Therefore, it was concluded that, "the MMPI–2–RF *T*–scores provide an adequate normative framework" for current use (Tellegen & Ben-Porath, 2011, Appendix C, p. 294).

What follows is a more detailed discussion of the development of the MMPI–2–RF scales as follows: validity scales, restructured clinical (*RC*) scales, higher-order (*H-O*) scales, specific problems (SP) scales, Interest (I) scales, and Personality Psychopathology Five (*PSY-5*) scales. Such discussion will clarify scale interpretation, along with use of the scoring and interpretation scales. It should be assumed that similar statistical methods and stratagems were employed in developing the restructured scales for the previously presented adolescent version.

Validity Scales   The MMPI–2–RF validity scales include those measuring inconsistency, overreporting, and underreporting. The *VRIN-r* and *TRIN-r* measure variable and fixed responding, respectively. Essentially, the strongest positively correlated items (i.e., *True–True*; *False–False*) were identified for *VRIN-r*, and the strongest negatively correlated items were targeted for *TRIN-r* (i.e., *True~False*; *False~True*). Therefore, answering these items in the direction opposite their correlated direction (e.g., *True~False* for *VRIN-r* and *True~True* for *TRIN-r*) earned a positive score on these scales. In essence, an excess of positive scores reflected that particular response tendency. Additionally, for the *TRIN-r* scale, the sum of the *False–False* inconsistencies are subtracted from the *True–True* inconsistencies to yield a difference score that shows the directional tendency of the fixed responding. This is denoted by a T or F adjacent to the *T*–score. Specifically, a 79T denotes fixed responding in the *True–True* or acquiescent (i.e., tendency to agree) direction, while a 79F denotes fixed responding in the counter-acquiescent (i.e., tendency to disagree) direction.

Overreporting on the MMPI–2–RF is measured by five scales, hence four greater than for the MMPI–A–RF. First, a brand new Infrequent Somatic Responses (*Fs*) scale was developed specifically for the MMPI–2–RF (Wygant, Ben-Porath, & Arbisi, 2004). Its 16 items include extremely uncommon somatic complaints that are endorsed by 25% or less of medical patients (Wygant, 2007). Second, a Fake Bad Scale (*FBS*) was initially developed to identify personality injury litigants who overreport symptoms (Lees-Haley, English, & Glenn, 1991). A meta-analysis done by Nelson, Sweet, and Demakis (2006) generally supported the ability of the *FBS* to function as designed, especially regarding the overreporting of both cognitive and somatic symptoms. The 43-item *FBS* scale was incorporated into the MMPI–2 in or around 2008 (Ben-Porath, Tellegen, & Graham, 2008). After its incorporation into the MMPI–2–RF, the label was changed to the Symptom Validity Scale. However, it was abbreviated *FBS-r* for purposes of continuity and 13 items were dropped, hence totaling 30. It effectively complements the other validity scales in detecting the overreporting of cognitive and somatic symptoms (Tellegen & Ben-Porath, 2011, p. 15).

Third, the 21-item Infrequent Psychopathology Responses (*Fp-r*) scale is strongly correlated with its counterpart *Fp* of the MMPI–2. It is effective in measuring exaggerated symptom responding in individuals manifesting severe psychopathology (i.e., in psychiatric samples). There is some evidence that the *Fp-r* outperforms *F-r* in detecting those who inflate the presence of abnormality (Arbisis & Ben-Porath, 1998). Fourth, a revised Infrequent Responses (*F-r*) scale was constructed by investigating which of the 338 total MMPI–2–RF items were only endorsed by 10% or less of the standardization sample and not yet assigned to other validity scales. A total of 32 items were selected for the *F-r* scale, which has shown to be perhaps the most effective of the overreporting scales). Fifth, the Response Bias Scale (*RBS*) was developed by Gervais, Ben-Porath, Wygant, and Green (2007), which was designed to identify symptom exaggeration among individuals being assessed for disability. The 28-item scale has been found to effectively discriminate between disability applicants who report their symptoms truthfully versus non-truthfully (i.e., in an inflated manner).

Finally, the MMPI–2–RF possesses two underreporting scales. They were developed by dint of a series of factor-analyses done on underreporting indicators on the MMPI–2, including the original MMPI *L* and *K* validity scales, the Superlative Self-Presentation (*S*) scale (Butcher & Han, 1995), and the Wiggins's social desirability (*Sd*) scale (Wiggins, 1959). Such analyses yielded two independent factors and, hence, as many underreporting scales. The first, labeled Uncommon Virtues, was assigned the abbreviation *L-r* because 11 of its 14 items appeared on the original MMPI/MMPI–2 *L* counterpart, all of which are keyed *False*. The remaining three items on *L-r* were derived from *Sd*, which are felicitously keyed *True*, hence guarding against fixed responding. The second underreporting scale was labeled adjustment validity, and abbreviated *K-r* because all 14 items also appeared on the original MMPI/ MMPI–2 *K* counterpart.

Restructured Clinical (RC) Scales As stated, the MMPI–2–RF was essentially a revision of the MMPI–2 (Ben-Porath & Tellegen, 2011; Tellegen & Ben-Porath, 2011). The cardinal purpose of this essential third iteration of the adult MMPI was to improve both the discriminant and convergent validity of the clinical scales by reducing scale intercorrelations, this being caused by remarkable item overlap characteristic of the MMPI–2 (see prior discussion and Butcher et al., 1989). The principal objective was to virtually eliminate the unacceptably high item-overlap and consequential inflated covariance among with clinical scales. The process followed several steps, which was also employed during MMPI–A–RF development. They are as follows.

The first step was to identify a common non-specific factor, which Tellegen (1985) termed *demoralization*,[7] which has been consistently found to be responsible for increasing intercorrelations among scales generally found in self-report inventories. An initial series of analyses effectively identified a set of "marker" items, which together represented a pleasant-to-unpleasant continuum of self-reported mood (Tellegen, Watson, & Clark, 1999a, 1999b; Watson & Tellegen, 1985). For the second step, items from each of the clinical scales were combined with the demoralization marker items and independently factor-analyzed. From these analyses, it was basically found that each clinical scale consisted of two factors; that is, a cluster of demoralization items, which belonged on a demoralization scale, and an independent cluster of non-demoralization items, which belonged on their originally assigned clinical scale. At this juncture, the grouping of non-demoralization items that remained on their original clinical scale were referred to as *seed scales*. This label was selected because such scales were not yet fully developed.

Step three focused on further modifying the seed scales such that they were even more distinctive or non-overlapping with the other clinical scales. This was accomplished by a combination of content item analyses, a series of item-scale correlations, and external item validity data. Regarding the correlational analysis, items that were highly correlated within each scale, yet minimally correlated with the other scales, were retained to further enhance item-scale uniqueness. This included identification of items from the MMPI–2 that were distinctively correlated with a particular seed scale, which were then added to such scale. The fourth and final step consisted of minor item adjustments that were made based upon correlations with external criteria, along with an extensive number of validation studies (i.e., external validation). See Tellegen et al. (2003) for more detail on *RC* construction and Ben-Porath and Tellegen (2011) for additional evidence of *RC* scale validity and utility. This four-step process resulted in the following nine Restructured Clinical (*RC*) scales: (a) Demoralization (*RCd*), (b) Somatic Complaints (*RC1*), (c) Low Positive Emotions (*RC2*), (d) Cynicism (*RC3*), (e) Antisocial Behavior (*RC4*), (f) Ideas of Persecution (*RC6*), (g) Dysfunctional Negative Emotions (*RC7*), (h) Aberrant Experiences (*RC8*), and (i) Hypomanic Activation (*RC9*). The broader higher-order (*H-O*) scales were derived from these *RC* scales, a topic to which the discussion now turns.

Higher-Order (H-O) Scales The objective of constructing more broadly defined measures for the MMPI–2–RF was to create a useful organizational structure of the test that would facilitate interpretation, analogous to the hierarchical organization and interpretive process espoused by the standardized cognitive tests of intelligence and achievement (see Chapters 7 and 8, respectively). These more general higher-order (*H-O*) scales were derived by conducting a series of factor analyses including all of the *RC* clinical scales. A reliable three-factor structure was discovered, representing the general constructs of (a) emotional dysfunction, (b) thought dysfunction, and (c) behavioral dysfunction (see Tellegen & Pen-Porath, 2011, Table 2–2, p. 17). Based on these data, and similar analyses using the standardization sample, the factor names and their highest RC clinical scale loadings were as follows: (a) emotional/internalizing dysfunction (*EID*), highest loadings *RCd*, *RC2*, *RC7*; (b) thought dysfunction (*THD*), highest loadings *RC6*, *RC8*; and (c) behavioral/externalizing dysfunction (*BXD*), highest loadings *RC4*, *RC9*. Subsequent factor and correlational analyses ensured that (a) virtually all items contributing to each H-O scale score came from the *RC* clinical scales with the highest factor loadings, and (b) the H-O scale items would be non-overlapping or unique. For example, all the selected items contributing to *THD* are derived from the *RC6* and *RC8* clinical scales.

Specific Problems (SP) and Interest Scales (I)   As noted, a secondary major objective of MMPI–2–RF development was to provide a comprehensive measure of psychopathology not limited to the *RC* scales. The additional scales discussed here were essentially developed in the same fashion as the *RC* scales. Specifically, item sets representing various constructs were factor analyzed to dichotomize items into demoralization and non-demoralization groupings. The demoralization items were dropped, and the non-demoralization items were retained in the form of initial seed scales representing each construct. A subsequent series of item-scale correlations identified those that were excessively correlated with other scales, which led to their being culled from the seed scales. In addition, some items from the large 567-item MMPI–2 pool were added to a particular seed scale if uniquely correlated with that scale and no others. Lastly, analysis of item-scale content was done by reviewers who were considered MMPI–2 experts, hence providing some degree of content validity to these additional substantive scales.

The result was the addition of 25 new substantive scales, 23 of which were denoted as Specific Problems (SP) scales, along with 2 representing Interest (I) scales. The SP scales were further subdivided into sets based on content and differential correlations with the *H-O* scales as follows: (a) somatic scales; (b) internalizing scales; (c) externalizing scales; and (d) interpersonal scales. These scales tend to possess fewer items, although as will be discussed subsequently when addressing *T*–scores, they have acceptable standard errors of measurement (*SEM*s) and an exceptional degree of external validation (see Ben-Porath & Tellegen, 2011; Tellegen & Pen-Porath, 2011).

Personality Psychopathology Five (PSY-5) Scales   Development of the Personality Psychopathology Five (*PSY-5*) scales was addressed previously when discussing how they were incorporated into the MMPI–A–RF. Therefore, they will be only briefly reviewed again here as the relate to the MMPI–2–RF and as a segue to the ensuing NEO inventories. The *PSY-5* were initially constructed by Harkness, McNulty, and Ben-Porath (1995), and were designed according to a model of personality proposed by Harkness and McNulty (1994). These scales were first incorporated into a revised edition of the MMPI–2 manual as follows: (a) aggressiveness (*AGGR*); (b) psychoticism (*PSYC*); (c) disconstraint (*DISC*); (d) negative emotionality/neuroticism (*NEGE*); and (e) introversion/low positive emotionality (*INTR*) (Butcher et al., 2001). Next, it was observed that there was increasing convergence between the *PSY-5* scales and both the NEO-PI-R and the *DSM–5* new dimensional model of diagnosing personality disorders (Harkness, Reynolds, & Lileinfeld, 2014), which made them especially pertinent to consider here with the MMPI–2–RF. This issue is delved into in much more detail when discussing the NEO–PI–3 (McCrae & Costa, 2010) subsequently, which will felicitously complete this chapter on personality inventory tests.

To construct *PSY-5* scales for the 338-item MMPI–2–RF, Harkness and McNulty (2007) took the 139 *PSY-5* items of the MMPI–2 and subjected them to an iterative process of item-scale and external item-criterion analyses. Of the 96 remaining items, 22 were deleted and 30 were added, which served to enhance scale discriminability. The result was five reconstructed *PSY-5* scales with the same labels, except with an appended lower case "*r*" denoting the reconstruction. Thereafter, analyses showed that the reconstructed *PSY-5* scales were comparable to their MMPI–2 counterparts (Harkness & McNulty, 2007). Because the derivation of these scales was discussed previously when presenting the MMPI–A–RF, no more will be mentioned here regarding the *PSY-5* scales, except to reiterate that they are comparable across both restructured MMPI tests.

Summary   This section provided an overview regarding the revision of the MMPI–2–RF and its various scales. The principal objective was to provide a background from which to better comprehend test structure, organization, scoring, and interpretation, along with a rationale as to why this third iteration is preferred over that of the MMPI–2. Next, a review of the MMPI–2–RF normative sample is presented to inform readers of its limits of generalizability.

NORM REFERENCE DATA

The standardization sample was virtually the same as for the MMPI–2, with the one major exception of non-gendered versus gender-based norms. This sample included 2,600 adults, including 1,462 women and 1,138 men. A minor modification in the MMPI–2–RF sample was the random elimination of 224 women such that the number of males and females were equalized at 1,138 each (Greene, 2011). When compared to population distribution of the United States according to the 1990 census, which was collected in proximity to the MMPI–2 norms, the standardization sample was considered a relatively good representation in terms of ethnic origin, age, and education (see Ben-Porath & Tellegen, 2011, Tables 3–1, 3–2, 3–3, p. 14).

More specifically, the age ranged from 18 years, 0 months to 85 years, 11 months. Concerning ethnicity, Whites were somewhat overrepresented at 81.8% versus the census 76.2%, which was attributed to the standardization requirement of being English-speaking. In addition, education level was also somewhat higher in the standardization group versus the population, including 27% versus 15.3% college graduate, and 18.8% versus 7% postgraduate, respectively. Regarding gender, because there were equal numbers of males and females, the single issue was whether to use non-gendered or gendered norms. For such analysis, the non-gendered *T*–scores were subtracted from gendered *T*–scores, including 118 comparisons. Results showed that few clinically significant differences were found. Further, those that were found were considered more stylistic versus substantive. Therefore, the MMPI–2–RF provides non-gendered norms, although gendered norms can be selected if desired. Finally, recall from the previous discussion regarding the comparability of the MMPI–2 and MMPI–2–RF, that the former test's norms were also deemed to be an adequate representation of the pertinent population demographics reported for 2008, at which time the MMPI-RF was published.

ADMINISTRATION

The MMPI–2–RF consists of 338 *True–False* items, which require an average reading level of sixth grade (Dahlstrom et al., 1994; Schinka & Borum, 1993). However, some items may require a seventh-grade reading level (Dahlstrom et al., 1994). Average administration time varies by type as follows: (a) computerized is 20–30 minutes and (b) booklet and answer sheet is 30–50 minutes. As stated, the MMPI–2–RF is normed on individuals 18 years, 0 months through 85 years, 11 months. Because the MMPI–A–RF also includes 18-year-olds, an examinee of such age can legitimately be administered either the latter test or the adult MMPI–2–RF. To determine which test is most appropriate, the principal consideration is the living circumstances of the individual. That is, if the prospective examinee is working, living alone or with a partner, and is showing other indicators of autonomy, the adult MMPI–2–RF is the more logical selection. In contrast, if the individual is enrolled in school, continues to live at home, and is showing other indicators of adolescence, then the MMPI–A–RF is the better choice.

During actual administration, the examiner or technician is encouraged to supervise the examinee, although such is not required to occur in the same room. Further, the examiner is permitted to provide dictionary definitions of any of the words if asked by the examinee, although without elaboration or "extended discussion" (Archer et al., 2016, p. 63; see also Ben-Porath & Tellegen, 2011).

Computerized administration and scoring is advisable for five reasons, including (a) convenience (i.e., reading individual items on a computer screen and entering responses by computer mouse point-and-click versus reading lists of items from a booklet and entering responses via a series of columns on a Scantron form), (b) efficiency (i.e., as much as 50% less administration time), (c) accuracy (i.e., automated step-by-step instructions and scoring), (d) optional audio administration of the items, and (e) increased likelihood of test validity (i.e., double True and False non-scorable responses and inadvertently entering responses to incorrect items are effectively precluded).

As for the previous personality inventories, it is advised that the MMPI–2–RF be administered via the Q-global (Pearson, 2021) online scoring and reporting platform. Once on Q-global (i.e., https://qglobal.pearsonclinical.com/qg/login.seam), the examinee's demographics are entered (viz., name, ID number, birth date, gender), "Assign New Assessment" is selected, and a list of all available Pearson tests appears. Once MMPI–2–RF is selected by means of a *radio button* (i.e., a computer listing of options in the form of circles that permits only one selection), the "Assign" option activates and should be selected by mouse click. An "Assessment Details" page appears with the examinee name and demographics. There are several entries here that are considered, such as examiner's name, administrative language (i.e., English or Spanish), and most importantly, "On-Screen Administration." Once selected, the examiner's email will appear, which later notifies the examiner that the test has been completed, and a "Launch with Test Session Lock" option is also available. Again, this option is strongly encouraged because this will lock the screen during administration such that examinees are precluded from minimizing the screen and surfing the Internet for personal use. The lock screen Pearson software needs only to be downloaded once to the computer and there is no added fee.

When administration is done, the screen can be unlocked by pressing Ctrl + Shift + Q. Subsequent to selecting "Start Assessment," a final "Notice" appears informing test administrators that, for purposes of security, they will be logged out of Q-global (Pearson, 2021) during the administration process. Clicking on "I Acknowledge" begins the actual administration.

Once in screen-locked mode, the instructions to examinees begin with selecting the preferred language, "English" or "Spanish." Next, a welcome screen appears, which indicates that instructions will begin. The ensuing screen asks examinees to read each statement and decide, using their own opinions, whether it is "true as applied to you" (i.e., true or mostly true) or "false as applied to you" (i.e., false or usually not true). Items appear individually on the screen, with the *True–False* options directly below. The examinee can advance without selecting *True* or *False*, although they are prompted once in the form by a "Request Response" instruction before advancing. Therefore, non-responsiveness is possible. When the test is completed, the administrator can unlock the screen and choose "Generate Report" to begin the scoring process or wait until a later opportunity for scoring. This brings us to the scoring section of the MMPI–2–RF presentation, wherein Figure 11.4 (see e-resources) and Form 11.6 will be referenced to facilitate the presentation.

SCORING

This scoring section deals with two topics. The first is apportioned into three subtopics as follows: (a) the Q-global computer reports and how the data is organized, (b) the MMPI–2–RF *UT*–scores derivation and meaning; and (c) the reported PRs and CIs in the tables designed for inclusion within a testing report. The second topic describes how to report and interpret the validity of the MMPI–2–RF protocol. Once the latter is reviewed, this sets the stage for interpreting this test's substantive scales, which are most commonly termed the diagnostic scales, as they are central to such objectives, namely, psychodiagnosis. They are presented in this order.

The MMPI–2–RF Data Yield   Once the MMPI–2–RF administration has been completed on Q-global (Pearson, 2021), the examiner will be emailed to that effect, along with a confirmation that the protocol is ready for scoring. Whether scoring is done immediately after administration or some time thereafter, the examiner locates the examinee's name, checks it, and mouse clicks upon the name. Next, the following information appears on a single line: (a) assessment identification number, (b) test name, (c) date of delivery, and (d) type of report (in this example, "On Screen Administration. Report Generated"). This line is also to be checked, followed by selecting "Generate Report." An options box opens with the report: "Please select . . ." Clicking on the down arrow in that box provides a number of options, most pertinently: (a) MMPI–2–RF Interpretative Report and (b) MMPI–2–RF Score Report. The latter provides all the information needed for presenting the data within a psychological assessment report using the form that has been prepared for this purpose (i.e., Form 11.6). The interpretive report provides the same data, although it adds computer-generated interpretive statements, which is not recommended because in many cases they are contradictory, do not provide data reference points, and lack a coherent interpretative strategy that uses contextual assessment information. On a more practical note, they are extremely expensive.

Within pages 2–6 of the MMPI–2–RF score report, the following is provided for each scale: (a) raw score, (b) *T*–score (also profiled in graphic format), and (c) percent of items answered. Unless a specific norm reference group is selected in terms of gender and setting, the default non-gendered entire standardization sample is used to derive the standard scores as described previously. However, the examiner may check, "Select Comparison Group," in which case further alternatives regarding a comparison norm reference group and gender (i.e., male or female) become available. On pages 2–6 of the score report, the scales are reported in clusters as follows: (a) validity scales; (b) *H-O* and *RC* scales; (c) somatic/cognitive and internalizing scales; (d) externalizing, interpersonal, and interest scales; and (e) *PSY-5* scales. On page 7, all scales and their *T*–scores are reported as organized by their assigned substantive domain as follows: (a) somatic/cognitive dysfunction; (b) emotional dysfunction; (c) thought dysfunction; (d) behavioral dysfunction; (e) interpersonal functioning; and (f) interests. The MMPI–2–RF possesses 51 scales in all, including 9 validity scales and 42 substantive scales (i.e., the diagnostic scales). The latter are further apportioned into 3 *H-O* scales, 9 *RC* scales, 23 SP scales, and 5 *PSY-5* scales.

As done for the MMPI–A–RF, the MMPI–2–RF utilizes uniform *T*–scores (*UT*) versus linear *T*–scores, the latter being used in the original MMPI. Although both possess the same metric of a mean of 50 and standard deviation 10, linear *T*–scores are reported to be less than optimal in this case because, from their inception, the MMPI clinical scale raw score distributions have been positively skewed to varying degrees. Therefore, the MMPI *T*–scores across the scales represented somewhat different percentile ranks, which hindered inter-scale comparisons. Although the *UT*–score process was introduced previously when presenting the MMPI–A–RF, it will be delineated here in more detail because (a) it was first used with the adult MMPI tests, (b) the process is rather intricate and bears repeating for

Table 11.1 Uniform T-sScore–Linear T–score Percentile Rank Comparisons

T–score	UT–PR	LT–PR
80	99	99
75	98	99
70	96	98
65	92	94
60	85	84
55	73	70
50	55	50
45	34	32
40	15	16
35	4	7
30	1	2

Note. UT = Uniform T–score; PR = percentile rank; LT = Linear T–score. LT–PRs assume a standard normal distribution. PRs were rounded to the nearest whole number.

Adapted from: Ben-Porath, Y. S., & Tellegen, A. (2011). *Minnesota Multiphasic Personality Inventory–2–RF (MMPI–2–RF): Manual for administration, scoring, and interpretation*. Minneapolis: MN: University of Minnesota Press, Table 3-4, p. 15.

clarification, and (c) some readers may focus their testing and/or interest on adult cases and therefore would benefit from being informed as to how this procedure was accomplished with this particular version of the test.

The UT–score procedure was actually first used with the MMPI–2 data and was thereafter continued without revision with the MMPI–2–RF. The UT–score sequence consisted of four basic steps (Tellegen & Porath, 1992). First, as typically done, clinical scale raw scores were transformed into linear T–scores by first computing their z–scores, then entering these values into the following formula:

$$T\text{–score} = \bar{x} + z(s) = 50 + z(10)$$

Equation 11.2

where $\bar{x}$ represents the preselected mean of a T–score, which is 50, z represents the computed z–score, and s represents the preselected standard deviation of the T–score distribution, which is 10. This was done across 16 individual distributions. Second, T–score values for percentiles 0.5, 1, 1.5, . . . 98, 98.5, 99, and 99.5 (i.e., in 0.5-unit increments) were derived by means of interpolation. Third, the T–score values and their associated percentiles were averaged across the 16 distributions. The average values and their percentile equivalents are presented in the MMPI–2–RF scoring manual (Ben-Porath & Tellegen, 2011, Table 3-4, p. 15). These "composite standard score" values reflected the expected positive skew and the UT–score/percentile prototype distribution; for instance, UT–score = 35 (percentile = 4); UT–score = 50 (percentile = 55); UT–score = 70 (percentile = 96), hence more extreme at the lower end and less extreme at the higher end. This trend is depicted more clearly in Table 11.1, which displays a representative set of UT–score/percentile rank (PR) values (middle column).

Table 11.1 also juxtaposes the linear T–score/PR values for comparison purposes. Scrutiny of the UT–score and linear T–score PRs are in the final analysis very similar. For example, the largest discrepancy is at the mean (i.e., five PR units), whereas most of the remaining comparisons are within one or two PR units. In terms of test interpretation, the differences in PR between the two types of standard scores are rather miniscule, namely, a statistical distinction without a meaningful clinical difference.

Fourth, all raw score distributions were transformed by means of linear regression so they would conform as closely as possible to the composite standard scores, namely, the prototypic UT–score/PR distribution. The same procedure was used to compute UT–scores for the remaining substantive scales. The end result was a prototype UT–score distribution that was consistent across all of the MMPI–2–RF substantive scales (see Tellegen et al., 2003; Ben-Porath & Tellegen, 2011, Figure 3–1, p. 16) and *PSY-5* scales (Harkness et al., 1995) in regard to T–score/PR values. However, linear T–scores continue to be used for the MMPI–2–RF validity scales and Interest (I) scales.

For the interested reader, raw–score to T–score conversions for all MMPI–2–RF scales are available in Appendix A of the test manual (Ben-Porath & Tellegen, 2011, p. 89–93). Supplemental analyses showed that the MMPI–2 and MMPI–2–RF counterpart UT–scores were comparable. However, what is missing from both the manual and computer score report, for the purposes of reporting MMPI–2–RF test results within the context of a psychological assessment report, are all the UT–score to PR conversions. Rather than not reporting such PRs in a testing report, it is best practice to at least estimate these values by reporting the PRs according to a standard normal distribution (see

Appendix A, Table A.1). As elucidated previously, the PR values for *UT*–score versus linear *T*–scores are reasonably close such that using the normal curve PRs would not significantly distort test interpretation. While the effort put forth by the test authors in the name of precision is commendable, the differences in PR values between the linear and uniform *T*–scores are not clinically significant, thus the former can be effectively utilized in test interpretation. Therefore, the data tables for all substantive scales (i.e., diagnostic scales) report PRs according to the standard normal distribution, which is clearly stated in relevant table notes. Also, as stated when discussing the MMPI–A–RF, the tables use the term *T*–scores and not *UT*–scores to avoid confusion.

In addition, the diagnostic scales all include a column for reporting CIs, here again with a 68% degree of certainty of including the examinee's true score. Although the computer reports and the pertinent test manuals do not report such CIs, the standard errors of measurement (*SEM*s) for all the scales are reported in the technical manual (Tellegen & Ben-Porath, 2011, Tables 3-3–3-6, pp. 24–25). For the normative sample, *SEM*s based on test–retest correlations (i.e., stability coefficients) were most important to consider versus measures of internal consistency. That is, CIs based on the constancy of the symptoms or traits over time was deemed to be most relevant to test interpretation. Therefore, the *SEM*s based on the normative test–retest correlations reported in the manual were entered into the CI column cell for each scale located immediately beneath the bracketed interval. The examiner merely adds and subtracts that value to obtain and enter the interval into the table (see Form 11.6, Tables 4–11). The entered *SEM* should then be deleted as no longer needed and to remove undesired clutter in the data table.

The reported *T*–score range in the computer score report graphs is from 20 to 120, although this varies among the scales within a narrower range, most typically between 30 and 100. Higher scores indicate greater degrees of either (a) aberrant test-taking response tendencies (validity scales) or (b) degrees of psychopathology according to the construct being measured by a particular diagnostic scale. This information is provided in each of the table notes. As a final note on scoring, the computer score report provides a list of critical items that have been endorsed by examinees in the deviant direction. Those relevant to the case, or that indicate a danger to self or other, should be noted in the narrative interpretation of the pertinent tables.

Determining MMPI–2–RF Validity   Consistent with generally accepted approaches in interpreting self-report inventories, presentation of the validity scales is done prior to scrutinizing the diagnostic scales. This is depicted in Figure 11.4 (see e-resources), which again presents a flowchart of the recommended MMPI–2–RF interpretive process. There are three classes of validity scales in the MMPI–2–RF, including non-responding (*n* = 3), underreporting (*n* = 2), and overreporting (*n* = 5). In Form 11.6, they are enumerated in three different tables in this order because each grouping has different interpretive score ranges.

Table 1 (Form 11.6) addresses non-responding, which occurs when the examinee fails to read, understand, or respond earnestly to the test items. The Cannot Say (*CNS*) scale relies on the number of items that were incapable of being scored, typically items that were not given a *True* or *False* response by the examinee. Because this scale utilizes a raw score metric, specific notes have been inserted identifying (a) the special raw score metric for this scale and (b) the interpretative ranges of valid, cautiously valid, and invalid. The cautiously invalid result refers to a less than 90% rule, which states that any scale with more than 10% omissions is potentially invalid. As stated, the Q-global score report prints the raw score, *T*–score, and percent of items answered for each scale. In addition, the MMPI–2–RF manual reports the number of items per scale (Ben-Porath & Tellegen, 2011, Appendix B, pp. 95–107). Note that scales with five or fewer items should be especially scrutinized in the case of high *CNS* scores (i.e., either 1–14, or N ≥ 15 requiring even greater scrutiny). They include (a) gastrointestinal complaints (*GIC*), (b) suicidal/death ideation (*SUI*), (c) helplessness/hopelessness, (d) self-doubt (*SFD*), and (e) anxiety (*ANX*).

The remaining scales in Table 1 (Form 11.6) measure various other types of non-responding. In particular, the Variable Response Inconsistency (*VRIN-r*) scale detects erratic or random responding (i.e., *True–False* or *False–True*) to items with similar content and which are worded and keyed in the same direction (i.e., *True–True* or *False–False*). The True Response Inconsistency (*TRIN-r*) scale contains items with similar content but worded and keyed in opposing directions, hence requiring a *True–False* or *False–True* pairing to show reliable responding. Repeatedly answering *True–True* or *False–False* irrespective of item content indicates the following possibilities: (a) *acquiescence response set* (i.e., a *True–True* agreement tendency), (b) *disagreement response set* (i.e., a *False–False* oppositional tendency), or (c) *fixed responding response set* (i.e., deliberately selecting *True* or *False* in stereotyped fashion without reading the items). Because this scale's score is computed in part by subtracting *False–False* pairs from *True–True* pairs, the directional pattern can be revealed. Therefore, a *T*–score with an adjacent "T" (e.g., 80T) or an adjacent "F" (e.g., 75F) indicates (a) the degree of fixed responding (i.e., the absolute *T*–score) and (b) the direction of such responding (i.e., T = fixed *True* responding; F = fixed *False* responding). Note that both the score metric and complete scale names appear in the general table notes, along with the interpretive score ranges, to assist the testing psychologist in interpretation and the subsequent reader in terms of comprehension. The added letter of T or F for the *TRIN-r* scale is listed and defined in the table notes. An absence of a designated letter means there is no true-response inconsistency direction detected in the examinee's response set. In addition, three narrative excerpts follow the table as follows: (a) valid interpretation, (b) cautious valid interpretation, and (c) invalid interpretation with an advisement to terminate test interpretation at that point. The astute reader may recognize that these non-responding scales function in similar fashion to that of the MMPI–A–RF, which is an advantage because one interpretive scheme can be easily applied to both tests, at least in terms of non-responding.

Table 2 (Form 11.6) measures underreporting, also known as defensiveness or minimization of problems. Uncommon Virtues (*L-r*) represents a rather unsophisticated denial of any shortcomings, while Adjustment Validity (*K-r*) represents a more sophisticated attempt to report more than adequate adjustment. Table notes identify the metric, the general meaning of high scores, scale names, and interpretive ranges. Because high *T*–scores for *K-r* can also indicate genuine healthy adjustment, the higher and more conservative *L-r* score ranges reported in the test manual (Ben-Porath & Tellegen, 2011, Table 5-10, p. 31) are adopted for both scales for purposes of efficiency. Again, narrative excerpts are composed for valid, cautiously valid, and invalid results. The cautiously valid interpretation includes both mild and moderate elevations for efficiency. This is because they are so interpretively close in degree that simply adding a few adjectives to the language can adjust for the difference.

Table 3 (Form 11.6) possesses fives scales designed to detect symptom overreporting or exaggeration. Because this validity grouping is relatively large, there is both redundancy and complementarity incorporated into this table. Taken together, symptom overreporting is measured in the following ways: (a) infrequent responses in the general population, (b) infrequent responses in a psychiatric population, (c) infrequent physical complaints in a medical patient population, (d) excessive physical and cognitive complaints, and (e) excessive memory complaints. These five scales possess somewhat variable *T*–score cut-offs in the test manual for purposes of interpreting validity, although they are reasonably comparable. Hence, it is more efficient to scrutinize the various advised cut-offs in the manual, and in effect average them to create a single scheme that efficiently applies to all five scales. This stratagem is also justified by interpreting the five scales together as a profile, rather than in isolation, to reliably detect any symptom exaggeration that would deleteriously compromise test validity. Most of these scales consider *T*–scores of 79 and below to be non-problematic responding (i.e., normal). Further, the 100–120 *T*–score range is typically associated with invalidity (i.e., marked overreporting). Finally, the intermediate ranges then can logically be filled in with mild overreporting (viz., *T*–scores 80–89) and moderate overreporting (viz., *T*–scores 90–99).

If the interpretation has not yet been terminated due to invalidity, this data should then be summarized prior to initiating interpretation of the substantive or diagnostic scales. This is to remind both the testing psychologist and the reader of the general approach to interpretation that is to be adhered to, contingent upon the measured test-taking approach of the examinee. A number of narrative interpretations have been drafted under the heading, "MMPI–2–RF Validity Conclusion." These include a valid result with a standard interpretive strategy, ensued by three cautiously valid outcomes with qualified interpretations for non-responsive set, underreporting set, and overreporting set. Therefore, the percentage of scored responses on each scale will be considered in the case of non-responding, and scale elevations will be interpreted as over- or underestimates of genuine psychopathology depending on the directional tendency of the examinee, especially those elevations that are statistically significant. Note that use of the terms "non-responsive," "underreporting," and "overreporting" are (a) close to the facts, (b) minimize subjectivity and the use of inference, and (c) are more neutral in terms of connotation. For instance, compare the aforementioned terms to language such as, minimizing, exaggerating, "cry for help," and defensiveness. Such terms tend to express negative connotation, may be inaccurate, and require extra test information for corroboration. Hence, the more neutral and fact-based terminology is inserted in the interpretive excerpts as the default language, which can be modified at the examiner's discretion based on the facts of the case.

Integrating cautiously valid results into the CI data of the diagnostic scales can be extremely useful and efficacious. For instance, if a moderate underreporting test-taking response pattern is evinced, then estimating the examinee's true score as falling at the higher end of the relevant CI is a much more precise interpretation than vaguely stating in a general manner that the profile underestimates psychopathology. In the case of moderate overreporting, the cautious interpretation would be toward the opposing lower end of the interval. The various cautiously valid excerpts are worded using such logic.

Referring back to Figure 11.4 (e-resources), which presents an interpretive scheme for the MMPI–2–RF scale clusters, the validity-related Tables 1–3 are located in the top box of the flowchart, hence titled "Validity Scales." Once the validity scale results have been construed, the next step begins interpretation of the substantive (or diagnostic) scales, initiated by determining the overall degree and general pattern of symptoms. This brings us to the end of the scoring section and the beginning of test interpretation, which assumes the validity analysis was either valid or cautiously valid.

INTERPRETATION: MMPI–2–RF SUBSTANTIVE SCALES

This interpretation section is apportioned into two subsections. First is an overview of the substantive scales and their general structure and organization. This is ensued by the interpretive process portrayed in Figure 11.4 (see e-resources).

General Organization and Structure   The MMPI–2–RF substantive scales are presented in Tables 4–11 (Form 11.6). They follow a logical pattern proceeding from the validity scales to the substantive scales (i.e., scales that provide diagnostic data). Further, the latter follow a logical sequence proceeding from the three general *H-O* scales, *EID* (i.e., emotion, affect, or feeling), *THD* (i.e., thought), and *BXD* (i.e., undercontrolled behavior patterns), to tables that show either (a) more narrowly defined constructs related to each of the aforementioned general types of dysfunction or (b) four additional areas of psychological functioning (i.e., dysfunction) related to differential diagnosis (viz., personality, interpersonal, and somatic/cognitive). The *EID* scale was split into two subsets of emotion, the first showing specific manifestations of depression (and the related mood construct of hypomanic/manic symptoms), and the second showing specific manifestations of anxiety (and the related constructs of OCD, stress, trauma, and fears/phobias). There are no scale redundancies. That is, each diagnostic scale appears only once among the tables, typically according to conceptual similarity and/or those manifesting the highest scale intercorrelations. They have a similar organization to that of the adolescent version, although with several added tables of data, some reflecting the greater number of areas of functioning found in adulthood.

Although this organization differs from that of the MMPI–2–RF Q-global computer score report, it is most conducive to detecting the presence of I diagnoses and answering many frequent differential diagnostic questions, such as (a) unipolar depression versus bipolar psychopathology (with or without psychotic features), (b) mood disorder with psychotic features versus schizoaffective disorder, (c) behavior (i.e., conduct) disorder versus clinical disorder, and (d) clinical disorder versus personality psychopathology. Hence, it is worth the extra time to locate the proper scales on the score report and input them into the scoring and interpretation tables in Form 11.6, primarily because interpretation will be both more efficient and accurate.

Interpretive Process   Once the overall interpretative strategy has been determined by validity scale analysis (see prior), proceeding to the diagnostic scales can occur, beginning with the broad *H-O* scales. This is portrayed in Figure 11.4 (e-resources) by the arrow exiting from the left side of the "Validity Scales" box, then turning down to the "Higher-Order (*H-O*) Scales" box. These scales are listed in Table 4 (Form 11.6). Their absolute and relative score elevations, along with the focus of the particular testing case (e.g., rule out the presence of bipolar disorder), should determine the subsequent interpretative approach. Note that the measured symptoms descriptions for each scale entered into the final column of Table 4 (Form 11.6) are based on reported item content and empirical correlates, both afforded by the test manual. The question for Table 4 is, "What general symptom cluster, if any, is predominant in the profile; emotional, thinking, or behavioral?" The absolute *T*–score elevations, along with their ipsative differences, are both key. Other questions are as follows: (a) "Do any of the scales reach or exceed marginal elevations, or especially moderately or markedly significant elevations?" (b) "If so, what are the relative differences in terms of CI comparisons? That is, to what degree do they overlap or are they divergent?" This analysis will serve as a guide as to which set of substantive scales will be highlighted in subsequent interpretation.

Each of the *H-O* scales has an assigned set of substantive scales, this according to the test manual's recommended structure (Ben-Porath & Tellegen, 2011, Table 5-1, p. 22). First, as was done for the MMPI–A–RF, the *EID H-O* scales are dichotomized into those conceptually and empirically (with an emphasis on the former) most related to the mood disorders (*EID-1*), including depression and (hypo)manic symptoms (see Table 5 in Form 11.6; see also Figure 11.4, first box on the bottom row), and those relating more to anxiety-type symptoms (*EID-2*), including generalized anxiety, obsessive and compulsive symptoms, stress-induced symptoms, trauma-related symptoms, and phobias in order of presentation (see Table 6; see also Figure 11.4, second box on the bottom row). The latter grouping is consistent with previous *DSM* editions in which these symptoms were listed under the more general class of anxiety disorders (e.g., see American Psychiatric Association, 2000) prior to the advent of *DSM–5*. Hence, they seemed to be sufficiently related constructs so as to integrate them into one table for purposes of MMPI–2–RF psychodiagnosis. Narrative summaries following the *EID-1* mood and *EID-2* anxiety tables have been prepared, including one excerpt that describes a negative or within normal limits (WNL) interpretation, and one describing positive or remarkable elevations of varying degrees. The positive version consists of three points of fact, including the particular symptoms that are present, the most likely clinical disorders or chief problems indicated, and an overall averaging of degree or symptom severity. The narrative excerpts are meant as a guide, with sufficient flexibility such that the interpretation can be easily modified to match the presence of unique symptom patterns.

Second, the *THD H-O* scale has only two specific manifestations, both related to psychotic-type symptoms and listed in Table 7 of Form 11.6 (see also Figure 11.4, box titled "Thought Dysfunction (*THD*): Psychosis"). Again, by *psychotic*, it is meant that such symptoms are profoundly severe, involve a breakdown in reality testing (i.e., a formal thought disorder), and require intensive intervention, typically implicating a consideration for psychiatric hospitalization. After the Table 7 scales (Firm 11.6) are similar pre-worded narrative interpretations or excerpts, which are intended to guide the interpretation of both negative and positive results.

Third, the *BXD* specific manifestations all involve some type of acting-out (i.e., under-controlled or externalizing) behavioral symptoms, including severe anger management problems, antisocial or conduct-disordered behavior, rule-breaking behavior, and substance misuse. Such symptoms can also be conceptualized as an emerging personality disorder with impulsive, acting-out, antisocial traits. The contextual assessment information, including mental status examination and behavioral observations, along with the presenting symptoms and course, assists in making a sound clinical judgment in determining which interpretation is most valid. Significant *BXD* elevations suggest the presence of personality dysfunction, hence the double arrows in the flowchart directed to the *PSY-5* scale cluster, and subsequently, to the interpersonal dysfunction (*ID*) scale cluster (see Figure 11.4, three boxes with double arrows).

Of note, it bears repeating that there are no scale redundancies among any of the substantive scales even though some of the scales could have been placed in more than one scale cluster (e.g., *PSYC-r* in Table 7 as thought dysfunction and in Table 9 as personality dysfunction). Interpretive narrations follow the table for describing positive and negative results.

Table 8 (Form 11.6) features the *PSY-5* scales as their original grouping associated with the five-factor model (FFM; Costa & McCrae, 1992) and the *DSM–5* proposed trait model (see APA, 2013, Section III, p. 761–781). As indicated previously, the *PSY-5* scales overlap sufficiently with the FFM (Harkness, Renolds, & Lilenfeld, 2014) and the new *DSM–5* dimensional model of personality disorders such that reporting them can facilitate personality disorder diagnosis. The association between the FFM and the *DSM–5* dimensional model of personality disorder is further explicated when presenting the NEO–PI–3 immediately subsequent. As reviewed prior, some of the original *PSY-5* scale trait labels have been reversed so that all are in the dysfunctional or abnormal direction (Harkness et al., 1995). Thus, the final column in Table 9 has been titled "Measured maladaptive traits," rather than "Measured symptoms."

Consistent with their original purpose and subsequent development, the *PSY-5* scales are here interpreted exclusively as enduring maladaptive traits suggestive of personality psychopathology, this despite the fact that the test manual also defines these scales as manifesting symptoms of clinical disorders (Ben-Porath & Tellegen, 2011; Tellegen & Ben-Porath, 2011). For example, significant elevations on *AGGR-r* and *DISC-r* strongly suggest an emerging antisocial personality. In addition, elevations on *NEGE-r* and *INTR-r* are indicative of borderline personality disorder, with a supplemental elevation on *PSYC-r* further showing a very disturbed borderline personality case with potential psychotic or severe dissociative episodes. Further, *AGGR-r* has been related to particularly *offensive aggression* (Moyer, 1987), while *DISC-r* correlates with disconstrained behavior patterns that are well-ingrained (Romney & Bynner, 1992). Such use of these scales takes advantage of the personality theory that led to their development and provide a very useful integration of empirical evidence bolstered by a robust theory. They are not used as indicators of clinical syndromes because (a) this diverges from their original development and primary use, and (b) such use causes unneeded redundancy with other scales.

Note that the interpretive flowchart depicted in Figure 11.4 (see e-resources) has arrows from both the *BXD* scale cluster (double arrows) and from the validity scale cluster. This denotes the option of prioritizing the personality and interpersonal functioning scales if called for by the referral question(s). Therefore, if personality disorder is of prime focus, then analysis of the substantive scales can be initiated with the *PSY-5* and supplemented by the interpersonal dysfunction scales, consistent with the rationale that maladaptive personality traits tend to have their most deleterious effects upon an individual's social relationships (see, e.g., Chronis et al., 2007; Kochanska, Aksan, & Joy, 2007). Thereafter, analysis can proceed through the *BXD* scales or back through the *H-O* scales and toward the clinical disorders symptoms, hence in effect reversing the priority of the interpretive process to be consistent with that of the Millon tests, namely, personality psychopathology first followed by clinical disorders.

Table 10 (Form 11.6) lists the interpersonal dysfunction (ID) scales identified in the test manual as part of the MMPI–2–RF structure, which is identical to the MMPI–A–RF adolescent counterpart.[8] It is an apposite complement to the *PSY-5* table, as such data can provide added support for various personality disorders listed in the current *DSM–5* categorical system, including paranoid (*RC3*), dependent (*IPP*), avoidant (*SAV*), and schizoid (*DSF*). As applied to the MMPI–A–RF, such data would more likely indicate the emerging or risk of such personality psychopathologies. This is portrayed by the double arrows between the two clusters of scales in Figure 11.4 (see e-resources). Hence, the MMPI–2–RF provides personality-related data relevant for the two available *DSM–5* models, both current and proposed.

Excerpts that delineate negative and varying positive results follow the *PSY-5* and ID scales, with language that indicates which personality disorders are best fits for the data (i.e., conceptually speaking). Again, the positive versions end with an overall estimate of degree or severity, which is becoming increasingly prominent within the *DSM–5* nosology and is ideal for continuous measurement scale data as provided by these personality tests. Of note, the two Interest scales are not included, as they are more pertinent to career-counseling endeavors.

Finally, Table 11 (Form 11.6) lists the somatic/cognitive dysfunction (*SCD*) scales. This grouping tends to be deemphasized in outpatient mental health testing referrals, whereas testing for mood, anxiety, psychotic, and personality disorders are much more prominent. This explains why they are listed in the final box on the bottom row in Figure 11.4 (see e-resources). Also, note that only one arrow is directed toward them from the validity scales, denoting that they can fit into the analysis as the case facts so indicate. They are most pertinent, however, when a referring psychiatrist or other mental health therapist desires an opinion on possible somatization or illness anxiety disorders that may be complicating the symptom picture. Additionally, they can become relevant in more specialized neuropsychological testing cases, or screening for neurocognitive or genuine medical disorders. Hence, these are placed last in the order of constructs that are addressed by the MMPI–2–RF. Once again, narrative summaries of negative and positive results follow the table and table notes.

SUMMARY

The newest of the MMPI tests is presented in the succeeding section. It may be conceptualized as a more contemporary version of the MMPI–2–RF, including updated norms, a subset reworded items to improve clarity, and added items to expand coverage without increasing test length. It was published just prior to this book being submitted for publication. Hence, the administrative and technical manuals represent the primary publications of the ensuing section.

Minnesota Multiphasic Personality Inventory, Third Edition

This section presents the newest of the MMPI tests, which is fundamentally a more contemporary version of the MMPI–2–RF. In consequence, the ensuing discussion is organized in similar fashion to the two previous restructured versions, although it is more abbreviated in that it highlights the MMPI–3's essential and unique features.

SYNOPSIS

The *Minnesota Multiphasic Personality Inventory, Third Edition* (*MMPI–3*; Ben-Porath & Tellegen, 2020a, 2020b) is a self-report personality inventory intended for individuals 18 years, 0 months through 80-plus years. It is designed as a broadband instrument (i.e., a multidimensional test) that principally measures the presence of abnormality in the form of both clinical disorders and personality psychopathology, although it incorporates some additional constructs that are either absent or less well represented by the MMPI–2–RF (e.g., eating problems, obsessive-compulsive symptoms, respectively). It contains a total of 335 items, 263 of which are culled from the MMPI–2–RF, along with 72 new items (Ben-Porath & Tellegen, 2020b, p. 33). Furthermore, 24 of the 263 MMPI–2–RF items have been amended to improve clarity. These item modifications, along with significant changes in the U.S. population since the mid-1980s, at which time the MMPI–2–RF was standardized, called for the development of updated norms for the MMPI–3. Next, a review of the MMPI–3's development is presented.

DEVELOPMENT OF THE MMPI–3

The principal objectives of the MMPI–3 were as follows: (a) expand coverage of clinically relevant constructs while avoiding an increase in test length, (b) improve the quality of the test (i.e., reliability, validity, utility), and (c) update the norm reference sample to reflect contemporary population demographics and trends. In general, the developers attempted to improve the precision, accuracy, and diagnostic coverage of the MMPI–2–RF predecessor while simultaneously maintaining its fundamental organization and structure. Achieving this delicate balance was necessary to avoid sacrificing the immense quantity of validity research done that established the external correlates of the MMPI–2–RF substantive scales. As will become apparent, the test authors very much succeeded in this task.

The construction of the MMPI–3 proceeded in several phases. First, an expanded MMPI–2–RF was created that included its 338 previous items, in addition to 95 trial items. Also, 39 of the 338 MMPI–2–RF items were reworded to improve comprehension. This resulted in an expanded experimental version of the test termed the MMPI–2–RF-EX. This version was administered to several developmental samples for a series of validation analyses, along with examination of how scores on the MMPI–3 compared with those of the MMPI–2–RF.

MMPI–3 scale development was initiated with the MMPI–2–RF *RC* scales (i.e., *RC1–RC9*). Item analyses were done to ensure the distinctiveness of the scales and internal consistency. Next, similar analyses were done on the SP scales. Updating the *H-O* scales began with the items remaining available after the *RC* and SP analyses were completed. Any items that detracted from the internal consistency of the *H-O* scale to which they were assigned were dropped from further use. In addition, items found to correlate in a discriminant manner with its assigned *H-O* scale, and which was also consistent with scale content, were retained. Hence, the test developers were utilizing an integration of empirical and conceptual methods to create the new scales, which was in contrast to employing a pure actuarial method of empirical criterion keying as defined prior. Finally, the *PSY-5* scales were developed in the same fashion as were the *H-O* scales using the remaining previous, redrafted, and new items by their original authors Harkness and McNulty. Prior to finalizing the item assignments, the new and redrafted items were investigated for their psychometric comparability using a bilingual Spanish–English sample of 57 individuals. Items that show less than 80% bilingual response agreement and insufficient item total score and internal consistency correlations were dropped from the MMPI–3. This resulted in the final 335 items that comprise the new MMPI–3 substantive scales.

The final phase regarded development of the MMPI–3 validity scales. Using the 335 items found for the substantive scales, the MMPI–3 validity scales were formulated using the identical strategies used in formulating the MMPI–2–RF validity scales (discussed previously). Consequently, the MMPI–3 possesses that same quantity and type of validity scales as for the MMPI–2–RF. Thus, there is no need to repeat the details here. (The interested the reader is referred to § Development of the MMPI–2–RF, subsection Validity Scales.)

The final version of the MMPI–3 consists of 335 items and 52 scales. The scale breakdowns are as follows (total number of scales in parentheses): (a) validity scales ($n = 10$); (b) H-O scales ($n = 3$); (c) *RC* scales ($n = 8$); (d) SP scales ($n = 26$); and (e) *PSY-5* scales ($n = 5$). The SP scales are further subdivided into (a) somatic/cognitive scales ($n = 5$); (b) internalizing scales ($n = 10$); (c) externalizing scales ($n = 7$); and (d) interpersonal scales ($n = 5$). Factor analyses and scale intercorrelations found significant associations among the internalizing, externalizing, and *PSY-5* scales with the broad-based H-O scales, which gave the test a hierarchical organization as seen in the MMPI–2–RF. This will be reviewed in more detail when discussing the MMPI–3 interpretive process subsequently.

There are also several modifications in the MMPI–3 scales as compared to the MMPI–2–RF scales that are worthy of mention. First, the *RC3* has been transformed into a cynicism scale (*CYN*), which is classified within the externalizing SP scales. Family problems (*FML*) remains in the MMPI–3 test, although it has been reclassified from the interpersonal SP scales to the externalizing SP scales. This is due to its stronger association with acting-out behavior and interpersonal conflict (Ben-Porath & Tellegen, 2020a). An impulsivity (*IMP*) scale has also been added to this externalizing classification, which is a symptom of many personality disorders (American Psychiatric Association, 2013). In a related matter, the interpersonal passivity (*IPP*) scale has been keyed in the reverse direction and relabeled dominance (*DOM*), although it remains classified with the interpersonal SP scales. Self-importance (*SFI*) is new and has also been added to the interpersonal SP scales and targets narcissism. The stress/worry (*STW*) scale has been dichotomized into two independent scales, which are titled stress (*STR*) and worry (*WRY*), although both remain with the internalizing SP scales. A more expansive anxiety scale has been added to the internalizing SP scales, which is appropriately termed anxiety-related experiences (*ARX*). Within the same class, multiple specific fears (*MSF*) was dropped due to insufficient items. Lastly, eating concerns (*EAT*) is new and classified with the somatic/cognitive SP scales, although gastrointestinal complaints (*GIC*) and head pain complaints (*HPC*) have been dropped due to insufficient quality.

NORM REFERENCE DATA

There were two standardization samples, including one for English and one for Spanish. In the interest of brevity, only the English normative sample will be reported here. Targets for the norm reference sample were based on the U.S. Census Bureau population proportion projections for age and ethnicity in the 2020 census (U.S. Census Bureau, 2017a). Criteria for education were based on reported 2017 education distributions with a correction that attempted to adjust such estimates for the 2020 projections (U.S. Census Bureau, 2017b), although such correction was not further explicated (Ben-Porath & Tellegen, 2020b, p. 33). The English standardization sample consisted of 810 males and 810 females, which were stratified according to age, education, and race/ethnicity as indicated by the aforementioned 2020 U.S. Census projections.

More specifically, the ages ranged from 18 years to more than 80 years. Concerning ethnicity, Whites represented at 60.3%, Hispanic 14%, Black 12.4%, Asian 5.1%, Mixed Race 4.5%, and Other 3.7%, most of which were comparable to the 2020 projections. The exception was a slight underrepresentation of the Hispanic subgroup. Education level consisted of 34.8% college graduate, 27.7% some college, 29% high school graduate, and 8.6% no high school. These figures were commensurate with 2020 projections, with a minor underrepresentation of the lowest education subgroup and an overrepresentation of those in the highest education subgroup. Finally, age bands and percentages were as follows: (a) 18–29 years (21.6%), (b) 30–59 years (55.7%), (c) 60–79 years (20.6%), and (d) 80+ years (2.1%). These figures indicate an underrepresentation of the older age subgroups, especially the 80-plus cohort. However, the MMPI–3 standardization sample overall showed a better match with its projected population figures than both the MMPI–2 and MMPI–2–RF did with their population demographics.

ADMINISTRATION

Not surprisingly, the MMPI–3 administration procedures mirror those for the MMPI–2–RF. Therefore, the information covered here will be limited to that which is essential and unique to the MMPI–3. Where the two tests overlap on vital features, these are presented in abbreviated fashion. For more detail, the reader is referred to the MMPI–2–RF administration section presented in prior.

The MMPI–3 consists of 335 *True–False* items, which require an average estimated reading level of between fourth and fifth grade (Ben-Porath & Tellegen, 2020a, p. 24). This is about one grade level lower than the MMPI–2–RF. It is interesting that the MMPI–3 test developers initially considered a four-point polytomous response format, consisting of *Definitely True, Mostly True, Mostly False,* and *Definitely False*. The objective was to enhance test precision (Ben-Porath & Tellegen, 2020b, p. 19). However, a study comparing the standard *True–False* versus the aforesaid polytomous format found only slight increases in test reliability in favor of the latter, which did not justify changing to the more discriminative response alternatives (see Finn, Ben-Porath, & Tellegen, 2015).

The MMPI–3 can be administered by the same modalities as the MMPI–2–RF. These include test booklet and answer sheet and by computer via the Q-global (Pearson, 2021) online platform. Once on Q-global (i.e., https://qglobal.pearsonclinical.com/qg/login.seam), the examinee's basic identifying information is entered (viz., name, ID number, birth date, gender), the appropriate test selected (viz., MMPI–3 English), and additional demographics checked (viz., relationship status, education, and ethnicity). The most common administrative mode is "In Person Online," wherein the examinee completes the inventory while on the Pearson web page. A "Screen Lock" function precludes examinees from using the computer to search the Internet or computer software and files. After "Launch Assessment" is selected, the instructions appear regarding how to use the *True–False* format and to answer all items. An "Enter Audio" function also appears on the initial instructions screen. If selected, the MMPI–3 items are read to the examinee. Other modes include "Paper Form Manual Entry" and "Send Link Via Email, Remote On-Screen." The former permits booklet responses to be entered by keyboard and scored by computer, while the latter permits an examinee to complete the test at a location outside the facility.

Average administration time varies by modality as follows: (a) computerized is 25–35 minutes and (b) booklet and answer sheet is 35–50 minutes. As indicated when discussing the MMPI restructured tests, an 18-year-old can be administered the MMPI–A–RF, MMPI–2–RF, or the MMPI–3. The principal consideration in determining which test to administer depends on the estimated degree of autonomy achieved by examinees of this age, which typically is indicated by their living circumstances, demonstrated judgment, and cognitive abilities as manifested during the initial assessment and mental status examination. That is, if prospective examinees are working, living alone or with a partner, and are showing other indicators of social maturity and autonomy, the adult MMPI–2–RF and MMPI–3 tests are more logical alternatives. In contrast, if individuals are enrolled in school, continue to live at home, and are showing other indicators of social immaturity more indicative of adolescence, then the MMPI–A–RF is the more felicitous choice. The choice between the MMPI–3 and MMPI–2–RF most likely depends on the degree to which scale differences address the diagnostic issues of a case and the comfort level and resources of the testing psychologist.

All other administrative rules are the same as for the MMPI–2–RF. For instance, all items should be answered, the examiner should be present and available during administration, and dictionary definitions of words can be provided to the examinee if needed. An advantage of computer administration is that double-marked answers, which are unscorable, are precluded by the administration software.

SCORING

Similar to administration, MMPI–3 scoring is virtually identical to that of the MMPI–2–RF. Therefore, the discussion here will be circumscribed to (a) highlighting facets that are unique to the MMPI–3 and (b) presenting vital features that are shared by the two instruments in abbreviated fashion. The purpose is to avoid unnecessary redundancy. The reader is referred to the scoring section of the MMPI–2–RF for more details regarding this aspect of testing.

The MMPI–3 Data Yield   The MMPI–3 can be scored by computer on the Q-global (Pearson, 2021) online platform or by hand using a series of plasticized scoring templates. In terms of efficiency and cost-effectiveness, computer scoring is clearly most favored. In addition to the advantages of reduced scoring error, the computerized data output provides the percentage of items responded to on each scale, which is vital for appraising validity, along with an enumeration of all critical items answered in the keyed direction. The latter includes affirmative responses to items with suicidal ideation or intent, which should be addressed with some degree of urgency.

As for the MMPI–2–RF, the MMPI–3 substantive scales (i.e., diagnostic scales) employ uniform *T*–scores (*UT*) versus linear *T*–scores. To reiterate, the purpose of *UT*–scores is to create standard scores that possess the same PRs across all diagnostically related scales. The composite standard score values that were statistically computed for both MMPI restructured forms, and which are used for the MMPI–3, are available in the MMPI–2–RF scoring manual (Ben-Porath & Tellegen, 2011, Table 3-4, p. 15). Furthermore, Table 11.1 juxtaposes the linear *T*–score/PR values for comparison purposes. Although the *UT*–score distribution is positively skewed, they are practically speaking very similar to the *T*–score PRs. Therefore, note that in Form 11.7, which consists of all the data tables designed for reporting MMPI–3 test results within a psychological assessment report, PRs enumerated within the tables are based on the standard normal distribution. Recall that this was done for both the MMPI–A–RF (Form 11.5) and MMPI–2–RF (Form 11.6). This practice also makes the standard score PR estimates for the MMPI–3 comparable to other tests that report PRs according to the normal distribution, which are considerable in number.

Regarding the MMPI–3 Q-global report options, there is the score report and interpretive report. Again, the score report provides all the data needed for using the MMPI–3 data tables presented in Form 11.7. In order of presentation, the score report provides the following data output: (a) validity scales; (b) *H-O* and *RC* scales; (c) somatic/cognitive and internalizing scales; (d) externalizing and interpersonal scales; (e) *PSY-5* scales; (f) MMPI–3 *T*–scores by domain; and (g) item level information (unscorable responses and critical responses). The validity and substantive scales are also graphed to facilitate interpretation (e.g., profile analysis).

Determining MMPI–3 Validity   As done for the other MMPI tests, Figure 11.5 is available for download on Routledge's e-resources website and provides a visual flowchart that outlines a recommended interpretive approach to the MMPI–3. Analogous to the MMPI–2–RF, test interpretation is initiated with examination of the validity scales. This is designated in Figure 11.5 (top box), and in Form 11.7 wherein data tables 1–3 contain three classes of validity scales, namely, non-responsive, overreporting, and underreporting. Table 1 comprises various types of non-responding that result in unscorable items. Three are identical to that of the MMPI–2–RF, whereas a scale new to the MMPI–3 already appears on the MMPI–A–RF (see Form 11.5), namely, Combined Response Inconsistency (*CRIN*). Because the interpretive approach to these scales is identical to both the MMPI–A–RF and MMPI–2–RF, it will not be repeated here. However, it is important to reiterate that the reason non-responding validity scales are interpreted first is that, if they are invalid, all other validity and substantive scales will result in the same fate.

Table 2 enumerates the overreporting validity scales (Form 11.7). Again, use of the objective "overreporting" terminology is intended to avoid both negative connotation and potential inaccuracy. Any embellished inferential statements, such as "faking bad," require evidence external to the test data and should be refrained from

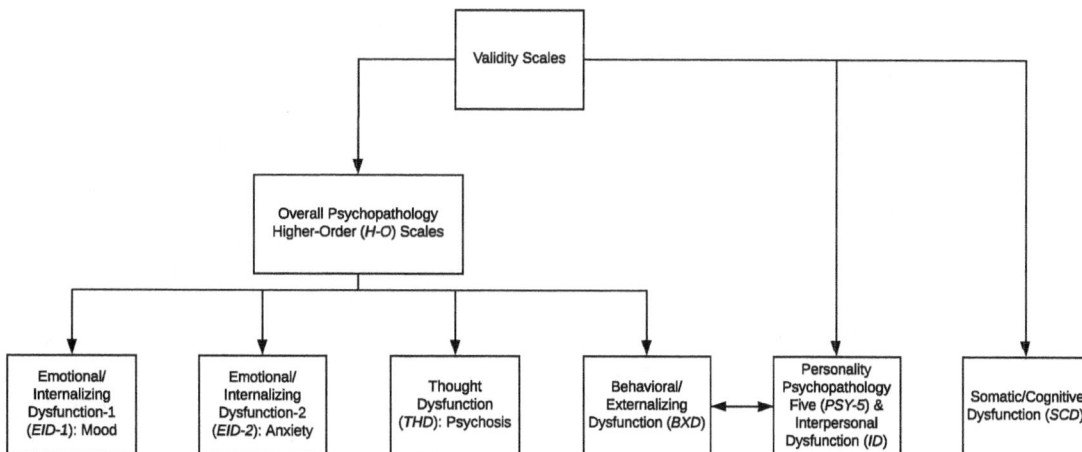

Figure 11.5 Minnesota Multiphasic Personality Inventory, Third Edition (MMPl-3) Interpretive Process

unless such evidence can be provided. These scales are virtually identical to those on the MMPI–2–RF, and thus should be utilized in similar fashion. It is noteworthy that that MMPI–3 manual lists somewhat different thresholds for interpreting the overreporting scales. Thus, to enhance test utility, these thresholds were averaged to render them uniform across all five scales, which consist of four levels of elevation as follows: (a) 20–79, normal; (b) 80–89, mild; (c) 90–99, moderate; and (d) 100–120, marked. These are listed in the specific table notes and are consistent with the recommendation by the test authors to use such thresholds in a heuristic manner and not as absolute markers.

Finally, Table 3 lists the two underreporting validity scales (Form 11.7). These are also identical to those used in the MMPI–2–RF and again should be interpreted in the same manner. Note that both general and specific notes follow each table, which define its principal contents, including data metrics, results, and test-taking sets measured by each scale. Perhaps most importantly, pre-drafted narrative interpretations of various results follow each table and their notes. These generally include versions for the following results: valid, cautiously valid, and invalid. If results are valid, the examiner should retain the valid interpretation, delete the remaining versions, and efficiently move on to the next table. If results are cautiously valid, the substantive scales should be interpreted in such manner that counters (or adjusts for) whatever atypical test-taking pattern was responsible for qualifying the validity results. For example, if an underreporting response set is detected, then the substantive scale scores should be interpreted as falling toward the higher ends of the reported CIs to offset likely underestimates of psychopathology. Following the three validity scales, an "MMPI–3 Validity Conclusion" appears wherein the validity results should be integrated and an overall interpretive approach to the substantive scales delineated. This approach should then be employed consistently throughout the remainder of the MMPI–3 interpretive process. As shown in Figure 11.5 (see e-resources), once validity of the test has been established, along with the interpretive approach for the ensuing substantive scales, diagnostically related test interpretation can begin in earnest. The reason validity analysis is relatively extensive on these personality inventory measures is that the diagnostic usefulness of the data output relies heavily on examinees' willingness and ability to report their symptoms honestly and accurately. Now begins interpretation of the MMPI–3 substantive scales.

INTERPRETATION: MMPI–3 SUBSTANTIVE SCALES

Figure 11.5 (see e-resources) serves as a visual guide for the MMPI–3 interpretive process, while Form 11.7 displays the more corresponding data tables. Hereafter, this part is divided into two subsections. The first examines the general organization and structure of the MMPI–3 as portrayed in Figure 11.5 (see e-resources). The second describes how the particular substantive scales can be effectively interpreted using Form 11.7.

General Organization and Structure   The MMPI–3 is organized in hierarchical fashion, analogous to the MMPI–2–RF. At the broadest level are the *H-O* scales, which are designed to measure the examinee's emotional, thinking, and behavioral functioning. This is portrayed in Figure 11.5 (see e-resources) by the mid-level box titled "Overall Psychopathology, Higher-Order (*H—O*) Scales." Thereafter, four arrows point downward toward the SP scales that contribute to (i.e., are most correlated with) one of the corresponding *H-O* scales. A higher score among an *H-O* scale indicates that there will tend to be higher elevations among its SP scales and vice versa. Note that in Figure 11.5, there are two *EID* subsets labeled mood (*EID-1*) and anxiety (*EID-2*). The former contains scales that are most conceptually similar to depressive and hypomanic/manic episodes; hence the term "mood." The latter consists of scales that are most conceptually similar to psychopathologies that were previously classified in the *DSM–IV–TR* as anxiety disorders (see American Psychiatric Association, 2000), including OCD, *post-traumatic stress disorder* (*PTSD*), and *GAD*; hence the term "anxiety." The reasons for this apportionment are both conceptual and quantitative. Keeping them together would have resulted in an excessive number of scales, making it an unwieldy table for purposes of test interpretation, while the division assists more effectively in differential diagnosis because it is more consistent with *DSM* nosology.

At the bottom level of Figure 11.5 (see e-resources) are two types of scales as follows: (a) SP scales and (b) *PSY-5* scales. The SP scales may be differentiated into those that are assigned to an *H-O* scale and those that are not. The latter consist of *ID* and *SCD* scales. This is portrayed in Figure 11.5 by the lack of any connective arrows between the *H-O* scales and the *ID* and *SMD* scales. The *PSY-5* scales are also independent of the *H-O* scales, which is consistent with the manner they were developed (see earlier in this chapter). As will become apparent next, this organizational structure affords the testing psychologist a number of flexible interpretive strategies, which is required in testing practice due to the significant variability in case facts and diagnostic issues. Next, Form 11.7 will be scrutinized in terms of the substantive data yield and interpreting the MMPI–3 results within the context of a psychological assessment report.

Interpretive Process   Prior to initiating this discussion, some preliminary comments are in order. First, all the data tables in Form 11.7 are designed in comparable fashion to those of both the MMPI–A–RF and MMPI–2–RF tests. More specifically, they include a sequence of columns for the scale abbreviated name, *T*–score, CI, PR, and a summary of the measured symptoms or traits. Within the CI column of each data table, an *SEM* value is inserted for each scale. The *SEM* was based on those reported in the MMPI–3 technical manual that were computed from each scale's test–retest stability coefficient (Ben-Porath & Tellegen, 2020b, Tables 3-3 through 3-6, pp. 47–48). In the case of the MMPI–3, separate *SEM* values were reported for men and women. Therefore, when such values differed between the sexes, they were averaged and rounded up to be more conservative in estimating the certainty of the true score value. As done for the two restructured MMPI tests, a 68% CI was selected such that the interval would not become excessively wide for effective ipsative analysis among an examinee's scale scores.

Second, the data tables are immediately ensued by general and specific table notes, which are devoted to delineating the score metrics, the directional meaning of the scores, the associated full-scale name, the meaning of table abbreviations, definitions of key statistics, and diagnostic meaning of various score elevations. Third, pre-drafted interpretive excerpts follow each data table, generally describing WNL results, along with the meaning of abnormal score elevations. The excerpts are meant as interpretive guides and may be modified to fit the particular test results. Fourth, it is noteworthy that the most detailed interpretive excerpts are found following Table 9, which address the *PSY-5* and *ID* scales. This is because the elucidation of personality psychopathology tends to be more intricate and complex than describing clinical syndromes.

The remainder of this discussion proceeds through the MMPI–3 data tables. The focus is on the basic scale content of each table and what they have to offer in terms of psychodiagnosis. Because the organization and structure of the MMPI–3 and MMPI–2–RF are remarkably similar, the presentation here will focus on highlighting the essential and unique aspects of the MMPI–3. Note that the MMPI–3 scale names no longer have the "r" appendage because they have been modified and updated from their original restructuring.

The standard approach to interpreting the MMPI–3 substantive scales is to begin at the most general level, then proceed to more specific scales contingent upon the particular preceding *H-O* scale profile. Table 4 (Form 11.7) lists the three *H-O* scales, including *T*–score, 68% CI, and PR, along with a summary of the measured symptoms. A 68% CI was selected to prevent the interval from becoming excessively large and imprecise for effective analysis. The initial focus should be on a norm-based analysis, which can then be ensued by an ipsative examination if needed. A spiked profile indicates that the symptoms are variable and of a particular kind, which assists in differential diagnosis. If all three *H-O* scales are high, then a relative analysis should help indicate which of the more narrowly defined scales can be prioritized. Here, the CIs would be the focus of an intraindividual or ipsative analysis. That is, intervals that do not overlap are interpreted as statistically different from each other, while overlapping CIs indicate a lack of differential score elevations. Following Table 4 (Form 11.7) are interpretive summaries for each of the *H-O* scales, ensued by excerpts that guide ipsative analysis. In all instances, however, the specific diagnostic issues of a case should supersede other considerations and guide the analysis. In fact, if the case diagnostic questions are sufficiently well defined and narrow in scope (e.g., "Rule out personality disorder, especially borderline"), the *H-O* scales can be circumvented and the examiner can proceed directly to the pertinent scales on the lowest, most diagnostically specific, level of Figure 11.5 (see e-resources). Following analysis at the broad *H-O* scale level, the next step is to proceed to the more narrowly defined SP, *PSY-5*, *ID*, and *SCD* scales, which are located at the lowest level in Figure 11.5. The ensuing discussion will cover these scales in said order.

In the event the *EID H-O* scale is significantly elevated and/or the diagnostic issues regard emotional-type symptoms, Tables 5 and 6 in Form 11.7 become the consequential focus of the analysis. Table 5 contains scales that are most conceptually similar to depressive (i.e., unipolar) and hypo/manic (i.e., bipolar) disorders. This table is also relevant in cases with questions regarding suicidal symptoms and risk of self-harm. Table 6 consists of scales that target anxiety, stress, apprehension, trauma-related disorder, dissociative phenomena, and both obsessions and compulsions. As compared to the MMPI–2–RF, the MMPI–3 has become more robust in detecting OCD-like symptoms, stress, GAD, and trauma.

Table 7 contributes to the thought dysfunction (*THD*) *H-O* scale and therefore covers psychosis, including delusions, hallucinations, and thought disturbance. These data should be given priority in the event the *THD H-O* scale dominates the broad-level profile. This table can also be used with Table 5 if there is a differential diagnostic question among a mood disorder with or without psychosis, schizophrenia, and schizoaffective disorder. In particular, the relative score elevations should assist in making such a diagnostic discrimination. Moderate elevations on Table 7 data can also identify a personality disorder or trauma-disorder with transient psychotic features.

Table 8 comprises the SP scales assigned to the behavioral/externalizing dysfunction (*BXD*) *H-O* scale. If this *BXD H-O* scale elevates above the others, whether norm based or ipsative based, this data table should become the focus of subsequent analysis. It contains scales that are associated with antisocial, aggressive, conduct-disordered, and impulsive behavior patterns, along with traits associated with interpersonal conflict. These data can also effectively supplement the *PSY-5* and *ID* data in the differential diagnosis of personality disorder, especially those with acting-out traits or defenses. Finally, Table 8 scales are relevant when the differential diagnosis includes a question about both the presence and degree of substance-use disorders, especially alcohol. If the substance abuse (*SUB*) scale elevates, examination of critical item content can reveal more specifically which drugs were identified among the items answered in the keyed direction. More specifically, items address use of alcohol, cannabis, prescription drugs, and general drug use associated with acting-out behaviors.

Table 9 integrates the *PSY-5* scales with the *ID* SP scales. There are several arguments in favor of this decision. First, conceptually they complement each other effectively, especially when interpreted in proximity rather than in separate tables. Second, personality psychopathology has its most deleterious effects upon interpersonal relationships (American Psychiatric Association, 2013). Hence, one can easily hypothesize these two variables as having a causal link. Third, these constructs may be found in several personality disorders as part of their listed criteria, hence facilitating diagnosis and treatment planning. As can be seen, the *PSY-5* and *ID* scales are interspersed rather than listed within their original groupings (e.g., *PSY-5* scales first, followed by *ID* scales). Rather, they are sequenced by conceptual similarity. Therefore, the first several scales cover aggression and dominance (i.e., antisocial traits), grandiosity (i.e., narcissism), and impulsivity (which is associated with many personality disorders), followed by emotional instability (i.e., neuroticism), psychoticism (i.e., schizotypal or transient psychotic episodes), disliking others (i.e., schizoid traits), and traits that indicate dependent and avoidant characteristics. Again, note the greater degree of interpretive detail following this table, the purpose of which is to facilitate the description of personality diagnosis and targets for treatment planning.

It is also noteworthy in Figure 11.5 (see e-resources) that the *PSY-5* and *ID* scales can be interpreted directly following the validity scales because they are not related to the broad-based *H-O* scales. This strategy is ideal in cases where personality differential diagnosis represents the core part of the testing case. Furthermore, as alluded to prior, the double arrows between the PSY-5/*ID* box and *BXD* SP scales in Figure 11.5 (see e-resources) denotes the close conceptual relationship between the two scale clusters. In particular, the *BXD* SP scales can assist in identifying personality disorders with acting-out defenses or traits, including the assessment of a risk for violence or danger to others.

Finally, Table 10 includes *SCD* SP scales that are also independent of all three *H-O* scales. Additionally, they are narrowly specialized in terms of measured constructs. In particular, these scales measure symptoms most consistent with the *DSM–5* general class of somatization disorders, which is evinced by the all-too-conspicuous presence of *RC1*. Recall that *RC1* can be historically traced back to the original MMPI clinical scale named hypochondriasis, currently known as *anxiety illness disorder*, although still classified under the somatization disorders in *DSM–5* nosology. This scale essentially indicates that the examinee manifests physiological symptoms in response to stress; that is, such clients somatize their psychological stress. Further, both neurological complaints (*NUC*) and cognitive complaints (*COG*) can be employed as screening data for possible neurocognitive dysfunction, which is evidence of medical necessity for neuropsychological testing. Lastly, as addressed before, the new scale EAT is indicative of an eating disorder. Subsequent item analysis can assist in narrowing the diagnostic alternatives by targeting key symptoms, including binging, purging, and restricting.

SUMMARY

This concludes a review of the contemporary MMPI restructured forms, both adolescent and adult, along with the newest adult MMPI–3 form. They are all very similar in structure and organization, largely due to their comparable development. That is, each test was developed based on an impressive series of (a) factor analyses, (b) internal consistency correlations, (c) temporal stability coefficients, (d) scale intercorrelations, and (e) external correlations. The last item was vital in terms of test validation, that is, providing empirical evidence that the vast number of scales measure the symptoms and problematic behavioral patterns and traits they claim to measure. Therefore, test interpretations based on their data output are founded on both conceptual and statistical methods of assessment and not solely, or even primarily, on empirical criterion keying. Scale content is also more conceptually pure in the sense that they measure more well-defined constructs with significantly less confounding. This is divergent from the predecessors MMPI, MMPI–2, and MMPI–A, which used scales that were seriously confounded and based on either statistical or conceptual methods of development. However, this is the direction of most contemporary personality inventories (see, e.g., Greene, 2011).

The MMPI–3 presentation was briefer in that it has been very recently published and is extremely comparable to its predecessor the MMPI–2–RF. Therefore, the discussion emphasized its most important facets, especially those that are unique to its design. The objective was to enable clinicians to determine which of the two to select for a particular adult testing case. Next, this chapter felicitously concludes by presenting the NEO–PI–3, which is currently being used as a measure of the *DSM–5* alternative personality disorders dimensional model. Therefore, presenting this final test represents an auspicious opportunity to introduce the FFM of personality, including its history and development, along with the *DSM–5* alternative dimensional model of personality disorders. In addition to being applied to a newly developed model of personality disorders, this test also affords both self-report and observer-report formats and is normed for both adolescents and adults.

The NEO Personality Inventory Series

This final major section of the chapter introduces a series of NEO Personality Inventories (NEO-PI) that originated from a broad-based dimensional model of normal personality (i.e., the *normal perspective*; see Ben-Porath, 1994), as opposed to the Millon and MMPI tests that have explicitly focused on abnormality and the *clinical perspective* from their inception. It is only more recently that the model upon which the NEO-PIs originated have been applied to the measurement of abnormality or psychopathology. Because of their unique history, this section will begin with the typical synopsis of the NEO-PI tests, followed by a review of the Five-Factor Model (FFM) upon which they were founded, and finally discussing the development the principal test used in the test inventory and the manner in which it can be effectively employed in mental health testing practice (viz., the NEO–PI–3). Thereafter, the typical sections follow, although the norm reference section necessarily includes information concerning its development, as the two topics are highly interrelated.

SYNOPSIS

The *NEO Personality Inventories* (*NEO-PI*; McCrae & Costa, 2010) consist of a group of structured self- and observer-report tests designed to measure the major dimensions or domains of personality for individuals aged 12 years, 0 months through 85 years, 11 months. The principal test is the *NEO Personality Inventory, Third Edition* (*NEO–PI–3*) because (a) it provides the most comprehensive data on personality and (b) it contains the most updated norms. In particular, the test consists of 240 items that may be responded to using a Likert-type scale and yields data on the 5 *domains* that comprise the FFM and their 30 *facets* of personality. Domains are broad-based dispositions, whereas *facets* are more narrowly defined aspects of personality that together define a domain.

The other two most relevant NEO Inventories are as follows: (a) NEO PI–R; and (b) *NEO Five-Factor Inventory, Third Edition* (*NEO–FFI–3*). The NEO PI–R is the immediate predecessor to the NEO–PI–3. Compared to the NEO–PI–3, it contains 37 different items that are now outdated and not as effectively written, along with older norms. The NEO–FFI–3 is a 60-item brief version of the NEO–PI–3 in that its data yield is limited to the five domains (i.e., no data are available concerning facets). Because accurate personality disorder diagnoses cannot be made when data are so limited, this precludes use of the NEO–FFI–3 for said purpose. For these reasons, the NEO PI–R and NEO–FFI–3 will be not discussed further as they are not appropriate for contemporary mental health testing practice.

All NEO Inventories have two versions, including Form S for self-report and Form R for observer-report. These are parallel forms of the test because they contain virtually the same items and personality data. The major modification is that Form R items are worded in the third person such that a peer, family member, expert (e.g., a psychotherapist), or other individual who possesses adequate knowledge of the examinee can be recruited to provide such personality data.

To provide a meaningful history of the NEO–PI–3, a brief review of the FFM of personality is needed. This is because the NEO–PI–3 is designed to operationalize or measure the broad domains and specific facets (i.e., traits) proposed by such a model. Research supporting the FFM will then provide a framework from which the development of the NEO–PI–3 can be understood in proper context. Thereafter, historical development of the NEO–PI–3 will be afforded, followed by the manner in which it is used in psychodiagnosis.

THE FIVE-FACTOR MODEL OF PERSONALITY

The *Five-Factor Model* (*FFM*), which is also referred to as the *Big Five*, consists of a taxonomy of personality constructs that to date has received the most attention, empirical support, and acceptance by personality researchers (Costa & McCrae, 1995; Goldberg, 1981; McCrae & John, 1992; Saucier & Goldberg, 1996). Development of the FFM began when personality researchers started investigating the following fundamental question: "What are the most important human traits?" Here, traits are defined as "pervasive consistencies in thoughts, feelings, and behaviors" (McCrae & Costa, 2010, p. 59). Such a question assumes human traits actually exist and hence was pursued by researchers practicing within the *dispositional domain* of personality theory, that is, the inherent tendency of people to behave in particular ways. As will be seen, the FFM evolved by means of two approaches in identifying the most important traits, that is, the lexical and statistical approaches.

Two well-known trait theorists, Allport and Odbert (1936), scrutinized the English dictionary and identified in excess of 17,000 trait terms and classified them as follows: (a) stable traits; (b) temporary states, moods, and activities;

(c) social evaluations; and (d) metaphorical, physical, and doubtful terms. Thereafter, Cattell (1943) analyzed the 4,500 stable traits and reduced them to 35 clusters or groupings of personality trait terms using a lexical approach.

The *lexical approach* to identifying the most important traits is based on the assumption that important individual differences in personality become encoded into our natural language over time (Goldberg, 1981; John, 1990; Ostendorf, 1990). The underlying reasoning here is that the terms used in written and spoken language become embedded into the lexicon because they maximize adaptation; that is, they assist people in understanding themselves and others and ultimately contribute to making wiser choices in terms of behavior. This approach includes the following two criteria for identifying important traits: (a) synonym frequency and (b) cross-cultural universality. *Synonym frequency* proposes that there is a positive relationship between the number of synonyms created for a trait and its importance in describing human personality; that is, the more synonyms, the more important that trait, and the fewer synonyms, the less important. Further, a trait that is codified into many different languages, and hence has high *cross-cultural universality*, indicates that it is more vital as regarding human affairs and overall adaptation.

The inception of the FFM arrived when Fiske (1949) was able to employ the newly available factor analysis (i.e., a *statistical approach* to identifying the most important traits). Succinctly, *factor analysis* is a statistical procedure that identifies which terms correlate with each other, although they tend not to correlate with other terms. When terms correlate in such a manner, they co-vary uniquely to form a factor or domain of personality. In that sense, factor analysis is also referred to as a data-reduction technique, which takes numerous interrelated terms and forms a smaller quantity of broad-based factors or dispositions. In essence, Fiske had a small sample of subjects rate themselves using 22 of Cattell's 35 trait clusters, factor analyzed their ratings, and discovered an inchoate five-factor solution. That is, Fiske (1949) was the first to discover a crude version of the model, which lacked more refined structure at that early point in development.

Subsequently, Tupes and Christal (1961) factor analyzed the same 22 trait clusters across 8 samples of people and evinced a more distinctive five-factor model consisting of the following broad domains: (a) surgency (i.e., extraversion), (b) agreeableness, (c) conscientiousness, (d) emotional stability (i.e., emotional instability or neuroticism), and (e) culture (i.e., openness). The labels for each factor were those that they believed best summarized the content of the terms to which they loaded (i.e., a factor loading). Briefly, a *factor loading* is the degree to which a specific term correlates with its assigned factor. The higher the factor loading, the more a term represents the presence of its factor. Also note that the terms denote one end of a bipolar dimension. Hence, for example, extraversion forms a bipolar dimension or continuum with introversion at the opposing end. Hence, the specific structure of the FFM was now identified.

The FFM has been subsequently replicated by numerous independent personality researchers (Botwin & Buss, 1989; Digman & Inouye, 1986; Goldberg, 1981; Norman, 1963; Rammstedt, Goldberg, & Borg, 2010). It also has been found to exist in different languages and cultures in every decade for the past approximately 50 years (Rammstetd at al., 2010). Lastly, and most significantly, the FFM, or Big Five, has most recently been espoused in somewhat modified form by the *DSM–5* as the alternative trait model for personality disorder diagnosis (American Psychiatric Association, 2013, Section III, Emerging Measures and Models, Alternative *DSM–5* Model for Personality Disorders, pp. 761–781). More specifically, the authors of the *DSM–5* refer to their alternative trait model as "a maladaptive variant" of the Big Five because, as will become clear subsequently when discussing test interpretation, the primary labels for each factor/domain and facet are on the psychopathological end of the dimension (e.g., antagonistic versus agreeable; irresponsibility versus responsibility). Lastly, it follows that the NEO–PI–3, which is specifically designed to measure the FFM, is by logical extension a standardized personality test capable of measuring the presence of the newly proposed *DSM–5* broad-based domains and more narrowly defined facets. This brings us to the NEO–PI–3 (McCrae & Costa, 2010).

THE NEO PERSONALITY INVENTORY, THIRD EDITION

By the mid-1970s, a number of trait models were developed using the aforementioned strategies and methods. Each claimed to best represent the structure of human personality (e.g., Buss & Plomin, 1975; Eysenck & Eysenck, 1975; Guilford, Zimmerman, & Guilford, 1976; Cattell, Eber, & Tatsuoka, 1970). Although there were discrepancies among these models, Costa and McCrae believed there was sufficient agreement on two higher-order factors or major domains so as to begin developing a reliable or consistent model of personality structure; these were labeled neuroticism (N) and extroversion (E).

Next, analysis proceeded from these general domains to more specific traits (i.e., *facets*) due to the growing recognition that the latter provided a more comprehensive and detailed understanding of human personality, rather than remaining at the broad-based domain level of analysis (Briggs, 1989). Indeed, mounting evidence showed that these facets, which comprised each of these broad domains, possessed impressive degrees of predictive validity that actually surpassed simple reliance on the broad five factors or domains (Paunoman & Ashton, 2001; Reynolds & Clark, 2001).

The first official version of the NEO–PI–3 was published in 1978 as the NEO Inventory, which included the first two identified factors neuroticism and extroversion, the addition of a third domain labeled openness to experience (O), and 18 related facet scales (Costa & McCrae, 1976, 1978). In 1983, agreeableness (A) and conscientiousness (C) were incorporated and the test was published in 1985 as the NEO-Personality Inventory (NEO-PI) (Costa & McCrae, 1985). In 1990, some item modifications were made to the original three domains, and facet scales were added to the newer A and C domains, hence resulting in the 1992 NEO Personality Inventory-Revised Edition (NEO PI–R) (Costa & McCrae, 1992). The ensuing ten years consisted of the NEO PI–R being used with individuals aged ten through adulthood (Baker & Victor, 2003; De Fruyt, Mervielde, Hoekstra, & Rolland, 2000). Finally, in 2005, 37 of the 240 items were modified to improve the test's psychometric properties, resulting in the contemporary *NEO Personality Inventory, Third Edition* (*NEO–PI–3*; McCrae & Costa, 2010). This edition included the aforementioned five broad domains, along with their 30 facet scales (i.e., 6 facets per domain). Once again, the facet scales represent more narrowly defined constructs that more effectively differentiate the five domains. As a final note, the NEO–PI–3 computer scoring software calculates the five domains as "factors," which are considered more accurate empirical measures of the FFM. This is discussed further subsequently.

USE OF THE NEO–PI–3 IN MENTAL HEALTH PRACTICE

As indicated, the NEO–PI–3 was initially developed as a measure of normal human personality. That is, it originated from the broad-based *normal perspective* of personality theory and measurement (Ben-Porath, 1994). However, due to its robust research support as a comprehensive model and measure of human personality, it was eventually integrated into the practice of both counseling and psychotherapy (Costa & McCrae, 2008; McCrae & Costa, 1986; Piedmont, 1998; Singer, 2005). More pertinently, this instrument has been used in clinical psychology practice (Costa, 1991; Costa & McCrae, 2009) and in diagnosing personality disorders (Costa & Widiger, 2002; McCrae, Löckenhoff, & Costa, 2005). For instance, many of the clinical syndromes as defined in the *DSM–5*, such as *persistent depressive disorder*, have been conceptualized as personality dispositions in experiencing various moods (Widiger & Trull, 1992). Furthermore, relationships among several *DSM* clinical syndromes and the FFM have been documented (Costa & Widiger, 2002; Wiggins & Pincus, 1989). Relevant associations among NEO–PI–3 scale scores and both *DSM* clinical syndromes and personality disorders will be detailed subsequently when discussing test interpretation.

NORM REFERENCE DATA AND TEST DEVELOPMENT

The majority of previous research on the NEO–PI (Costa & McCrae, 1985) and NEO PI–R (Costa & McCrae, 1992) were based on two longitudinal samples. The latter version of the test contained a standardization sample that was selected to match the U.S. census projections for 1995 (U.S. Census Bureau, 1984). In contrast to the previous two versions, however, the NEO–PI–3 was designed to cover a larger age span. Therefore, new and more contemporary samples were obtained to develop and establish such norms for the NEO–PI–3. Norming and test development were done simultaneously and in three phases as follows: (a) adolescent sample, (b) adult sample, and (c) middle school sample. Prior to selecting these three samples, however, some vital item analyses were done on the test, which are described next.

To initiate item analysis, the NEO PI–R items were administered to 1,959 high school students. A total of 48 items were targeted for replacement due to low item-facet correlations and/or low readability. For each of three 48 items, two alternatives were written. The NEO PI–R and the new alternative items were first administered to the Phase I adolescent sample (McCrae, Costa, & Martin, 2005), then to the Phase 2 adult sample (McCrae, Martin, & Costa, 2005). They found that 37 of the 48 new items lowered readability and increased the median item-facet correlation; that is, the test was improved in terms of being readable and enhancing internal consistency. Consequently, the new items were incorporated into the test. The three phases of test development with the aforesaid samples were then initiated.

In Phase 1, previous NEO PI–R and new trial items were administered to 500 individuals ages 14–20 from 26 U.S. states, this being for the self-report Form S. Additional sibling pairs and ratings of anonymous targets were done for the observer-report Form R norms (McCrae Costa et al., 2005). In Phase 2, previous NEO PI–R and new trial items were administered to 635 men and women across 29 U.S. states, ranging in age from 21 to 91, who were asked to rate themselves for the norming of Form S. In addition, participants were recruited in pairs so as to permit them to rate each other for the norming of Form R (McCrae, Martin et al., 2005). Phase 3 consisted of 424 children ages 12–13 years, who were asked to either rate themselves for the further norming of Form S or rate an anonymous target for the further norming of Form R. Finally, the new test was administered to the Phase 3 boys and girls ages 12–13 (Costa, McCrae, & Martin, 2008). Analyses supported the use of the new test with this youngest age sample, both in terms of factor structure and internal consistency. After completion of these three phases, the test authors made the decision that the NEO–PI–3 norms would be based on the aforementioned Phase 1 and Phase 2 samples. Therefore, they essentially scored their responses to the NEO PI–R with the new and more effective 37 items. For adults, norms for the age range of 21–85 are based on the respondents for Form S and the targets of observer ratings for Form R. The NEO–PI–3 also has adolescent norms based on respondents or targets ages 14–20.

For each adult and adolescent norm group, the raw score means and standard deviations for the domain and facet scales for both Form S and Form R are presented in the professional manual (McCrae & Costa, 2010, Appendix B, pp. 111–119). The data are further broken down into gender-specific and gender-combined groupings. For adults, data are based on adults ages 21–90, including 279 males and 365 females ($N = 635$). Norms are provided for both gender-specific and combined groupings. For adolescents, norms are based on 242 males and 258 females ($N = 500$). Again, norms are given for both gender-specific and combined groupings. Research on middle-school samples indicates that the adolescent NEO–PI–3 norms are appropriate for both Form S and R (McCrae, Costa et al., 2005). Therefore, the adolescent norms are considered applicable to individuals ages 12–20 (McCrae & Costa, 2010), pp. 68 and 112).

ADMINISTRATION

Administration will focus on use of the NEO software system (Costa, McCrae, & PAR Staff, 2010), which loads by means of CD-ROM onto the testing psychologist's personal computer for purposes of electronic administration, scoring, and provision of an interpretive report. The score reports must be purchased from Psychological Assessment Resources (PAR) and downloaded to the NEO software system. The last two functions are done together and will be described later in this chapter. This section focuses only on the administrative process using this system.

At the opening screen, the examinee's demographics are entered, including name, office file or record number, birth date, and gender. The NEO–PI–3 is selected from the list, which also includes the NEO PI–R (i.e., the immediate predecessor to the NEO–PI–3) and NEO–FFI–3 (i.e., screening version, domains only). Next, a blank electronic answer sheet that resembles a large Scantron appears, after which Form S (i.e., self-report form) or Form R (i.e., observer-report form) can be selected. If Form R is selected, the rater's information is input, including "Rater Gender" immediately beneath the "Test Form" selection. The "Administer" button immediately beneath "Rater Gender" is then selected, which is ensued by (a) the number of available administrations in the psychologist's inventory and (b) a "continue" prompt.

The instructions ask the informant to select one of the following alternatives as applied to either oneself (Form S) or the examinee (Form R): 1 = *Strongly Disagree* (i.e., definitely false); 2 = *Disagree* (i.e., mostly false); 3 = *Neutral* (i.e., cannot decide or equally true and false); 4 = *Agree* (i.e., mostly true); and 5 = *Strongly Agree* (i.e., definitely true). Three sample items follow. Selecting a response automatically forwards to the next item, although "Previous" and "Next" selections permit moving back and forth. Items appear on the screen one at a time. After responding to the final item, a "Testing is complete . . . Call the administrator," prompt appears. Prior to saving and scoring, an electronic answer key once again appears. However, at this juncture, it is filled in with all the examinee's responses, along with a prompt to remind testing psychologists of the number of purchased administrations remaining in their test inventory).

Administration time is estimated to be 30–40 minutes (McCrae & Costa, 2010, p. 7). As a general rule, definitions of words the examinee does not understand can be provided. To facilitate the process of providing standardized definitions of words, a glossary of commonly asked terms by examinees is provided in the manual (McCrae & Costa, 2010, Table 3, p. 8). This glossary consists of words most frequently identified by middle school participants in Phase 3 of test development as problematic (see prior). Such definitions were drafted in consultation with middle school faculty. In cases where examinees continue to be confused as to (a) the item's meaning or (b) how to answer an item, an instruction to select the "3 = Neutral" alternative is permitted. A total of 41 or more omissions invalidates the protocol. For 1–40 omissions, the neutral alternative can be entered by the examiner for each such item, after which the protocol can be scored.

SCORING

The NEO–PI–3 can be scored manually or by either of two computerized versions. The latter include the following: (a) a professional report service in which a scannable (*SS*) answer sheet must be submitted to the publisher (PAR) for scoring and interpretation and (b) the NEO software system in which scoring and interpretation can be done

Table 11.2 NEO Personality Inventory, Third Edition (NEO–PI–3) T–score Range and Qualitative Descriptions

T–score Range	Percent of Sample[a]	Qualitative Description
66–100	7	Very high
56–65	24	High
45–55	38	Average
35–44	24	Low
0–34	7	Very low

Note. *T*–score mean = 50, standard deviation = 10; range = 0–100.
[a]Percent of the standardization sample that fell within the associated *T*–score range.

any time after the examinee completes the inventory (Costa, McCrae, & PAR Staff, 2010). As stated, the latter is the preferred and most convenient alternative. Irrespective of method, scoring is initiated by computing the facet scale raw scores. Again, facet scales measure the more specific traits that contribute to the Big Five domains or broad-based dispositions. For manual scoring, facet scale raw scores assigned to one of five domains scales are summed, hence resulting in five domain total raw scores. *Domain scales* consist of clusters of intercorrelated facets; hence they represent the more general or broad-based dispositions. Third, raw scores for all facets and domains are then transformed into standardized *T*–scores, with a mean of 50 and standard deviation of 10, range 0–100.

Computerized scoring employs the same computational sequence as does manual scoring, although it diverges in the calculation of the Big Five. Here, factor scales are computed in lieu of the domain scales. *Factor scales* represent the same broad-based constructs as domain scales; however, they are computed from a weighted combination of raw scores from *all 30* facet scales rather than simply from the raw scores derived from a single domain. Why the difference in calculation? In factor analyzing the data, many of the facet scale scores were found to possess secondary loadings on domains other than their principal one. When all 30 are considered in a weighted fashion consistent with their primary and secondary loadings, it leads to more accurate and pure measures of the FFM (McCrae & Costa, 1989; McCrae et al., 2008). This is why they are referred to as factor scales versus domain scales. Hence, domain scales are considered to be only approximations of the factor scales, which is another cogent reason for using the NEO software system. Although the weighted formulas are provided in the NEO Inventories manual (McCrae & Costa, 2010, Table 4, p. 8), they are complex and extremely time consuming to employ manually and thus are most efficiently scored by means of computer.

Table 11.2 summarizes the *T*–score ranges, the associated percent of the standardization sample that fell within each range, and the assigned qualitative description for each range provided by the test authors (McCrae & Costa, 2010, p. 17). The qualitative descriptions were chosen based on the following rationale: (a) they captured the expected percentages of the standardization sample consistent with characteristics of a normal distribution, and (b) the five qualitative descriptors were logically consistent with the five response alternatives for each item, ranging from "strongly disagree" to "strongly agree" (see prior).

Note that these are linear *T*–scores, which makes the assumption that such personality traits tend to be normally distributed in the population. In addition, the scales represent continuous dimensions with bipolar opposites (e.g., extraversion–introversion). Therefore, scores on such scales represent degrees of particular personality traits or tendencies. Specifically, the more extreme the score on a factor or facet scale (e.g., a *T*–score of 75 on extraversion), the greater likelihood that such an individual will show the trait's distinctive features. As a corollary, the less extreme or more average (i.e., centered) the score (e.g., a *T*–score of 52 on extraversion), the less likely the individual will show the trait's distinctive features; that is, that individual will most probably show a combination of extraverted and introverted proclivities, also known as "ambiverts" (McCrae & Costa, 2010, p. 17).

Although percentile ranks (PRs) are not provided by the interpretive report, the professional manual includes a conversion chart, listing *T*–scores ranging from 20 to 80 and their associated PR values (McCrae & Costa, 2010, Appendix F, p. 136). It is nearly identical to the standard score conversion table located in Appendix A, Table A.1 and referenced in previous chapters. It does provide more precise conversions among some of the *T*–scores, listing PRs to the hundredths place (i.e., one decimal place) rather than rounding only to the nearest whole PR number with no decimals. Therefore, for testing psychologists who wish to be as precise as possible where indicated, these more precise PRs were incorporated from the professional manual into the PRs previously obtained from MedFriendly (2020). As a result, examiners now have these two resources from which to insert the PR conversions, with the choice of being more or less precise contingent upon their discretion.

The final type of data, which is not provided in the NEO–PI–3 professional manual, are confidence intervals (CIs). A consistent theme of this book is that such data are vital in (a) communicating to the reader the degree of accuracy of a reported score and (b) assisting in the interpretation of significant differences among scale scores in the process of ipsative (i.e., intraindividual analysis); in other words, the analysis of relative differences in scale scores within the profile to supplement the initial normative comparisons with the general population of peers. In computing CIs, one needs an estimate of each scale's *standard error of measurement* (*SEM*). Although *SEM*s are not reported in the manual, reliability coefficients are reported from which *SEM*s can be computed using the following equation:

$$SEM = SD\sqrt{1 - r_{xx}}$$

Equation 11.3

where *SD* is the standard deviation of the pertinent metric being used, and r_{xx} represents one of several possible reliability coefficients for that scale. Because the metric being used here is a *T*–score, the *SD* value would be 10.

Additionally, selection of the most appropriate reliability coefficient (*r*) to insert into Equation 11.2 must be made. In this case, personality traits are being measured, which by definition should be relatively consistent or enduring over time. Based on this consideration, test–retest reliability coefficients (i.e., temporal stability coefficients) supersede that of internal reliability coefficients. One problem is that there are no data on test–retest reliability for the NEO–PI–3 in the professional manual. However, there is robust evidence showing that the NEO PI–R and NEO–PI–3 are equivalent, evincing very high equivalence among the correlations of virtually all scale scores, ranging from 0.98 to 0.99 for the factor scales and 0.83 to 0.99 for the facet scales (McCrae & Costa, 2010, p. 66), along with evidence of structural equivalence (e.g., McCrae, Zonderman, Costa, Bond, & Paunonen, 1996; De Fruyt, De Bolle, McCrae, Terracciano, Costa, & Collaborators of the Adolescent Personality Profiles of Cultures Project, 2009).

As such, empirical evidence supports using test–retest reliability data on the NEO PI–R as estimates for the NEO–PI–3, then using such correlations in Equation 11.2 to compute the 95% CIs for both factor and facet scales. Test–retest coefficients were computed for the NEO PI–R in a sample of 132 participants (Kurtz & Parrish, 2001). Results showed test–retest coefficients ranging from 0.91 to 0.93 (*Mdn* = 0.92) for the five factor scales, and 0.70 to 0.91 (*Mdn* = 0.83) for the 30 facet scales. Inserting the *Mdn* values into the formula, with a *SD* of 10 for *T*–scores, the *SEM*s are as follows:

Factor scales: $SEM = SD\sqrt{1 - r_{xx}} = 10\sqrt{1 - .92} = 2.83 \approx 3$;

Facet scales: $SEM = SD\sqrt{1 - r_{xx}} = 10\sqrt{1 - .83} = 4.12 \approx 4$.

Therefore, the 68% CI for factor scales would be the observed score plus and minus one *SEM* (i.e., the obtained *T*–score ± 3). Further, the 68% CI for facet scales would be the observed score plus and minus one *SEM* (i.e., the obtained *T*–score ± 4). Note that these are reflected within the scoring and interpretation table notes. Next, the NEO–PI–3 interpretive report is discussed, focusing on the preferred NEO software system output, and whose data are key to the data tables that have been prepared for reporting and interpreting the results of this measure (Forms 11.8 and 11.9). Because the interpretation process is more detailed than for other personality inventories, this topic has been deferred to this final section. Here will be introduced the forms designed for reporting the NEO–PI–3 data within an assessment report. Additionally, the validity checks are more item based and integrated with the diagnostic scales. Therefore, they will be discussed in the ensuing interpretation section versus here under scoring, as has been routinely done in most other test presentations.

INTERPRETATION

As indicated previously, the interpretive process delineated here focuses on the NEO software system. However, the output is virtually the same irrespective of scoring method, with the single major exception of domain scales being calculated when using manual scoring versus factor scales when using computer scoring. After this initial part of the interpretation section are two further subsections, the first discussing the NEO–PI–3 validity scales and the second the factor and facet scales.

Once administration is complete using the NEO software system, the file is saved for reporting any time thereafter. To score a completed administration, a "View Report" button must be selected, after which there are two options, that is, a summary report and an interpretive report. The summary report only provides a three-page description of the examinee's personality on the FFM, or Big Five (i.e., N, E, O, A, C), beginning with the examinee's most prominent to least prominent domain according to the score results. Hence, this report is insufficient for interpretation purposes.

In contrast, the interpretive report, titled "NEO Personality Inventory-3: Interpretative Report," (hereafter "Interpretative Report") is a detailed 22-page output available in electronic form, which can be printed out as a hard copy. This is the version to be selected, as it includes all the data needed for the scoring and interpretation tables designed for use within an assessment report (see Forms 11.8 and 11.9). In particular, it provides the following information: (a) *T*–score profile (i.e., a one-page graph of scores for all factors and facets); (b) a data table (i.e., a one-page table with raw scores, *T*–scores and the descriptive ranges for all factors and facets); (c) an interpretation of the factors and facets, along with personality correlates found in research, the applicability of various *DSM* disorders, and treatment implications; (d) NEO style graphs (i.e., a series of *circumplex models* or circular diagrams of personality based on an examinee's standing on one factor relative to another factor when placed at 90° angles); and (e) a NEO problems in living checklist. These are discussed in turn, including which data to select and integrate into the data tables presented in Forms 11.8 and 11.9.

Note also that here two versions of the data tables for the NEO–PI–3 have been prepared. They include (a) one that is designed for personality assessment as originally intended (hereinafter titled the "Personality" version; see Form 11.8), and (b) one modified to more exclusively detect and diagnose the presence of psychopathology (hereinafter titled the "Psychopathology" version; see Form 11.9). The latter incorporates constructs from the newly proposed *DSM–5* alternative dimensional model for diagnosing personality disorders, along with some of the clinical syndromes suggested by the data (e.g., ADHD). The personality (Form 11.8) and psychopathology (Form 11.9) data tables will be discussed together, with some emphasis where needed on the added information provided by the psychopathology version. However, the difference is only one of emphasis. That is, the personality version may also be used to detect both normal and abnormal personality simply by integrating some of the language used in the psychopathology version. In fact, it is likely that work will soon be initiated on designing one integrated form that uses the most effective components of both versions. This will also be consistent with this model being a work in progress in the *DSM–5*.

Finally, both versions can be used for the self-report format (viz., Form S) and the observer-report format (viz., Form R), which is identified by the examiner deleting the version letter that does not apply in the title of the test located prior to Table 1 (i.e., NEO–PI–3, Form S/R). The "S" precedes "R" in anticipation that the self-report format will be selected most often in mental health testing practice. Using either Form S or R for the same data tables is made possible because the scales are identical. Therefore, there is no need to create separate tables in selecting and denoting the type of informant used to provide the data. If Form R is used, however, the examiner may want to enter the informant's relationship to the examinee immediately prior to Table 1. If Form S is used, or Form R is used and the examiner does not wish to include respondent information, this entry can be deleted in its entirety. The remainder of the presentation applies to both self-report and observer-report formats.

NEO–PI–3 Validity Scales   As in all *explicit personality tests*, validity of the measure must be first considered. Because validity is not directly relevant to diagnosis, the personality and psychopathology versions possess identical validity

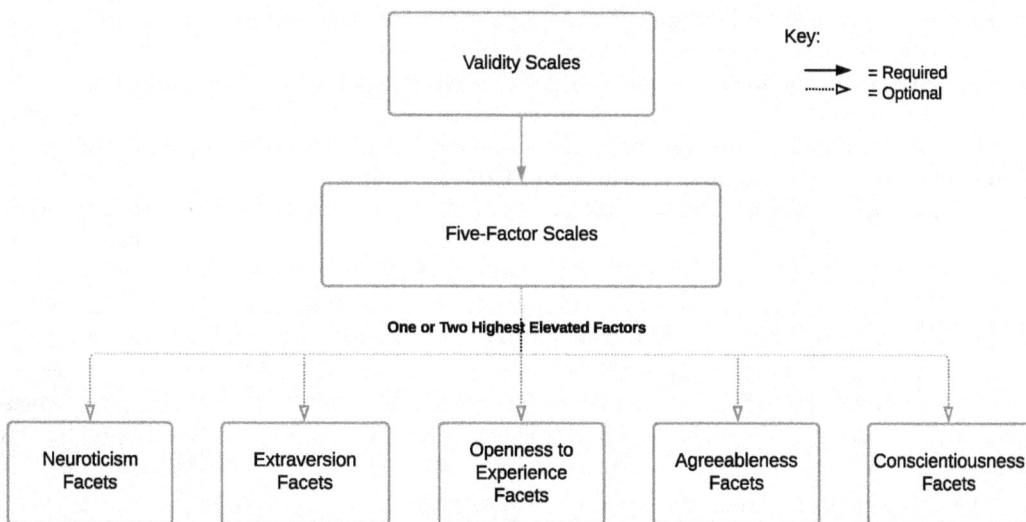

Figure 11.6 NEO Personality Inventory, Third Edition (NEO-PI-3) Interpretive Process

tables. Hence, there will be no distinction between the two at this early point in the analysis. Interestingly, the NEO–PI–3 does not offer the typical types of validity checks found on most other personality inventories (cf. MMPI–2–RF; Ben-Porath & Tellegen, 2011; Tellegen & Ben-Porath, 2011). That is, the authors argue that excessive validity items, scales, and corrections (i.e., score adjustments) can actually subvert their intended effect in the following ways: (a) by frustrating examinees with repeated items designed to check response consistency, (b) by lengthening the test thus causing unnecessary fatigue, and/or (c) by adjusting scores in an inaccurate direction or by overcorrecting. They also go on to cite empirical evidence that validity scales are either ineffectual for their intended purposes or actually reduce test validity (Piedmont, McCrae, Riemann, & Angleitner, 2000). Therefore, Forms 11.8 and 11.9 both begin with each of the NEO–PI–3 rather simple and straightforward validity checks integrated into the measure, beginning with items directly relevant to this issue. This is depicted in Figure 11.6, which is available for download on Routledge's e-resources website. Similar to other such flowcharts, it presents an interpretive stratagem for assigning meaning to the NEO–PI–3 data yield beginning with the validity scales (top box).

First, Table 1 consists of the most explicit validity-type items (Forms 11.8 and 11.9). They include (a) omissions and (b) three items directly asking if the examinee was accurate and honest, responded to all items, and marked items correctly. The interpretive report provides these data within the NEO–PI–3 item responses section. Here, the entire answer sheet can be examined, including the selected alternative for each item and any omissions, answers to all three validity items, and the computed percentages of each alternative selected (e.g., Neutral N: 9.17%). These data can be easily incorporated into Table 1 (Forms 11.8 and 11.9). Narrative excerpts for valid and invalid results follow the table, which can be selected in whole or in part with discretionary modifications. The invalid version is drafted in a manner such that the causes of such outcomes are listed. The invalid reasons that apply should be retained, while those that do not apply should be deleted. Additionally, the narrative ends with proposals for corrective action (e.g., administer an implicit personality test that is less affected by test-taking response sets).

Second, Table 2 (Forms 11.8 and 11.9) is designed to analyze both *acquiescence* and *nay-saying response sets*, indicating tendencies to agree or disagree with items irrespective of their content, respectively. The NEO–PI–3 attempts to mitigate such threats to validity by balancing the direction of the items, approximately half of which are worded in the positive direction and are directly scored (e.g., "I often feel depressed" on a depression scale), and half of which are worded in the negative or opposing direction and are reversed scored (e.g., "I rarely feel depressed," or I often feel happy," on a depression scale). Both tendencies are measured by combining the percentage of agree and strongly agree responses. Although these response sets do not invalidate the results, they necessarily qualify the interpretive approach.

One note, however, is that the professional manual provides the criteria for identifying these tendencies in terms of frequency counts, while the interpretive report provides such data in percentages. Therefore, the frequency counts criteria have been converted into percentages. For example, the manual indicates that 50 or fewer agree and strongly agree responses reveals a nay-saying response set. Thus, (50 ÷ 240) x 100 = 20.83%, which in the table note begins the nay-saying range that extends all the way to 0%. The examiner simply inputs the separate percentages, sums them, and enters the result in the final column. Table notes list the criteria in terms of percentages. Lastly, narrative excerpts for valid and cautiously valid results are provided. Note again that the second validity table results do not invalidate the test results, although they may qualify them. The cautious narratives mention the strategy of interpreting the diagnostic data as falling toward the end of the confidence intervals opposite that of the detected response set (i.e., nay-saying set toward the higher end of the CIs; acquiescence set toward the lower end of the CIs), which is designed to counterbalance the response set distortion. How far within the CI to counterbalance interpretation is contingent upon the degree to which the response set is manifest. Finally, note that the language used in the cautious interpretation can be easily modified to describe a "clear" response set or simply its presence, hence integrating degrees of its measured presence.

Finally, Table 3 (Forms 11.8 and 11.9) is a third validity-related cluster of evidence that is designed to detect any evidence of random fixed responding, this in the form of excessive invariant response sequences (e.g., a sequence of 20 agree responses). Such streaks can be identified by visually scanning the NEO–PI–3 item responses table, which provides the examinee's selection for each item. According to the authors, the following response sequences invalidate the report: (a) strongly disagree ($N \geq 7$), (b) disagree ($N \geq 10$), (c) neutral ($N \geq 11$), (d) agree ($N \geq 15$), and (e) strongly agree ($N \geq 10$). Therefore, the rows in Table 3 enumerate these five alternatives, the criteria signifying invalidity for each, a *no* or *yes* result, and the interpretation (i.e., valid or invalid, once again favoring the former). Entering the examinee's actual or observed invalid sequence is unnecessary, as a simple affirmative result is sufficient for dichotomous validity purposes. As for the prior two validity tables, Table 3 data are followed by both valid and invalid excerpts. The invalid version lists the objective reason for test invalidity (viz., fixed random responding), ensued by hypotheses as to why this may have occurred. The hypotheses can be deleted or modified in whole or in part as deemed proper by the examiner, especially because these hypotheses require inference and supporting facts.

This ends the NEO–PI–3 validity analysis, which included the three aforementioned tables. In review, Tables 1 and 3 contain results that may invalidate the entire test. If such a result is evinced, all tables thereafter should be immediately deleted. This interpretation section now proceeds to the diagnostic data, which consists of the both the broad-based factor scales and more narrowly defined facet scales. Here, the personality (Form 11.8) and psychopathology (Form 11.9) versions begin to diverge.

NEO–PI–3 Factor and Facet Scales   To begin the diagnostic analysis, the key data must be located and culled from the rather extensive 22-page interpretive report produced by the NEO software system (Costa, McCrae, & PAR Staff, 2010). The most advantageous place to begin is the NEO–PI–3 *T*–score profile located on page 2 of the interpretive report. To reiterate, this output provides a one-page visual graph of scale score elevations on all 5 factors and 30 facets, the latter organized by the factor to which each set belongs. Although it does not afford the detail and precision needed for the data tables (Form 11.7 and 11.9), it represents an efficient pictorial summary of all scale elevations. Thus, a cursory examination of the entire data set will initially reveal the presence of any extreme scores.

Next, and most importantly, the NEO–PI–3 data table on page 3 of the interpretive report provides (a) raw scores for all facet scales, and (b) *T*–scores and descriptive ranges for all factor scales and facet scales. It is here where analysis of personality begins in earnest. The NEO–PI–3 consists of a hierarchical test structure, proceeding from the general factors to the more specific facets. Therefore, the interpretative strategy proceeds in a similar and familiar fashion, that is, general to specific.

An interpretive flowchart is presented in Figure 11.6, although it is not vital here because the steps are rather straightforward as follows: (a) validity scales, (b) factor scales, and (c) facet scales of the one or two most extreme factor scales. That is, if there is only one elevated factor scale outside the average range, then only those facet scales need be reported and interpreted. If there are two or more factor scales elevated outside the average range, then the facet scales of the two most extreme factor-level scores are reported. Finally, if all factor scales fall within the average range, then none of the factor scales need to be reported. This is elaborated upon later in this chapter. Figure 11.6 reflecting this interpretive strategy applies to both the personality (Form 11.8) and psychopathology (Form 11.9) versions.

Table 4 of both versions of the data tables consists of all five NEO–PI–3 factor scales, with columns for the factor name; *T*–scores; 68% CIs computed by plus and minus one SEM (i.e., 3 points), with the amount to add and subtract inserted within each cell as a quick reminder of the value; PRs; qualitative descriptions (i.e., descriptive ranges for *T*–scores); and a summary of measured tendencies referred to as *dispositions* due to their broad-based nature. The measured disposition descriptions are worded in the direction of the factor label (i.e., higher scores indicate a greater presence of the label and its measured dispositions); for example, higher scores for extraversion mean greater degrees of extraversion. In contrast, lower scores outside the average ranges indicate increasing dispositions in the opposite direction (e.g., lower scores on extraversion indicate an increasing disposition to be introverted). Table notes delineate the *T*–score metric, statistical symbols, *T*–score ranges associated with qualitative descriptions (i.e., for rapid reference), SEM values and how they were computed, definitions of CI and PR, and finally, the manner in which PRs were determined.

Here, the testing psychologist can identify which (if any) factors are most extreme and represent distinctive personality dispositions. It is analogous to interpreting composite scores for IQ tests, providing a general profile of broad-based strengths and weaknesses. The two distinctions are (a) a lack of an overall personality quotient (cf., a full-scale IQ score) and (b) the measuring of personality stylistic traits in which both extreme ends of the dimension can lead to psychopathology (cf. ability traits in which the higher extreme is increasingly desirable, while the other extreme denotes increasing degrees of disability). For example, although being highly closed minded on the openness factor scale would predictably contribute to difficulties adapting to new circumstances, being excessively open-minded would trend into an abuse of fantasy and a concomitant disregard for reality. A third distinction between the NEO–PI–3 and the typical IQ test structure, this one being more empirical in nature, is that the more narrowly defined facet scales possess the same *T*–score metric as the broader factor scales, hence averting any reduction in measured precision, in contrast to IQ scores which proceed from standard scores (mean = 100; $SD = 15$) to scaled scores (mean = 10; $SD = 3$). At this point, Form 11.8 will be reviewed in terms of the FFM personality factors and how they may be interpreted. This will be followed by a description of how to use the psychopathology version.

Form 11.8 is designed to interpret the NEO–PI–3 as designed by its authors (McCrae & Costa, 2010). Table 4 lists the five factor names, the associated data, qualitative description, and a summary of the measured broad-based dispositions. The qualitative descriptions are defined in Table 11.2. Note that there are two higher ranges and two lower ranges that enclose the average range. Any elevations outside of the mid-average range is a remarkable elevation.

Table 11.3 NEO–PI–3 Factor and DSM–5 Domain Counterparts

NEO–PI–3 Factor[ab]	DSM–5 Domain[a]	NEO–PI–3 Scoring Direction for DSM–5[c]
Neuroticism (vs. Emotional stability)	Negative affectivity (vs. Emotional stability)	+
Extraversion (vs. Introversion)	Detachment (vs. Extraversion)	–
Openness to experience (vs. Closed minded)	Psychoticism (vs. Lucidity)	+
Agreeableness (vs. Disagreeableness)	Antagonism (vs. Agreeableness)	–
Conscientiousness (vs. Non-conscientious)	Disinhibition (vs. Conscientiousness)	–

Note. NEO–PI–3 = NEO Personality Inventory, Third Edition; *DSM–5* = *Diagnostic and Statistical Manual of Mental Disorders, 5th Edition*; pairings are made by conceptual similarity and supported by clinical experience.

[a]Each factor and domain lists the primary label first, followed by its polar opposite in parentheses. [b]Higher scores on the NEO–PI–3 indicate a greater presence of the primary label's distinctive traits, whereas lower scores indicate their lesser presence, absence, or opposite. [c]The third column shows the direction of scoring on the NEO–PI–3 as it pertains to the *DSM–5* domain primary label; i.e., "+" indicates that *higher scores* on the NEO–PI–3 show a greater presence of the *DSM–5* domain primary label's distinctive traits, while "–" indicates that *lower scores* on the NEO–PI–3 show a greater presence of the *DSM–5* domain primary label's distinctive traits.

Narrative interpretations are drafted following Table 4 (Form 11.8), the first five describing results for each factor. An effective interpretive strategy is to identify the two most extreme factor scales, whether high or low, by their deviation from the mean (i.e., *T*–score = 50). The first and second most extreme factor scales represent the most and second most prominent or distinctive dispositions in the examinee's personality profile.

Thereafter, ipsative analyses should be done, comparing the two most extreme elevations to the average (mean = 50, 68% CI = 47–53). A lack of overlap (i.e., discrepancies) between the factor scale CI and the average CI indicate the difference is statistically significant and meaningful, which can be described as mild, moderate, or marked, borrowing language from the MMPI series. Next, the facet scales of each of the two most extreme factor scales should be reported and interpreted. Excerpts follow the facet scale Tables 5–9. In the unlikely event all five factor scales fall in the average range, the "All Scales–Average" excerpt should be employed. In such circumstance, none of the facet scales need be reported; that is, the broad-based dispositions provide a sufficient description of the NEO–PI–3 profile results. All data tables and excerpts that are not used should be deleted to shorten and focus the report. All italicized headings should also be deleted, as they are intended only as guides.

Next, the discussion moves to the psychopathology version in Form 11.9. It contains identical data tables concerning the diagnostic scales (viz., Tables 4–9). The principal difference regards the interpretive excerpts inserted after each table, which focus on (a) detecting personality psychopathology and (b) integrating the *DSM–5* alternative dimensional model that is based on the FFM.

While the previously presented personality version (Form 11.8) can incorporate abnormal and normal aspects of personality functioning, the psychopathology version (Form 11.9) is designed to have a near exclusive focus on detecting abnormality, largely personality disorders, although also some selected clinical disorders. As such, it incorporates cross-references among the NEO–PI–3 factors that are direct representations of the FFM to their *DSM–5* domain counterparts, the latter as defined in the *DSM–5* alternative dimensional model. In identifying a taxonomy of pathological personality traits that are dimensional in nature, the contributors of the *DSM–5* relied on meta-analytic reviews and empirical data showing relationships between trait models in the personality literature and those of the *DSM–IV* categorical personality disorder diagnoses (American Psychiatric Association, 1994). Definitions of the *DSM–5* personality disorder trait domains and facets, which are modeled after the FFM, are listed in Section III, Emerging Measures and Models, of the *DSM–5* (American Psychiatric Association, 2013, Table 3, pp. 779–781). What resulted was an integration of the traits of the FFM, including both the broader factors/domains and the more narrowly defined facets, with criteria from some of the previous *DSM–IV–TR* categorical personality disorders (American Psychiatric Association, 2000), including antisocial, avoidant, borderline, narcissistic, obsessive-compulsive, schizotypal, and personality disorder–trait specified (PD–TS). The PD–TS may include any of the previous categorically defined personality disorders enumerated in the *DSM–IV* and which have been once again espoused as the principal model in the *DSM–5* (American Psychiatric Association, 2013, pp. 645–684). As the NEO–PI–3 measures the FFM, it is now linked to measuring disorders in the new *DSM–5* alternative dimensional model.

Table 11.3 shows a convenient summary among the NEO–PI–3 factors and the *DSM–5* domain counterparts, both with the primary pole of the dimension labeled first, followed by the opposing pole of each in parentheses. These pairings have been converted based on the conceptual similarity among the constructs, supplemented by clinical experience. The primary pole is the end of the dimension that is being directly measured for its degree of presence (i.e., higher scores indicate a greater presence of the distinctive traits as defined by the primary label), while lower scores may be construed as (a) a lesser presence, (b) an increased absence, or (c) an opposite manifestation of such traits. The third and final column in Table 11.3 indicates the directional relationships among the NEO–PI–3 factor scale scores as applied to their *DSM–5* domain counterparts; that is, a "+" sign shows a positive relationship, wherein higher NEO–PI–3 scores show a greater degree of the *DSM–5* domain primary label, whereas a "—" sign shows a negative or inverse direction such that high NEO–PI–3 factor scale scores show a lesser degree of presence of the *DSM–5* domain primary label and vice versa.

This somewhat awkward set of circumstances is because personality inventories, such as the NEO–PI–3, were initially designed to identify a taxonomy of universal or typical personality traits that were a natural component of being human, which were manifested in all people to varying degrees (i.e., on a dimension) and that could be measured quantitatively (viz., the psychometric approach). Because it was found that these traits were normally distributed in the population (i.e., analogous to intellectual traits), a statistical definition of abnormality becomes a viable objective. Hence, as pointed out previously, scoring on either extreme of agreeableness may be interpreted as propensities toward maladjustment. For instance, too little agreeableness may result in antagonistic individuals who are egocentric and excessively competitive. In contrast, excessive agreeableness may result in ingenuous and gullible individuals, who are overly trusting, continually suppressing their own needs in deference to others, and easily manipulated. As the *DSM–5* researchers began espousing this dimensional approach to the diagnosis of personality disorders, they understandably identified the primary label of each domain scale in the psychopathological direction, whereas the NEO–PI–3 is more of a mixture (see Table 11.3). Hence, the examiner must attend closely to the directional relationships between NEO–PI–3 factor scale scores and their *DSM–5* counterparts.

To facilitate test interpretation, Table 4 of the psychopathological version of the data tables (Form 11.9) incorporates the relationship direction of the NEO–PI–3 factor scale scores with each of the *DSM–5* domain scale counterparts, which are located conveniently within the table notes (the *DSM–5* labels in italics). For example, the NEO–PI–3 extraversion (E) factor has an inverse relationship with the *DSM–5* detachment domain. In this case, low or very low scores would indicate high or very high degrees of detachment. As before, summary labels of the alternate *DSM–5* personality disorders follow each excerpt that indicates their presence. Continuing the previous example, high or very high detachment may indicate avoidant, obsessive-compulsive, or schizotypal personality, depending on the facet scale score results. This should facilitate psychological test interpretation and psychodiagnosis using this new dimensional model, which also provides much more useful descriptions of problems that may be targets for intervention.

To further facilitate test interpretation, narrative excerpts have been drafted for each of the five factor–domain scale pairings (denoted in italics) when the data are in the direction of psychopathology, including the personality disorder(s) that may be implicated in italics. The narrative pairings are enumerated in the same order they are presented in the table and are based on the *DSM–5* descriptions of each domain when showing the presence of psychopathology. In the event factor scale scores are all well within normal limits, a "Negative Results" excerpt is provided, which either indicates a recommendation to scrutinize case relevant facet scale scores or no further analysis.

Table 11.4 NEO–PI–3 Facet and DSM–5 Facet Counterparts

NEO–PI–3 Facet	DSM–5 Facet	NEO–PI–3 Scoring Direction for the DSM–5[a]	Facet–Domain Match[b]
Anxiety (N)★	Anxiousness (NA)[†]	+	Yes
Angry hostility (N)★	Hostility (NA)[†]	+	Yes
Depression (N)★	Depressivity (E)[†]	+	No
Self-consciousness (N)★	Intimacy avoidance (DET)[†]	+	No
Impulsiveness (N)★	Impulsivity (DIS)[†]	+	No
Vulnerability (N)★	Emotional lability (NA)[†]	+	Yes
Warmth (E)★	Callousness (ANT)[†]	–	No
Gregariousness (E)★	Withdrawal (DET)[†]	–	Yes
Assertiveness (E)★	Submissiveness (NA)[†]	–	No
Activity (E)★	Restricted affectivity (DET)[†]	–	Yes
Excitement (E)★	Risk-taking (DIS)[†]	+	No
Positive emotions (E)★	Anhedonia (DET)[†]	–	Yes
Fantasy (O)★	Cognitive-perceptual dysregulation (PSY)[†]	+	Yes
Aesthetics (O)★	---	---	---
Feelings (O)★	---	---	---
Actions (O)★	Perseverations (NA)[†]	–	No
Ideas (O)★	Unusual beliefs and experiences (PSY)[†]	+	Yes

(Continued)

Table 11.4 (Continued)

NEO–PI–3 Facet	DSM–5 Facet	NEO–PI–3 Scoring Direction for the DSM–5[a]	Facet–Domain Match[b]
Values (O)★	Eccentricity (PSY)[†]	+	Yes
Trust (A)★	Suspiciousness (DET)[†]	−	No
Straightforwardness (A)★	Deceitfulness (ANT)[†]	−	Yes
Altruism (A)★	Callousness (ANT)[†]	−	Yes
Compliance (A)★	Manipulativeness (ANT)[†]	−	Yes
Modesty (A)★	Grandiosity (ANT)[†]	−	Yes
Tender-mindedness (A)★	Attention-seeking (ANT)[†]	−	Yes
Competence (C)★	Separation anxiety (NA)[†]	−	No
Order (C)★	Rigid perfectionism (DIS)[†]	+	Yes
Dutifulness (C)★	Irresponsibility (DIS)[†]	−	Yes
Achievement striving (C)★	Distractibility (DIS)[†]	−	Yes
Self-discipline (C)★	Distractibility (DIS)[†]	−	Yes
Deliberation (C)★	Impulsivity (DIS)[†]	−	Yes

Note. NEO–PI–3 = NEO Personality Inventory, Third Edition; *DSM–5* = *Diagnostic and Statistical Manual of Mental Disorders, 5th Edition*; pairings are made by conceptual similarity and supported by clinical experience. ★ denotes the NEO–PI–3 factor to which that facet belongs as follows: N = Neuroticism; E = Extraversion; O = Openness to Experience; A = Agreeableness; C = Conscientiousness. [†] denotes the *DSM–5* domain to which that facet belongs as follows: NA = Negative Affectivity; DET = Detachment; ANT = Antagonism; DIS = Disinhibition; PSY = Psychoticism.

[a]The third column shows the direction of scoring on the NEO–PI–3 as it pertains to the *DSM–5* facet primary label; i.e., "+" indicates that *higher scores* on the NEO–PI–3 show a greater presence of the *DSM–5* facet primary label's distinctive traits, while "−" indicates that *lower scores* on the NEO–PI–3 show a greater presence of the *DSM–5* facet primary label's distinctive traits. [b]The fourth and last column indicates whether the NEO–PI–3 facet and corresponding *DSM–5* facet are derived from the matched NEO–PI–3 factor–*DSM–5* domain pairs listed in Table 15.3.

In contrast, evidence in the pathological direction on one or more of these unequivocally indicates the need for further analysis of the facet scale scores. The excerpt denoted as "Potential Psychopathology Detected—Further Analysis Indicated," provides such language. In such circumstances, analysis of the facet scale score summary tables should be rearranged by prioritizing those showing the most to least potential psychopathology. Their prearranged order is as follows: (a) neuroticism facets, (b) extraversion facets, (c) openness facets, (d) agreeableness facets, and (e) conscientiousness facets. This sequence mirrors the order of the factor scales in Table 4 and in Figure 11.6 (see e-resources).

Before moving on to the facet scales, there has been some relevant research showing relationships between NEO–PI–3 factor scale scores and several *DSM–5* clinical syndromes. First, low factor scale scores on conscientiousness, which would be equivalent to high disinhibition (see Table 4, Form 11.9) is associated with *attention-deficit/hyperactivity disorder* (*ADHD*; Nigg et al., 2002). Thus, this disorder was added to the conscientiousness/disinhibition narrative excerpt. Second, Widiger and Trull (1992) found strong links between high neuroticism factor scale scores and chronic depression and anxiety. This would be equivalent to being high in the *DSM–5* negative affectivity domain and indicative of *persistent depressive disorder* (i.e., pure dysthymic disorder) and *GAD* (see Table 4, Form 11.9). Therefore, these disorders have been added to the "Neuroticism/Negative Affectivity" narrative excerpt to alert examiners of this correlation and diagnostic potential. Also added is a depressive personality disorder, as this psychopathology is consistent with psychoanalytic diagnosis (McWilliams, 1994).

Analysis now moves to the NEO–PI–3 facet scale scoring and interpretation Tables 5–9 of the psychopathology version (Form 11.9), which present the facet scale score summaries for each broad-based factor. Note that they are presented in the same sequence in which they appear in Table 4. More specifically, each facet table is named by its factor's primary label, is ensued by the corresponding *DSM–5* primary label in parentheses and is designed similarly to the factor scale score summary. For convenience, Table 11.4 shows a summary of the conceptually similar pairings and the proper directional relationship between the NEO–PI–3 facet scale scores and the presence of the *DSM–5* facet primary trait labels. Such pairings are also supported by clinical experience. Examiners can refer to this table for a rapid reference of all the NEO–PI–3 facet scales, as they have been paired conceptually with the *DSM–5* facet scales, and the relationship direction among the NEO–PI–3 facet scale scores and their *DSM–5* facet counterparts (i.e., positive or negative/inverse). Furthermore, as applied to the facet scale pairings, examiners can determine whether the facets match their corresponding factor–domain groupings. In Table 11.4, note that while most of the facets are derived from the previous factor–domain pairings (see Table 11.3), some do not. This indicates that there is some divergence between the NEO–PI–3 factor/domain–facet structure and that of the *DSM–5* domain–facet structure. Several illustrations will be provided for clarification.

First, impulsiveness is a facet of neuroticism in the NEO–PI–3 structure, whereas in the *DSM–5*, the virtually identical facet impulsive is associated with disinhibition (i.e., conscientiousness). Second, note that (a) some NEO–PI–3 facets have no obvious conceptual *DSM–5* counterparts, and (b) some are showing redundancy. Regarding the latter, the *DSM–5* distractibility facet is conceptually similar to both NEO–PI–3 achievement striving and self-discipline facets. Third, the conceptual association is implied versus direct. For instance, the NEO–PI–3 tender-minded facet consists of sympathy, concern, and an unequivocal focus on the needs of others, whereas the *DSM–5* attention-seeking facet includes an insatiable need for others to focus on the self. Both implicate the self, although one with an outward focus and the other with an inward focus.

Fortunately, the majority of the pairings are both conceptually similar and factor–domain consistent (e.g., the angry hostility–hostility facet pairing both derived from the neuroticism–negative affectivity factor–domain pairing; see Tables 11.4 and 11.3, respectively). Admittedly, the most difficult, and therefore the most tenuous pairings are those among the openness to experience NEO–PI–3 factor–domain facets and the *DSM–5* psychoticism domain facets. In fact, conceptually similar pairings could not be found for aesthetics and feelings that were rationally justifiable. Therefore, interpretations here regarding evidence of psychoticism should be made cautiously and supported by either assessment information or other pertinent test data, such as from the MMPI–2–RF (see prior) or Rorschach Inkblot Test (see Chapter 12).

As for the factor–domain data in Table 4 (Form 11.9), drafted narrative excerpts for each of the facet scale score summary tables (label headings in italics) when the data are in the direction of psychopathology, including the personality disorder(s) that may be implicated (in italics). The narrative pairings are enumerated in the same order they are presented in their respective tables and are based on the new *DSM–5* alternative model descriptions of each facet when showing the presence of maladaptive traits.

Note, however, that the new *DSM–5* alternative model incorporates the categorical personality disorders from previous *DSM* editions via the *personality disorder–trait specified (PD–TS)* diagnosis. Therefore, it is diagnostically more comprehensive to utilize the analogous pairings among the NEO PI–R facets and the categorically defined *DSM–III–R* personality disorders (American Psychiatric Association, 1987). These are provided in the professional manual in tabular format (McCrae & Costa, 2010, Table 5, p. 51), which in turn, was reprinted from the Revised NEO Personality Inventory (NEO PI–R) and NEO Five-Factor Inventory (NEO–FFI) professional manual (Costa & McCrae, 1992, p. 34).

In such a table, NEO PI–3 facets that are related to *defining traits* (i.e., essential features) of each personality disorder are distinguished from those related to each personality disorder's *associated features* (i.e., non-essential variations). In addition, these links are based on (a) conceptual similarity, (b) clinical experience, and (c) research on personality disorders. Similar analyses using *DSM–IV* criteria showed virtually the same results (Dyce & O'Conner, 1998; Widiger, Trull, Clarkin, Sanderson, & Costa, 1994). To maximize diagnostic validity, only NEO associations with defining traits are incorporated into the interpretive excerpts inserted after each of the facet scale Tables 5–9 of the psychopathology version (Form 11.9). Furthermore, when the NEO–PI–3 score direction is the reverse of that shown for that narrative excerpt, the opposite sign follows the personality trait label in parentheses.

In cases where a particular facet has no pairing, a positive sign is shown because a variable is always positively associated with itself, followed by the narrative interpretation for high scores. If a personality disorder is listed adjacent to these narratives, and its presence is indicated by low NEO–PI–3 scores, a "–" sign appears after the trait label. For example, schizoid follows the excerpt for the openness to experience facet feelings (viz., O3). The "–" sign denotes that low scores on this facet are consistent with the presence of *schizoid personality disorder*, although in such cases narrative language in the opposing direction is also needed (i.e., a deficit in experiencing deep and differentiated emotions). Of note, there are a number of consistent pairings in personality disorders that appear in both the previous categorical models and the new alternative model (e.g., high angry hostility [N2] is linked with antisocial personality as defined by both models). The high redundancy among the categorical personality disorders is due to their problematic overlap and comorbidity, which represents the principal reason the new alternative model is being proposed. Hence, the examiner is free to delete these, although they should be retained for now, at least until the alternative model gains more empirical support, acceptance, and use in clinical practice.

Following each of the facet scale score summary tables (Tables 5–9, Form 11.9) are narrative excerpts indicating the presence of maladaptive personality traits as defined by the new *DSM–5* alternative model. Finally, a "Negative Results" excerpt is provided for each of the five facet scale score summary tables in the event these data are in need of being reported and do not show evidence of psychopathology.

Lastly, optional supplementary analyses are available for both the NEO–PI–3 personality and psychopathology versions (Forms 11.8 and 11.9). Specifically, the NEO–PI–3 interpretive report yields a series of NEO style graphs that are based on a *circumplex model of personality* (i.e., a circular model), which was made popular by several prominent trait theorists (see, e.g., Di Blas, 2007; Wiggins, 1979). Such a model pairs selected traits on two-dimensional planes that are orthogonal or perpendicular to each other (i.e., at 90° angles), one being vertical and the other horizontal,

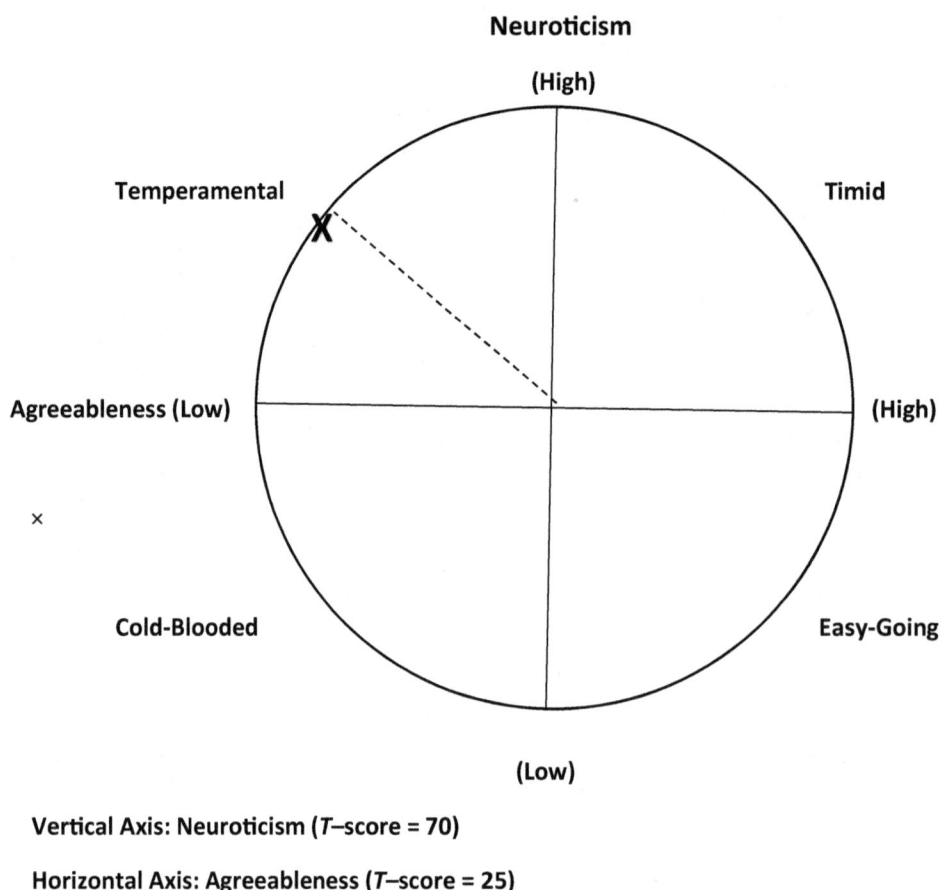

Vertical Axis: Neuroticism (*T*–score = 70)

Horizontal Axis: Agreeableness (*T*–score = 25)

Figure 11.7 NEO Style Graph: Style of Anger Control

Note. The graph depicts a circumplex model of personality, which pairs two trait dimensions at 90° angles. The 90° angles symbolize that these traits are independent of each other. The **X** shows the examinee's score on neuroticism in relation to the score on agreeableness, which is located in the upper-left quadrant (a) far from the center of the circle and (b) proximate to the dashed diagonal that passes through the center of that quadrant (i.e., relatively high on neuroticism and low on agreeableness). This is interpreted as the near ideal model of a *temperamental type* in terms of managing anger. This type is described as easily angered and tending to express this emotion directly. Such individuals can show abrupt episodes of rage that are in clear excess of situational circumstances and manifest long periods of anger. There is a measurable risk for both verbal and physical violence toward others.

which denotes that they are completely independent of each other (i.e., where examinees score on one trait is fully independent of where they score on the other trait). This arrangement permits the measurement of an examinee's position on one trait (i.e., low or high) relative to the other trait (i.e., low or high) for the purpose of determining if there exists evidence of a distinctive personality type in a purely descriptive sense (Block & Ozer, 1982).

For example, one NEO style graph pairs extraversion with agreeableness, resulting in four potential "Style of Interaction" quadrants or types. They include (a) leaders (i.e., high extraversion–low agreeableness: (b) welcomers (i.e., high extraversion–high agreeableness); (c) the unassuming (i.e., low extraversion–high agreeableness); and (d) competitors (i.e., low extraversion–low agreeableness). Each type provides a summary description involving a cluster of personality tendencies. The graph provides the examinee's *T*–scores on each of the two traits, along with an "X" that locates where two scores intersect within the *circumplex* or circular graph. Summary descriptions are most distinctive or present under the following criteria: (a) the "X" is far from the center, (b) the "X" is proximate to the diagonal passing through the central of the quadrant, and (c) all facet scale scores making up each of the factors are of comparable value. There are ten such NEO style graphs.

Figure 11.7 illustrates one of the more interesting NEO style graphs pertaining to anger control, which is a common and vital issue in mental health practice. Here, neuroticism and agreeableness are placed at 90° angles, thus creating four quadrants. The examinee in this example scores relatively high on neuroticism (i.e., emotional instability) and low on agreeableness (i.e., highly disagreeable). If employing the *DSM–5* labels, the latter would be interpreted as high on antagonism. The position of the "X" is noteworthy in that it is far from the circumplex's center and proximate to an imaginary diagonal that divides that particular quadrant in half. This renders the examinee as representing an ideal version of that type (i.e., a prototype), which here is labeled "Temperamental." As one can imagine, being both chronically angry and emotionally unstable represents a virulent combination, one that possesses a risk of violence toward others. Hence, identifying a prominent NEO style and providing a summary description can effectively supplement test interpretation, especially if the identified style is distinctive and pertinent to the diagnostic issues of a case.

SUMMARY

This completes presentation of the NEO Personality Inventories, the majority of which focused on the NEO–PI–3. This personality test is unique in several important aspects. First, it originated from models that examined normal personality traits. Hence, it can currently be used to measure both normality and abnormality. Second, it is recognized as one of the tests that can measure personality disorders according to the newly proposed dimensional model of personality disorders in the *DSM–5*. Thus, it may be the principal test going forward as far as diagnosing *DSM* personality disorders via a dimensional model versus the currently accepted categorical model. Third, it can be used with both adolescents and adults. Fourth, and finally, it is the only one of the personality inventories in this chapter to offer an observer-report version. This can be vital in cases where the examinee does not possess the ability or willingness to complete a self-report inventory (e.g., an individual with neurocognitive impairment who is showing personality changes). These aspects are primarily responsible for incorporating the NEO–PI–3 both in clinical testing practice and in this book.

Recapitulation

This chapter was devoted to personality inventories. More specifically, it consisted of three prominent and influential series of tests, including Millon, MMPI, and the NEO inventories. Each series afforded different aspects that assist in the diagnosis of personality psychopathology and clinical disorders. The Millon tests are theory based and further developed by empirical methods. These tests view personality psychopathology as primary and clinical disorders as embedded within the former. There are three versions of similar format and data, which together cover from preadolescence through adulthood. The MMPI series emerged from empirical criterion keying and thus were statistically based. This book focused on the two restructured adolescent and adult versions, along with the newest adult third edition, which all rely on content-oriented test interpretation using scales with significantly less item overlap, hence construct-purer scales, which also have extensive empirical support for their validity. Although these tests are still largely atheoretical, the Personality Psychopathology Five (*PSY-5*) scales do incorporate theoretical notions that were refined by empirical methods. Finally, the NEO Personality Inventories were introduced, although with an emphasis on the NEO–PI–3. This measure is founded upon the FFM, which originated from investigations of universal normal human traits. It has recently been adopted by *DSM–5* as a bona fide measure of the newly proposed dimensional model of diagnosing personality disorders. Hence, the NEO–PI–3 can be used to measure human personality using both normal and abnormal personality models, in contrast to the former two personality tests that focus more on measuring abnormality. Finally, data tables for all personality inventories presented in this chapter were provided so that their results can be effectively reported within a formal psychological assessment report. The sheer length of this chapter informs the degree to which personality testing is reliant on this format. The next chapter also discusses personality testing, although using a much different format. Briefly, these are performance-based tests that tend to be more open ended in terms of response format and implicit, the latter referring to the fact that examinees are much less cognizant of the meaning of their responses.

Key Terms

- acquiescence
- acquiescence response set
- actuarially based psychodiagnosis
- adjustment disorder with anxiety
- adjustment disorder with depression
- adjustment disorders
- alternative *DSM–5* model for personality disorders
- antisocial personality disorder (APD)
- associated features

- attention–deficit/hyperactivity disorder (ADHD)
- avoidant personality disorder
- axis I clinical disorders
- axis II personality psychopathology
- bariatric surgery
- Big Five
- *BR–scores*
- circumplex
- circumplex model of personality
- clinical disorder
- clinical perspective
- clinical syndrome
- clinically significant personality traits
- codetypes
- content-based interpretation
- coping styles
- cross-cultural universality
- cross-validation sample
- defining traits
- demoralization
- *Diagnostic and Statistical Manual of Mental Disorders, Third Edition, Revised (DSM–III–R)*
- diagnostic specifier
- dimensional approach
- disagreement response set
- dispositional domain
- disruptive behavior disorders
- disruptive mood dysregulation disorder
- emerging
- empirical criterion-keying
- empirically based codetype interpretation
- epileptoid
- error variance
- essential symptoms
- explicit personality test/s
- facet scales
- factor-analysis
- Five-Factor Model (FFM)
- fixed-responding response set
- formal thought disorder
- generalized anxiety disorder (GAD)
- hypersomnia
- illness anxiety disorder
- implicit personality test
- insidious onset
- insomnia
- *International Classification of Diseases, 10th Revision, Clinical Modification (ICD–10–CM)*
- interpersonal
- lexical approach
- major depressive disorder (MDD)
- major depressive disorder, severe
- major depressive disorder, severe, with anxious distress, moderate
- Millon Adolescent Clinical Inventory, Second Edition (MACI–II)
- Millon Adolescent Personality Inventory (MACI)
- Millon Behavioral Health Inventory (MBHI)
- Millon Behavioral Medicine Diagnostic (MBMD)
- Millon Behavioral Medicine Diagnostic, Bariatric Norms (MBMD, Bariatric)

Notes

1. In retrospect, the Conners CBRS employs a similar novel combined dimensional (i.e., interval *T*–scores) and categorical (i.e., *DSM–5* symptom counts) measurement approach in the diagnosis of clinical disorders among children and adolescents (see Chapter 10). The increasing use of this combined measurement approach in contemporary psychological testing and psychodiagnosis is testament to the increasingly apparent false dichotomy between dimensional and categorical variables. At a minimum, this indicates that the two approaches are complementary and thus not mutually exclusive. After all, scrutiny of specific *DSM–5* clinical and personality disorders reveal frequent references to dimensional aspects of its prototypically classified symptoms, including, for example, some of the following intensity and frequency descriptors: (a) *often*, (b) *easily*, (c) *severely*, (d) *in excess*, (e) *markedly*, (f) *persistent*, (g) *excessive*, (h) *repeated*, and (i) *almost always* (American Psychiatric Association, 2013). Furthermore, severity and course specifiers are unambiguously ordinal/interval or dimensional in nature.
2. A paper-and-pencil response sheet version can be administered, although it must be mailed in for computer scoring. This is a rather unappealing procedure since it leads to dilatory results. Hand scoring is no longer available.
3. If this section was overly pedantic, rather than attempting to reread it, one can probably skip this section. Just accept that *BR*–scores attempt to adjust for the estimated prevalence rate of a personality construct and syndrome in the population. A noble effort, although there is not much advantage over *T*–scores, especially since psychological diagnoses have such large symptom overlap, and considering the robustness of the normal distribution in the measurement of human traits in the population (e.g., see Gravetter & Wallnau, 2017).
4. For those clinicians who continue to use the prior editions of the adult and adolescent tests, including the Millon Adolescent Clinical Inventory (MACI; Millon et al., 2006a), and Millon Clinical Multiaxial Inventory-III (MCMI–III; Millon, 2006b), they may be referenced in this book's first edition (Spores, 2012).
5. *Psychasthenia* was a term for a mental health disorder characterized by an amalgamation of phobias, obsessions, compulsions, and/or excessive anxiety. While the term itself is antiquated, it continues to be associated with Clinical Scale 7 of the MMPI and MMPI–2.
6. Because the discussion has proceeded through many tests that can be computer scored on the Pearson Q-global platform, it should be mentioned here that there is an alternate computer-scoring option. It is referred to as the Pearson Q-local software. It functions identically in terms of scoring and reporting to that of Q-global except that the purchased score reports are downloaded onto a USB thumb drive that is essentially a counter key, which in turn is inserted into the selected personal computer. However, Q-global is more advisable because administration can be done at any location that has a computer with Internet access, while the latter is limited to a single computer onto which the Q-local software build must be loaded, along with the purchased tests on the aforesaid USB counter key. Other disadvantages of the Q-local selection is (a) an annual rental fee for the Q-local software and (b) loss of purchased tests in the event the counter key is lost or destroyed (which can be extremely expensive). The only palpable disadvantage to the Q-global option is the requirement of Internet access; that is, if Internet access is interrupted or unavailable, testing is precluded for that period of time. This being the only disadvantage argues strongly for the Q-global option.
7. Demoralization was initially proposed by Jerome Frank (1973, 1974a, 1974b, 1985), who applied it to people who described themselves as discouraged, low in self-esteem, and with expectations of failure and despair.
8. It may be apparent that the Minnesota Multiphasic Personality Inventory-2 (MMPI–2) (Butcher et al., 1989) is not among the tests in the selected inventory. The immediate implications are that this author's psychological testing practice does not include (a) the traditional MMPI/MMPI–2 codetype interpretation strategy and (b) more than 50 years of research and development of the many MMPI–2 content and supplementary scales (Greene, 2011). However, the MMPI–2–RF is (a) remarkably shorter in length and administration time, thus making it more amenable for patients to complete accurately (i.e., 338 items/35–50 minutes versus 567 items/60–90 minutes, respectively), and (b) is comprised of scales with remarkably reduced item overlap. It is therefore superior in terms of facilitating *DSM–5* differential diagnoses, irrespective of the analysis being exclusively content oriented.

References

Aegisdottir, S., White, M. J., Spengler, P. M., Maugherman, A. S., Anderson, L. A., Cook, R. S., . . . Rush, J. D. (2006). The meta-analysis of clinical judgment project: Fifty-six years of accumulated research on clinical versus statistical prediction. *The Counseling Psychologist, 34*, 341–382.

Allport, G. W., & Odbert, H. S. (1936). Trait-names: A psycho-lexical study. *Psychological Monographs, 47* (1, Whole No. 211).

American Psychiatric Association. (1987). *Diagnostic and statistical manual of mental disorders* (3rd ed. rev.; DSM—III—R). Washington, DC: Author.

American Psychiatric Association. (1994). *Diagnostic and statistical manual of mental disorders* (4th ed.; DSM—IV). Washington, DC: Author.

American Psychiatric Association. (2000). *Diagnostic and statistical manual of mental disorders* (4th ed., text rev.; DSM—IV—TR). Washington, DC: Author.

American Psychiatric Association. (2013). *Diagnostic and statistical manual of mental disorders* (5th ed.; DSM—5). Arlington, VA: Author.

American Psychological Association, American Educational Research Association, & National Council on Measurement in Education. (1974). *Standards for educational and psychological tests*. Washington, DC: Author.

Arbisis, P. A., & Ben-Porath, Y. S. (1998). Characteristics of the MMPI—2 F(P) scale as a function of diagnosis in an inpatient VA sample. *Psychological Assessment, 10*, 221–228.

Archer, R. A., Handel, R. W., Ben-Porath, Y. S., & Tellegen, A. (2016). *Minnesota multiphasic personality inventory, adolescent, restructured form (MMPI—A—RF): Administration, scoring, interpretation, and technical manual*. Minneapolis, MN: University of Minnesota Press.

Arnett, P. A., Smith, S. S., & Newman, J. P. (1997). Approach and avoidance motivation in psychopathic criminal offenders during passive avoidance. *Journal of Personality and Social Psychology, 72*, 1413–1428.

Baker, S. R., & Victor, J. B. (2003, August). *Adolescent self-reports of personality and temperament: NEO PI—R and TPQ*. Paper presented at the XIth European Conference on Developmental Psychology, Milan, Italy.

Benjamin, L. S. (1996). *Diagnosis and treatment of mental disorders. Interpersonal diagnosis and treatment of personality disorders* (2nd ed.). New York, NY: Guilford Press.

Ben-Porath, Y. S. (1994). The MMPI and MMPI—2: Fifty years of differentiating normal and abnormal personality. In S. Strack & M. Lorr (Eds.), *Differentiating normal and abnormal personality*. New York, NY: Springer.

Ben-Porath, Y. S., & Butcher, J. N. (1989). Psychometric stability of rewritten MMPI items. *Journal of Personality Assessment, 53,* 645–653.

Ben-Porath, Y. S., & Tellegen, A. (1995). How (not) to evaluate the compatibility of MMPI and MMPI—2 profile configurations: A reply to Humphrey and Dahlstrom. *Journal of Personality Assessment, 65,* 52–58.

Ben-Porath, Y. S., & Tellegen, A. (2011). *Minnesota multiphasic personality inventory—2—restructured form (MMPI—2—RF): Manual for administration, scoring, and interpretation.* Minneapolis: MN: University of Minnesota Press.

Ben-Porath, Y. S., & Tellegen, A. (2020a). *Minnesota multiphasic personality inventory—3 (MMPI—3): Manual for administration, scoring, and interpretation.* Minneapolis: MN: University of Minnesota Press.

Ben-Porath, Y. S., & Tellegen, A. (2020b). *Minnesota multiphasic personality inventory—3 (MMPI—3): Technical manual.* Minneapolis: MN: University of Minnesota Press.

Ben-Porath, Y. S., Tellegen, A., & Graham, J. R. (2008). *The MMPI—2 symptom validity scale (FBS).* Minneapolis, MN: University of Minnesota Press.

Bernreuter, R. G. (1933). The theory and construction of the personality inventory. *Journal of Social Psychology, 4,* 387–405.

Blair, R. J. R., Sellars, C., Strickland, I., Clark, F., Williams, A. O., Smith, M., & Jones, L. (1995). Emotion attributions in the psychopath. *Personality and Individual Differences, 19,* 431–437.

Block, J. (1971). *Lives through time.* Berkeley, CA: Bancroft Books.

Block, J. (1977). Advancing the psychology of personality: Paradigmatic shift or improving the quality of research. In D. Magnusson & N. S. Endler (Eds.), *Personality at the crossroads* (pp. 37–63). Hillsdale, NJ: Erlbaum.

Block, J., & Ozer, D. J. (1982). Two types of psychologists: Remarks on the Mendelsohn, Weiss, and Feimer contribution. *Journal of Personality and Social Psychology, 42,* 1171–1181.

Botwin, M. D., & Buss, D. M. (1989). Structure of act-report data: Is the five-factor model of personality recaptured? *Journal of Personality and Social Psychology, 56,* 988–1001.

Boudry, F. (1983). The evolution of the concept of character in Freud's writings. *Journal of the American Psychoanalytic Association, 31,* 3–31.

Briggs, S. R. (1989). The optimal level of measurement for personality constructs. In D. M. Buss & N. Cantor (Eds.), *Personality psychology: Recent trends and emerging directions* (pp. 246–260). New York, NY: Springer-Verlag.

Buchwald, H., Avidor, Y., Braunwald, E., Jensen, M., Pories, M., et al. (2004). Bariatric surgery: A systematic review and meta-analysis. *Journal of the American Medical Association, 292,* 1724–1737.

Buss, A. H., & Plomin, R. (1975). *A temperament theory of personality development.* New York, NY: John Wiley & Sons.

Butcher, J. N., & Han, K. (1995). Development of an MMPI—2 scale to assess the presentation of self in a superlative manner: The S scale. In J. N. Butcher & C. D. Spielbeger (Eds.), *Advances in personality assessment* (Vol. 10, pp. 25–50). Hillsdale, NJ: Erlbaum.

Butcher, J. N., Dahlstrom, W. G., Graham, J. R., Tellegen, A., & Kaemmer, B. (1989). *Minnesota multiphasic personality inventory, second edition (MMPI—2): Manual for administration, and scoring.* Minneapolis, MN: University of Minnesota Press.

Butcher, J. N., Dahlstrom, W. G., Graham, J. R., Tellegen, A., & Kaemmer, B. (2001). *Minnesota multiphasic personality inventory, second edition (MMPI—2): Manual for administration, and scoring* (rev. ed.). Minneapolis, MN: University of Minnesota Press.

Butcher, J. N., Graham, J. R., Ben-Porath, Y. S., Tellegen, A., Dahlstrom, W. G., & Kaemmer, B. (2001). *MMPI—2 (Minnesota multiphasic personality inventory—2) manual for administration, scoring, and interpretation* (Rev. ed.). Minneapolis, MN: University of Minnesota Press.

Butcher, J. N., Graham, J. R., Williams, C. L., & Ben-Porath, Y. S. (1990). *Development and use of the MMPI—2 content scales.* Minneapolis: University of Minnesota Press.

Butcher, J. N., Williams, C. L., Graham, J. R., Archer, R. P., Tellengen, A., Ben-Porath, Y. S., & Kaemmer, B. (1992). *Minnesota multiphasic personality inventory, adolescent, (MMPI—A): Administration, scoring, and interpretation.* Minneapolis, MN: University of Minnesota Press.

Carlson, J., & Maniacci, M. P. (2012). *Alfred Adler revisited.* New York, NY: Routledge, Taylor & Francis.

Carver, C. S., & Antoni, M. H. (2004). Finding benefit in breast cancer during the year after diagnosis predicts better adjustment 5 to 8 years after diagnosis. *Health Psychology, 26,* 595–598.

Caspi, A., & Roberts, B. W. (2001). Personality development across the life course: The argument for change and continuity. *Psychological Inquiry, 12,* 49–66.

Caspi, A., Elder, G. H., Jr., & Bem, D. J. (1987). Moving against the world: Life-course patterns of explosive children. *Developmental Psychology, 23,* 308–313.

Cattell, R. B. (1943). The description of personality: Basic traits resolved into clusters. *Journal of Abnormal and Social Psychology, 38,* 476–507.

Cattell, R. B., Eber, H. W., & Tatsuoka, M. M. (1970). *The handbook for the sixteen personality factor questionnaire.* Champaign, IL: Institute for Personality and Ability Testing.

Centers for Disease Control and Prevention (CDC). (2021a). *Weight loss & obesity.* Retrieved from www.hhs.gov/programs/prevention-and-wellness/healthy-lifestyle/index.html

Centers for Disease Control and Prevention (CDC). (2021b, January 28). *Healthy weight* [Web log post]. Retrieved from www.cdc.gov/healthyweight/assessing/bmi/adult_bmi/index.html

Chamorro-Premuzic, T. (2011). *Personality and individual differences* (2nd ed.). Chichester, West Sussex, UK: British Psychological Society & Blackwell Publishing.

Chronis, A. M., Lahey, B. B., Pelham, W. E., Jr., Williams, S. H., Baumann, B. L., Kipp, H., . . . & Rathouz, P. J. (2007). Maternal depression and early positive parenting predict future conduct problems in young children with attention-deficit/hyperactivity disorder. *Developmental Psychology, 43*, 70–82.

Cohen, J. (1988). *Statistical power analysis for the behavioral sciences.* Hillsdale, NJ: Lawrence Erlbaum Associates.

Costa, P. T., Jr. (1991). Clinical use of the five—factor model: An introduction. *Journal of Personality Assessment, 57*, 393–398.

Costa, P. T., Jr., & McCrae, R. R. (1976). Age differences in personality structure: A cluster analytic approach. *Journal of Gerontology, 31*, 564–570.

Costa, P. T., Jr., & McCrae, R. R. (1978). Objective personality assessment. In M. Storandt, I. C. Siegler, & M. F. Elias (Eds.), *The clinical psychology of aging* (pp. 119–143). New York, NY: Plenum Press.

Costa, P. T., Jr., & McCrae, R. R. (1985). *The NEO Personality Inventory manual.* Odessa, FL: Psychological Assessment Resources (PAR).

Costa, P. T., Jr., & McCrae, R. R. (1992). *Revised NEO personality inventory (NEO PI—R) and NEO five-factor inventory (NEO-FFI) professional manual.* Odessa, FL: Psychological Assessment Resources (PAR).

Costa, P. T., Jr., & McCrae, R. R. (1995). Solid ground in the wetlands of personality: A reply to Block. *Psychological Bulletin, 117*, 216–220.

Costa, P. T., Jr., & McCrae, R. R. (2008). The NEO inventories. In R. P. Archer & S. R. Smith (Eds.), *Personality assessment* (pp. 213–246). New York, NY: Routledge, Taylor & Francis.

Costa, P. T., Jr., & McCrae, R. R. (2009). The five-factor model and the NEO inventories. In J. M. Butcher (Ed.), *Oxford handbook of personality and clinical assessment* (pp. 299–322). New York, NY: Oxford University Press.

Costa, P. T., Jr., & Widiger, T. A. (Eds.). (2002). *Personality disorders and the Five-Factor Model of personality* (2nd ed.). Washington, DC: American Psychological Association.

Costa, P. T., Jr., McCrae, R. R., & Martin, T. A. (2008). Incipient adult personality: The NEO—PI—3 in middle-school-aged children. *British Journal of Developmental Psychology, 26*, 71–89.

Costa, P. T., Jr., McCrae, R. R., & PAR Staff. (2010). *NEO software system* (Version 3.01) [Computer software, CD-ROM]. Psychological Assessment Services (PAR).

Craig, R. J. (1999). *Interpreting personality tests: A clinical manual for the MMPI—2, MCMI—III, CPI—R, and 16PF.* New York, NY: John Wiley & Sons.

Dahlstrom, W. G., Archer, R. P., Hopkins, D. G., Jackson, E., & Dahlstrom, L. E. (1994). *Assessing the readability of the Minnesota multiphasic personality inventory instruments: The MMPI, MMPI—2, MMPI—A.* Minneapolis: MN: University of Minnesota Press.

Dahlstrom, W. G., Welsh, G. S., & Dahlstrom, L. E. (1972). *An MMPI handbook: Vol.1. Clinical interpretation* (Rev. ed.). Minneapolis, MN: University of Minnesota Press.

De Fruyt, F., De Bolle, M., McCrae, R. R., Terracciano, A., Costa, P. T., Jr., & Collaborators of the Adolescent Personality Profiles of Cultures Project. (2009). Assessing the universal structure of personality in early adolescence: The NEO—PI—R and NEO—PI—3 in 24 cultures. *Assessment, 16*, 301–311.

De Fruyt, F., Mervielde, I., Hoekstra, H. A., & Rolland, J. P. (2000). Assessing adolescents' personality with the NEO PI—R. *Assessment, 7*, 329–345.

Di Blas, L. (2007). A circumplex model of interpersonal attributes in middle childhood. *Journal of Personality, 75*, 863–897.

Digman, J. M., & Inouye, J. (1986). Further specification of the five robust factors of personality. *Journal of Personality and Social Psychology, 50*, 116–123.

Drake, L. E. (1946). A social I.E. scale for the Minnesota multiphasic personality inventory. *Journal of Applied Psychology, 30*, 51–54.

Dyce, J. A., & O'Conner, B. P. (1998). Personality disorders and the five-factor model: A test of facet-level predictions. *Journal of Personality Disorders, 12*, 31–45.

Ehrenworth, N. V., & Archer, R. P. (1985). A comparison of clinical accuracy ratings of interpretive approaches for adolescent MMPI responses. *Journal of Personality Assessment, 49*, 413–421.

Eysenck, H. J., & Eysenck, S. B. (1975). *Manual of the Eysenck personality questionnaire.* London, England: Hodder and Stoughton.

Finn, J. A., Ben-Porath, Y. S., & Tellegen, A. (2015). Dichotomous versus polytomous response options in psychopathology assessment: Method or meaningful variance? *Psychological Assessment, 27*, 184–193.

Fiske, D. W. (1949). Consistency of the factorial structures of personality ratings from different sources. *Journal of Abnormal and Social Psychology, 44*, 329–344.

Frank, J. D. (1973). *Persuasion and healing.* Baltimore: The John Hopkins University Press.

Frank, J. D. (1974a). Common features of psychotherapies and their patients. *Psychotherapy and Psychosomatics, 24*, 368–371.

Frank, J. D. (1974b). Psychotherapy, The restoration of morale. *American Journal of Psychiatry, 131*, 271–274.

Frank, J. D. (1985). Further thoughts on the anti-demoralization hypothesis of psychotherapeutic effectiveness. *Integrative Psychiatry, 3*, 17–20.

Friedman, M., & Rosenman, R. H. (1974). *Type A behavior and your heart.* New York: Knopf.

Funder, D. C. (2006). Towards a resolution of the personality triad: Persons, situations, and behaviors. *Journal of Research in Personality, 40*, 21–34.

Gardner, J., & Oswald, A. J. (2004). How is mortality affected by money, marriage, and stress? *Journal of Health Economics, 23*, 1181–1207.

Gervais, R. O., Ben-Porath, Y. S., Wygant, D. B., & Green, P. (2007). Development and validation of a response bias scale (RBS) for the MMPI—2. *Assessment, 14*, 196–208.

Gilberstadt, H., & Duker, J. (1965). *A handbook for clinical and actuarial MMPI interpretation.* Oxford, England: Saunders.

Glenn, A. L., Raine, A., Mednick, S. A., & Venables, P. (2007). Early temperamental and psychophysiological precursors of adult psychopathic personality. *Journal of Abnormal Psychology, 116*(3), 508–518.

Goldberg, L. R. (1981). Language and individual differences: The search for universals in personality lexicons. In L. Wheeler (Ed.), *Review of personality and social psychology* (Vol. 2, pp. 141–165). Beverly Hills, CA: Sage.

Gonzalez, J. S., Penedo, F. J., Antoni, M. H., Durán, R. E., Fernandez, M. I., McPherson-Baker, S., . . . Schneiderman, N. (2004). Social support, positive states of mind, and HIV treatment adherence in men and women living with HIV/AIDS. *Health Psychology, 23*, 413–418.

Graham, J. R., Timbrook, R. E., Ben-Porath, Y. S., & Butcher, J. N. (1991). Code-type congruence between MMPI and MMPI—2: Separating fact from artifact. *Journal of Personality Assessment, 57*, 205–215.

Gravetter, F. J., & Wallnau, L. B. (2017). *Statistics for the behavioral sciences* (10th ed.). Boston, MA: Wadsworth, Cengage Learning.

Green, R. L. (2011). *The MMPI—2/MMPI—2—RF: An interpretative manual.* Boston, MA: Pearson.

Grossman, S. D., & Amendolace, B. (2017). *Essentials of MCMI—IV assessment.* Hoboken, NJ: John Wiley & Sons.

Guilford, J. S., Zimmerman, W. S., & Guilford, J. P. (1976). *The Guilford-Zimmerman temperament survey handbook: Twenty-five years of research and application.* San Diego, CA: Edits.

Harkness, A. R. (1992). Fundamental topics in the personality disorders: Candidate Trait dimensions from lower regions of the hierarchy. *Psychological Assessment, 4*, 251–259.

Harkness, A. R., & McNulty, J. L. (1994). The personality psychopathology five (PSY—5): Issues from the pages of a diagnostic manual instead of a dictionary. In S. Strack & M. Lorr (Eds.), *Differentiating normal and abnormal personality* (pp. 291–315). New York, NY: Springer.

Harkness, A. R., & McNulty, J. L. (2007). An overview of personality: The MMPI—2 personality psychopathology five scales (PSY—5). In James N. Butcher (Ed.), *Oathways to MMPI—2 use: A practitioner's guide to test usage in diverse settings.* Washington, DC: American Psychological Association.

Harkness, A. R., McNulty, J. L., & Ben-Porath, Y. S. (1995). The personality psychopathology five (PSY—5): Constructs and MMPI—2 scales. *Psychological Assessment, 7*, 104–114.

Harkness, A. R., Reynolds, S. M., & Lileinfeld, S. C. (2014). A review of systems for psychology and psychiatry: Adaptive systems, personality psychopathology five (PSY—5), and the DSM—5. *Journal of Personality Assessment, 96*, 121–139.

Haslam, C., Cruwys, T., Milne, M., Kan, C.-H., & Haslam, S. A. (2016). Group ties protect cognitive health by promoting social identification and social support. *Journal of Aging and Health, 28*(2), 244–266.

Hathaway, S. R. (1947). A coding system for MMPI profile classification. *Journal of Consulting Psychology, 11*, 334.

Hathaway, S. R., & Mckinley, J. C. (1943). *The Minnesota Multiphasic Personality Schedule.* Minneapolis, MN: University of Minnesota Press.

Hathaway, S. R., & McKinley, J. C. (1940). A multiphasic personality schedule (Minnesota). I: Construction of the schedule. *Journal of Psychology: Interdisciplinary and Applied, 10*, 249–254.

Hathaway, S. R., & McKinley, J. C. (1942). *The Minnesota Multiphasic Personality Schedule.* Minneapolis: University of Minnesota Press.

Hinshaw, S. P., & Stier, A. (2008). Stigma as related to mental disorders. Annual Review of *Clinical Psychology, 4*, 367–393.

Holt-Lunstad, J., Uchino, B. N., Smith, T. W., Cerny, C. B., & Nealey-Moore, J. B. (2003). Social relationships and ambulatory blood pressure: Structural and qualitative predictors of cardiovascular function during everyday social interactions. *Health Psychology, 22*, 388–397.

https://www2census.gov/programs-surveys/demo/tables/2017/educational-attainment/2017/cps-detailed-tables/table-1–1.xlsx

https://www2census.gov/programs-surveys/popproj/datasets/2017/2017-popproj/np2017_d1.csv

Humm, D. G., & Wadsworth, G. W., Jr. (1935). The Humm-Wadsworth temperament scale. *The American Journal of Psychiatry, 92*, 163–200.

Janus, M. D., de Groot, C., & Toepfer, S. M. (1998). The MMPI—A and 13-year-old inpatients: How young is too young? *Assessment, 5*, 321–332.

John, O. P. (1990). The "Big Five" factor taxonomy: Dimensions of personality in the natural language and questionnaires. In L. A. Pervin (Ed.), *Handbook of personality* (pp. 66–100). New York: Guilford Press.

Kamp, J., & Tringone, R. F. (2008). Development and validation of the Millon Pre—Adolescent Clinical Inventory (M—PACI). In T. Millon & C. Bloom (Eds.), *The Millon inventories: A practitioner's guide to personalized clinical assessment* (2nd ed., pp. 528–547). New York, NY: The Guilford Press.

Kendler, K. S., Czajkowski, N., Tambs, K., Torgersen, S., Aggen, S. H., Neale, M. C., & Reichborn-Kjennerud, T. (2006). Dimensional representations of DSM–IV cluster A personality disorders in a population-based sample of Norwegian twins: A multivariate study. *Psychological Medicine, 36*, 1583–1591.

Kernberg, O. (1967). Borderline personality organization. *Journal of the American Psychoanalytic Association, 15*, 641–685.

Kernberg, O. F. (1975). *Borderline conditions and pathological narcissism.* New York: Jason Aronson.

Kernberg, O. F. (1984). *Severe personality disorders.* New Haven, CT: Yale University Press.

Kochanska, G., Aksan, N., & Joy, M. E. (2007). Children's fearfulness as a moderator of parenting in early socialization: Two longitudinal studies. *Developmental Psychology, 43*, 222–237.

Korkman, M., Kirk, U., Kemp, S. (2007a). *NEPSY—II: Administrative manual.* San Antonio, Texas: The Psychological Corporation-Pearson.

Korkman, M., Kirk, U., Kemp, S. (2007b). *NEPSY—II: Clinical and interpretative manual.* San Antonio, Texas: The Psychological Corporation-Pearson.

Kraeplin, E. (1921). *Manic-depressive insanity and paranoia.* Edinburgh, Scotland: Livingstone.

Kral, J., Sjostrom, L., & Sullivan, M. (1992). Assessment of quality of life before and after surgery for severe obesity. *American Journal of Clinical Nutrition, 55,* 6115–6145.

Kroenke, C. H., Quesenberry, C., Kwan, M. L., Sweeney, C., Castillo, A., & Caan, B. J. (2012). Social networks, social support, and burden in relationships, and mortality after breast cancer diagnosis in the Life After Breast Cancer Epidemiology (LACE) study. *Breast Cancer Research and Treatment, 137,* 261.

Kulik, J. A., & Mahler, H. I. M. (1989). Social support and recovery from surgery. *Health Psychology, 8,* 221–238.

Kulik, J. A., & Mahler, H. I. M. (1993). Emotional support as a moderator of adjustment and compliance after coronary bypass surgery: A longitudinal study. *Journal of Behavioral Medicine, 16,* 45–63.

Kurtz, J. E., & Parrish, C. L. (2001). Semantic response consistency and protocol validity in structured personality assessment: The case of the NEO PI—R. *Journal of Personality Assessment, 76,* 315–332.

Landis, C., & Katz, S. E. (1934). The validity of certain questions which purport to measure neurotic tendencies. *Journal of Applied Psychology, 18,* 343–356.

Larsen, R. J., & Buss, D. M. (2021). *Personality psychology: Domains of knowledge about human nature* (7th ed.). New York, NY: McGraw-Hill.

Lees—Haley, P. R., English, L. T., & Glenn, W. J. (1991). A fake bad scale on the MMPI—2 for personal injury claimants. *Psychological Reports, 68,* 203–210.

Livesley, W. J. (Ed.). (1995). *Diagnosis and treatment of mental disorders. The DSM—IV personality disorders.* Guilford Press.

Lykken, D. T. (1995). *The antisocial personalities.* Hillsdale, NJ: Erlbaum.

Marks, P. A., & Seeman, W. (1963). *The actuarial description of abnormal personality: An atlas for use with the MMPI—2.* Baltimore: Williams & Wilkins.

Marks, P. A., Seeman, W., & Haller, D. L. (1974). *The actuarial use of the MMPI with adolescents and adults.* Baltimore: Williams & Wilkins.

Martinez, A. G., Piff, P. K., Mendoza-Denton, R., & Hinshaw, S. P. (2011). The power of a label: Mental illness diagnoses, ascribed humanity, and social rejection. Journal of *Social and Clinical Psychology, 30,* 1–23.

Mason, J., Southwick, S., Yehuda, R., Wang, S., Riney, S., Bremner, D., . . . Zhou, G. (1994). Elevation of serum free triiodothyronine, total triiodothyronine, thyroxine-binding globulin, and total thyroxine levels in combat-related posttraumatic stress disorder. *Archives of General Psychiatry, 51,* 629–641.

McCann, J. T. (1999). *Assessing adolescents with the MACI; Using the Millon adolescent clinical inventory.* New York, NY: John Wiley & Sons.

McCann, J. T. (2008). Using the Millon Adolescent Clinical Inventory (MACI) and its facet scales. In T. Millon & C. Bloom (Eds.), *The Millon inventories: A practitioner's guide to personalized clinical assessment* (2nd ed., pp. 494–519). New York, NY: The Guilford Press.

McCrae, R. R., & Costa, P. T., Jr. (1986). Clinical assessment can benefit from recent advances in personality psychology. *American Psychologist, 41,* 1001–1010.

McCrae, R. R., & Costa, P. T., Jr. (1989). Rotation to maximize the construct validity of factors in the NEO personality inventory. *Multivariate Behavioral Research, 24,* 107–124.

McCrae, R. R., & Costa, P. T., Jr. (2003). *Personality in adulthood: A five-factor theory perspective* (2nd ed.). New York: Guilford Press

McCrae, R. R., & Costa, P. T., Jr. (2010). *NEO inventories for the NEO personality inventory—3 (NEO—PI—3), NEO five factor inventory—3 (NEO—FFI—3), NEO personality inventory—revised (NEO PI—R): Professional manual.* Lutz, FL: Psychological Assessment Services (PAR).

McCrae, R. R., & John, O. P. (1992). An introduction to the five-factor model and its applications. *Journal of Personality, 60,* 175–215.

McCrae, R. R., Costa, P. T., Jr., & Martin, T. A. (2005). The NEO—PI—3: A more readable revised NEO personality inventory. *Journal of Personality Assessment, 84,* 261–270.

McCrae, R. R., Löckenhoff, C. E., & Costa, P. T. (2005). A step towards DSM—V: Cataloging personality-related problems in living. *European Journal of Personality, 19,* 269–270.

McCrae, R. R., Martin, T. A., & Costa, P. T., Jr. (2005). Age trends and age norms for the NEO personality inventory—3 in adolescents and adults. *Assessment, 12,* 363–373.

McCrae, R. R., Yamagata, S., Jang. K. L., Riemann, R., Ando, J., Ono, Y., . . . Spinath, F. M. (2008). Substance and artifact in the higher-order factors of the bi five. *Journal of Personality and Social Psychology, 95,* 442–455.

McCrae, R. R., Zonderman, A. B., Costa, P. T., Jr., Bond, M. H., & Paunonen, S. V. (1996). Evaluating replicability of factors in the revised NEO personality inventory: Confirmatory factor analysis versus Procrustes rotation. *Journal of Personality and Social Psychology, 70,* 552–566.

McKinley, J. C., & Hathaway, S. R. (1940). A multiphasic personality schedule (Minnesota). II: A differential study of hypochondriasis. *Journal of Psychology: Interdisciplinary and Applied, 10,* 255–268.

McKinley, J. C., & Hathaway, S. R. (1942). A multiphasic personality schedule (Minnesota). IV: Psychasthenia. *Journal of Applied Psychology, 26,* 614–624.

McKinley, J. C., & Hathaway, S. R. (1944). Minnesota multiphasic personality inventory. V: Hysteria, hypomania, and psychopathic deviate. *Journal of Applied Psychology, 28,* 153–174.

McNulty, J. L., Harkness, A. R., Ben-Porath, Y. S., & Williams, C. L. (1997). Assessing the personality five (PSY—5) in adolescents: New MMPI—A scales. *Psychological Assessment, 9,* 250–259.

McWilliams, N. (1994). *Psychanalytic diagnosis.* New York, NY: The Guilford Press.

McWilliams, N. (2011). *Psychoanalytic diagnosis: Understanding personality structure in the clinical process* (2nd ed.). New York: The Guilford Press.

MedFriendly. (2020). *Standard score to percentile conversion.* Retrieved June 6, 2020, from www.medfriendly.com/standardscoretopercentile conversion.html

Millon, T. (1990). *Toward a new personology: An evolutionary model.* New York, NY: John Wiley & Sons.

Millon, T. (2011). *Disorders of personality: Introducing a DSM/ICD spectrum from normal to abnormal.* Hoboken, NJ: John Wiley & Sons.

Millon, T., & Davis, R. D. (1996). *Disorders of personality: DSM—IV and beyond.* New York: John Wiley & Sons.

Millon, T., & Grossman, S. D. (2005). Personology: A theory based on evolutionary concepts. In M. F. Lenzenweger & J. F. Clarkin (Eds.), *Major theories of personality disorder* (2nd ed., pp. 332–390). New York, NY: The Guilford Press.

Millon, T., & Millon, C. M. (2008). Scientific grounding and validation of the MCMI. In T. Millon & C. Bloom (Eds.), *The Millon inventories: A practitioner's guide to personalized clinical assessment* (pp. 3–45). New York, NY: The Guilford Press.

Millon, T., Antoni, M., Millon, C., Minor, S., & Grossman, S. D. (2006). *Millon behavioral medicine diagnostic, manual. (MBMD, General medical norms;* 2nd ed.). Minneapolis, MN: NCS Pearson.

Millon, T., Antoni, M., Millon, C., Minor, S., & Grossman, S. D. (2007). *Millon behavioral medicine diagnostic, manual supplement: Bariatric report (MBMD, bariatric norms).* Minneapolis, MN: NCS Pearson.

Millon, T., Antoni, M., Millon, C., Minor, S., & Grossman, S. D. (2010). *Millon behavioral medicine diagnostic, manual supplement: Pain patient reports (MBMD, pain norms).* Minneapolis, MN: NCS Pearson.

Millon, T., Green, C., & Meagher, R. (1979). The MBHI: A new inventory for the psychodiagnostician in medical settings. *Professional Psychology, 10,* 529–539.

Millon, T., Grossman, S. D., & Millon, C. (2015). *Millon clinical multiaxial inventory, fourth edition (MCMI—IV) manual.* Minneapolis, MN: Pearson Assessments.

Millon, T., Millon, C., & Davis, R. D. (1993). *Millon adolescent clinical inventory (MACI) manual* (1st ed.). Minneapolis, MN: National Computer Systems (NCS).

Millon, T., Millon, C., Davis, R. D., & Grossman, S. D. (2006a). *Millon adolescent clinical inventory (MACI) manual* (2nd ed.). Minneapolis, MN: NCS Pearson.

Millon, T., Millon, C., Davis, R. D., & Grossman, S. D. (2006b). *Millon clinical multiaxial inventory, third edition (MCMI—III) manual.* Minneapolis, MN: NCS Pearson.

Millon, T., Tringone, R., Grossman, S, & Millon, C. (2020). *Millon adolescent clinical inventory, second edition (MACI—II) manual.* Minneapolis, MN: NCS Pearson.

Millon, T., Tringone, R., Millon, C., & Grossman, S. D. (2005). *Millon pre—adolescent clinical inventory (M—PACI) manual.* Minneapolis, MN: NCS Pearson.

Moskowtiz, D. S., &, Fournier, M. A. (2015). The interplay of persons and situations: Retrospect and prospect. In L. Cooper and R. J. Larsen (Eds.), *Handbook of personality and social psychology: Personality processes and individual differences.* Washington, DC: American Psychological Association.

Moyer, K. E. (1987). *Violence and aggression: A physiological perspective.* New York: Paragon House.

Myers, I. B. (1998). *Introduction to type* (6th ed.). Palo Alto, CA: Consulting Psychologists Press.

Myers, I. B., McCaulley, M. H., Quenk, N. L., & Hammer, A. L. (1998). *MBTI manual: A guide to the development and use of the Myers—Briggs type indicator* (3rd ed.). Palo Alto, CA: Consulting Psychologists Press.

Nelson, N. W., Sweet, J. J., & Demakis, G. J. (2006). Meta-analysis of the MMPI—2 fake bad scale: Utility in forensic practice. *The Clinical Neuropsychologist, 20,* 39–58.

Newman, J. P. (1987). Reaction to punishment in extraverts and psychopaths: Implications for the impulsive behavior of disinhibited individuals. *Journal of Research in Personality, 21,* 464–480.

Nigg, J. T., & Goldsmith, H. H. (1994). Genetics of personality disorders: Perspectives from personality and psychopathology research. *Pathological Bulletin, 115,* 346–380.

Nigg, J. T., John, O. P., Blaskey, L. G., Huang-Pollock, C. L., Willcutt, E. G., Hinshaw, S. P., & Pennington, B. (2002). Big five dimensions and ADHD symptoms: Links between personality traits and clinical symptoms. *Journal of Personality and Social Psychology, 83,* 451–469.

Norman, W. T. (1963). Toward an adequate taxonomy of personality attributes: Replicated factor structure in peer nomination personality ratings. *Journal of Abnormal Psychology, 66,* 574–583.

Oldenburg, J. C. (1997). *The relation between age and MMPI—A scale scores and correlates in a clinical population* (Unpublished doctoral dissertation). Kent State University, Kent, OH.

Ostendorf, F. (1990). *Language and personality structure: Towards the validity of the five-factor model of personality.* Regensburg, Germany: Roderer-Verlag.

Parcesepe, A. M., & Cabassa, L. J. (2013). Public stigma of mental illness in the United States: A systematic literature review. *Administration and Policy in Mental Health and Mental Health Services Research, 40,* 384–399.

Patrick, C., Drislane, L. E., & Strickland, C. (2012). Conceptualizing psychopathy in Triarchic terms: Implications for treatment. *The International Journal of Forensic Mental Health, 11,* 253–266.

Paunoman, S. V., & Ashton, M. C. (2001). Big five factors and facets and the prediction of behavior. *Journal of Personality and Social Psychology, 81,* 524–539.

Pearson. (2021). *Q—global: Better insights. Anytime. Anywhere.* [Internet Web-Based Computer Scoring]. Retrieved from https://qglobal.pearsonclinical.com/qg/login.seam.

Piedmont, R. L. (1998). *The revised NEO personality inventory: Clinical and research applications.* New York, NY: Plenum.

Piedmont, R. L., McCrae, R. R., Riemann, R., & Angleitner, A. (2000). On the validity of validity scales: Evidence from self-reports and observer ratings in volunteer samples. *Journal of Personality and Social Psychology, 78*, 582–593.

Pollock, V. E., Briere, J., Schneider, L., Knop, J., Mednick, S., & Goodwin, D. W. (1990). Childhood antecedents of antisocial behavior: Parental alcoholism and physical abusiveness. *American Journal of Psychiatry, 147*, 1290–1293.

Rammstedt, B., Goldberg, L. R., & Borg, I. (2010). The measurement equivalence of Big-Five factor markers for persons with different levels of education. *Journal of Research in Personality, 44*, 53–61.

Reichborn-Kjennerud, T. (2008). Genetics of personality disorders. *Psychiatric Clinics of North America, 31*, 421.

Reichborn-Kjennerud, T., Czajkowski, N., Neale, M. C., Orstavik, R. E., Torgersen, S., Tambs, K., . . . Kendler, K. S. (2007). Genetic and environmental influences on dimensional representations of DSM–IV cluster C personality disorders: A population-based multivariate twin study. *Psychological Medicine, 37*, 645–653.

Reynolds, S. K., & Clark, L. A. (2001). Predicting dimensions of personality disorder from domains and facets and the five-factor model. *Journal of Personality, 69*, 199–222.

Romney, D. M., & Bynner, J. M. (1992). A simplex model of five DSM—III personality disorders. *Journal of Personality Disorders, 6*, 34–39.

Rosanoff, A. J. (1927). *Manual of psychiatry and mental hygiene* (6th ed.). Hoboken, NJ: John Wiley & Sons.

Santry, H., Gillen, D., & Lauderdale, D. (2005). Trends in bariatric surgical procedures. *Journal of the American Medical Association, 294*, 1909–1917.

Saucier, G., & Goldberg, L. R. (1996). The language of personality: Lexical perspectives on the five-factor model. In J. S. Wiggins (Ed.), *The five-factor model of personality: Theoretical perspectives* (pp. 21–50). New York, NY: The Guilford Press.

Schinka, J. A., & Borum, R. (1993). Readability of adult psychopathology inventories. *Psychological Assessment, 5*, 384–386.

Seara-Cardoso, A., & Viding, E. (2015). Functional neuroscience of psychopathic personality in adults. *Journal of Personality, 83*, 723–737.

Shedler, J., & Westen, D. (2004). Dimensions of personality pathology: An alternative to the five-factor model. *American Journal of Psychiatry, 161*, 1743.

Singer, J. A. (2005). *Personality and psychotherapy: Treating the whole person.* New York, NY: The Guilford Press.

Stevens, S. S. (1946). On the theory of scales of measurement. *Science, 103*, 677–680.

Strack, S. (2002). *Essentials of Millon inventories assessment* (2nd ed.). New York, NY: John Wiley & Sons.

Super, D. E. (1942). The Bernreuter Personality Inventory: A review of research. *Psychological Bulletin, 39*, 94–125.

Sutcliffe, N., Clarke, A. E., Levinton, C., Frost, C., Gordon, C., & Isenberg, D. A. (1999). Associates of health status in patients with systemic lupus erythematosus. *Journal of Rheumatology, 26*, 2352–2356.

Tellegen, A. (1982). *Brief manual for the Differential Personality Questionnaire.* Unpublished manuscript. Minnesota: University of Minnesota.

Tellegen, A. (1985). *Structure of mood and personality and their relevance to assessing anxiety with an emphasis on self-report.* Hillsdale, NJ: Erlbaum.

Tellegen, A. (1988). The analysis of consistency in personality assessment. *Journal of Personality, 56*, 621–663.

Tellegen, A., & Ben-Porath, Y. S. (1992). The new uniform T scores for the MMPI—2: Rationale, derivation, and appraisal. *Psychological Assessment, 4*, 145–155.

Tellegen, A., & Ben-Porath, Y. S. (2011). *Minnesota multiphasic personality inventory—2 restructured form: Technical manual.* Minneapolis: MN: University of Minnesota Press.

Tellegen, A., Ben-Porath, Y. S., McNulty, J. L., Arbisi, P. A., Graham, J. R., & Kaemmer, B. (2003). *The MMPI—2 restructured clinical (RC) scales: Development, validation, and interpretation.* Minneapolis, MN: University of Minnesota Press.

Tellegen, A., Watson, D., & Clark, L. A. (1999a). Further support for a hierarchical model of affect: Reply to green and Salovey. *Psychological Science, 10*, 307–309.

Tellegen, A., Watson, D., & Clark, L. A. (1999b). On the dimensional and hierarchical structure of affect. *Psychological Science, 10*, 297–303.

Termin, L. M., & Miles, C. C. (1936). *Sex and personality: Studies in masculinity and femininity.* New York, NY: McGraw Hill.

Torgersen, S., Czajkowski, N., Jacobson, K., Reichborn-Kjennerud, T., Roysamb, E., Neale, M. C., & Kendler, K. S. (2008). Dimensional representations of DSM–IV cluster B personality disorders in a population-based sample of Norwegian twins: A multivariate study. *Psychological Medicine, 38*, 1617–1625.

Trull, T. J., Useda, J. D., Costa, P. T., Jr., & McCrae, R. R. (1995). Comparison of the MMPI—2 personality psychopathology five (PSY—5), the NEO—PI, and the NEO—PI—R. *Psychological Assessment, 7*, 508–516.

Tupes, E. C., & Christal, R. C. (1961). *Recurrent personality factors based on trait ratings* (USAF ASD Technical Report, No. 61–97, U.S). Air Force, Lackland Air Force Base, TX: US Air Force.

U.S. Census Bureau, Department of Commerce. (1984). *Projections of the population of the United States, by age, sex, and race: 1983 to 2080* (Series P-25, No. 952). Washington, DC: U.S. Government Office.

U.S. Census Bureau. (2017a). *Table 2. Projected population by single year of age, sex, ace, and Hispanic origin: 2016 to 2060 [Data file].* Washington, DC: U.S. Government Office.

U.S. Census Bureau. (2017b). *Table 1. Educational attainment of the population 18 years and over, by age, sex, race, and Hispanic origin: 2017 [Data file].* Washington, DC: U.S. Government Office.

Vaillant, G. E. (2002). Adaptive mental mechanisms: Their role in a positive psychology. *American Psychologist, 55*, 89–98.

Wadden, T., Brownwell, K., & Foster, G. (2002). Obesity: Responding to the global epidemic. *Journal of Consulting and Clinical Psychology, 70*, 510–525.

Warner, R. M. (2021a). *Applied statistics I: Basic bivariate techniques* (3rd ed.). Thousand Oaks, CA: Sage.

Warner, R. M. (2021b). *Applied statistics II: Multivariable and multivariate techniques* (3rd ed.). Thousand Oaks, CA: Sage.

Watson, D., & Tellegen, A. (1985). Toward a consensual structure of mood. *Psychological Bulletin, 98*, 219–235.

Westen, D. (1990). Psychoanalytic approaches to personality. In L. A. Pervin (Ed.), *Handbook of personality: Theory and research* (pp. 21–65). New York: Guilford Press.

Widiger, T. A. (Ed.). (2012). *Oxford library of psychology. The Oxford handbook of personality disorders.* New York, NY: Oxford University Press.

Widiger, T. A., & Trull, T. J. (1992). Personality and psychopathology: An application of the Five-Factor Model. *Journal of Personality, 60*, 363–393.

Widiger, T. A., Trull, T. J., Clarkin, J. F., Sanderson, C., & Costa, P. T., Jr. (1994). A description of the DSM—III—R and DSM—IV personality disorders with the five-factor model of personality. In P. T. Costa, Jr. & T. A. Widiger (Eds.), *Personality disorders and the five-factor model of personality* (pp. 41–56). Washington, DC: American Psychological Association.

Widiger, T., & Trull, T. J. (2007). Plate tectonics in the classification of personality disorder: Shifting to a dimensional model. *American Psychologist, 62*, 71.

Wiggins, J. S. (1959). Interrelations among the MMPI measures of dissimulation under standard and social desirability instructions. *Journal of Consulting Psychology, 23*, 419–427.

Wiggins, J. S. (1966). Substantive dimensions of self-report in the MMPI item pool. *Psychological Monographs: General & Applied, 80*, 42.

Wiggins, J. S. (1979). A psychological taxonomy of trait-descriptive terms: I. The interpersonal domain. *Journal of Personality and Social Psychology, 37*, 395–412.

Wiggins, J. S., & Pincus, A. L. (1989). Conceptions of personality disorders and dimensions of personality. *Psychological Assessment: A Journal of Consulting and Clinical Psychology, 1*, 305–316.

Woodworth, R. S. (1920). *Personal data sheet.* Chicago: Stoelting.

World Health Organization (WHO). (1992). *The ICD–10 classification of mental and behavioral disorders: Clinical descriptions and diagnostic guidelines.* Geneva, Switzerland: Author.

Wygant, D. B. (2007). *Validation of the MMPI—2 infrequent somatic complaints (Fs) scale* (Unpublished doctoral dissertation). Kent State University, Kent, OH.

Wygant, D. B., Ben-Porath, Y. S., & Arbisi, P. A. (2004, May). *Development and initial validation of a scale to detect somatic over-reporting.* Paper presented at the 39th Annual Symposium on Recent Developments in the Use of the MMPI—2 and MMPI—A, Minneapolis, MN.

Yasgur, B. S. (2017, November). Borderline personality disorder: Not just an adult condition. *Psychiatry Advisor.* Retrieved from www.psychiatryadvisor.com/home/topics/child-adolescent-psychiatry/borderline-personality-disorder-not-just-an-adult-condition/

Zimmerman, M., Rothschild, L., & Chelminski, I. (2005). The prevalence of DSM—IV personality disorders in psychiatric outpatients. *American Journal of Psychiatry, 162*, 1911–1918.

See Routledge's e-resources website for forms. (www.routledge.com/9780367346058)

12 Performance Personality Tests

Overview

This chapter is the second of two that focuses principally on the measurement of personality functioning and secondarily on the presence of clinical psychopathology. The rationale for presenting them within a separate chapter was due to their remarkably divergent format and data yield. Another discrepancy is that the performance personality tests selected for inclusion in this book are much fewer in quantity (viz., three). So, an immediate question to address is why are there so few performance personality tests in the book's test inventory for clinical practice? The chief reason is that they are more labor intensive and consume much of the precious time insurers are willing to *preauthorize* (PA) for a single testing case within outpatient mental health care. They are equally demanding in terms of training and becoming competent in their use. Irrespective of these less-than-desirable features, they retain a vital role in testing practice, which will become increasingly apparent as this chapter unfolds. If this was not the case, there would be no need for this chapter, and personality testing would be circumscribed to the personality inventories. Because the construct of personality is once again the cardinal focus of measurement in this chapter, a reiteration of its definition will be afforded here; especially one that is drafted in a manner that is more accordant with performance personality testing.

Here, *personality* can be defined as comprising a collection of organized and relatively enduring internal *traits* and *mechanisms* that influence behavioral interactions and *adaptation* to the environment (Larsen & Buss, 2021). There are several key concepts within this particular definition that require elaboration. First, traits are *average tendencies* that define the manner in which people are both different from and similar to each other. This aspect of the definition is also relevant to personality inventory tests (discussed in Chapter 11). This is because both performance personality tests and personality inventories provide data concerning description and prediction. Hence, if it is known that an individual is highly extroverted (i.e., description), it can also be predicted with reasonable accuracy that she will tend to seek out and gravitate toward relationships and people. Likewise, if an individual is highly neurotic (i.e., description), it can be predicted that he will be vulnerable to a variety of clinical disorders (e.g., depression or anxiety) and will most likely develop unstable relationships with others. Additional psychological traits include such variables as self-esteem, narcissism, and hypervigilance, all of which describe an individual and permit predictions of future outcomes.

Second, *mechanisms* refer to the underlying processes of personality, most of which comprise perceptual or information-processing actions. Mechanisms consist of three stages, including (a) encoding, (b) cognitive reasoning and decision-making, and (c) behavioral output. It will soon become apparent that the performance personality tests focus principally on measuring the underlying mechanisms of personality from which inferences regarding personality traits (i.e., descriptors) can be constructed. In turn, inferences regarding personality traits leads to diagnostic decisions as to whether an individual currently has, or is at risk for, one or more clinical disorders. The latter diagnostic strategy is also used by the Millon inventories discussed in Chapter 11. More specifically, two of the tests in this chapter attempt to formulate inferences that are proximate to the response process or behavioral test data, hence reducing the reliance upon inference, while one test relies on the projective hypothesis and is thus more dependent on theoretical notions.

The ensuing section delineates the principal components that define the performance personality tests later described, which is facilitated in part by contrasting them with the personality inventories previously presented. This is followed by a section that considers the conditions under which such performance personality tests best contribute to a psychological test battery, including the consideration of potential insurance coverage issues. Finally, the three selected performance personality tests are presented in sequence, which represents the core part of this chapter.

DOI: 10.4324/9780429326820-14

Performance Personality Tests: A Conceptualization

What constitutes a performance personality test? This broad question can be further apportioned and narrowed in scope into the following: (a) What are the main characteristics of the performance personality tests of this chapter, and (b) how are they divergent from the personality inventory tests presented in Chapter 11? These questions will be addressed next in such sequence. They are intended for those tests that are later described in this chapter and not necessarily more generally. This is because performance personality tests consist of a wide array of features. To refer to them all would require a good deal of abstraction and generalization or, if detail were given, would consume excessive space. Hence, it is more economical to remain circumscribed to the three tests later described and will also consequently be more comprehensible. Although many of the ensuing comments may be apposite to other performance tests and thus generalize effectively, some many not, and the reader should be aware of this.

Different Formats

Performance personality tests and personality inventories have quite different formats. More specifically, the performance personality test stimuli consist of visual images printed on cards. These stimuli are semi-ambiguous (i.e., both suggestive and evocative) and are accompanied by instructions that together encourage the examinee to produce open-ended responses. The manner in which the examinee responds to this task is assessed using a coding and accompanying scoring system designed to reveal the underlying mechanisms and traits that together constitute personality. This coding and scoring system requires judgment or inference on the part of the examiner.

In contrast, the personality inventories employ a forced-choice, closed-ended format to a listing of standardized statements. Scoring requires minimal inference and typically consists of aggregating or summing responses to statements on scales, each of which is designed to measure a psychological construct. This is evidenced by the fact that personality inventories can be completely scored via automated computer software, whereas coding verbal responses, as done in performance personality tests, always requires human judgment and inference. Once the coding is completed, computer software can then be employed. Concerning performance tests, the degree of inference required once coding and scoring is completed varies depending on how proximate inferences are to the actual response process (i.e., the psychological processes that led to the recorded response). Performance personality tests that rely more on theory require more inference. It will soon become apparent that the three performance personality tests presented subsequently run the gamut, from interpreting close to the response process or observable behavior to relying more heavily on theory.

Explicit Versus Implicit Measures

Recall that the personality inventories are *explicit measures* in that the informant is directly asked to assess the presence of traits, feelings, thoughts, and other aspects of examinees' personalities, whether it be self-report or observer-report. This explains the heavy reliance on validity scales, the purpose of which is to detect a variety of potential response sets that may distort the meaning of the diagnostic data. In contrast, the performance personality tests used here are *implicit measures*, which means they assess aspects of examinees' personalities without asking them directly (Greenwald, McGhee, & Schwartz, 1998). They accomplish this by tapping into examinees' personality mechanisms, directly appraising (a) unconscious aspects of personality via *projection* (A. Freud, 1946), (b) *perceptual sets*, and (c) *social-cognitive abilities*, all of which may be identified, quantified, and/or reliably associated with various psychological traits, emotional states, moods, beliefs, reality testing capability, thought process and content, and overall psychological adjustment.

Like all measures, the implicit personality tests incorporated into this book have both assets and liabilities. First, a distinct asset of such tests is that they do not require the examinee to possess the ability to introspect. That is, they are based on performance, not psychological insight or psychological mindedness. Second, it is difficult for examinees to intentionally distort the results (also known as *impression management*). This represents a near essential feature in *high-stakes testing*, which is defined as any testing circumstance in which a key decision will be rendered, usually one which will have vital consequences for the examinee or the examinee's significant others. Examples of high-stakes testing include parents undergoing personality testing in custody evaluations, personal injury litigants completing testing for compensation, and testing criminal defendants in competency examinations. In such cases, the testee has compelling reasons to distort the results in a manner that favors a desired outcome. When using an implicit test, it is significantly more difficult (although not impossible) to distort such results because the method of scoring and interpretation is sufficiently disguised. Finally, especially for children, they can be less threatening, as they resemble play activities versus an actual test that might be administered when in the formal classroom.

However, there are also liabilities. First, these implicit tests require much more time and effort, especially concerning the examiner, typically doubling the time needed for completion of a self-report inventory. Analogously, such tests require significantly more training, supervision, and practice for the examiner. This is typically due to the more intricate coding and scoring systems employed by such tests. Second, insurance carriers infrequently provide a sufficient number of testing hours and time for use of such tests. Therefore, the examiner needs to be especially adept at administering, scoring, interpreting, and reporting the data yield and to be selective in using the data needed in a particular case. The data tables that have been created for reporting the results of these tests will assist greatly in this endeavor. Third, their face validity is de minimis by virtue of them being implicit. Recall that *face validity* represents the degree to which a psychological test on the surface looks like what it claims to measure. Although not a genuine aspect of validity, face validity is believed to potentially enhance an examinee's motivation to complete the test because it appears relevant (Hogan, 2019, p. 124). Contrary to this, absent face validity can have a deleterious effect on such motivation because an examinee may not believe the test has the ability to provide the intended results. Therefore, the implicit nature of these tests can cut both ways as does a double-edged sword. Of course, the remedy is to properly prepare the examinee for such testing (e.g., explaining the reason for testing, establishing adequate trust and rapport with the examinee).

Fourth, and finally, by being performance based, such personality tests yield *signs* of psychopathology (i.e., not merely reported *symptoms*), which may be indicative of an array of personality and clinical disorders. For example, an excess of distorted form responses on the Rorschach Inkblot Test (i.e., *F*—), irrespective of the scoring system used, shows that the individual likely perceives the external world in a similarly distorted manner. The challenge regards *differential diagnosis*. That is, "Does this sign indicate the presence of schizotypal personality disorder, schizophrenia, amphetamine psychosis, or a mood disorder with psychotic features?" To address this question adequately, the testing psychologist must consider (a) the remaining Rorschach data profile, (b) other available test data, and (c) the clinical interview information (including mental status examination results). The point here is that, while performance personality tests detect actual signs of psychopathology, they do not provide a direct correspondence with major diagnostic systems, such as the *Diagnostic and Statistical Manual of Mental Disorders, Fifth Edition* (*DSM–5*; American Psychiatric Association, 2013), and the *ICD–10 Classification of Mental and Behavioural Disorders* (*ICD–10*; World Health Organization or WHO, 1992/2004). Hence, differential diagnosis using such measures is more complicated, inferential, and labor intensive, that is, if they are being used for such purpose. However, the task is much easier if attempting to answer certain specified referral questions that are addressed by such tests, such as "How impaired is this person's reality testing?" or "How sophisticated is this child's social cognition or social problem-solving?"

Different Types of Data

The third and final facet of the performance personality tests, as contrasted with the personality inventories, is the disparate type of data yielded by these two classes of measures. Recall that the personality inventories provide mostly self-report data (i.e., *S-data*), along with one also affording observer-data (i.e., *O-data*). The advantage of gathering data via self-report is that it capitalizes on the fact that individuals have access to unique thoughts, feelings, and other personality information that is available to no one else. In addition, O-data derives from one or more third-person perspectives that are capable of detecting behaviors and traits to which the examinee may not be aware. Further, because more than one observer can contribute information, the data can also reveal perspectives on the examinee's personality in a variety of environmental contexts.

In contrast, performance personality tests provide test data (i.e., *T-data*). Such data are based on the examinee's elicited behavior observed and measured under standardized and controlled conditions, which are then used as reliable and valid indicators of personality (Block, 1977; Megargee, 1969). T-data are vital in that they are very difficult to garner in the real world where there is a lack of control of extraneous variables. Furthermore, because T-data are yielded under such controlled experimental-like conditions, they can be used to reliably test a multitude of specific hypotheses that effectively address the diagnostic and treatment issues presented in an assessment case (Elfenbein, Curhan, Eisenkraft, Shirako, & Baccaro 2008). Next examined are the circumstances under which a performance personality test should be considered as part of an assessment battery.

Reasons for Including a Performance Personality Test Within a Test Battery

This section describes the general circumstances in which the performance personality tests of this chapter should be incorporated as part of a test battery. It is apportioned into two more specific topics. The first focuses on referral issues conducive to performance personality tests. The second refers to insurance coverage issues that may assist or hinder PA for the requested hours.

Referral Issues Conducive to Performance Personality Tests

To reiterate, the performance personality tests (a) are more labor intensive, (b) necessitate greater diagnostic inference, and hence (c) require approximately twice the number of testing hours as compared to the more direct and explicit personality inventories. Therefore, their inclusion within a test battery should be sufficiently justified. What follows are three of the most frequent issues in which these tests are especially apposite. They include (a) examinees who lack introspection (i.e., poor psychological mindedness), (b) examinees who are likely to attempt to manipulate test results (i.e., during high-stakes testing), and (c) the presence of diagnostic issues that require the measurement of underlying personality mechanisms as defined earlier. These issues shall be expounded upon in this sequence.

First, performance personality tests are imperative when the examinee's ability to introspect is deficient or likely to be severely impaired, thus precluding the use of explicit measures. Of course, this assumes there are no available observer-report measures that would be viable substitutes. An example includes testing an adolescent who has a confirmed premorbid diagnosis of autism spectrum disorder (ASD) for the presence of clinical levels of depression and any suicidal tendencies. An analogous circumstance is when the examinee is to be tested for a disorder that, by definition, hinders the ability to introspect and report one's symptoms accurately. Examples here include testing for *obsessive-compulsive disorder with poor insight* and some psychotic symptoms that hinder the ability to recognize abnormality (e.g., delusions of persecution). By employing such tests in these cases, the examiner can effectively use *T*-data to assess specific hypotheses as to whether signs of such a disorder are present. Finally, performance personality tests should be used when clinical assessment or prior information indicates a very high likelihood of a response set that would distort test results (e.g., *acquiescence* or *social desirability*; see Chapters 10 and 11). Although this is technically not synonymous with deficient introspection or lack of insight, it would also result in an invalid outcome due to inaccurate reporting.

Second, performance personality tests may be effectively used when there exist circumstances that foster a distinct likelihood that the examinee will intentionally attempt to manipulate test results, most especially in high-stakes testing as defined previously. Such situations include an application for disability, the presence of unresolved custody issues, forensic criminal competency and insanity cases, and personal injury cases. Similarly, impression formation may occur as the direct result of the suspected disorder that is the target of testing, especially when the referring clinician already strongly suspects the disorder's presence but simply wants empirical confirmation. Examples consist of disorders that, by definition, involve defensiveness and manipulation. Apposite examples of the latter include *antisocial personality disorder (APD)*, *conduct disorder (CD)*, *paranoid personality disorder (PPD)*, and *histrionic personality disorder (HPD)*. This particular use capitalizes on the implicit nature of these tests wherein face validity is nebulous and obscure, hence obfuscating the examinee's ability to intentionally manipulate results.

Third, and finally, such tests are both informative and valuable when direct performance-based measures of underlying personality mechanisms are desired or needed. Examples of key mechanisms include perception and thinking, cognitive processing, self-perception, perception of others, social-cognitive problem-solving abilities, ego strength (i.e., coping skills), and experienced distress. Once again, this is predicated upon the T-data characteristic of these tests, that is, the examinee actually showing signs of the trait under controlled, standardized conditions versus the trait being reported by the examinee.

Insurance Coverage Issues

As with the personality inventories, obtaining PA for these performance personality tests is typically viable assuming that (a) medical necessity has been established and (b) the test is properly standardized with up-to-date and representative norms. Looking ahead, the first of the three tests presented subsequently (viz., the Children's Apperception Test) may have the greatest degree of difficulty obtaining PA due to a lack of contemporary norms. Hence, once an examinee reaches the age that matches the norms of the other two tests discussed in this chapter (viz., Rorschach Inkblot Test and Roberts–2), which is age six, then the latter two should supplant the former.

Once one of the aforementioned measures has been selected, however, a second crucial issue regards the number of test hours insurance companies will typically approve. Based on clinical experience, third-party payers will approve no more than two hours per such test, which they typically classify as projective despite that fact that this is an incorrect designation for the latter two tests. Thus, if the testing psychologist does not employ an extremely efficient means of administering, scoring, and interpreting these tests, the outcome shall be virtually the same as an outright denial; that is, they will be rendered impractical for want of utility. That is, in clinical testing practice, a clinician cannot afford to repeatedly select and administer tests in which only a fraction of the time to use it is preauthorized. This rule applies irrespective of the effectiveness of the particular test. Over time, testing clinicians will become increasingly frustrated and demoralized, hence not performing to their potential, which is deleterious to the client, clinician, and to the field of psychological testing. On the bright side of this issue, the data tables that have been created for these tests are designed to assist the examiner in effectively using them within a two-hour duration, which will typically match the number of hours insurance carriers will allot for their employment. As evidence for this, all three tests have been consistently utilized in actual clinical practice, especially the Rorschach, within a two-hour duration, and with effective and extremely gratifying results. They are also more interesting to give because they help us examine our clientele from the inside out and discover mechanisms and their resulting traits that would not otherwise have been detected by any of the personality inventories.

Next begins the core part of this chapter; that is, the performance personality tests. In addition to presenting them as all the other tests in previous chapters, their developmental histories and rationale for including them in the book's inventory are covered. The presentation begins with the test designed for the youngest age group and progresses from that point to the tests intended for older age cohorts, which is consistent with all previous chapters.

The Performance Personality Tests

Overview

This section presents three performance personality tests and represents the core section of this chapter. It begins with the *Children's Apperception Test* (*CAT*; Bellak & Abrams, 1998) for two reasons. First, it provides performance personality data for the youngest age group, including children under six years of age. This test was specifically included in this book's inventory because there was otherwise a salient void. In particular, nowhere was there a measure that garnered personality test information (i.e., *T-data*) directly from the examinee in individuals younger than six years of age. Both the Rorschach and Roberts–2 begin their norms at age six and thus are inappropriate for such young examinees. In the absence of such a measure, assessment data for clinical disorders and personality issues would be circumscribed to observer-report measures (i.e., *O-data*). Essentially, it seemed odd to assess and individual's psychological functioning without obtaining some data directly from that individual.

So why was the CAT selected and not the Thematic Apperception Test (Morgan & Murray, 1935), which has a much longer history of use and development? In particular, the CAT was chosen because (a) it is especially designed for younger populations, and (b) it is accompanied by a manageable and comprehensible empirical scoring system. A major caveat is that it is designed as a projective test based on psychodynamic principles. Therefore, reliability and validity may be questionable, and clinicians who do not subscribe to either the projective hypothesis or psychodynamic theory may not accept the interpretations yielded by such test results. However, without such a test, there would be no opportunity to gather T-data to measure personality development and functioning in the young child. Additionally, a history of the CAT's development is provided with references so that interested readers can investigate this test in more detail, hence increasing their expertise in the use of such test.

Next, the *Roberts–2* (Roberts & Gruber, 2005) is presented because it covers a mid-range population in terms of *chronological age* (*CA*). In terms of targeted constructs, this test provides data regarding social-cognitive problem-solving abilities, which impact social skills, and in ancillary fashion includes empirical scales that are intended to identify the presence of several common clinical disorders (e.g., anxiety and depression). The Roberts–2 was nearly dropped from the inventory and book due to lack of use. However, it can still be very useful in testing referrals that question the examinee's social-cognitive problem-solving abilities with a secondary focus on detecting clinical disorders. If the sole purpose is detecting clinical psychopathology, however, the R–PAS is likely the test of choice with its greater empirical support and usage. It also addresses many more personality mechanisms than does the Roberts–2. The Roberts–2 cards can be used as a projective test, as in the TAT and CAT; however, it was specifically not designed as such (Roberts & Gruber, 2005, pp. 4–5).

Finally, the section and chapter ends with the most contemporary scoring system currently developed for the Rorschach Inkblot Test; namely, the *Rorschach Performance Assessment System* (*R–PAS*; Meyer, Viglione, Mihura, Erard, & Erdberg, 2011, 2012). This system comes with updated form quality (*FQ*) tables and norms and converts coded results into standard scores using the same metric as do the intelligence tests. Those clinicians who still prefer to use the *Rorschach, Comprehensive System* (*R–CS*; Exner, 2001, 2003) may do so by consulting the first edition (Spores, 2012, Chapter 9). Continued use of the R–CS is understandable because there are some significant changes with the R–PAS, such as dropping the distinctions in emphasis among form–shading and form–achromatic determinants (e.g., *FY, YF,* or *Y* and FC', C'F, or C'). For these reasons, some of the author's testing colleagues have either continued using the R–CS in its entirety or have used the R–CS with the updated FQ tables. In any case, only the updated R–PAS will be found here in its entirety, although a complete history is presented to afford the reader valuable context.

Children's Apperception Test, Ninth Edition, Revised, Color Version

There are actually different versions of the CAT stimulus card sets, the original consisting of ten black-and-white animal drawings, along with a human figures set of ten cards of the same interpersonal scenes. The one focused on here is the original animal drawings that were revised to be in color versus black and white. Otherwise, they are identical to the original set of cards. It will become apparent that there is no evidence the color and black-and-white versions yield significantly different results. Hence, because anecdotal evidence showed that the colored cards tended to elicit more interest on the part of young examinees, the colored set is typically preferred. Therefore, the ensuing presentation is meant to be applied to either pack of animal cards: the original black-and-white set or the more recent revised colored version of the original animal set.

Synopsis

As stated, it became apparent there was a vacuity in personality testing for very young children in the author's clinical practice; that is, a test in which the personality data were produced by the child clients themselves. By young, reference is made to those under the age of six. This was disconcerting because it seemed to be in direct contravention of the testing principle that argues for the use of converging evidence in rendering reliable and valid diagnostic results. Although there were a copious number of observer-based measures for this age group in the author's test inventory (e.g., parent, teacher, caregiver), there were none that were produced by the most central person in the assessment; namely, the actual client.

As this conundrum was being pondered, it became increasingly apparent that this paucity was understandable for at least two reasons. First, it is well recognized that personality emerges gradually over a period of years, beginning with fundamental, biologically based, emotional, and behavioral dispositions referred to as *temperament* (Strelau, 1998). An excellent example includes fear reactions and inhibited behavior, which have been studied in detail (see, e.g., Fox, Henderson, Marshall, Nichols, & Ghera, 2005). Other examples are activity level, general mood, attention span, and persistence (Thomas & Chess, 1977). Second, young children lack the ability to effectively introspect and accurately report their true and genuine inner feelings, beliefs, behavior patterns, symptoms, and traits. This effectively eliminates self-report rating scales or personality inventories.

Therefore, the investigation began by researching performance personality tests for this young population, which led to projective methods that were founded upon psychoanalytic theories of personality and psychopathology. Within this genre of performance personality measures, the *Children's Apperception Test, Ninth Edition, Revised* (*CAT– 9–R*; Bellak & Abrams, 1998), along with its *Color Version* (*CAT–9–RC;* Bellak & Abrams, 2012), were found to be the most felicitous selections for reasons that will be further explained. As stated, this instrument is classified as a projective test, although it is also accompanied by a promising quantitative scoring system designed to measure ego or personality functioning and development in children aged 3 years, 0 months through 10 years, 11 months (Bellak & Abrams, 1998, 2012; Bellak & Bellak, 1949; Bellak, Hurvich, & Gediman, 1973).

More specifically, the CAT–9–RC consists of ten cards depicting animals in a variety of different social circumstances. The various situations are more specifically designed to elicit responses related to (a) issues concerning dependency and autonomy (i.e., referred to dynamically as oral problems), (b) sibling rivalry, (c) attitude toward parental figures and authority (i.e., referred to dynamically as the *oedipal complex* and the related *primal scene*), (d) aggression toward self and others, (e) fears of being left alone at night (i.e., related to the dynamic issues of masturbation, toileting, and parents' response to these behaviors), and (f) acceptance by the adult world. To fully comprehend the CAT–9–RC, it is most prudent to be cognizant of the concepts upon which it is based, along with its derivation as a storytelling test of apperception.

Therefore, a detailed history setting the stage for emergence of the CAT–9–RC is next provided. This history is further apportioned into (a) an overview of the subtopics covered in this section, (b) the general assumptions and principles of projective testing, (c) a classification of projective tests, (d) a review of the storytelling technique and the TAT (i.e., the forerunner of the CAT), (e) reliability of the TAT and storytelling as a technique, (f) validity of the TAT and storytelling technique, (f) limitations of the TAT and storytelling technique, and finally, culminating in (h) the development of the CAT–9–RC.

History Contributing to Development of the CAT–9–RC

In this section, a succinct history of projection and the projective hypothesis as applied to personality testing is first presented. Second, the manner in which projective tests have been classified is discussed, including tests of apperception. Third, the *Thematic Apperception Test* (*TAT*) is presented as a prelude to the CAT–9–RC, which was originally designed to correct the proposed limitations of the TAT as regarding young children. Fourth, and finally, the CAT–9–RC is delineated in terms of design, assumptions, and the personality constructs it is intended to measure in a quantitative versus qualitative manner.

PROJECTIVE TESTING: ASSUMPTIONS AND PRINCIPLES

When Frank (1939) introduced the concept of *projection*, he assumed that when examinees were asked to respond to ambiguous stimuli (e.g., inkblots, interpersonal scenes), they in essence cast or transmit aspects of their personality into their interpretation of them, including such things as feelings, beliefs, self-perception, and perception of the external environment (e.g., other people, relationships among events and objects). In that sense, projective tests may be understood as unstructured in both design and purpose. Projection is related to the principle of *psychological determinism* or the *law of causality*, which contends that everything said or written as a response to some circumstances or stimuli has a dynamic or meaningful internal cause. Hence, projection and projective tests have always had strong psychoanalytic roots (Freud, 1919).

Murray (1938) and Bellak (1954) preferred to use the related term of *apperception*, which they defined as the meaningful interpretation of a stimulus. More specifically, apperception involves the use of learned or acquired memory traces to make sense out of a stimulus that is ambiguous to some degree. This explains why this term is salient in the titles of the tests they developed. A final principle related to projective test interpretation is that of *apperceptive distortion*. This occurs when an examinee's interpretation of a stimulus is to some extent discrepant from consensual reality. That is, such a phenomenon manifests itself in degrees relative to pure perception; specifically, the more discrepant a response is from consensual reality, the more it reflects something unique and meaningful about an examinee's personality. Gross distortion is unequivocally maladaptive and in extremes indicates the presence of a psychotic process.

THE CLASSIFICATION OF PROJECTIVE TESTS

Frank was the first theorist to classify projective tests based on certain characteristics. However, Lindzey's (1959) system is considered to be more effective in that the categories are more clearly defined and distinct. They are as follows: (a) tests based on theory versus empirical evidence, (b) formal interpretation of symbols or signs versus a more holistic content-focused interpretation, (c) measurement of general personality versus specific variables, (d) group versus individual administration, and (e) type of elicited response. Of all these categories, the last one is considered the most vital. The various types of responses include the following: (a) association (e.g., a word-association test; Hill, 1975), (b) completion (e.g., sentence-completion tests; Holaday, Smith, & Sherry, 2000); (c) choice or order (e.g., Q-sort technique; Stephenson, 1953), (d) expression (e.g., describing an inkblot; Rorschach, 1921/1942), and (e) construction (e.g., storytelling; Murray, 1943). The CAT–9–RC is best classified as a constructive apperceptive test. That is, children are asked to create or manufacture an imaginational or fantastic story about animal characters in various social situations. The ambiguous properties in the card stimuli effectuate a projective process wherein examinees reveal unconscious aspects of their personality functioning, which can be assessed either quantitatively or qualitatively.

STORYTELLING AND THE THEMATIC APPERCEPTION TEST (TAT)

Storytelling in response to pictures was actually first introduced by Alfred Binet, who is best known for inaugurating the formal measurement of intelligence (Binet & Henri, 1896). Later, this technique was employed within the context of psychological experimentation (Brittain, 1907; Clark, 1926; Libby, 1908; Schwartz, 1932). However, H. A. Murray was the first to incorporate a storytelling format into personality testing.

Called the *Thematic Apperception Test* (*TAT*; Morgan & Murray, 1935), this instrument was first used to elicit fantasies from patients who, for either monetary or other reasons, needed to proceed more quickly through psychoanalysis. Later, the scope of the test was broadened to measure various facets of personality, including unconscious drives, sentiments, unresolved conflicts, and complexes. The test itself consists of 30 black-and-white cards, each depicting a variety of social situations (Jahnke & Morgan, 1997; Morgan, 1991, 1995a, 1995b, 1995c, 1996, 1998a, 1998b, 1999a, 1999b; 1999c; Murray, 1943). Although the test stimuli present people and objects that are easily identified, there remains sufficient ambiguity in the scenes to permit the manifestation of apperception as defined prior. In Murray's words, the test capitalizes on "the tendency of people to interpret an ambiguous human situation in conformity with their past experiences and present wants" Murray, 1943, p. 1). In addition, many of the cards are designated for boys, girls, men, women, or some combination of these. There are also some general cards, including a blank card that is the most ambiguous of all.

Regarding administration, the examinee is instructed that the TAT is a test of imagination, defined as one form of intelligence, and to make-up "as dramatic story" as possible for each scene, including (a) what is currently happening in the scene, (b) what the particular characters are feeling and thinking, (c) what led up to the scene, and (d) how the story ends or the outcome (Murray, 1943, p. 3). Rather than a formal inquiry, the examiner can use prompts (a) to ensure the examinee covers most or all of that afforded in the instructions and (b) to help the examinee elaborate on themes that appeared diagnostically important (e.g., providing more information about a character that was added to the scene by the examinee). Although there are 31 cards, administration is limited to a subset of 20 cards, which are to be given to examinees in two separate sessions not to exceed 10 cards per session, approximately five minutes per card, and with a minimum of one intervening day between sessions. While the testee reported each story, the tester would typically create a written, verbatim record, which represents the raw data for interpretation. Other modes of administration that are more infrequently employed include using a stenographer or having examinees compose their stories in written form.

Murray's original interpretive scheme was qualitative (i.e., narrative) and fundamentally consisted of identifying three key aspects of the stories, including *needs* (i.e., characterological or internal forces of behavior), *presses* (i.e., external or environmental forces of behavior acting upon the characters), and *thema* (i.e., the interaction between needs and presses, together with the outcomes in terms of the hero's success or failure). Furthermore, the test was initially designed to appraise a number of variables (see Table 12.1), some of which are analogous to those of the discussed henceforth. As can be seen in Table 12.1, assessment of these variables relies principally on the projective hypothesis, including analysis of both apperception and any apperceptive distortion reflected in the story content.

Although the TAT was initially slow to gain acceptance within the psychological community, by the 1960s it was equal in extent to the Rorschach Inkblot Test (Buros, 1965; Sundberg, 1961), first by clinical psychologists in practice, then followed by research-oriented psychologists. In fact, in years past, professors taught that the TAT and Rorschach were excellent complementary tests to employ within the same battery. Specifically, it was purported that the TAT focused on revealing interpersonal aspects of personality functioning, while the Rorschach tapped into more of an intrapsychic X-ray of the mind and personality.[1]

Simultaneously, criticisms and problems concerning the TAT began to accumulate. Some of these were more general while others were targeted more specifically to young children. First, and more broadly speaking, a proliferation of both qualitative and quantitative scoring and interpretive systems were developed for the TAT, none of which gained clear prominence as was done for the Rorschach Inkblot Test by the Rorschach, Comprehensive System (R–CS; Exner, 2003). In part, this was attributed to Murray's qualitative scheme (see Table 12.1), which was vague and without much elaborative guidance (Kleinmuntz, 1967).[2] In addition, the test was non-technical, produced simple verbal content as raw data, and could be interpreted according to a variety of personality theories. Although these characteristics may seem to represent assets, an inadvertent result was that many clinical psychologists produced their own unique interpretive schemes without developing a standardized scoring and interpretative system (Kleinmuntz,

Table 12.1 Thematic Apperception Test (TAT) Variables: Content Analysis

Variable Name	Thematic Content
The hero	Which character does the examinee most resemble, identify with, show the most interest in, or adopt his or her point of view?
The hero's motives, trends, and feelings	What does the hero tend to think, feel, and do? Note personality type, mental disorder, anything unusual or unique, or common but extreme in intensity or frequency.
Forces in the hero's environment	What situations, chiefly human situations, confront the hero, especially those that are unique, intense, or frequent (i.e., repetitive).
Outcomes	What is the comparative strength of the forces emanating from the hero (i.e., needs) and the forces emanating from the environment (presses)?
Themes	Interaction of the hero's needs and environmental presses, together with the outcome (viz., a simple thema). Complex themas are a sequence of interlocking simple themas.
Interests and sentiments	Positive and negative *cathexis* of older women (i.e., mother figures), older men (father figures), and same-sex characters (i.e., sibling figures).

Note. The hero can be more than one character. *Cathexis* = the investment of emotional significance in a person, object, or situation.

1967). Notwithstanding these drawbacks, the selective review presented subsequently is intended to illustrate the following: (a) the promising features of a storytelling test (such as used in the TAT), (b) an analogous storytelling test that is arguably more appropriate for young children (viz., the CAT–9–RC), and (c) a quantitative scoring system designed to measure key aspects of a young child's developing personality (viz., ego functioning). This will be done by examining the reliability and validity of the TAT.

Reliability of the TAT   Recall that reliability concerns both the consistency and accuracy of a psychological test. Interrater reliability is the most pertinent type of reliability for a projective measure such as the TAT, primarily because such a test utilizes a complex scoring system that must be applied consistently by examiners. This is contrasted with ostensibly "objective" methods of personality assessment in which an examinee must select one of a number of alternative responses (e.g., *True* or *False*), which is scored in such a manner with minimal subjective judgment on the part of the examiner. In terms of how interrater reliability is measured, the most common method is the use of the correlation coefficient. For years, the experts have advised that interrater *reliability coefficients* reach the high 0.80s to achieve feasible degrees of consistency (Cohen & Swerdlik, 2018; Gulliksen, 1950; Kleinmuntz, 1967; Murstein, 1963) and in the 0.90s if test results are to be used to make vital decisions, which is frequently done with personality test data (e.g., see Warner, 2013, p. 907).

As concerning the TAT, interrater reliabilities have invariably reached or exceeded 0.90 (a) when examiners are properly trained in the use of a particular system (including reasoning practice) and (b) when the system's variables or categories are diligently defined with detailed instructions and case examples (Cramer, 1987, 1999; Kagan & Moss, 1959; McClelland, Clark, Roby, & Atkinson, 1949; Veroff, Atkinson, Feld, & Gurin, G., 1960). For instance, McClelland's empirical or quantitative TAT scoring system, which measures the *implicit needs* for achievement (n-Ach), affiliation or intimacy (n-Int), and power (n-Pow), have yielded interrater reliability coefficients that have consistently fallen within this accepted range (Ackerman, Clemence, Weatherhill, & Hilsenroth, 1999; Atkinson, 1957; McClelland, Atkinson, Clark, & Lowell, 1953; Ornduff, Freedenfeld, Kelsey, & Critelli, 1994); Westen, Ludolph, Lener, Ruffins, & Wiss, 1990). In contrast, interrater reliabilities for more poorly defined scoring systems, with vaguely defined variables, have been predictably low (Clark, 1944; Veroff, Atkinson, Feld, & Gurin, 1960; see also Jenkins, 2008).

Test–retest reliability is also relevant concerning the TAT. In addition to measuring temporal stability, this analysis also provides evidence as to whether the intended construct being measured is sufficiently consistent to be considered a personality trait. Murray's original needs–presses scoring system has shown the following stability coefficients (with the time interval between test and retest noted in parentheses); (a) $r = 0.08$ (2 months); (b) $r = 0.60$ (6 months); (c) $r = 0.50$ (10 months); and (d) $r = 0.46$ (12 months). These stability coefficients are generally moderate in magnitude or strength, with an expected downward trend as the time interval increases or widens (Kleinmuntz, 1967, p. 313). Other kinds of test reliability, especially internal stability reliability, have been deemed inappropriate for the TAT. This is attributed to the fact that the card stimuli pull or evoke a variety of themes (e.g., aggression), hence by definition precluding any expectation of within-test (i.e., between card) consistency. However, the overall evidence reported here demonstrates that a projective storytelling technique, assuming the scoring principles are properly designed and examiners are sufficiently trained, has the capacity to accurately measure personality traits.

Validity of the TAT   Validity of the TAT addresses three vital issues, including differential diagnosis, describing personality, and predicting behavioral outcomes. The first regards the ability of the TAT to identify an individual's disorder within a particular nosological system, whether it be that proposed by the *DSM–5* (American Psychiatric Association, 2013), the *Psychodynamic Diagnostic Manual, Second Edition* (*PDM–2*; Lingiardi & McWilliams, 2017), or some other recognized scheme. However, similar to other projective tests, the TAT has never been known or even expected to perform such function effectively, especially concerning purportedly atheoretical diagnostic systems such as the *DSM–5* (Abt & Bellak, 1950; Bellak et al., 1973).

In terms of describing personality, Harrison initially found some of the greatest degrees of success for the TAT. In essence, he demonstrated that his personality descriptions, which were based on participants' TAT stories, were congruent with 83% of their biographical data garnered by independent judges. In addition, Harrison's diagnostic inferences were correct in 75% of the cases. Finally, his estimation of subjects' IQ scores based on their TAT stories correlated 0.78 with their obtained IQ scores. More recent evidence indicates that the TAT can effectively discriminate between people high and low in the need for achievement (Kwon, Campbell, & Williams, 2001; Tuerlinckz, De Boeck, & Lens, 2002), along with evidence demonstrating a direct relationship between aggressive fantasies in TAT stories and overt acting-out violence (Megargee & Cook, 1967).

Regarding predictive validity, participants measured as being high in achievement motivation implicitly (i.e., unconsciously) on the TAT by means of storytelling was effective in predicting their long-term success as business managers (Chen, Su, & Wu, 2012; McAdams, 2008). Of more general and greater significance, measuring motives by means of implicit tests (such as the TAT) has been found to be superior in making long-term predictions of behavior as compared to using explicit or conscious measures (Chen, Su, & Wu, 2012; Koestner & McClelland, 1990; McAdams, 1990; Woike, 1995). That is, explicit measures are more accurate in making short-term predictions of behavior. Finally, the TAT has been shown to be useful as a treatment outcome measure (Kempler & Scott, 1972). To recapitulate, these results show that storytelling tests, such as the TAT, can achieve the following: (a) the measurement of important unconscious aspects of personality, (b) the ability to make reasonably accurate predictions regarding long-term behavioral outcomes, and (c) the capability of being more accurate in making behavioral outcome predictions compared to using explicit self-report tests.

It was this kind of evidence that supported the addition of the CAT to the test inventory for purposes of measuring young examinee's personalities. It also provided an auspicious opportunity to incorporate projective testing into this book, which many practitioners continue to support and use in both assessment and treatment. However, prior to discussing development of the CAT–9–RC, it is important also discuss some of the principal limitations of this approach to testing, which is provided next.

Limitations of the TAT   Although the previous review illustrates that the TAT, and by extension the storytelling technique, possesses reliability and validity as a measure of personality, some caveats are in order. In particular, when such assessment systems are content oriented and not quantitative, and when their variables and classifications lack detail and definition, both reliability and validity suffer considerably (Clark, 1944; Lillenfeld, Wood, & Garb, 2000; Veroff et al., 1960). Thus, it can be contended that a storytelling technique, such as the TAT, can be an effective personality test, but only if it is used with a properly refined, detailed, and quantitative (i.e., empirical) scoring system. However, another more narrowly defined potential limitation when it comes to young children concerns a key stimulus feature of the TAT cards, that is, the fact that they are reliant on human figures.

Dr. Ernest Kris, a colleague of Leopold Bellak, is credited with first proposing that the TAT stimulus cards are likely to be insufficiently useful to younger children aged ten and younger due to the fact that they rely exclusively on human figures (Bellak, 1975; Bellak & Abrams, 1998, 2012; Bellak et al., 1973). In particular, human figures have been considered too large in physical size, authoritarian in symbolism, and thus excessively intimidating to young children, thus impeding both identification with the characters and the projective process itself.

Therefore, based largely on theoretical or conceptual considerations, animal figures were hypothesized to be more appropriate for younger children. The underlying rationale is as follows: (a) animals are generally smaller in size relative to children, as children are to adults, hence children will identify much easier and more naturally with animals in the role of the "underdog"; (b) animals are more ambiguous relative to human figures in terms of gender, age, and role, hence facilitating the projective process; and (c) animals are more neutral regarding family customs and culture, hence minimizing any impediment to identification with the figures. For these reasons, it was hypothesized that animal figures would better facilitate the process of identification, projection, and apperception, the last including a greater potential for apperceptive distortion, which all translated into obtaining more meaningful interpretations of young children's developing personality or ego functioning. Next, development of the CAT–9–RC is discussed, ensued by a presentation of this test as a standardized method of measuring young children's personality by means of T-data.

Development of the CAT–9–RC

The original set of 18 CAT–9–RC cards were drawn in black and white by a professional illustrator of children's books, Violet La Mont, according to suggestions made by its original authors Bellak and Bellak (1949). Each card depicted animals in various situations deemed fundamental to children aged 3–10. The final number was reduced to ten cards, based on pilot test cases conducted by the authors, along with protocols shared by psychologists working with young children responding to the original set. Many of the latter were Bellak's students who were enrolled in his TAT courses and who provided feedback regarding the 18 cards. Much later, the same ten cards were colorized (Bellak & Abrams, 2012), which is the version principally used here, as it appears to be more effective in initiating and maintaining young children's interest, focus, and attention (not to mention that of the examiner).[3]

In the most recently published manual, Bellak and Abrams identify the CAT–9–RC as a "direct descendant" of Henry Murray's TAT, which is chiefly why this test is reviewed prior in some detail as it provides useful context. These authors further describe the CAT–9–RC as an "*apperceptive method of investigating personality by studying the dynamic meaningfulness of individual differences in the perception of standard stimuli*" (Bellak & Abrams, 2012, p. 1). The original focus was on revealing the nature of young children's relationships with major attachment figures in their lives, especially parental and authority figures, along with siblings and peers, and the children's primary drives. The design included an emphasis on psychoanalytic theory, such as the *Oedipal complex* and the related *primal scene*

Table 12.2 Children's Apperception Test, Ninth Edition, Revised, Color Version (CAT–9–RC): Card Descriptions and Themes

Card #	Description	Themes
1	Baby chicks seated at table with large bowl of food; adult chicken in background.	Food privation or deprivation; sibling rivalry; food as reward or punishment; oral-dependent issues.
2	Tug-of-war upon hill between one large bear pulling on rope against one large and baby bear pulling on opposing side.	Aggression; autonomy; identification with mother or father figure; rope as source of concern (e.g., rope breaking; castration fears).
3	Adult lion seated with pipe and cane; little mouse appears in hole in lower right.	Father figure; aging/ailing figure or strong figure (benign or dangerous); identification with mouse and/or lion.
4	Adult kangaroo carrying basket and milk bottle with baby in pouch holding balloon; larger kangaroo child in proximity on bike.	Sibling rivalry; concerns of origin of babies; identification with older (autonomy) or younger (regression) child kangaroo; flight from danger.
5	Crib with two baby bears and empty large adult bed in background; darkened nighttime scene.	Concerns of primal scene (i.e., what goes on between parents in bed); mutual manipulation and exploration between children.
6	Darkened cave with one small bear in foreground and two adult bears in background.	Concerns of primal scene; jealousy; problems of masturbation at bedtime.
7	Tiger with observable fangs and claws jumping at a monkey, who is trying to jump away.	Aggression; anxiety related to aggression; defense against aggression by card rejection or innocuous story; can monkey outsmart the tiger; animal tails may symbolize castration fears.
8	Adult monkey sitting and talking with baby monkey in foreground; two adult monkeys in background sitting and talking on sofa and drinking tea.	Child's role in the family system; identifies dominant foreground monkey as mother or father figure, and as benign or admonishing/inhibiting one.
9	View from darkened room through open door into a lighted room, including a child's bed with baby white rabbit looking directly at doorway.	Fear of darkness and being left alone; desertion by parents; curiosity regarding what occurs in the adjoining room.
10	Baby dog lying on the lap of an adult dog sitting on a stool in the foreground, with toilet seat, towel and rack, and partial bathtub in background.	Crime and punishment; child's internal moral conceptions; toilet training and masturbation issues; regressive trends.

(i.e., children's fantasies regarding their parents' sexual activities in the bedroom), in addition to an analysis of drives such as aggression (i.e., *intra-aggression* and *extra-aggression*). However, because the CAT–9–RC is primarily concerned with the production and analysis of content, as is the TAT (Bellak, 1944, 1949), it is actually conducive to conceptualizing a case by application of a variety of personality theories and notions concerning psychopathology (e.g., Adler, 1969; Rogers 1942). This will be illustrated when the ego functions are named and interpreted later.

Table 12.2 provides a complete listing of the ten CAT–9–RC cards, including succinct descriptions of the scenes and their targeted themes and relationship issues. Although key psychoanalytic concepts can be identified, such as sexual and aggressive drives, castration fears, and Oedipal issues, the thematic pull of the cards can easily be expanded to issues common to other personality theories. These include interpersonal relationships with parents, authority figures, siblings, peers, and one's perceived role in the family, along with more intrapsychic issues, such as autonomy, dependency needs, moral values, antisocial character tendencies (Schaefer & Norman, 1967), anxiety and fears, and personality development (Nolan, 1959). As expected, CAT–9–RC has demonstrated an enduring ability of providing rich sources of insight as a clinical tool, especially with young children. Hence, it was selected to fill the lack of a performance personality test for young children, especially because it is accompanied by a rather detailed quantitative scoring system (see Bellak et al., 1973, pp. 73–351).

Norm Reference Data

Although this test is designed for children ranging in age from 3 to 10 years, the CAT–9–RC manual does not provide norms for this test. Therefore, in lieu of providing norms afforded by a standardization sample, as was done for the majority of previous measures in this book, this section delineates the metrics upon which such norms could be developed. The reason for a lack of norms is principally due to this test's original design mirroring that of the TAT, which assesses variables based on ego psychology using a qualitative thematic content analysis approach (see Table 12.1; see also Bellak, 1955/1992, Short Form, pp. 1–4). Therefore, it will be examined how the CAT–9–RC was modified into a quantitative scoring system upon which norms may be formulated.

Ego psychology is classified as a *depth theory* versus *trait theory*. As such, from its inception the CAT–9–RC was created to measure the dynamic dimensions of personality (i.e., the mechanisms of personality as defined earlier in this chapter). When taking a depth approach to personality assessment, the focus is on ascertaining internal personality patterns and integrating processes (Kleinmuntz, 1967, p. 58). An example would be garnering evidence that a testee has a tendency to be *intropunitive* due to the presence of a *harsh superego introject*. Therefore, this is consistent with the broader term personality mechanism, which accounts for the presence of particular observable or overt traits. Elaborating on the aforesaid example, someone who is measured to have a strong intropunitive mechanism, such as a harsh superego, is predicted to show masochistic, self-defeating, or melancholic traits. Therefore, depth theory is ambitious in the sense that it attempts to explicate both the what (i.e., a description) and the why (i.e., an underlying explanation) of personality, which is more conducive to treatment planning.

This is contrasted with *trait theory*, which attempts to identify how many independent dimensions of traits exist, along with the manner in which these are organized within the individual to describe that person's profile of relatively consistent patterns of behavior. Whereas trait theory espouses a psychometric (i.e., measurement) approach focused strictly on description (and by logical extension prediction), depth theorists are more attuned to the internal dynamics of the total personality, thus explanation. However, because the assessment of dynamic dimensions of personality is more intricate and challenging to measure quantitatively, depth theorists tend to utilize qualitative analysis that relies more upon theory than tests norms. This does not mean, however, that the two are mutually exclusive.

As will become more apparent in subsequent sections, Bellak et al. (1973) have developed a scoring system that can be used to quantitatively measure a number of dynamic dimensions of personality functioning as applied to young children.[4] This system has been further refined in a number of research studies using various samples, examining issues such as reliability and validity (Bellak & Goldsmith, 1984). Furthermore, a more scrupulously written ego function assessment manual was made available several years later, including the following: (a) discussions concerning scaling; (b) suggested interview questions, test stimuli, supplemental inquiries and responses to guide scoring accuracy; (c) optional id and superego variables, questions, and responses for scoring; and (d) a detailed revised rating manual for each ego function (Bellak, 1989). The latter provides descriptions of how each ego function would manifest itself at each interval on the seven-point scale, with higher numbers showing more adaptive functioning. This portion of the manual is a revised version of what was used in the original study that identifies the 12 ego functions and the scoring metric (Bellak at al., 1973). Regarding scaling, this manual also provides formulas for converting scores on the 7-point scale into proportionate scores on a 13-point scale (i.e., multiplying the number by two and subtracting one (e.g., a score of 5 on the 7-point scale would be 5 x 2 = 10–1 = 9). Hence, although there are no national norms available, such a system at minimum brings the analysis into the quantitative or psychometric arena. If a proper norm reference sample was ever garnered, this scoring metric could be employed to devise standard scores for subsequent test interpretation. Next, CAT–9–RC administration will be presented, ensued by a more detailed discussion of the quantitative scoring system and, finally, test interpretation.

Administration

CAT–9–RC administration begins by introducing the test to the child as, "a story game" (Bellak & Abrams, 1998, p. 2). The objective is to create a positive attitude in the young examinee, which in turn leads to increased productivity (Lyles, 1958). More specifically, the child is asked to make up a pretend story to each card, including what led up to the scene, what is occurring in the picture, what comes next, and then how it ends or its outcome (i.e., a beginning, middle, and end). The cards should be administered one at a time and in their numbered sequence. Non-leading prompts are encouraged if the child is having difficulty (e.g., if the testee is merely describing the picture or ends the story prematurely), including, "and then what happens next," or "now how does the story end?" (Bellak & Abrams, 1998). The examiner creates a written verbatim record of the examinee's responses, as in the TAT, including diagnostically relevant side remarks, physical activity, gestures, facial expressions, and posturing (Blatt, Engel, Mirmow, 1961).

After the administration of all ten cards, an optional inquiry may be done in which the child is asked to elaborate on points of significance to scoring and interpretation (see the following Scoring and Interpretation sections). As frequently observed in performance personality testing, practice and experience with the scoring and interpretive principles facilitates knowing when and how to prompt for the pertinent information. Estimated time of administration is 20–45 minutes (Encyclopedia of Children's Health, 2021). The variability in durations is due to the open-ended nature of this test and individual differences due to both age and temperament.

Scoring

As previously indicated in the Norm Reference Data section, the quantitative scoring system that is applied to the CAT–9–RC is theoretically based on ego psychology (Bellak et al., 1973), in essence, an updated version of Freud's original drive-reduction psychoanalytic theory (Freud, 1900/1913, 1915/1957), with emphasis on ego functioning. Although a large portion of the assessment system is qualitative in nature, paralleling that of the TAT (see also Table 12.1), Bellak et al. (1973) proposed a quantitative scoring scheme that measures 12 dimensions of *ego functioning* (i.e., personality functioning and development). The 12 ego functions are operationally defined according to general propositions, along with their major subfunctions referred to as components, all of which are based on a comprehensive literature review of previous ego functions and scales designed to measure them (e.g., Bellak, 1958; Bellak & Hurvich, 1969; Bellak, Hurvich, Silvan, & Jacobs, 1968; Beres, 1956; Hurvich & Bellak, 1968). Therefore, the 12 ego functions and their components need to be defined first because scores for each must be inferred from examinee's CAT–9–RC stories and test behavior, supplemented by clinical interview and other assessment information as done for all psychological test data. As shown by previous TAT reliability and validity studies, the more clearly these are defined, the more *accurate* will be the scoring and interpretations upon which they are based.

Moving forward, this scoring section is broken down into three subtopics. First, a review of ego psychology is offered, with a particular focus on the personality structure as defined by this theory. These concepts are vital to comprehend because they represent the theoretical context upon which the CAT–9–RC is based. Second, the 12 ego functions, the superego, and ego strength are all diligently defined because it is these personality constructs that are measured by this test. Finally, the ego function assessment (EFA) scoring procedure will be explained, including its scoring metric and the data table designed for presenting CAT–9–RC score results as part of a psychological assessment report.

EGO PSYCHOLOGY AND THE PERSONALITY STRUCTURE

Ego functions were first defined by Freud in the 1895 ego functions "project." The initial structural model of psychoanalytic theory was later delineated as consisting of the famous triad, id, ego, and superego (Freud, 1923), wherein all psychic energy derived from the id instincts. Later, ego functions were conceptualized by theorists such as Erikson (1950/1963) as independent from that of id, with its own reservoir of psychic energy variously termed *autonomous ego functions* or the *conflict-free ego sphere*. The major implication was that many ego functions were no longer considered defensive in nature and preoccupied with conflict, but rather were also growth oriented and adaptive. In general, the ego is now considered the component of the personality designed to cope with the external environment and its demands (American Psychological Association, 2015), including perception, thinking, problem-solving, reasoning, reality testing, regulation of affect, reconciliation of conflicting ideas and impulses, intelligence, memory, self-awareness, and motor functions. Because these mechanisms essentially represent what most mental health workers think of as core components of personality, these theoretical notions can be generalized to other theories of personality as well (e.g., self-concept).

Of further relevance, ego functions were thought to gradually develop from a simple undifferentiated form into a more differentiated, integrated, and more complex form by means of a salutatory (i.e., stage-like) process (e.g., see Erikson, 1950/1963). Such formation represented the infant's growing awareness of being an individual who was separate, distinct, and autonomous from others, especially parents. More specifically, this development proceeded from the preconscious stage, in which the ego was only partially formed, to the conscious stage from which all the ego functions discussed subsequently emerge to help the individual cope with both threats and challenges posed both internally and externally.

In their study of ego functions, Bellak and colleagues (Bellak et al., 1973) intended to (a) discover the principal ego functions that could be identified using comprehensive interviews and other available diagnostically relevant information about their patients and (b) explicitly define their components such that they could be measured quantitatively in a reliable and valid manner. In doing so, they espoused the aforementioned ego psychological approach to personality. To reiterate, this approach emphasizes the functions of the ego in controlling such things as impulses, forethought, planning, and adaptation to the external environment. It also assumes that the ego possesses its own energy source, hence permitting it to pursue objectives independent of satisfying the instinctual drives in socially acceptable ways. Lastly, it moves personality functioning and analysis beyond biological drive states and into a more psychosocial view of human development as exemplified by Erikson.[5]

In addition to espousing an ego psychology approach to personality assessment, Bellak et al. (1973) made several additional assumptions. First, they proposed that ego functions are continuous dimensions, as opposed to characteristics that are either dichotomously present or absent. Second, as stated prior, they also conceptualized them as unfolding with escalating sophistication in a stage-like (i.e., salutatory) sequence (Bellak, 1975). These facets rendered the various ego functions as akin to personality mechanisms and associated behavioral dispositions, which can be measured or quantified as done in a pure trait descriptive approach to personality assessment, although with age as a consideration due to the proposed developmental aspect. For example, degrees of separation or independence would be expected to become more differentiated with age maturation, along with conscious awareness and behavioral control over impulses. Next, the 12 ego functions identified in the Bellak at al. (1973) original study is summarized, including their definitions and components, along with one dimension of superego functioning. The latter was incorporated because it seemed to represent a very important aspect of personality functioning (i.e., moral development), despite it representing a qualitatively different construct within the theory (i.e., superego versus ego). Lastly, ego strength is a composite variable of the 12 ego functions.

THE 12 EGO FUNCTIONS, SUPEREGO, AND EGO STRENGTH

There are 12 ego functions that make up the *ego function assessment* (*EFA*; Bellak & Abrams, 1998, p. 11). They are enumerated in Form 12.1, along with columns for entering scores, qualitative descriptions, and their components. The focus of this section is on clarifying the descriptions and components for purposes of maximizing scoring reliability. The components are provided by the manual (Bellak & Abrams, 1998), although they are more elaborated in Bellak (1989), Bellak et al. (1973), and Bellak and Goldsmith (1984). Such elaboration will be incorporated here with examples of story themes and reactions of the examinee that denote impairment within each ego function. It is important to note that evidence of each of these ego functions can derive from both (a) the content of each story (i.e., examinee responses) and (b) the process of storytelling (i.e., test administration behavior). Furthermore, other assessment information, including other test data and especially that garnered by the initial clinical interview, can provide meaningful context for CAT–9–RC test interpretation. In that sense, CAT–9–RC test interpretation should typically appear last within a test battery, as other test data can facilitate the scoring and interpretive process.

Test observations should target both verbal (e.g., aside commentary, thought process and content, sophistication of vocabulary and imagination) and nonverbal (e.g., physical activity, gestures, facial expressions, posturing, voice tone) evidence analogous to information garnered during a mental status examination. Lastly, both normal and abnormal aspects of each ego function are mentioned for a more comprehensive understanding of each; that is, being cognizant of what defines abnormal personality deepens one's knowledge of what normal personality represents (see Larson & Buss, 2021). The remainder of this section presents the ego functions and their elaborated descriptions, both individually and in sequence. For more information regarding these constructs, the reader is referred to the manual and supplemental resources (Bellak, 1989; Bellak & Abrams, 1998; Bellak & Goldsmith, 1984; Bellak et al., 1973).

Reality Testing and Judgment   *Reality testing* and *judgment* are more common constructs, hence need less elaboration. *Reality testing* refers to psychological mindedness or the ability to introspect. The question here is how well individuals examine their own feelings and internal mental states. Impairments include evidence of delusions, disorientation, and limited reflective awareness in the story thematic content and/or process. *Judgment* essentially refers to how well the story characters can anticipate or discern the likelihood of danger, being censured by others, engaging in behavior considered to be inappropriate by others, or being subject to disapproval.

Sense of Reality   *Sense of reality* addresses both external events and internal experiences. Impairments include characters that show a sense of alienation within the self and from others, and any evidence of dissociation, depersonalization, derealization, emotional isolation, identity diffusion, déjà vu experiences, and trances. Regarding internal experience, this functioning also includes characters' development of individuality, along with uniqueness, and sense of self and self-esteem. These features can be assessed by the degree of the separation of self or main character from principal object representations or other story characters. Compared to reality testing, which addresses the presence of any psychotic disturbances, sense of reality regards one's conscious awareness of both self and the world and from that perspective would reveal more dissociative types of psychopathology.

Regulation and Control of Drives, Affects, and Impulses   *Regulation and control of drives, affects, and impulses* focuses on the general ability to self-regulate, which consists of impulse control, delay of gratification, and the management of affect, emotion, and behavior, such as frustration tolerance and anger management. Evidence of impairment here includes story themes of temper outbursts, conduct disturbance, bad habits, low frustration tolerance, acting-out behaviors, suicide or homicide, rage, irritability, or in contrast, excessive control over these impulses.

Object Relations　*Object relations* addresses the nature and quality of one's interpersonal relationships or attachment patterns. The word "object" refers to a living, animate person or being, including the self, versus an inanimate entity (see Kernberg, 1975, 1984). Therefore, relationships among the story characters are the focus of analysis, especially attachments between the main character and others. Degree of investment, aims of the relationship, the ability to sustain a relationship, and the ability to tolerate separation from significant relationships are all key components. Themes of social overactivity, withdrawal or detachment, narcissistic self-concern, *symbiotic attachments*, and difficulties perceiving others as separate from oneself all demonstrate evidence of psychopathology. A symbiotic attachment constitutes a relationship in which there is no interpersonal boundary between the two individuals. Although this may be considered normal in very early infant–caregiver relationships, it denotes a pathological relationship soon thereafter because the two individuals are functioning psychologically as a single personality or ego state. Hence, this usually indicates a lack of separation-individuation in personality development, even in early childhood.

Thought Processes　*Thought processes* refer to both the process and content of storytelling. Key aspects are the examinee's ability to sustain attention and concentration and to manifest thinking that is logical, sequential, relevant, and coherent. The following questions should be considered: (a) Do associations flow in a logical manner? (b) Is thinking realistic and relevant? Evidence of impairment includes magical thinking, inattention, illogical reasoning, poor immediate and intermediate memory, and disturbed communication patterns, such as the failure to develop *syllogistic thinking* (Bateson, Jackson, Haley, & Weakland, 1956). Briefly, syllogistic thinking consists of a major premise (e.g., all boys are aggressive), a minor premise (e.g., Joey is a boy), and a conclusion (e.g., Joey is aggressive). If the examiner is familiar with Rorschach scoring principles, *deviant verbalizations* (DV) and *deviant responses* (DR) constitute impairments in thought processes (see subsequently).

Adaptive Regression in the Service of the Ego (ARISE)　*Adaptive regression in the service of the ego* (*ARISE*) is perhaps the most vaguely defined ego function and is thus difficult to score accurately. According to ego psychology, there is a normal and expected oscillating process that occurs in which the ego occasionally relaxes its perceptual and conceptual acuity, along with other ego controls, which permits an integration of creativity and ultimately an increase in adaptive potential. In other words, the ego temporarily regresses by relaxing its controls and defenses, which actually leads to greater ego integration and ego strength. From this perspective, individuals with weak egos fail to develop properly because such regression may be unmanageable and therefore too threatening. If permitted to occur in such instances, it risks ego disintegration and severe psychopathology rather than growth. In the context of CAT–9–RC storytelling, ARISE is manifested when examinees effectively employ their imaginations to create a unique and truly imaginary story pursuant to instructions. Succinctly put, ARISE is a type of controlled regression that is paradoxically necessary for growth and further integration (i.e., working together) of ego functions (Rabin, 1960). Psychopathology here is illustrated by one of two extremes. First, abnormal functioning can be shown by the presence of rigid, stereotyped thinking, in which characters and scenes are concretely described, with little (if any) imagination, even with prompting by the examiner. In effect, this trend demonstrates a psychological escape from the task because it is threatening to a weak ego. Second, psychopathology is also demonstrated by the antithetical extreme involving eccentric, overideational thinking. Here, thought processes may be loose, fragmented, bizarre, peculiar, alogical, and vague.

Defensive Functioning　*Defensive functioning* essentially refers to how effective ego defense mechanisms (i.e., coping skills) are working for the hero (i.e., main character) and other characters. That is, are thinking and behavior used adaptively by the characters in the story, especially concerning the identified hero? Also, this addresses the extent to which defenses employed by the story characters have succeeded or failed, symptomatically speaking. Some key defenses identified by Bellak (1975) include *repression* (i.e., the unconscious forgetting of something threatening), *denial* (i.e., something remembered, although in the absence of its significance), *regression* (i.e., moving to an earlier, more pleasant, and less threatening time in development, albeit immature), *displacement* (i.e., expression of an unacceptable thought or feeling onto a nonthreatening target), *projection* (i.e., perceiving in others an unacceptable feeling or belief that resides in oneself), *reaction formation* (i.e., expressing the opposite of one's true feelings), *undoing* (i.e., reaction formation with an additional step that reverses the undesired behavior), and *isolation* (i.e., removing from conscious awareness the emotional significance of an event). Common examples of isolation are (a) when an examinee states after telling an emotional story, "But I don't really care," and (b) when an examinee remains unusually calm when discussing an emotional event. *Intellectualization*, which is a coping mechanism whereby the individual uses reasoning and logic to avoid emotionally threatening feelings, can be conceptualized as a form of isolation. The latter will also be addressed when discussing the Rorschach Inkblot Test later in this chapter. Psychopathology here is generally evidenced by unconscious contents that trigger anxiety, panic, impaired concentration and memory, vulnerability, and a substantial emotional withdrawal to prevent the uncontrolled expression of these feelings.

Stimulus Barrier   *Stimulus barrier* refers to the examinees' sensory processing thresholds in all modalities, primarily external, including vision, audition, touch, and *proprioception* (i.e., body awareness), although also pain, and their effects on functioning. In the event thresholds are too low, hypersensitivity results, causing withdrawal-type physical symptoms, along with irritability. On the other hand, excessively high thresholds are associated with under-responsiveness to stimuli, hence causing impoverished aesthetic sensibilities in CAT–9–RC stories. The latter may be a sign of autism if sufficiently pervasive.

Autonomous Functions   Autonomous functions (Loewenstein, 1954, 1967, 1972) generally involve the ability to conduct oneself independently. Based on psychoanalytic theorizing, the ego consists of primary and secondary autonomous functioning. The former refers to basic sensory-perceptual apparatuses (e.g., vision, audition) that lead to independent functioning, while the latter refers to higher-order operations, including habit patterns, complex learned skills, work routines, hobbies, and interests. Examples of impairments include functional blindness or deafness, poor daily living skills, disturbed will or motivation, interference with automatized (i.e., overlearned) behaviors, and the expenditure of intense effort during tasks. Normalcy in this ego function is defined by default or the absence of any evidence of impairment. Most frequently, secondary autonomous functioning is of primary concern in psychological testing cases. Hence, the degree to which the child functions in an autonomous manner is of principal concern and should be adjusted for age. Hence, more autonomy would be expected of a five-year-old than a three-year-old.

Synthetic-Integrative Functions   Synthetic-integrative functions refer to whether an individual's attitudes, beliefs, feelings, values, affects, behaviors, and self-representation are sufficiently congruent and consistent such that identity formation is developing normally. It is analogous to Erikson's stages of psychosocial development (1950/1963), which is essentially a life-span delineation of ego development and Marcia's (1966) elaboration of this construct into four statuses, including *identity achievement* and *identity diffusion* as the healthiest and unhealthiest outcomes, respectively. It is also consistent with Roger's (1942, 1951) *self-concept*, which consists of both the *real self* and *ideal self*, and especially the degree of congruence between the two as defining psychological health versus psychopathology. Evidence of psychological disturbance would include stories with incongruity among thoughts and feelings, disorganized behavior, absence of goal-directed behavior, poor planning, little or no effort to relate different areas of experience, and fluctuating emotional states, especially without an awareness of such vacillation. This explanation of synthetic-integrative functions also illustrates how such constructs can be assimilated into various conceptualizations of personality mechanisms and traits.

Mastery–Competence   Finally, *mastery–competence* reflects people's ability to perform effectively relative to their stated capacities to actively interact with and successfully cope with environmental forces. However, this also refers to one's subjective sense of competence, hence it includes aspects of the personality such as self-confidence, *self-esteem*, and *self-efficacy*, or one's expectancy of success if effort is properly put forth (Bandura, 1982). The degree of discrepancy between one's objective and subjective sense of competence is measured at face value. That is, there are three possible relative outcomes as follows: (a) negative (i.e., one's actual or objective competence exceeds one's subjective sense of competence; a low self-concept), (b) equivalence or congruence (i.e., accurate self-perception), and (c) positive (i.e., one's actual or objective competence is below one's sense of competence; a high self-concept and potential narcissism if excessive). An additional tendency to investigate here is the degree of consistency of one's sense of competence juxtaposed with one's actual or objective competence, especially considering that the CAT–9–RC is measuring child personality that is in the midst of emerging or developing. One example of psychopathology is a main character who does nothing to alter affect or interact with the environment to resolve difficulties. Excessive passivity and feeling powerless to act are both indicative of an absent sense of competence.

Superego   Although little if any mention is made regarding the id in most versions of ego psychology (e.g., Erikson, 1950/1963), superego functioning continues to play a significant role in personality conceptualization (Bellak et al, 1973; Bellak & Abrams, 1998, 2012). In part, this is because the superego is considered a derivative of the ego and represents both the conscience (i.e., internalized moral standards) and the ego ideal (i.e., the portion of the psyche that imposes perfection into one's behavior and forces the abandonment of infantile narcissism). Appraisal of superego functioning is also relatively straightforward in a child's CAT–9–RC stories and can be addressed by answering the question "Does the punishment fit the crime?" That is, whatever transgression is manifested in the stories, the central analysis is the degree of punishment (if any) imposed on the culprit in relation to the severity of the crime. This analysis is comparable to that regarding one's actual or objective competence versus one's subjective sense of competence, with three possible outcomes as follows: (a) retributive justice (i.e., the punishment is warranted; healthy superego), (b) the punishment is excessive (i.e., harsh superego; tendency to be *intropunitive*), and (c) the punishment is insufficient or absent (i.e., weak superego; tendency to be *extrapunitive*). However, analogous to self-competency, an additional aspect of superego functioning is the consistency with which punishment is meted out, typically manifested across several CAT–9–RC stories rather than simply within a single story. Finally, the timing of punishment (i.e., immediate versus delayed) should be considered, as it can affect its quality and effectiveness (Miltenberger, 2012; Speigler, 2016).

Ego Strength Bellak et al. (1973) also considered "a sum total of ego functions as ego strength" (p. 336), analogous to a full-scale IQ score denoting a complex general *g* factor (Spearman, 1904, 1927) that subsumes all the subtest and index scores of an individually administered intelligence test. *Ego strength* has been defined as the ability "to tolerate frustration and stress, postpone gratification, modify selfish desires when necessary, and resolve internal conflicts and emotional problems before they lead to neurosis" (American psychological Association, 2015, p. 355). This definition is conceptually consistent with the 12 ego functions as previously delineated by Bellak et al. (1973).

The final subtopic regards the ego function assessment (EFA) process, scoring metric, and data table. Here, it is explained how each ego function is to be quantified and the scale of measurement involved. Data entry into Form 12.1 is also to be reviewed. This information will then set the stage for CAT–9–RC interpretation.

EGO FUNCTION ASSESSMENT (EFA): SCORING METRIC AND TABLE

Bellak at al. (1973) provide a manual for scoring the ego and related functions (pp. 74–284, 334–350), which was modified by Louis N. Gruber and published in the *Ego Function Assessment (EFA)* manual (Bellak, 1989, pp. 29–41). These sources also include the superego function. Each recommend utilizing either a 7-point scale with halfway points between whole numbers or a 13-point scale using all whole numbers. On both scales, higher scores denote more effective ego functioning; in their words, "13 signifies the very best functioning," (Bellak et al, 1973, p. 336), this referring to the 13-point alternative. The short form (Bellak, 1955/1992), which is essentially a record form that an examiner may use in scoring the CAT–9–RC both qualitatively and quantitatively, utilizes the 13-point scale option in graphic format.

More specifically, the graph lists each ego function at the top identified with Roman numerals I–XII (proceeding from left to right), the scale 1–13 on the left vertical axis (i.e., proceeding from lower numbers at the bottom to higher numbers toward the top), the hypothesized score ranges for each of four diagnostic groups on the right axis (i.e., proceeding from lowest to highest as follows: psychotic, borderline, neurotic, and normal), and with a grid in the middle wherein data points can be placed for each ego function score, then connected to form an ego function profile (Bellak, 1955/1992, p. 5; Bellak, 1989, p. 44; Bellak & Abrams, 1998, p. 14). On the same page of the short form (Bellak, 1955/1992), there is a table that lists the same 12 ego functions, their components, and sample interview questions for each, including two added personality constructs, superego and (primary) drives.

When first constructed, the EFA rating scale was considered to be a continuous variable on an ordinal (i.e., rank-order) measurement scale (see Stevens, 1946; Figure 12.1). Technically, this means that, although higher numbers denote increasingly adaptive levels of ego functioning, intervals between numbers are not considered to be equivalent. Interpreted in this manner, the numerical scale does not provide information as to how much greater one ranking is than another ranking. This interpretation of such a rating scale in psychology is one type of accepted practice. For example, it has been contended that intelligence, achievement, aptitude, and personality tests technically measure more or less accurately the rank-order position of individuals on a test and not the amount of the construct they possess (see, e.g., Kerlinger, 1973; Trochim, 2006). However, it is also common practice for psychologists to interpret such assessment data as representing an equal interval measurement scale because it permits (a) the application of a greater number of statistical manipulations (e.g., the computation of means and standard deviations) and (b) the analysis of individual and group differences (Nunnally, 1978).

Consistent with the latter, Bellak et al. (1973) did compute means on this 13-point scale for 3 of 4 of their diagnostic categories as follows: (a) schizophrenia ($M = 5.86$; range = 2–9); (b) neurotic ($M = 7.42$; range = 4–10); and (c) normal ($M = 5.86$; range 2–9). Although they ultimately modified these numbers to render more theoretically consistent discriminations among these diagnostic groups, including a borderline category, they continued to employ statistics that assume an interval scale of measurement, including references to standard deviations. Therefore, to be consistent with the manner in which Bellak et al. (1973) used this EFA scale, and which is accepted practice in

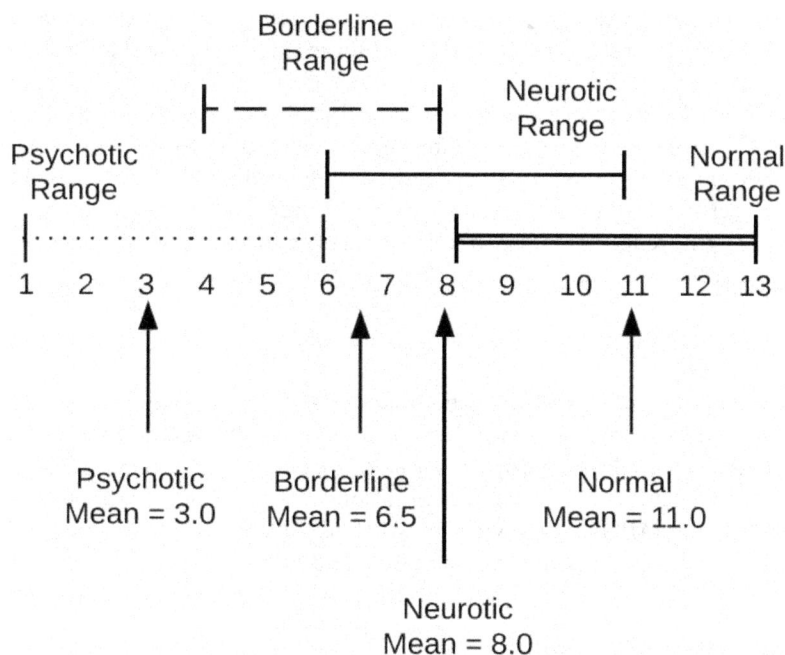

Figure 12.1 Ego Function Assessment (EFA) Scale

Note. The hypothetical distribution range is from 1 to 13, with a midpoint of 7. Means and ranges for each diagnostic category are shown. These ranges are hypothesized to permit those with a psychotic disorder to regress down to 1, incorporate a borderline diagnostic range, and permit "normals" to extend up to 13 (i.e., very best functioning). These adjustments are deemed necessary due to range restriction within the psychotic and normal subgroups and an insufficient number of those with a borderline diagnosis.

interpreting psychological test scores (Kline, 2000; Cohen & Swerdlik, 2018), these numbers are interpreted as representing an equal interval scale of measurement.

Scrutiny of Figure 12.1 illustrates the hypothetical diagnostic scheme Bellak et al. (1973) devised to rate each of the 12 ego functions, including means and score ranges. Of note are the following two characteristics: (a) the overlap among the score ranges and different diagnostic categories; and (b) the conceptualization of a continuum of ego functioning. By interpreting this scale as representing equal interval measurement, both intra- and inter-individual comparisons become possible, especially the former as it permits profile interpretation.

In their original study, these researchers used the mean ego function score as a general or overall measure of ego strength, analogous to the full-scale IQ score for intelligence, thus theoretically implying a hierarchical structure. Therefore, rather than simply summing the other ego functions for an overall ego strength score, they divide this sum or aggregate by the number of ego functions scores contributing to that total; hence, the total score divided by 12. The advantage of using an averaging type of aggregate measure is that the overall score falls on the same 13-point scale as do the specific ego functions. This renders comparisons between overall functioning and more specific aspects of ego functioning much more straightforward and associated with the same diagnostic score ranges. Note from Figure 12.1 two key characteristics: (a) the concept of a continuum or degree of ego functioning; and (b) some degree of overlap among the diagnostic categories and their score ranges. The intent of the latter is to provide flexibility in diagnostic practice (e.g., an individual who is neurotic although trending into the normal range in response to treatment). Furthermore, it simultaneously acknowledges some degree of measurement error consistent with the reporting of confidence intervals, which cannot be computed here. This flexibility is also advantageous when integrated with data from other measures employed within a test battery, including those with different formats and respondents (e.g., standardized rating scales completed by parents and teachers), and further supplemented by clinical interview information.

Form 12.1 shows the single scoring and interpretation table for EFA reporting. Although Bellak et al. devised an interview guide (1973, Appendix A, pp. 422–435) and accompanying scoring manual (Appendix B, pp. 436–491), which would elicit information and guide the scoring of each of the ego function, they also employed other psychological test data, such as the TAT, in contributing to the final EFA scores for any one particular case. Consistent with this practice, the updated EFA manual incorporates other kinds of psychological test data into the interpretive scoring guide to facilitate EFA scoring.

A similar approach is advocated here. First and foremost, the scoring process should focus on young children's responses to the CAT–9–RC. In particular, scoring considers the within and between story content and process elicited from the child during administration and is analyzed for evidence pertinent to each ego function and single superego function.[6] It is also strongly advised that the CAT–9–RC and EFA be done last after all other data within an assessment and test battery have been interpreted. This will facilitate EFA scoring and interpretation analogous to what Bellak et al. (1973) have done by actively integrating other data into the EFA. Once scores for each ego function are entered, they are to be summed or aggregated and divided by 12 for an overall *ego strength* score. The *superego* function is scored separately in the same manner as are the independent ego functions, although it should not be included in the overall ego strength score because it represents a qualitatively different construct or mechanism within the personality structure. Interpretation is the next and final step.

Interpretation

Interpretation requires an explication of psychoanalytic diagnosis and the meanings of the previously referenced categories *psychotic, borderline, neurotic,* and *normal* (in order of increasing psychological health). At present, contemporary psychoanalytic diagnosis as delineated in the *Psychodynamic Diagnostic Manual, Second Edition* (PDM–2; Lingiardi & Bornstein, 2017), makes use of three systems or axes of diagnosis as applied to children, including *personality syndromes (P) axis, mental functioning (M) axis,* and symptom patterns (S) axis. Of most relevance here are the P and M axes, both of which will be elaborated upon in this section in said order.

THE PDM–2 PERSONALITY SYNDROMES (P) AXIS

The personality syndromes (P) axis consists of two components: (a) personality organization (i.e., a spectrum of personality functioning) and (b) personality style or pattern. It is the former that comprises the four diagnostic categories psychotic, borderline, neurotic, and normal (i.e., healthy). A succinct history regarding these levels of personality, also referred to as severities of disturbance, will assist in clarifying these diagnostic terms.

During the later years of the 19th century, psychoanalytic classification consisted of two categories of pathology. One was termed *neurosis,* which referred to both minor and major types of disorder wherein reality testing remained intact. The other and more disturbed type was termed *psychosis,* in which there existed a severe impairment in the perception of consensual reality (McWilliams & Shedler, 2017). Gradually, clinicians began to distinguish two subtypes of neurosis, one in which symptoms were more isolated and situational, whereas the other involved more pervasive symptoms that caused dysfunction in numerous life areas. The former was considered to be a *symptom neurosis,* whereas the latter was afforded the name *character neurosis;* the contemporary analogues would be adjustment disorder and personality disorder (American Psychiatric Association, 2013), respectively.

During the 20th century, clinicians began to identify a group of patients who were simultaneously too disturbed to be considered neurotic and insufficiently disturbed to be considered psychotic, hence the naissance of the category *borderline* (Adler, 1985; Frosch, 1964; Grinker, Werble, & Drye, 1968; Gunderson & Singer, 1975; Hartocollis, 1977; Kernberg, 1975, 1983, 1984; Knight, 1953; Main, 1957; Masterson, 1972, 1976; Stern, 1938; Stone, 1980, 1986). Therefore, from a psychoanalytic viewpoint, the current categories of normal, neurotic (symptom, character), borderline, and psychotic represent varying types of personality organization that are located on a continuum of severity (listed here from normal to increasingly disturbed) and constitute the first component of the P axis.

The second component comprising the P axis is referred to interchangeably as personality styles, patterns, types, and most frequently, syndromes. As such, they represent varying constellations of traits an individual will tend to display, analogous to contemporarily recognized personality disorders (e.g., dependent and obsessive-compulsive personalities). Note that the word "disorder" is intentionally avoided when referring to this component because the other P axis component determines the severity level or degree of psychopathology. Although contemporary psychoanalytic diagnosis recognizes the *DSM–5* version of borderline personality disorder, it is strictly for pragmatic convenience due to the voluminous amount of research done on this use of the construct (McWilliams & Shedler, 2017).

Because childhood is being considered, the first component of personality organization or functioning is most relevant. That is, conceptually speaking, there has been insufficient personality development for a discernable personality style to have been formed. Therefore, the focus here is on assessing overall personality organization or functioning that is in the process of emerging.

Table 12.3 provides a cross-reference or crosswalk among various diagnostic categories, general EFA score ranges, corresponding levels of specific mental abilities that define overall personality organization or functioning

Table 12.3 Ego Strength Diagnosis and Levels of Personality Functioning (P) Axis

Ego Strength Diagnostic Category	Score Range	Level of Mental Functioning	Description
Normal	11–13	Healthy/optimal	Optimal or very good functioning in all or most mental capacities; modest, expectable variations in flexibility and adaptation across contexts.
Neurotic-to-normal	8–11	Mild impairments to appropriate mental functioning	Mild constrictions and areas of inflexibility (e.g., self-esteem, regulation of affect and impulses, self-observing); appropriate functioning with some areas of difficulty.
Borderline-to-neurotic	6–8	Major to moderate impairments to appropriate mental functioning	Tendencies toward fragmentation and difficulties in self–object differentiation, along with limited feelings and thoughts; moderate constrictions affecting stability of relationships and sense of identity.
Psychotic-to-borderline	4–6	Significant defects in basic functions	Significant defects in most domains of mental functioning, along with problems in the organization and integration–differentiation of self and objects.
Psychotic	1–4	Major/severe defects in basic functions	Impaired reality testing; fragmentation and difficulties in self–object differentiation; disturbed perception, integration and regulation of affect and thought; defects in motor and memory abilities and judgment.

Source. Lingiardi, V., & Bornstein, R. F. (2017). Profile of mental functioning M Axis. In V. Lingiardi & N. McWilliams (Eds.), Psychodynamic diagnostic manual (2nd ed., pp. 118–119). New York: The Guilford Press.

Note. Interpretation scheme that facilitates diagnostic decision-making between ego function score and suggested level and description of personality functioning.

(i.e., regarding the P axis), and descriptive summaries of each level. The last two are also provided in the PDM–2 (Lingiardi & Bornstein, 2017, pp. 118–119), although the pairings were created between the ego function severity categories based on a 13-point scale and the ratings in the PDM–2 based on a 48-point scale (i.e., 12–60); for both scales, higher scores denote greater degrees of healthy adaptation. Obviously, the pairings are not precise, as they are based on both deductive and inductive logic as opposed to empirically derived correlations. Its imprecision notwithstanding, this table is pragmatically useful for purposes of test interpretation.[7] As indicated in Form 12.1, the examiner merely notes the diagnostic category shown by the examinee's ego strength score, then inserts the appropriate description from that column and row provided by Table 12.3 (see last column labeled "Description") into the interpretive excerpt in Form 12.1. The point of insertion in Form 12.1 for this interpretive description is highlighted in red font for easy detection and can be changed back to black when completed. Analysis then proceeds to the specific ego functions, their separate scores, and their interpretations.

Looking to the future, the creation of norms for the CAT–9–RC and young children's personality development as measured by EFA would be of great value to contemporary psychological testing. In particular, such data would inform us as to average age-related changes in the measured ego functions, hence permitting analysis of whether a particular child's ego functions are developing normally, are delayed, or are advanced. Currently, all that is available is theory and expert judgment as to what can be developmentally expected.

THE PDM–2 MENTAL FUNCTIONING (M) AXIS

The mental functioning (M) axis is relevant here because it considers a number of more narrowly defined capacities that contribute to general personality organization and functioning reviewed previously. The capacities are schematically organized into four domains, including (a) cognitive and affective processes, (b) identity and relationships, (c) defense and coping, and (d) self-awareness and self-direction. Because young children's personalities are still in the process of forming, the M axis capacities, which are highly developmental in nature, become the prominent target of analysis. Table 12.4 lists the 12 mental capacities, including their names and succinct descriptions of each, which are provided in more detail in the *Psychodynamic Diagnostic Manual, Second Edition* (*PDM–2*; Lingiardi & Bornstein, 2017, pp. 76–79). Scrutiny of this table reveals (a) the developmental aspect of each ability and, most importantly, (b) their conceptual similarity to the various ego functions.

Table 12.4 Mental Functioning (M) Axis Capacities

Capacity Name	Capacity Definition
1. Regulation, attention, and learning	Ability to attend to and process information, regulate attentional focus, divide attention to multitask, filter information from consciousness when needed, and learn from experience.
2. Affective range, communication, and understanding	Ability to experience, express, and comprehend the full range of affects in ways that are appropriate to the situation and consistent with social norms.
3. Mentalization and reflective functioning	Ability to refer and reflect on one's own and others' mental states and to use this in personal and social interactions; mentalization is a form of imagination used in understanding behavior.
4. Differentiation and integration	Ability to distinguish self from other, fantasy from reality, internal representations from external objects and circumstances, and present from past and future.
5. Relationships and intimacy	Depth, range, and consistency (i.e., stability) of a person's relationships and the ability to adjust interpersonal distance/closeness as needed for different relationships.
6. Self-esteem regulation and quality of internal experience	Level of confidence and self-regard that characterizes an individual's relationship to self, others, and the larger world; self-esteem realistically based on actual accomplishments.
7. Impulse control and regulation	Ability to modulate impulses and express them in adaptive, culturally appropriate ways; frustration tolerance; ability to recognize and describe impulses as a means of self-regulation.
8. Defensive functioning	Ability to cope and express wishes, affect, and other internal experiences; ability to modulate anxiety from internal conflict, external challenge, or threat to self without excessive distortion.
9. Adaptation, resiliency, and strength	Ability to adjust to unexpected events and changing circumstances; ability to cope effectively and creatively when confronted with uncertainty, loss, stress, or challenge.
10. Self-observing capacities	Ability to observe one's internal life mindfully and realistically and use this information adaptively; ability and interest in being introspective (psychological mindedness).
11. Construct and use internal standards and ideals	Ability to form internal values and ideals; ability to make mindful decisions based on a set of coherent, flexible, and internally consistent underlying moral principles.
12. meaning and purpose	Ability to construct a personal narrative that gives coherence and meaning to personal choices, a sense of directedness and purpose, and a spirituality that imbues one's life with meaning.

Source. Lingiardi, V., & Bornstein, R. F. (2017). Profile of mental functioning M Axis. In V. Lingiardi & N. McWilliams (Eds.), *Psychodynamic diagnostic manual* (2nd ed., pp. 76–79). New York: The Guilford Press.

Note. Domains and capacities: (a) cognitive and affective process (capacities 1–3); (b) identity and relationships (capacities 4–6); (c) defense and coping (capacities 7–9); (d) self-awareness and self-direction (capacities 10–12).

For example, the ego function *reality testing* and mental capacity *differentiation and integration* both address the individual's ability to perceive consensual reality unequivocally or accurately. In addition, object relations and relationships and intimacy both refer to the nature and quality of one's interpersonal relationships. The essential point here is that there is considerable similarity between the variously defined (a) ego functions (Bellak et al., 1973) and (b) PDM–2 mental capacities (Lingiardi & Bornstein, 2017). Consequently, Table 12.4 can be employed as a pragmatic guide for the dual purpose of (a) proofing the validity of the assigned ego function scores and (b) providing more elaborate interpretive statements of these functions within a psychological assessment report.

As can be seen in Form 12.1, additional interpretive excerpts focus on describing lower scores on the various ego functions, followed by a complementary excerpt describing higher scores. The examiner simply lists the lower and higher functions, then inserts the matching defined capacities from Table 12.4. The points of insertion into Form 12.1 are again highlighted in red font for easy detection. Although there is not a clean one-to-one correspondence between the ego functions and mentalization capacities, they are conceptually similar and some can address combinations of ego function results.

Finally, there is an excerpt designed to interpret the superego function result, whether it is high, average, or low. This can be effectively interpreted according to developmental expectations, hence the degree to which the score is below or above the expected level, along with the implications of the outcome on predicted behavior, such as impulse control, affective regulation, and comporting one's behavior according to generally accepted social rules.

Summary

This concludes the first of three performance personality tests presented in this book and test inventory. It fills an important void in offering test data (T-data) regarding a young child's developing personality functioning from the age of 3–10, although especially for ages 3–5 for which there would be no other such personality test. It is the only one that is explicitly designed as a projective test, and founded upon the projective hypothesis and psychoanalytic principles, especially ego psychology. However, it measures a grouping of personality mechanisms that can be generalized to other conceptualizations of personality and assist in accounting for child behavioral and emotional disorders, including contributing to treatment planning. Form 12.1 provides a data table for reporting the quantitative test results of the CAT–9–RC, and two supplementary tables (viz., 12.3 and 12.4) for inserting the proper interpretive statements, thus expediting the process of test scoring and interpretation.

Of note, this scoring and interpretive scheme can be employed with TAT cards and examinees of all ages. This is important to realize, as there may be occasions when an added implicit test of personality will be needed in adolescent and adult cases, along with card stimuli that are more conducive to older age cohorts.

The remaining two performance tests are not designed as projective tests, although they similarly measure personality mechanisms and traits by implicit means that contribute to psychodiagnosis and treatment planning. The Roberts–2 will be presented next because it is limited to childhood and adolescence. In contrast, the Rorschach Inkblot Test and its newest scoring system contain norms that begin as do the Roberts–2 in childhood, although it continues through adulthood.

The Roberts, Second Edition

The Roberts, Second Edition (Roberts–2) is foremost a performance personality test of social reasoning that is assumed to influence psychological adjustment. Secondarily, this test affords data that helps in detecting the presence of various types of psychological disturbance. Unlike the CAT–9–RC, it has a norm reference sample and standard scores typically found for the personality inventories and rating scales. The subsequent presentation shall follow the typical outline used in previous chapters for presenting tests, including synopsis, norm reference sample, administration, scoring, and interpretation, along with data tables designed to present the Roberts–2 data yield efficiently within the context of a psychological assessment report.

Synopsis

The Roberts–2 is principally designed as a measure of social-cognitive ability as exhibited in expressive language (Roberts & Gruber, 2005, p. 4). More specifically, its developmental/adaptive scales assess social and emotional intelligence; that is, the level of mastery of knowledge relevant to interpersonal and intrapersonal functioning and adjustment (Cantor & Kihlstrom, 1987; Goleman, 1995). To link such social-cognitive ability to actual personality and behavioral functioning, the following three assumptions must be met: (a) there exist individual differences in this ability, (b) such differences can be reliably measured, and (c) those individuals with greater ability will predictably display more effective and adaptive interpersonal skills in real life and thus personality functioning (Cantor & Kihlstrom, 1987; Friedman & Schustack, 2012; Goleman, 1995; Roberts & Gruber, 2005); that is, this test has *ecological validity*. In addition, however, the Roberts–2 consists of emotion, unusual, and atypical clinical scales, which are statistically associated with personality maladjustment and clinical disorders (Roberts & Gruber, 2005).

The Roberts–2 is a revision of the *Roberts Apperception Test for Children* (RATC; McArthur & Roberts, 1982), neither of which are designed as projective tests as the authors argue in detail in the test manual (Roberts & Gruber, 2005, pp. 4–5). This is illustrated in the dropping of the term "Apperceptive" from the title of the updated revision of this test. Several characteristics of the Roberts–2 differentiate it from a projective test such as the CAT–9–RC presented previously. These characteristics include, but are not limited to, the following: (a) pictures of social scenes that deliberately present structured social circumstances that are commonly recognized real-life occurrences (i.e., stimulus cards with "high press"); (b) use of examinees' expressive language production as an indication of their social-cognitive abilities; (c) a comprehensive scoring system with an attendant nationally representative norm reference sample; (d) use of an assortment of scales that measure children's capacity to recognize, reason, and resolve common social themes and situations rather than examining their internal moods and emotional conflicts; and (e) supporting evidence of test–retest reliability and validity. Next examined is the Roberts–2 standardization sample to determine the limits of generalizability, including a brief examination of test reliability and validity. The latter is added because such data substantiates the claim of the authors that this performance personality test is not projective in nature or design.

Norm Reference Sample, Reliability, and Validity

This section is further apportioned into three subparts. First, the basic demographics of the norm reference sample are presented. This is followed by succinct examinations of reliability and validity evidence to establish the Roberts–2 as a standardized, non-projective, performance personality test.

SAMPLE DEMOGRAPHICS

The norm reference sample totaled 1,060 non-clinical individuals ranging in age from 6 years, 0 months through 18 years, 11 months; including 1st–12th grades. Data were garnered among 29 sites, across 15 states, and representing 4 major regions of the United States. More specifically, there were about equal percentages of males and females. Each year of age included an average of about 80 individuals, with the largest group being 11 years ($n = 98$) and the smallest group 18 years ($n = 39$). Regarding race/ethnicity, 72.7% were White, 12.8% Black, 10.4% Hispanic/Latino, and 3.4% Asian. Percentage breakdowns among the four U.S. regions included 48% from the South, 23.5% from the West, 15.5% from the Midwest, and 13% from the East. Finally, parents' educational level was used as an index of socioeconomic status, which was divided into four classes (with proportionate breakdowns in parentheses) as follows: (a) less than high school graduate (12.8%); (b) high school graduate (36.2%); (c) some college (24.7%); and (d) four or more years of college (26.3%).

The majority of these sample demographics were matched to figures reported by the U.S. Census Bureau (U.S. Bureau of the Census, 2004) based on the population of adults aged 25–54 who were most likely to be parents of school-age children. The single exception was gender, which was based on children aged 5–18. Comparison of the norm reference sample demographics with the aforesaid population figures showed an acceptable match for all variables (see Roberts & Gruber, 2005, Table 5, p. 128).

RELIABILITY

Recall that reliability addresses test consistency and accuracy. Because the Roberts–2 uses an intricate scoring system that relies on examiner judgment, sufficient interrater or interscorer agreement is important to demonstrate. Furthermore, by virtue of the fact that this test measures personality traits in the form of social-cognitive abilities and clinical disorders, which are both relative consistencies in people's behavior, there should also be evidence that demonstrates temporal stability of the Roberts–2 scales. Both will be reviewed in such order.

Interrater Reliability   A study was done which ten Roberts–2 tests (i.e., 16 stories) were completed, five by a nonclinical group and five by a clinical group. Children in both groups varied in age from 6 to 16. A total of ten experienced clinicians completed a four-hour workshop in learning to score the Roberts–2 according to instructions. Following this, the ten Roberts–2 tests were first scored by the senior author (viz., Glen Roberts), followed by the ten trained clinicians. Correlations were all accomplished on a scale-by-scale basis, with each of the trained clinician's scale scores correlated with the senior author's scale scores. The median of the ten correlations between each trained clinician and the senior author for each scale was reported for the nonclinical group, the clinical group, and the combined group. The vast majority of inter-scorer correlations for all scales were in the middle 0.80 to high 0.90 range, with very few falling below 0.80. In particular, all the scales measuring the presence of psychopathology were above 0.85. These data provide evidence that experienced clinicians can learn to score the Roberts–2 in a consistent and accurate manner subsequent to a four-hour workshop.

Test–Retest Reliability   A study of test–retest reliability was also done using both nonclinical and clinical samples. The nonclinical sample consisted of 30, including 15 males and 15 females, and an age range of 6–18. The clinical sample also included 30 participants between the ages of 6 and 18, although consisted of a disproportionate subgroup of males (i.e., 73.3%) versus females (i.e., 26.7%). Once again, stability coefficients were done on a scale-by-scale basis. Although the interval between test and retest was not reported, the vast majority of coefficients ranged again from the middle 0.80 to high 0.90 range, which is more than sufficient to show adequate temporal stability. Certainly these data show superior test–retest reliability as compared to other major projective storytelling tests, such as the TAT, which typically show stability coefficients in the range of 0.30 (see, e.g., Lilienfeld, Wood, & Garb, 2000).

VALIDITY

In addition to the aforementioned nonclinical standardization sample used to establish the Roberts–2 norms, a referred clinical sample was also garnered for purposes of examining test validity. However, the demographics of this sample were deigned to match those children who were referred for public mental health services as opposed to the general population. This clinical sample totaled 467. The majority were males (68%), and ages ranged from 6 years through 18 years. Subgroups apportioned by one-year intervals showed some variability in number, ranging from 5 for the 18-year-old cohort to a high of 59 for the 14-year-old cohort. Most cohorts contained between 30 and 50 participants. Finally, the race/ethnic background proportions mirrored that of the nonclinical norm reference sample.

Validity analysis focused on two principal functions of the Roberts–2, that is, the ability to measure developmental differences in social-cognitive ability and the ability to discriminate between nonclinical and clinical groups in both social-cognitive ability and degree of adjustment. Regarding the former, the statistical analyses focused primarily on the Roberts–2 developmental scale scores and age. The hypothesis was that as chronological age (CA) increased, so would scores on the Roberts–2 developmental scales. Indeed, this was what was consistently found among the various developmental scales. A few examples will be presented.

First, The Roberts–2 Available Resources Scales measure the social-cognitive ability to understand the effective use of various intrapersonal and interpersonal resources to resolve a problem feeling or situation. Analysis of variance (ANOVA) was conducted using chronological age (CA) as one nonmanipulated independent variable (viz., age in years as follows: 6–7, 8–9, 10–13, 14–18), and sample type as a second nonmanipulated independent variable (viz., norm reference sample versus referred clinical sample), with mean available resources scale score as the dependent variable. The results showed the expected interaction effect. For the norm reference group, there was a clear simple effect in that, as CA increased, so did the available resources scale scores. However, the clinical group scores were significantly lower than for the norm reference sample, as expected, and did not show the clear increase with CA. Thus, the developmental increase in social-cognitive ability was contingent upon whether the group was nonclinical or clinical. Similar results were found for the theme overview scales, which measure general social-cognitive competence or ability.

Taken together, these data, along with similar additional results reported in the test manual, demonstrate that the Roberts–2 can detect the expected increase in social-cognitive sophistication with age among normally developing children and adolescents. Furthermore, it can discriminate between nonclinical and clinical groups, with the former showing greater degrees of social-cognitive ability as predicted. In contrast, clinical groups manifest consistently lower social-cognitive ability irrespective of age. Additional studies will not be reported due to space limitations, although they generally show similar trends.

SUMMARY

This concludes the norm reference sample section for the Roberts–2. It was deemed necessary to also include a representative sample of reliability and validity data to bolster the contention that the Roberts–2 is not a projective test, but rather a performance personality test that yields standardized data principally concerning an examinee's social-cognitive sophistication and secondarily the degree of personality adjustment or maladjustment in the form of psychological problems. Next, the Roberts–2 administration process will be reviewed, followed by scoring and interpretation.

Administration

The Roberts–2 test stimuli consist of a grand total of 16 cards in a set, which together present a structured and representative sample of key intrapersonal and interpersonal scenes using characters in achromatic drawings. Each scene involves specific emotions, behaviors, and/or problem situations that require sophisticated problem-solving for purposes of effective resolution. Some examples include family and peer interaction scenes, along with fearful and aggressive situations. There are 6 different 16-card sets from which to purchase, obtain, and use, including those with White, Black, and Hispanic characters, each consisting of male and female versions. Eleven of the cards are administered to one gender only, while five cards are administered to both males and females.

The 16 cards in each set are standardized in that they are specifically designed to present common structured social situations from which examinees principally (a) demonstrate their social cognitive ability and secondarily (b) manifest maladaptive emotions and reactions. Specifically, the card numbers and designated social situations are as follows: Card 1—Family Interaction (Parents and Child), Card 2—Maternal Support, Card 3—Schoolwork, Card 4—Peer Support, Card 5—Parental Affection, Card 6—Peer or Racial Interaction, Card 7—Anxiety or Illness, Card 8—Family Interaction, Card 9—Physical Aggression, Card 10—Sibling Rivalry, Card 11—Fear, Card 12—Maternal Depression or Illness, Card 13—Aggression Release, Card 14—Maternal Limit Setting, Card 15—Female in Bath, Card 16—Paternal Support.

All 16 cards are to be administered in their designated sequence. Respondents are instructed to make up a complete story to each card using their *imagination*, including what led up to the scene, what occurs, and how it ends, while in the process addressing the thoughts, feelings, and actions of the character(s) (Roberts & Gruber, 2005, p. 11). Although the stories do not need to be long, they must be complete by addressing all elements included in the instructions. Specifically, these elements are what occurred (a) before the picture (i.e., a beginning), (b) during the picture (i.e., a middle), and (c) after the picture (i.e., an ending or outcome). In addition, at each phase of the story, the respondent is asked to address what the characters are doing (i.e., behavior), feeling (i.e., emotion), and thinking (i.e., cognition).

Special structuring questions are permitted on Cards 1 and 2, which are designed to acclimate the respondent to the task and to help ensure that the instructions are sufficiently understood. Thereafter, prompting is circumscribed to (a) clarifying any vague or indefinite terms in a story whose meaning is vital to scoring and (b) clarifying any continuing confusion on the part of the examinee regarding test administration. Hence, further inquiry and leading questions are prohibited on Cards 3–16. In the event the examinee refuses to create a story to one or several cards, they are to be presented a second time after the first administration of all other cards. If the examinee continues to reject one or more cards such that further efforts will damage rapport or be fruitless, the examiner is to mark them as "refused" and record any associated behavioral observations that may be diagnostic.

The examiner's verbatim written record of each story represents the data base from which raw scores are derived, and thereafter transformed into standard scores on multiple scales classified as either (a) developmental/adaptive or (b) clinical (discussed subsequently). The former primarily measures social-cognitive abilities and includes the following four scale clusters: (a) theme overview (i.e., general social-cognitive competence or ability), (b) available resources (i.e., ability to understand the effective use of various intrapersonal and interpersonal resources to resolve a problem feeling or situation), (c) problem identification (i.e., ability to comprehend interpersonal problems and feelings), and (d) resolution (i.e., ability to resolve interpersonal problems and feelings) (Roberts & Gruber, 2005). The last item measures the presence of personality pathology or clinical disorders and includes the following three scale clusters: (a) emotion (i.e., the presence of maladaptive emotions and behaviors), (b) outcome (i.e., the presence of various types of undesirable or ineffective outcomes), and (c) unusual or atypical responses (i.e., the presence of severe neurocognitive and psychological dysfunction) (Roberts & Gruber, 2005). In addition to the verbatim transcript, behavioral observations should be made, especially those that are diagnostically relevant and/or atypical. Estimated administration time is 30–40 minutes. Thus, this test can be administered comfortably within a one-hour session.

Scoring

The scoring section is divided into two related subtopics. First, the Roberts–2 data metrics are reviewed, including the standard scores, score ranges, and ancillary scores, along with the manner in which they are transformed. The second subtopic reviews the data tables that have been created for purposes of reporting these data within a psychological assessment report. These subtopics set the stage for discussing Roberts–2 test interpretation.

THE ROBERTS–2 DATA YIELD AND METRICS

The Roberts–2 employs standardized *T*–scores (mean = 50; standard deviation = 10; range 20–90) for all the developmental/adaptive and clinical scales. Separate norms are available for the following age groups by year: (a)6–7; (b)8–9; (c)10–13; and (d) 14–18 (Roberts & Gruber, 2005). Separate norms were justified for these four groups due to the aforesaid validity results that showed a consistent effect for age as manifested by the nonclinical standardization sample. Thus, transforming raw scores into *T*–scores may be done directly on the Roberts–2 Record Form (Roberts & McArthur, 2005) or by the available Roberts–2 unlimited-use CD (Western Psychological Services, 2005).

The record form consists of (a) a coding protocol sheet wherein frequencies of different responses per card are recorded (e.g., complete meaning), (b) separate scoring profile sheets for the aforementioned age cohorts, and (c) a sheet for taking notes of behavioral observations. The scoring profile sheets include tables for marking raw scores and finding their associated *T*–scores for each of the Roberts–2 scales. The computer scoring software transforms all entered raw scores into *T*–scores automatically. Thereafter, the software lists all scales, raw scores, and *T*–scores, along with a graphic profile of the latter. However, it does not report confidence intervals (CIs) or percentile ranks (PRs). It is advisable to use the computer software because (a) it is much faster, (b) it minimizes scoring error, and (c) it represents a one-time purchase.

The *T*–score range noted in the test manual's "Normative Score Tables" is from 20 (i.e., 3 standard deviations below the mean) to 90 (i.e., 4 standard deviations above the mean), which is intended to cover the low frequency and positive skewness of some of the more extreme raw scores found in the standardization sample data (see Roberts &

Gruber, 2005, p. 149). Of note, there are some minor discrepancies in raw score to *T*–score conversions when using the manual and record form compared to the computer software. That is, the computer software occasionally reports higher and more accurate *T*–scores because the record form truncates the *T*–score range from 30 to 80, likely due to space limitations. The data tables that have been designed for reporting and interpreting the Roberts–2 results follow these minimum and maximum scores (see Form 12.2).

Using the Roberts–2 record form as a guide, the *T*–score ranges and associated qualitative descriptions concerning the developmental/adaptive scales are as follows: (a) 20–39 is a *low* elevation, (b) 40–59 is an *average* elevation, (c) 60–69 is a *high* elevation, and (d) 70–90 is an *extremely high* elevation (Roberts & Gruber, 2005. pp 156–160). One and two asterisks are appended to high and extremely high elevations because they are statistically significant and effectively rule out chance as an explanation for such results; that is, it is a diagnostically meaningful result. These *T*–score ranges and qualitative descriptions are listed in the specific notes of all tables that list developmental/adaptive scales. The objective is to facilitate test interpretation once the scores have been entered into the appropriate tables (see the Interpretation section).

Using the record form to determine the score ranges and qualitative descriptions as applied to the clinical scales resulted in a modified scheme. This is in part due to the consistent focus on measuring the presence of psychopathology, with higher scores reflecting increasing signs of maladaptive clinical disorders (viz., anxiety and depression), personality traits (i.e., unresolved issues of rejection and aggression), and severe dysfunction (i.e., neurocognitive dysfunction and psychotic signs). They are as follows: (a) 20–59 is *within normal limits* or *absence of psychopathology*, (b) 60–69 is *mild to moderate psychopathology*, and (c) 70–90 is *severe psychopathology*. Note that these are this author's recommended qualitative descriptors, as the test manual does not provide such information. Note also that the general term "psychopathology" has been selected because it is sufficiently broad to capture clinical disorder, personality disorder, and unusually severe abnormality suggesting brain dysfunction and psychosis. Next, the results and interpretation tables that have been prepared for the Roberts–2 are reviewed.

THE ROBERTS–2 DATA TABLES FOR PSYCHOLOGICAL ASSESSMENT REPORTS

Figure 12.2 is available for download on Routledge's e-resources website, which provides a visual representation of how the Roberts–2 scales are organized and also introduces the manner in which they are enumerated in Form 12.2. That is, Form 12.2 comprises all the tables within which the Roberts–2 scores are to be input and presented within a formal psychological assessment report. Form 12.2 begins with a validity table (viz., Table 1), which is fairly basic and straightforward in its design. Namely, it scrutinizes whether the examinee provided a sufficient number of stories (i.e., ample data) from which valid interpretations can be derived. Tables 2–5 enumerate the various developmental/adaptive scales, all of which measure various aspects of an examinee's social-cognitive abilities. Finally, Tables 6 and 7 list the clinical scales, which are devoted to measuring (a) perceptual sets that reflect the presence of a certain type of clinical or personality psychopathology and (b) signs of severe neurocognitive or psychotic disorder.

Regarding the developmental/adaptive scales, the tables consist of five columns listing the scale name, *T*–score, 68% CI, PR, and a summary description of the measured social-cognitive ability. The CIs are based upon the reported *SEM*s for each scale afforded by the combined nonclinical standardization sample and clinical sample used to establish test validity (Roberts & Gruber, 2005, Table 10, p. 134). The *SEM* for some scales were not reported due to low frequency. For these scales, the average *SEM* for that particular group of developmental/adaptive scales was used. These values are inserted beneath the brackets for the CI and should be added to and subtracted from the examinee's obtained *T*–score to rapidly compute the interval, then deleted as no longer needed. The PR is based on the standard normal distribution as listed in Appendix A (Table A.1) in this book. The CIs are for analyzing

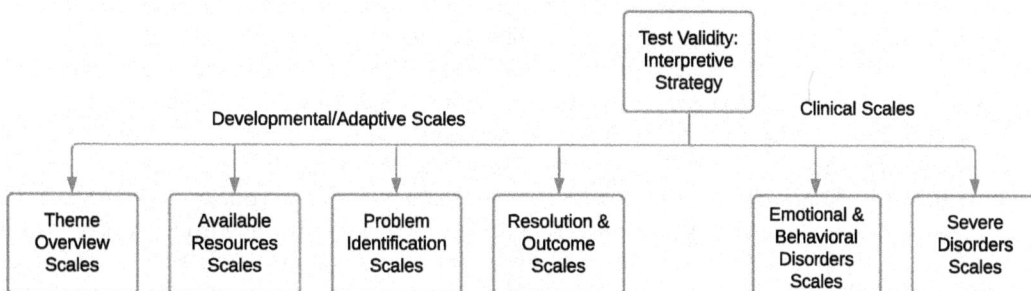

Figure 12.2 Roberts, Second Edition (Roberts-2) Performance Personality Test Interpretive Process

intraindividual differences and to account for test error. The PRs are more easily understood by laypersons, which is the prime reason they are included.

This concludes the section on Roberts–2 scoring. Next, an interpretive strategy for the Roberts–2 will be presented. Repeated references to Figure 12.2 (see Routledge's e-resources website) will be made to clarify the recommended interpretive process, which is designed to emphasize both efficiency and flexibility, especially in the way the various scales are organized and presented.

Interpretation

This final section focuses on interpretation of the Roberts–2, although is apportioned into three subtopics as follows. First, the original test structure has been reorganized to render them to be (a) more conducive to testing clinical populations in mental health practice and (b) more applicable to detecting *DSM–5* disorders. The first subtopic discusses four separate modifications that contribute to this revised test structure. Second, interpretation of Roberts–2 data that pertains to validity is reviewed because it is contingent upon raw score data rather than standard scores. Third, the diagnostic-relate scales (viz., developmental/adaptive and clinical) are presented. All subtopics make use of both Figure 12.2 and Form 12.2 to further clarify the narrative presentation.

ROBERTS–2 REVISED TEST ORGANIZATION

As stated, four adjustments have been made to the original organization of Roberts–2 diagnostic scales and the manner in which they are scored, which was guided by clinical testing experience and by *DSM–5* applicability. First, and most palpably, the clinical outcome scales are reported immediately subsequent to the developmental/adaptive resolution scales and within the same data table (viz., Table 5; Form 12.2) for two reasons. First, they are conceptually more similar to each other and serve as effective complements; specifically, together they measure the tendency to produce resolutions and outcomes that are potentially (a) more effective *and* (b) more problematic. Second, outcome scales show evidence of an inverse or negative relationship with resolution scales (Roberts & Gruber, 2005). Therefore, the resolution scales measure increasing degrees of sophistication, and thus effectiveness in formulating resolutions to intrapersonal and interpersonal problems, while the outcome scales measure various types of undesirable resolutions. Hence, they all address the ability to resolve interpersonal problems, with some being more or less adaptive or desirable. Using such rationale, the outcome scales were moved from their clinical classification to the developmental/adaptive classification and incorporated into Table 5 (Form 12.2) with the resolution scales.

The second adjustment is more minor in that it involves moving the limit setting available resources scale to the same data table that combines the resolution and outcome scales (viz., Table 5; Form 12.2). This is because a statistically high score on limit setting indicates that the respondent believes behavioral control requires *external* disciplinary consequences (e.g., scolding, spanking, time out, losing privileges, paying for damage) as opposed to utilizing internal coping resources, such as emotional self-regulation (Roberts & Gruber, 2005). In this sense, high scores on limit setting represent a developmentally immature, and hence maladaptive, strategy for problem resolution and outcome (Fox & Calkins, 2003; Rothbart, Posner, & Kieras, 2006). Following this rationale and from a diagnostic perspective, this available resources scale is more accordant with the resolution and outcome scales. Hence, it is placed last behind the outcome scales in Table 5 (Form 12.2). The three types of scales incorporated into Table 5 (Form 12.2) are denoted by different symbols, which are defined in full within general table notes.

The third adjustment concerns the unusual scale listed in Table 7 (Form 12.2), which comprises the following three separate scores: (a) refusal (i.e., rejecting a card), (b) no score (i.e., rote physical description of the card stimulus scene), and (c) antisocial (i.e., violations of social norms and laws) (Roberts & Gruber, 2005). Refusals and antisocial story content are not scored on this scale because the former is accounted for in measuring test validity (see later in this chapter), whereas the latter is largely redundant with the aggressive clinical scale listed in Table 6 (Form 12.2). Excessive "no score" responses (i.e., simple physical scene descriptions) (Roberts & Gruber, 2005) are analogous to *mechanical perseverations* (see Exner, 2003), which are a sign of neurocognitive dysfunction (Exner, 2002, 2003). Hence, the modified "unusual–no score" scale *T*–score located in Table 7 (Form 12.2) represents a standardized quantitative measure of such mechanical perseverations and can effectively lead to a cogent argument for auxiliary neuropsychological testing is indicated.

The fourth and final modification from the original Roberts–2 scale organization concerns the "Atypical Categories Scale," which is an amalgamation of nine more specific aberrant score responses ranging from excessive violence (viz., ATYP4) to sexual content (viz., ATYP8) (Roberts & Gruber, 2005). The one that has been most useful regarding a *DSM–5* diagnosis is "ATYP1—Illogical," which measures the presence of cognitive distortions and loosening of associations (Roberts & Gruber, 2005, p. 125), that is, thought disorder or psychosis. By scoring the modified "Atypical—Illogical Scale" in this manner, the resulting standard score represents a quantitative measure of psychotic disturbance or formal thought disorder. Raw scores on the eight other Roberts–2 atypical categories can be otherwise noted by the testing psychologist and interpreted qualitatively in the narrative, which would be required even in the absence of such modification because all these responses are integrated into one scale. The simple objective was to limit this datum to the most useful kind of atypical response, here one that would be a near pathognomonic sign for psychosis.

This concludes the four modifications to the Roberts–2 test structure that were made to render this test more conducive to mental health testing. Next, the Roberts–2 validity check is presented.

ROBERTS–2 VALIDITY ANALYSIS

Roberts–2 interpretation begins with an examination of validity or whether the subsequent data is sufficient for purposes of deriving inferences regarding personality functioning. This is designated in Figure 12.2 (e-resources) with the top box titled "Test Validity: Interpretive Strategy." This title is apposite because the results here determine whether the ensuing data are valid, which justifies the general interpretive strategy to be employed.

More specifically, Table 1 (Form 12.2) initiates the analysis with validity indicators analogous to the Rorschach (discussed next), particularly in terms of whether the respondent has provided a sufficient amount or quantity of data for subsequent scoring. In columnar order of appearance, the table presents the (a) validity result, (b) rationale for each result, and (c) interpretation strategy to be employed for the subsequent diagnostic scales. There are three potential validity results most commonly found in testing practice (i.e., *valid*, *qualified valid*, and *invalid*) from which the psychologist selects contingent upon the data. Pursuant to test instructions, administration is to be summarily halted for cases in which the examinee manifests a card refusal to one of the first two cards (Roberts & Gruber, 2005, p. 12). This represents the invalid version in the third and last row of Table 1 as it is a rare outcome, especially if the examinee has been properly prepared for the testing procedures and rapport has been established.

The qualified valid version was inserted within the second row because there have been cases, especially involving very young children (e.g., ages 6–8), wherein examinees become progressively more fatigued in the process of creating 16 stories. Consequently, they begin providing cursory, and hence non-scorable, stories. Because the test instructions do not stipulate precisely how many non-scorable stories should prompt a cautious interpretation (see Roberts & Gruber, 2005), the testing psychologist must employ clinical judgment in the use of this version. The actual number of non-scorable stories, which includes card refusals, should be recorded in the reason for result section ($N = \#\#$). In such instances, a conservative approach to interpretation should be espoused. That is, high scores should be interpreted as valid but likely underestimates of whatever is being measured simply due to a lack of quantity, usually toward the higher end of the reported CIs contingent upon the extent of the scarcity of the raw data. The testing psychologist may also insert a unique and less typical validity result into one of the rows. Usually this will involve the qualified result row. Because the retained result within Table 1 is self-explanatory, there is no need for table notes or narrative summaries.

As stated, however, the valid result is the most common outcome. In such cases, the first row is retained while simply deleting the other two versions. Interpretation then rapidly moves to the diagnostic scales where a decision point must be made. This is addressed next.

DETERMINING THE OVERALL ROBERTS–2 INTERPRETIVE STRATEGY

As depicted in Figure 12.2 (e-resources), the directional arrows do not differentiate those that are required from those that are optional. This symbolizes the fact that the testing psychologist may use only those scales that are relevant to a specified case and ignore the remaining scales in other tables. In most cases, reporting all the scales within a table makes the most sense because they are interrelated. Therefore, if an examinee's social-cognitive abilities are expected to be deficient or otherwise ineffectual, and a contributor to the presence of clinical disorder and/or emerging personality disorder, then both developmental/adaptive and the clinical scales would be utilized. The interpretive progression in such instances would begin at the far left of Figure 12.2 with the theme overview scales and continue across all remaining scales.

On the other hand, if the referral only called for a measurement of an examinee's social-cognitive abilities, the interpretive strategy would begin with the theme overview scales and end with the resolution and outcome scales, hence omitting the two clinical clusters. A third possibility would be an exclusive interest in detecting psychopathology, therefore initiating the interpretive process with the emotional and behavioral disorders scales, ending with the severe disorders scales, and omitting the developmental/adaptive scales. Finally, a testing psychologist may be interested in scoring and interpreting both the developmental/adaptive scales and clinical scales, although reverse the sequence, thus affording priority to the latter. The flexibility of the general interpretive approach to the Roberts–2 is explicitly noted in the notes to Figure 12.2. The remainder of this section on Roberts–2 interpretation assumes that all the scales are to be employed in their typical order as portrayed in both Figure 12.2 and Form 12.2, namely, from the developmental/adaptive scales through the clinical scales.

DEVELOPMENTAL/ADAPTIVE SCALES

Tables 2–5 (Form 12.2) include the Roberts–2 developmental/adaptive scales and together provide a measure of the examinee's various social-cognitive abilities. Table titles identify both the broad class (viz., developmental/adaptive scales) and more specific categories from which the specific scales are derived (e.g., theme overview). The more specific categories are designated in the title of each of the boxes in Figure 12.2 (e-resources). As introduced in the prior section on scoring, these tables are similarly designed and include the following columns: (a) scale name, (b) *T*–score, (c) 68% CI, (d) PR based on the standard normal distribution, and (e) a succinct description of the social-cognitive ability being measured.

Regarding interpretation, the scales enumerated within each cluster are either interpreted (a) as separate concepts or (b) as part of a hierarchy of increasing degrees of social-cognitive reasoning concerning a single content area. In Form 12.2, the former includes theme overview scales (Table 2), available resources scales (Table 3), and outcome scales (Table 5). That is, each of these scales is interpreted independent of the others. For example, the degree to which an examinee understands the use of one's own positive emotions in resolving an interpersonal problem (i.e., support self—feeling) is scored completely independent of the examinee's understanding of the importance of consulting appropriate others to help resolve interpersonal problems (i.e., reliance on other).

In contrast, the problem identification scales (Table 4; Form 12.2) represent a hierarchy of related and increasingly sophisticated social-cognitive reasoning that shows how well an examinee is able to detect an interpersonal problem and its causes. For example, the degree to which an examinee can describe a problem situation in detail, including internal and external contributing factors (i.e., clarification), is inversely related to simply detecting an interpersonal problem (i.e., recognition) and describing some of the associated feelings (i.e., description). Here, the ability to clarify the causes of an interpersonal problem by definition incorporates (a) the ability to simply recognize that the problem exists in the first place, and (b) the feelings related to the recognized problem. This will be reflected in the scoring, as higher numbers will be earned on the clarification scale, which then diverts points from the recognition and description scales.

Therefore, in all developmental/adaptive scales that are hierarchically organized in this manner, achieving a greater *T*–score on more sophisticated scales automatically reduces scores on less sophisticated scales along the hierarchy. This is because more of the raw data, which is the verbatim story, will reflect reasoning at a certain level, hence reducing scores at other levels. In consequence, the key to interpreting these hierarchical scales is to identify the highest-level scale that represents the examinee's degree of reasoning, which by definition incorporates all lower levels. In the previous example, an examinee whose principal level of reasoning is clarification will be assumed to also be capable of reasoning using description and recognition. This is because the clarification scale subsumes the abilities measured by the scales lower on the hierarchy (viz., recognition and description). Therefore, the succinct descriptions of all measured social-cognitive abilities were carefully composed based on their more elaborate descriptions and numerous examples provided within the test manual (Roberts & Gruber, 2005, pp. 25–41, 50–53). In fact, the descriptions are of sufficient detail that the reader can easily discern whether the scales are independent of each other or related within a hierarchy.

All these developmental/adaptive scale tables also include general and specific notes listing the *T*–score metric and the directional meaning of higher scores, along with standard score ranges and their associated qualitative descriptors, respectively. These are afforded for purposes of facilitating test interpretation and reader comprehension. Finally, narrative excerpts immediately follow each table, which succinctly define the measurement focus of the Roberts–2 category or categories included in each table (Roberts & Gruber, 2005, pp. 25–41, 50–53), along with an elaboration based on the type of scales used in that specific grouping.

More particularly, Table 2 (Form 12.2) consists of the two *theme overview scales* that concern the most general abilities. They include (a) *popular pull*, which measures the ability to understand emotion, behavior, and problem situations of an interpersonal nature, and (b) *complete meaning*, which measures the ability to understand and effectively resolve a sequence of problematic interpersonal interactions and feelings (Roberts & Gruber, 2005 pp. 25–27). Not infrequently, these two general measures of social intelligence assist in addressing *DSM–5* differential diagnostic issues; for example, helping to differentiate between *autism spectrum disorder* and *social (pragmatic) communication disorder*. In most cases, however, providing a more detailed analysis of the examinee's social-cognitive deficits is indicated, especially for the purposes of targeting specific treatment goals. The excerpt following Table 2 first addresses the examinee's overall measured social-cognitive ability level, ensued by a follow-up ipsative analysis examining any relative difference between the two measured abilities.

Table 3 (Form 12.2) enumerates the four *available resources scales*, which generally measure the examinee's ability to understand the effective use of various intrapersonal and interpersonal assets to resolve a problem feeling or situation (Roberts & Gruber, 2005). They include the following specific scales and measured abilities: (a) *support self—feeling*, defined as the ability to understand the effective use of one's own positive emotions (e.g., happiness); (b) *support self—advocacy*, defined as the ability to understand the effective use of one's own resources (e.g., problem-solving, perseverance); (c) *support other—feeling*, defined as the ability to understand the effective use of others' emotional responsiveness (e.g., caring, affection); (d) *support other—help*, defined as the ability to understand the effective use of others' unsolicited instrumental assistance (e.g., accepting another's offer of help on a task); and (e) *reliance on other*, defined as the ability to understand the effective use of proactively seeking assistance from appropriate others (e.g., parents, teachers) (Roberts & Gruber, 2005, pp. 27–34).

The interpretive excerpt that follows Table 3 is apportioned into two parts. First, the overall score profile is interpreted, whether the scores tend to fall within one or a few levels or whether they are significantly more variable. This is ensued by a more detailed analysis in which the testing psychologist can assume an ipsative comparison or continue with a norm-based analysis, as these scales are independent of each other in terms of interpretive significance. In the event an ipsative comparison is desired, all references to the population of same-aged peers should be deleted.

Table 4 (Form 12.2) includes the Roberts–2 *problem identification scales*. These scales measure a continuum of social-cognitive abilities directly related to comprehending interpersonal problems and feelings, ranging in degree of sophistication from vague and simplistic to elaborate and differentiated. Greater degrees of elaboration and differentiation are associated with a greater likelihood of developing more effective resolutions or outcomes. Therefore, these scales clearly form a hierarchy of increasing degrees of sophisticated reasoning reflecting the capacity to identify interpersonal problems.

They specifically include the following scales and their associated level of social-cognitive problem identification abilities: (a) *recognition*, defined as the simple detection of a current problem feeling or situation expressed in vague terms and without explanation of preceding factors; (b) *description*, defined as the description of a specific problem with associated feelings, although with poorly defined preceding factors and lack of an internal cognitive process (e.g., wondering about); (c) *clarification*, defined as the elaborated description of a problem situation, with identification of an internal cognitive state (e.g., cannot understand), but limited description of preceding factors; (d) *definition*, defined as the description of a problem and its cause, including reasons for feelings and behavior, some mention of prior circumstances, and elaboration of an internal process; and (e) *explanation*, defined as the complete description of the problem situation, including full identification and elaboration of feelings, with clear reference to, and processing of, preceding causal factors (Roberts & Gruber, 2005, pp. 35–38). The latter two rarely occur and are therefore not scored for the two youngest age groups (viz., 6–7 and 8–9 years) (Roberts & Gruber, 2005). This necessitated an additional "--" general table note symbol denoting that the score type is not available or computed for the respondent's age.

The excerpt following Table 4 uses language that considers the hierarchical nature of these scales. This is accomplished by using statements that identify the highest level of an examinee's reasoning that manifests the highest scores. This effectively summarizes the principal level of reasoning the examinee is capable of employing to detect an interpersonal problem or problematic feelings. Of note, this may include more than one level in the event two adjacent scales are approximately equally elevated. The language in the excerpt can be easily modified to describe such results.

Table 5 (Form 12.2) is the final, longest, and most elaborate of the developmental/adaptive scale data. In order of appearance, it includes the *resolution scales*; the *outcome scales*, which as stated were reallocated from their original clinical scale designation; and finally, one available resource scale (viz., *limit setting*). Analogous to the problem identification scales, the resolution scales generally measure a continuum of social-cognitive abilities, although in this case those directly related to solving interpersonal problems and feelings. Greater degrees of sophistication are assumed to be associated with the development of more effective outcomes. Hence, the inversely related outcome scales measure the presence of various types of undesirable or ineffective outcomes, which are associated with ineffective social-cognitive reasoning. As argued previously, the limit setting scale similarly represents an immature resolution strategy, hence its placement immediately following the outcome scales.

The particular resolution scales and their associated social-cognitive problem-solving abilities include the following: (a) *simple closure*, defined as an easy ending, consisting of an abrupt and poorly defined outcome, along with a lack of problem-solving process or mediating steps; (b) *easy positive outcome*, defined as an ending with a positive outcome, although being devoid of a descriptive process or explanation as to how the solution was achieved; (c) *constructive resolution*, defined as an elaborated description of a problem situation, with identification of an internal cognitive state (e.g., cannot understand), and limited description of preceding factors; (d) *constructive resolution of feelings and situation*, defined as a description of a problem and its cause, including reasons for feelings and behavior, some mention of prior circumstances, and elaboration of an internal process; and (e) *elaborated process with insight*, defined as a complete description of the problem situation, including full identification and elaboration of feelings, with clear reference to, and processing of, preceding causal factors (Roberts & Gruber, 2005, pp. 38–41). Again, the latter two are not scored for 6–9-year-olds, thus requiring a score-not-available symbol to be added to the general table notes.

The outcome scales and their undesirable conclusions are as follows: (a) *unresolved outcome*, defined as a clear absence of an ending or resolution, such that the problem feelings and circumstances remain completely unprocessed and unmodified; (b) *nonadaptive outcome*, defined as problem feelings and circumstances processed, but the coping strategy does not solve the problem adequately; (c) *maladaptive outcome*, defined as a coping strategy that exacerbates the situation and often includes externalizing behavior; and (d) *unrealistic outcome*, defined as a coping strategy that is unequivocally unrealistic and represents both fantasy and wishful thinking, thus rendering it ineffectual despite its putative positive quality (Roberts & Gruber, 2005, pp. 50–53). Again, Table 5 ends with the limit setting scale, which indicates that coping and adjustment are dependent on external disciplinary consequences and control (e.g., scolding, spanking, time-out, losing privileges, paying for damage) (Roberts & Gruber, 2005, pp. 34–35). Furthermore, general table notes have been added that identify each scale as either resolution, outcome, or available resource.

Lastly, a number of narrative interpretations follow Table 5, due to the fact that it contains a significant amount of related data that must be clarified in terms of diagnostic meaning and implications. The first excerpt addresses the first five interrelated resolution scales by locating the examinee's most prominent and sophisticated level(s) of reasoning. In the event two adjacent scales are the most prominent, with little discrepancy between the two (i.e., significantly overlapping CIs), the language can be easily modified to identify the two most sophisticated levels. From this evidence, inferences can be made regarding the examinee's ability to formulate solutions to interpersonal problems.

What follows is an excerpt that transitions from the resolution scales interpretation, which presents a developmental sequence from less to more sophisticated reasoning, to the outcome scales, which are independent of both the resolution scales and among themselves. That is, it is made clear here that more sophisticated reasoning among the resolution scales does not necessarily translate into a lack of undesirable outcomes. This is followed by three interpretive narrations. The first lists the type and degree of undesirable outcomes that are detected by the data. The second integrates the outcome scales data with those of the resolution scales wherein the results are consistent. The third integrates the same data, although in this case the results are inconsistent in the form of sophisticated problem resolution reasoning juxtaposed with unfavorable and ineffectual outcomes. These excerpts may be modified as the unique case facts require and are designed to significantly increase the speed of test interpretation. Interpretation now moves to the final clinical scales.

CLINICAL SCALES

The final two tables in Form 12.2 consist entirely of clinical scales, which are designed to detect the presence of various types of psychopathology. These scales are also depicted in Figure 12.2 (e-resources) as the final two boxes to the right under "Clinical Scales." The Table 6 title elaborates on the original Roberts–2 label of emotion scales and reads, "Emotional and Behavioral Disorders," so as to be more applicable to the *DSM–5* nosology. It should be noted, however, that behavior disorders are relatively consistent patterns of acting out that can also be conceptualized as emerging personality traits if sufficiently rigid and inflexible.

The table bodies are designed as are the developmental/adaptive scales, although interpretation of the clinical scales data differs in three major ways. First, the *T*–score interpretive scheme consists of only three, rather than four, ranges. Second, the *T*–score ranges consistently reflect greater degrees of abnormality as scores become progressively higher, whereas for the developmental/adaptive data, the meaning of higher scores varied depending on the particular scale. Third, all the clinical scales data are independent, whereas some of the developmental/adaptive scales represented a hierarchical sequence. To facilitate test interpretation, a specific tabular note lists information as to how the clinical scale *T*–score ranges should be interpreted and designated within the table. They are as follows: (a) no asterisk for a *T*–score of 30–59, which is within normal limits or indicates an absence of psychopathology; (b) one asterisk for a *T*–score of 60–69, which shows the presence of mild to moderate psychopathology; and (c) two asterisks for a *T*–score of 70–90, which shows the presence of severe psychopathology. Entries in the final column are again based on the more detailed narrative descriptions provided in the test manual (Roberts & Gruber, 2005, pp. 41–56). General table notes define the *T*–score metric and directional meaning of higher scores.

Examining the targeted content, Table 6 (Form 12.2) clinical scales generally measure the presence of maladaptive emotions and behaviors as reflected in Roberts–2 story content. *T*–score elevations falling within the disordered range are interpreted as representing an internal social-cognitive perceptual set of the respondent, which leads to the inference that such a disorder is actually present. More specifically, Table 6 includes the following emotional and behavioral disorders clinical scales and their associated symptoms: (a) *anxiety*, defined as a state of trepidation and fear, including worry, guilt, embarrassment, and apprehension about environmental demands; (b) *depression*, defined as misery, sadness, unhappiness, sorrow, crying, disappointment, apathy, fatigue, and an inability to cope with situational factors or problems; (c) *rejection*, defined as jealousy, being ostracized, feeling unloved or disliked, and including major disruptions in attachment (e.g., abandonment, loss of primary object relations), separation, or emotional distancing; and (d) *aggression*, defined as angry feelings (e.g., madness, rage, frustration), along with verbal aggression (e.g., arguing, teasing, belittling), and physical aggression (e.g., bullying, destroying property) (Roberts & Gruber, 2005, pp. 41–50).

The concluding Table 7 (Form 12.2) employs the terms "Severe Disorders" to reflect its content and to distinguish it from Table 6. That is, they consist of the two modified scales discussed prior and include the following: (a) *unusual—no score*, which represents signs of concrete, stereotyped, rigid, and inflexible descriptions of the card stimuli scenes indicative of mechanical perseveration and thus neurocognitive dysfunction, and (b) *atypical—*

illogical, which represents signs of severe cognitive and perceptual distortions, *bizarre mentation*, looseness of thought, and formal thought disorder or psychosis (Roberts & Gruber, 2005, pp. 53–56). Therefore, rather than measuring perceptual sets indicative of psychopathology, these scales measure actual *signs* of psychopathology, which is consistent with the format of the Roberts–2 being a performance personality test.

Both Tables 6 and 7 are ensued by comparable excerpts designed to expedite interpretation of the clinical scales. First, interpretation is initiated by a statement that addresses the overall clinical profile, including the general range of scores and whether they tend to be consistent or variable. The second excerpt delves into the particular scale elevations, including what type of psychopathology appears to be present, the degree, and language that can address either ipsative (i.e., relative) comparisons or norm-based comparisons. Again, if ipsative comparisons are desired, the language addressing the population of same-aged peers should be deleted as unnecessary.

Summary

This completes the presentation of the Roberts–2. It is a unique test in that it measures an examinee's social-cognitive abilities, perceptual sets from which the presence of psychopathology can be inferred, and actual signs of severe psychopathology, including neurocognitive dysfunction and psychosis. Considering that the Roberts–2 is labor intensive and yields a rather significant amount of data to report and interpret, these data tables have been designed with accompanying interpretive excerpts to maximize its utility in mental health practice. This leads to the third and final performance personality test of this chapter, one with the longest and most fascinating history of development.

Rorschach Performance Assessment System

This chapter concludes with the last of the three performance personality tests. This is appropriate for a number of reasons. First, it is perhaps the most enduring, influential, and controversial personality test the field of psychology has to offer. Second, it has stimulated and provoked a substantial quantity of research, and thus, irrespective of where psychologists stand on whether they consider this test as being acceptable, it unequivocally possesses heuristic value. However, the most compelling reason for including it here is that it provides a rather comprehensive measure of an individual's personality in action. That is, rather than asking people to tell us what they are like, this test asks examinees to demonstrate what they are like. Therefore, when people cannot report their personality accurately, for whatever reason, the Rorschach test fills the gap. It is for this reason the Rorschach should be part of every psychologist's test inventory.

Synopsis

The *Rorschach Performance Assessment System* (*R–PAS;* Meyer, Viglione, Mihura, Erard, & Erdberg, 2011) is an examiner-administered, performance, standardized test of personality functioning, which is normed on individuals aged 6 years, 0 months through 86 years, 11 months. As indicated prior, the raw data are garnered by directly observing and measuring personality in action (Meyer et al., 2011, p. 1). Meyer et al. (2011) aptly describe the nature of the Rorschach data as follows:

> Rorschach behavior and variables demonstrate how people filter and organize information, what they attend to, how they make sense of and apply meaning to stimuli and situations, how conventionally or idiosyncratically they perceive, and how logically or effectively they think and communicate with another person.
>
> (Meyer et al., 2011, p. 317)

The R–PAS specifically measures the following aspects of personality functioning: (a) perceptual-cognitive ability (i.e., reality testing); (b) problem-solving ability; (c) coping style; (d) information processing and thinking ability; (e) interpersonal behavior; (f) representations of self and other, along with internalized schemas regarding interpersonal interactions; and (g) salient concerns and preoccupations. The coded responses represent a microcosm of an individual's behaviors and abilities, which can then be generalized to the real world. The R–PAS is the most contemporary system available following the *Rorschach Comprehensive System* (*R–CS;* Exner, 2001, 2003). Because the test itself is 100 years old, first developed and published by Hermann Rorschach (1921/1942), a succinct history is in order to provide useful context.

History of the Rorschach Inkblot Test

Why Hermann Rorschach initially chose inkblot stimuli for purposes of psychodiagnosis is a matter of some conjecture. As a child, he frequently played a popular game of that era termed *Klecksographie*, or *Blotto*, in which inkblot stimuli, preprinted by a manufacturer or created by the individual player, were employed in various ways, for example, creating poem-like associations to such stimuli (Kerner, 1857).

Years later, in 1908, the Swiss psychiatrist Eugene Bleuler first proposed a new syndrome he ultimately termed *schizophrenia*, initially identified as dementia praecox (Bleuler 1908; Fusar-Poli & Politi 2008). Soon thereafter, Rorschach, likely influenced by his artistically trained father and previous childhood experience with the Blotto game, created and refined the now famous ten standardized inkblots. In particular, the inkblots were initially designed to elicit meaningful responses to discriminate patients manifesting symptoms of schizophrenia from those without such symptoms, especially those with comparable forms of psychoses that were organically based. In 1921, Rorschach published his now well-known monograph *Psychodiagnostic*, including the currently used ten standardized inkblots. This monograph provided supporting empirical evidence that the clustering of various responses to the inkblot stimuli were effective in detecting distinctive types of psychological and behavioral characteristics, particularly in identifying signs of schizophrenia (Rorschach, 1921). Unfortunately, his premature death precluded Rorschach from further developing his incipient but promising personality test.

Thereafter, five distinct and independent scoring systems emerged in the United States, each of which elaborated Rorschach's initial work, although in significantly contrasting ways. They included systems in the United States by Samuel Beck (Beck, 1944, 1945, 1952; Beck, Beck, Levitt, & Molish, 1961), Marguerite Hertz (Hertz, 1939, 1952, 1970), Bruno Klopfer (Klopfer, Ainsworth, Klopfer, & Holt, 1954; Klopfer & Kelly, 1942; Klopfer, Meyer, Brawner, & Klopfer, 1970), Zygmunt Piotrowski (Piotrowski, 1950, 1957), and David Rapaport (Rapaport, D., Gill, M., & Shafer, R., 1946). All five Rorschach systems were well established by 1957. The immediate problem was that these segregated systems were strikingly different in administration, scoring, and interpretation. Exacerbating this fact is that there existed a paucity of cooperation among these systems' authors, which unfortunately also included a somewhat adversarial relationship between Beck and Klopfer. To seek a resolution to this unfortunate state of affairs, John Exner completed and published a comparative analysis of the five systems (Exner, 1969). His chief conclusion was that these systems shared only one essential feature, namely, the ten inkblots. Otherwise, he found them to be foundationally unique and independent.

The ensuing major development was the founding of the *Rorschach Research Council* (RCC; Exner, 1997), which had the ultimate goal of integrating the most empirically supported features of the five systems into one, which was felicitously called the Rorschach Comprehensive System (R–CS; Exner, 2001, 2003). The CS quickly became the dominant system used in the United States, including norm reference data ranging from as young as 5 years to as old as 86 (Hilsenroth & Handker, 1995; Mihura & Weinle, 2002).

However, an emerging criticism was that the R–CS scoring criteria, and the norms upon which test interpretations were based, possessed a propensity to overestimate the degree of individuals' true psychopathology (Wood, Nezworski, Garb, & Lilienfeld, 2001a, 2001b). Some attributed this to the form quality (FQ) standards being excessively stringent, including too many poor form or minus responses (Meyer et al., 2011). However, subsequent accumulating evidence increasingly showed that the system's tendency to overestimate abnormality was due to a much broader array of R–CS variables than simply strict FQ criteria, especially as applied to children and adolescents (e.g., see Meyer et al., 2011; Viglione & Giromini, 2016).

In response, efforts began to improve the R–CS norms by gathering updated and more representative international samples for this scoring system. Although such efforts would culminate in a special publication of updated R–CS norms (Shaffer, Erdberg, & Meyer, 2007), Dr. Exner passed and the RCC was consequently disbanded. Legal rights of the R–CS were left to Dr. Exner's family. After deliberation, the family chose to honor his legacy by proscribing further changes to the R–CS, thereby leaving the system intact as Dr. Exner had so developed it.

Following these events, four members of the prior RRC used the R–CS as a foundation for developing what now represents the most ambitious and contemporary empirically based system for use of the Rorschach, namely, the R–PAS (Meyer, Viglione, Mihura, Erard, & Erdberg, 2011, 2012). Fundamental improvements in the R–PAS include the following: (a) impressive validity-focused meta-analyses for individual scores exceeding that for all other major psychological tests (e.g., see Graceffo, Mihura, & Meyer, 2014); (b) expanded, more contemporary, and better-matched norm reference samples in terms of demographic variables (Viglione & Giromini, 2016), including the use of non-gendered international norms (Meyer, Giromini, Viglione, Reese, & Mihura, 2015); (c) decreased variability in the number of responses per protocol (e.g., see Meyer, Viglione & Giromini, 2014); (d) reduced examiner effects (Meyer et al., 2011); and (e) enhanced accuracy and precision in variable interpretation (Meyer et al., 2011). The importance of the latter requires some elaboration considering the Rorschach has had a controversial existence virtually since its inception.

Briefly, improvements in Rorschach variable interpretation can be largely attributed to two components incorporated into the R–PAS system, including the usage of (a) standard scores and (b) response-based interpretations. First, standard scores (mean = 100, standard deviation = 15) represent familiar units of measurement for psychologists (see Table A.1) and are applied consistently to all Rorschach variables in terms of both measurement and ultimate interpretation. In consequence, they are superior to the previous use of raw scores in the R–CS, which differ considerably across the Rorschach variables and require examiners to either memorize or repeatedly reference the interpretive criteria for over 60 variables. In the designed Rorschach R–CS scoring and interpretation tables, an attempt to increase utility was done by juxtaposing the interpretive criteria of each R–CS variable and then organizing them according to the principal psychological construct they appeared to measure (e.g., mood, stress) (see Spores, 2012).[8] However, interpretation is much less cumbersome and time consuming when all variables are linearly transformed to a common metric, as when standard score conversions are employed. Although converting Rorschach variables via linear transformations can be problematic because many possess inherently skewed distributions, the R–PAS systems employed a number of statistical strategies that attempted to account for this (see later in this chapter). Furthermore, the effort was laudable because of the enormous enhancement in convenience and utility that resulted from the standardization of test data.

Second, the *response process* refers to psychological operations that lead to an answer to the Rorschach question "What might this be?" during administration of the ten standardized inkblots. Stated another way, the response process is a behavioral representation of the coded score and may be generalized from the microcosm of the test environment to the real world environment, which lies at the core of measuring personality in action. Hence, a perception of a human, who is crying and feeling sad, would generate a morbid thematic code (*MOR*) within the test environment. The response process leading to such a perception in the test environment would reflect a propensity to view objects in the real world through a theme of sadness, a pessimistic outlook, damage, injury, and/or imperfection. Many such *MOR* responses produced by the examinee would be interpreted as an individual who possesses such a melancholic and despondent view of the real world, including perhaps themselves and other people. Thus, the R–PAS now closes the link or relationship between the coded behavior and the inference to which it leads. Moving the interpretation so it is more proximate to the empirical raw data improves both interpretive accuracy and credibility; that is, the interpretations become both more comprehensible and believable.

These authors are continuing to improve the system, including collecting additional norm reference data based directly on R–PAS procedures. Next, the R–PAS standardization samples are presented such that the limits of generalizability of this system can be elucidated. This is ensued by the now familiar sequence of sections covering administration, scoring, and culminating with interpretation, the last of which includes a review and description of the newly designed R–PAS data tables provided in Form 12.3, supplemented by a flowchart diagraming the recommended interpretative process. The latter is available for download on Routledge's e-resources website, which is labeled as Figure 12.3 and strongly recommended for reference throughout the ensuing presentation. These data tables seek to further maximize the clinical utility of this system and have been developed by means of actual clinical practice, as have been all the data tables offered in this book.

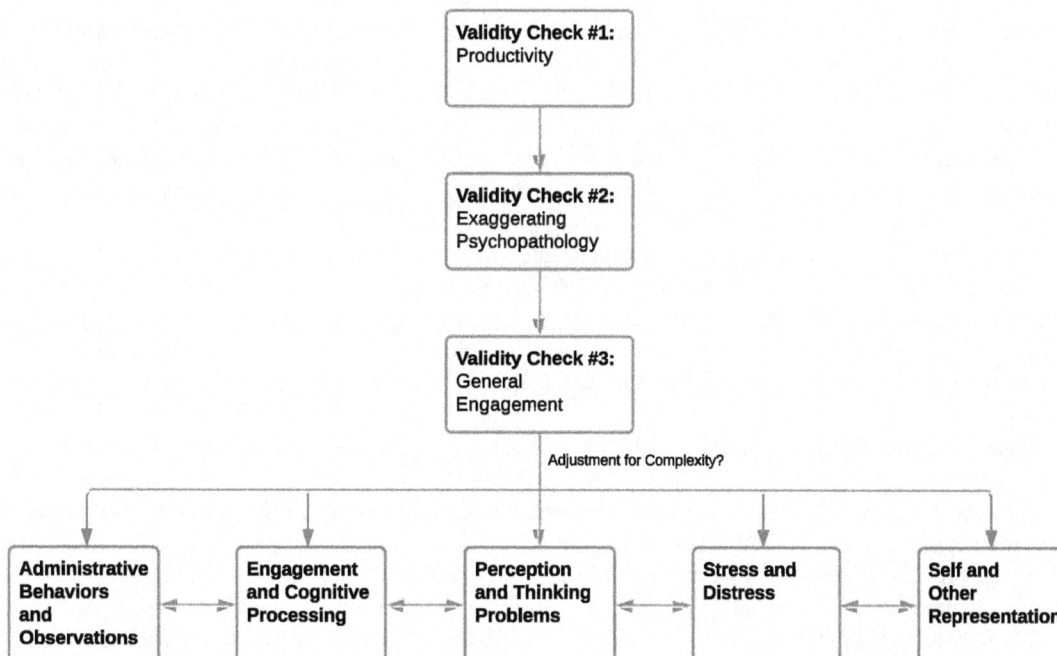

Figure 12.3 Rorschach Performance Assessment System (R-PAS) Interpretive Process

Norm Reference Samples

Norm reference data sets the standards upon which all other individuals taking a particular test will be compared. As will be seen, the R–PAS norming process proceeded through a series of iterations, with the objective of producing more accurate scoring and interpretation compared to the R–CS, the most commonly used and accepted predecessor to the R–PAS. Updates were made to both (a) the FQ standards and (b) the standardization samples to which current and future examinees will be compared. Additionally, the norms that were initially based on raw scores were then transformed into standard scores (*SS*), with a mean of 100 and standard deviation of 15 (range 50–150) to further facilitate interpretation. This section covers the norming process, which was rather complex and protracted in and of itself. The raw score transformation process will be more aptly covered under the scoring and interpretation sections. It will become apparent that the R–PAS was normed beginning with adults, then expanding to children and adolescents. The end result of the ensuing process, which can be divided into four phases, is that the R–PAS is standardized on individuals aged 6 years, 0 months through 86 years, 11 months. Interestingly, the technical portion of the manual provides data regarding gender, ethnicity, and marital status, but no details regarding age. This section is subsequently apportioned into norm development for adults, which occurred first, ensued by norms for children and adolescents ages 6–17, inclusive.

R–PAS ADULT NORMS

First, the norming process began with an original adult, "Non-Modeled Reference Sample." This sample of 1,396 individuals served as the basis for converting R–CS variables to R–PAS variables. The non-modeled aspect of the sample title denotes that these protocols and variables therein were all derived from R–CS administration and scoring criteria. Sampling procedures were as follows. Fifteen subsamples were identified from as many nations. A maximum 100 protocols or fewer were randomly selected from each subsample. The grand total international sample was ultimately 1,396 adults ages 18 and older, with no further specifics regarding age breakdowns or an upper limit. Descriptive data for this non-modeled sample of 1,396 adults are provided in the R–PAS manual in Tables 9.6 and 9.7 (Meyer et al., 2011, pp 310–315), which report descriptive statistics for each R–PAS variable, and in Table 16.8 (Meyer et al., 2011, p. 476), which reports data regarding gender, ethnicity, and marital status. The Table 16.8 data are as follows: (a) gender (males = 44.2%; females = 55.8%), (b) ethnicity (White = 63.1%; Black 1.9%; Hispanic 15%; Asian = 1.3%; Other/Mixed = 18.8%), and (c) marital status (single = 36.7%; with partner = 2.7%; married = 52%; separated 0.8%; divorced = 5.5%; widowed = 2.3%). It is likely that no specifics regarding age were provided because numerous studies have shown that it is uncorrelated with Rorschach variables from the point of middle adolescence through adulthood (Exner & Weiner, 1995; Weiner, 2003), although this inference is speculative.

Second, an additional "Target Base Sample" of 123 adult protocols (i.e., ages 18–86) was obtained using R–PAS administration and scoring. The term target base denotes that this sample served as a comparison group to that of the original 1,396 international sample. That is, they wanted to identify those protocols in the larger more representative original sample, which were sufficiently similar to the target base sample for purposes of justifying their use as a norm reference group for the new R–PAS. In consequence, a total of 640 records from the 1,396 Non-Modeled Reference Sample were deemed sufficiently similar to the target base sample to be considered adequate models for the new R–PAS system. That is, these data served as a reliable estimate of norm reference data that would have been obtained if R–PAS administration procedures and coding guidelines were employed.

Hence, this group of 640 was named the "R-Optimized Modeled Reference Sample" because it represents the R–CS variables that are now adopted by the new R–PAS for adults aged 18 and older. These data are presented in two tables in the R–PAS manual. The first table includes such descriptive statistics as means, modes, standard deviations, measures of skew and kurtosis, ranges, percentiles (5th, 25th, 50th, 75th, and 95th), and percentages of the 640 sample in which each variable was scored. The latter is a consequence of some low base rate variables that do not appear within every protocol (see Meyer et al., 2011, Table 9.4, pp. 304–308). The second table lists frequency counts for these variables (Meyer et al., 2011, Table 9.5, p. 309).

A third step involved incorporating non-R–CS variables into the new R–PAS, which were previously found to be empirically useful in Rorschach interpretation although never included in the R–CS. Descriptive data for these variables are not reported in the R–PAS manual, although the process of how they were incorporated is described. In particular, the process began with a sample of 145 adult protocols that were derived by using R–CS principles. A total of 118 of these were deemed sufficiently similar to the aforementioned target base sample of 123 to justify their use. The new non-R–CS variables were then scored per their uniquely devised scoring principles (e.g., aggressive content, or *AGC*, and oral dependent language, or *ODL*).

Fourth, both the R–CS and non-R–CS variable descriptive raw score data were combined. These data represent the source of the current adult norms used for the R–PAS, at least until new norms can be collected using pure R–PAS administration and scoring principles. Although the upper age limit for the 640 R-Optimized Modeled Reference Sample (and their R–CS adopted variables) and the 118 matched protocols (and their non-R–CS variables) is not provided, it can be reasonably inferred to be 86 years, as reported for the Target Base Sample; hence 18 years through 86 years, 11 months. Now, how were the current R–PAS norms established for children and adolescents ages 6 years, 0 months through 17 years, 11 months?

Norming for individuals under 18 years occurred in several steps (Meyer, Viglione, & Giromini, 2014). First, a sample of 310 records using R–PAS administration and scoring guidelines were collected from individuals aged 6–17 years residing in the United States and Brazil. This sample was referred to as the "R-Optimized Modeled Reference Sample for Children 6 Years through 17 Years." Second, an additional 35 records were obtained from children in the United States and Italy. Although these were obtained using R–CS principles, such protocols were deemed sufficiently similar to the aforementioned target base adult sample ($N = 123$) for inclusion in the child/adolescent sample. Thus, there was a grand total of 345 child and adolescent protocols that were used to begin establishing norm reference data for 6–17 years.

Third, there was a need to adjust for developmental differences between adults and children from 6 to 17 years. The adult target base protocols using R–PAS guidelines were used to *anchor* developmental expectations at the adult end of the age continuum, which was divided into young adults (i.e., ages 18–26), middle adults (i.e., 27–54), and older adults (i.e., 55–86). Developmental normative adjustments for R–PAS-derived variables for ages 6 were then accomplished by two complementary methods, the first statistical and the second logical as follows: (a) *continuous norming* that uses regression analyses to predict developmental ages curves (i.e., analogous to developmental age curves in height and weight) and (b) *inferential norming* that uses expert judgments of developmental trajectories to further refine the empirically derived regression curves, thus resulting in the most reasonable and logically expected developmental trends (see also Meyer, Vigilione, & Ginomini, 2014).

Now that international norms had been established for individuals 6 years, 0 months through 86 years, 11 months, two objectives remained in order to enhance R–PAS accuracy and precision in scoring and interpretation. They included (a) transforming the raw score norms into *SS* units and (b) updating the FQ tables (i.e., tables that delineate the fit and frequency of content on various blots and blot locations). Both of these issues will be covered in the section on scoring. In the interim, R–PAS administration will be described.

Administration

R–PAS administration is referred to as the *R-Optimized Procedure*. This terminology may be familiar, as it was used just previously when discussing the manner in which the contemporary R–PAS norms were established. This procedure is dichotomized into the following: (a) *response phase* (*RP*) and (b) *clarification phase* (*CP*). In the RP, the examinee is to answer the question "What might this be?" Here, the examiner asks for a minimum of two different responses, or perhaps three, although he or she pulls the card in the event the examinee provides four independent scorable responses. Card rejections are prohibited, otherwise the data are considered invalid. Prompts (i.e., *Pr*) and pulls (i.e., *Pu*) are recorded and are part of scoring and interpretation (discussed presently). Card orientation is also recorded, including "<" (i.e., card top pointed left), ">" (i.e., card top pointed right), and "@" denoting that the examinee has turned the card but ultimately made a response within the original card upright direction. No symbol is used for responses to cards held in the upright position without turning. Such responses are scored because they are considered clinically meaningful indications of an examinee's productivity and engagement in the task. It is also consistent with the performance aspect of this test. Succinctly, the RP administration instructions are stated as "*prompt for two, pull after four*" (Meyer et al., 2011, p. 13). However, only one such prompt is permitted per card.

In contrast to the R–CS, if the examinee provides a total of 15 or fewer scorable responses, the examiner is permitted to readminister the cards in the correct numerical sequence without additional prompts, although cards with the maximum permitted four responses during the initial RP are not readministered. Taken together, these procedures are designed to produce valid profiles, ranging from a minimum of 16 to a maximum of 40 separate scorable responses, including an optimum range identified as 18–27 responses (see Meyer et al., 2011, p. 9). That is, short and long protocols are considered less than 18 and more than 27, respectively. Controlling and targeting the total number of responses (i.e., *R*) to this optimal range enhances score reliability because many of the variables are directly influenced by this quantity. It also renders administration time more predictable (i.e., one hour or less) and avoids having to readminister the entire test starting from the first response, which is done in CS administration.

The CP immediately follows the RP. The cardinal objective is to garner only that information needed to resolve any remaining ambiguities in coding from the RP (e.g., "Does the examinee mean one response that is synthesized or two separate responses?" "Is a response vista or diffuse shading?" "Is form dominant over color or vice-versa?"). Such a process is less demanding and tedious as compared to that of the R–CS, primarily because the examiner is not required to see the percept exactly as did the examinee. The principal CP instruction reads as follows: "I will read your responses back to you and I want to know where on the card you were looking and what about the inkblot made it look like that to you" (Meyer et al., 2011, p. 16). As indicated prior, total estimated administration time is more predictably under 60 minutes (Meyer et al., 2011, p. 6). This less ambitious approach to clarification (a) reduces the probability of invoking leading questions that bias the examinee's responses and (b) avoids instigating a form-dominated response set on the part of the examinee. Both of these interfere with the desired examinee-directed approach to R–PAS administration. That is, the overall objective is to permit examinees to guide the process as much as practicable because then the response process will maximally reveal their true personalities.

There are a number of reasons for the aforementioned R–PAS modifications in administration as contrasted with the R–CS system. All generally serve to enhance reliability, validity, and especially from a practice perspective, clinical utility. First, the excessively open-ended nature of R–CS administration rules that set no limits on the number of responses given by examinees resulted in extensive variability in this influential variable, which ultimately confounded test interpretation. In particular, excessively short protocols (e.g., $R = 14$) increased the likelihood of false-negative results by reducing the chances of capturing pathological responses, hence risking an underestimate of the true degree of psychopathology. In contrast, excessively long protocols (e.g., $R = 50$) increased the likelihood of capturing more pathological responses, hence tending to risk an overestimate of psychopathology. Therefore, the R–PAS administration instructions, including those guiding the RP and CP, maximize the odds that the examinee will produce an *optimal range of scorable responses*, operationally defined as *18 to 27*. Empirically, it has been shown that this range of scores produces an ideal degree of test reliability and validity (i.e., neither over- nor underestimating the level of psychopathology in a particular case). Next examined is the R–PAS coding and scoring procedures.

Scoring

R–PAS scoring fundamentally includes three issues as follows: (a) the rules for coding examinee's verbatim responses elicited in both the RP and CP into what essentially represent raw score data, (b) the process of transforming the raw score codes into standard scores as a necessary prelude to interpretation, and (c) understanding how to read the R–PAS computer-scoring printout. At this juncture, preference for use of computer scoring when available has been made clear. However, for this test, it is imperative because of the extensive computations required, along with a number of variables using complex algorithms that render hand-scoring both impractical and unwise (e.g., *TP-Comp*). This section is apportioned into these three subtopics and in said sequence.

R–PAS CODING

As in the R–CS, each of the examinee's responses garnered from the RP and CP are first transformed into a sequence of codes, which are subsequently used to compute the major variables for purposes of test interpretation (see Form 12.3, especially the diagnostic variable listed in Tables 4–8). In order, the questions that are asked, along with their associated coding categories that provide the answers (in parentheticals and italics font), include the following: (a) "What is the card angle?" (*card orientation*); (b) "Where is it seen?" (*location*); (c) "Is white space used, and if so, how?" (*space reversal and space integration*); (d) "What is seen?" (*contents*); (e) "Are any objects meaningfully related?" (*synthesis*); (f) Are all objects in the percept vague?" (*vagueness*); (g) "Are there two identical objects?" (*pair*); (h) "How well does it fit the inkblot?" (*form quality*); (i) "Do many people see it?" (*popular*); (j) "What features of the inkblot make it look like that?" (*determinants*); (k) "Are there issues with thought processes?" (*cognitive codes*); (l) "What special themes are present?" (*thematic codes*); and (m) "Were steps taken by the examiner to manage the number of scorable responses?" (*prompts* and *pulls*) (see Meyer et al, 2011, Table 3.1, p. 37).[9] These can be answered in such order on the R–PAS online computer scoring program, which is described in the third subtopic of this section.

How well an examinee's perception fits an inkblot location concerns form quality, which has been a key variable in virtually all Rorschach systems, including the R–PAS. Although virtually the same locations and location numbers for each of the ten inkblots remains unmodified from that of the R–CS, the R–PAS FQ tables and coding criteria have been updated to reflect more contemporary standards. Therefore, derivation of the current R–PAS FQ tables will be expanded upon here (see Meyer at al., 2011, pp. 179–253; see also Meyer et al, 2012).

There were a number of distinct steps taken in the process of updating the FQ coding. First, the following five general content classifications were defined: (a) distinctly human-related, (b) human- or animal-related, (c) distinctly animal-related, (d) biologically-related, and (e) other objects. Within these broad classifications, a total of 5,060 objects were identified for each card by location, that is, whole blot (*W*), common detail (*D*), and unusual detail (*Dd*). Second, the FQ for each object by location was appraised by two components of perceptual accuracy, including (a) *fit* (i.e., the estimated degree of match between the identified object with that of the inkblot contours at the location in which it is perceived) and (b) *frequency* (i.e., the rate at which an object is perceived by the general population at a particular location). Regarding the latter, the greater the frequency or rate at which an object is perceived at an inkblot location by people in general, the greater the inferred accuracy (i.e., consensual reality). In order from most to least accurate, the objects by location were ultimately coded as either *ordinary form quality* (viz., *FQo*; the percept is seen quickly and easily), *unusual form quality* (viz., *FQu*; the percept is less frequent and less accurate, but not grossly contrary with respect to the blot contours), or *minus form quality* (viz., *FQ—*; the percept is infrequent or rare and clearly inaccurate, distorted, or arbitrary).

Three sources were used to determine the final FQ codes for each object by location. They consisted of (a) a computed average perceptual form accuracy (FA) rating made by an international panel of experts (viz., form fit), (b) the frequency with which the response object was reported by five international samples of examinees (i.e., minimum frequency to be included was 1.5% of the sample), and (c) historical FQ codes assigned by the most recent and empirically well-established systems, including most especially those provided by the R–CS (Exner, 2003), Beck et al. (1961), and Hertz (1970).

Why the minimum 1.5% frequency criterion? The majority of response object frequencies follow a positively skewed distribution, with large differences between percentile ranks. These distributions are called *Zipf* (1932, 1949), *Pareto, zeta, rank size*, or *power-law distributions*, wherein certain objects are perceived very frequently while others are perceived much less frequently, with an enormous gap in frequency counts. This is illustrated by comparing the frequency of circadian rhythm-related events (e.g., sleeping) to extremely rare catastrophic-type events (e.g., earthquakes). By analogy, there occurs a precipitous decline in the frequency of perceiving some very typical objects (e.g., bat, human) in certain common inkblot locations to most others manifesting a much lower frequency (e.g., drill). Hence, the 1.5% criterion was purposely chosen to be sufficiently low to capture a wider variety of objects to be included in the final R–PAS FQ tables, including those that are extremely rare. This guideline effectively averted the risk of resulting in too few objects, or a restricted range of objects, to be scored. On the other hand, to avoid an overly lengthy and cumbersome list, very similar objects falling at the same locations on the inkblots were combined (e.g., "winged insect" or "bird" versus a listing of ten specific examples unless it had distinctive features), thus effectively reducing both the redundancy and length of the R–PAS FQ tables. Hence, a balance between overly scarce and excessively inundating was the sought-after objective. Next, raw score code to SS transformations are discussed.

R–PAS RAW SCORE TO STANDARD SCORE TRANSFORMATIONS

As indicated, the R–PAS data proceed through several transformations. First, examinee's responses are coded. Thus, technically examinee's verbatim verbal and nonverbal communications recorded during the RP and CP administration process represent the original data, comparable to that of the Roberts–2. These communications are transformed into codes that answer the 11 questions enumerated prior. For each response, codes addressing the 11 questions are entered in a row, including one row for each response, which creates an R–PAS code sequence. Each column of the code sequence represents a different coding category. Second, numerous counts and calculations are performed on the aforesaid code sequence, hence resulting in the derivation of key variables with interpretive value, varying from simple frequencies to complex equations, referred to at this juncture as raw quantitative scores; that is, none of these scores have yet been linearly transformed into standard scores (SSs). These initial raw scores are then transformed into percentiles or percentile ranks, with a median of 50 and a range from 0 to 99. Lastly, these percentiles are converted into SS equivalents, with a mean of 100, standard deviation of 15, and range of 50–150. It is instructive to examine further precisely how the raw scores were transformed into PRs and SSs.

First, norm reference code derivations, frequencies, and percentages were converted into their corresponding empirically-based percentiles; that is, *percentiles derived from the sample statistics*, not the theoretical normal curve (Meyer at al., 2011; Meyer & Erdberg, 2018). An immediate complication was how to assign a PR to Rorschach-type low base-rate variables, which are notoriously numerous in this test. A *low base-rate variable* is operationally defined as, "those that occur 5 times or less in every 100 responses" (Mihura & Meyer, 2018; Chapter 2, 2018, p. 30), or a proportion of 0.05 of all responses. The average number of responses on the R–PAS is 24; hence, 24 x 0.05 = 1.20. This means that low base-rate scores on a typical R–PAS protocol have a mean of 1.20 or less. Such variables have very limited distributions. In consequence, a single raw score on such a variable can be associated with an unusually wide range of PR values. For example, a texture (*T*) response is one such variable in which 55% of all people taking the test have a raw score of 0. That means that in this case, a single raw score of 0 is associated with 55 PR values, namely, 0–55. So, which value is this raw score's PR equivalent? Another way to ask this question is, "How does one decide on a single PR value that would most accurately represent a raw score of 0 on this variable?" The test authors decided to resolve this conundrum by taking the average or midpoint of such a PR range. Hence, for the T variable, a PR of 27.5 would be assigned (i.e., the range of PR values is from 0 to 55, hence 55 ÷ 2 = 27.5).

Second, all such PRs were then converted into *SS* equivalents based on the theoretical standard normal distribution. For example, a PR of 50 equals a *SS* of 100, a PR of 16 equals a *SS* of 85, and a PR of 84 equals a *SS* of 115 (see also Table A.1). Of note, and with due diligence, the authors do caution that fitting area transformation–type PRs to linearly based SSs according to the normal distribution has the effect of exaggerating PR changes in the middle of the distribution closer to the mean, while minimizing PR changes within the distribution extremes or farther from the mean. For example, a small two–point *SS* change from 100 to 102 is associated with a four–point PR change (viz., 51 to 55), whereas a much larger ten–point *SS* change farther from the mean, such as 65 to 75 (i.e., five times as large), is associated with the same four–point PR change (viz., 1 to 5). This is because PRs are clustered tightly in the middle of the normal distribution while being increasingly disbursed as one moves toward the extremes. However, the authors go on to justify this type of transformation by arguing that all R–PAS variables could now be quantified according to a common metric, including a mean of 100 and standard deviation of 15. Therefore, Rorschach users are no longer required to memorize varying raw score ranges and their interpretive meanings for over 60 variables. This has never before been achieved in Rorschach testing and has the beneficial effect of significantly simplifying and objectifying Rorschach interpretation.

The implication for R–PAS scoring is that the *SS* and associated PR values for each Rorschach variable reported in the final results may be slightly different. For example, in one of the author's recent cases, an 8-year-old girl earned the same *SS* score of 97 on the *Blend* and *FQo%* variables, although their PRs were 42 and 41, respectively. This is not an error but is a consequence of (a) the inconsistency of the raw score distributions manifested by the many Rorschach variables and (b) the manner in which the *SS* equivalents were derived (i.e., from the changeable Rorschach variable raw score distributions, exacerbated by their low base-rate variables). This phenomenon repeatedly manifests itself throughout the R–PAS data output. Thus, it was important that this facet of R–PAS score results be made explicit.

As stated, the SSs and PRs can be adjusted for complexity, which impacts test validity because it measures the degree to which an examinee is engaged in the task. It also accounts for the majority of the variance in Rorschach variables, analogous to *demoralization* accounting for the majority of variability in MMPI clinical scale variables (see Tellegen, Ben-Porath, McNulty, Arbisi, Graham, & Kaemmer, 2003; see also Chapter 11). Too little complexity is thought to risk missing psychopathology, whereas too much complexity is thought to risk detecting more abnormality than is actually present. For example, an examinee who provides a greater number of responses and whose responses are more complex (e.g., more blends or multiple determinants within a single response) is more likely to provide at least some problematic codes, which may show more abnormality than is actually present. In contrast, an examinee who provides a minimum number of responses that are simplistic and unadorned, is likely to show little psychopathology. Another way to frame this is that, excessively low complexity has high positive predictive power. That is, any evidence for abnormality in this context can be afforded greater significance because of the simplicity of the protocol and the lower likelihood of showing psychopathology. In contrast, excessively high complexity has high negative predictive power. That is, an absence of abnormality has greater credence in the context of a protocol in which the probability of showing abnormality would be greater than average. This issue will be revisited when discussing interpretation.

Because R–PAS variables contain a mixture of normal and non-normal (i.e., skewed or kurtotic) distributions, the test authors employed a special quantile regression technique to predict what examinees' scores would be if they had an average or optimal (i.e., median) level of complexity. A *quantile* is a value on a distribution that has been segmented into equal units. The unit size chosen was 100 (i.e., percentiles), consistent with the *SS* metric. This divides each variable's distribution into 100 units of equal size. For complexity adjusted scores, the median or 50th percentile was predicted (versus the mean as in standard regression), using the *complexity* score as the single predictor.

> . . . Protocol level Complexity is an aggregate measure involving information from . . . three response components that contribute to the aggregate score. . .: (1) Location, Space, Synthesis, and Vagueness sections, (2) Contents, and (3) Determinants.
>
> (Meyer et al., 2011, pp. 295)

Subsequent to predicting the median value for every complexity *SS*, parameters of the regression model were saved to derive equations for the slope and intercept for optimally predicting the expected value given the examinee's measured level of complexity. Next, to calculate the complexity adjusted normative values, a difference score was computed by taking the observed minus the expected value, termed a residual score. The residual score is added to the median value for that variable, and the result is the *complexity adjusted* score.[10] If this explanation is too complex in and of itself, simply focus on the interpretative meaning of a complexity adjusted score: namely, it represents examinees' predicted PRs and SSs assuming they had an average (i.e., median) level of complexity. If complexity-adjusted scores are not requested in the computer scoring, they are reported but electronically printed in light gray font and they are not profiled or graphed. To utilize the R–PAS data tables that have been created (see Form 12.3), the graphed data are not needed as they are unnecessarily redundant and slow the process of test interpretation; that is, only the listed SSs and PRs adjacent to each variable are needed.

What about confidence intervals (CIs)? Unfortunately, these data are not provided anywhere in the manual. This is unfortunate because, as has been contended throughout this book, CIs effectively communicate that a test, or any measure, is not completely accurate. They also contribute to test interpretation, both in terms of ipsative analyses and accurately describing SSs that straddle two qualitative categories. The R–PAS manual also does not report measures of temporal consistency in the form of test–retest reliability coefficients to estimate the standard errors of measurement (SEMs) for the R–PAS variables (see Meyer at al., 2011, pp. 439–440). However, the manual does report the median interrater reliability for the R-Optimized Administration as follows: $N = 50$ protocols; $N = 59$ variables; Median $r = 0.92$ (see Meyer at al., 2011, Table 14.3, p. 435). Therefore, the following formula was used to compute a uniform 68% CI for the R–PAS variables:

$$SEM = SD\sqrt{1 - r_{xx}}$$

Equation 12.1

where *SD* is the standard deviation of the pertinent metric being used, and r_{xx} represents the interrater reliability coefficient for the Rorschach variables. Because the metric being used here is a *SS*, the *SD* value is 15 and the reported coefficient is 0.92. Therefore:

$$SEM = SD\sqrt{1 - r_{xx}} = 15\sqrt{1 - .92} = 4.24 = 4$$

Hence, the 68% CI = 1 x 4 = 4 *SS* points, which is reported for all variables in the scoring and interpretation tables (see Form 12.3).

At this juncture, R–PAS coding and their transformation to SSs have been presented. The latter included an optional adjustment for complexity. The final subtopic regards the R–PAS online scoring program, which is essential to know if this test is to be used in mental health testing, where test efficiency is essentially mandated. The focus will be on the computer-scoring output and the manner in which it is organized so the data can be rapidly input into the data tables for inclusion within a psychological assessment report. This will provide the context for test interpretation.

R–PAS ONLINE SCORING AND DATA OUTPUT   Using the Internet-based R–PAS computer scoring program is essential to its utility. It saves valuable coding and computing time while reducing human error. Respectively, the home page title and address is *Rorschach Performance Assessment System*® (R–PAS®; 2021) and www.R–PAS.org/Default.aspx. There are different protocol types that can be purchased (e.g., research only), although the most comprehensive one for psychological testing practice is "Clinical (all functions)." The remainder of this subtopic is apportioned into the following: (a) data entry and (b) data output. The former reviews the information needed to enter the examinee identifying information section and code sequence section. The latter reviews the data output and how it is organized by the R–PAS program.

DATA ENTRY   The patient identifying information needed to create a protocol is the client file number or name (C-ID), chronological age, gender, and years of education (completed or current grade). The default administration is R-Optimized (versus CS). Similarly, the default FQ table is R–PAS (versus CS). Both defaults should be retained for the new R–PAS system. Also required is the administration date. The data may be input by either keyboard or computer mouse click. The latter permits coding directly from the examinee's recorded responses without the need for manual coding; hence, it is the preferred one for increasing efficiency. Each response is typically scored in its entirety before advancing to the next response. Within each response, the process begins by entering in the codes that are explicit and obvious, then proceeding to those that are more difficult to discern. Finally, prior to moving to the next response, scanning across all the potential codes is done to ensure that nothing has been inadvertently overlooked. The authors refer to this scoring approach as *coding horizontally* (i.e., across all the coding categories row by row, with each representing a single response). In contrast, coding vertically means proceeding by code category versus by response. For example, the examiner would code all responses first for orientation, then location, and likewise until all the coding categories have been entered. The latter is referred to as *coding vertically* (i.e., down the coding sequence rows, category by category), and is extremely slow and cumbersome because it requires rereading each response for each new code. Of note, purchasing and using the convenient portable guide also increases coding efficiency (Meyer et al., 2012), which is highly recommended.

Databases are encrypted and password protected to ensure confidentiality. The database employs a. NET platform using server-sided processing; that is, all calculations are processed on the server and results are sent directly to the user's computer screen. Appendix G (pp. 502–516) in the main R–PAS manual affords a succinct guide on how to use the online scoring system (Meyer et al., 2011), although much of the scoring system is self-explanatory.

DATA OUTPUT   The online computer-scoring output is six pages long. Table 12.5 lists all six pages, their titles, and a summary description accompanied by the primary use for which they are designed. Page 1 reports the *R–PAS code sequence*, which consists of a listing of coded responses in the order they occurred per card. The responses are scored according to standardized principles detailed in the manual (Meyer et al., 2011, pp. 31–177). Such information was referred to in the R–CS as the sequence of scores. This represents the sequence of codes per response. In order, the code categories are card (Cd, listed by Roman numerals), # (response number, listed by Arabic numerals), orientation (Or), location (card location), location #, SR (space reversal), SI (space integration), Content, Sy (synthesis) Vg (vague); 2 (pair), FQ (form quality), P (popular), determinants, cognitive (cognitive codes), thematic (thematic codes), HR (human representation), ODL (oral dependent language), and R-Opt (R-optimized). At the top of Page 1 is basic identifying information, including identification number, age, gender, and education. This page can be reviewed for any errors or patterns that may be diagnostically useful later in the interpretive process. It also provides the total number of responses given by the examinee and any card rejections (which would actually invalidate the protocol).

Page 2 presents an *R–PAS Protocol Level Counts & Calculations* report. Here, all codes entered into the sequence on Page 1 of the output are tallied in the form of frequency counts, percentages, proportions, and algorithms. Note that, as in the R–CS, there are a number of proportionally based scores (e.g., PHR/GPHR) that, per R–PAS interpretation guidelines, are not to be reported due to unreliability when their data is based on fewer than four raw scores. Here, the online program will simply insert "N/A" in place of an actual percent score on this page. These proportional variables are identified by a specific table note in the data tables designed for reporting the R–PAS scores within a psychological assessment report. This page is a prelude to the principal variables used for nomothetic interpretation and also yields some of the information that investigates test validity discussed later in the interpretation section.

Table 12.5 Rorschach Performance Assessment System (R–PAS) Computer Program Data Output

Page #	Page Title	Page Summary Description and Primary Use
1.	R–PAS Code Sequence	Listing of all responses (rows) and their 19 code categories (columns). Used for overview of examinee's protocol, including total number of responses and any card rejections.
2.	R–PAS Protocol Level Counts & Calculations	Frequency counts and calculations derived from the aforesaid code sequence, some of which represent final R–PAS variables and some as a prelude to computing final variables for interpretation.
3.	R–PAS Summary Scores and Profiles—Page 1	Listing of all final R–PAS variables with the greatest amount of research support, organized by domain, including raw scores, SSs, and Ps, which are also profiled. Used for primary nomothetic interpretation.
4.	R–PAS Summary Scores and Profiles—Page 2	Listing of all final R–PAS variables with a lesser amount of research support, organized by domain, including raw scores, SSs, and PRs, which are also profiled. Used for secondary nomothetic interpretation.
5.	EII-3 and Composite Calculations	Illustrated complex computations for the *EII-3* and all composites. Informs of the elements contributing to these composite variables to facilitate interpretation.
6.	R–PAS Profile Appendix—Summary Scores for All Variables	Tabled summary of all R–PAS variables organized by code section. Miscellaneous use but especially for research purposes.

Note. SSs = standard scores; Ps = percentiles; *EII-3* = Ego Impairment Index.

The next page is titled *R–PAS Summary Scores and Profiles—Page 1*. This page reports the most empirically validated variables in the R–PAS system, including each variable's (a) raw scores, (b) SSs and percentiles (Ps), (c) complexity-adjusted SSs and Ps, (d) a graphic profile of the non-adjusted SSs in different colored circles depending on their deviation from the mean of 100, and (e) variable abbreviations. These variables are listed in five conceptually organized domains designed to facilitate test interpretation, including (a) administration behaviors and observations, (b) engagement and cognitive processing, (c) perception and thinking problems, (d) stress and distress, and (e) self and other representation. Their meanings will be scrutinized in the interpretation section since that is their chief function, although they are introduced here as they serve to organize the data output. By default, the program will show everything except the minimum and maximum scores for each variable (they vary, although are all within the 50–150 range), and the *complexity adjustment* data will be in light gray. The ensuing fourth page in the sequence is titled *R–PAS Summary Scores and Profiles—Page 2*, which provides all the remaining clinical variables organized in the same five domains but having less empirical support.

Some comments concerning the page 3 and 4 data output are in order. First, as introduced prior, there are seven variables that are computed as proportions. For these variables, the online scoring program will not print the result unless there are a minimum of four total raw scores. Otherwise, this would risk reporting signification proportions that are based on tenuous quantities, which of course vitiates test reliability and validity. In the event there are four or more raw scores, the program will print the raw score ratio in lighter gray font within brackets between the variable name and the computed raw score. For example, take the color dominance proportional variable. The sufficient output could read as follows: CF + C)/SumC [3/4] 75%. Here, the name is listed first, CF + C)/SumC, the raw score proportion in brackets, [3/4], and the computed raw score, 75%. This shows that there are seven total raw scores in the proportion (3 + 4 = 7). Hence, this meets the criterion of being reported with ample reliability (i.e., the minimum of four raw scores). If there were only three raw scores, [1/2], the proportion would be 50%; however, this result would be supplanted by an "N/A" sign. Similarly, any proportion with a zero denominator would automatically receive an "N/A" sign because a number cannot be divided by 0; for example, M/MC [0/0] 50%, would obviously fail to meet the criterion because it is based on zero in the denominator (i.e., 0 + 0 = 0). Hence, for all such unreliable proportions with fewer than four reliable codes, "N/A" is reported.

The aforesaid data output for both R–PAS Summary Scores and Profiles—Page 1 and R–PAS Summary Scores and Profiles—Page 2 is the result of the two default "Profile shows" selections, which are located at the bottom of the R–PAS Protocol Level Counts & Calculations page. These two default selections are *Raw Scores*, which is responsible for inserting the variable raw scores, along with their non-adjusted SS and PR scores, and *Units*, which is responsible for inserting the raw score ranges in the graphic profile in light gray. However, there are two additional data output options to consider. The first is *Min/Max in Norms*, which will locate the minimum and maximum scores in the graphic profile by graying out values that exceed the range of scores for that variable. This can be helpful if the examiner wishes to assess how extreme a score is on a particular variable in graphic form. In addition, there is a "Complexity Adjusted" option, which will (a) show SS scores adjusted for the examinee's measured complexity now in regular black font (i.e., no longer in lighter gray font), and (b) graph the adjusted SSs in square shapes if they differ from the non-adjusted scores (designated by circles) by eight or more SS points.

Page 5 of the printout is titled *EII-3 and Composite Calculations*. It essentially provides all the underlying equations for the composite variables. This information can assist in terms of variable interpretation, although it is most likely used in conducting clinical research. Lastly, Page 6 of the printout is titled *R–PAS Profile Appendix—Summary Scores for All Variables*. It essentially includes all the same clinical variables and data, although organized according to code category. Again, it is likely that researchers would be most interested in this manner of organizing the data.

Summary   To recapitulate, the R–PAS computer output consists of six pages of data, which are summarized in Table 12.5 for review. However, the principal ones to focus on are the following (page number in parentheses): (a) R–PAS Code Sequence (page 1); (b) R–PAS Protocol Level Counts & Calculations (page 2); (c) R–PAS Summary Scores and Profiles—Page 1 (page 3); and (d) R–PAS Summary Scores and Profiles—Page 2 (page 4). Succinctly, the first two provide data for the validity tables (Form 12.3), while the last two provide data for the remainder of the data tables designed for including them within the context of a psychological assessment report.

The final section reviews the data tables that have been prepared for inserting and interpreting the R–PAS test results within a psychological assessment report. The discussion begins with data that examine test validity. Next, the diagnostic data are presented in a sequence of tables that follow the aforesaid five domains. A stratagem for interpretation is also presented that diverges somewhat from the authors' approach. However, these tables are sufficiently flexible, so the testing psychologist can modify the interpretive scheme presented here if desired.

Interpretation

The interpretive approach delineated here is supplemented by the flowchart presented in Figure 12.3 (e-resources), which illustrates the advised process of deriving meaning from the R–PAS scores, and Form 12.3, which includes three tables that address test validity (Tables 1–3), and five diagnostic-related tables that measure various aspects of personality functioning (both assets and liabilities) and the presence of any clinical psychopathology (Tables 3–8). To further facilitate the process, interpretive excerpts follow each table, which also provide guidance on how to approach and organize the inferences and conclusions based on the data output. The discussion is hereafter apportioned into two subtopics, including R–PAS validity analysis and R–PAS diagnostic interpretation. Throughout the process, remember that the prime objectives are efficiency and utility.

R–PAS VALIDITY ANALYSIS

Figure 12.3 (e-resources) initiates the interpretive scheme with three validity checks, each denoted by a separate box. These three boxes correspond to Tables 1, 2, and 3 in Form 12.3, which is designed for reporting and interpreting R–PAS results within a psychological assessment report. In sequence, the three validity checks scrutinize the examinee's productivity (Validity Check #1), any evidence of an attempt to exaggerate psychopathology (Validity Check #2), and the degree of engagement in the Rorschach task. The first results in a dichotomous valid or invalid outcome, while the latter examines whether statistical adjustments should be made in the interpretive process. While three validity tables may seem rather involved and potentially time consuming, they are designed to be interpreted rapidly. Let us take these in sequence.

Validity Check #1: Productivity   Table 1 (Form 12.3) contains two variables that determine whether the examinee has been sufficiently productive. Both are raw scores and include total responses (R) and card rejections, the latter defined as an examinee who refuses to provide at least one scorable response to any one or more of the ten standardized Rorschach inkblots. Concerning these two variables, the R–PAS guidelines are as follows: (a) R less than 16 scorable responses is invalid (i.e., a range between 16 and 40 is required); (b) *card rejections* greater than 0 is invalid. Both can be easily found on the R–PAS Code Sequence page (page 1). R is also recorded on both R–PAS Protocol Level Counts & Calculations (page 2) and R–PAS Summary Scores and Profiles—Page 1 (page 3). Table 1 (Form 12.3) provides the variable name, the raw score, criteria for a valid result, the result, and the measured response process. General table notes further define the variables and what is meant by response process. Since productivity is essential, such data should always be reported first to show the reader that all other variables, with the exception of the proportional scores as previously discussed, have sufficient scorable data for subsequent interpretation. However, it is rare that the R–PAS will be invalid at this early point, especially if the examinee has been properly prepared. Thus, typically the valid interpretive excerpt following Table 1 (Form 12.3) can be retained and the invalid version deleted. However, if it is invalid at this juncture, the examiner simply enters the data into Table 1, then deletes the valid excerpt while retaining the invalid version. The remainder of the tables are then deleted.

Validity Check #2: Exaggerating Psychopathology   If Table 1 data are valid, Figure 12.3 (e-resources) illustrates that the analysis then moves to Table 2 (Form 12.3). It is organized in similar fashion as Table 1, including the same five columns. The two variables here are designed to detect deliberate efforts on the part of the examinee to exaggerate the presence of psychological disturbance (i.e., feigning). They include FQ—% from R–PAS Protocol Level Counts & Calculations (page 2) and CritCont% (critical contents) from R–PAS Summary Scores and Profiles—Page 1 (page 3). The first variable and rule are actually borrowed from the R–CS. It is a deceptively simple datum and inference. Specifically, if $FQ-\% \geq 70$, per R–CS guidelines, the examinee would manifest such a profound degree of psychopathology that standardized administration would be precluded (Exner, 2003). Considering that the R–PAS FQ criteria are less stringent than that used in the R–CS (Meyer et al, 2011), it would be more difficult for the examinee to reach this degree of distortion. Therefore, this interpretation would be bolstered even further. Hence, such data evinces the logical conclusion that the examinee has feigned or intentionally exaggerated abnormality. The reason for such behavior must be determined by additional assessment information, usually from the clinical interview or collateral information. For example, is there an identifiable external motivation for such feigning? If so, a case can be argued for a *DSM–5* diagnosis of malingering.[11]

Second, an extremely high *CritCont%* score, which is based on content analysis, indicates that the examinee has produced an excessive quantity of conspicuously crude, dramatic, and disturbing responses that tend to evoke shock, which also supports a hypothesis of feigning psychopathology (Meyer et al., 2011; see also Mihura & Meyer, 2018, p. 35). The empirical question is "What should be considered a sufficiently high *CritCont%* score?" In the absence of more specific guidance on this question, perhaps scrutinizing the R-Optimized Modeled Reference Sample ($N = 640$) data would assist in establishing some logically sound threshold. According to this sample data, *CritCont%* scores of 3.1, 10, 19, 28, and 45.9 represent percentile ranks of 5, 25, 50 (i.e., the median), 75, and 95, respectively (see Meyer et al., 2011, Table 9.4, p. 307). Hence, a score of about 46% and above would represent the top 5% of the norm reference sample (i.e., the population) and would be one reasonable threshold to at least trigger a content analysis of such responses for possible feigning and malingering. In practice, however, this has resulted in a number of false-positive conclusions in valid cases of severe *post-traumatic stress disorder* (*PTSD*). An alternative is to estimate a more conservative criterion, operationally defined as a PR of 99. Using interpolation, the remaining 5 PRs (i.e., 95–100) represents 54.1% of the sample (i.e., 100–45.9). Assuming each PR covers an equal portion of the sample, then 1 PR would equal 10.82. To reach a PR of 99, 4 PRs would be 43.28. Adding 43.28 to 45.9 equals 89.18. Rounding, a *CritCont%* score of 89 or greater would represent a PR equal to or greater than 99% of the sample and would be interpreted as exaggerating psychopathology. This criterion has a greater risk of false-negative results, although when it does occur the conclusion of feigning has more credible empirical support. Hence, this criterion is now entered into the Table 2 validity check (Form 12.3).

Of course, because these data are produced by an adult sample, extra caution should be taken when applying such a threshold to examinees under 18 years of age. However, considering that such a threshold would merely trigger further content analysis of such scores and by itself would not be determinative, the risk of faulty conclusions seems to be sufficiently mitigated. In any case, it appears to be prudent to include this in the validity analysis since there are so few variables in R–PAS that measure aspects of test validity. Of course, examiners are always free to delete this variable from the analysis or raise the criterion, especially if a false-positive result appears to be likely. In fact, this has been done several times in this author's clinical practice in cases where complex PTSD was corroborated by other evidence and this variable was as much as 75%. Therefore, this score should also be deleted from the table if it is highly elevated but still deemed valid by the clinician due to the presence of severe trauma in the history or other bona fide causes. In such a circumstance, retaining this variable here in the validity analysis would be perplexing to the reader because it would by itself suggest invalidity.

General notes to Table 2 provide the names of the variable abbreviations, along with their basic formulas. The latter is inserted especially for the testing psychologist to expedite test interpretation. That is, the formulas are a felicitous reminder as to what content or thematic codes are included in composite variables, similar to the EII-3 and composite calculations computer printout (page 5; see also Table 12.5). Of note, this strategy is used throughout the data tables, as it speeds the interpretation process and simultaneously informs the reader as to what the variable fundamentally represents. Once again, two narrative interpretations follow the table, one version for a valid result, the other for an invalid result. In the event results are deemed to be invalid due to probative evidence of feigning, the remainder of the data tables should be simply deleted. In this case, the examiner may add evidence that supports a hypothesis of feigning, including behavioral observations, other test data, external health records, and collateral information from the clinical interview.

Validity Check #3: Complexity   Assuming the results of Tables 1 and 2 are both valid, Figure 12.3 (e-resources) illustrates that the analysis moves to Table 3, which is titled in Form 12.3 as "Validity Check #3: R–PAS General Engagement Score Summary." It contains a single composite variable appositely termed *complexity*. Succinctly, the fundamental purpose of Table 3 is to empirically determine if statistical adjustments are needed to improve test interpretation. Hence, a review of this variable is needed to describe accurately the validity issue that is here being addressed.

To review, *complexity* represents the degree of sophistication, productivity, and resources reflected in an examinee's protocol. More specifically, this variable considers such aspects as location, use of space (i.e., both space integration and reversal), object qualities, contents, determinants, and the *density* of responses. *Density* reflects the degree to which a response consists of multiple codes and determinants that are integrated or synthesized in meaningful ways. At the most concrete level of description, *complexity* is an aggregate score that consists of a weighted sum of three components as follows: (a) location, space, and object qualities; (b) contents; and (c) determinants.

The issues of prime concern here are as follows. In the event an examinee's measured complexity is too high or too low, this may distort some of the variables that are affected by this principal feature. In terms of assessing for abnormality, which is the typical focus of psychological testing, increased complexity is associated with a commensurate increase in such variables as cognitive codes and poor human representations (PHR), both of which are indicators of psychopathology (viz., perceptual and thinking disturbances and impairment in interpersonal relationships, respectively). In fact, a substantial number of R–PAS variables are highly correlated with complexity (see Meyer wet al., 2011, p. 349) and thus will be influenced in similar fashion. Excessively high *complexity* increases the risk of *false-positive results* of abnormality, namely, diagnosing more psychopathology than is actually present.

In complementary fashion, in cases where an examinee's *complexity* is remarkably low, simplistic, crude, or basic, the likelihood of obtaining anomalous scores is commensurately lower. This results in a risk of false-negative results, that is, missing or underestimating the presence of true psychopathology. However, there is an optimal range of *complexity* in which such risks are minimized or virtually eliminated (Meyer et al., 2011). Hence, complexity-adjusted scores are advised when the *complexity SS* exceeds one standard deviation above or below the mean compared to the examinee's same age group. In measurement terms, this means the authors are advising that complexity-adjusted scores be consulted when (a) *SS* is less than 85 (i.e., too low) or (b) *SS* is greater than 115 (i.e., too high). In contrast, use of the non-adjusted scores is recommended when *complexity* is optimal, operationally defined as SSs anywhere within a range of 85–115, inclusive. Now, the design of Table 3 will be examined to illustrate how it manages this issue.

The organization of Table 3 (Form 12.3) resembles those of the diagnostic tables to follow rather than the previous validity Tables 1 and 2. This is done for two reasons. First, *complexity* can be used as a dual-purpose variable in that (a) it correlates with many other diagnostic variables (hence, it is related to their ultimate values), and (b) it is a diagnostic-related personality variable classified within the engagement and cognitive processing domain (see Table 5, Form 12.3). In particular, Table 3 lists the variable name, *SS*, 68% CI, PR, qualitative description, and measured response process. The qualitative description varies from that of the ensuing diagnostic variables in that it contains the aforesaid three interpretively meaningful ranges from lower to higher as follows: (a) *SS* of 50–84 is a low elevation, (b) *SS* of 85–115 is an average or optimal elevation, and (c) *SS* of 115–150 is a high elevation. Note that the different symbols are appended to designate low (viz., †) and high (viz., ★) elevations. Table 3 also has a generous amount of information listed in general and specific tabular notes, including definitions of the employed metrics, response process, SEM and the manner in which it was estimated, the *SS* interpretive scheme, and definitions of statistical symbols. The interpretive scheme assists both the examiner and reader in comprehending the ensuing narrative interpretations. Finally, there are three interpretive excerpts for as many possible outcomes, which are identified by an italicized term that leads off the narrative descriptions. The examiner need only retain the indicated result and delete the rest, including the leading italicized term. This is meant to speed interpretation.

The Issue of Adjusting for Complexity   Before moving on, it is important to briefly examine the decision to adjust for complexity. Doing so is essentially the same as conducting an analysis of covariance, with *complexity* representing the covariate. The resulting adjustments show what the examinees' R–PAS variables would be if their complexity were average or optimal. While that may be informative, *complexity* is also an indication of examinees' personalities. Namely, it is the result of a response process that reflects the amount of differentiation, integration, sophistication, and productivity displayed by individuals in answering the question "What might this be?" If this variable is modified to be average or typical, thus adjusting the other correlated variables, the proper interpretation for each adjusted variable would be as follows: Mr. Smith's *M* is 85, given his level of complexity (Meyer et al., 2011, p. 326). A principal question is, are we not changing aspects of the individual's personality by reporting complexity-adjusted scores? In cases where psychopathology is over- or underestimated, this practice can be justified. Therefore, as is frequently the case in psychology, the answer to whether complexity-adjusted scores should be reported is "It depends on the case facts and objectives."

For this reason, Table 3 was included so examiners have the option to adjust for the *complexity* variable and may exercise their discretion accordingly. So, what is this author's typical practice? In cases where the diagnostic issues are more pertinent to the presence or absence of a clinical disorder, especially psychotic, mood, anxiety, trauma, or stress-related psychopathology, the complexity-adjusted scores are consistently reported and interpreted. For example, complexity-adjusted scores are routinely used in competency-to-stand-trial examinations where psychosis is an issue. However, if the case being considered directly relates to the client's degree of complexity, then both the *complexity* variable and the scores that are impacted by it should be preserved in their unadjusted quantities. An example would be if the examinee's problem-solving approach to people and the world is a principal objective of testing, then it and all associated variables should not be adjusted. Increasingly, however, this author is using the complexity-adjustment option in actual testing practice. One thing is clear, a distinct advantage of the R–PAS program is that the examiner does have such an option, whereas the R–CS and prior systems do not offer this alternative analysis.

Of note, the *complexity* variable is never itself adjusted. Therefore, if it is used as a diagnostic variable in Table 5 when other scores have been so adjusted, then a specific table note should be attached that clearly indicates this fact. Otherwise, readers may misunderstand and believe the *complexity* variable is also somehow being modified. Of course, if *complexity* is not reported at all in Table 3 for considering whether to adjust the remaining scores, then such a table note is unnecessary. It is preferable to use *complexity* either as an adjustment factor or as a diagnostic variable but not both, as it may be confusing to readers. Further, even in its absence, there is a more than sufficient quantity of engagement and cognitive processing variables for effective interpretation.

Summary   This concludes a review of the three validity checks incorporated into R–PAS interpretation. They consist of checks on whether there exists (a) sufficient productivity, (b) any evidence of feigning, and (c) atypical degrees of complexity in the protocol that may require statistical adjustments to maximize the usefulness of interpretation. Although this validity analysis may seem involved, in actual practice the process moves rapidly. This is because there is actually little if any drafting that needs to be added. That is, the data can be quickly inserted and the proper narrative excerpts retained while the rest is deleted. The process should actually take little more than five minutes and thereafter end with the decision of whether include adjustments for *complexity*, which is depicted in Figure 12.3 (e-resources). It is now time for R–PAS diagnostic interpretation.

R–PAS DIAGNOSTIC VARIABLES ANALYSIS: THE FIVE DOMAINS

Figure 12.3 (e-resources) portrays the diagnostic R–PAS variables, which are organized by the domain to which they are assigned. Each box on the bottom row of Figure 12.3 represents a separate domain. They are listed in order from left to right as they appear in the data tables in Form 12.3 (viz., Tables 4–8). The double arrows inserted between the boxes or domains symbolize that the examiner may change the order to suit the diagnostic issues of the particular case. Although the authors discuss an interpretive process that is comprehensive and likely effective for those new to the Rorschach (viz., scan, sift, synthesize, and summarize; Meyer et al., 2011, pp. 323–328), next offered is one that is more efficient and conducive to mental health testing.

General Approach   Form 12.3 (e-resources) lists the diagnostic R–PAS variables according to their assigned domain. Thus, the only redundancy is the *complexity* variable (also in Table 3), which appears again among the engagement and cognitive processing domain (Table 4). The variables are listed in the tables in the order they appear on R–PAS Summary Scores and Profiles—Page 1 (i.e., variables with a greater amount of research support) and R–PAS Summary Scores and Profiles—Page 2 (i.e., variables with a lesser amount of research support). Note that they are not apportioned in separate data tables in Form 12.3 according to the amount of research support. However, they are differentiated more subtly by a different font color, with typical black font for the variables with greater support and purple for variables with lesser research support. The rationale for not organizing them into different tables is that all these variables have the potential of showing key results depending on the case facts.

Therefore, the most pragmatic approach can be delineated in the following three steps. First, a cursory examination of all five domains is done to determine if any can be deleted as being completely irrelevant. This issue should be resolved quickly and efficiently because it was at least partly considered when first making the decision to include the R–PAS as part of the test battery immediately after the completion of the initial assessment. Those domains that are deemed irrelevant can then be deleted in full. Second, the remaining domains should be reordered from most to least pertinent to the case. Third, the variables within each domain can be interpreted as the scores are being entered and the qualitative descriptions determined. During this process, the examiner should be noting which variables are higher than average and which are lower than average. If the variables deemed most supported by research provide the needed interpretations (i.e., those in black font), the examiner can delete the ones less supported (i.e., purple font) to save time. If this is done, the examiner should also delete the secondary variable names from the table notes. Fourth, the third step is done for all remaining domains. Although the R–PAS authors identify some R–PAS variables as not possessing as much research support, one should not be surprised at the frequency with which they assist in resolving the case diagnostic issues. This is why they have been retained in the same tables as the ones with greater support.

Before moving on, the discussion will temporarily revert to the third step reviewed earlier. Once all the data have been entered within a domain, the examiner proceeds to the narrative excerpts following each table. Invariably, the interpretation section begins with a definition of the variables within that particular domain, which also reminds the examiner of what essentially is being measured. There are three narratives that follow the domain definition as follows: (a) an excerpt that lists variables that are either high average, very high, or extremely high; (b) an excerpt that lists variables that are either low average, very low, or extremely low; and (c) a listing of all response processes, signs, and personality traits as measured by each variable in the domain, *in the order they appear in the data table*.

Once the examiner reaches this juncture, the scores that are trending toward the higher end should be referenced, either within a qualitative descriptor if most or all variables fall within that category, or within a range (e.g., from high average to extremely high). Thereafter, the data pattern should be interpreted by listing the distinctive response processes, signs, and traits. Remember that the higher the score, the more distinctive and present that response process, sign, and trait. Next, the same steps should be done for variables that are trending low; that is, either low average, very low, or extremely low. The overall data pattern should first be summarized, again either within a qualitative descriptor or within a range (e.g., from low average to very low). Next, the data pattern should be interpreted by listing the response processes, signs, and personality traits that are distinctive *in the opposing direction*. It is vital to remember that the variables here should be interpreted as being distinctively less present or absent, not necessarily in the opposing direction. Thus, for example, if aggressive content (*AGC*) is very low, it shows an absence of a preoccupation with aggression, not necessarily a passive orientation. Similarly, an extremely low score on the thought and perception composite (*TP-Comp*) means an absence of thought disorganization, impaired reality testing, and psychotic process.

Finally, an interpretive excerpt has been inserted for average or typical elevations. Although the primary analysis is usually focused on extreme elevations, especially those in the high range, and to a lesser extent the lower range, there are circumstances in which average or typical variables will be important to highlight. This is especially the case where specified signs or traits are expected, such as disordered thought and impaired reality testing. For such instances, the normal or within normal limits interpretive language has been integrated following each major set of variables and their tables.

Of note, the interpretive statements for variables with lesser research support are once again presented in purple font to differentiate them from the variables with more scientific backing in black font. The purple color for these variables and their interpretive statements can then be easily changed to black after they are inserted in the proper high or low excerpt.

In summary, then, the examiner is systematically formulating a list of high and low response processes, sign, and traits for each relevant domain, thus creating a personality profile. Those which are especially relevant to the diagnostic issues of a case should be highlighted (e.g., ruling out a psychotic process). Integrating the results from all reported domains can occur at three points as follows: (a) after each domain (see the interpretive insert for integration after each table in Form 12.3), (b) after all R–PAS domains have been interpreted (which must be entered by the examiner after the final table of variables reported in the assessment report), and (c) in the final summary of results section of the entire psychological assessment report. In this manner, only the most relevant and distinctive elements (both present and absent) of an examinee's personality structure are thus interpreted, first in the form of a listing, then integrated with each other and with the diagnostic issues of a case. Next, the interpretive scheme for the SSs will be presented.

The Standard Score (SS) Interpretive Scheme First to be presented is the principal *SS* qualitative description scheme suggested by the test authors in the R–PAS manual. The purpose is to compare it with the one now used by this author. Although this author began using the R–PAS authors' interpretive suggestions, change to the alternative scheme one was done because it (a) is more discriminative, (b) is more commonly used with SSs that have a mean of 100 and a standard deviation of 15 (see, e.g., Chapters 7 and 8), and (c) is also reported as an optional scheme in the R–PAS test manual (Meyer et al., 2011, Appendix G, p. 498). First, Table 12.6 displays the primary interpretation guide recommended in the R–PAS manual. Essentially, the *SS* ranges are apportioned into three categories of low, average, and high, analogous to the one utilized for analysis of the *complexity* variable in Table 3 (Form 12.3). However, the

Table 12.6 Rorschach Performance Assessment System (R–PAS) Primary Interpretation Scheme

Variables	Interpretation of Obtained Standard Score (SS) and Percentile Rank (PR)		
	Low	*Average*	*High*
R–PAS Summary Scores and Profiles—Page 1	SS = 50–90 PR = 0.04–25	SS = 91–109 PR = 26–73	SS = 110–150 PR = 75–99.96
R–PAS Summary Scores and Profiles—Page 2	SS = 50–85 PR = 0.04–16	SS = 86–114 PR = 18–82	SS = 115–150 PR = 84–99.96

Source. Interpretation guidelines for Page 1 and Page 2 variables in Meyer, G. J., Viglione, D. J., Mihura, J. L., Erard, R. E., & Erdberg, P. (2011). *Rorschach Performance Assessment System (R–PAS): Administrative, coding, interpretation, and technical manual.* Toledo, OH: Rorschach Performance Assessment System, L.L.C., pp. 347 and 366, respectively.

Note. *SS* = standard score, *SS* mean = 100, standard deviation = 15, range = 50–150.

Table 12.7 Rorschach Performance Assessment System (R–PAS) Alternative Interpretation Scheme

Standard Score (SS) Range	Percentile Rank (PR) Range	Qualitative Description
130–150	98–99	Extremely high
120–129	91–97	Very high
110–119	75–90	High average
90–109	25–74	Average (typical)
80–89	9–24	Low average
70–79	3–8	Very low
50–69	0–2	Extremely low

Source. Meyer, G. J., Viglione, D. J., Mihura, J. L., Erard, R. E., & Erdberg, P. (2011). *Rorschach Performance Assessment System (R–PAS): Administrative, coding, interpretation, and technical manual.* Toledo, OH: Rorschach Performance Assessment System, L.L.C., Appendix G, p. 498.

Note. Percentile rank ranges are rounded so all values fit within only one standard score range and qualitative description category.

ranges differ according to whether the variables appear on R–PAS Summary Scores and Profiles—Page 1 or R–PAS Summary Scores and Profiles—Page 2, with more extreme scores required of the latter to reach the more extreme low and high ranges. However, this scheme has proved to be insufficiently discriminative and cumbersome because of the different score ranges used for the two sets of variables.

Rather, the test manual offers an ancillary interpretive scheme that is used more frequently with major psychological tests that employ SSs with the aforementioned metrics, one that is more discriminative, hence retaining more diagnostic information, and more familiar to psychologists in general. This alternative scheme is depicted in Table 12.7 and is based on a table of SS and PR score ranges and associated qualitative labels or categories (Meyer et al., 2011, Appendix G, p. 498). The fact that this scheme is more discriminative is shown by the seven categories, including an average (i.e., typical) range, surrounding by three high levels and three low levels. This scheme has worked well in practice in terms of differentiating the degrees of a response process that are present. The term "typical" was added to the average category to clarify that this means "normal" or "adequately adjusted." For example, the *TP-Comp* variable indicates a response process that includes impaired reality testing. An average score here with the added "typical" clarifies that an average score here means normal functioning. In any case, the examiner may modify the scheme in Form 12.3 and insert the primary interpretive scheme espoused by the test authors. The next and final subtopic reviews each domain and tables of variables to clarify what they are measuring and how they may best be used in practice.

The R–PAS Domains and Variables　This final subtopic reviews each major R–PAS domain and their assigned variables, which are listed in separate tables in the order they appear in the computer data output. After the pertinent domains are selected for a case in the initial step of the general approach, and any domains are deleted as being irrelevant, the remaining domains must be ordered in terms of priority. As stated previously, domain order is determined by the case diagnostic issues and facts. In the event the testing case is seeking a general personality assessment, then interpreting all domains in their original order is most viable and should be considered the default mode unless the case facts deem otherwise. This has been done, for example, when providing personality assessments for family courts to help them decide which parent is to be awarded custody. Once the domain order is selected, almost invariably all variables are ultimately reported within a domain.

Within each domain, the authors recommend that *aggregate* variables be interpreted first, followed by single variables, some of which may comprise the former (Meyer et al., 2011, p. 325). *Aggregate R–PAS variables* are those in which several more narrowly defined elements, usually other scored variables, contribute to the total combined score. For example, *SevCog* is the summation of six cognitive codes (viz., *DV2* + *INC2* + *DR2* + *FAB2* + *PEC* + *CON*). In this example, *SevCog* is the aggregate variable, while *CON* is a single variable that contributes to the former. However, the simpler approach is to first peruse the profiles provided by the computer output to formulate an idea of where the most extreme scores lie. Then the variable scores are entered in sequence, making note of statistically high and low scores, including their degree (e.g., high average, very high, or extremely high). To facilitate the simultaneous score reporting and interpretation process, the interpretive scheme is listed in a specific table note. Once the examiner reaches the end of the table, the listed traits and signs that correspond to the variables' response processes can be moved systematically to either the high and low scores excerpt, omitting the average scores as being unremarkable. In such manner, a profile of the examinee's distinctive traits and signs has been systematically created. These results should at some later juncture be integrated with themselves within the table, between R–PAS tables, and/or with other data. This will depend on the needs and facts of the case.

The discussion thus far has provided an overall strategy regarding (a) selecting the proper domains to report, (b) determining their order, and finally, (c) the manner in which the variable scores are to be entered and subsequently interpreted. Next, each domain is reviewed in terms of the general personality constructs they tap into and some of the diagnostic issues for which they may be especially useful. This is meant only as an overview to afford the reader an idea of the content that defines each of the five R–PAS domains and their variables.

First, the *administration behaviors and observations variables* are listed in Table 4 (Form 12.3; see also Figure 16.3, e-resources) and represent task-relevant behaviors that provide interpretive context for the remaining R–PAS variables (viz., Tables 5–8). These data measure the degree to which the examinee has been sufficiently productive in response to the situational demands of the Rorschach task. They include the number of times the examiner has had to prompt the examinee for more than one response, pull the card after four responses, and the frequency with which card-turning behavior has been manifested for each card. Frequent card turning has variable interpretations, including curiosity, flexibility, anxiety, defiance, and compulsivity, which must be judged by behavioral observations. These variables provide further data regarding the examinee's motivation and cooperation during the testing.

Second, the *engagement and cognitive processing variables* listed in Table 5 (Form 12.3; see also Figure 12.3, e-resources) are related to an individual's complexity, productivity, sophistication, and psychological resources, along with motivation and degree of active involvement in the Rorschach test. This domain addresses the cognitive and problem-solving aspects of test behavior, including information about coping styles and ways of adapting to the world. High scores on many of these variables (e.g., *complexity*) are associated with personality traits such as intelligence, creativity, curiosity, attention to detail, openness to experience, and coping resources, the latter including *intellectualization*, which is the use of thinking and reasoning to repress or avoid threatening feelings. Low scores can be indicative of characterological constriction or rigidity, depressive withdrawal, anxiety that causes emotional constriction, traumatic numbing, and discomfort and insecurity with ambiguity. Some of these variables are useful to examine in cases of suspected *attention-deficit/hyperactivity disorder (ADHD)*, and *obsessive-compulsive disorder (OCD)* because they tap into information-processing styles. However, many variables can be identified that provide insight as to an examinee's ability to modulate feelings, the potential for dissociation, and the use of fantasy to avoid dealing with reality.

Third, the *perception and thinking problems variables* are listed in Table 6 (Form 12.3; see also Figure 12.3, e-resources) and are related to an individual's problems in thinking, judgment, and perception, along with those involved with conventionality and seeing the world as do others in the Rorschach test. This domain incorporates variables that reflect the perceptual distortions and thought disturbance that are signs of psychosis, including indicators of disturbances in the organization and content of thought. These variables are indispensable when testing examinees for a psychotic disorder, who manifests *alexithymia* and does not appreciate the seriousness of their symptoms. Hence, administering a personality inventory would be ineffective and likely produce a false-negative result. These variables are capable of detecting psychosis in action, hence signs versus symptoms. They are also useful for detecting all degrees of psychotic disturbance, including schizophrenia, mood disorders with psychotic features (i.e., in combination with stress and distress variables in Table 7, Form 12.3), schizotypal personality, borderline personality with transient psychotic features, and schizoid personality with negative features of schizophrenia, which represents only a partial listing. Furthermore, many of these variables are aggregate in nature and thus possess more reliability than most other R–PAS variables.

Fourth, the *stress and distress variables* are listed in Table 7 (Form 12.3; see also Figure 12.3, e-resources). They are related to past and current environmental events, which are experienced as threats and out of one's control, along with various feelings of dysphoria. This domain has implications for affective discomfort and emotional disarray that may be experienced implicitly by an individual (i.e., outside of conscious awareness). They are especially useful in detecting anxiety disorders, depressive disorders, implicit risk of suicide or self-harm, experienced dysphoria, and trauma-related disorders. The last item includes all adjustment disorders, PTSD, and attachment disorders (i.e., in conjunction with the self and other representation variables in Table 8, Form 12.3). These variables are defined as if they are explicit or conscious to the individual. Hence, a caveat is that these variables are being measured implicitly. *Implicit measures* of variables indicate that they are likely to be nonconscious or out of the person's awareness. For example, if Gigi informs Frank that he smiles when anxious, a propensity for which Frank was previously unaware, then such behavior was up to that point implicit to him. Hence, these variables, along with all other R–PAS variables, should understood as implicit to the individual. It is here where the variables appear to be explicit in their descriptive summaries that this issue is best clarified.

Lastly, the *self and other representation variables* are enumerated in Table 8 (Form 12.3; see also Figure 12.3, e-resources) and relate to individuals' ways of understanding themselves, other people, and their social relationships as a foundation of their interpersonal relatedness. This domain addresses object relations and interpersonal and self-schema, with implications for self-image, self-experience, and interpersonal competency and relationships. Because interpersonal relatedness is a core element of human adaptation, these variables directly impact overall psychological and personality functioning. These variables are also pertinent to detecting maladaptive and adaptive personality traits and signs, relationship patterns, internalized object-relations, and attachment styles. As such, it should make sense that this is one of the largest domains in the R–PAS arsenal. Lastly, the *Sx* (viz., *sexual content*) responses have been inserted here despite the fact that this variable does not appear in any of the domains. In particular, high frequency counts on this variable show an implicit preoccupation with sexual matters. Therefore, reporting *Sx* responses has been useful in psychosexual examinations, with the objective of estimating the risk of recidivism for convicted sexual offenders, along with psychological assessments for victims of sexual molestation. It was inserted within this domain because it seemed most closely associated with interpersonal relationships.

Summary   This concludes the presentation of the R–PAS. As a performance personality test that covers an age range from 6 to 86 years, it represents an invaluable instrument as part of a psychological test inventory. It is capable of directly measuring both situational and characterological personality traits and signs that can facilitate psychodiagnosis and effectively identify targets for psychotherapeutic and biomedical intervention. However, it requires a significant amount of training and is more labor intensive that the personality inventories. Thus, it is vital to increase the utility of this measure as much as possible so that it can be used in mental health practice. The presented data tables for the R–PAS (Form 12.3), along with the recommended interpretive process (Figure 13.3, e-resources), and standard score interpretive scheme (Table 12.7), will assist in this endeavor.

Recapitulation

This chapter focused on personality testing using performance measures (i.e., the measurement of personality in action). The chapter began by defining what constitutes performance personality tests and comparing and contrasting them to personality inventories, including their different formats, implicit versus explicit measures, and the different types of data they yield. Reasons for including performance personality tests within a test battery, along with likely insurance coverage issues, was then briefly discussed. The core of the chapter, however, consisted of the presentation of three performance personality tests. The CAT–9–RC was presented first because it covers the youngest age group. Because it was the only one of the three that was projective by design, a review of its development was provided, which also included assumptions of projective testing and the projective hypothesis. The data tables for this test included a scoring system based on psychodynamic principles and personality development in young children. The Roberts–2 was next presented as a performance personality test that measures a range of social-cognitive abilities, in addition to scales intended to detect the presence of psychological and personality problems. Data tables designed to report and interpret Roberts–2 data within a psychological assessment report were then provided. Finally, the R–PAS was presented, including a history of how this test and various scoring systems evolved over a 100-year span. Data tables designed to report R–PAS results with a psychological assessment report was then provided, including a more discriminating interpretive scheme than that espoused by the test authors. The subsequent and final chapter of Part II presents two psychological measures specifically designed to detect the feigning of psychopathology, one for psychiatric symptoms and disorders and the other for neuropsychological disorders. These tests are deemed vital to have as part of a psychological test inventory because of the high stakes testing that is increasingly done in outpatient mental health practice.

Key Terms

- accurate
- acquiescence (yea saying)
- adaptation
- Adaptive Regression in the Service of the Ego (*ARISE*)
- administration behaviors and observations variables
- aggregate R–PAS variables
- alexithymia
- antisocial personality disorder (APD)
- apperception
- apperceptive distortion
- attention-deficit/hyperactivity disorder (ADHD)

- autism spectrum disorder (ASD)
- autonomous ego functions
- autonomous functions
- average tendencies
- bizarre mentation
- borderline
- card rejections
- cathexis
- Children's Apperception Test (CAT)
- Children's Apperception Test, Ninth Edition, Revised, Color Version (CAT–9–RC)
- chronological age (CA)
- clarification phase (CP)
- coding horizontally
- coding vertically
- complexity adjusted
- complexity adjustment
- conduct disorder (CD)
- conflict-free ego sphere
- continuous norming
- defensive functioning
- denial
- depth theory
- deviant responses (DR)
- deviant verbalizations (DV)
- *Diagnostic and Statistical Manual of Mental Disorders, Fifth Edition (DSM–5)*
- differential diagnosis
- displacement
- ecological validity
- ego function assessment (EFA)
- ego strength
- EII-3 and composite calculations
- engagement and cognitive processing variables
- explicit measures
- extra-aggression
- extrapunitive
- face validity
- fit
- frequency
- harsh superego introject
- high-stakes testing
- histrionic personality disorder (HPD)
- ICD–10 Classification of Mental and Behavioural Disorders (ICD–10)
- ideal self
- identity achievement
- identity diffusion
- imagination
- implicit measures
- implicit needs
- impression management
- inferential norming
- intellectualization
- intra-aggression
- intropunitive
- isolation
- judgment
- law of causality

- low base-rate variable
- mastery–competence
- mechanical perseverations
- mechanisms
- mental functioning (M) axis
- minus form quality (*FQ–*)
- needs
- neurotic
- normal
- object relations
- obsessive-compulsive disorder (OCD)
- obsessive-compulsive disorder with poor insight
- O-data
- Oedipal complex
- ordinary form quality (*FQo*)
- paranoid personality disorder (PPD)
- pareto distributions
- perception and thinking problems variables
- perceptual sets
- personality
- personality mechanisms
- personality syndromes (P) axis
- power-law distributions
- presses
- primal scene
- projection
- "prompt for two, pull after four"
- proprioception
- *Psychodynamic Diagnostic Manual, Second Edition (PDM–2)*
- psychological determinism
- psychotic
- rank size distributions
- reaction formation
- real self
- reality testing
- regression
- regulation and control of drives, affects, and impulses
- reliability coefficient/s
- repression
- response phase (RP)
- response process
- Roberts–2
- R-optimized procedure
- Rorschach Performance Assessment System® (R–PAS®)
- Rorschach, Comprehensive System (R–CS)
- R–PAS Code Sequence
- R–PAS Profile Appendix—Summary Scores for All Variables
- R–PAS Protocol Level Counts & Calculations
- R–PAS Summary Scores and Profiles—Page 1
- R–PAS Summary Scores and Profiles—Page 2
- S-data
- self and other representation variables
- self-concept
- self-efficacy
- self-esteem
- sense of reality

- sexual content (*Sx*)
- signs
- social desirability
- social (pragmatic) communication disorder
- social-cognitive abilities
- stimulus barrier
- stress and distress variables
- superego
- syllogistic thinking
- symbiotic attachment/s
- symptom neurosis
- symptoms
- synthetic-integrative functions
- T-data
- temperament
- thema
- Thematic Apperception Test (TAT)
- thought processes
- trait theory
- traits
- undoing
- unusual form quality (*FQu*)
- zeta distributions
- Zipf distributions

Notes

1. In the summer of 1980, while matriculating within a terminal Master's degree program in clinical psychology at Illinois State University, this author was first trained to use the Rorschach according to what his professor Samuel Hutter, M.S., referred to as a *modified Beck System* (Beck, Beck, Levitt, & Molish, 1961; Beizmann, 1966/1970). It was one of the most empirically based systems available at the time and was effective in measuring reality testing, a key ego (i.e., personality) function.
2. This is perhaps best illustrated by the fact that his test manual is so atypically succinct (Murray, 1943).
3. Of a historical note, the CAT has proceeded through several iterations from its inception in 1949. Specifically, a supplemental *CPT-S* version was first created (Bellak & Bellak, 1952), which consisted of pictures of children in typical family circumstances (e.g., chronic illness, death, birth, and separation from parents). This was ensued by a version that included human figures in the exact same social scenes as in the original set (*CAT-H*; Bellak & Hurvich, 1966), produced in response to evidence that some children created more productive stories to such figures (e.g., see Lawton, 1966).
4. Here, a rapprochement between depth and trait theory is realized, namely, a depth theory approach that also measures personality mechanisms and consequential traits quantitatively.
5. Bellak et al. (1973) actually did incorporate several id scales (viz., libidinal drive, aggressive drive, and sublimation), along with supplemental superego scales pertinent to Freud's original drive theory and structural model (e.g., interference with ego functions). Therefore, they did not completely abandon the traditional structural model and, in fact, devoted a chapter each to defining both the id and superego constructs. The superego construct was retained and incorporated because it is useful in measuring a young child's developing internalized moral standards and behavioral controls (i.e., executive functions and emotion regulation abilities), especially the latter considering that externalizing behavior problems are frequent presenting symptoms among this young clinical population.
6. Some researchers have attempted to create quantifiable subscales by measuring more specific components of each ego function, then aggregating them for an average score for each of the 12 ego functions. In doing so, they have increased the hierarchy to three levels, proceeding from specific to general as follows: (a) ego function component scores, (b) ego function scores, and (c) ego strength overall score. The objective here was to enhance scoring reliability and validity, which has not yet been realized (e.g., Bellak & Goldsmith, 1984).
7. The relationship among the various ego functions and specific mental abilities (M axis) that affect overall personality functioning would also represent an interesting research project, especially in measuring personality development in young children.
8. The previously designed and published R-CS scoring and interpretation tables are not included here because (a) they are available in the first edition (see Spores, 2012), (b) there have since been no substantive changes to the R-CS, and (c) this reserves space in this edition for more contemporary testing materials.
9. For an explication of the specific codes within each general category, their definitions, and their abbreviations, the reader is referred to the R–PAS administrative, coding, interpretation, and technical manual, especially Chapters 3 and 4, which cover basic and advanced coding (Meyer et al., 2012 pp. 31–177).
10. See Meyer et al., 2011, pp. 481–484 for a more detailed explanation and examples.
11. The author admits to being nonplussed as to why R–PAS has not adopted this variable as an indicator of feigning because it can be measured by the administration procedures and seems to be logically sound. In any case, this measure is useful for such purposes, including in competency-to-stand-trial examinations.

References

Abt, L. E., & Bellak, L. (Eds.). (1950). *Projective psychology.* New York, NY: Alfred A. Knopf.

Ackerman, S. J., Clemence, A. J., Weatherill, R., & Hilsenroth, M. J. (1999). Use of the TAT in the assessment of DSM–IV cluster B personality disorders. *Journal of Personality Assessment, 73,* 422–448.

Adler, A. (1969). *The practice and theory of individual psychology.* Totowa, NJ: Littlefield, Adams, and Company.

Adler, G. (1985). *Borderline psychopathology and its treatment.* New York, NY: Aronson.

American Psychiatric Association. (2013). *Diagnostic and statistical manual of mental disorders* (5th ed., DSM—5). Arlington, VA: Author.

American Psychological Association. (2015). *American psychological association (APA) dictionary of psychology* (2nd ed.). Washington, DC: Author.

Atkinson, J. W. (1957). Motivational determinants of risk-taking behavior. *Psychological Review, 64,* 359–372.

Bandura, A. (1982). Self-efficacy mechanisms in human agency. *American Psychologist, 37,* 122–147.

Bateson, G., Jackson, D. D., Haley, J., & Weakland, J. (1956). Toward a theory of schizophrenia. *Behavioral Science, 1,* 251–264.

Beck, S. J. (1944). *Rorschach's test I: Basic processes.* New York, NY: Grune & Stratton.

Beck, S. J. (1945). *Rorschach's test II: A variety of personality pictures.* New York, NY: Grune & Stratton.

Beck, S. J. (1952). *Rorschach's test III: Advances in interpretation.* New York, NY: Grune & Stratton.

Beck, S. J., Beck, A. G., Levitt, E. E., & Molish, H. B. (1961). *Rorschach's test: Basic processes* (3rd ed.). New York, NY: Grune & Stratton.

Beizmann, C. (1966/1970). *Handbook for scoring Rorschach responses* (Samuel J. Beck Translation). Appliquee, Paris: Centre de Psychologie.

Bellak, L. (1975). *The thematic apperception test (TAT), the children's apperception test (CAT), and the senior apperception technique (SAT) in clinical use* (3rd ed.). New York, NY: Grune & Stratton.

Bellak, L. (1944). The concept of projection: An experimental investigation and study of the concept. *Psychiatry, 7,* 353–370.

Bellak, L. (1949). A multiple-factor psychosomatic theory of schizophrenia. *Psychiatric Quarterly, 23,* 738–755.

Bellak, L. (1954). *TAT and CAT in clinical use.* New York, NY: Grune & Stratton.

Bellak, L. (1955/1992). *Short form: For recording and analyzing thematic apperception test, children's apperception test, & senior apperception technique.* Englewood, NJ: C.P.S.

Bellak, L. (1958). *Schizophrenia: A review of the syndrome.* New York, NY: Grune & Stratton.

Bellak, L. (1989). *Ego function assessment (EFA) manual.* Larchmont, NY: C.P.S.

Bellak, L., & Abrams, D. M. (1998). *A manual for the children's apperception test (animal figures)* (9th ed. Rev.). New York, NY: C.P.S. Publishing Corporation.

Bellak, L., & Abrams, D. M. (2012). *A manual for the children's apperception test (animal figures)* (9th ed. Rev., color ed. Rev.). New York, NY: C.P.S. Publishing Corporation.

Bellak, L., & Bellak, S. S. (1949). *A manual for the children's apperception test.* Larchmont, NY: C.P.S. Publishing Corporation.

Bellak, L., & Bellak, S. S. (1952). *The supplement to the children's apperception test (CAT—S).* Oxford, England: C.P.S. Publishing Corporation.

Bellak, L., & Goldsmith, L. A. (Eds.). (1984). *The broad assessment of ego function assessment.* New York, NY; John Wiley.

Bellak, L., & Hurvich, M. S. (1966). A human modification of the children's apperception test (CAT—H). *Journal of Projective Techniques & Personality Assessment, 30,* 228–242.

Bellak, L., & Hurvich, M. S. (1969). A systematic study of ego functions. *Journal of Nervous and Mental Disease, 148,* 569–585.

Bellak, L., Hurvich, M. S., & Gediman, H. K. (1973). *Ego functions in schizophrenics, neurotics, and normals: A systematic study of conceptual, diagnostic, and therapeutic aspects.* New York, NY: John Wiley & Sons.

Bellak, L., Hurvich, M. S., Silvan, M., & Jacobs, D. (1968). Towards an ego psychological appraisal of drug effects. *American Journal of Psychiatry, 125,* 45–56.

Beres, D. (1956). Ego deviation and the concept of schizophrenia. *The Psychoanalytic Study of the Child, 11,* 164–235.

Binet, A., & Henri, V. (1896). La psychologie individuelle [Individual psychology]. *L'Année Psychologique, 2,* 411–465.

Blatt, S. L., Engel, M., & Mirmow, E. (1961). When inquiry fails. *Journal of Projective Techniques, 25,* 32–37.

Bleuler, E. (1908). Die prognose der dementia praecox (schizophreniegruppe). *Allgemeine Zeitschrift Fur Psychiatrie, 65,* 436–464.

Block, J. (1977). Advancing the psychology of personality: Paradigmatic shift or improving the quality of research. In D. Magnusson & N. S. Endler (Eds.), *Personality at the crossroads* (pp. 37–63). Hillsdale, NJ: Erlbaum.

Brittain, H. L. (1907). A study in imagination. *Pedagogical Seminary, 14,* 137–207.

Buros, O. K. (Ed.). (1965). *The sixth mental measurements yearbook.* Lincoln, NE: Buros Center for Testing.

Cantor, N., & Kihlstrom, J. F. (1987). *Personality and social intelligence.* Englewood Cliffs, NJ: Prentice-Hall.

Chen, S., Su, X., & Wu, S. (2012). Need for achievement, education, and entrepreneurial risk-taking behavior. *Social Behavior and Personality: An international journal, 40,* 1311–1318.

Clark, L. P. (1926). The fantasy method of analyzing narcissistic neuroses. *Medical Journal Review, 123,* 154–158.

Clark, R. M. (1944). A method of administering and evaluating the thematic apperception test. *Genetic Psychological Monographs, 30,* 3–55.

Cohen, R. J., & Swerdlik, M. E. (2018). *Psychological testing and assessment* (9th ed.). New York, NY: McGraw-Hill Education.

Cramer, P. (1987). The development of defense mechanisms. *Journal of Personality, 55,* 597–614.

Cramer, P. (1999). Future directions for the thematic apperception test. *Journal of Personality Assessment, 72,* 74–92.

Elfenbein, H. H., Curhan, J. R., Eisenkraft, N., Shirako, A., & Baccaro, L. (2008). Are some negotiators better than others? Individual differences in bargaining outcomes. *Journal of Research in Personality, 42,* 1463–1475.

Encyclopedia of Children's Health. (2021). *Children's apperception test.* Retrieved from www.healthofchildren.com/C/Children-s-Apperception-Test.html

Erikson, E. H. (1950/1963). *Childhood and society* (2nd ed.). New York: Norton.

Exner, J. E. & Weiner, I. B. (1995). *The Rorschach a comprehensive system: Assessment of children and adolescents* (2nd ed., Vol. 3). New York: John Wiley & Sons.

Meyer, G. J., Viglione, D. J., & Giromini, L. (2014). An introduction to Rorschach-based performance assessment. In R. P. Archer & S. R. Smith (Eds.), *Personality assessment* (pp. 301–369). New York, NY: Routledge/Taylor & Francis Group.

Exner, J. E. (1969). *The Rorschach systems.* New York, NY: Grune & Stratton.

Exner, J. E. (1997). *Rorschach research study group mission statement.* Unpublished Manuscript.

Exner, J. E. (2001). *A Rorschach workbook for the comprehensive system* (5th ed.). Asheville, NC: Rorschach Workshops.

Exner, J. E. (2002). *A primer for Rorschach interpretation.* Asheville, NC: Rorschach Workshops.

Exner, J. E. (2003). *The Rorschach a comprehensive system: Basic foundations and principles of interpretation* (4th ed., Vol. 1). Hoboken, NJ: John Wiley & Sons.

Fox, N. A., & Calkins, S. D. (2003). The development of self-control of emotion: Intrinsic and extrinsic influences. *Motivation and Emotion, 27,* 7–26.

Fox, N. A., Henderson, H. A., Marshall, P. J., Nichols, K. E., & Ghera, M. M. (2005). Behavioral inhibition: Linking biology and behavior within a developmental framework. *Annual Review of Psychology, 56,* 235–262.

Frank, L. K. (1939). Projective methods for the study of personality. *Journal of Psychology, 8,* 389–413.

Freud, A. (1946). *The ego and the mechanisms of defence.* International Universities Press.

Freud, S. (1900/1913). *The interpretation of dreams.* New York: Macmillan.

Freud, S. (1915/1957). The unconscious. In J. Strachey (Ed. and Trans.), *The standard edition of the complete psychological works of Sigmund Freud* (Vol. 14, pp. 166–204). London: Hogarth Press.

Freud, S. (1919). *Totem and taboo.* New York: Moffatt, Yard.

Freud, S. (1923). *The Ego and the Id.* In J. Strachey et al. (Trans.), *The standard edition of the complete psychological works of Sigmund Freud* (Vol. 19). London: Hogarth Press.

Friedman, H. S., & Schustack, M. W. (2012). *Personality: Classic theories and modern research.* Boston, MA: Pearson.

Frosch. J. (1964). The psychotic character: Clinical psychiatric considerations. *Psychiatric Quarterly, 38,* 91–96.

Fusar-Poli, P., & Politi, P. (2008). Paul Eugene Bleuler and the birth of schizophrenia (1908). *American Journal of Psychiatry, 165,* 1407.

Goleman, D. (1995). *Emotional intelligence: Why it can matter more than IQ.* New York: NY: Bantam.

Graceffo, R. A., Mihura, J. L., & Meyer, G. J. (2014). A meta-analysis of an implicit measure of personality functioning: The mutuality of autonomy scale. *Journal of Personality Assessment, 96,* 581–585.

Greenwald, A. G., McGhee, D. E., & Schwartz, J. L. K. (1998). Measuring individual differences in implicit cognition: The implicit association test. *Journal of Personality and Social Psychology, 74(6),* 1464–1480.

Grinker, R. R., Werble, B., & Drye, R. C. (1968). *The borderline syndrome: A behavioral study of ego functions.* New York, NY: Basic Books.

Gulliksen, H. (1950). *Wiley publications in psychology. Theory of mental tests.* Hoboken, NJ: John Wiley & Sons.

Gunderson, J. G., & Singer, M. T. (1975). Defining borderline patients: An overview. *American Journal of Psychiatry, 133,* 1–10.

Hartocollis, P. (1977). *Borderline personality disorders: The concept, the syndrome, the patient.* New York, NY: International Universities Press.

Hertz, M. R. (1939). On the standardization of the Rorschach method. *Rorschach Research Exchange, 3,* 120–133.

Hertz, M. R. (1952). The Rorschach: Thirty years after. In D. Brower & L. E. Abt (Eds.), *Progress in clinical psychology.* New York, NY: Grune & Stratton.

Hertz, M. R. (1970). *Frequency tables for scoring Rorschach responses with code charts, normal and rare details, F+ and F—responses, and popular and original responses* (5th ed.). Cleveland, OH: The Press of Case Western Reserve University.

Hill, J. (1975). Individuation and the association experiment. *Annual of Archetypal Psychology,* 145–151.

Hilsenroth, M. J., & Handler, L. (1995). A survey of graduate students' experiences, interests, and attitudes about learning the Rorschach. *Journal of Personality Assessment, 64,* 243–257.

Hogan, T. P. (2019). *Psychological testing: A practical introduction* (4th ed.). Hoboken, NJ: John Wiley & Sons.

Holaday, M., Smith, D. A., & Sherry, A. R. (2000). Sentence completion tests: A review of the literature and results of a survey of members of the Society for Personality Assessment. *Journal of Personality Assessment, 74,* 371–383. Retrieved from www.social-researchmethods.net/kb/scalgen.php

Hurvich, M., & Bellak, L. (1968). Ego function patterns in schizophrenics. *Psychological Reports, 22,* 299–308.

Jahnke, J., & Morgan, W. G. (1997). A true TAT story. In W. G. Bringmann, H. E. Lück, R. Miller & C. E. Early (Eds.), *A pictorial history of psychology* (pp. 376–379). Carol Stream, IL: Quintessence Publishing.

Jenkins, S. R. (Ed.). (2008). *A handbook of clinical scoring systems for thematic apperceptive techniques.* New York, NY: Lawrence Erlbaum Associates.

Kagan, J., & Moss, H. A. (1959). Stability and validity of achievement fantasy. *The Journal of Abnormal and Social Psychology, 58,* 357–364.

Kempler, H. L., & Scott, V. (1972). Assessment of therapeutic change in antisocial boys via the TAT. *Psychological Reports, 30,* 905–906.

Kerlinger, F. N. (1973). *Foundations of behavioral research* (2nd ed.). New York: Holt.

Kernberg, O. F. (1975). *Borderline conditions and pathological narcissism.* New York: Jason Aronson.

Kernberg, O. F. (1983). Object relations theory and character analysis. *Journal of the American Psychoanalytic Association, 31,* 247–271.

Kernberg, O. F. (1984). *Severe personality disorders.* New Haven, CT: Yale University Press.

Kerner, J. (1857). *Klexographien: Part VI.* In R. Pissen (Ed.), *Kerners Werke.* Berlin: Boag.

Kleinmuntz, B. (1967). *Personality measurement: An introduction.* Homewood, IL: The Dorsey Press.

Kline, P. (2000). *Handbook of psychological testing* (2nd ed.). New York, NY: Routledge.

Klopfer, B., Ainsworth, M. D., Klopfer, W. G., & Holt, R. R. (1954). *Developments in the Rorschach technique* (Vol. 1). New York, NY: Harcourt, Brace & World.

Klopfer, B., & Kelly, D. (1942). *The Rorschach technique.* Yonkers-on-Hudson, NY: World Book.

Klopfer, B., Ainsworth, M. D., Klopfer, W. G., & Holt, R. R. (1954). *Developments in the Rorschach technique I: Technique and theory.* Yonkers-on-Hudson, NY: World Book.

Klopfer, B., Meyer, M. M., Brawer, F. B., & Klopfer, W. G. (1970). *Developments in the Rorschach technique III: Aspects of personality structure.* New York, NY: Harcourt Brace Jovanovich.

Knight, R. (1953). Borderline states in psychoanalytic psychiatry and psychology. *Bulletin of the Menninger Clinic, 17,* 1–12.

Koestner, R., & McClelland, D. C. (1990). Perspectives on competence motivation. In L. A. Pervin (Ed.), *Handbook of personality: Theory and research* (pp. 527–548). The Guilford Press.

Kwon, P. S., Campbell, K. G., & Williams, M. (2001). Sociotropy and autonomy: Preliminary evidence for construct validity using TAT narratives. *Journal of Personality Assessment, 77,* 128–138.

Larsen, R. J., & Buss, D. M. (2021). *Personality psychology: Domains of knowledge about human nature* (7th ed.). New York, NY: McGraw-Hill Education.

Lawton, M. (1966). Animal and human CAT's with a school sample. *Journal of Projective Techniques, 30,* 243–246.

Libby, W. (1908). The imagination of adolescents. *American Journal of Psychology, 19,* 249–252.

Lillenfeld, S. O., Wood, J. M., & Garb, H. N. (2000). The scientific status of projective techniques. *Psychological Science in the Public Interest, 1,* 27–66.

Lindzey, G. (1959). On the classification of projective techniques. *Psychological Bulletin, 56,* 158–168.

Lingiardi, V., & Bornstein, R. F. (2017). Profile of mental functioning M Axis. In V. Lingiardi & N. McWilliams (Eds.), *Psychodynamic diagnostic manual* (2nd ed., pp. 76–79). New York, NY: The Guilford Press.

Lingiardi, V., & McWilliams, N. (Eds.). (2017). *Psychodynamic diagnostic manual, second edition* (PDM—2). New York, NY: The Guilford Press.

Loewenstein, R. (1954). Some remarks on defenses, autonomous ego and psychoanalytic technique. *International Journal of Psycho-Analysis, 35,* 188–193.

Loewenstein, R. (1967). On the theory of the superego: A discussion. In R. Lowenstein, L. Newman, M. Schur, & A. Solnit (Eds.), *Psychoanalysis—A general psychology.* New York, NY: International Universities.

Loewenstein, R. (1972). Defensive organization and autonomous ego functions. *Journal of the American Psychoanalytic Association, 15,* 795–809.

Lyles, W. (1958). *The effects of examiner attitudes on the projective test responses of children* (Unpublished doctoral dissertation). New York University, New York.

Main, T. F. (1957). The ailment. *British Journal of Medical Psychology, 30,* 129–145.

Marcia, J. E. (1966). Development and validation of ego-identity status. *Journal of Personality and Social Psychology, 35,* 118–133.

Masterson, J. F. (1972). *Treatment of the Borderline Adolescent: A developmental approach.* New York, NY: Wiley-Interscience.

Masterson, J. F. (1976). *Psychotherapy of the borderline adult: A developmental approach.* New York, NY: John Wiley & Sons.

McAdams, D. P. (1990). Motives. In V. Derlega, B. Winstead, and W. Jones (Eds.), *Contemporary research in personality* (pp. 175–204). Chicago: Nelson-Hall.

McAdams, D. P. (2008). Personal narratives and the life story. In O. John, R. Robins, & L. A. Pervin (Eds.), *Handbook of personality: Theory and research* (pp. 241–261). New York: Guilford Press.

McArthur, D. S., & Roberts, G. E. (1982). *Roberts apperception test for children (RATC) manual.* Los Angeles, CA: Western Psychological Services (WPS).

McClelland, D. C., Atkinson, J. W., Clark, R. A., & Lowell, E. L. (1953). *The achievement motive.* New York, NY: Appleton-Century-Crofts.

McClelland, D. C., Clark, R. A., Roby, T. B., & Atkinson, J. W. (1949). The projective expression of needs. IV. The effect of the need for achievement on thematic apperception. *Journal of Experimental Psychology, 39,* 242–255.

McWilliams, N., & Shedler, J. (2017). Personality syndromes—P Axis. In V. Lingiardi & N. McWilliams (Eds.), *Psychodynamic diagnostic manual* (2nd ed., pp. 15–67). Silver Spring, MD: Guilford Press.

Megargee, E. I. (1969). Influence of sex roles on the manifestation of leadership. *Journal of Applied Psychology, 53,* 377–382.

Megargee, E. I., & Cook, P. E. (1967). The relation of TAT and inkblot aggressive content scales with each other and with criteria of overt aggression in juvenile delinquents. *Journal of Projective Techniques and Personality Assessment, 31,* 48–60.

Meyer, G. J., & Erdberg, P. (2018). Using R–PAS norms with an emphasis on children and adolescents. In J. L. Mihura & G. J. Meyer (Eds.), *Using the Rorschach performance assessment system® (R–PAS®)* (pp. 46–61). New York, NY: The Guilford Press.

Meyer, G. J., Giromini, L., Viglione, D. J., Reese, J. B., & Mihura, J. L. (2015). The association of gender, ethnicity, age, and education with Rorschach scores. *Assessment, 22,* 46–64.

Meyer, G. J., Viglione, D. J., & Giromini, L. (2014, January 29). *Current R–PAS transitional child and adolescent norms.* Retrieved from R—PAS Website http://R–PAS.org/CurrentChildNorms.aspx

Meyer, G. J., Viglione, D. J., Mihura, J. L., Erard, R. E., & Erdberg, P. (2011). *Rorschach performance assessment system (R—PAS): Administrative, coding, interpretation, and technical manual.* Toledo, OH: Rorschach Performance Assessment System, L.L.C.

Meyer, G. J., Viglione, D. J., Mihura, J. L., Erard, R. E., & Erdberg, P. (2012). *Rorschach performance assessment system (R—PAS): Portable form quality tables and coding guide.* Toledo, OH: Rorschach Performance Assessment System, L.L.C.

Mihura, J. L., & Meyer, G. J. (2018). Introduction to R-PAS. In J. L. Mihura & G. J. Meyer (Eds.), *Using the Rorschach Performance Assessment System® (R-PAS®)* (pp. 3–22). The Guilford Press.

Mihura, J. L. & Weinle, C. A. (2002). Rorschach training: Doctoral students' experiences and preferences. *Journal of Personality Assessment, 79*, 39–52.

Miltenberger, R. G. (2012). *Behavior modification: Principles and procedures* (5th ed.). Belmont, CA: Wadsworth Cengage Learning.

Morgan, C. D., & Murray, H. A. (1935). A method for investigating phantasies: The Thematic Apperception Test. *Archives of Neurology and Psychiatry, 34*, 289–306.

Morgan, W. G. (1991, March). *The art of testing: The history and development of the TAT images*. A paper presented at the 37th Annual Meeting of the Southeastern Psychological Association, New Orleans, LA.

Morgan, W. G. (1995a). Origin and history of the thematic apperception test images. *Journal of Personality Assessment, 65*, 237–254.

Morgan, W. G. (1995b, March). *The thematic apperception test (TAT) paintings*. A paper presented at the 1995 Midwinter Program of the Society for Personality Assessment, Atlanta, GA.

Morgan, W. G. (1995c, March). *Thematic apperception test (TAT) images with photographic origins*. A paper presented at the 41st Annual Meeting of the Southeastern Psychological Association, Savannah, GA.

Morgan, W. G. (1996, August). *The art of the TAT: The history of TAT images originating as prints*. A paper presented at the 104th Annual Convention of the American Psychological Association, Toronto, Ont., Canada.

Morgan, W. G. (1998a, February). *Early versions of the TAT: History and correspondence of images*. A paper presented at the Midwinter Meeting of the Society for Personality Assessment, Boston, MA.

Morgan, W. G. (1998b). TAT zuban no kigento rekishi. [Origin and history of the thematic apperception test images.] (F. Saito & H. Urata, Trans.). *The Faculty of Humanics Review, 6*, 29–51.

Morgan, W. G. (1999a). Test developer profile: Christiana D. Morgan. In R. J. Cohen & M. E. Swerdlik, *Psychological testing and assessment: An introduction to tests and measurement* (4th ed.). Mountain View, CA: Mayfield Publishing.

Morgan, W. G. (1999b, March). *Picture C: Its origin and development*. A paper presented at the 1999 Midwinter Meeting of the Society for Personality Assessment, New Orleans, LA.

Morgan, W. G. (1999c). The 1943 TAT images: Their origin and history. In M. T. Gieser & M. I. Stein (Eds.), *Evocative images: The thematic apperception test and the art of projection* (pp. 65–83). Washington, DC: American Psychological Association.

Murray, H. A. (1943). *Thematic apperception test (TAT): Manual*. Cambridge, MA: Harvard University Press.

Murray, H. A. (1938). *Explorations in personality*. New York: Oxford University Press.

Murstein, B. I. (1963). *Theory and research in projective techniques (emphasizing the TAT)*. Hoboken, NJ: John Wiley & Sons.

Nolan, R. A. (1959). *A longitudinal comparison of motives in children's fantasy stories as revealed by the children's apperception test* (Unpublished doctoral dissertation). The Florida State University, Tallahassee, FL.

Nunnally, J. O. (1978). *Psychometric theory*. New York, NY: McGraw-Hill.

Ornduff, S. R., Freedenfeld, R. N., Kelsey, R. M., & Crtitell, J. W. (1994). Object relations of sexually abused female subjects: A TAT analysis. *Journal of Personality Assessment, 63*, 223–238.

Piotrowski, Z. (1950). A Rorschach compendium: Revised and enlarged. In J. A. Brussel et al, *A Rorschach training manual*. Utica, NY: Macmillan.

Piotrowski, Z. (1957). *Perceptanalysis*. New York, NY: Macmillan.

Rabin, A. I. (1960). Projective methods and projection in children. In A. I. Rabin & M. R. Haworth (Eds.), *Projective techniques with children* (pp. 2–11). New York, NY: Grune & Stratton.

Rapaport, D., Gill, M., & Shafer, R. (1946). *Diagnostic psychological testing*. Chicago, IL: Year Book.

Roberts, G. E., & Gruber, C. (2005). *Roberts—2: Manual*. Los Angeles, CA: Western Psychological Services (WPS).

Roberts, G. E., & McArthur, D. S. (2005). *Roberts—2 record form*. Los Angeles, CA: Western Psychological Services (WPS).

Rogers, C. (1942). *Counseling and newer concepts in practice*. Boston, MA: Houghton Mifflin.

Rogers, C. (1951). *Client-centered therapy*. Boston, MA: Houghton Mifflin.

Rorschach, H. (1921/1942). *Psychdiagnostik* (H. Huber, Trans.). Bern, Switzerland: Rorschach Archives.

Rorschach Performance Assessment System® (R–PAS®). (2021). *Rorschach performance assessment system (R—PAS)*. [Internet Web-Based Computer Scoring]. Retrieved from https://R–PAS.org/.

Rothbart, M. K., Posner, M. I., & Kieras, J. (2006). Temperament, attention, and the development of self-regulation. In K. McCartney & D. Phillips (Eds.), *Blackwell handbook of early childhood development* (pp. 338–357). Malden, MA: Blackwell.

Schaefer, J. B., & Norman, M. (1967). Punishment and aggression in fantasy responses of boys with antisocial character traits. *Journal of Personality and Social Psychology, 4*, 237–240.

Schwartz, L. A. (1932). Social-situation pictures in the psychiatric interview. *American Journal of Orthopsychiatry, 2*, 124–133.

Shaffer, T. W., Erdberg, P., & Meyer, G. J. (2007). Toward international normative reference data for the comprehensive system. *Journal of Personality Assessment, 89*, 201–216.

Spearman, C. E. (1927). *The abilities of man: Their nature and measurement*. New York: Macmillan.

Spearman, C. E. (1904). "General intelligence" objectively determined and measured. *American Journal of Psychiatry, 15*, 201–293.

Spiegler, M. D. (2016). *Contemporary behavior therapy* (6th ed.). Boston, MA: Cengage Learning.

Spores, J. M. (2012). *Clinician's guide to psychological assessment and testing: With forms and templates for effective practice*. New York, NY: Springer Publishing.

Stephenson, W. (1953). *The study of behavior: Q-technique and its methodology*. Chicago: University of Chicago.

Stern, A. (1938). Psychoanalytic investigation and therapy in borderline group of neuroses. *Psychoanalytic Quarterly, 7*, 467–489.

Stevens, S. S. (1946). On the theory of scales of measurement. *Science, 103*, 667–680.

Stone, M. H. (1980). *The borderline syndromes: Constitution, personality, and adaptation*. New York, NY: Mcgraw-Hill,

Stone, M. H. (Ed.). (1986). *Essential papers on borderline disorders: One hundred years at the border.* New York, NY: New York University Press.

Strelau, J. (1998). *Perspectives on individual differences. Temperament: A psychological perspective.* New York, NY, US: Plenum Press.

Sundberg, N. D. (1961). The practice of psychological testing in clinical services in the United States. *American Psychologist, 16*(2), 79–83.

Tellegen, A., Ben-Porath, Y. S., McNulty, J. L., Arbisi, P. A., Graham, J. R., & Kaemmer, B. (2003). *The MMPI—2 Restructured clinical (RC) scales: Development, validation, and interpretation.* Minneapolis, MN: University of Minnesota Press.

Thomas, A., & Chess, S. (1977). *Temperament and development.* Oxford, England: Brunner/Mazel.

Trochim, W. M. K. (2006). *General issues in scaling.* Conjoint.ly. https://conjointly.com/kb/general-issues-in-scaling/

Tuerlinckx, F., De Boeck, P., & Lens, W. (2002). Measuring needs with the Thematic Apperception Test: A psychometric study. *Journal of Personality and Social Psychology, 82,* 448–461.

U. S. Bureau of the Census. (2004). *Statistical abstract of the United States: 2004* (124th ed.). Washington, DC: U. S. Government Printing Office.

Veroff, J., Atkinson, J. W., Feld, S. C., & Gurin, G. (1960). The use of thematic apperception to assess motivation in a nationwide interview study. *Psychological Monographs: General and Applied, 74,* 1–32.

Viglione, D. J., & Giromini, L. (2016). The effects of using the international versus Comprehensive System Rorschach norms for children, adolescents, and adults. *Journal of Personality Assessment, 98*(4), 391–397.

Warner, R. M. (2013). *Applied statistics: From bivariate through multivariate techniques* (2nd ed.). Los Angeles, CA: Sage Publications.

Weiner, I. B. (2003). *Principles of Rorschach interpretation* (2nd ed.). Mahwah, NJ: Lawrence Erlbaum Associates, Publishers.

Westen, D., Ludolph, P., Lerner, H., Ruffins, S., & Wiss, C. W. (1990). Object relations in borderline adolescents. *Journal of the American Academy of Child and Adolescent Psychiatry, 29,* 338–348.

Western Psychological Services (WPS). (2005). *Roberts—2 scoring CD.* [CD-ROM & USB Key Computer software]. Torrance, CA: Author.

Woike, B. A. (1995). Most memorable experiences: Evidence for a link between implicit and explicit motives and social cognitive processes in everyday life. *Journal of Personality and Social Psychology, 68,* 1081–1091.

Wood, J. M., Nezworski, M. T., Garb, H. N., & Lilienfeld, S. O. (2001a). The misperception of psychopathology: Problems with norms of the comprehensive system for the Rorschach. *Clinical Psychology: Science & Practice, 8,* 350–373.

Wood, J. M., Nezworski, M. T., Garb, H. N., & Lilienfeld, S. O. (2001b). Problems with the norms of the comprehensive system for the Rorschach: Methodological and conceptual considerations. *Clinical Psychology: Science & Practice, 8,* 397–402.

World Health Organization (WHO). (1992/2004). *The ICD–10 classification of mental and behavioral disorders: Clinical descriptions and diagnostic guidelines.* Geneva, Switzerland: Author.

Zipf, G. K. (1932). *Selected studies of the principles of relative frequency in language.* Cambridge, MA: Harvard University Press.

Zipt, G. K. (1949). *Human behavior and the principles of least effort.* Cambridge, MA: Addison-Wesley.

See Routledge's e-resources website for forms. (www.routledge.com/9780367346058)

13 Malingering Tests

Overview

This chapter concludes Part II of this book, which is devoted to a detailed presentation of all the psychological tests included in the inventory introduced in Chapter 1. For each test, tables have been provided within forms such that the data yield can be reported and interpreted efficiently within a formal psychological assessment report. Furthermore, each test focused on detecting the presence of various clinical and/or personality disorders and addressing a variety of diagnostic issues and questions commonly encountered in mental health practice. This chapter continues this focus with one major exception. Namely, it concerns the identification of *feigning* the presence of a psychological disorder, including both clinical or psychiatric disorders and neurocognitive disorders. So, what does it mean to feign the presence of psychopathology?

Some synonyms for *feign* include dissimulate, fabricate, bluff, simulate, pretend, dissemble, fake, invent, sham, give appearance of, make show of, put on an act, put up a front, and play possum. Thus, *feigning* is here defined as "the deliberate fabrication or gross exaggeration of psychological or physical symptoms without any assumptions about its goals" (Rogers, 2008a, p. 6). In terms of *DSM–5* nosology, the disorders that are most conceptually similar to feigning are (a) *malingering* (code Z is defined 76.5) and (b) *factitious disorder* (code F68.10).

As a *Z code*, malingering is not considered to be a genuine mental health disorder but more of a condition or problem that can otherwise affect the prognosis, course, or treatment of a psychiatric or neurocognitive disorder. Specifically, *malingering* is defined as (a) the intentional or volitional production of "false or grossly exaggerated" symptoms (i.e., feigning) that are (b) motivated by identifiable external incentives (American Psychiatric Association, 2013, pp. 726–727). In legal terms, this is a two-pronged test, both of which must be met to constitute malingering. The first prong meets the definition of feigning, which, as will become apparent, can be detected by standardized testing. What testing cannot do is provide evidence for the second prong, which is evidence of an external incentive. This must be discovered by means of clinical interviewing and/or supplemented by external records.

Factitious disorder is considered a bona fide mental disorder, which is classified in the *DSM–5* under the general rubric of *somatic symptom and related disorders*. In broad terms, these are psychiatric clinical disorders that principally consist of physical symptoms with no identifiable medical etiology. In the specific case of *factitious disorder*, the criteria include (a) the intentional falsification of symptoms (i.e., feigning) (b) in the absence of any identifiable external rewards. So, once again we have a two-pronged test, although the second prong implies that a thorough investigation has been done, which resulted in negative findings. Therefore, in both cases, standardized testing can address the first prong; however, clinical interviewing and external records (or an absence thereof) must determine the second prong.

This chapter contains two standardized tests. Both are specifically designed to detect the presence and/or likelihood of feigning. In this sense, a more accurate title for this chapter would be, "Feigning Tests." However, in mental health practice, their cardinal purpose is to assist in detecting whether an individual is malingering. A secondary consideration is to render a differential diagnosis between malingering and factious disorder. Figure 13.1 provides the typical referral that invokes the need and ultimate request for malingering testing. This is depicted either by (a) an initial referral for testing that specifically requests the ruling out of malingering or (b) an initial clinical interview that produces the suspicion, by means of garnering historical information and/or mental status examination, that malingering is likely to be occurring.

As indicated in Figure 13.1, the first issue to resolve is whether a determination of feigning is empirically supported. In the event there is insufficient evidence of feigning, the diagnostic decision is that whatever psychopathology is present is indeed genuine. This is shown in Figure 13.1 going down the far-left arrow to "Genuine Psychiatric or Neurocognitive Disorder." On the other hand, if there is probative evidence of feigning symptoms, hence resulting in an affirmative inference or conclusion of the same, the analysis continues down the far-right arrow of Figure 13.1 to whether there is an identifiable external reward or goal. This issue can only be resolved by data garnered

DOI: 10.4324/9780429326820-15

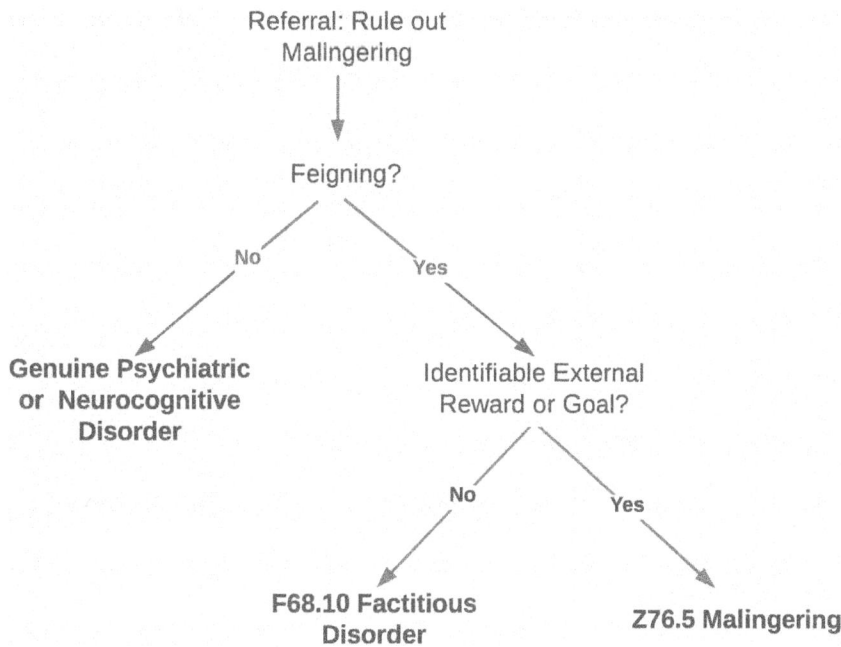

Figure 13.1 Malingering Diagnostic Decision Tree

Note. Feigning is defined as the deliberate fabrication or gross exaggeration of psychological or physical symptoms without any assumptions about its goals. Malingering is defined as the feigning of such symptoms for an identifiable external reward or goal. Feigning can be detected by standardized psychological testing. The identification of an external reward or goal is determined by clinical interviewing and external records. Factitious disorder is the feigning of symptoms in the absence of an external reward or goal after adequate investigation. Bold text denotes a final determination.

by the clinical interview or external records that have been obtained, all of which are peripheral to the testing results. If there is probative evidence for the presence of such rewards or goals, malingering is found. If not, a diagnosis of factitious disorder is made. Again, this is depicted in the second prong of Figure 13.1. In actual practice, however, the external reward or goal typically leads to testing for malingering and not vice versa, although additional probative evidence can be garnered after testing to corroborate the findings.

As denoted in Figure 13.1, there are two general categories of disorders that can be feigned: psychiatric and neurocognitive. Because psychiatric disorders are typically diagnosed by clinical interviewing, the first measure to be presented utilizes this method of administration to detect the feigning of psychiatric symptoms (e.g., anxiety disorder, mood disorder, psychotic disorder). The second test is principally designed to detect the feigning of a neurocognitive disorder and to some extent a neurodevelopmental disorder, especially intellectual impairment. Because these disorders are chiefly diagnosed by performance testing, this feigning measure employs a performance-type administration.

Together, these two instruments are vital for testing psychologists to possess in their inventories because their primary objective is to detect the feigning of psychiatric and neurocognitive psychopathology. As psychological testing has continued to expand, *high-stakes testing* has increased in commensurate fashion. Briefly, high-stakes testing occurs anytime the results will be used to influence subsequent decisions that significantly affect the examinee's life. If we were to consider a psychological diagnosis as, by definition, significantly affecting an individual's life, then all testing would be considered high stakes. More realistically, however, high-stakes testing is probably more effectively defined as on a continuum, with "significantly affecting a person's life" being conceptualized as more of degree than of kind. Hence, diagnoses with short-term implications, such as adjustment (i.e., stress-related) disorders, would be lower on the continuum, and longer-term disorders and/or very severe disorders, such as autism spectrum disorder (ASD), intellectual disability (ID), schizophrenia, and serious personality disorders (e.g., psychopathy) representing greater significance. Also, the decisions that will be made, such as being competent to stand trial, being awarded custody, and being determined as eligible for special education or disability services, are relevant, as many of these will have long-term implications. Because such high-stakes testing has continued to increase, so has the second prong of the malingering analysis (Figure 13.1), namely, an identifiable external incentive for having severe psychopathology. Thus, possessing measures with the prime objective of detecting feigning or its likelihood are vital in contemporary mental health testing.

A question to address before presenting these two tests is, why not simply use the many exaggeration or over-reporting validity scales and variables available on the various rating scales and personality tests? The brief answer is because these scales do not always elevate when an individual is feigning. For example, many of the overreporting scales on even the most sophisticated personality inventories can elevate significantly in the case of genuine severe psychopathology (see, e.g., Arbisis & Ben-Porath, 1998, regarding the *F-r* scale). This would lead to a false-positive determination of feigning, which would be unfortunate because valuable treatment may be withheld, delayed, or diminished in such instances. Furthermore, the opposite result can occur in the form of a feigner escaping detection. For instance, even on the implicit R–PAS the *critical contents percent* (*CritCont%*) variable may not elevate to suspicious levels (i.e., *CritCont%* > 89%) for an examinee who is deliberately feigning (Meyer, Viglione, Mihura, Erard, & Erdberg, 2011). This may be attributed to the fact that such contents are a more obvious feature of the R–PAS Response Process (e.g., blood, explosions, morbid and aggressive responses). Consequently, such contents can be more easily manipulated by an examinee such that they elevate to clinical levels, but not excessively high so as to trigger the detection of feigning by the examiner. This would result in a false-negative determination or a missed detection of feigning. In such instances, an individual may be provided unneeded treatment or, more likely, undeserved benefits.

In contrast to these single scales and variables, the tests presented in this chapter are much more disguised, sophisticated, and better validated for the detection of feigning. First, they appear to be genuine tests that fit nicely within a typical test battery. Second, they incorporate refined and empirically supported methods of detecting feigning or its likelihood, either by statistical logic and reasoning or by empirical evidence. The reviews of the two tests to follow provide more detailed support of their superiority compared to relying on one or several validity scales and variables that yield higher degrees of incorrect decisions on this matter.

The Malingering Tests

As stated, there are two malingering tests that will be presented. They are both normed largely for adults, most likely because the majority of malingering referrals for testing involve this largest population. The first is the *Structured Interview of Reported Symptoms, Second Edition* (*SIRS–2*; Rogers, Sewell, & Gillard, 2010), which is administered by means of a structured clinical interview. This is consistent with the manner in which psychiatric disorders are most commonly diagnosed; that is, via clinical interviewing. The second is the *Test of Memory Malingering* (*TOMM*; Tombaugh, 1996), which is more narrowly focused on the malingering of a neurocognitive disorder and, to some extent, any disorder involving cognitive dysfunction as a principal component (e.g., intellectual impairment, attention deficits). The TOMM has a slightly lower age range, beginning at 16 years and extending through most of adulthood.

Structured Interview of Reported Symptoms

Synopsis

The Structured Interview of Reported Symptoms, Second Edition (SIRS–2; Rogers et al., 2010) is designed to detect the feigning of mental health disorders in individuals 18 years and older (Lally, 2003). The detection of feigning can be dichotomized into two general categories of reporting symptoms, including the reporting of symptoms that are unlikely and those that are amplified (Rogers, 2008a, 2008b). *Unlikely detection strategies* identify individuals who are feigning by their reporting of improbable symptoms and bogus complaints. It is based on the assumption that people with genuine disorders do not report or endorse any such symptoms, that is, the mode being essentially zero. In contrast, *amplified detection strategies* identify individuals who are feigning by virtue of their magnification of symptoms and associated features. It is based on the assumption that there exists a marked discrepancy in the levels of reported plausible symptoms between those who feign and those who are being genuine; that is, the former report measurably higher numbers of reasonable symptoms than do the latter. In summary, the unlikely strategy relies on the simple reporting of improbable symptoms, whereas the amplified strategy relies on a quantitatively higher amount of reasonable or common symptoms.

Hence, the SIRS–2 essentially consists of eight primary scales, along with secondary supplemental scales, that detect feigning by identifying various more specific types of unlikely and amplified strategies that the respondent is using and, at least hopefully, fails to recognize such is being recorded and aggregated by the examiner. Briefly reviewing them here provides a useful framework prior to describing the SIRS–2 in more detail. They include (a) the *rare symptoms* (i.e., symptoms and associated features that do not often occur), (b) *symptom combinations* (i.e., otherwise common independent symptoms and features that are rarely paired or occur contemporaneously), (c) *improbable or absurd symptoms* (i.e., preposterous symptoms and features), (d) *blatant symptoms* (i.e., reporting most key symptoms as representing major issues), (e) *subtle symptoms* (i.e., reporting most common problems as representing major issues), (f) *selectivity of symptoms* (i.e., indiscriminately reporting a vast array of possible symptoms), (g) *severity of symptoms* (i.e., reporting most symptoms to be unbearable), and (h) *reported versus observed symptoms* (i.e., consistently reporting more pathology than is clinically observed).

Construct drift is the gradual broadening of an operationalized clinical construct beyond its clearly defined parameters. This phenomenon must be avoided in using the SIRS–2. That is, of itself, the SIRS–2 is designed to detect the feigning of symptoms as defined prior and not malingering. Again, this is depicted in Figure 13.1, which defines malingering as consisting of the feigning of symptoms as representing only the first factor of a two-pronged test. Put simply, then, upon positive SIRS–2 results of feigning, the testing psychologist must look to additional assessment procedures (e.g., clinical interview data, examination of archival records) to establish the external objective or goal of feigning (see Figure 13.1). Stated another way, establishing the presence of feigning with the SIRS–2 is necessary but not sufficient in concluding that the condition of malingering as defined is present.

Another related clinical construct is important to consider when using the SIRS–2. The term *disengagement* delineates a rare response style that occurs when respondents are minimally involved in the assessment process. More succinctly, this is also referred to as a *disengaged response pattern*. So, why would a respondent disengage in such a manner? This strategy is typically employed by an individual for the purpose of avoiding the detection of feigning. It is for this reason that such is incorporated into the SIRS–2 structured interview process (see subsequent).

The final question that bears consideration in this synopsis section is, which explanatory model should be adopted when using the SIRS–2 in general outpatient clinical practice? Such explanatory models make different assumptions about why an individual is feigning or malingering. There are three such models: (a) pathogenic, (b) criminological, and (c) adaptational. The *pathogenic model* argues that those who feign and malinger psychopathology possess genuine symptoms, which they intentionally exaggerate in an attempt to control them. The *criminological model* views feigning and malingering as simply one component among an array of conduct-disordered traits, which together define the presence of *antisocial personality disorder (APD)*.

Lastly, the *adaptational model* defines feigning and malingering as a reasoned choice for the purpose of either avoiding negative outcomes or obtaining positive outcomes, such as losing or gaining disability financial support or being declared insane at the time of the offense. Essentially, the person makes a reasoned decision to intentionally feign symptoms because this will enhance one's adjustment to environmental stressors. Such behavior is conceptualized as a manner of coping. The adaptational model tends to be the most apposite as applied to outpatient psychological testing cases, especially those that are high stakes in nature (e.g., disability, personal injury awards, custody, competency to stand trial, insanity, being prescribed psychostimulants for ostensible ADHD, appropriateness for bariatric surgery). It is also the most logically consistent with the premise that all abnormal behavior represents a way of coping, or people's attempt to adapt the best they can with the skills and resources they possess at the time. An additional virtue of explaining feigning and malingering in this manner is that it views people within a positive framework, irrespective of its accuracy. Hence, if anything else, it promotes empathy and rapport between examiner and examinee, and likely contributes to malingering test interpretation that is objective, factual, and ethical; an issue taken up near the conclusion of this chapter.

Norm Reference Sample

Development and validation of the SIRS–2 was done on individuals 18 years, 0 months and older. The SIRS–2 was standardized on a total sample of 2,298 protocols. Of these, 2,131 SIRS–2 protocols were administered under standard instructions, and 167 under simulation instructions (i.e., respondents were instructed to feign symptoms of a variety of mental disorders). The total sample was apportioned in terms of type of case and consisted of two clinical and two nonclinical groups as follows: (a) 236 clinical-general; (b) 1,232 clinical-forensic; (c) 613 nonclinical-correctional; and (d) 217 nonclinical-community-college. Demographic characteristics among these four groups varied and are reported in terms of age (i.e., younger than 20 through older than 40), gender (16% male and 84% female), ethnicity (i.e., 8.9% African American, 81.4% European American, 2.5% Hispanic American, 3.8% Biracial/Other, and 3.4% Unknown), education (i.e., 2.6% less than 9th grade, 20.8% 9th–12th grade, 76.6% greater than 12th grade), and employment status (19.6% Employed, 80.4% Unemployed, 0% Student, and 4.8% Unknown) (Rogers et al., 2010, pp. 60–61). The percentages in parentheses are from those in the clinical-general sample, as they most resemble those who are examined in mental health practice settings.

Of note, although the clinical-general sample is heavily weighted in favor of females, this is counterbalanced by higher percentages of males in the other three samples. This includes 77.4% male in the clinical-forensic sample, 100% in the nonclinical-correctional sample, and 47.9% in the nonclinical-community-college sample. Three age cohorts for the general sample are reported as follows (percentage of the sample in parentheses): (a) younger than

20 years (1.7%); (b) 20–40 years (48.9%); and (c) older than 40 years (49.4%). Therefore, the actual upper age limit is not reported. However, the mean age is reported as 39.42 (standard deviation = 11.05). If we assume the SIRS02 included people up to 4 standard deviations from the mean, which is typical of many standardized tests in terms of score norms, the upper age limit would be 84 years, 11 months (i.e., 39.42 + [11.05 x 4] = 83.62~84). This seems like a reasonable estimate and is coincidently the same upper limit as the other test to be presented in this chapter. Therefore, 84 years, 11 months will be reported as the SIRS–2 upper age limit estimate, as opposed to a vague "through adulthood" descriptor. Moving forward, the mean education in years is reported as 14.24 (standard deviation = 2.28). Together, this sample was deemed as providing a "broad representation of patients spanning different age groups, educational levels, and employment categories." In addition, the SIRS–2 standardization sample protocols, "do not mirror any norm-based criteria. Instead they are intended to provide broad representation of sociodemographic variables" (p. 62).

Administration

The SIRS–2 is administered using the 16-page interview booklet. Administration time is estimated to be from a more typical 30 minutes (i.e., involving a well-functioning individual who is not feigning) to as much as 45 minutes (i.e., involving an impaired individual who is feigning). The administrative format is identified unequivocally as a *structured interview*, which means the items are to be presented as written, in the exact order as described, and scored as it is being administered; that is, the interview process is essentially invariant, with minimal clinical discretion. Hence, interviewers are absolutely prohibited from intercalating their own questions or modifying the questions in any manner. Test standardization is maintained by (a) disallowing idiosyncratic questions and (b) minimizing feedback regarding performance.

The front cover of the interview booklet essentially summarizes the respondent's performance. In particular, it includes all the SIRS–2 scale scores (viz., primary scales, classification scale, and supplementary scales) and a profile for plotting the SIRS–2 primary scales into one of four interpretive classifications as follows: genuine, indeterminate, probable feigning, and definite feigning. The back of the front cover of the interview booklet (i.e., page 2) consists of the SIRS–2 decision model, which is a flowchart that guides interpretive conclusions after all the scoring has been completed. Pages 3–14 of the interview booklet include the verbatim interview administrative instructions to be given to the interviewee, the verbatim test questions and their range of potential ratings, procedural instructions the examiner must follow, and structured inquiries contingent upon the interviewee's particular response.

The interview booklet also includes six principal sections that are apportioned into two parallel sequences. Each sequence consists of the following: (a) detailed inquiries, (b) repeated inquiries, and (c) general inquiries. Detailed inquiries focus on four amplified detection strategies as delineated in the previous synopsis section, including (a) selectivity of symptoms (SEL), (b) severity of symptoms (SEV), (c) blatant symptoms (BL), and (d) subtle symptoms (SU). Here, examinees are required to respond to very specific symptoms, and further estimate whether they are major or extreme. Repeated inquiries present identical questions as afforded in the detailed inquiries and are designed to measure the degree of discrepancy between the two on the inconsistency of symptom (INC) scale. Here, individuals who are feigning are presented with a demanding cognitive load, which is intentional in that it (a) effectively diverts their attention from primary detection strategies and (b) reduces the odds that they can counter or avoid them.

General inquiries represent the majority of SIRS–2 questions, and each is designed to use a single detection strategy. More specifically, the SIRS–2 primary scales emphasize an unlikely detection strategy, asking examinees about extremely infrequent symptoms, including rare symptoms (RS), symptom combinations (SC), improbable or absurd symptoms (IA), and reported versus observed symptoms (RO). General inquiries also consist of four supplemental scales, including (a) direct appraisal of honesty (DA) or interest in being cooperative and accurate with mental health clinicians, (b) defensive symptoms (DS) or degree of denial or symptom minimization (which also reduces item transparency), (c) improbable failure (IF; or screening for feigned cognitive impairment), and (d) overly specified symptoms (OS; or common symptoms reported with an unrealistic degree of precision).

Scoring

In general, SIRS–2 scoring is done simultaneously with administration. Specific instructions are given for (a) detailed and repeated inquiries and (b) general inquiries. The overall tenor of such instructions is in the conservative direction to minimize *false-positive conclusions* (i.e., concluding that a genuine responder is feigning). For example, lower scores in the direction of not feigning are assigned to ambiguous responses. This scoring section is apportioned into three subsections. The first delineates the structured interview procedure, including the between and within question-block sequence, along with the response and scoring alternatives. The second is a discussion of how the SIRS–2 scales are computed and its final classification scheme, including how the data can be reported in a table designed to be incorporated as part of a psychological assessment report. The third is a brief section that describes two alternate data tables that provide percentile rank scores (i.e., PRs) for comparison of the test results to a sample who is feigning psychopathology and to a sample who presents with genuine mental disorders.

THE SIRS–2 INTERVIEW AND SCORING PROCEDURE

The interview begins in earnest with "Detailed Inquiries I," which regards whether some common or reasonable symptoms (e.g., feelings of self-doubt or restlessness) are major problems (viz., questions 1–16). The questions are organized into four blocks of four questions each, which are scored during administration as either X (*No Answer*), 0 (*No, symptom is not a major problem*), or 1 (*Yes, symptom is a major problem*). After completing the initial four blocks, the examiner returns to any symptoms reported as major problems (i.e., initially scored as 1) and asks, whether each is *unbearable* (i.e., too painful to stand or something the individual cannot handle). Affirmative responses change the initial score for that question from 1 to 2; hence, scores of 2 denote major problems that are unbearable, while scores remaining at 1 denote major problems that are not unbearable or that can be handled.

The interview then moves to "General Inquiries I" (viz., questions 17–70), which are largely straightforward and easy to administer. Scoring for the majority of these questions is as follows: X (*No Answer, the examinee does not understand the question*); 0 (*No, the examinee does not agree*); 1 (*Qualified Yes/Sometimes, the examinee shows substantive agreement with some limitation*); or 2 (*Definite Yes, the examinee gives a clear affirmative response without limitation*). A minority of General Inquiries I questions are multiple-choice format and are classified as either (a) divided questions or (b) rule-out questions. Divided questions are designed to camouflage the purpose of the SIRS–2. They attempt to accomplish this by asking an initial question without bizarre content, which, if answered negatively, is scored 0 without a follow-up; for instance, having any unusual beliefs about cars.

Alternatively, if answered by either a Definite or Qualified Yes, a follow-up is asked, including either an unlikely content or an odd combination of symptoms across the two paired questions; for instance, believing that cars have their own religion. Such questions are scored as X (*No Answer*), 0 (*No to the initial question*), 1 (*Qualified Yes/Sometimes to both questions, or Qualified Yes/Sometimes to one question combined with a Definite Yes to the other question*), or 2 (*Definite Yes to both questions*). Rule-out questions are designed to ensure that unusual perceptions or experiences are not due to an explainable external source, such as the use of drugs or severe sleep deprivation. If the rule-out question is answered in the affirmative, it is scored as 0, otherwise it is scored in the standard manner (see prior).

Additionally, reported versus observed Symptoms (RO) and improbable failure (IF) in the General Inquiries I section require special scoring. Regarding the former, the examiner scores any discrepancies between the examinee's observed behavior during the interview compared to the examinee's self-report of that same behavior, e.g., eye blinking more than the average person. Scoring alternatives are X (*No Answer*), 0 (*Consistent, a general consistency is found between the clinical observation and self-report*), 1 (*Inconsistent, an obvious inconsistency is observed*), or 2 (*Suddenly Worse, the inconsistent behavior is observed to become more prominent after asking the question*). The Suddenly Worse score applies only to behaviors that indicate impairment; for example, losing one's train of thought more than most people versus eye blinking more than most people.

The IF scale (viz., items 57 and 58) asks the examinee to report a series of five single-word opposites and five single-word rhymes, respectively, as quickly as possible; for example, asking, "What is the opposite of boy?" or "What rhymes with ham?" Points are given for obvious errors. Because these items should produce perfect scores of 0, earned points here are interpreted as screen positive for feigning cognitive dysfunction, with a follow-up recommendation for a more comprehensive examination to detect exaggerating neurocognitive impairment; for instance, use of the TOMM (Tombaugh, 1996; see subsequently).

After the General Inquiries I sequence is completed, the interview moves to the Repeated Inquiries I section (viz., questions 71–86), which asks the same four blocks of four questions of reasonable symptoms used in the Detailed Inquiries I section and is scored identically as representing major and unbearable symptoms. However, one additional scale is available here following completion of this section of the SIRS–2, namely, computation of an inconsistency score. The focus here is on detecting any discrepancies between reporting the simple presence or absence of a symptom and not so much on the degree of inconsistency. Hence, inconsistency scores of 1 (INC = 1) are given for either of the following: 0 (*No, symptom is not a major problem*) versus 1 (*Yes, symptom is a major problem*) or 0 (*No, symptom is not a major problem*) versus 2 (*Yes, symptom is a major problem and is unbearable*). The direction of the discrepancy is irrelevant; that is, reporting "yes" then "no" or reporting "no" then "yes" are both scored as INC = 1.

Once this sequence is completed, it is repeated, although with different specific items. Therefore, the interview proceeds through Detailed Inquiries II (viz., questions 87–102), General Inquiries II (viz., questions 103–156, including special RO and IF questions), and Repeated Inquiries II (viz., questions 157–172). This completes the interview process and sets up final tallies on the SIRS–2 primary scales, classification scale, and supplementary scales.

Once the structured interview is completed, calculation of the SIRS–2 scale scores can proceed. The primary scales are listed in Table 1, Form 13.1, which is designed to report the SIRS–2 scale scores, their interpretive classifications, and clinical descriptions in summary format within the context of a psychological assessment report. The succeeding discussion delineates the manner in which the primary scales are computed.

First, the General Inquiries section yield scores for four primary scales, along with one classification scale and four supplementary scales. The primary scales are listed in Table 1 (Form 13.1) and include (a) rare symptoms (RS), (b) symptom combinations (SC), (c) improbable or absurd symptoms (IA), and (d) reported versus observed symptoms (RO). Respectively, the classification scale (listed in Table 1, Form 13.1) and supplementary scales (listed in Table 2, Form 13.1) include (a) rare symptoms total (RS-T), (b) direct appraisal of honesty (DA), (c) defensive symptoms (DS), (d) improbable failure (IF), and (e) overly specified symptoms (OS). The Detailed/Repeated Inquiries provide scores for the remaining four primary scales (listed in Table 1, Form 13.1) and one supplementary scale (listed in Table 2, Form 13.1), respectively, including (a) blatant symptoms (BL), (b) subtle symptoms (SU), (c) selectivity of symptoms (SEL), (d) severity of symptoms (SEV), and (e) inconsistency of symptoms (INC).

All scoring is done manually within the interview and scoring booklet and is facilitated by typically summing the scores on questions associated with assigned indicators or symptoms. Therefore, all final scores reported in Table 1 (i.e., Form 13.1) represent an aggregation of the item raw scores for each scale. For example, scores on questions associated with a red circle in the booklet are summed together for the SC primary scale score. Also, scores on the Detailed Inquiries questions are shaded in the booklet, which are summed for the BL primary scale score. The two exceptions to summing the scores for the scale score total are SEL and SEV, wherein scores of 1 and 2 are *counted* as 1 point. Therefore, the scale scores for SEL and SEV technically reflect the total absolute frequency count versus the total summed score. Because it is such a technicality, it seemed unnecessary to indicate this aspect in the SIRS–2 data table (see Table 1, Form 13.1). That is, the information gained does not justify the increase in complexity in the scoring and interpretation Table 1 in Form 13.1.

The final step prior to interpretation involves deriving scores for two indexes, both of which are incorporated into Table 1 (Form 13.1). Specifically, these include (a) the Modified Total Index (MT Index), and (b) the Supplementary Scale Index (*SS* Index). An *index* is computed by summing a defined series of SIRS–2 scale scores, rather than a summation of the raw scores or counts. Therefore, the MT Index is computed by adding together the following primary scales: RS, SC, IA, and BL. Next, the *SS* Index is computed by summing the following supplementary scales: DA, DS, IF, and OS. Finally, the Rare Symptoms-Total (RS-T) scale (Table1, Form 13.1) consists of 11 items from the RS primary scale, along with 4 items from the IF supplementary scale that meet the following two objectives: (a) 92.1% of false positives had SIRS–2 ratings of 0 and (b) 33.6% of true positives had SIRS–2 ratings above 0. That is, these items best discriminated between genuine responders and feigning responders.

The principal objective here, and in general, is to minimize false positives (i.e., accusing genuine responders that they are deliberately faking) because this result is considered the most aversive and deleterious to both clients and to the reputation of psychological testing in general. This is analogous to the U.S. criminal justice system, which is designed to minimize the declaring of innocent people as being guilty of criminal behavior and subsequently punished without cause. Once all the aforementioned scale scores and index scores have been totaled and placed on the front cover of the interview booklet, and entered into Table 1, Form 13.1, the SIRS–2 is ready for interpretation.

Raw score percentile ranks (PRs) are available for those feigning psychopathology and clinical groups that genuinely report psychopathology. Hence, an examinee's results may be compared to a group that was proven to be feigning psychological symptoms and a sample in which genuine psychopathology was shown to be present. If either of these norms are used, it is recommended that examinees be compared with the norms that match their final classification. For example, examinees whose SIRS–2 results indicate a positive classification of feigning should be compared to the feigning sample that represents said population of individuals. On the other hand, results that show genuine responding should be compared to the genuine clinical sample and population of peers. In indeterminate cases, either can be employed depending on the goals of the examiner.

However, it is vital to recognize that PR scores do not have any impact on the accuracy of the SIRS–2 classification scheme, which is the cardinal objective when using the SIRS–2. Additionally, the meaning of PR scores can be perplexing unless they are in accord with the final classification, otherwise reporting them has the potential of paradoxically obfuscating the interpretation of the SIRS–2 data (see next). Therefore, the testing psychologist must be judicious in deciding whether to report them because more information in this instance can obscure matters more than clarify them.

As a consequence of these optional data and norms, three SIRS–2 data tables have been prepared. The first was presented previously as the principal data table (see Form 13.1). This one includes only the basic scale scores that are juxtaposed with the response style classification column for purposes of interpretation (see subsequently). The other two data tables incorporate the PRs compared to genuine responders (see Form 13.2) and to those who feign psychopathology (see Form 13.3). These data tables are designed and organized in the exact same fashion, the single exception being the inclusion of the PR scores of the particular norm reference sample, including both Table 1 and 2 scales and indexes. The testing psychologist can thus select the most felicitous form in considering the circumstances of the case, the results, and time considerations, the latter because the PR scores will consume more time on the psychologists' part. Next, we examine how these data are to be efficiently and objectively interpreted.

Interpretation

The interpretation process focuses on the classification scheme. This means that, although Forms 13.2 and 13.3 add PRs to the data yield, the prime analysis is exactly the same. Therefore, the ensuing discussion will reference only Form 13.1 for purposes of efficiency. However, it should be understood that the principal analysis applies to all Forms 13.1 through 13.3 unless otherwise specified.

As introduced in the scoring section, there are two scoring and interpretation tables that facilitate the analysis (see Form 13.1). Table 1 contains the data for the principal analysis, namely, deriving the ultimate response style classification that determines the probability that the respondent is feigning mental disorder. This initial table includes the eight primary scales, two indexes, and the RS-T (which is actually a Rare Symptoms or RS subscale). As such, this table is absolutely required, as it forms the core of the analysis. In contrast, Table 2 consists of the five supplementary scales and are discretionary because they simply contain information that may or may not be useful to the analysis.

To begin, the examiner follows a flowchart on the back of the front cover of the interview booklet, which delineates the SIRS–2 Decision Model. This model considers all the scale and index scores in Table 1 of the SIRS–2 data tables (Form 13.1). The psychologist should first fill in all the data in the "Score" column of Table 1. Next, all the response style classifications noted from the SIRS–2 profile on the interview booklet front cover should be found and inserted into the "Response style classification" column of Table 1 (Form 13.1). Because each scale and index score has different ranges for the four different classes (viz., genuine, indeterminate, probable feigning, and definite feigning), it is most efficient simply to enter them into the juxtaposed "Response style classification" column, rather than listing all the different score ranges and classes. Although the latter would provide all the needed information for interpretation, the excessive amount of information that would be required would undoubtedly obfuscate the meaning of the scores. After all the scores and classifications have been entered, the decision process can be initiated.

The first consideration is whether feigning can be concluded. There are actually three algorithms that are classified as positive for feigning as follows: (a) three or more primary scales fall in the *probable range*, plus the RS-T is greater than a score of 4 or the MT Index is greater than a score of 45; (b) one or more primary scales fall in the *definite range*, plus the RS-T is greater than a score of 4 or the MT Index is greater than a score of 45; or (c) one or two primary scales fall within the *probable range* and the MT Index is greater than 45. Respectively, these represent the first two narrative interpretations listed under Table 1, including description of the permutation and the interpretive conclusion (see Form 13.1). The very low false-positive rate of 2.5%, which is denoted throughout the SIRS–2 Decision Model, is incorporated into the narrative interpretation so that this is made explicit to the reader. In these cases, reporting of the SIRS–2 supplementary scales are not necessary. That is, vis-à-vis such an outcome, the SIRS–2 analysis has done its job in the clearest and most confident manner possible. Thus, in the interests of time and efficiency, the SIRS–2 interpretation process can summarily terminate at this juncture, and the additional consideration of an external incentive needed to determine the presence of malingering can begin. A practical guideline to interpretation is that feigning should be first established, then scrutiny for an extraneous motivation can be pursued (i.e., to further corroborate malingering). This is because, in the absence of feigning, no further exploration in the assessment report is necessary. That is, even if there exists an external reward, if feigning is not found, then malingering is immediately ruled out irrespective of any incentive to do so.

The second consideration regards two potential indeterminate results and includes the aforesaid one or two primary scales in the *probable range* plus (a) an MT Index between 22 and 45 (i.e., *indeterminate-evaluate*) or (b) an MT Index between 13 and 21 (i.e., *indeterminate-general*). The subsequent two narrative interpretations follow these two semi-positive feigning versions. Regarding the former, analysis of the supplementary scales is advised because the likelihood of feigning in this category exceeds 50%; that is, feigning is more likely present than absent. Hence, the supplementary scales can be employed to further clarify the ultimate classification.

In contrast, if the indeterminate-general result is found, the determination of feigning, and its companion malingering, are unlikely to be present because the rate of feigning among this group is only 34.3%. This figure is not significantly different than the prevalence rate of 31.8% found in the SIRS–2 norm reference sample as a whole. If this issue is further sought after, then additional psychological tests are needed (e.g., MMPI–2–RF) and likely will not be deemed medically necessary as the odds are against such finding. Reporting the supplementary scales in this instance, then, is at the psychologist's discretion. It is likely to be a good idea if wanting to establish medical necessity for an additional test for feigning or malingering. However, as stated, it is most likely that further testing will not add much to the analysis, and a lack of evidence for feigning and malingering is probably the most practical conclusion to the case. The narrative interpretation for this classification is stated in these terms.

The third consideration concerns whether *disengagement* has occurred. Once again, *disengagement* is a form of a lack of investment for the purpose of disguising the presence of feigning. In terms of the score algorithm, there are no primary scales that fall in either the *definite* or *probable range*, and the *SS* Index is less than a score of 4. This outcome falls within the *disengagement: indeterminate-evaluate* classification, hence it possesses the same recommendation to examine the supplementary scales for any additional evidence of feigning (see prior).

Fourth, and finally, is the *genuine* classification, which indicates that the examinee was truthful and accurate in reporting symptoms of psychopathology. The majority of genuine responders show an absence of statistical elevations on the primary scales and the MT Index. They also provide an expected degree of symptoms on the *SS* Index, which shows adequate involvement within the SIRS–2 interview process. The *negative predictive power* (*NPP*) for this classification is 0.91; that is, there is 91% accuracy in the conclusion that this examinee is truly not feigning the presence of psychopathology. This last statement is integrated as part of the interpretive excerpt for the genuine classification conclusion.

Next are the supplementary scales, which in many instances will be optional and used at the discretion of the testing psychologist. In any case, they are presented in Table 2 (Form 13.1) for use only when the time and effort is justified for two reasons: (a) once again they are not involved in the principal decision-making and (b) their interpretation is more tenuous regarding the detection of feigning (e.g., a positive result on IF is to be interpreted only as an initial screen positive for feigning cognitive impairment). Hence, these data are suggestive only and need additional supporting evidence or corroboration. Note also that although they are dimensional, they are interpreted by use of a recommended threshold score that varies for each scale. Any score below such threshold indicates an absence of the response style and above which it is present. The particular response style is defined in the final "Interpretation of a positive result column" in Table 2. Again, because these scales are ancillary in both nature and quality, their results require further supporting evidence.

An interpretive excerpt follows Table 2 that lists all response styles measured. Hence, the examiner only needs to delete those that are negative and retain the interpretations that are positive, as designated in the "Result" column. The "Negative range" column is inserted into the table such that the examiner can rapidly and easily determine the dichotomous result; that is, positive or negative. Again, as noted in the interpretive excerpt, even strong positive results require corroboration by one or more external data sources. Therefore, in most cases, these scales will not add much to the ultimate analysis unless more evidence is available.

Finally, the identical interpretive scheme delineated prior is to be used for Forms 13.2 and 13.3. Of note, there are no supplementary interpretive statements that address the PR data. This is because their use is highly contingent upon the objectives of the psychologist in making the decision to use them. For example, the PRs for genuine responders can be reported to show that the examinee is more similar to this classification as evidenced by some relatively high rankings. However, such interpretations must be afforded with due diligence because the PRs are not part of the various algorithms employed. Furthermore, they have not been used as of this writing, hence advice based on actual experience is precluded. What can be advised is that in most cases they are not needed, and they risk subverting the chief objective in completing this test, which is to determine if the examinee is feigning psychopathology and, if the data are in the positive direction, the likelihood thereof. Lastly, any conclusions can be bolstered by any useful qualitative test observations (see later in this chapter).

Summary

This concludes the first of two tests principally designed to measure the presence and likelihood that an examinee is feigning the presence of psychopathology. This first measure is in structured interview format because this administrative procedure is accordant with the manner in which mental health clinicians typically diagnose psychiatric disorders, such as anxiety, depression, bipolar, and psychotic disorders. The SIRS–2 is scored during the administrative process, and the data tables that have been designed to report and interpret the results add to test utility. They include three forms, including a principal form for reporting the basic scale and index scores (Form 13.1), along with supporting ancillary scales and two supplemental forms that integrate PRs based on a standardization sample of genuine responders (Form 13.2) and one that incorporates PRs provided by a normative sample of feigners (Form 13.3). They are all to be interpreted using the same interpretive scheme and algorithms. The sophistication of the SIRS–2 in detecting the presence of feigning should unequivocally show its superiority compared to the use of single validity scales and variables. Finally, the SIRS–2 includes a screening for the feigning of neurocognitive dysfunction, which can be followed up with the ensuing performance test to be presented.

Test of Memory Malingering

Synopsis

The Test of Memory Malingering (TOMM; Tombaugh, 1996) is normed on individuals ranging in age from 16 years, 0 months to 84 years, 11 months and is principally designed to discriminate between bona fide cases of neurocognitive memory impairment and those who fake or exaggerate such dysfunction (i.e., feigning) for personal gain (i.e., malingering). For neuropsychological test data to be valid, examinees must give their maximum effort during the administrative process. Hence, although in this instance individuals cannot manufacture high scores that show normal or higher than normal results (i.e., a fake-good profile), they can fabricate low scores (i.e., a fake-bad profile). When such occurs, individuals may be awarded benefits that they neither deserve nor need, which would then constitute malingering as defined previously, and that consequently consumes or negates the support that should be going to those who are genuinely in need. So, how does the TOMM go about discriminating between those who feign neurocognitive impairment versus those who are genuine responders?

The TOMM is a 50-item test of recognition memory, consisting of two learning and two immediate testing trials, along with one optional delayed retention trial. Essentially, examinees are required to point to one of two pictures that they recognize from each of the prior learning phases and once again engage in this exercise without further learning and subsequent to a 15-minute delay. Unique features of the TOMM include (a) a memory task that appears difficult on its face (viz., exposure to a sequence of 50 pictures that are presented one-by-one during a learning trial) (b) but is in reality a readily achievable task in the process of identifying which of two pictures was seen prior (i.e., scores lower than 45 of 50 items are extremely rare for both nonclinical and neurocognitively impaired clinical samples) and (c) is supplemented by explicit feedback as to the correctness or incorrectness of each response for the purpose of widening the gap between those who feign and those who are genuine (i.e., examinees who intend to fake bad are enticed to use such feedback such that their feigning is more readily detected). Broadly speaking, then, the TOMM is designed to be sensitive to feigning impairment while being insensitive to genuine neurocognitive dysfunction. In other words, both nonclinical and clinical genuine responders achieve significantly high TOMM scores, whereas individuals who feign or are under suspicion of feigning obtain very low TOMM scores.

Based on this introduction, let us examine how the TOMM is both similar to and different from the SIRS–2. In terms of similarity, both the TOMM and SIRS–2 are designed to detect the feigning of psychopathology. Therefore, they both focus on the first prong of the malingering test delineated in Figure 13.1, which is the reason for presenting them in the same chapter. In this sense, the TOMM and SIRS–2 require additional evidence of an external reward or incentive to prove the presence of malingering (see Figure 13.1). Although the TOMM manual employs the terms malingering and non-malingering when discussing its norm reference and test validation groups, along with its decision rules (see later), the more precise terms would be feigning versus non-feigning neurocognitive functioning groups. However, to be consistent with the TOMM manual and its published decision rules, the malingering terms will be employed. Therefore, the reader should be aware of this discrepancy to avoid confusion.

In terms of how the TOMM and SIRS–2 diverge, one need look no further than (a) the administration procedure and (b) the type of psychopathology being feigned. First, the TOMM is a performance test that relies on examinees' effort versus a structured interview procedure that relies on examinees' self-report. Second, the TOMM is a test of both immediate and short-term recognition memory, which falls within the more narrowly defined domain of neurocognitive functioning versus the more general domain of psychological functioning (i.e., thinking, perception, personality, anxiety, and mood). Therefore, the TOMM is a measure designed chiefly to detect the feigning of neurocognitive disorders (see Chapter 9). It may also be relevant to detecting disorders with a clear cognitive component, including attention (e.g., *attention-deficit/hyperactivity disorder* or *ADHD*) and intellectual ability (e.g., *intellectual disability* or *ID*).

So, when is the TOMM typically administered? Most typically, it is given to examinees who have at some prior or proximate point in assessment demonstrated the presence of neurocognitive dysfunction and have responded in a manner that triggers a suspicion of feigning. This may have occurred within the context of a formal mental status examination (see Chapter 3), a neuropsychological test battery (see Chapter 9), an intelligence test (see Chapter 7), or any other examination that involves cognitive functioning. The use of *qualitative analysis* can be employed as a screening for feigning neurocognitive dysfunction, thus initiating a referral to empirically test for this response style. Qualitative analysis is discussed in detail in an ensuing section (viz., Approaches to Detecting the Malingering of Neurocognitive Dysfunction).

Because of the aforesaid differences between the SIRS–2 and the TOMM, a history of psychological measures designed to detect the feigning neurocognitive dysfunction is provided next. This will provide valuable context regarding the development and structure of the TOMM.

A History of Neurocognitive Malingering and Its Assessment

This section presents a brief history of the malingering of neurocognitive dysfunction, including psychological tests and assessment measures designed to detect this response style. The first subtopic focuses on the act of malingering and reasons therefore, while the second shifts the focus to prior approaches designed to help detect its presence.

THE ACT OF MALINGERING NEUROCOGNITIVE DISORDER

Malingering was previously defined as the intentional faking or exaggeration of symptoms of a disorder for personal gain. In cases where test scores determine whether an individual receives financial or personal gain (i.e., high-stakes testing), it must be determined whether full effort is being exerted. Malingering was originally a military term applied to soldiers who were attempting to evade duty by faking symptoms of an illness (Nies & Sweet, 1994). It has also been relevant in medicine (Ruff, Wylie, & Tennant, 1993) and in criminal competency and insanity cases (Rogers & Shuman, 2000; Vitacco, Rogers, Gabel, & Munizza, 2007; Zapf, Roesch, & Pirelli, 2014). In the 1980s, neuropsychological tests were increasingly used to measure the degree of disability in medical-legal cases of brain injury. However, it was not simply the test scores per se that was key, but rather their interpretation that was the determining factor in resolving whether such cases reflected genuine impairment or were instead the product of malingering (Larrabee, 1990). For example, where neuroimaging evidence was either unremarkable, ambiguous, or equivocal, which occurred quite frequently, judgments concerning the legitimacy of an individual's complaint and putative disability relied heavily upon both the neuropsychological test scores and the manner in which they were interpreted, especially the latter. The ability of neuropsychologists to determine bona fide brain dysfunction has since been rigorously debated (see, e.g., Arkes, Faust, & Guilmette, 1990; Matarazzo, 1991; Schmidt, 1989).

Because these were performance ability measures and not of the self-report variety, the validity of test scores depended principally on examinees giving their maximum effort. The failure to do so was conceptualized as a disorder of motivation, which included, but was not limited to, malingering. For instance, insufficient effort could be due to such things as a cry for help, a non-neurocognitive disorder (e.g., anxiety, depression), and unconscious motives, such as in *conversion disorder* or a desire to adopt a "sick role," as in *factitious disorder* described previously. Therefore, malingering was considered one form of motivational disorder.

This brings us to contemporary times and the *DSM–5* definition of malingering presented in Figure 13.1. In essence, malingering is differentiated from all other mental health disorders by its "intent to deceive" and the "identifiable external incentives." However, many view the "false or grossly exaggerated" component of the malingering definition as being too constrictive and as actually falling on a continuum ranging from mild exaggeration to flagrant fabrication. From a measurement perspective, the continuum approach makes the most sense versus a dichotomous all or none phenomenon (Millis, 1992; Resnick, 1988; Rogers, 1988; 1990; Zielinski, 1994). Yet, a certain threshold must be somehow delineated to maximize correct decisions. Next, a historical perspective on approaches designed to help detect the presence of malingering neurocognitive disorder is provided, which represents a nice segue into further examining the TOMM and how it is employed in clinical practice. It will become apparent that it offers its own set of decision rules analogous to the SIRS–2.

APPROACHES TO DETECT THE MALINGERING OF NEUROCOGNITIVE DYSFUNCTION

Two approaches used by psychologists to help detect the malingering of neurocognitive dysfunction include (a) *qualitative analysis* of an examinee's behavior and responses during formal test administration and (b) *performance-based tests* designed to detect malingering (e.g., the TOMM). It will become apparent that the former falls short of a valid test for feigning and malingering, although it can be employed as a screening method. A third general approach used to help detect malingering general psychopathology is the use of overreporting validity scales on self-report inventory tests. This latter approach was addressed briefly earlier in this chapter and at length in Chapter 11, and thus will not be further considered here.

First, *qualitative analysis* relies on the psychologist's clinical experience, skill, and judgment in detecting potential signs of feigning dysfunction. In essence, these are facets that contribute to a clinician's overall diagnostic ability. Some of the most common signs of feigning can be detected during the process of one-on-one test administration. They include (a) recognition scores being lower than recall scores (i.e., recall is more difficult because no clues are given during attempted retrieval), (b) attention scores being significantly lower than learning and memory scores (i.e., the latter which represent a more demanding cognitive load), (c) failing easier items while passing more difficult items (i.e., usually earlier items on a cognitive subtest, which are typically listed in order of increasing difficulty to reach administration discontinue points during the process of *adaptive testing*; see also Chapter 6), (d) atypically repetitive "I don't know" responses or decreasing effort in response to more difficult items, (e) inconsistent scores on tests measuring comparable abilities, (f) discrepancies between memory complaints and test behavior (e.g., when an examinee makes language comprehension complaints while immediately and consistently understanding verbal test instructions), (g) excessive near misses or approximate answers, (h) excessive impairments in delayed recall, and (i) a pattern of scores that are discordant from those expected based on the examinee's reported neurological injury or disease process (see Tombaugh, 1996).

However, not all of these may apply to any one case. Furthermore, such qualitative signs tend to be infrequent and few in number (Trueblood & Schmidt, 1993), can be manifested by individuals with other bona fide mental and neurodevelopmental disorders (Mittenberg, Azrin, Millsaps, & Heilbronner, 1993), and have proven to be unreliable in assisting psychologists in discriminating between those with a known brain injury from those instructed to simulate such a condition (Faust, Hart, & Guilmette, 1988). Taken together, qualitative analysis lacks both reliability and validity and is questionable as a technique for conclusively identifying the feigning, and thus malingering, of neurocognitive disorder. It is, however, an effective screening strategy that justifies a request for the formal testing of feigning neurocognitive disorder.

Moving to *performance-based tests*, the earliest such instruments employed a memory recognition paradigm. The first one of these that achieved some degree of success was in the detection of sensory impairment using a procedure called *symptom validity testing* (*SVT*; Pankratz, Fausti, & Peed, 1975). Essentially, the examinee heard a tone and, after a delay, was asked to identify the target tone from that of a distractor. Feigning was indicated by a lower than chance performance. This was based on the logic that a 50% correct score could be obtained by simple random guessing without knowledge of the previously presented tones. Because this and similar tests resulted in high false-positive results (see, e.g., Prigatano & Amin, 1993), other norm-based criteria have since been used, including (a) scores falling below the lowest score of a sample of known brain-damaged individuals (Binder & Willis, 1991), (b) scores falling more than 1.3 standard deviations below the mean of those with documented traumatic brain injury (TBI) (Greiffenstein, Baker, & Gola, 1994), and (c) scores falling below a certain percentage correct (Guilmette, Hart, & Guiliano, 1993). All were marked by significant limitations, although their underlying rationale and recognition-type memory procedures led to development of the TOMM (Tombaugh, 1996).

Next, we will delve further into the TOMM by first examining its norm reference samples, administration procedure, scoring process, and finally, interpretation by means of decision rules. A data table for reporting and interpreting its results within a psychological assessment report is also presented.

Norm Reference Samples

The TOMM norm reference data consists of two nonclinical samples collected during a series of as many phases. The first sample included 405 individuals ranging in age from 16 to 84, which were administered an initial four-choice, no feedback TOMM version. Prior to each test phase, participants were asked to estimate their performance. This was followed by actual administration of the final version of the test, with the two exceptions including (a) three distractors during the test phases versus one and (b) no performance feedback versus feedback (i.e., which would have confounded performance estimation). The second sample included 70 individuals with an age range of 17–73, which were administered the final two-choice TOMM version. Data from both showed the following unambiguous trends: (a) consistently perfect or near perfect performance and (b) substantial underestimations of actual test performance.

Follow-up validation studies were done with clinical samples, a sample of malingerers, and a sample of "at-risk malingerers" (Tombaugh, 1996). The "at risk malingerers" were in litigation at the time of testing. Therefore, they were deemed to be prone to this type of responding. As indicated previously, the malingering groups in the validity studies were more accurately feigning according to the definition presented previously (see also Figure 13.1), although malingering will be used here to be consistent with terms used in the cited research. The results provided by the clinical samples demonstrated that individuals who score within the severely impaired range on standardized tests of learning and retention perform extremely well on the TOMM, many of which are comparable to those with normal neurocognitive function. The latter two samples demonstrated that the TOMM sufficiently discriminates between those who simulate malingering versus controls and those who were in litigation and deemed at-risk for malingering versus controls. Taken together, the norm reference and follow-up validity data show that the TOMM can be used as a face valid test of memory functioning for those aged16–84, which assists in discriminating between examinees (both nonclinical and clinical) who genuinely give maximum effort from those who intentionally underperform and thus feign the presence of neurocognitive impairment. Next, we will examine how the TOMM is administered.

Administration

The TOMM is administered in two required learning and immediate recognition trials, along with an optional, although extremely useful, retention trial. More specifically, Trial 1 is initiated with a sample item. This involves the learning of two line-drawings of common objects presented singly on two separate cards (e.g., a pen, then a coin). This is immediately ensued by the presentation of two *panels*, which are cards with two objects drawn upon them (e.g., a pen and a cell phone, and a coin and a dog). One of the objects is the same as previously presented, which is referred to as a *target* (e.g., here, the pen and the coin). The new object is referred to as a *distractor* (e.g., here, the cell phone and the dog). The examinee is to point to the target on each panel, showing that she can correctly identify the two sample targets and that she comprehends the instructions. This process is repeated as needed until mastery, although this is typically accomplished on the first attempt.

Once the two sample items are done correctly, Trial 1 begins with the presentation of 50 line drawings of common objects, each presented singly on separate cards for three seconds of exposure, along with a one-second interval between pictures. The first test phase follows immediately, during which time the examinee is presented a sequence of 50 panels that have two line drawings upon which a target and distractor are printed. The examinee must identify the target versus a distractor on each of the 50 panels. Noteworthy are the following: (a) the Trial 1, Trial 2, and retention stimuli are in three separate spiral-bound booklets, which consist of 50 target line drawings and 50 recognition panels that are easily flipped during the process of administration; (b) the two line drawings (i.e., target and distractor) on each panel are randomly presented vertically to avoid confounding for examinees who may be suffering from *hemiplegia* (i.e., ignoring the left or right visual fields due to brain dysfunction or damage in one cerebral hemisphere; see Chapter 9, Figure 9.1); (c) the examinee is prompted to respond within ten seconds to each panel to enhance administrative efficiency and to remain consistent with standardized procedures; and (d) feedback as to the correctness of the examinee's response is afforded.

In terms of providing continuous feedback regarding test performance, the examiner is to clearly state "Correct" or an acceptable synonym for accurate recognition, and "No, that's not correct, it is this one," accompanied by the examiner pointing to the target for an incorrect response. This facet of test administration is artfully designed to maximize the divergence in performance between those motivated to do well versus those motivated to do poorly or feign impairment. Specifically, the presentation of 50 line drawings of objects in a long sequence appears to be a very difficult task, therefore rendering it a face valid test of memory or neurocognition to the examinee. Furthermore, Trial 2 follows immediately and includes identical learning and testing phases, with the following two exceptions: (a) the pictures are presented in a different order and (b) target pictures are paired with new and thus unique distractors.

Lastly, an optional retention trial (viz., Trial-Retention) can be administered 15 minutes after Trial 2 has been concluded. This interval is to be filled with "non-visual tests," which would include items administered aurally, such as asking an examinee to define words, solve math word problems, or provide answers to factual questions, all without the use of visual aids. Trial-Retention is extremely brief to administer because it consists of only a test phase, which is given identically to those of the first two trials, including prompting for a reply after ten seconds have elapsed.

Total administration time without including the optional Trial-Retention is about 15–20 minutes, which is commensurate with that of a typical subtest on a formal measure of memory or intelligence. As a practical matter, the TOMM can be inconspicuously inserted into a test administration session that includes formal tests of intelligence, neurocognition, and achievement. From most examinees' perspectives, the majority of whom are laypeople, the TOMM appears as a subtest that is a natural part of the battery. To further disguise the real objective of this test, the three administrative booklets have the acronym TOMM printed on the front covers, which conceals the full title that includes the term "Malingering." Finally, incorporating the Trial-Retention into the TOMM administration will add about 25 minutes to the task (i.e., 15 minutes of wait time plus about 8 minutes of maximum time for Trial-Retention stimuli).

Scoring

The TOMM can be scored by hand during the process of administration by simply summing the total number of correct responses (i.e., by aggregation). The TOMM: Score Sheet (Tombaugh, 1996) consists of a face sheet for entering examinee identifying information, a summary of test instructions, and space for entering observations of examinee test-taking behaviors that may be diagnostic, a Trial 1 score sheet, a Trial 2 score sheet, and a Trial-Retention score sheet. Each score sheet provides a listing of the 50 panels, with object names in pairs for each item, with the target in bold font and the distractor in regular font. Each item is to be checked when administered and the response circled. Finally, the correct responses (i.e., the circled bold font object names) are summed for a total score at the bottom of the sheet. Thus, the fundamental results comprise three total correct raw scores (hereinafter, scores), one each for Trial 1, Trial 2, and Trial-Retention, including a possible range from 0 to 50, with higher scores indicating better performance. A single scoring and interpretation data table has been prepared for the TOMM, wherein the three aforementioned scores can be respectively inserted (see Table 1, Form 13.4).

By column from left to right, Table 1 (Form 13.4) indicates the trial name, examinee's score, maximum possible score, and the two decision rules employed by this test. Because what is being measured here contains a high likelihood of being contentious, namely, a determination of feigning and the implication of malingering, the major table notes describe the administration process in sufficient objective detail so as to illuminate the test's underlying logic, stratagem, and empirical support. This provides useful context to the narrative explanation of the malingering rules that ensue the table and precedes the ultimate determination of the particular examinee's obtained scores. The adjacent final two columns in the table present the interpretive results of the obtained scores in a pithy fashion, which is expanded upon in the narrative excerpts following the tabular notes. Thus, the TOMM scoring represents perhaps the simplest and most straightforward process reported in this book. However, it is the interpretive logic that is much more intricate, along with the potential controversial nature of the conclusions rendered. These issues are addressed next.

Interpretation

In testing for the feigning of neurocognitive impairment, it is best practice that the results be clearly presented, and the logic for test interpretation be both sound and supported by the garnered facts. This is how Form 13.4 is designed, including a single data table, the judicious use of general and specific tabular notes, the interpretive scoring scheme, the most fundamental results appearing in bold font for highlighting the key facts, defining the key psychological constructs, including both malingering and feigning, defining the decision rules and the scientific data from which they are derived, and finally, interpretive excerpts for positive results and negative results. The psychologist merely inserts the data, which leads to the appropriate interpretation and conclusion, and afterwards deletes the statements that do not apply. There are two basic algorithms for interpreting evidence indicative of malingering, namely, Malingering Rule 1 and Malingering Rule 2. The subsequent two subtopics elaborate on these two rules as they form the basis of TOMM interpretation. This section concludes with a review of the narrative interpretations that have been drafted for this measure.

MALINGERING RULE 1

Malingering Rule 1 is termed the *scoring lower than chance rule*. It is based on the statistical fact that a person possesses a 1 in 2 chance of choosing the correct option on each panel by means of mere guessing, namely, a 50% probability. Therefore, on average, a person would achieve a total raw score of 25–50 selections by random guessing. Any score below this indicates a willful attempt or intention to score poorly (i.e., unlikely due to chance). This initial rule applies to all three trials. To increase precision, the interpretation of Malingering Rule 1 has been apportioned into three score ranges, proceeding from lowest to highest as follows: (a) very positive (i.e., 0–17), positive (i.e., 18–24) and negative (i.e., 25–50). The 0–17 range was created by reasoning that such scores fall far below the lowest threshold of the 95% confidence interval for the binomial score distribution computed by Siegel (1956). That is, it can be stated with a 95% degree of confidence that (a) an individual guessing which of two options is correct (i.e., "a" or "b"), (b) for a total of 50 guesses, (c) will select the correct option anywhere from 18 to 32 times, (d) with an overall average of 25 times. Hence, a score lower than this 95% CI would logically enhance an interpretation of malingering sufficient to justify the term "very positive" versus a lesser emphatic "positive," the latter being reserved for the remaining score interval that suggests malingering, which would work out to a range of 18–24 and is just below the average 25–50 for guessing correctly. Of course, any score 25 and above is assigned a negative interpretation. These ranges are listed in the specific table note to Malingering Rule 1 for ease of application.

The statistical logic of Malingering Rule 1 just described is presented following clear definitions of the related constructs of feigning and malingering as set out in Form 13.4. Therefore, the reader of the report, including the examinee, will be fully apprised of the quantitative reasoning behind this algorithm, whatever the ultimate results. Although Malingering Rule 1 applies to all three trials, the author admits it is rare that any examinee would be so presumptuous or naïve as to score so egregiously low to trigger the first rule on any of three administrations. That is, without a supplementary decision rule, this test would likely produce an excessive number of false-negative determinations. For this reason, the second rule was formulated and is relied upon for more accurate detections of true feigning.

MALINGERING RULE 2

The final column of the TOMM interpretation table regards *Malingering Rule 2*, which although it appears as a definitive, bright-line, threshold-based principle, is actually intended as a guideline or as based on degree versus kind. Specifically, the lower an obtained score falls below 45, the greater likelihood of feigning (and malingering) on the part of the examinee. Thus, in contrast to relying on statistically based logic as does Malingering Rule 1, Malingering Rule 2 is founded upon past performance data garnered from both neurologically intact nonclinical and clinical samples, the latter consisting of those manifesting various forms of traumatic brain injury (TBI), borderline and mild intellectual disabilities (i.e., cognitive impairment), severe aphasia (i.e., any language impairment attributed to brain dysfunction), and *major neurocognitive disorders* (previously known as *dementias*).

In essence, a 97% or higher accuracy rate was achieved by all groups with one exception, namely, patients with major and advanced neurocognitive disorders manifesting a severe degree of impairment. However, even the latter group typically performed at 92% or better accuracy.

Additionally, nonclinical examinees most frequently obtained perfect or near-perfect scores of 49 or 50 of 50 maximum possible points (i.e., an impressive 99–100% accuracy rate). Lastly, validity studies show that a cut-off of 45 maximizes the TOMM's sensitivity, that is, correctly classifying 95% of nonclinical and 91% of all clinical individuals as not feigning or malingering. Hence, Table 1 in Form 13.4 contains specific notes for Malingering Rule 2 that explicitly define the positive range as 0–44 and the negative range as 45–50.

As was similarly done for Malingering Rule 1, empirical evidence buttressing the use of Malingering Rule 2 is presented. Rather than being based on statistical logic, however, the scientific results that bolster this decision rule are delineated. By definition, Malingering Rule 2 does not apply to Trial 1, hence the double-dash symbol is inserted into the Trial 1, Malingering Rule 2 cell of Table 1 (Form 13.4). The last specific table note informs the reader that Trial-Retention is optional, consistent with administration instructions and the author's enigmatic advice that it is required, "only if the score on Trial 2 is less than 45" (Tombaugh, 1996, p. 18). By puzzling, this refers to the fact that if such advice was followed religiously, the consequence would have been a miss in detecting the presence of feigning and malingering in at least four cases.

NARRATIVE INTERPRETATIONS

The final conclusions are either positive or negative for feigning. If any one or more of the decision rules are positive, the final conclusion is that feigning, and thus likely malingering, has occurred. Of course, certain data patterns can trigger positive results in more than one decision rule. For example, imagine that an examinee scores 16 on Trial 1, 42 on Trial 2, and 48 on Retention. What decision rules (if any) would be triggered as positive, and how confident would you be? Here, we would have a very positive result for Trial 1, Rule 1, and a positive result for Trial 2, Rule 2, with the remaining results being negative. The point is that the examiner must first fit the data and examine (a) how many positive results are present and (b) how strong the data are, the latter especially as applied to Rule 2 because it is also a dimensional score. That is, once the threshold of 45 is breached, the lower the score falls under 44, the more confident the examiner can be in the determination that feigning has occurred. Rule 1 is more purely categorical, although with the positive range bifurcated into two classifications based on principles of probability.

To facilitate this analysis, both a positive and negative version of the TOMM test interpretation has been drafted. The first is positive and, after inputting the proper score, guides the examiner as follows: (a) Trial 1, Rule 1 result; (b) Trial 2, Rule 1 result; (c) Trial 2, Rule 2 result; (d) Retention, Rule 1 result; and (e) Retention, Rule 2 result. Note that Rule 2 does not apply to Trial 1. The second version is negative and proceeds systematically through all permutations. The second version is to be used *only* when all applicable trials and rules are negative. In concluding, each version has a final summary statement.

As a final note, drafting the narrative interpretations was done in a manner that emphasizes objectivity. For example, the positive interpretation in Form 13.4 carefully avoids attributing the response style of feigning to the character of the individual, despite this practice requiring longer interpretive statements. Consider the following wording that should be strictly avoided even in cases of near certain feigning: "There is evidence that Mr. Smith is a feigner of neurocognitive impairment." Rather, "There is evidence that the feigning of neurocognitive impairment has occurred, this according to Malingering Rule 1." Such practice comports with never assigning a psychological diagnosis to the individual (e.g., "Ms. Smith is a persistently depressive individual"), but rather a condition that is currently afflicting the individual (e.g., "John meets the criteria for a persistent depressive disorder").

SUMMARY

This concludes the second of as many tests designed to detect the feigning of psychopathology. This particular test, the TOMM, focused on the detection of examinees providing less than the required maximum effort on a neurocognitive task of memory. Such detection is founded upon two algorithms, the first based on indisputable statistical probability, although infrequently found even among known malingers and simulated malingerers, and one based on scientific evidence, which is more dimensional in that once the positive threshold is reached and surpassed, more extreme scores show steadily increasing degrees of confidence that feigning indeed has occurred (i.e., a continuous measurement scale). Before concluding this chapter, along with Part III of this book, a brief section on the ethics of testing for feigning is in order, principally because such practice invariable requires the use of deception.

Testing for Feigning and Malingering: Ethical Considerations

As briefly stated in a prior section of this chapter, formal testing for the feigning and malingering of psychopathology is typically preceded by suspicion by either the testing psychologist or a referral source that such a response style is occurring. What differentiates this type of testing from more standard testing circumstances is the need to employ deception and unobtrusive procedures for such a response style to be accurately detected. These facets can best be appreciated after having examined two tests that are specifically designed to detect feigning and malingering, which is why forbearance was employed and this issue was deferred until the closing sections of this chapter to be broached. More specifically, if examinees are aware that they are being tested, in whole or in part, for evidence of feigning by means of faking and/or the exaggeration of symptoms, and by extension malingering, then obviously they would be more capable of effectively disguising or concealing such behavior, along with withholding any information and/ or records that would otherwise reveal the presence of external incentives that might be obtained by the presence of severe psychopathology. By using deception and unobtrusive procedures, however, the ethical principle of *informed consent* is, by definition, contravened.

Informed consent was introduced in Chapter 3 and was in pertinent part defined as an agreement by clients to partic-ipate in an assessment procedure after being fully apprised of all the information needed to render a knowledgeable, educated, and intelligent decision regarding their active involvement (see Corey, 2017; Welfel, 2016). This issue is analogous to experiments conducted in behavioral research that use human participants and employ deceptive tac-tics, especially frequent in social psychology (see, e.g., Milgram, 1963, 1964, 1974). Within the realm of research, the use of deception is permitted under certain specified conditions. They include the following: (a) the stated research hypothesis will provide valuable information, (b) the importance and value of the information that will be obtained is deemed to outweigh any foreseeable risks to participants, (c) the information cannot be obtained without the use of deception (i.e., the deception must be justified), (d) the participants will be fully *debriefed* following the study, and (e) any unforeseen negative reactions of participants will be addressed by a preplanned intervention process. *Debriefing* is a process whereby the participants are completely apprised of the true nature of the study, including the hypothesis, the reason(s) why deception was required, the expected results, and permission from participants to use their data to be reported in the aggregate.

Fortunately, these criteria can be applied rather easily to the deception used in psychological testing when attempting to detect the feigning and malingering of psychopathology. Let us address these conditions in the afore-said sequence. First, the hypothesis being investigated in psychological testing is generally differential diagnosis; that is, accurately identifying the presence of a certain type of psychopathology among several potential disorders, along with adequately addressing any related issues and questions. Valid differential diagnosis leads to timely and effective treatment recommendations. In contrast, inaccurate psychodiagnoses and answers to questions can have an array of deleterious outcomes, ranging from a simple waste of testing resources to missing the detection of an imminent risk for violence or self-harm, resulting in increased morbidity and/or mortality. Thus, the hypothesis that there are one or more disorders afflicting the individual, along with their predicted detection by means of psychological testing, will provide extremely valuable information, and thus its importance outweighs any foreseeable risk to the client undergoing testing procedures. Furthermore, logically speaking, testing for feigning and malingering cannot proceed effectively without the use of deception and unobtrusive testing techniques.

Next, the debriefing will occur in the form of written feedback, represented by the complete final psychological assessment report and usually supplemented by oral feedback conducted by either the testing psychologist or from the original referral source, many of whom will provide the follow-up treatment, in whole or in part. At minimum, the written report should include the following: (a) a rationale justifying the need for such testing, including the need for deception and unobtrusive measures; (b) any external incentives for malingering identified by the clinical interview and/or other records; (c) the key empirical data from the malingering test and further supplemented by clear, complete, and comprehensible test interpretation (see, e.g., Forms 13.1–13.4); and (d) recommendations for remediation. Finally, the tenor of the report should be strictly factual and objective. The data tables and forms that have been created in reporting and interpreting the SIRS–2 and TOMM will assist in this endeavor.

In summary, testing to detect feigning and malingering can and should be done, but in an ethical manner. Such testing cannot be done without the use of deception and unobtrusive procedures, which necessarily infringe upon the ethical principal of informed consent. However, if pursued according to the aforesaid criteria, such testing can provide a valuable, respectful, and overall ethical service to examinees, their referral sources, their treatment providers, and finally, to the psychological-testing profession.

Recapitulation

This chapter introduced a special kind of psychological testing that is formally designed to detect the presence of feigning psychopathology for the purposes of an external reward, namely, malingering. Feigning was defined as the deliberate fabrication or exaggeration of symptoms, which can be detected by formal testing. The presence of external reward that is contingent upon such psychopathology must be produced by clinical interviewing and/or the identification of external records. An absence of feigning effectively rules out malingering. Two tests were presented that were similar in their objective of detecting feigning, although the administration process and types of symptoms being feigned differed. Specifically, the SIRS–2 is administered by structured interview and is designed to detect the feigning of clinical disorders, whereas the TOMM is designed to detect the feigning of neurocognitive impairment and disorders that capture this type of dysfunction. The SIRS–2 does have a screening of neurocognitive impairment component, although this must be followed- up by further testing if present. For both measures, data tables were presented for the purpose of incorporating their results within a psychological assessment report in a clear, objective, and ethical manner. Finally, ethical issues involved in the testing for feigning and malingering were discussed because such special testing requires the use of deception and unobtrusive procedures and therefore infringes upon the principle of informed consent to assessment and treatment. In particular, the manner in which such testing can be done in an ethical manner was reviewed.

This also concludes Part II of this book, the objective of which was to review all psychological tests that presented in the introductory chapter inventory (Table 1.1), including the provision of data tables designed to be incorporated into a formal psychological assessment report. The remaining materials are available on Routledge's e-resources website, including the following: (a) test interpretive flowcharts; (b) case examples; and (c) modifiable electronic versions of all the practice forms, report forms, and test data tables presented throughout the book. These are listed in the detailed table of contents.

Key Terms

- adaptational model
- amplified detection strategies/strategy
- antisocial personality disorder (APD)
- attention-deficit/hyperactivity disorder (ADHD)
- blatant symptoms
- construct drift
- conversion disorder
- criminological model
- critical contents percent (*CritCont%*)
- debriefing
- definite range
- dementia/s
- disengaged response pattern

- disengagement
- disengagement: indeterminate-evaluate
- distractor
- factitious disorder
- false-positive conclusions
- feign
- feigning
- genuine
- high-stakes testing
- improbable or absurd symptoms
- indeterminate-evaluate
- indeterminate-general
- informed consent
- intellectual disability (ID)
- major neurocognitive disorders
- malingering
- Malingering Rule 1
- Malingering Rule 2
- negative predictive power (NPP)
- observed symptoms
- panel/s
- pathogenic model
- performance-based tests
- probable range
- qualitative analysis
- rare symptoms
- scoring lower than chance rule
- selectivity of symptoms
- severity of symptoms
- somatic symptom and related disorders
- structured interview
- Structured Interview of Reported Symptoms, Second Edition (SIRS–2)
- subtle symptoms
- symptom combinations
- symptom validity testing (SVT)
- target
- Test of Memory Malingering (TOMM)
- unbearable
- unlikely detection strategies
- Z code

References

American Psychiatric Association. (2013). *Diagnostic and statistical manual of mental disorders* (5th ed., DSM—5). Arlington, VA: Author.

Arbisis, P. A., & Ben-Porath, Y. S. (1998). Characteristics of the MMPI—2 F(P) scale as a function of diagnosis in an inpatient VA sample. *Psychological Assessment, 10*, 221–228.

Arkes, H. R., Faust, D., & Guilmette, T. J. (1990). Response to Schmidt's (1988) comments on Faust, Hart, Guilmette, and Arkes (1988). *Professional Psychology Research and Practice, 21*, 3–4.

Binder, L. M., & Willis, S. C. (1991). Assesment of motivation after financially compensable minor head trauma. *Psychological Assessment: A Journal of Consulting and Clinical Psychology, 3*, 175–181.

Corey, G. (2017). *Theory and practice of counseling and psychotherapy* (10th ed.). Belmont, CA: Thomson.

Faust, D., Hart, K., & Guilmette, T., J. (1988). Pediatric malingering: The capacity of children to fake believable deficits on neuropsychological testing. *Journal of Consulting and Clinical Psychology, 56*, 578–582.

Greiffenstein, M. F., Baker, W. J., & Gola, T. (1994). Validation of malingered amnesia measures with a large clinical sample. *Psychological Assessment, 6*, 218–224.

Guilmette, T. J., Hart, K. J., & Guiliano, A. J. (1993). Malingering detection: The use of a forced-choice method in identifying organic versus simulated memory impairment. *The Clinical Neuropsychologist, 7*, 59–69.

Lally, S. J. (2003). What tests are acceptable for use in forensic evaluations? A study of experts. *Professional Psychology: Research and Practice, 34*, 491–498.

Larrabee, G. J. (1990). Cautions in the use of neuropsychological evaluations in legal settings. *Neuropsychology, 4*, 239–247.

Matarazzo, J. D. (1991). Psychological assessment is reliable and valid: Reply to Ziskin and Faust. *American Psychologist, 46*, 882–884.

Meyer, G. J., Viglione, D. J., Mihura, J. L., Erard, R. E., & Erdberg, P. (2011). *Rorschach performance assessment system (R–PAS): Administrative, coding, interpretation, and technical manual.* Toledo, OH: Rorschach Performance Assessment System, L.L.C.

Milgram, S. (1963). Behavioral study of obedience. *The Journal of Abnormal and Social Psychology, 67*, 371–378.

Milgram, S. (1964). Issues in the study of obedience: A reply to Baumrind. *American Psychologist, 19*, 848–852.

Milgram, S. (1974). *Obedience to authority: An experimental view.* New York, NY: Harper & Row.

Millis, S. R. (1992). The recognition memory test in the detection of malingering and exaggerated memory deficits. *The Clinical Neuropsychologist, 6*, 406–414.

Mittenberg, W., Azrin, R., Millsaps, C., & Heilbronner, R. (1993). Identification of malingered head injury on the Wechsler memory scale-revised. *Psychological Assessment, 5*, 34–40.

Nies, K. J., & Sweet, J. J. (1994). Neuropsychological assessment and malingering: A critical review of past and present strategies. *Archives of Clinical Neuropsychology, 9*, 501–552.

Pankratz, L., Fausti, S. A., & Peed, S. (1975). A forced-choice technique to evaluate deafness in the hysterical or malingering patient. *Journal of Consulting and Clinical Psychology, 43*, 421–422.

Prigatano, G., & Amin, K. (1993). Digit Memory Test: Unequivocal cerebral dysfunction and suspected malingering. *Journal of Clinical and Experimental Neuropsychology, 15*, 537–546.

Resnick, P. L. (1988). Malingering of posttraumatic disorders. In R. Rogers (Ed.), *Clinical assessment and deception* (pp. 84–103). New York, NY: Guilford Press.

Rogers, R. (1988). *Clinical assessment of malingering and deception.* New York, NY: Guilford Press.

Rogers, R. (1990). Models of feigned mental illness. *Professional Psychology: Research and Practice, 21*, 182–188.

Rogers, R. (2008a). An introduction to response styles. In R. Rogers (Ed.), *Clinical assessment of malingering and deception* (3rd ed., p. 6). New York: NY: Guilford Press.

Rogers, R. (2008b). Detection strategies for malingering and defensiveness. In R. Rogers (Ed.), *Clinical assessment of malingering and deception* (4th ed., pp. 18–41). New York, NY: Guilford Press.

Rogers, R., & Shuman, D. W. (2000). *Conducting insanity evaluations* (2nd ed.). New York, NY: Guilford Press.

Rogers, R., Sewell, K. W., & Gillard, M. S. (2010). *Structured interview of reported symptom* (2nd ed.). Lutz, FL: Psychological Assessment Resources (PAR).

Ruff, R. M., Wylie, T., & Tennant, W. (1993). Malingering and malingering-like aspects of mild closed head injury. *Journal of Head Trauma Rehabilitation, 8*, 60–73.

Schmidt, J. P. (1989). Why recent researchers have not assessed the capacity of neuropsychologists to detect malingering. *Professional Psychology: Research and Practice, 20*, 140–141.

Siegel, S. (1956). *Nonparametric statistics for the behavioral sciences.* New York, NY: McGraw-Hill.

Tombaugh, T. N. (1996). *Test of memory malingering (TOMM).* North Tonawanda, NY: Multi-Health Systems (MHS).

Trueblood, W., & Schmidt, M. (1993). Malingering and other validity considerations in the neuropsychology evaluation of the mild head injury. *Journal of Clinical and Experimental Neuropsychology, 15*, 578–590.

Vitacco, M. J., Rogers, R., Gabel, J., & Munizza, J. (2007). An evaluation of malingering screens with competency to stand trial patients: A known-groups comparison. *Law and Human Behavior, 31*, 249–260.

Welfel, E. R. (2016). *Ethics in counseling and psychotherapy: Standards, research, and emerging issues* (6th ed.). Boston, MA: Cengage Learning.

Zapf, P. A., Roesch, R., & Pirelli, G. (2014). Assessing competency to stand trial. In I. B. Weiner & R. K. Otto (Eds.), *The handbook of forensic psychology* (4th ed., pp. 281–314). Hoboken, NJ: John Wiley & Sons.

Zielinski, J. J. (1994). Malingering and defensiveness in the neuropsychological assessment of mild traumatic brain injury. *Clinical Psychology: Science and Practice, 1*, 169–183.

See Routledge's e-resources website for forms. (www.routledge.com/9780367346058)

Appendix A

Table A.1 Standard Score to Percentile Rank Conversion Guide

z–score[a] $\bar{x} = 0.00; s = 1.00$	Standard score[a] $\bar{x} = 100; s = 15$	Scaled score[a] $\bar{x} = 10; s = 3$	T–score[a] $\bar{x} = 50; s = 10$	Percentile rank (PR)[b]
+3.70	155	20	87	99.99
+3.65	155	20	86.5	99.99
+3.60	154	20	86	99.98
+3.55	153	20	85.5	99.98
+3.50	153	20	85	99.98
+3.45	152	20	84.5	99.97
+3.40	151	20	84	99.97
+3.35	150	20	83.5	99.96
+3.30	150	20	83	99.96
+3.25	149	20	82.5	99.95
+3.20	148	20	82	99.93
+3.15	147	19	81.5	99.91
+3.10	147	19	81	99.91
+3.05	146	19	80.5	99.89
+3.00	145	19	80	99.87
+2.95	144	19	79.5	99.83
+2.90	144	19	79	99.83
+2.85	143	18	78.5	99.79
+2.80	142	18	78	99.74
+2.75	141	18	77.5	99.69
+2.70	141	18	77	99.69
+2.65	140	18	76.5	99.62
+2.60	139	18	76	99.53
+2.55	138	17	75.5	99
+2.50	138	17	75	99.4[†]
+2.45	137	17	74.5	99
+2.40	136	17	74	99.2[†]
+2.35	135	17	73.5	99
+2.30	135	17	73	98.9[†]
+2.25	134	17	72.5	99
+2.20	133	17	72	98.6[†]
+2.15	132	16	71.5	98
+2.10	132	16	71	98.2[a]
+2.05	131	16	70.5	98
+2.00	130	16	70	97.7[†]
+1.95	129	16	69.5	97
+1.90	129	16	69	97.1[†]
+1.85	128	16	68.5	97
+1.80	127	15	68	96.4[†]
+1.75	126	15	67.5	96
+1.70	126	15	67	95.5[†]
+1.65	125	15	66.5	95
+1.60	124	15	66	94.5[†]
+1.55	123	14	65.5	94
+1.50	123	14	65	93.3[†]
+1.45	122	14	64.5	93
+1.40	121	14	64	91.9[†]

(Continued)

Table A.1 (Continued)

z–score[a] $\bar{x} = 0.00; s = 1.00$	Standard score[a] $\bar{x} = 100; s = 15$	Scaled score[a] $\bar{x} = 10; s = 3$	T–score[a] $\bar{x} = 50; s = 10$	Percentile rank (PR)[b]
+1.35	120	14	63.5	91
+1.30	120	14	63	90.3[†]
+1.25	119	14	62.5	90
+1.20	118	14	62	88.5[†]
+1.15	117	13	61.5	87
+1.10	117	13	61	86.4[†]
+1.05	116	13	60.5	86
+1.00	115	13	60	84.1[†]
+0.95	114	13	59.5	82
+0.90	114	12	59	81.6[†]
+0.85	113	12	58.5	81
+0.80	112	12	58	78.8[†]
+0.75	111	12	57.5	77
+0.70	111	12	57	75.8[†]
+0.65	110	12	56.5	75
+0.60	109	12	56	72.6[†]
+0.55	108	12	55.5	70
+0.50	108	11	55	69.2[†]
+0.45	107	11	54.5	68
+0.40	106	11	54	65.5[†]
+0.35	105	11	53.5	63
+0.30	104	11	53	61.8[†]
+0.25	104	11	52.5	61
+0.20	103	11	52	57.9[†]
+0.15	102	10	51.5	55
+0.10	102	10	51	54.0[†]
+0.05	101	10	50.5	53
0.00	100	10	50	50.0[†]
−0.05	99	10	49.5	47
−0.10	98	9	49	46.0[†]
−0.15	98	9	48.5	45
−0.20	97	9	48	42.1[†]
−0.25	96	9	47.5	39
−0.30	96	9	47	38.2[†]
−0.35	95	9	46.5	37
−0.40	94	9	46	34.5[†]
−0.45	93	8	45.5	32
−0.50	93	8	45	30.8[†]
−0.55	92	8	44.5	30
−0.60	91	8	44	27.4[†]
−0.65	90	8	43.5	25
−0.70	90	8	43	24.2[†]
−0.75	89	8	42.5	23
−0.80	88	8	42	21.2[†]
−0.85	87	7	41.5	19
−0.90	87	7	41	18.4[†]
−0.95	86	7	40.5	18
−1.00	85	7	40	15.9[†]
−1.05	84	7	39.5	14
−1.10	84	7	39	13.6[†]
−1.15	83	6	38.5	13
−1.20	82	6	38	11.5[†]
−1.25	81	6	37.5	10
−1.30	81	6	37	9.7[†]
−1.35	80	6	36.5	9
−1.40	79	6	36	8.1[†]
−1.45	78	6	35.5	7
−1.50	78	6	35	6.7[†]
−1.55	77	5	34.5	6
−1.60	76	5	34	5.5[†]
−1.65	75	5	33.5	5
−1.70	75	5	33	4.5[†]

$z\text{–score}^a$ $\bar{x} = 0.00; s = 1.00$	Standard score^a $\bar{x} = 100; s = 15$	Scaled score^a $\bar{x} = 10; s = 3$	$T\text{–score}^a$ $\bar{x} = 50; s = 10$	Percentile rank (PR)^b
−1.75	74	5	32.5	4
−1.80	73	5	32	3.6[†]
−1.85	72	5	31.5	3
−1.90	72	5	31	2.9[†]
−1.95	71	4	30.5	3
−2.00	70	4	30	2.3[†]
−2.05	69	4	29.5	2
−2.10	69	4	29	1.8[†]
−2.15	68	4	28.5	2
−2.20	67	3	28	1.4[†]
−2.25	66	3	27.5	1
−2.30	66	3	27	1.1[†]
−2.35	65	3	26.5	1
−2.40	64	3	26	0.8[†]
−2.45	63	3	25.5	1
−2.50	63	3	25	0.6[†]
−2.55	62	3	24.5	1
−2.60	61	2	24	0.47
−2.65	60	2	23.5	0.38
−2.70	60	2	23	0.38
−2.75	59	2	22.5	0.31
−2.80	58	2	22	0.26
−2.85	57	1	21.5	0.21
−2.90	57	1	21	0.21
−2.95	56	1	20.5	0.17
−3.00	55	1	20	0.13
−3.05	54	1	19.5	0.11
−3.10	54	1	19	0.11
−3.15	53	0	18.5	0.09
−3.20	52	0	18	0.07
−3.25	51	0	17.5	0.05
−3.30	51	0	17	0.05
−3.35	50	0	16.5	0.04
−3.40	49	0	16	0.03
−3.45	48	0	15.5	0.03
−3.50	48	0	15	0.03
−3.55	47	0	14.5	0.02
−3.60	46	0	14	0.02
−3.65	45	0	13.5	0.01

Note. $\bar{x}$ = mean; s = standard deviation. Standard scores, scaled scores, T–scores, and percentile ranks are all positive values. All listed scores are derived from the theoretical standard normal distribution. Percentile rank is the percentage of the norm reference sample (which is representative of the corresponding population) falling at and below a particular linearly transformed test score. [†] denotes that the more precise PR value was provided by McCrae and Costa (2010, Appendix F, p. 136).
[a]Derived by means of linear transformation. [b]Derived by means of area transformation.
Sources. (a) McCrae, R. R., & Costa, P. T. (2010). *NEO Inventories for the NEO Personality Inventory-3 (NEO–PI–3), NEO Five Factor Inventory-3 (NEO–FFI–3), NEO Personality Inventory-Revised (NEO PI–R): Professional manual*. Lutz, FL: Psychological Assessment Services (PAR); (b) Adapted from website MedFriendly. *Standard score to percentile conversion*. Retrieved June 6, 2020, from www.medfriendly.com/standardscoretopercentile conversion.html.

Glossary

A

ability achievement discrepancy (AAD) analysis. Statistically significant difference between intelligence, as measured by an overall IQ score, and an individual's measured proficiency in basic academic subjects or skills, not attributable to other factors, such as lack of access to adequate education, sensory impairment, disease, or other mental or neurodevelopmental disorders.

ability deficit. Behavior that is absent or deficient because the person lacks the necessary skills.

ability memory discrepancy (AMD). Statistically comparing an individual's measured intellectual competence with their measured memory abilities.

accountability. Principle that made school systems responsible for their product, which referred to student learning, application of which was the impetus for standardized achievement testing in the United States.

accuracy. (1) The degree to which a test measures what it claims for its stated purpose (i.e., test validity). In clinical psychology, this frequently refers to the validity of a diagnosis that has been formulated based on test data. (2) The difference between what a test indicates is true and what is known to be or is actually true.

accuracy disability. Impairment in reading words correctly, which is one of the three fundamental skills needed for effective reading, the other two being reading rate and comprehension.

accurate. The degree to which test results are truthful or valid.

achievement batteries. Name sometimes used for tests that measure learning due to the fact that they typically comprise subtests or independent tests, each of which measure a specific academic skill (e.g., numerical computation, word reading, sentence composition).

achievement test/s. A psychological measure of an individual's learning and mastery of fundamental academic subjects, including oral communication, reading, written expression, and mathematics.

achievement view. Conceptualization of intelligence as representing the degree to which an individual has accumulated knowledge taught in the formal academic classroom.

achievement. The degree of previous learning or accomplishment in various types of subject matter or specifically defined academic areas.

acquiescence (or yea saying). Response set in which individuals simply agree with test items irrespective of their content.

acquiescence response set. Tendency of a test taker to agree with items irrespective of their content, especially occurring on explicit personality inventory tests and rating scales tests.

actuarial assessment. See *actuarially based psychodiagnosis*; *statistical method*.

actuarially based psychodiagnosis. Diagnostic results that are based exclusively on a profile or pattern of standardized scores without the employment of clinical expertise or judgment.

acute stressors. Threats or challenges that confront individuals that have an abrupt onset and are severe in degree.

adaptation. The process of coping with threats and challenges posed by the environment.

adaptational failure/s. Inability to master or progress in achieving developmental milestones, typically increasing the risk for mental or personality disorder.

adaptational model. Theory that feigning and malingering represent a reasoned choice for the purpose of either avoiding negative outcomes or obtaining positive outcomes.

adaptive behavior. The execution of daily activities that are required for self-sufficiency or autonomous functioning and that consists of the following three domains: (a) conceptual (e.g., language, reading, number concepts), (b) practical (e.g., daily living skills, occupational skills), and (c) social (e.g., interpersonal relationships, responsibility, conforming to rules and laws). Also known as *adaptive functioning*.

Adaptive Behavior Assessment System, Third Edition (ABAS–3).   Measure of an individual's performance of daily activities required for personal sufficiency, typically completed by an observer-report rating scale format, used for individuals ranging in age from 1 month through 89 years, 11 months.

Adaptive Behavior Assessment System, Third Edition (ABAS–3) Scoring Assistant.   Unlimited-use scoring software CD ROM for the ABAS–3 measure.

adaptive behavioral functioning.   See *adaptive behavior.*

Adaptive Regression in the Service of the Ego (ARISE).   Paradoxical relaxing of ego functions to permit the individual to become creative and use imagination productively and in a growth-oriented manner.

adaptive skills.   Defined by the Bayley–III developmental test as, "those practical, everyday skills required for children to function and meet environmental demands, including effectively and independently taking care of oneself and interacting with other people" (Bayley, 2006b, p. 10).

adaptive testing.   Standardized test administrative procedure typically employed when measuring ability traits in which items are presented in increasing order of difficulty, which incorporates start points, reversal rules, stop points, and discontinuation rules. The objectives are to (a) shorten administration time, (b) enhance measurement precision, and (c) maintain test-taker motivation.

adjunctive service/s.   Ancillary assessments and interventions designed to provide a client with a more comprehensive and efficacious mental health treatment plan. As used in this book, any professional service other than psychotherapy that is used to treat mental health disorders.

adjustment disorder with anxiety.   Clinical syndrome defined by a clearly excessive reaction to identifiable environmental stressors, principally including symptoms of anxiety, which cause dysfunction and which should dissipate within six months of stressor resolution.

adjustment disorder with mixed anxiety and depressed mood.   Psychological syndrome involving co-occurring symptoms of anxiety and depression caused by identifiable environmental stressors.

adjustment disorders.   Subset of *DSM–5* trauma-related disorders that are all triggered by psychosocial stressors, including variable symptom clusters (e.g., depression, anxiety, conduct problems), with the assumption that such symptoms will dissipate within six months of symptom resolution.

administration behaviors and observations variables.   In the R–PAS system, data that measure the degree to which the examinee has been sufficiently productive in response to the situational demands of the Rorschach task.

admissions (intake).   Process in which an individual's demographic information and principal symptoms are reviewed to (a) activate the case for subsequent mental health services and (b) assign the client to the most appropriate type of service to begin treatment (e.g., psychotherapy, psychological testing).

admissions specialist.   Individual responsible for gathering the information needed for (a) activating cases for subsequent mental health services and (b) assigning clients to the most appropriate type of service to initiate treatment (e.g., psychotherapy, psychological testing).

ADOS–2 algorithms.   Code ratings transformed into an empirically supported scoring scheme that predicts the presence and severity of autism.

adult ambivalent attachment style.   Emotional style of bonding that individuals form in their adult relationships, which manifests as becoming excessively dependent and demanding of significant others. Also known as a *preoccupied style.*

adult avoidant attachment style.   Emotional style of bonding that individuals form in their adult relationships, which manifests as a lack of trust and a fear of making commitments in relationships. Also known as a *dismissing style.*

adult disorganized-disoriented attachment style.   Emotional style of bonding that individuals form in their adult relationships, which manifests as an absence of a coherent plan for developing genuine emotional attachments with others. Also known as a *fearful style.*

adult secure attachment style.   Emotional style of bonding that individuals form in their adult relationships, which manifests as a healthy balance between being intimate and freedom to be independent.

affect.   Situational variation in feelings assessed by a client's objective visible emotional reactions.

affect recognition.   The ability to interpret basic universal emotions from various nonverbal facial expressions, including happiness, sadness, anger, fear, disgust, surprise, and contempt.

Affordable Care Act.   U.S. federal law that requires health insurance companies to cover preexisting conditions, such as autism.

age equivalent (AE) score.   Median raw score for a particular age, usually reported in terms of years and months.

age scale.   Test that groups items primarily by the age group that can master such items versus item content, which leads directly into the derivation of a mental age. Compare with *point scale.*

aggregate R–PAS variables.   R–PAS variables in which several more narrowly defined elements contribute to the total combined score.

agnosia.   Failure to interpret objects accurately despite normal sensory function that can be attributed to brain damage or dysfunction.

agraphia.   Any difficulties in written expression or language that can be attributed to brain damage or dysfunction.

alcohol use disorder.   Substance use disorder involving the problematic consumption of alcohol, defined as causing dysfunction in major areas of an individual's life.

alexithymia.   Condition in which an individual suffers from a severe deficit in experiencing, expressing, and describing emotional responses.

alpha level.   In hypothesis testing, the selected probability for rejecting the prediction of no effect, no difference, or no relationship.

alternative *DSM–5* model for personality disorders.   Dimensional model of personality psychopathology that adopts a variation of the Five-Factor Model (FFM), which emphasizes different profile extremes as indicating different personality disorders, including antisocial, avoidant, borderline, narcissistic, obsessive compulsive, schizotypal, and trait-specified variants. The maladaptive extremes include antagonism, detachment, disinhibition, negative affectivity, and psychoticism.

Alzheimer's disease.   Progressive and terminal major cognitive disorder in which there is profound memory loss due to continuing brain atrophy; the dead neurons are replaced by plaques and neurofibrillary tangles.

ambivalent attachment.   Style of emotional bonding in which the child shows mixed positive and negative reactions toward the major caretaker; considered an insecure style.

American Association on Intellectual and Developmental Disabilities (AAIDD).   Organization that provides leadership in the field of intellectual and developmental disabilities, which was inaugurated in 1876.

American Association on Mental Retardation (AAMR).   Previous name of the American Association on Intellectual and Developmental Disabilities. See *American Association on Intellectual and Developmental Disabilities (AAIDD)*.

amnesia.   Any loss of memory, usually by means of a physical trauma or injury to the head region. If due to emotional trauma, it is described as *psychogenic*.

amplified detection strategies.   Interview responses given by individuals who are feigning psychopathology by virtue of their magnification of symptoms and associated features.

amplified detection strategy.   Approach to identifying feigners of psychopathology by giving them an opportunity to magnify the presence of reasonable symptoms typically reported by those with genuine disorders.

amygdala.   Subcortical structure within the limbic system of the brain, which controls motivational behaviors, such as response to reward, aversion, fear conditioning, anger, emotional memories, and appetite.

analog clock.   Device that displays an approximate time by means of hands that revolve around a dial and point to particular locations.

anhedonia.   Profound inability in experience pleasure, typically a symptom associated with a severe major depressive disorder or a negative symptom of schizophrenia spectrum disorder.

anosognosia.   An inability to perceive the severity of one's condition due to profound mental disturbance and/or brain dysfunction; a complete absence of self-awareness.

anoxia (asphyxia).   Loss or shortage of oxygen; risk of brain damage if it occurs during childbirth. Also known as *asphyxia*.

anterograde amnesia.   Loss of memory for events after occurrence of head trauma or injury; inability to form new memories after an injury or trauma.

antisocial personality disorder (APS).   Character pathology including a gross disregard for the welfare and safety of others, major rule violations of social norms and laws, verbal and physical aggression, impulsivity, irresponsible behavior, a minimum age of 18 years, and the presence of conduct disorder prior to the age of 15; similar to *psychopathy*.

anxiety disorders.   General class of disorders involving apprehension, tension, difficulty relaxing, and irritability.

Apgar test.   Rapid screening assessment of a neonate's overall functioning, including the following five variables: (a) heart rate, (b) respiratory effort, (c) muscle tone, (d) color, and (e) reflex irritability. Each variable is scored from 0 to 2; range 0–10. Total scores lower than 4 need immediate medical attention.

aphasia.   Any language impairment that can be attributed to brain damage, injury, or dysfunction.

apperception.   The meaningful interpretation of a stimulus, including the use of learned or acquired memory traces.

apperceptive distortion.   Occurs when an examinee's interpretation of a stimulus is to some extent divergent from consensual reality; indicates that said interpretation has personal meaning.

apraxia.   Impairment of movement caused by brain dysfunction.

aptitude view. Conceptualization of intelligence as an individual's cognitive competency or measured potential to benefit from a formal training program (i.e., ability to learn).

area transformations. Raw score conversion process that modifies the original unit of measurement in a manner that changes the location of scores along a distribution. Such conversions in a standard normal distribution results in exaggerating deviation changes near the mean or central tendency and deemphasizing such changes in the extremes. Common examples are the *percentile* (*P*) and *percentile rank* (*PR*), both of which are more comprehensible to laypeople.

Asperger's disorder or syndrome. *DSM–IV–TR* pervasive developmental disorder that includes repetitive behaviors, along with a severe and widespread inability to bond effectively with people. In contrast to more disturbed degrees of autism spectrum disorder (ASD), language and cognitive functioning are normal and intact. This diagnosis has more recently been classified under the heading of ASD, with the following two specifiers (a) with or without accompanying intellectual impairment and (b) with or without accompanying language impairment.

associated environmental stressors. Diagnostic dimension that includes situational or external factors that either trigger the onset or affect the progression of psychological disorders.

associated features. Nonessential maladaptive trait variations of the newly proposed dimensional personality disorders in the *DSM–5*; that is, these may be present but are not indispensable in terms of actual diagnosis.

association areas. Cortical regions that are not tied to any one sensory modality, which permit the combined analysis or integration of all sensory information (i.e., cross-modal sensory-perception); thought to contain long-term memory.

associative play. Parallel play with more interaction (e.g., sharing items, such as paper to draw on), although it lacks a mutual objective.

attachment. The strong emotional bond or tie that develops between an individual and an intimate companion, especially one who is perceived by the individual to be irreplaceable. The most reliable indicators of attachment are proximity seeking and evoked feelings of security.

attention. The ability to focus on specific activities and suppress irrelevant stimuli.

attention (selective). Willful or volitional focusing while effectively excluding competing irrelevant stimuli.

attention to novelty. Span of time infants focus on a new stimulus.

attention-deficit/hyperactivity disorder (ADHD). Neurodevelopmental disorder that consists of (a) hyperactive/impulsive and (b) inattentive symptom clusters, along with three types of presentation, one for each symptom cluster and a combined manifestation. Required age of onset is currently prior to age 12, and all types are graded as mild, moderate, or severe.

auditory (or echoic) sensory memory. Memory for what one initially encodes through hearing, which lasts a duration of two to four seconds in the absence of attention.

Autism Diagnostic Observation Schedule (ADOS). Performance-based test designed to detect signs of autism; immediate predecessor to the ADOS–2.

Autism Diagnostic Observation Schedule (ADOS–2). Performance-based test designed to detect signs of autism by means of coding an examinee's responses to interpersonal situations, which for each case yields an overall classification (i.e., non-spectrum, autism spectrum, or autism), along with a comparison score that measures the degree of symptoms adjusted for both age and language ability.

Autism Diagnostic Observation Schedule, Second Edition (ADOS–2) Unlimited-Use Computer Scoring Software. Unlimited-use scoring software CD ROM for the ADOS–2 measure.

autism spectrum disorder (ASD). Neurodevelopmental disorder consisting of impairments in both social communication and restricted/repetitive behavior clusters of symptoms, with onset in early childhood and with an attendant risk of other deficits, such as intellectual and language dysfunction.

autobiographical memory. Recollections that are a significant part of a person's life, which require the development of vocabulary and a sense of self.

autonomic nervous system. Part of the nervous system that controls the involuntary muscles and glands of the body (e.g., heart, sweat glands, digestive system).

autonomous ego functions. Aspects of this structure of the personality that are not devoted to conflict resolution and hence are growth oriented (e.g., intelligence, perception). Proposed by more contemporary versions of psychoanalytic theory, such as ego psychology.

autonomous functions. See *autonomous ego functions*.

average tendencies. The probability of showing particular traits over time and across different situations.

avoidant attachment. Style of emotional bonding in which the child shows indifference toward the major caretaker; considered an insecure style.

avoidant personality disorder. Characteristic inhibition, feelings of inadequacy, and excessive sensitivity to negative evaluation by others, resulting in unwanted social isolation.

Axis I clinical disorders. In previous *DSM* manuals, the first dimension of the multiaxial diagnosis involving acute syndromes that usually precipitate the request for treatment.

Axis II personality psychopathology. In previous *DSM* manuals, the second dimension of the multiaxial diagnosis involving enduring traits or conditions, with an insidious onset that requires longer-term treatment.

B

babbling. The infant's use of repeated syllables without real meaning, usually including consonant-vowel combinations (e.g., "dadadada").

bariatric surgery. Term applied to a group of related surgical procedures done for purposes of weight loss, including gastric bypass, sleeve gastrectomy, and duodenal switch, each of which works by modifying the anatomy or position of the stomach and small intestines.

Barnum statements. Information about personality that is so vague as to be worthless, which people tend to accept as being true about themselves, especially when the information is positive.

basal rules. A standardized test's principles that indicate how many items to administer to reach a point where it is assumed that the examinee will pass all previous items.

base rate (BR). The frequency of occurrence of an obtained score or result in that test's norm reference sample. It is often reported as a percentage and generalized to the population represented by the standardization sample.

baseline functioning. A measured beginning level of ability or performance used for comparison with values representing one of the following: (a) response to an environmental stimulus or intervention or (b) progression of a disease, disability, or dysfunction.

Bayley Scales of Infant and Toddler Development (BSID). Developmental test standardized on young individuals ranging in age from 1 to 42 months; immediate predecessor to the BSID–II.

Bayley Scales of Infant and Toddler Development, Fourth Edition (Bayley–4). Developmental test standardized on young individuals ranging in age from 1 to 42 months; immediate successor to the Bayley–III.

Bayley Scales of Infant and Toddler Development, Second Edition (BSID–II). Developmental test standardized on young individuals ranging in age from 1 to 42 months; immediate predecessor to the Bayley–III.

Bayley Scales of Infant and Toddler Development, Third Edition (Bayley–III.) Infant test of development, which measures cognitive, language, motor, and social-emotional development, along with adaptive behavior, normed on individuals from age 1 month through 3 years, 6 months).

Bayley Scales of Infant Development, Third Edition, Scoring Assistant. Unlimited-use scoring software CD ROM for the Bayley–III measure.

behavioral health evaluation. Comprehensive initial clinical interview, which was required prior to requesting any follow-up psychological testing; CPT Code 90801 prior to January 1, 2019.

behavioral medicine. The application of psychological science to the diagnosis, treatment, and prevention of physical problems.

best ADOS–2 item. Test items that are scored based on the examinee showing the most sophisticated form of a response rather than the majority of relevant responses.

best interests of the child. General rule of law in which the court makes family-related determinations by principally considering the needs of the minor child, which has been criticized for being excessively vague and vulnerable to subjectivity.

Big Five. Alternate name for the Five-Factor Model. See the *Five-Factor Model (FFM)*.

binding. Method of assimilating new information into previously learned information within the brain.

Binet-Simon Intelligence Scale. First formal intelligence test in 1905 designed by Binet and Simon, which was initially used to diagnose learning disorders in children within the French school system.

bipolar disorder. Disorder of emotion consisting of unpredictable vacillations, cycles, or mixtures of mood, including predominantly depression and mania, although also irritability, agitation, and anxious distress to varying intensities and frequencies, and possibly exhibiting psychotic features. Previous terms were manic-depression, bipolar affective disorder, and manic-depressive psychosis.

bipolar I disorder. *DSM–5* mood disorder that includes cycling or mixtures of full manic and full depressive episodes. When rendering such a diagnosis, the type of current episode must be identified (i.e., manic, depressed, mixed), along with severity level.

bizarre mentation. Thought content that consists of beliefs that are implausible; delusional thinking.

blatant symptoms.   Feigning strategy in which individuals report ordinary symptoms as representing major problems.

Block Design Partial Score (BDp).   Process score that is based on the total number of correctly placed single blocks across all items, including any time bonus, in contrast to the Block Design subtest in which points are only earned for completed designs within the time limit.

Block Design Rotation Errors.   Block Design incorrect responses in which the internal design is accurately assembled as a gestalt, but as a whole the design is improperly rotated such that no credit is earned.

body mass index (BMI).   Indicator of body fat defined as people's weight in kilograms/pounds divided by the square of their height in meters/inches; that is, people's weight in relation to their height.

borderline.   Based on psychodynamic theory, level of functioning on a continuum between neurotic and psychotic. An individual functioning at this level typically has intact reality testing, although they may temporarily manifest psychotic symptoms when under sufficient stress.

borderline intellectual functioning.   Intellectual functioning measured between standard scores of 70 and 79, with a mean of 100 and standard deviation of 15.

borderline personality disorder (BPD).   Disorder of character consisting of significant instability in all major areas of functioning, including interpersonal relationships, attachment patterns, emotions, and sense of self, along with intropunitive symptoms, such as self-mutilation and suicidal symptoms. Originated from psychoanalytic theory, referring to an individual who was conceptualized as not clearly neurotic or psychotic and hence represented a transitional condition, including some degree of ego integration, although of sufficient disturbance to manifest transient psychotic episodes.

brisk administration.   Refers to giving a test to an examinee so the pace is steady, consistent, and smooth and with an absence of unnecessary hiatuses or gaps during which time examinees can become bored, distracted, or impatient.

broadband measure.   Psychological test that addresses the primary construct, along with additional symptoms, conditions, or problems that typically accompany the psychopathology of interest; a comprehensive or thorough measure of the principal construct.

Broca's area.   Brain region, usually in the frontal lobe, left hemisphere, that controls the production of speech or expressive language.

BR–scores.   Base rate standard scores used by the Millon personality inventories, which adjust for the estimated frequency of occurrence of a personality disorder or clinical disorder in the population.

C

California First-Year Mental Scale.   Contributing measure to the Bayley Scales, published in 1933.

California Infant Scale of Motor Development.   Contributing measure to the Bayley Scales, published in 1936.

California Preschool Mental Scale.   Contributing measure to the Bayley Scales, published in 1934.

cancellation task.   Activity that requires an examinee to select a specific target among similar distractors, usually within a specified time limit, namely, a controlled search paradigm.

card rejections.   During R–PAS administration, an examinee who refuses to provide at least one scorable response to any one or more of the ten standardized Rorschach inkblots.

cardinality.   Quantitative or numerical measure of elements of a set.

Caregiver Questions.   On the Bayley-4, items in which the caregiver can be asked to rate the frequency with which the examinee can successfully perform a task when the child does not respond.

careless responding.   Response set that occurs when a respondent is unmotivated to complete the test and consequently answers the items rapidly and in a haphazard or random manner.

case manager.   Mental health clinician who provides a variety of usually behavioral interventions designed to improve a client's activities of daily living (ADLs), typically including lower-functioning individuals with disabilities (e.g., intellectual) and including in-home services.

cathexis.   In psychoanalysis, the investment of emotional significance (or libido in classic drive theory) in a person, object, or situation.

Cattell-Horn-Carroll (CHC) theory of intelligence.   Contemporary theory of intelligence that retains the Stratum III global *g* factor, along with 16 Stratum II broad factors and Stratum I specific abilities.

ceiling rules.   A standardized test's principles that indicate how many items to administer to reach a point where it is assumed the examinee will fail all subsequent items.

cell assembly.   Cluster of neurons that habitually fire in sequence and represent a memory, first proposed by Hebb.

central nervous system (CNS).   Portion of the nervous system including the brain and spinal cord.

central sulcus.   Large division of the brain running vertically down between the frontal lobe and parietal lobe.

cephalocaudal.   General trend in development from the head to the tail.

cerebellum.   Circular structure at the base of the brain (or hindbrain), which coordinates incoming senses with outgoing motor movement, largely for body balance; also known as the *old brain*, thought to be one of the first structures that evolved.

cerebral cortex.   Outermost covering of the brain that controls the most complex neurocognitive functions that make people distinctly human (e.g., abstract thinking).

change-sensitive scores (CSS).   Test data that indicate an examinee's degree of change in various cognitive abilities.

Chicago Tests of Primary Mental Abilities.   Measure based on Thurstone's multifactor theory that includes his seven proposed independent chief mental abilities, namely, reasoning, comprehension, perceptual speed, word fluency, numerical ability, spatial visualization, and associative memory.

Children's Apperception Test (CAT).   See *Children's Apperception Test, Ninth Edition, Revised, Color Version (CAT–9–RC).*

Children's Apperception Test, Ninth and Revised Edition, Color Edition (CAT–9–RC).   Projective storytelling test, consisting of ten stimulus cards with animal figures in various interpersonal scenes, designed to measure various components of ego (i.e., personality) functioning, along with detecting primary defense mechanisms, in children ranging in age from 3 years, 0 months through 10 years, 11 months.

chronic stressors.   Threats or challenges that an individual faces, which tend to be moderate in degree and of long duration.

chronological age (CA).   A person's computed age in calendar-based units of time from birth (as compared to mental or psychological age). Represents a readily quantifiable variable defined as the time elapsed since the event or act of birth. In psychological testing, CA is typically computed as follows: test year (xxxx), month (xx), day (xx) minus birth year (xxxx), birth month (xx), birth day (xx). If borrowing is necessary within the computations, each year is valued at 12 months, and each month is valued at 30 days. For example, an individual born on February 27, 2001 (i.e., 2001–02–27), who is being tested on January 4, 2016 (i.e., 2016–01–04), would have a computed chronological age of 14 years, 10 months, 7 days. The younger the testee, the more likely all three units will be reported, while the more common practice is to report the years and months.

circumplex.   Refers to a circular model of personality that places two independent traits at 90^0 angles with a circular boundary, hence creating quadrants, each representing combinations of each trait in terms of degrees (i.e., high-high; high-low; low-high; and low-low).

circumplex model of personality.   Circular model of personality that graphs two trait dimensions perpendicular to each other (i.e., at 90° angles or orthogonally), hence denoting their independence, and creating four quadrants, one of which the examinee will fall into depending on her scores on each trait dimension.

circumstantiality.   Responses that consist of digressive extraneous detail in which the point is finally made or the question is answered.

civil commitment.   Circumstances in which individuals can be legally declared to have a mental illness and be placed against their will in a hospital for treatment.

Clarification Phase (CP).   Second and final part of R–PAS administration in which the examinee is given the inkblot card back and each initial response given is repeated. The objective is to obtain sufficient information in which to code the inkblot location and determinants for each response, including any special cognitive codes or hematic codes.

Clinical Assessment of Behavior (CAB).   Multidimensional screening measure designed to indicate whether an array of psychological disorders and other problems may be present and in need of further testing, normed on individuals ranging in age from 2 years, 0 months through 18 years, 11 months. Data are observer based and provided by a parent or primary caregiver.

Clinical Assessment of Behavior, Parent Form (CAB–P).   Reliable observer-based rating scale, completed by parents or primary caregivers, for objectively identifying the presence of a variety of behavioral and emotional disorders in children and adolescents ages 2 years, 0 months through 18 years, 11 months.

Clinical Assessment of Behavior Scoring Program (CAB–SP).   Computer scoring program for the CAB, which loads onto the testing psychologist's personal computer for unlimited scoring.

clinical assessment.   See *clinical judgment.*

clinical disorder/s.   A clustering or covariance of essential and nonessential psychological symptoms that cause dysfunction and typically exhibit the following characteristics: (a) identifiable onset, (b) acute presentation, (c) precipitant for professional intervention, and (d) amenability to treatment.

clinical interview. Face-to-face meeting between a clinician and examinee, during which time information is garnered by question-and-answer format about the examinee, which is used to formulate initial diagnostic impressions and objectives for either further assessment and testing or treatment.

clinical judgment. Deriving diagnostic conclusions based on expert training and experience.

clinical method. Use of expert training and experience in rendering psychological diagnosis.

clinical perspective. Personality inventories developed with a focus on detecting abnormal behavior or psychopathology.

clinical social worker. Licensed Clinical Social Worker (LCSW) who provides individual counseling or therapy, group therapy, and/or family and couples therapy in the mental health field.

clinical syndrome/s. See *clinical disorder/s*.

clinically significant personality traits. As applied to the Millon personality inventories, *BR*–score (75–84), which indicates the presence of characteristics that cause problems.

code ratings. ADOS–2 quantitative scheme in which a continuous series of numbers (i.e., codes), usually 0–1–2, are to be scored (i.e., rated) on each item according to the degree of autism signs exhibited by the examinee.

codetypes. A cookbook style of MMPI test interpretation in which the highest two or three scales determine the personality type, based on research showing the external correlates of such profile pattern (e.g., code 8–6–7 or psychotic valley profile).

coding horizontally. On the R–PAS, the coding of an examinee's verbatim responses across all coding categories within each response independently, as opposed to coding vertically downward within each category.

coding rotation error/s. Type of error wherein the examinee repeatedly writes a code that is an exact reversal or mirror image of the correct code symbol.

coding vertically. On the R–PAS, the coding of an examinee's verbatim responses downwards according to coding category versus horizontally within each response.

coefficient alpha. Statistic that measures the extent to which items on a test measure the same psychological construct.

cognition. Refers to internal or covert mental actions, such as thinking, reasoning, problem-solving, formal intelligence, memory, and language, in contrast emotions.

cognitive flexibility. The ability to modify one's behavior, problem-solving strategy, or approach to a task or social circumstance.

cognitive. See *cognition*.

collaborative therapeutic assessment. Approach to psychological testing that integrates assessment and treatment throughout the process and focuses on helping the examinee gain greater self-discovery and new understandings.

collaterals. Individuals who are part of the psychological assessment and testing process who are intimately familiar with the examinee, typically caregivers and/or close family members.

commitment. One of Marcia's dimensions in developing an identity, which refers to when an individual has settled on a clear objective and is working toward its attainment.

communication disorder/s. Class of neurodevelopmental disorders that involve some kind of impairment in verbal and/or nonverbal behavior, designed and intended to influence others.

comorbidity. The presence of coexisting disorders.

completion technique. Class of projective techniques in which examinees are required to finish a partial stimulus in the manner they deem appropriate.

complex attention. Multifaceted attention, including sustained attention (i.e., maintaining attention over time), selective attention (i.e., maintaining attention in the presence of competing or distracting stimuli), and divided attention (i.e., paying attention to two tasks simultaneously).

complex PTSD (c-PTSD). Post-traumatic stress disorder (PTSD) with added symptoms that significantly complicate the symptom profile and treatment, including such symptoms as adopting a hostile or distrustful attitude toward the world and people or manifesting significant problems with emotional self-regulation, and usually is caused by repeated, severe, and prolonged trauma.

complexity-adjusted. In the R–PAS, scores modified to represent what they would have been if the examinee's complexity was average or optimal.

complexity adjustment. R–PAS statistical alteration for protocols that do not possess the optimal degree of measured productivity and involvement in the task.

composite equivalent scores. Standard scores (mean = 100, standard deviation = 15) that were linearly transformed from a scaled score metric (mean = 10, standard deviation = 3).

computer test interpretive software. Program that typically transforms raw scores into standard scores according to a test's norms, although it also provides statements as to the diagnostic meaning of the data.

computer test scoring software.   Program that typically transforms raw scores into standard scores according to a test's norms, although it does not provide interpretive statements.

conception.   The uniting of a male with a female reproductive cell (i.e., sperm and ovum, respectively) to form a fertilized egg (i.e., zygote), which initiates the development of a life form.

conditional probability.   Measure of the likelihood that one event will occur given (or if) some other event has occurred; $p(A \mid B)$ = the probability of A given B.

conditioned emotional responses.   Affective reactions that are elicited automatically by conditioned stimuli via principles of classical conditioning.

conduct disorder (CD).   Disorder that features the violation of the fundamental rights of others and/or major societal norms, including the following four symptom clusters: (a) aggression toward people and animals, (b) destruction of property, (c) deceitfulness and/or theft, and (d) serious rule violations. Minimum criteria include three symptoms from any cluster during the prior 12 months, along with one symptom within the past 6 months.

confabulation.   Symptom wherein a person fills in gaps in memory with fantastical stories caused by neurocognitive dysfunction, first proposed by German psychiatrist Karl Bonhoeffer in 1900.

confidence interval (CI).   Range within which an examinee's true score is expected to fall, which is accompanied by a specified percent of certainty.

Confidentiality of Substance Use Disorder, 42 C.F.R. Part 2.   Federal law that provides those with a substance use disorder added protection from prosecution when they release information regarding their involvement with illicit drugs. The objective is to encourage people with substance abuse problems to admit their problem to obtain effective treatment.

confirmatory factor analysis (CFA).   Advanced factor analytic statistical procedure that measures the degree of fit (i.e., goodness-of-fit) between the empirical or observed data and a proposed structural model for a psychological test. The familiar chi-square statistic can be used to test the (null) hypothesis that the observed set of item intercorrelations is no different from the proposed model or factor structure. Used to provide evidence that a psychological test is measuring what it claims it is measuring (i.e., construct validity).

conflict-free ego sphere.   See *autonomous ego functions*.

confounding variable.   An extraneous third variable that is not controlled and thus coexists with the independent variable; undesirable in the context of an experiment because it may be equally responsible for a measured changed in the dependent variable.

Conners 3, ADHD Index Version, Parent Form (Conners 3–AI–P).   Screening measure designed to indicate whether attention-deficit hyperactivity disorder (ADHD) may be present and in need of further testing in individuals ranging in age from 6 years, 0 months through 18 years, 11 months; data are observer based and provided by a parent or primary caregiver.

Conners 3rd Edition (Conners 3).   Behavioral rating scale instrument for measuring the presence of attention-deficit hyperactivity disorder (ADHD), along with common co-occurring problems and disorders in individuals ranging in age from 6 to 18 years.

Conners 3rd Edition, ADHD Index Version (Conners 3–AI).   Observer-based screening measure designed to indicate whether attention-deficit hyperactivity disorder (ADHD) may be present and in need of further testing in individuals ranging in age from 6 years, 0 months through 18 years, 11 months.

Conners' Adult ADHD Rating Scales (CAARS).   Group of rating scale forms designed to help measure and facilitate a diagnosis of attention-deficit hyperactivity disorder (ADHD) in adults, including the type of presentation (i.e., inattentive, hyperactive/impulsive, or combined), and symptom level or degree (i.e., mild, moderate, or severe). Data are both self-report and observer-report.

Conners' Adult ADHD Rating Scales, Long Version (CAARS–L).   Rating scale measure consisting of all items designed to facilitate the diagnosis of attention-deficit hyperactivity disorder (ADHD) in adults, including the type of presentation (i.e., inattentive, hyperactive/impulsive, or combined), and symptom level or degree (i.e., mild, moderate, or severe). Data are both self-report and observer-report.

Conners' Adult ADHD Rating Scales, Screening Version, Self-Report Form (CAARS–S–SR).   Brief screening measure designed to indicate whether attention-deficit hyperactivity disorder (ADHD) may be present in adults and in need of further testing. Data are self-report and thus provided by the examinee.

Conners Comprehensive Behavior Rating Scales (Conners CBRS).   Standardized rating scale instrument designed to measure a variety of neurodevelopmental, behavioral, and emotional disorders, as determined by observations made by parent and teachers, normed on individuals ranging in age from 6 years, 0 months through 18 years, 11 months, along with a self-report form for individuals ranging in age from 8 years, 0 months through 18 years, 11 months.

Conners Continuous Auditory Test of Attention (Conners CATA). Computer-administered test in which the testee must persist in responding to auditory-based target stimuli (i.e., low-tone and high-tone pairings) and withholding responses to an auditory-based nontarget stimulus (i.e., single high tone presentations), over an extended period without rest periods or breaks. This test provides multiple measures of attention and impulse control for individuals aged 8 years, 0 months through adulthood.

Conners Continuous Performance Test, Third Edition (Conners CPT–3). Computer-administered test in which the examinee must persist in responding to visually based target stimuli (i.e., all letters of the alphabet except "X") and withholding responses to a visually based nontarget stimulus (i.e., the letter "X") over an extended period without rest periods or breaks. This test provides multiple measures of attention and impulse control for individuals aged 8 years, 0 months through adulthood.

Conners CPT–II. Immediate predecessor to the CPT–3.

Conners Early Childhood (Conners EC). Standardized rating scale instrument designed to measure a variety of behavioral and emotional problems, along with any delays in major developmental milestones, as determined by observations made by primary caretakers and teacher/childcare workers, for individuals ranging in age from 2 years, 0 months through 6 years, 11 months.

Conners Early Childhood, Behavior, Short Version (Conners EC–BEH–S). Observer-based screening measure designed to indicate whether attention-deficit hyperactivity disorder (ADHD) may be present in young children and in need of further testing. This measure is normed on individuals ranging in age from 2 years, 0 months through 6 years, 11 months.

Conners Early Childhood, Behavior Short Version, Parent Form (Conners EC–BEH–S–P). Screening measure designed to indicate whether attention-deficit hyperactivity disorder (ADHD) may be present in young children and in need of further testing. Data are observer based and provided by a parent or primary caregiver. This measure is normed on individuals ranging in age from 2 years, 0 months through 6 years, 11 months.

Conners K–CPT. Immediate predecessor to the K–CPT 2.

Conners Kiddie Continuous Performance Test, Second Edition (Conners K–CPT 2). Computer-administered test in which the examinee must persist in responding to visually based target stimuli (i.e., pictures of objects other than a ball) and withholding responses to a visually based nontarget stimulus (i.e., a ball) over an extended period without rest periods or breaks. This test provides multiple measures of attention and impulse control for individuals aged 4 years, 0 months through 7 years, 11 months.

co-norming. Two or more related measures that are administered and standardized simultaneously using the same norm reference sample, which eliminates individual differences errors when such scores are compared to determine any score differences.

conservative response style. Decision-making approach by the respondent who tends toward claiming that a stimulus was not present when uncertain.

consolidation. Dendritic modifications in the neurons of the brain, which represent the strengthening of memory traces and the prevention of forgetting.

consolidation system. Proposed group of brain structures responsible for encoding information into long-term memory, especially including the hippocampus and thalamus.

construct drift. The gradual broadening of the meaning of a clinical construct beyond its originally defined parameters, which contributes to confusion and error as to how the construct is applied.

construct/s. Abstract idea used to organize, interpret, and explain observed facts. Many psychological symptoms and disorders (e.g., anxiety) represent constructs.

construct validity. Quality of a psychological test that determines the degree to which it measures the intended characteristic for a specifically defined use.

constructive processing theory. Concept that long-term memories are assembled and recreated each time they are encoded, retrieved, reworked, and encoded again to incorporate new information and/or exclude previous details, which accounts for why memories are not perfect replicas of prior experiences.

content-based interpretation. Interpretation of test data based on the content of the pertinent scales as opposed to codetype profile interpretation.

continuity of care. Process by which a team of health care professionals from various relevant specialties cooperate in the ongoing treatment and management of an individual, with the shared objective of high-quality and cost-effective care; succinctly, the provision of high-quality care over time.

continuous norming. Method of estimating the relationship between raw scores and norm values based on various types of mathematical models. Compare with traditional norming in which raw scores and norm values are based on the standard normal distribution.

continuous performance test/s (CPTs).   Computer-automated test that presents the individual with a tedious and repetitive task and without the opportunity for respite or rest periods; typically measures immediate and sustained attention, along with immediate and sustained impulse control associated with neurocognitive and neurodevelopmental disorders, such as attention-deficit hyperactivity disorder (ADHD).

contralateral.   Opposite; usually referring to the fact that the cerebral hemispheres in the human brain control the opposite side of the body.

contrast effects.   Response tendency that increases error variance in observer-based ratings, defined as current ratings being influenced in the opposing direction by prior ratings or experiences in the contrary direction; for example, previous positive ratings inflating current negative ratings, and previous negative ratings inflating current positive ratings.

convergent validity.   Regarding psychometrics, the degree to which two tests that purportedly measure the same or similar constructs are themselves correlated with each other. As applied to psychological test results, the degree to which two tests that measure the same or similar constructs, especially those targeting the same or similar kinds of psychopathologies, yield comparable results; for example, an implicit and explicit personality test both showing evidence that the examinee has a major depressive disorder.

conversion disorder.   Somatoform disorder in which a physical symptom, typically neurological in form, is manifested in the absence of an identifiable medical cause, the assumption being that an unresolved psychological or emotional factor is causing the symptom to occur.

cooing.   An infant's repetition of vowel sounds (e.g., ahahahah); predecessor to babbling.

cooperative play.   Children interacting to achieve a common goal or objective.

coping styles.   A construct used by the Millon Behavioral Medicine Diagnostic (MBMD) that involves cognitive, behavioral, and interpersonal strategies individuals employ to obtain rewards and avoid discomfort in both medical settings and in general; some may facilitate and some may hinder medical treatment progress.

corpus callosum.   Subcortical band of fibers (i.e., axons) that permits the two hemispheres to communicate.

cortex.   See *cerebral cortex*.

CPT Code 90791.   Psychiatric diagnostic evaluation (no medical services) designation for billing purposes, which is an initial clinical interview with mental status examination provided by a mental health clinician that is not medically trained (e.g., clinical psychologist, clinical social worker).

CPT Code 90792.   Psychiatric diagnostic evaluation with medical services designation for billing purposes, which is an initial clinical interview with mental status examination provided by a mental health clinician that is medically trained (e.g., psychiatrist).

CPT Code 90801.   Prior to January 1, 2019, CPT code for "behavioral health evaluation" or comprehensive initial clinical interview designation for billing purposes, which was a requirement prior to making a request for follow-up testing.

CPT Code 90832, 16–37 minutes.   CPT code for billing individual psychotherapy sessions lasting anywhere between 16 and 37 minutes, which is designed according to the time-rule.

CPT Code 90834, 38–52 minutes.   CPT code for billing individual psychotherapy sessions lasting anywhere between 38 and 52 minutes, which is designed according to the time-rule.

CPT Code 90837, 53 or more minutes.   CPT code for billing individual psychotherapy sessions lasting 53 minutes or longer, which is designed according to the time-rule.

CPT Code 96101.   Prior to January 1, 2019, CPT code for billing psychological test services, including the psychodiagnostic assessment of emotionality, intelligence, personality, and psychopathology, per hour, including administration (face-to-face), interpretation, and report writing (additional time other than face-to-face).

CPT Code 96112.   Effective January 1, 2019, new CPT code for billing the administration, scoring, data interpretation, and report generation of developmental tests, first 60 minutes.

CPT Code 96113.   Effective January 1, 2019, new CPT code for billing all added 30-minute units needed to complete developmental test services as defined prior.

CPT Code 96118.   Prior to January 1, 2019, CPT code for billing neuropsychological test services, including the psychodiagnostic assessment of neurocognitive abilities, such as attention, memory, language, and visual-spatial, along with executive functioning and other types of cognitive functioning related to the diagnosis of brain damage or dysfunction, and secondarily, the assessment of personality and adaptive behavior functioning considered to be related to neurocognitive impairment.

CPT Code 96130.   Effective January 1, 2019, CPT code for billing psychological test evaluation services by a physician or qualified health care professional (e.g., licensed psychologist), first hour (i.e., first 60-minute unit).

CPT Code 96131.   Effective January 1, 2019, CPT code for billing all added 60-minute units needed to complete psychological test-evaluation services.

CPT Code 96132.   Effective January 1, 2019, CPT code for billing neuropsychological test evaluation services by a physician or qualified health care professional (e.g., licensed psychologist), first 60 minutes.

CPT Code 96133.   Effective January 1, 2019, CPT code for billing all added 60-minute units needed to complete neuropsychological test-evaluation services.

CPT Code 96136.   Effective January 1, 2019, CPT code for billing a psychological test or neuropsychological test administration and scoring by a physician or qualified health care professional (e.g., licensed psychologist), consisting of two or more tests, any method, first 30 minutes (i.e., a minimum of 16–30 minutes).

CPT Code 96137.   Effective January 1, 2019, CPT code for billing each additional 30 minutes of psychological or neuropsychological test administration and scoring, two or more tests, and any method needed to complete such services.

criminological model.   Theory that feigning and malingering psychopathology are simply symptoms of a more general diagnosis of antisocial personality disorder (ASD).

crisis.   One of Marcia's two dimensions that refers to when individuals are actively confronting identity questions and investigated alternatives; typically around the age of 18.

criterion.   (1) A predetermined standard, objective, or outcome (e.g., falling within the top 10% of all test takers). (2) Within the context of regression analyses, the variable to be predicted by one or more other variables; also referred to as the dependent variable.

criterion-based approach.   Measuring an individual's ability by comparing his or her performance to a preset standard (e.g., passing 80% of the items).

criterion-based test.   Measure in which an examinee's scores are compared to a predetermined standard (e.g., passing 80% of the items).

critical contents percent (CritCont%).   R–PAS variable computed as $An + Bl + Ex + Fi + Sx + AGM + MOR/R$, which at high levels is associated with a trauma history, dissociation, crude cognitions, and lapses in ego function, although at extraordinarily high levels (i.e., > 45%) it gives evidence of symptom exaggeration or feigning psychopathology.

critical value.   The minimum difference between two scores needed to conclude that they are statistically different, typically reported with a degree of probability (usually less than 5% or 1%).

cross-cultural universality.   Assumption that if a trait term is being used in a greater number of languages around the world, the more important that trait has become in describing and predicting human behavior.

cross-validation.   Determining the degree to which initial test-validity results generalize to samples of new individuals for which the test is intended.

cross-validation sample.   Second subgroup of individuals upon which a test is used to determine if it yields results comparable to the initial standardization group.

cry for help.   A wish to communicate to others that one is in a dire situation, usually by means of a suicidal gesture.

crystalized intelligence.   The store of knowledge or information of a given society (e.g., history facts, vocabulary). Type of cognitive ability that includes one's fund of acquired knowledge, vocabulary, and skills based on experience, education, and learning.

cued recall.   Retrieving information with the assistance of hints or clues.

cumulative percentages.   The sum of percentages in a data set.

Current Procedural Terminology (CPT).   Uniform numerical coding system, published and maintained by the American Medical Association, that defines an array of health procedures and is used for billing third-party payers for remuneration.

cut-off score.   Established value or quantity on a diagnostic or screening test that represents a dividing point on a continuous measurement scale, which is designed to apportion results into different categories; usually positive versus negative results.

cyclothymic disorder.   *DSM–5* chronic, although milder, form of bipolar disorder, which comprises alternations or mixtures of hypomanic and minor depressive symptoms. For children, the minimum duration of symptoms is one year without evidence of symptom remission.

D

data.   As defined by the Current Procedural Terminology (CPT) guidelines effective January 1, 2019, consists of both quantitative raw and transformed standard scores, whether linear or area transformations, qualitative classifications or descriptions (e.g., high average, borderline), and diagnostically relevant clinical interview facts and information.

debriefing.   Process whereby participants are completely apprised of the true nature of a research, assessment, or treatment procedure within which they were involved, including the hypothesis, the reasons why any deception was required if so used, the expected results, and permission from participants to use their data to be reported in the aggregate.

decay theory.   Explains forgetting as the weakening of a memory trace due a lack of re-exposure to or use of the pertinent information over time.

decision-making.   Part of executive functioning that involves choosing the correct action in the face of several alternatives.

declarative episodic memory (explicit memory).   Consciously remembering novel information that is bound by the testing situation; the type of memory measured by the WMS–IV.

decussation.   Refers to the fact that neural tracts from each cerebral hemisphere cross at the base of the neck and control the opposite side of the body.

deductive reasoning.   Logic proceeding from a general premise or hypothesis to a specific conclusion that is held to be true.

defensive functioning.   Refers to ego operations (mostly the defense mechanisms) that are targeted toward resolving conflict that is an inherent part of the personality.

deficits.   A lack of traits, skills, or abilities an individual should possess by a certain age or point in development.

defining traits.   Essential features of the newly proposed alternative dimensional model of personality disorders in the *DSM–5*; such features must be present or the diagnosis fails.

definite range.   On the SIRS–2, score pattern that ascertains the presence of feigning.

delay.   Occurs when a growing child is measured as being significantly behind in a particular line of development.

delayed memory.   The recall of learned information after an elapsed interval (e.g., 20 minutes) after exposure.

delinquent acts.   Violation of the law by a minor child or adolescent, either representing a crime if done by an adult (e.g., theft) or an adult legal act that is not permitted simply due to being younger than majority age (e.g., underage consumption of alcohol, violation of curfew), the latter being referred to a status offense.

delusional.   Referring to ideas and beliefs that are in contravention of reality.

dementia.   Neurocognitive disorder that deleteriously affects primarily cognitive functioning, including memory, attention, language (i.e., aphasia), visual-spatial ability, executive functioning, social perception, and sensory-motor functioning (i.e., ataxia). Use of this term in the *DSM–5* is significantly circumscribed due to accumulated negative connotation.

demographically corrected norms.   Standardization sample based on variables that have the most impact on the measured construct versus matching the sample according to general population statistics (usually using census data). In neuropsychological testing, these include age, education level, and sex.

demonstration items.   Test items done by the examiner that are designed to explain and illustrate via modeling the manner in which the items are completed.

demoralization.   Construct initially proposed by Jerome Frank, who applied it to people who described themselves as discouraged, low in self-esteem, and with expectations of failure and despair.

denial.   Something remembered although without being aware of its significance.

dependent variable.   The measured outcome that represents the predicted effect or association in an experiment or quasi-experiment, respectively.

depth theory.   Proposes that the human psyche is divided into a conscious level, semi-conscious level, and unconscious level and that human behavior must be understood in terms of exploring people's underlying motives and needs.

descriptive statistics.   Quantitatively summarizes data so meaningful or useful trends can be discerned for practical purposes.

detectability (d').   Specific measure on a Current Procedural Terminology (CPT) test that quantifies the ability of the examinee to discriminate targets from nontargets.

developmental coordination disorder.   Neurodevelopmental motor disorder in the *DSM–5* involving the inability to acquire and execute motor skills, which ultimately interferes substantially with the execution of daily activities. Also known as *childhood dyspraxia*.

developmental milestone/s.   Phylogenetic checkpoints in human development that determine what the average individual is able to do at a particular age. The measured average age and age range for the manifestation of various fundamental physical and cognitive skills during infancy and early childhood.

developmental norms.   Typical skills and achievement expected at particular ages; also known as *age norms*.

developmental psychopathology.   The study of abnormal behavior, which takes into account age as a key variable when describing, predicting, and explaining the onset and course of various neurodevelopmental disorders, mental health disorders, and personality disorders.

developmental psychopathology model. Paradigm in which childhood disorders are conceptualized as adaptational failures involving delay, fixation, regression, and/or deviance; i.e., childhood psychopathology is generally defined as a significant discrepancy from what is deemed developmentally normal or typical.

developmental test/s. Standardized age-related instrument that assesses fine and/or gross motor, language, cognitive, social, memory, and/or executive functions.

deviance. Adaptational failure in which some individual manifests thoughts, feelings, and/or behaviors deemed to be aberrant by statistical and/or social norms (e.g., IQ score in the bottom 2% of the population; a 20-year-old who hears ongoing voices not physically present and commanding self-destructive behavior).

deviant responses (DRs). R–PAS cognitive code of language and reasoning consisting of loosening of associations, incomprehensible explanations or elaborations, fluid and rambling responses, and fusion of contradictory connotations.

deviant verbalizations (DVs). R–PAS cognitive code of language and reasoning that occurs when the examinee uses incomprehensible, internally inconsistent, and contradictory words or phrases that result in communication failures and condensation of mutually exclusive elements.

deviation IQ. Intelligence measured by how many standard deviation units an individual's obtained score falls from the average of same-aged peers.

diagnoses to be ruled in/confirmed. A listing of one or more disorders that are already part of the working diagnoses but are now in question and in need of corroborating evidence.

diagnoses to be ruled out. A listing of one or more disorders that are suspected but not yet corroborated by supporting evidence.

diagnoses to be screened for. A listing of one or more disorders that are suspected, although usually to a lesser extent than those to be ruled out because only a brief examination is being requested.

diagnosis (psychodiagnosis). The practice of determining if an individual's reported, observed, and measured signs and symptoms are of sufficient frequency and/or intensity to meet the defined criteria of a clinical syndrome, neurodevelopmental disorder, or personality disorder. Such information determines treatment planning and intervention and is required when billing for mental health services rendered.

Diagnostic and Statistical Manual of Mental Disorders, Fifth Edition (DSM–5). The current official nosological system of mental disorders, neurodevelopmental disorders, and personality disorders adopted in the United States and published in 2013 by the American Psychiatric Association.

Diagnostic and Statistical Manual of Mental Disorders, Fourth Edition, Text Revision (DSM–IV–TR). The immediate predecessor to the *DSM–5* that was the official nosological system of mental disorders and personality disorders in the United States from 2000 through 2013 and published by the American Psychiatric Association. This was the last edition to include the multiaxial system of psychodiagnosis, most especially distinguishing clinical syndromes (i.e., Axis I) from personality disorders (Axis II).

Diagnostic and Statistical Manual of Mental Disorders, Third Edition, Revised (DSM–III–R). Predecessor to *DSM–IV* and *DSM–IV–TR* classification of mental disorders that was one of the initial editions to employ the multiaxial system of diagnosis.

Diagnostic Classification of Mental Health and Developmental Disorders of Infancy and Early Childhood (DC:0–5). Nosology of mental health and developmental disorders published by Zero to Three, which covers psychopathology that emerges any time from birth through age five.

diagnostic specifier. Added descriptor to a primary diagnosis, which is relevant to prognosis, course, and treatment.

differential. On the Conners CBRS forms, validity score that computes the absolute frequency of occurrence of discrepant ratings on similar items; measures the degree to which a respondent was inconsistent in providing ratings as one indication of possible invalidity.

differential diagnosis. The process of distinguishing the presence of one psychological disorder weighed against the probability of other disorders accounting for a client's presenting signs and symptoms.

diffusion. One of Marcia's four proposed identity statuses, which refers to an individual who is devoid of both crisis and commitment and is the most maladaptive.

digital clock. Device that represents a more exact time (versus an analog clock) by means of a numeric display.

dimensional approach. System of diagnosis in which psychological disorders are defined in terms of degrees of essential symptoms, each quantifiably measured on a continuum of severity and together forming a profile. An underlying assumption is that all individuals possess such symptoms to some extent, and those deemed "abnormal" possess excessive manifestations of the stated criteria.

disagreement response set. See *nay-saying response set.*

discharge. Termination process that renders an entire case inactive from the facility or practice in which professional services were provided.

discontinue rules. In adaptive standardized testing of cognitive abilities or skills, recommended rules for terminating the administration of a test or subtest, with the assumption that the examinee would no longer pass any further items.

discriminant analysis (DA). Statistical procedure that predicts group membership on a Y outcome variable (e.g., nonclinical or clinical) from a combination of numerical scores on several X predictor variables.

disengaged response pattern. A rare response style that occurs during a clinical interview when respondents are minimally involved in the assessment process, usually designed to intentionally mask their motive to feign the presence of psychopathology.

disengagement. A rare response style that occurs when respondents are minimally involved in the assessment process, typically for the purpose of avoiding the detection of feigning.

disengagement: indeterminate-evaluate. On the SIRS–2, classification indicating a lack of investment for the purpose of disguising the presence of feigning.

disinhibited social engagement disorder. Trauma- and stressor-related disorder in which the child manifests the presence of indiscriminate attachment, as evidenced by interacting with unfamiliar adults with an absence of due caution.

disorganized-disoriented attachment. Style of bonding in which the child shows an absence of emotional bonding and even fear of the major caretaker; considered the most disturbed of all the known emotional styles of bonding and is associated with pathogenic care (i.e., abuse and neglect).

displacement. Expression of an unacceptable thought or feeling onto a nonthreatening target.

dispositional domain. Major area of personality psychology theory and research that focuses on the inherent tendency of people to behave in a particular way; also known as the *study of human traits*.

disruptive behavior disorders. In earlier editions of the *DSM*, general cluster of clinical syndromes first evident in childhood and adolescence, which largely included externalizing, under-controlled, impulsive, acting-out symptoms or defenses as essential to the diagnosis.

disruptive mood dysregulation disorder (DMDD). Newly proposed *DSM–5* depressive disorder defined by (a) severe temper outbursts or rages (verbal and/or physical) in excess of situational circumstances, (b) minimum frequency of three times per week for one year manifested in at least two environments, (c) continuing irritable or angry mood between outbursts, and (d) appearance of symptoms between 6 and 18 years of age.

dissociation. Alternation or detachment in conscious awareness, memory, or identity, which is commonly found in trauma- and stressor-related disorders, although they can also appear under more commonly experienced conditions, including sleep deprivation, and other psychological disorders, including especially borderline personality disorder.

distractibility. An impairment in sustained attention within the context of extraneous stimuli (i.e., actions, sounds).

distractor. On the TOMM, line drawing that appears on a stimulus card paired with another line drawing referred to as the target; examinees are asked to point to the one they recognize from a prior learning phase (i.e., the target).

disuse. Another term for decay theory. See *decay theory*.

divided attention. Paying attention to two tasks simultaneously.

domain. As applied to the measurement of personality traits, the more general or broad-based disposition to behave in a particular manner. When measured or quantified, a domain consists of clusters of more narrowly defined and interrelated facets.

dopamine. Neurotransmitter produced primarily in the substantia nigra that is responsible for multiple functions, including motor control and response to reward and pleasure.

double-coding. Activities prompted during test administration that are intended to evoke examinee behaviors and reactions that can apply to multiple items, the effect of which is to speed administration time; typically observed in infant tests.

Draw-A-Family (DAF). Projective predecessor to the Kinetic Family Drawing in which examinees draw an akinetic drawing of themselves and their families. Thought to be limited due to the inert aspect of such productions.

***DSM* symptom counts (*DSM* count).** Categorical measure on the Conners CBRS that indicates whether criteria are met for a particular *DSM* clinical disorder or syndrome.

DTS. Abbreviation for "developmental test services," which includes developmental test administration, scoring, data interpretation, and report generation, defined within a 60-minute unit.

DTSA. Abbreviation for "developmental test services additional," which includes the added developmental test administration, scoring, data interpretation, and report generation services required in a developmental testing case, defined as added 30-minute units.

due care. Duty of care defined as the manner in which a reasonably prudent person would act in the same or similar circumstances; considered an objective standard in the law.

duty of care. The manner in which a reasonably prudent person would act in the same or similar circumstances; an objective legal standard that is applied to determine whether negligence has occurred. Those with professional education have the added duty to act as a reasonable person with that type of specialized training.

dysgraphia. Impairment in the ability to write, including problems with spelling, writing one's thoughts in a coherent manner, and motor difficulties in handwriting, all associated with neurological dysfunction. Also known as *agraphia*.

dyslexia. Impairment in the ability to read associated with an inability to make connections between letters and their sounds, which is also often associated with difficulties in spelling; impairment learning the sound-symbol system of language, thought to be caused by underlying neurological dysfunction.

Dyslexia index. New screening measure available on the WIAT-4.

dyspraxia (apraxia). The inability to perform intentional actions as the result of brain dysfunction, damage, or injury.

E

echolalia. Automatic repetition of someone else's speech or word phrases; a sign of autism.

ecological validity. The degree to which one can generalize psychological test results to the real-world environment.

effect size. Measure of the strength or magnitude of one variable's influence on another variable. The percentage of variability in one variable that can be accounted for or explained by another variable, which is a common type of effect size measure.

efficiency. As regarding psychological testing, use of the minimum number of tests, testing services, and units (or time) to sufficiently address the diagnostic issues in a particular case.

effortful control. Temperament dimension that includes the ability to focus, shift attention, inhibit responses, and appreciate activities that are low in stimulus intensity; to continue working until goal attainment.

ego dystonic. Behaviors, feelings, beliefs, or psychological symptoms that are viewed by the person as being inconsistent with his or her personality, hence implying an internal desire or motivation for change; considered a favorable prognostic sign for treatment. Also known as *ego alien*.

ego function assessment (EFA). Evaluation of an individual's personality development and adjustment according to 12 ego functions, which when aggregated and averaged, contribute to an overall ego strength score.

ego syntonic. State in which individuals perceive their psychological symptoms as acceptable and not foreign or distressing and are thus more difficult for clinicians to modify by means of therapeutic intervention.

EII-3 and Composite Calculations. Illustrated complex computations for the EII-3 and all composites on the R–PAS. Informs of the elements contributing to these composite variables to facilitate interpretation.

elaborative rehearsal. Expanding the meaning of specified information for the purpose of improving memory for such material (e.g., applying a new concept to one's own life circumstances).

emerging. Descriptor that precedes a personality disorder diagnosis to denote that it is still in its incipient stages and not yet fully developed (e.g., emerging borderline personality disorder).

emotion. Within the context of a mental status examination, observations of two aspects of a client's feelings, that is, affect and mood.

emotion regulation. The ability to manage and modulate feelings, affect, and arousal level, especially for negative feelings (e.g., anger); the processes involved in initiating, maintaining, and modifying affective responses according to situational demands.

emotional competence. The ability to manifest effective patterns of affective expression, increased comprehension of emotions (both self and others), and more efficacious emotion-regulation skills.

empathy. The ability to understand other people's thoughts, feelings, and symptoms from their own perspective.

empirical criterion keying. Statistical method that seeks to find items that best discriminate between a sample who has a particular disorder and a nonclinical sample, irrespective of the item content.

empirically based codetype interpretation. See *codetypes*.

empiricism. Belief that knowledge can be best gained by the collection of facts.

encoding. The process of transferring information into long-term memory storage.

encryption. Process that encodes data so that only select people who possess the correct password or secret key can read it.

engagement and cognitive processing variables.   In the R–PAS system, a cluster of scores that measure the thinking, reasoning, and problem-solving aspects of test behavior, including information about coping styles and ways of adapting to the world.

engram.   An alternate term for a physical memory trace in the brain.

epileptoid.   Personality trait that consists of being achievement oriented and meticulous.

episodic LTM.   Relatively permanent recall of eventful information.

episodic memory.   Refers to the recollection of events that occur in people's lives.

equivalent forms.   See *parallel forms*.

error score/s.   Score that quantifies the frequency of a particular type of incorrect response that has diagnostic value (e.g., letter reversals indicative of dyslexia).

error utilization.   Part of executive functioning that involves the ability to benefit from feedback.

essential symptoms.   Those features that represent the sine qua non of a clinical disorder; that is, without their presence, that disorder is deemed absent.

etiological variables.   Factors considered to be the origin or cause of particular psychological or mental disorders.

exact administration.   Providing instructions to the examinee that are identical to those given in a test's manual without any diversion.

executive functioning.   Ability to self-regulate, including paying attention, organizing, planning, prioritizing, focusing, managing emotions, and self-monitoring, which is principally located in the prefrontal cortex of the brain.

executive system (central executive system).   Theoretical component of human memory that provides key supervisory actions, including information flow, selective and sustained attention, and engagement of the long-term memory system.

experimentwise error rate.   See *familywise error rate*.

explicit measures.   Personality tests in which the informant is directly asked to assess the presence of certain specified traits, feelings, thoughts, and other aspects of examinees' personalities, whether it be self-report or observer-report.

explicit personality test/s.   Instruments that measure traits and symptoms in a direct and thus efficient manner, although makes it easy for examinees to intentionally distort the results by means of test-taking response sets involving impression formation.

explicit theories.   Explanatory models of intelligence that have empirical or scientific support.

exploratory factor analyses.   (1) Data reduction statistical procedure that reveals previously unknown clusters of inter-item correlations in a set of data referred to as factors, which represent latent variables that have potential explanatory power (e.g., quantitative reasoning). These factors are assigned summary terms based on the correlated item content. (2) Specific factor analytic statistical method employed when the internal structure of a psychological test is either completely unknown or theoretically proposed though not yet empirically investigated. See also *factor analysis*

expressive language.   Speech production.

extended battery.   In general, refers to an instrument's test or subtests that measure one or more supplemental constructs that add to test interpretation, although they are considered optional. As applied to the Woodcock–Johnson achievement test battery, refers to tests 12–20.

extended percentile ranks.   Added percentile rank values at both extreme ends of a distribution for the purpose of adding discriminatory power in those locations.

external referral.   Case sent for assessment and testing services by a health care provider affiliated with a facility outside of that where the testing psychologist is practicing.

extra-aggression.   Anger turned or directed toward outside forces or objects as opposed to oneself.

extracurricular.   Refers to activities that are outside the normal or expected course or career.

extrapunitive.   Tendency of an individual to direct blame or punishment toward persons other than oneself.

extraversion (or surgency).   Personality trait super-factor and temperament dimension that includes being active and confident, approaching novel situations with positive emotions, and easily and frequently interacting with people.

F

face validity.   Superficial appraisal that determines whether a test appears to measure what it purports to measure; also known as *logical validity*.

facet scales.   More narrowly defined traits that are part of a more broad-based personality domain, factor, or disposition.

face-to-face service. Psychological encounter (e.g., assessment, treatment) in which the client is physically present during a formally scheduled appointment.

factitious disorder. The intentional falsification of symptoms (i.e., *feigning*) in the absence of any identifiable external rewards.

factor analysis. Data reduction statistical procedure that identifies intercorrelated clusters of test items that represent latent variables or important psychological constructs.

factor loading. A correlation between an item and its factor that shows the amount of variance in the factor for which the item can account.

faking. Deliberate attempt on the part of respondents to distort the presence of symptoms when completing a psychological test, which can manifest as either exaggerating (i.e., *faking bad*) or minimizing (i.e., *faking good*) the presence of symptoms.

false negative (results). Regarding clinical psychological testing, a result that indicates the absence of a clinical syndrome or personality disorder when in fact it is present, that is, an *incorrect decision*.

false positive (results). Regarding clinical psychological testing, a result that indicates the presence of a clinical syndrome or personality disorder when in fact it is not present, that is, an *incorrect decision*.

false positive conclusions. Inference that renders a determination that something is present when in fact it is not; for example, determining that examinees are feigning psychopathology when in truth they are not.

familywise error rate. The accumulation of a *Type I error* rate (i.e., rejecting a true null hypothesis) with multiple hypothesis tests done within the same case or experiment. Also known as the *experimentwise error rate*.

feedback. A form of information-giving that works to confirm, modify, or broaden another's perspective.

feign. The deliberate fabrication or gross exaggeration of psychological or physical symptoms without any assumptions about its goals.

feigning. The deliberate fabrication or gross exaggeration of psychological and/or physical symptoms.

felonies. Serious crimes, frequently involving violence, and punishable by imprisonment within a penitentiary for more than one year and potentially by death.

fetus. Developing human from approximately the eighth week of gestation through birth at 38–40 weeks, considered to be full term, during which time all the major organs become increasingly refined by means of rapid growth until the final month of gestation.

final common pathway. Reference to memory because it represents the culmination of perception, attention, and executive functioning.

fine motor skills. Refers to physical abilities involving small or refined muscle movements, for instance, writing or drawing, typically developing later than *gross motor skills* or larger movements.

fissure. Term for a large sulcus or crease that usually forms a natural section of the brain.

fit. Regarding R–PAS coding of *form quality*, the estimated degree of match between the identified object with that of the inkblot contours at the location in which it was perceived, namely, poor, unusual, or ordinary.

Five-Factor Model (FFM). Trait theory that posits the presence of five broad dimensions of personality, including openness, conscientiousness, extraversion, agreeableness, and neuroticism, which was discovered by a combination of the lexical approach (i.e., that trait terms are embedded in our language) and statistical approach (i.e., factor analysis). Also known as the *Big Five*.

fixation. Adaptational failure in which an individual remains at an age-inappropriate immature stage of development. For example, a seven-year-old child who continues to show separation anxiety is considered abnormal, although this same reaction is considered indicative of secure (i.e., normal) attachment between 6 and 24 months.

fixed battery approach. Administration strategy that uses all tests or subtests that comprise a psychological or neuropsychological test battery without modifications.

fixed responding response set. Deliberately selecting consistently "True" or "False" response alternatives in stereotyped fashion without reading the items.

flash drive. See *thumb drive*.

flexible battery approach. Administration strategy that uses only those tests or subtests in a psychological or neuropsychological test battery needed to address the unique issues of a case.

flight of ideas. Pressure to continue talking with abrupt, rapid, and frequent topic shifts without elaboration, including words that impulsively trigger ensuing thoughts, associated with distractibility, and that does not answer the question posed.

fluency. The facility, smoothness, speed, and accuracy of completing a task.

fluent speech. Discourse that is smooth, forward moving, without hesitation, and seemingly effortless; antonym is *dysfluency*.

fluid intelligence.   Fundamental mental capacity that controls abstract problem solving and reasoning, which is considered culture free, independent of acquired knowledge, and genetically influenced; the ability to think logically and solve novel problems.

fluid reasoning.   Solving novel problems using abstract logical thinking.

Flynn effect.   Phenomenon in which IQ scores increase in the population by 3–5 points every decade, which means intelligence test norms must be updated every five years to avoid overestimating their examinees' intelligence.

forced choice.   Test items in which respondents must choose which of two or more alternatives best describe themselves.

foreclosure.   One of Marcia's four proposed identity statuses, which refers to an individual who has made a usually premature commitment in the absence of a crisis; a less favorable outcome.

form quality (FQ).   Rorschach scoring system codes designed to measure the accuracy of perceived objects according to both fit (i.e., the degree of match with the inkblot location) and frequency (i.e., the percentage of people in the norm group that perceived that object at that inkblot location).

formal thought disorder.   Diagnostic term used to designate the presence of extremely disturbed thinking, usually indicative of schizophrenia or another psychotic disorder.

frequency.   *Form quality (FQ)* component that measures how often the perceived object was reported at a particular inkblot location by those in the norm reference sample that is representative of the population; generally, the higher the frequency, the more favorable the FQ code.

functional emotional developmental capacities (FEDCS).   See *functional emotional milestones (FEMS).*

functional emotional milestones (FEMS).   Fundamental affective patterns that represent healthy psychological adjustment and provide purpose to an array of mental processes; also known as *functional emotional developmental capacities (FEDCS).*

functional systems model.   Complex interaction of brain regions, with each contributing a specialized role (i.e., a sub-role), first proposed by Luria and expanded upon in contemporary theorizing on brain functioning.

G

g.   Second-order latent variable used to explain a pattern of responses obtained by computing a full-scale IQ score.

g **factor.**   A proposed complex cognitive ability that is a component of many more narrowly defined cognitive abilities.

GABA (gamma-Aminobutyric acid, or γ-aminobutyric acid).   Inhibitory neurotransmitter in the central nervous system that reduces excitability.

general intelligence.   Overall complex mental ability defined as the capacity to acquire knowledge and information, to learn from experience, to use resources effectively in adapting to the environment, to comprehend, and to accurately use thought and reason to adapt to life's circumstances.

generalized anxiety disorder (GAD).   Anxiety disorder principally consisting of chronic apprehension, along with irritability, difficulty concentrating, muscle tension, and sleep disturbance.

genuine.   On the SIRS–2, classification indicating that the examinee was truthful and accurate in reporting symptoms of psychopathology.

Gf-Gc model of intelligence.   Two-factor theory of intelligence in which crystallized and fluid types of abilities comprise quantifiable lower-level or more specific abilities within a hierarchical organization.

Gilliam Asperger's Disorder Scale (GADS).   Observer-report unidimensional rating scale designed to detect symptoms of Asperger's syndrome, including an overall quotient, along with subscales that cover more specific areas of impairment. The measure is normed on individuals with documented diagnoses of Asperger's, ranging in age from 3 years, 0 months through 22 years, 11 months.

Gilliam Autism Rating Scale, Third Edition (GARS–3).   Observer-report unidimensional rating scale designed to detect symptoms of autism as defined by the *DSM–5*, including an overall index, along with subscales that cover more specific areas of impairment. The measure is normed on individuals with documented diagnoses of autism, ranging in age from 3 years, 0 months through 22 years, 11 months, including data for both verbal and nonverbal cases.

glial cells.   Another type of nerve cell in the central nervous system and brain that provides support, nourishment, and the protection of neurons.

gnosis.   The perceptual integrity of awareness and recognition (e.g., of faces).

grade equivalent (GE).   Median raw score for a particular grade level, usually reported in terms of grade and month of the academic year. Also known as a *grade score.*

grade scores. See *grade equivalent (GE)*.

Greenspan Social-Emotional Growth Chart: A Screening Questionnaire for Infants and Young Children. Delineates the functional emotional milestones identified by Greenspan, including six stages (or capacities) for children from birth through 42 months.

gross motor skills. Refers to physical abilities involving large muscle movements, for instance, running and jumping, typically developing earlier than fine motor skills or smaller movements.

growth scale values (GSVs). Scores that permit the tracking of an individual's progress on particular skills over time (i.e., over grades or ages). It compares individuals' growth regarding their own previous skill level and not to those of their peers as do norm-based standard scores.

guardian. Adult authorized by a court to have a legal decision-making power and a corresponding duty of care to an individual who is not autonomous by law and/or due to incapacity.

guardianship. Exists when the court authorizes a legal relationship between an adult and another individual who is not autonomous by law and/or due to incapacity, wherein the former has decision-making power and a corresponding duty of care to the latter.

gyri (gyrus, singular). Protuberances that form part of the convolutions of the cerebral cortex.

H

habituation. Diminution of an infant's response to repeated presentations of the same stimulus, that is, learning to be bored.

halo effect. Phenomenon wherein a prior global impression created in one area influences succeeding impressions in other areas, either in a positive or negative direction.

haptic. The sense of touch and proprioception.

harsh superego introject. In psychoanalytic theory, the internalization of excessively stringent morals and principles by means of one's relationship with a severely strict parental figure. Such an individual would be considered prone to anxiety and depression due to possessing excessively austere internal standards.

hassles. Small frustrations, annoyances, aggravations, or minor disagreements that occur on a daily basis or fairly frequently and which can cause some degree of irritation or distress.

Head Start. U.S. government-funded program with the objective of facilitating early childhood education, which includes a special focus on children deemed to be high-risk up to age five.

Health Insurance Portability and Accountability Act of 1996 (HIPPA). U.S. federal law designed to assist people in maintaining their health insurance, safeguard the confidentiality and security of their health care information, and control administrative costs.

hemispheres. Left and right halves of the brain that are specialized for different functions in humans, which control the contralateral (i.e., opposite) side of the body.

heritability. The proportion of individual differences in an observed or measured trait that is due to genetic variance.

hierarchical model of intelligence. Theory in which intelligence was thought to be composed of the three levels or strata of factors, with the *g* factor at the top (Stratum III), broad factors at the mid-level (Stratum II), and specific abilities at the bottom level (Stratum I).

hierarchy of presses. A multiphasic item subdivided into a ranked stepwise series of related activities, which together are designed to elicit progressively more sophisticated or complex responses on the part of the examinee.

high school certificate of completion. Signifies that the student has passed an alternate plan of study that does not include all the curricular requirements for graduation.

high school diploma. Signifies that the student has met all the curriculum and examination requirements for graduation.

high-stakes testing. Psychological testing used to render vital decisions about people.

hindbrain. Lowest set of brain structures located just above the spinal cord that regulate survival functions, including body balance, breathing, and arousal.

hippocampus. Horseshoe-shaped structure within the limbic system that is vital for the formation and storage of new memories, along with learning and emotions.

historical diagnosis. Disorder that has been assigned to a client at some point prior to the current assessment, which remains pending any subsequent contradictory evidence; designation indicating that such a disorder was not the target or focus of a current test battery.

histrionic personality disorder. Cluster B characterological diagnosis in which the individual expresses dramatic, shallow, rapidly shifting, and exaggerated emotions, manifests an insatiable need to be the center of attention, is ostentatious and seductive in physical appearance, is suggestive, and considers relationships to be more intimate than reality dictates.

Hit Reaction Time (HRT).   Specific measure on a Current Procedural Terminology (CPT) test that quantifies the examinee's mean or average reaction time to stimuli.

holophrases.   Single-word utterances usually accompanied by gestures; part of normal language milestones in early development.

HRT ISI Change.   Specific measure on a Current Procedural Terminology (CPT) test that quantifies the degree to which examinees remain consistent with longer inter-stimulus intervals (ISIs) versus impulsively responding prior to stimulus presentation.

hypersomnia.   Sleeping more than is typical without feeling rested, usually a symptom of a mood disorder.

hypervigilance.   Excessive preoccupation and alertness to potential danger in the environment, typically associated with severe trauma-related disorders, such as post-traumatic stress disorder (PTSD), along with paranoid personality disorder if such becomes an ingrained and inflexible trait.

hypothalamus.   Small brain region that controls basic kinds of motivation (e.g., hunger, thirst, sleep) and activates the sympathetic nervous system (i.e., the fight-or-flight response) in coping with stress.

I

ideal self.   The manner in which individuals define who they would like to become in terms of their fullest potential.

identity achievement.   Marcia's elaboration of Erikson's adolescent stage of identity versus role confusion, wherein the individual makes a commitment and has put forth sufficient effort in meeting such a pledge; considered to be the healthiest of identity outcomes.

identity diffusion.   Marcia's elaboration of Erikson's adolescent stage of identity versus role confusion, wherein the individual fails to make a commitment and is not even making such effort; considered to be the most pathological of identity outcomes.

identity versus role confusion.   Erikson's proposed fifth stage of psychosocial development covering the teenage years (i.e., ages 12–18), which focuses on the task of self-definition and developing a clear direction in life.

illness anxiety disorder.   Psychopathology in which people continue to grossly exaggerate the meaning of bodily sensations, such that they believe they are suffering from a variety of serious medical diseases and in which reassurance is fruitless. Previous term was *hypochondriasis*.

image degradation techniques.   Continuous performance test task that present stimuli according to graded levels of blurring to determine if this has a differential impact on sustained and selective attention.

imagination.   The creativity or fantasy needed to generate projective stories to interpersonal scenes, such as those presented in the TAT and CAT card stimuli, which is considered part of the autonomous functioning of the ego (i.e., the conflict-free or non-defensive sphere of the ego, according to the tenets of ego psychology).

immediate memory.   The recall of information instantly after exposure.

implicit measures.   Personality tests that measure particular characteristics of the examinee without asking them directly; for example, by measuring how the examinee reacts to certain stimuli.

implicit needs.   Internal desires of an individual, which are measured indirectly by means of a performance personality test.

implicit personality test/s.   Instrument that measures traits and symptoms in an indirect manner, which makes it more difficult for examinees to intentionally distort the results by means of test-taking response sets, although it measures constructs in a more indirect manner and thus requires more time and effort on the part of both the examiner and examinee.

implicit theories.   Subjective conceptualizations of intelligence or other psychological constructs used by laypeople according to their experiences in real life.

impression management.   Attempt made by examinees to control the manner in which they are perceived by others.

improbable or absurd symptoms.   Feigning strategy in which individuals report symptoms that are preposterous, outlandish, or of dubious probability.

incidental learning (automatic learning).   The gaining of knowledge without intention.

inconsistent responding.   Response set that occurs when an individual answers similar items in contradictory ways.

independent variable.   Any manipulated condition or characteristic in an experiment or quasi-experiment, which is the proposed cause of, or that is correlated with, a predicted outcome.

indeterminate-evaluate. On the SIRS–2, classification indicating that the likelihood of feigning exceeds 50%; that is, feigning is more likely than not.

indeterminate-general. On the SIRS–2, classification indicating that there is only a 34.3% likelihood of feigning; that is, feigning is more likely to be absent than present.

Individualized Education Plan (IEP). Synonym for Individualized Education Program (IEP) that is used in the United Kingdom and Canada.

Individualized Education Program (IEP). Document that delineates a child's special academic needs and strategies to meet those needs, along with any reassessments and noted progress. Required for all children with a documented learning disability or handicap pursuant to the Individuals with Disabilities Act [IDEA], Public Law 104–446. Synonym for *Individualized Education Plan* used in the United Kingdom and Canada. See also *Individualized Education Plan.*

Individuals with Disabilities Education Improvement Act (IDEA). U.S. federal law mandating that all individuals be afforded access to educational services, including the provision of any special interventions and accommodations that make this possible.

Individuals with Disabilities Education Improvement Act of 2004 (IDEA, 2004). Law designed to ensure that all children with disabilities are entitled to a free appropriate public education (FAPE) to meet their unique needs.

inductive reasoning. Logic proceeding from specific instances or facts to general laws.

industry versus inferiority. Erikson's proposed fourth stage of psychosocial development of school age (i.e., ages 6–11) in which children focus on mastering both cognitive and social skills, largely by means of social comparison.

inferential norming. A quantitative process in which a standardization sample's basic score distribution characteristics (i.e., mean, variance, skewness) are used to estimate the same characteristics for an entire representative population, which are then used as standards for examinees who subsequently complete the test or measure.

inferential statistics. Quantitative methods performed on representative samples of data that permit one to draw conclusions about populations.

information processing (multistore model). Model that analogizes the workings of human cognition to that of a computer, including the flow of data through a series of hypothetical storage compartments that differ in terms of capacity and duration.

information processing tasks. Actions that manipulate data to accomplish some kinds of objectives or goals, including such things as problem solving, learning, and recalling material previously stored.

information-giving. Counseling microskill in which the clinician provides needed education to a client about a pertinent topic or issue.

informed consent. An individual's voluntary agreement to participate in a procedure after being fully apprised of its nature, potential benefits and risks, and any alternatives, including the right to withdraw at any point. Comprises the following five elements: (a) authority to consent, (b) having the requisite information and knowledge, (c) understanding the information, (d) voluntariness, and (e) documentation.

inhibitory control. The ability to resist urges to engage in enticing behavior and to consciously stop automatic (i.e., overlearned or habitual) behaviors when so desired.

initial clinical interview. See *clinical interview.*

initiation. The ability to begin a task effectively and in a timely fashion.

insidious onset. Extremely gradual development of symptoms such that the disorder in question is initially masked and not detected until its later stages. Typically, such disorders are progressive and severe (e.g., Alzheimer's dementia).

insomnia. Any inability to sleep an average 8 hours within a 24-hour circadian cycle, including sleep onset type, intermittent wakening, poor-quality sleep, and early morning waking, typically secondary to another more major mental disorder, such as major depression. In the absence of another mental disorder and causing dysfunction, sleep problems are diagnosed as "primary insomnia," in which case situational stress factors are usually contributory.

institutional review board (IRB). A group comprising university faculty and at least one member from the community who have the responsibility for reviewing proposals for human and animal research to ensure the safety of the participants.

instructional zone. A continuum of development for learning apportioned into zones ranging from easy (i.e., the independent level) to difficult (i.e., the dependent-on-others level).

intellectual disability (ID). Neurodevelopmental disorder showing significant impairment or delay in (a) intelligence and (b) adaptive behavior, with onset prior to the age of 18. Adaptive behavior now determines ID severity level. Previous term for such a disorder was mental retardation (MR). Also known as *intellectual developmental disorder (IDD)*.

intellectualization.   Psychoanalytic defense mechanism in which thinking and reasoning are used to block threatening emotions from conscious awareness; a form of *isolation*.

intelligence quotient (IQ).   Began as the ratio of mental age divided by chronological age, then multiplied by 100 to drop any decimal places. Currently used as a generic term for an individual's IQ composite or factor scores irrespective of their method of computation.

intelligence.   The ability to learn from experience, acquire knowledge, and use resources effectively in adapting to new situations or solving problems. This construct is typically measured by the full-scale IQ score, which represents the *g* factor or latent variable derived from factor analysis.

intelligence test/s.   A psychological measure of an individual's mental competence.

interactive feedback.   Face-to-face oral feedback regarding psychological test results, which is now considered a billable service.

interference.   Loss of memory due to competing information.

interference theory.   Explanation of forgetting due to similar competing information presented within a short period of time.

internal consistency reliability.   Degree to which items that comprise a psychological test are intercorrelated.

internal referral.   Case that is transferred to a testing psychologist from a mental health clinician within the same agency or group practice. Also known as a *transfer*.

internal working model/s.   Covert mental representations of the self in relationship to others, formed through a child's early experiences with primary caregivers, which sets expectations regarding (a) worthiness of the self and (b) others' reactions to the self.

International Classification of Diseases, 10th Revision (ICD–10), Classification of Mental and Behavioural Disorders.   Nosology of all recognized diseases, which includes a section devoted to mental and behavioral disorders, published by the World Health Organization (WHO). The *DSM* system is becoming increasing compatible with the ICD system.

International Classification of Diseases, 10th Revision, Clinical Modification (ICD–10–CM).   International nosology of diseases that includes a classification of mental and behavioral disorders recognized by the World Health Organization (WHO).

interpersonal.   Refers to relations between people that affect the individual's behavior.

interpolation.   Statistical procedure in which established or known values along a sequence are used to estimate unknown values along that same sequence.

interrater reliability.   Degree to which individuals who provide separate ratings of an examinee are consistent with each other.

inter-stimulus interval (ISI).   The time between repeated presentations of a stimulus.

intra-aggression.   Anger turned or directed toward the self.

introject.   The mental incorporation of parts of previous significant people such that those dynamics continue to manifest themselves in some form in the present day (e.g., a client's intropunitive behavior stemming from an introjected abusive parent). Also referred to as *introjection*.

intropunitive.   Tendency of an individual to direct blame or punishment inward toward oneself. In psychoanalytic theory, an excessively harsh superego introject. See also *introject*.

introspection.   The process of scrutinizing one's own thoughts and feelings to better understand oneself and the reason for one's reactions and behaviors; psychological mindedness.

Iowa Assessments (Iowa Test of Basic Skills).   Standardized test of achievement that is group administered and employed by school systems to show evidence of student learning.

ipsative analysis.   Intraindividual examination of a person's test scores to determine relative strengths and weaknesses. Relative comparisons among an individual's scores within a multidimensional test designed to identify strengths and weaknesses, typically by means of pairwise comparisons or deviations from the examinee's average score. Compared with *norm-based comparisons*.

ipsative.   (1) Forced-choice measurements in surveys; the respondent must choose between two items of equivalent social desirability. (2) Refers to a comparing of an examinee's own test scores with themselves versus those provided by a norm reference sample. Reveals an examinee's relative strengths and weaknesses.

IQ.   Conventional abbreviation for Intelligence Quotient. Typically denotes a major score on a formal intelligence test at the full-scale or index level of measurement.

isolation.   Removing from conscious awareness the emotional significance of an event. See also *intellectualization*.

item response theory (IRT). Psychometric approach in which individuals' degree of possessing a particular characteristic is related to the likelihood that they will pass an item of a specified level of difficulty; the more of the characteristic individuals possesses, the more likely they will pass an item of greater difficulty.

item sets. Groups of items that denote a particular difficulty level, typically done with skills that are most easily measured in sets (e.g., five questions examining comprehension of a reading passage of a particular difficulty level).

J

Journal of Social and Personal Relationships. Peer-reviewed, multidisciplinary journal that focuses on the development of interpersonal relationships by drawing material from the fields of social psychology, clinical psychology, communication, developmental psychology, and sociology.

judgment. As an ego function, refers to how well one can anticipate or discern the likelihood of danger, being censured by others, engaging in behavior considered inappropriate by others, or being subject to disapproval.

juvenile delinquency. Regards a minor child or adolescent, typically between the ages of 10 and 18, who has committed an act that has violated the law in some way.

K

Kappa statistic (k). Quantitative measure of interrater reliability for qualitative (i.e., categorical) variables (e.g., psychiatric diagnosis), which is more accurate than simple percent agreement between judges because it accounts for chance. Values range from less than 0.00 to 1.00, with less than 0.00 indicating less than chance agreement and 0.81 to 1.00 indicating almost perfect agreement. Also known as *Kappa coefficient.*

Kinetic Drawing System for Family and School (Kinetic Drawing System). Projective technique in which examinees are asked to draw a picture of themselves and their families doing something together, which is later analyzed in terms of frequencies of various characteristics that have interpretive meaning.

Kinetic-Family-Drawing (KFD). Part of the Kinetic Drawing System that focuses on examinees' dynamic projective drawings of themselves and their families.

Kinetic-School-Drawing (KSD). Part of the Kinetic Drawing System that focuses on examinees' dynamic projective drawings of themselves, teacher, and one or two friends at school.

L

La Psychologie Individuelle. Publication in 1895 by Binet and Henri that proposed one of the first models of intelligence.

language. Communication system in which a limited number of signals (i.e., sounds, letters, gestures) can be integrated according to rules, which are capable of generating an infinite number of messages.

language disorder. Impairment in receptive and/or expressive communication that causes significant dysfunction.

lateral sulcus (Sylvian fissure). Large division of the brain running horizontally between the frontal–parietal lobes and the temporal lobe.

lateralization (of function). Refers to the left and right hemispheres of the brain being specialized for different functions.

law of causality. Principle in philosophy proposing that every change in nature is produced by some kind of etiology; in psychology, belief that every behavior has an underlying meaningful cause.

learning and memory. The ability to acquire, retain, and access newly stored information.

learning disabilities (LD). Conditions with an underlying neurological dysfunction associated with impairments in acquiring various academic skills, especially those in reading, written expression, and mathematics.

left hemisphere. In most people, the side of the brain that is specialized for language, sequential processing, logical reasoning (e.g., mathematics and science), and control of the right side of the body.

legal custody. Authority by law afforded a primary caretaker to make major decisions for a minor child; may be shared between separated or divorced parents.

lexical approach. Strategy used to identify the most important traits, based on the assumption that vital individual differences in personality become encoded into our natural language over time because they maximize adaptation.

liberal response style. Tending toward stating that a stimulus was present when uncertain.

Likert-type (rating) scale. Test item beginning with a statement regarding a psychological symptom, trait, behavior, attitude, or belief, ensued by a five-point scale to which respondents indicate the extent to which they agree or disagree with the statement. Such a scale is typically considered to represent an interval scale of measurement, hence permitting the addition of all such items on a test to compute a total or composite score.

limbic system. Network of subcortical structures that generally controls emotion, motivation, learning, and memory in humans.

linear transformation/s. Raw score to standard score conversions in which the exact positions of scores in a distribution are both preserved and made explicit to facilitate test interpretation, although this tends to be more difficult for laypeople to comprehend. Such transformations are generally performed by adding, subtracting, multiplying, or dividing by a constant and is analogous to converting units of measurement for purposes of interpretive convenience (e.g., inches to feet).

lobes. Additional divisions of the cerebral hemispheres into four sections, each having different functions, including frontal, temporal, occipital, and parietal.

localization of function approach. Theory that defines brain functioning according to which area is being focused on (e.g., left versus right hemisphere).

logistic regression. Statistical procedure that analyzes whether several continuous variables can accurately predict an individual's classification within a nominal type variable.

longitudinal fissure. Major natural division that divides the brain into left and right hemispheres.

long-term memory (LTM). Concerning the information-processing model of human memory, the storage compartment that theoretically consists of recollections of unlimited capacity and duration.

long-term potentiation. The enduring modifications in electrical potential between neurons that make up a lasting circuit or relatively permanent memory trace.

loosening of associations. Breakdown of meaningful connections between ideas that is considered more pathological than circumstantiality.

low base-rate variable. As applied to the R–PAS, variables that occur in only a small fraction of all protocols.

M

maintenance rehearsal. Method of retaining memory by simply repeating or paying attention to the information indefinitely such that it does not decay or fade.

major depressive disorder (MDD). *DSM–5* depressive disorder that consists of a major depressive episode and an absence of prior or current manic or hypomanic episodes. Principal specifiers include those for severity level, with anxious distress, with mixed features, and with atypical features.

major depressive disorder, severe. A major depressive episode that includes most or all criteria, although without psychotic features.

major depressive disorder, severe, with anxious distress, moderate. A major depressive episode that includes most or all criteria, although without psychotic features and with a DSM–5 specifier "anxious distress of moderate severity," which indicates a more guarded prognosis. See also *specifier*.

major depressive disorder, with melancholic features. Severe depressive disorder marked by an absence of reactivity, lost pleasure, vegetative symptoms, profound despondency, and excessive guilt.

major depressive episode (MDE). Characterized by a minimum of five of the following symptoms for at least a two-week duration and must include either one of the first two enumerated here: (a) sad or irritable mood, (b) lost interest or anhedonia, (c) sleep disturbance, (d) appetite disturbance, (e) agitation or slowed movements, (f) fatigue, (g) low self-esteem, (h) excessive guilt, (i) thoughts or attempts to kill oneself, and (j) impaired concentration or decision-making.

major neurocognitive disorder/s. Acquired brain dysfunction due to a possible or probable etiology and consisting of the following: (a) subjectively reported severe decline in functioning from previous levels, (b) neuropsychological test standard scores falling two or more standard deviations below the normative mean (i.e., a *PR* of 3 and below), and (c) such decline interfering with at least some degree of independent functioning.

major neurocognitive disorder due to Parkinson's disease. Acquired severe impairment in mental abilities secondary to Parkinson's disease, which is a progressive neurological disorder due to the brain's inability to produce sufficient dopamine, largely causing motor dysfunction.

major neurocognitive disorder due to traumatic brain injury. Acquired severe impairment in mental abilities due to physical injury to the brain.

majority of examples ADOS–2 items. Items that are scored based on the relevant behaviors that dominate the examinee's responses.

malingering. The deliberate fabrication or gross exaggeration of signs or symptoms of a disorder or disability for personal gain.

Malingering Rule 1. On the TOMM, feigning rule based on a 50% probability of obtaining a correct response by random guessing; any score below 50% (i.e., below 25 of 50 selections) is positive evidence of feigning. Also known as the *scoring lower than chance rule*.

Malingering Rule 2. On the TOMM, feigning rule based on empirical evidence that the lower an obtained score falls below 45, the greater the likelihood of feigning (and malingering) on the part of the examinee.

masochistic personality syndrome. Individuals who manifest behaviors that undermine their own well-being and are unconsciously attracted to pain and suffering. Also known as *self-defeating personality syndrome*.

Mastery–competence. People's ability to perform effectively relative to their stated capacities to actively interact and successfully cope with environmental forces.

math fluency. The rate or speed of recalling fundamental math facts with automaticity and without hesitation.

maze-tracing paradigm. Model in which examinees must trace their way out of mazes of increasing complexity, typically timed, and prohibiting the lifting of the writing utensil from the page once the mazes are begun.

mean (M or $\bar{x}$). The arithmetic average of a set of scores. It is the most common measure of central tendency in a set of data. Its principal strengths are that (a) it represents the best estimate of the corresponding population mean and (b) it can be algebraically manipulated.

mechanical perseveration. Responses that are repeated in stereotyped fashion without intervening responses of a different quality.

mechanisms. Underlying processes of personality, most of which comprise perceptual or information-processing actions and consist of the following three stages: (a) encoding, (b) cognitive reasoning and decision-making, and (c) behavioral output.

medical necessity. The general standard used by health care insurance companies to determine whether a testing procedure or treatment is warranted and thereby covered under the patient's health care plan. The specific criteria vary depending on (a) the insurance carrier and (b) the particular health care plan offered and selected by the patient.

medical record. Systematic written documentation of an individual's psychological and physical history, presenting symptoms, diagnoses, tests and test results, treatment recommendations and interventions, and progress over time and under a health care provider's jurisdiction.

medically necessary. Phrase used that refers to the criteria employed by health insurance companies to determine if a procedure is justified and should be preauthorized (PA) or approved.

melancholy. Form of severe and chronic depression characterized a notable absence of reactivity, lost pleasure, vegetative symptoms, profound despondency, and excessive guilt.

memory. The ability to recall information to which one has been previously exposed; the process of retaining and retrieving information.

memory for sound patterns (UM). Recollection of auditory types of information, including both non-speech and speech sounds.

memory stick. See *thumb drive*.

memory trace/s (engram/s). Stable neural connection in the brain thought to represent a long-term memory. Physical changes in the brain associated with neuron activity, which form when a person is exposed to various kinds of information.

menarche. The first menstrual cycle or first menstrual bleeding, often considered to represent a central element of puberty.

mental age (MA). The highest age-level items that examinees could pass, usually with a pre-specified proportion.

mental development. Typically refers to the progression of cognitive abilities, including thinking, reasoning, language, and memory.

mental disorder due to another medical condition. Psychopathology that is caused by a bona fide medical disorder or disease process.

mental flexibility. Part of executive functioning that involves the ability to shift to different rules, such as naming the correct arrow direction followed by naming the opposite direction.

Mental Functioning (M) Axis. In psychodynamic diagnosis, a dimension that consists of a number of more narrowly defined capacities that contribute to general personality organization and functioning, which are organized according to four domains as follows: (a) cognitive and affective processes, (b) identity and relationships, (c) defense and coping, and (d) self-awareness and self-direction.

mental health and developmental disorders. Diagnostic dimension that includes clinical syndromes, neurodevelopmental disorders, and personality disorders.

mental health parity laws. Legislation passed by most states that together require health insurance carriers to cover mental health disorders as equivalent to physical illnesses, diseases, or injuries.

mental status examination (MSE). Observation of the manner in which a patient thinks, feels, and behaves during an initial clinical interview, which helps determine the likelihood that one or more psychological disorders are present.

metric system. Units of measurement utilized by countries outside of the United States, which applies the idea that measurements become smaller and larger by a power of 10 (e.g., kilometer, meter, decimeter, centimeter, and millimeter).

middle responding. Response set in which an individual tends to answer toward the center of the scale; that is, neutral or moderate responses.

Millon Adolescent Clinical Inventory (MACI). Self-report personality inventory that facilitates the diagnosis of emerging or present personality disorders, along with related clinical syndromes and concerns, normed on individuals ranging in age from 13 years, 0 months through 19 years, 11 months; predecessor to the MACI–II.

Millon Adolescent Clinical Inventory, Second Edition (MACI–II). Self-report personality inventory for adolescents, consisting of 24 clinical scales that are presented in three sections as follows: (a) personality patterns (i.e., stable patterns of characteristics), (b) clinical syndromes (i.e., acute and transient clinical disorders), and (c) expressed concerns (i.e., distress in self-oriented and interpersonally based areas).

Millon Behavioral Health Inventory (MBHI). Immediate predecessor to the MBMD, which was developed from 1974 through 1983 and used frequently over the approximate 20 years of its existence.

Millon Behavioral Medicine Diagnostic (MBMD). Self-report inventory for individuals aged 18 years, 0 months through 85 years, 11 months, principally designed to assess psychological factors that can potentially influence the course of treatment for medical patients.

Millon Behavioral Medicine Diagnostic, Bariatric Norms (MBMD, Bariatric). Self-report inventory for individuals aged 18 years, 0 months through 85 years, 11 months, which is principally designed to assess psychological factors that can potentially influence the course of treatment for candidates of bariatric weight-loss surgery.

Millon Behavioral Medicine Diagnostic, Pain Norms (MBMD, Pain). Self-report inventory for individuals aged 18 years, 0 months through 85 years, 11 months, which is principally designed to evaluate psychological factors that can potentially influence the course of treatment for chronic pain patients.

Millon Clinical Multiaxial Inventory, Fourth Edition (MCMI–IV). Self-report personality inventory that facilitates the diagnosis of emerging or present personality disorders, along with related clinical syndromes, normed on individuals aged 18 years, 0 months through adulthood. This is the newest version of the adult MCMI series, with some added personality disorders (e.g., turbulent personality) and modifications to render this edition more conducive to *DSM–5* nomenclature (e.g., persistent depressive disorder versus dysthymia).

Millon Clinical Multiaxial Inventory, Third Edition (MCMI–III). Self-report personality inventory that facilitates the diagnosis of emerging or present personality disorders, along with related clinical syndromes, normed on individuals aged 18 years, 0 months through 88 years, 11 months. The immediate predecessor to the MCMI–IV.

Millon Pre-Adolescent Clinical Inventory (M–PACI). Self-report personality inventory that facilitates the diagnosis of emerging or present personality disorders, along with related clinical syndromes and concerns, normed on individuals aged 9 years, 0 months through 12 years, 11 months.

Millon's biosocial learning evolutionary theory. Theory proposing that people's behavior is influenced by an integration of learned strategies to (a) secure reinforcement and (b) minimize punishment for purposes of adaptation to the environment.

Mini-Mental State Examination (MMSE). Performance-based screening measure designed to indicate whether a neurocognitive disorder may be present in adults. Predecessor to the MMSE–2 and item content is equivalent to the MMSE–2 standard version.

Mini-Mental State Examination, Second Edition (MMSE–2). Screening measure designed to indicate whether a neurocognitive disorder may be present in adults. Data are performance based.

Mini-Mental State Examination, Second Edition, Brief Version, Blue/Red Form (MMSE–2–BV–BF). Performance-based screening measure designed to indicate whether a neurocognitive disorder may be present in adults. Consists of only 4 of the 13 items in the expanded version of this measure for a maximum of 16 points, with a cut-off raw score of 14 or less indicating a positive result for neurocognitive dysfunction. There are parallel blue and red forms.

Mini-Mental State Examination, Second Edition, Expanded Version, Blue/Red Form (MMSE–2–EV–BF/RF). Performance-based screening measure designed to indicate whether a neurocognitive disorder may be present in adults. Consists of 13 items for a maximum of 90 points, with a cut-off raw score of 50 or less indicating a positive result for neurocognitive dysfunction. There are parallel blue and red forms.

Mini-Mental State Examination, Second Edition, Standard Version, Blue/Red Form (MMSE–2–SV–BF/RF). Performance-based screening measure designed to indicate whether a neurocognitive disorder may be present in adults. Consists of 11 of the 13 items in the expanded version of this measure for a maximum of 30 points, with a cut-off raw score of 27 or less indicating a positive result for neurocognitive dysfunction. There are parallel blue and red forms.

Minnesota Multiphasic Personality Inventory (MMPI). First edition of this personality test that was initially distributed in 1940 and consisted of eight basic clinical scales developed according to the diagnostic nosological system of the 1930s and originally published across a number of articles.

Minnesota Multiphasic Personality Inventory, Adolescent (MMPI–A). Self-report personality inventory that facilitates the diagnosis of clinical syndromes and emerging or present personality disorders, which is normed on individuals aged 14 years, 0 months through 18 years, 11 months. Disadvantages include its long length and excessive inter-scale item overlap, the latter reducing its ability to discriminate among various *DSM–5* disorders.

Minnesota Multiphasic Personality Inventory, Adolescent, Restructured Form (MMPI–A–RF). Self-report personality inventory normed on individuals aged 14 years, 0 months through 18 years, 11 months. It was developed through a multivariate factor reanalysis of MMPI–A items using the same standardization sample, is significantly shorter in length, and possesses superior discriminant and convergent validity due to a significant reduction in scale intercorrelations.

Minnesota Multiphasic Personality Inventory, Second Edition (MMPI–2). Self-report personality inventory that facilitates the diagnosis of clinical syndromes and personality disorders, normed on individuals aged 18 years, 0 months through 89 years, 11 months. Disadvantages include its long length and excessive inter-scale item overlap, the latter reducing its ability to discriminate among various *DSM–5* disorders.

Minnesota Multiphasic Personality Inventory, Second Edition, Restructured Form (MMPI–2–RF). Self-report personality inventory normed on individuals aged 18 years, 0 months through 89 years, 11 months. It was developed through a multivariate factor reanalysis of MMPI–2 items using its standardization sample. Its two main advantages over the MMPI–2 are (a) a significantly shorter length and (b) a superior degree of discriminant and convergent validity due to a significant reduction in scale intercorrelations.

Minnesota Multiphasic Personality Inventory, Third Edition (MMPI–3). Newest of the MMPI self-report personality inventories normed on individuals aged 18 years, 0 months through 80-plus years according to 2020 U.S. census projections. It possesses a structure very similar to the MMPI–2–RF, although with some expansion of construct coverage while maintaining the same approximate length at 335 items.

minor neurocognitive disorder/s. Lesser severe acquired dysfunction in mental abilities due to a possible or probable etiology and consisting of the following: (a) subjectively reported modest decline in functioning from previous levels, (b) neuropsychological test standard scores falling between one and two SDs below the normative mean (i.e., PR between 3 and 16), and (c) such decline reducing the quality of life, although not interfering with independent functioning.

minus form quality (FQ–). In R–PAS coding, the percept is infrequent or rare and clearly inaccurate, distorted, or arbitrary in terms of fit.

mirror neuron systems. Proposed group of specialized nerve cells that fire in a parallel manner to the actions and behaviors of others, thought to facilitate empathy, social cognition, language, and the learning of skills through observation.

misdemeanors. Lesser crimes or minor offenses, punishable by fines or local incarceration for up to one year.

moments. Basic parameters of a score distribution, which together provide a complete picture of its characteristics, most frequently including the mean and variance.

mood. The overall emotional tone or general emotional trend as expressed by a client during the course of an entire clinical interview.

mood disorders with psychotic features. Disorders in which emotional disturbance is principal, with secondary symptoms indicating some disconnection from reality, such as the presence of delusions and hallucinations.

moratorium. One of Marcia's four proposed identity statuses, which refers to an individual who is in the midst of a crisis but has not yet reached a genuine commitment; assumed to be favorable in the sense that a commitment would eventually be obtained assuming that the person perseveres toward goal attainment.

morbid special score (MOR). Coded response in the Rorschach-CS and R–PAS, which includes damage, injury, disease, or death, and is interpreted as a sign of depression.

morphosyntactic development. Progression of the ability to understand how word forms change and are assembled within a sentence to establish meaning.

motor coordination. Muscle groups that work together to produce accurate manual output.

motor disorders. *DSM–5* neurodevelopmental disorders generally involving problems in movement, usually behavioral, although may also include some vocal symptoms.

multiaxial diagnostic summary. Psychiatric diagnoses and related information presented along five independent but related dimensions as instructed by the previous *DSM–IV–TR*. Axis I was devoted to clinical disorders that typically showed an identifiable onset and limited course. Axis II listed more chronic disorders with an insidious onset, including personality disorders and degrees of intellectual disability. Axis III consisted of any medical disorders that were deemed to be related to the diagnosed disorders on either of the two previous axes. Axis IV enumerated categories of psychosocial stressors judged to either precipitate or exacerbate the diagnosed Axis I and II disorders. Finally, Axis V was a dimensional rating of a patient's overall functioning, termed Global Assessment of Functioning (GAF). It ranged from 1 to 100, with lower scores indicating greater degrees of impairment or dysfunction, and 0 denoting inadequate information.

multiaxial system. See *multiaxial diagnostic summary*.

multidimensional tests. Tests consisting of items that form independent clusters, each measuring separate and distinct psychological constructs. Also known as *heterogeneous tests*.

multiple intelligences. Howard Gardner's theory in which he argues that there exist nine independent types of abilities, many of which are not measured by formal tests and are based on, or controlled by, different brain regions.

multi-score systems. Collection of related instruments that act as parallel forms, usually found in standardized rating scales.

multitrait-multimethod. Approach to investigating construct validity by examining correlations among psychological tests using different methods and measuring different traits. The strongest correlations are expected for tests using the same methods for similar traits, whereas the weakest correlations are expected for tests using different methods and measuring different traits.

multitrait-multimethod matrix (MTMM). Logic proposed by Campbell and Fiske (1959) that was developed to provide a research methodology for the theoretically based notion of the nomological network.

myelination. The growth of a fatty substance on the axons of neurons, which acts as an insulator that increases the speed of neural transmission.

N

naming. The ability to assign verbal labels to objects, people, events, and actions.

nay-saying response set. Tendency to disagree with or oppose items on a personality inventory or rating scale irrespective of item content.

needs. Characterological or internal forces of behavior as manifested in storytelling projective testing techniques.

negative affectivity. Temperament dimension that includes a tendency to manifest sadness, fearfulness, and irritability, along with exhibiting low frustration tolerance and being difficult to soothe and calm.

negative psychotic symptoms. Abnormal absences of behavior and functioning (e.g., lack of affect).

negative predictive power (NPP). Percentage of individuals correctly identified as not having the disorder or condition. Also known as *negative predictive value (NPV)*.

NEO Five-Factor Inventory, Third Edition (NEO–FFI–3). A 60-item brief version of the NEO–PI–3 in that its data yield is limited to measuring the five broad-based domains (i.e., no data are available concerning facets).

NEO Inventories. Series of structured self- and observer-report tests designed to measure the major dimensions or domains of personality for individuals aged 12 through 85 years.

NEO Personality Inventories (NEO–PI). See *NEO Inventories*.

NEO Personality Inventory, Revised (NEO–PI–R). Immediate predecessor to the NEO–PI–3 in which modifications were made to the original three domains of neuroticism, extraversion, and openness and the final two domains, agreeableness and conscientiousness, were added, this occurring in 1992.

NEO Personality Inventory, Third Edition (NEO–PI–3). Self-report inventory designed to measure the Five-Factor Model (FFM) taxonomy of personality traits, including openness, conscientiousness, extraversion, agreeableness, and neuroticism.

NEPSY–II. Comprehensive neuropsychological test battery for individuals aged 3 years, 0 months through 16 years, 11 months that measures all major abilities necessary in diagnosing major and minor neurocognitive disorders, including attention and executive functioning, language, learning and memory, sensorimotor functioning, social perception, and visuospatial processing.

NEPSY–II Full Battery. See *NEPSY–II*.

NEPSY–II General Battery. Comprehensive neuropsychological test battery for individuals aged 3 years, 0 months through 16 years, 11 months that measures major abilities necessary in diagnosing major and minor neurocognitive disorders. The general battery includes only those subtests that are best able to predict the presence of brain dysfunction or damage.

neurocognitive disorder/s. Mental disorders in which the cardinal dysfunction is in cognition, including attention, memory, language, spatial, executive functioning, and social perception, after a period of normal development and functioning in these areas. Specific diagnosis depends on the identified etiology (e.g., Alzheimer's disease or vascular disease). Previous term was *dementia*.

neurocognitive screening tests. Brief performance-based measures of various brain-behavior abilities designed to detect low-functioning cases in which more comprehensive follow-up assessment is needed.

neurodevelopmental disorder/s. In the *DSM–5*, broad class of disorders that, by definition, must have their onset prior to age 18, hence implicating underlying nervous system growth factors. Previously known as disorders first evident in infancy, childhood, and adolescence in *DSM–IV–TR*.

neurologist. Physician who specializes in diseases of the brain, nerves, and nervous system.

neuron. Basic nerve cell designed specifically for sending signals for purposes of communication.

Neuropsychological Assessment Battery (NAB). Comprehensive test battery that measures neurocognitive abilities needed to diagnose major and minor neurocognitive disorders in individuals ranging in age from 18 years, 0 months through 97 years, 11 months, including attention, memory, language, spatial, and executive functioning.

neuropsychological test/s. Specialized psychological instrument that measures key brain–behavior relationships. Such testing reveals what examinees can and cannot do according to their brain functioning, as contrasted with neuroimaging that assesses the physical structure and functioning of the brain.

neuropsychological testing. Specialized psychological testing that measures brain-behavior relationships in order to determine the extent and nature of brain damage or dysfunction. Performance on mental and behavioral tasks that are direct indicators of underlying neurological or organic brain integrity. Also known as *neurocognitive testing*.

neuropsychology. The study of brain–behavior relationships, or how the brain functions to produce human thought and behavior.

neurotic. Based on psychodynamic theory, an individual who is manifesting psychological symptoms due to either excessive use of typical defense mechanisms (e.g., rationalization), or use of more primitive defense mechanisms that distort reality to a greater extent (e.g., projective identification), although reality testing remains intact.

nominal scale. Scale of measurement consisting of the single property of identity, in which arbitrarily assigned numerical values simply represent discrete category labels.

nomological network. Lawful organization of psychological constructs and their observable manifestations, which together provide evidence that a psychological test is actually measuring the trait it purports to measure (i.e., construct validity).

non-autism developmental testing. Test battery that focuses on identifying delays in principal skill areas, typically during infancy and early childhood, including language, cognitive, motor, social-emotional, communication, and play, although not concerned with autism spectrum psychopathology.

nonessential variations. Those features of a clinical disorder that may be part of the symptom picture but are not indispensable for purposes of making the particular diagnosis.

nonorganic mental disorders. In earlier editions of the *DSM*, a general class of disorders that were not principally caused by brain damage or dysfunction; also known as *functional mental disorders*.

non-psychometric theories. Theories of intelligence that are not measurement oriented (e.g., Piaget's cognitive-developmental theory).

non-suicidal self-injury (NSSI). The act of deliberately inflicting harm on one's body as a means of coping with emotional pain, intense anger, and/or frustration, although without the intention of dying. Also known as *self-injurious behavior (SIB)*.

nontarget stimulus. An object or event in which an examinee is instructed to ignore or inhibit a response.

norepinephrine (or noradrenaline). Neurotransmitter and hormone that mobilizes the body for action.

norm reference sample. Selected groups of individuals who determine what is average, above average, and below average for a particular standardized psychological test. All other individuals who complete such a test are compared to these set criteria or norms. It is thus essential that these groups are truly representative of all subsequent individuals who are evaluated by such tests.

normal.   As used in psychodynamic diagnosis, an individual who is utilizing ego defense mechanisms temporarily and effectively, or defense mechanisms that are mature (e.g., sublimation), such that functioning is uninhibited; that is, the individual is able to love and work.

normal curve equivalent (NCE).   Scores with an equal interval scale of measurement that are derived from the formula $50 + 21.063 \times z$, where z is a standardized z–score with a mean of 0.00 and standard deviation of 1.00, and that have a mean of 50, standard deviation of 21.06, and a range of 1–99.

normal perspective.   Personality inventories developed with a focus on discovering normal or typical traits that comprise the human condition.

norm-based test.   Measure in which an examinee's scores are compared to those of a sample of individuals with the same basic characteristics who have previously taken the same measure under identical circumstances.

NTEV.   Abbreviation for "neuropsychological test evaluation," which includes neuropsychological data interpretation, integration, decision-making, treatment planning, report generation, and interactive feedback.

nurse practitioner (DNP or NP).   Doctor of Nursing Practice who may prescribe medications under the supervision of a licensed physician (i.e., MD or DO).

O

object relations.   In psychoanalytic theory, refers to relationships formed with emotionally significant people in the early life of an individual, which are internalized and affects how the individual treats oneself and relates to others going forward.

objective descriptors.   Within the context of a mental status examination, observations of a client's appearance and behavior that are based on observable facts upon which most people agree.

observed symptoms.   Feigning strategy in which individuals consistently report more pathology than is overtly manifested.

obsessive-compulsive and related disorders.   New *DSM–5* general class of disorders that features driven, repetitive, and intrusive behavioral and/or mental actions on the part of the individual.

obsessive-compulsive disorder (OCD).   Psychopathology that principally consists of obsessions and/or compulsions (most typically both), occurring a minimum of one hour per day and which cause dysfunction.

obsessive-compulsive disorder with poor insight.   Obsessive-compulsive disorder (OCD) in which the individual possesses very little awareness or acknowledgement that their particular obsessions or compulsions pose no real danger or threat.

O-data.   Scores obtained by means of observe-report.

Oedipal complex.   In psychoanalysis, the boy identifies with his father to share the unconscious sexual love he has for his mother, the result being the internalization of a superego, including both the conscience (i.e., internal moral principles) and ego ideal (i.e., an admired individual that one internalizes as a model).

olfaction.   The sense of smell.

omission errors.   The failure of an examinee to correctly respond or react to target stimuli, which is a sign of inattention.

one-to-one correspondence.   Counting each object in a set only once, sometimes facilitated by one touch per object; a crucial step in learning number concepts.

onlooker play.   Involves a child closely attending to a peer's activity, along with making meaningful comments about what is observed.

operational definition.   Providing the meaning of a psychological variable or construct in terms of how it will be either measured or manipulated.

operationally defined.   Giving meaning to a variable in terms of how it will be measured or manipulated.

oppositional defiant disorder (ODD).   Consists of the following three symptom clusters: (a) angry or irritable mood, (b) argumentative or defiant behaviors, and (c) vindictiveness. Minimum criteria include (a) four symptoms from any cluster, (b) duration of six months, and (c) frequency of once per week (two in the past month pertaining to the vindictive cluster).

orderliness.   Assumption of science that the world operates in a lawful manner.

ordinary form quality (FQo).   In R–PAS coding, the percept is seen quickly and easily by a significant number of people and reflects a reasonable fit to the inkblot location to which it is attributed.

organic.   Relating to a physical matter.

organic mental disorders.   In earlier editions of the *DSM*, general class of syndromes involving brain damage, disease, or dysfunction as the primary etiology, principally including neuropathology, such as dementia and delirium.

organogenesis. The beginning of the formation and functioning of the embryo's major organ systems during prenatal development.

orientation. Awareness of oneself in relation to one's environment.

orthographic mapping. The formation of letter-sound connections needed to read words by sight, spell words from recall, and for building vocabulary.

orthographic skills. Pertains to the ability to utilize a formal writing system, including the conventions of spelling.

other disorders of psychological development. ICD–10 disorder that is equivalent to an atypical neurodevelopmental disorder in the *DSM–5*.

other sensory-processing disorder. DC:0–5 sensory-processing disorder in which the child experiences atypical reactions to incoming sensory stimuli that does not meet the criteria for sensory under- or over-responsivity disorders and which causes significant distress or dysfunction.

other specified anxiety disorder. General diagnosis of anxiety wherein the clinician is uncertain as to the more specific diagnosis and chooses to share the reasons therefore.

other specified communication disorder. General diagnosis of communication difficulty wherein the clinician is uncertain as to the more specific diagnosis and chooses to share the reasons therefore.

other specified diagnostic alternatives. See *other specified disorder*.

other specified disorder. *DSM–5* diagnosis in which the full criteria for a recognized and well-defined bonafide disorder are not met (e.g., generalized anxiety disorder), the atypical symptoms are in need of clinical attention, and the mental health professional chooses to list the reasons why the criteria are not met.

other specified neurodevelopmental disorder. Most felicitous *DSM–5* diagnosis of any of the ensuing DC:0–5 diagnoses, although with the particular symptom presentations properly delineated: (a) sensory under-responsivity disorder, (b) sensory over-responsivity disorder, and (c) other sensory-processing disorder.

outliers. Observations that lie significantly outside an overall distribution pattern. As applied to psychological testing, extreme scores that significantly contradict the majority of test data in a particular case.

over-responsivity. An abnormally low sensory threshold to environmental stimuli.

overriding habits/inhibition. Part of executive functioning that involves the ability to select a more complex solution, such as naming the color of a word's font rather than the word itself.

P

panel. On the TOMM, stimulus card in which both target and distractor line drawings are printed; examinees are asked to point to the line drawing they recognize from the prior learning phase.

parallel forms. Two versions of the same test in which the observed scores are shown to possess the same mean, variance, and standard deviation. Also referred to as *equivalent forms*.

parallel play. Consists of children playing in proximity, mirroring each other in terms of engaging in the same activity, although with little if any interaction.

parallel tests. Different versions of the same test that contain the same content information and of equivalent difficulty level (i.e., same mean and standard deviation), although consisting of different items.

parens patriae. Power of the state to act as a surrogate or replacement parent for a minor child or disabled adult.

pareto distributions. See *Zipf distributions*.

parietal lobe. Area at the top of the brain behind the frontal lobe that controls sensation perception (i.e., temperature, taste, touch, and movement) and higher-level sensory integration.

Parkinson's disease. Neurological disorder caused by the loss of neurons that produce dopamine in the brain, which results in motor symptoms and possible neurocognitive impairment.

pathogenic. Capable of causing or increasing the risk for psychopathology.

pathogenic care. Serious deficiency in providing for those in a dependent role what is necessary for their health, welfare, maintenance, and protection.

pathogenic model. Explanatory theory that those who feign and malinger psychopathology possess genuine symptoms, which they intentionally exaggerate in an attempt to control them.

pattern of strengths and weaknesses (PSW). Multiple intraindividual comparisons between test scores to their overall average score to determine relative high and low points; assists in detecting the presence of specific learning disorders.

Paul Wellstone-Pete Domenici Mental Health Parity and Addiction Equity Act of 2008. Mental health equality federal law that precluded insurance companies from charging more for mental health services versus physical health services.

pediatrician. Physician who is trained to treat medical disorders in infancy, children, and adolescence.

percent delay. The amount of delay shown by a child as a proportion (or percent) of chronological age (CA), computed as, $Percent\ Delay = 100\% - \dfrac{AE}{CA} \times 100$.

percent-correct classification (PCC). Overall accuracy of classification irrespective of error type; that is, (True Positive + True Negative)/(True Positive + True Negative + False Positive + False Negative).

percentile (P). The point at or below which a specified percentage of scores fall. *P* scores are area transformations that do not preserve the original scores' location in the distribution. See also *percentile rank*.

percentile rank (PR). The percent of the norm reference sample that falls at or below a particular score, including a median of 50 and range from 1 to 99. PR scores are area transformations that do not preserve the original scores' location in the distribution. See also *percentile*.

perception and thinking problems variables. R–PAS data that are related to an individual's problems in thinking, judgment, and perception, along with variables involved with conventionality and seeing the world as do others on the Rorschach test.

perceptual sets. A predisposition to interpret events and objects in specified ways; also an anticipation of a certain event or outcome.

perceptual-motor. Integrating perception with intentional or volitional movement.

performance deficit. An individual who has acquired an ability yet does not display it consistently or reliably.

performance personality test/s. Standardized set of stimuli to which an examinee responds using an open-ended format, which are scored according to a set of uniform test instructions, and which provides information about different aspects of an individual's characteristic patterns of behavior, perception, affect, cognition, interpersonal style, and intrapersonal functioning. Such a test can be used as a microcosm for how examinees respond in the real world.

perseveration. Repetition of the same behavior without it being socially relevant or appropriate, which is typically caused by brain injury or dysfunction.

persistent depressive disorder. Moderate degree of depressive symptoms that are chronic, which decrease the quality of life but do not severely impair functioning; minimum duration is two years for adults and one year for children. Also known as *dysthymic disorder*.

Personality Assessment Screener (PAS). Brief 22-item self-report inventory that provides standardized screening data for a wide range of psychological symptoms, issues, and psychopathology for ages 18 through adulthood.

personality change due to another medical condition. *DSM–5* psychopathology in which a medical disease process or physical injury alters brain function and, therefore, personality traits.

personality coherence. Phenomenon in which a personality trait is maintained longitudinally throughout a person's life, although the manner in which it is expressed behaviorally changes predictably with chronological age (e.g., temper outbursts as a child may include stomping, refusing to move, and throwing objects, whereas in adulthood, these may manifest in the form of a tirade).

personality disorder/s. Continuing pattern of aberrant thinking, feeling, and behavior, which is inflexible and pervasive, especially manifesting temporal consistency and, to a lesser extent, cross-situational consistency, and which causes dysfunction.

personality disorder-trait specified (PD-TS). In the new alternative *DSM–5* dimensional model of personality disorders, this diagnosis is intended for personality psychopathology that is significant, although atypical, analogous to previously termed not otherwise specified diagnoses.

personality inventories. See *personality inventory test/s*.

personality inventory test/s. Catalogue of statements about habitual patterns of behavior to which an informant responds, usually using a forced-choice format (e.g., *True* or *False*), and which yields standardized scores on multiple scales that measure traits, clinical symptoms, attitudes, emotions, and other psychological aspects about an individual for purposes of psychodiagnosis.

personality mechanisms. Unconscious aspects of personality via projection, (b) perceptual sets, and (c) social-cognitive abilities, all of which may be identified, quantified, and/or reliably measured by implicit personality tests and are associated with various psychological traits, emotional states, moods, beliefs, reality testing capability, thought process and content, and overall psychological adjustment.

Personality Psychopathology Five (PSY-5) scales. Scales incorporated into many of the MMPI inventories designed to address issues commonly confronted by mental health clinicians as follows: (a) degree of aggressiveness and danger to others (*AGGR-r*), (b) degree of reality testing and any presence of psychosis (*PSYC-r*), (c) degree of impulsiveness and risk-taking or sensation-seeking (*DISC-r*), (d) degree of subjective distress and negative affect (*NEGE-r*), and (e) degree of anhedonia or lack of positive feelings or pleasure (*INTR-r*).

Personality Syndromes (P) Axis.   In psychodynamic diagnosis, a dimension that consists of two components: (a) personality organization (i.e., a spectrum of personality functioning ranging from normal to psychotic) and (b) personality style or pattern (i.e., certain specified traits).

personality trait/s.   Average tendency to think, feel, or behave in a particular way that is relatively enduring across time and situations, especially the former, and which can be measured for individual differences analyses and prediction.

pervasive developmental disorder (PDD).   Previous broad classification of severe, early onset, chronic psychopathology, which deleteriously affects all areas of an individual's functioning.

Phoneme–grapheme correspondence.   The association between speech sounds and their written representation in a particular language.

phonic decoding.   Responding orally to items that require the manipulation of sounds within words.

phonological abilities.   Concerns skills in utilizing speech sounds appropriately and consistently.

phonological awareness.   The ability to recognize and discriminate the basic sounds used in spoken language.

phonological disorder.   Now antiquated term for *speech sound disorder*.

phonological loop.   Component of working memory that retains information by means of maintenance rehearsal and is based on acoustic and phonemic elements that utilize speech-planning motor circuits.

phonological processing.   The ability to decode sounds associated with words.

phonological recoding.   Transforming written symbols into letter sounds, syllables, and words in the process of reading.

Phonological–orthographic relationships.   Associations between the basic spoken sounds of words in a language and composing these in written form, which is essential when learning to spell.

phrase speech.   Flexible use of non-echoed, three-word utterances, which sometimes involve a verb and are spontaneous, meaningful word combinations.

physical custody.   Authority by law afforded to a primary caretaker to have the child reside with him or her when caretakers are separated or divorced.

planning.   Part of executive functioning in which thinking is done to achieve an end objective, such as finding one's way out of a maze.

plasticity.   Ability of the brain to modify its structure, and thus functioning, in response to training, intervention, stimulation, and/or experience.

play.   Activities that are freely sought and pursued solely for the sake of enjoyment.

point scale.   Test in which items of similar content are grouped together, usually in order of increasing difficulty.

polytomous models.   Measurement that possesses more than two possible scores, as contrasted with dichotomous models, which possess only two possible scores.

polytomous scoring approach.   See *polytomous models*.

positive predictive power (PPP).   Percentage of individuals correctly identified as having the disorder or condition. Also known as *positive predictive value (PPV)*.

postcentral gyrus.   Protuberance located immediately subsequent to the central sulcus, commonly referred to as the primary sensory cortex or sensory strip.

post-traumatic stress disorder (PTSD).   Exposure to a catastrophic event or series of events, ensued by some combination of the following four symptom clusters: (a) intrusion; (b) avoidance of trauma-related stimuli (internal and/or external), including amnesia; (c) negative mood changes; and (d) changes in arousal and reactivity. Duration of symptoms must be, at minimum, six months from the point of trauma exposure.

power test.   Measure in which the items form a sequence of increasing difficulty and complexity, including those that are extremely difficult to pass.

power-law distributions.   See *Zipf distributions*.

pragmatic context.   The purpose or intention of a given vocalization or utterance evinced within a particular situation (e.g., making a request, sharing enjoyment, directing attention, seeking emotional comfort).

praxis.   Sensation that involves the ability to plan and organize movement.

preauthorization (PA).   Formal approval by a third-party payer or insurance company that (a) the type of professional service being asked for is covered by a client's health care policy and (b) it is deemed to be medically necessary. This does not necessarily mean the service is reimbursable by the insurance company because the client may not have yet met the policy's deductible.

precentral gyrus.   Protuberance located immediately prior to the central sulcus, commonly referred to as the primary motor cortex or motor strip.

precision.   The degree to which test results are consistent, dependable, repeatable, or reliable.

predicted-difference discrepancy analyses.   Statistically comparing individuals' measured intellectual competence with their measured achievement, which is done by subtracting each achievement standard score predicted by the selected intelligence test composite score from the actual or obtained achievement standard score.

predicted-difference method.   Ability–memory or ability–achievement discrepancy procedure wherein each index standard score predicted by the selected intelligence test index score is compared to the examinee's actual or obtained memory or achievement index standard score.

predictor.   Within the context of regression analyses, the variable used to forecast the outcome of a second variable or criterion; the predictor is also referred to as an independent variable.

preference for novelty.   Proclivity of infants to divert attention to a novel stimulus when compared to a stimulus they have become familiar with through repetition.

prefrontal cortex.   Anterior region of the frontal lobe that controls the most sophisticated types of executive functioning.

prehension.   The act of taking hold, grasping, or seizing.

premorbid level of functioning.   An estimation of an individual's ability to cope and adapt prior to the onset of psychopathology.

prenatal.   The entire period of development prior to birth, that is, from conception to birth, which normally spans 38–40 weeks. Considered a critical period for central nervous system (CNS) or brain development.

presence of a disorder.   As applied to the Millon personality inventories, a *BR*–score (75–84) that indicates a syndrome is present but is either secondary or subthreshold.

presenting symptoms.   The problematic emotions, thoughts, and behaviors that are subjectively reported by clients, which brought them in to seek professional mental health counseling services.

presses.   During administration of some performance tests, activities designed to elicit certain social interactions and communications from the examinee. In projective storytelling testing, external or environmental forces of behavior acting upon the characters.

pretend play.   Activities in which individuals act as if something or someone is real; that is, a situation is created in which more is occurring than what is literally happening. This requires abstract thinking consistent with Piaget's preoperational stage of cognitive development.

prevalence.   The total number of cases manifesting a particular disorder in a population for a defined duration (e.g., one year, a lifetime).

prevalence scores (PS).   Standard score metric used in the Millon Behavioral Medicine Diagnostic, Bariatric Norms inventory, which adjusts for the estimated frequency of occurrence of a medical disorder or related issue in the population, akin to the *BR*–score.

primal scene.   In psychoanalysis, children's fantasy of sexual relations between their parents.

primary care physician (PCP).   Physician who practices family medicine, pediatrics, or internal medicine; who provides general care at the point of first contact; and who usually is responsible for the patient's continuing comprehensive care.

primary mental abilities.   Seven mental abilities proposed by Louis Thurstone, which he believed were independent of each other, including reasoning, comprehension, perceptual speed, word fluency, numerical ability, spatial visualization, and associative memory.

primary motor cortex.   Part of the brain that controls voluntary movement throughout the body. Also known as the *motor strip*.

primary scores.   On the NEPSY–II, data that measure key clinical neurocognitive abilities, as evinced by such terms as "Total" or "Combined" in the subtest name. In the NAB, such scores measure the fundamental neurocognitive abilities that contribute to the more broad-based module index scores.

primary sensory cortex.   Part of the rain that registers tactile or haptic senses (i.e., touch, pain) throughout the body. Also known as the *sensory strip*.

priming.   Phenomenon wherein the introduction of a prior stimulus prepares an individual to respond in a particular way to a subsequent stimulus.

principal diagnosis.   The most prominent diagnosis, usually determined according to it being the most severe or impairing, and/or it representing the greatest focus of the particular service being provided.

proactive interference.   Forgetting that occurs when previously learned information competes with information learned at a future point in time.

probable range.   On the SIRS–2, a score pattern that shows a high likelihood of feigning or a determination of feigning if sufficient primary scales are so elevated.

probe.   As applied to a test involving structured interviewing, a prompt designed to acquire information necessary to score a particular item not yet scorable with the given information elicited by the original question.

problem-solving. Process by which people attempt to resolve difficulties, achieve objectives, or derive conclusions by means of higher-order processing or reasoning.

procedural (nonconscious) memory. Automatic or overlearned motor tasks that are engaged in without awareness.

process scores. (1) On the NEPSY–II, data that measure more narrowly defined neurocognitive abilities to qualify the primary scores. (2) Qualitative data based on some modification of standardized administration that can provide unique information concerning an examinee's performance and ability.

proficiency. Degree of capability in a skill or area of knowledge.

prognosis. Any evidence-based prediction or forecast. As applied to clinical psychological practice, the expected course and outcome of a mental disorder based on scientific evidence.

projection. (1) The assumption that when people respond to ambiguous stimuli (e.g., inkblots, interpersonal scenes), they cast or transmit aspects of their personality into their interpretation of them, including such things as feelings, beliefs, self-perception, and perception of the external environment (e.g., other people, relationships among events and objects). (2) Perceiving in others an unacceptable feeling or belief that resides in oneself. (3) The unconscious apperceptive distortion of stimuli predicated on all previous memory traces that an individual has stored through experience.

projective tests. Techniques that present a series of relatively ambiguous stimuli, which are designed to elicit unique responses that reflect the examinee's emotions, thoughts, needs, conflicts, and personality characteristics

prominence of a disorder. As applied to the Millon personality inventories, a *BR*–score (85–115) that indicates a syndrome is clearly detected and a candidate for being the principal diagnosis in a case.

"prompt for two, pull after four". Succinct label for the R–PAS R-Optimized Procedure instructions to the examinee during the initial response phase (RP).

prompt. (1) Brief verbal inducement for an examinee to respond and is employed to either (a) provide a reminder as to how to perform the task or (b) afford a cue to elicit a response. (2) Verbal cue by examiner used when the examinee shows no further response and needs encouragement or used for bolstering the examinee's confidence and continued motivation throughout test administration.

proposition speech output. Measures of language production in terms of quantified units of content.

proprioception. Sensation that involves body position awareness; the ability to sense the position of one's body from the input of muscular movement.

prototypical approach. Classification system wherein psychological disorders are defined by categories within which specified mandatory (i.e., essential) symptoms must be detected for the disorder to be considered existent, followed by a listing of supplementary symptoms (i.e., nonessential variations) from which a certain minimum number is required. Onset and durational criteria may also be components of selected disorders. Such a system conceptualizes psychological disorders in terms of kind or type and results in dichotomous affirmative (i.e., the disorder is present) or negative (i.e., the disorder is not present) diagnostic decisions.

provisional. See *provisional diagnosis*.

provisional diagnosis/es. A listed disorder that is (a) imprecise to some degree and in need of refinement, (b) usually based on insufficient or conflicting information, (c) intended to be temporary or time-limited, and (d) anticipated to change pending the addition of diagnostically pertinent data.

proximal stability. Good mobility and strength along the midline or spine.

proximodistal. General trend in development from near to far or from the center to the periphery.

P–score (probability score). Measures the likelihood that a respondent manifests a particular type of psychopathology; for example, a *P*–score greater than 50 indicates that it is more likely than not that an examinee has a clinically significant psychological disorder.

pseudowords. Non-words or nonsense words that consist of the basic sounds or phonemes in a language, used to test phonological awareness.

psychiatrist (MD or DO). Physicians who specialize in the treatment of mental health disorders, typically utilizing biomedical interventions.

psychoactive substances. Chemicals that principally alter mood, cognition, and behavior.

Psychodynamic Diagnostic Manual, Second Edition (PDM–2). Nosology of mental and personality disorders based on psychodynamic theory, consisting of a multiaxial system that attempts to consider the "whole" individual as follows: *P Axis* for personality syndromes, *M Axis* for mental functioning, and *S Axis* for the subjective experience of symptoms.

psychogenic. Having an emotional cause or origin in contrast to a medical one.

psychological assessment. The systematic use of multiple techniques or methods that are designed to gather and integrate data about an individual who is suspected of having one or more psychological disorders.

psychological assessment and testing process.   The five-stage sequence of psychological assessment and testing as delineated in this book, including the following: Stage 1—initial referral for testing, Stage 2—initial psychological assessment report, Stage 3—scheduling test administration appointments, Stage 4—final psychological assessment report, and Stage 5—communication of the results.

psychological determinism.   (1) The assumption that everything said or written in response to some situation has a dynamic cause or meaning. Originated within psychoanalytic theory. (2) The philosophical position that all psychological phenomena are necessarily the result of certain antecedent causes; that is, all behavior is fixed and free will is simply an illusion.

psychological disorder/s.   A disorder principally of the mind (versus body) recognized in one or more of the major nosological systems of psychopathology. Synonyms include mental disorders, mental health disorders, behavior disorders, developmental disorders, neurodevelopmental disorders, personality disorders, and personality psychopathology.

psychological mindedness.   The ability to examine and understand one's own thoughts, motives, desires, and feelings. Thought to be requisite for accurately completing a self-report personality inventory or symptom rating scale for purposes of psychodiagnosis and for amenability to insight-oriented psychotherapeutic intervention. Also known as the ability to introspect, many consider this ability to be one facet of emotional intelligence.

psychological test.   As defined by the Current Procedural Terminology (CPT) guidelines, refers to a psychodiagnostic assessment of emotionality, intelligence, personality, and psychopathology (excluding testing for neurocognitive disorders involving brain damage, dysfunction, or disease).

psychological testing.   Collecting samples of behavior from individuals, under standardized or controlled conditions, which provides information about their characteristics, including emotional, cognitive, behavioral, and/or personality functioning, all for purposes of diagnosis, prediction, explanation, and/or treatment planning.

psychometric g.   Charles Spearman's early term for the *g* factor, to which many specific abilities (*s* factors) were correlated in his two-factor theory.

psychometric theories.   Theories of intelligence and other psychological constructs derived largely from factor analyses and analogous statistical procedures (e.g., principal components analysis).

psychomotor.   Manner in which the brain's mental process affects an individual's physical movements (e.g., fidgeting, mania).

psychomotor agitation.   Physical restlessness, heightened tension, and elevated level of arousal, all of which are psychically determined (versus externally determined).

psychomotor retardation.   Generalized physiological slowing and extremely low level of arousal, all of which are psychically determined (versus externally determined).

psychopath.   See *psychopathy*.

psychopathology.   The scientific study of abnormal behavior or psychological disorders.

psychopathy.   Cleckley's theoretical definition of antisocial personality using more psychologically defined traits, including glibness and superficial charm, a grandiose sense of self, pathological lying, being cunning and manipulative, showing an absence of guilt and remorse, and a callous absence of empathy.

psychosis.   (1) A psychological construct that denotes the presence of one or more of the following: (a) lost contact with reality, (b) formal thought disorder, and (c) symptom severity requiring inpatient hospitalization for purposes of stabilization. (2) Disconnection from consensual reality (i.e., lost contact with reality).

psychotherapy.   The use of clinical methods and the professional relationship, both of which are founded upon established psychological principles, to assist people in changing their behaviors, cognitions, emotions, and personality traits to relieve symptoms and improve their functioning in the world.

psychotic.   See *psychosis*.

psychotic disorder.   See *psychosis*.

psychotic disorder due to another medical condition.   A medical disease process that causes severe psychological symptoms wherein the individual becomes disconnected from reality.

psychotropic medications.   Class of drugs that are capable of affecting people's minds, emotions, thoughts, and behavior.

Q

Q-global.   Online scoring and reporting platform created by Pearson Assessments, which is capable of computer administration, scoring, and interpretation of many major psychological tests.

qualitative analysis.   Use of a psychologist's clinical experience, skill, and judgment in detecting potential signs of feigning dysfunction during a clinical interview and/or psychological test administration.

qualitative classification. Nominal scale of measurement or class associated with a particular range of standardized test scores; useful in interpreting the general or diagnostic meaning of test score results, although with a loss of information (i.e., less precision).

qualitative descriptor. Test variable measured on a nominal–ordinal scale of measurement, which classifies examinees' standard scores as categories ranging from extremely low to extremely high, which is easier for laypeople to comprehend.

R

radio button. A computer listing in the form of circles that permits only one selection from a particular group of alternative options.

rank size distributions. See *Zipf distributions*.

rapport. The trust between clinician and client necessary to garner needed information for accurate assessment and positive behavior change in treatment.

rare symptoms. Feigning strategy in which individuals report symptoms with a very low frequency of occurrence.

rate disability. Impairment in reading words rapidly, which is one of the three fundamental skills needed for effective reading, the other two being accuracy and comprehension.

rating scale/s. Measures that perform similarly to surveys in that respondents assess either themselves or others according to the degree behaviors, traits, or clinical symptoms. Typically rating scales use norm reference samples that adjust for age, education, and other demographic variables that may affect test scores.

rational item selection. Use of raters with expertise concerning a personality theory to choose test items that conceptually have the greatest degree of compatibility with the personality constructs that comprise such a theory.

rationalism. Belief that knowledge can best be gained by logical reasoning.

raw score. The original or observed quantitative value on a psychological test prior to any subsequent transformations.

reaction formation. Expressing the opposite of one's true feelings.

reactive attachment disorder (RAD). Disturbance in emotional bonding characterized by a child who rarely seeks or responds to comfort when distressed and is accompanied by at least two of the following: (a) lack of social and emotional responsiveness; (b) relative absence of any positive feelings; and/or (c) non-provoked irritability, sadness, and fear. That such symptoms are the direct consequence of insufficient care is an essential criterion without which this diagnosis cannot be made.

real self. The manner in which individuals define who they are in objective terms.

reality testing. (1) Generally, the objective evaluation of emotion or thought, or the ability to interpret a situation as it actually exists. (2) As an ego function, refers to an individual's psychological mindedness or the ability to introspect and understand one's thoughts and feelings accurately.

recall task. Memory undertaking in which the individual is not provided with any hints or clues; sometimes referred to as a *free recall task*.

receptive language. Decoding speech for purposes of comprehension.

reference W. The chosen criterion (e.g., 90% proficiency) to which the examinee's measured ability (e.g., 50% proficiency) will be compared.

reflection of content. Counseling microskill in which psychotherapists paraphrase back to clients what they said, which helps to establish trust and rapport and encourages the client to provide more information.

reflection of feeling. Counseling microskill in which psychotherapists repeat to clients the emotion they have expressed in the therapy process, which helps establish trust and rapport and assists clients in gaining insight.

refractory epilepsy. Seizure disorder that is resistant to drug therapy.

reframing. Counseling microskill in which interviewers provide an alternative perspective that modifies, restructures, or gives a new perspective for the client that leads to positive behavior change.

regression. (1) Adaptational failure in which individuals return to an age-inappropriate immature stage of development, usually as the result of significant psychological stress. An example would be an adult who expresses a temper tantrum similar to a two-year-old child. (2) Moving to an earlier, more pleasant, and less threatening time in development, albeit immature.

regulation and control of drives, affects, and impulses. As an ego function that refers to a general ability to self-regulate, including impulse control, delay of gratification, and the management of affect, emotion, and behavior.

related medical variables and conditions. Diagnostic dimension that includes historical medical conditions and current medical variables that may impact (i.e., cause, maintain, and/or exacerbate) any diagnosed psychological disorders.

relative proficiency index (RPI).   Measure of a person's mastery or capability in a skill or area of knowledge compared with average age- or grade-level peers.

release of information (ROI).   Document that gives a provider permission to communicate certain specified health information to another provider, agency, or entity that is otherwise protected pursuant to both law and ethical principles.

reliability.   The degree of consistency of a psychological test with itself over time (i.e., test–retest), within itself (i.e., internal consistency), or with two versions of itself (i.e., parallel forms), interpreted as the extent to which such a test is a precise measure of a psychological construct.

reliability coefficient/s.   Correlation statistic employed within the context of a study designed to measure the consistency or accuracy of a psychological test.

repetitions.   Reiterations of test items or their attendant instructions, the purpose of which is to redirect examinees' attention, ensure their understanding of the task, or measure the extent to which they are paying attention and responding consistently.

repression.   (1) The unconscious forgetting of something threatening. (2) The unconscious inhibition of a feeling, thought, or memory that would otherwise cause anxiety; a defense mechanism.

resilience.   A person's ability to withstand remarkable stress, or readily recover from adversity, without succumbing to a psychological or neurodevelopmental disorder. Protective factors represent the core of this characteristic.

response anchors.   Items on self-report and observer-report rating scales, which consist of alternatives whose meaning is denoted by (a) verbal descriptors (e.g., *Not True*) and (b) assigned locations on a physical continuum (e.g., extreme right); especially without the use of numbers, at least until scoring begins.

response phase (RP).   Initial stage of R–PAS administration in which the examinee answers the question "What might this be?" The examinee is asked to provide two or three independent responses to each of the ten Rorschach inkblots.

response process.   Denotes the psychological operations or behavioral representations that lead to a response coded score in the R–PAS; may be generalized from the microcosm of the test environment to the real-world environment

response sets.   The tendency of people to respond to test items in a manner that is unrelated to their content, which may threaten validity of the data.

response style analysis.   Within the context of CPT testing, the approach an examinee employs when deciding whether a physical stimulus is present and whether to respond to it.

reticular activating system.   Band of fibers that traverse the brain stem through the thalamus located within the limbic system, which regulates general arousal of the cortex and preventing a comatose state.

retrieval.   The ability to extract information from long-term memory when needed.

retroactive interference.   Forgetting that occurs when later learned information competes with earlier learned information.

retrograde amnesia.   Loss of memory for events prior to head trauma or injury.

reversal rules.   As applied to a standardized test or subtest, directives to go back toward easier items until the examinee successfully earns full credit on a predetermined number of consecutive items (usually two or three in a row), with the assumption that all prior items would be passed.

reverse rules.   In adaptive standardized testing of cognitive abilities or skills, recommended rules for reverting to easier items of a test or subtest when the examinee is unable to successfully pass items at the age or grade-appropriate start point.

reverse scoring.   Wording items in opposite directions then adjusting the scoring such that both items show the same valence (e.g., higher scores mean more of the construct being measured).

right hemisphere.   In most people, the side of the brain that is specialized for visual spatial and holistic processing, interpretation of emotion and implied meaning (i.e., connotation), and control of the contralateral or left side of the body.

Roberts, Second Edition (Roberts–2).   Performance personality measure of social-cognitive ability as reflected in expressive language, normed on individuals ranging in age from 6 years, 0 months through 18 years, 11 months. The test stimuli consist of 16 stimulus cards of key intrapersonal and interpersonal scenes from which the examinee is asked to formulate a complete story. This test also consists of clinical scales that measure the presence of psychological disorders (e.g., illogical thinking).

R-optimized procedure.   Administrative principles used in the R–PAS that are designed to elicit an ideal number of scorable responses that neither underestimates nor overestimates the presence of complexity and thus psychopathology, namely, "prompt for two, pull after four."

Rorschach Inkblot Test, Comprehensive System (R–CS).   Performance-based standardized personality test normed on individuals ranging in age from 5 years, 0 months to 86 years, 0 months. This test is an implicit measure that directly appraises (a) perceptual sets and expectancies and (b) social-cognitive abilities, both of which may be quantified and reliably associated with various psychological traits, emotional states, moods, beliefs, reality testing ability, thought process and content, and overall psychological adjustment.

Rorschach Performance Assessment System (R–PAS). Performance-based standardized personality test normed on individuals ranging in age from 6 years, 0 months through adulthood. It represents a continuation and more contemporary version of the Rorschach-CS, retaining variables that have showed the greatest degree of validity, updating the form quality (FQ) tables and norms, and transforming the previous raw scores into standard scores with a mean of 100 and standard deviation of 15.

Rorschach Performance Assessment System® (R–PAS®). Web-based computer coding and scoring platform for the R–PAS system.

rote memory. The simple verbatim recall of presented information.

routing. The practice of using core subtests that measure vital mental abilities, which effectively determine the start points (i.e., appropriate beginning difficulty levels) of subsequent subtests in the battery.

R–PAS code sequence. Listing of all responses (rows) and their 19 categories of codes (columns). Provides a summary overview of the examinee's protocol, including the total number of responses and any card rejections.

R–PAS Profile Appendix—Summary Scores for All Variables. Tabled summary of all R–PAS variables organized by code section. Miscellaneous use but especially for research purposes.

R–PAS Protocol Level Counts & Calculations. Frequency counts and calculations derived from the code sequence, some of which represent final R–PAS variables and some of which represent a prelude to computing final variables for interpretation.

R–PAS Summary Scores and Profiles—Page 1. Listing of all final R–PAS variables with the greatest amount of research support, organized by domain, including raw scores, standard scores, and percentiles, which are also profiled. Used primarily for nomothetic interpretation.

R–PAS Summary Scores and Profiles—Page 2. Listing of all final R–PAS variables with a lesser amount of research support, organized by domain, including raw scores, standard scores, and percentiles, which are also profiled. Used for secondary nomothetic interpretation.

rule/d in/confirmed. Term denoting that a diagnosed psychological disorder is being questioned and needs more formal measurement to determine its status, most especially psychological testing.

rule/d out (r/o). Term indicating that a particular psychological disorder is suspected and needs more formal measurement to determine its status, most especially psychological testing.

S

s factors. In Charles Spearman's two-factor hierarchical theory of intelligence, refers to an array of specific intellectual abilities that are all partially related to a more complex and broad-based general or *g* factor.

sample items. Easy to complete demonstration items on a test or subtest that show how they are to be successfully answered or solved.

scaled scores. Standardized data with a mean of 10 and standard deviation of 3, usually appearing on the subtests of a more complex measure.

schizoid personality disorder. *DSM–5* Cluster A odd and eccentric character psychopathology that consists of a social detachment from people, a restricted range of emotional expression, and an absence of interest in pursuing life goals and interpersonal relationships.

schizophrenia. The most common of the psychotic disorders, consisting of two or more of the following essential symptom clusters that have been continuously present for a minimum of six months: (a) hallucinations, (b) delusions, and (c) disorganized speech. Catatonia and negative symptoms are nonessential variations.

score/s. Quantitative code or summary statement that represents a level of performance, or amount of a behavior or trait, which is provided by a test.

scoring lower than chance rule. See *Malingering Rule 1*.

screen for. Term indicating that a particular psychological disorder is suspected and the clinician referring for psychological assessment desires a brief standardized measure to determine if more comprehensive testing for such psychopathology is indicated.

screening battery approach. Administration strategy that uses only partial tests or subtests from a battery to determine if more comprehensive testing is necessary.

screening measure. See *screening test/s*.

screening test/s. Brief measures designed to determine if more comprehensive testing for a particular disorder is needed.

S-data. Scores obtained by means of self-report.

secondary gain. The maintaining of symptoms because they provide the individual with attention not otherwise given.

secure attachment. Style of emotional bonding in which the individual has basic trust in significant others and is considered the healthiest style.

seed scales. Restructured MMPI clinical scales consisting only of non-demoralization items (i.e., the demoralization items being factored out) although in need of further statistical development.

selective attention. Being able to focus on only the most important information from among all the competing sensory inputs.

selectivity of symptoms. Feigning strategy in which examinees indiscriminately report a vast array of potential symptoms.

self and other representation variables. R–PAS data that are related to an individual's way of understanding oneself, other people, and social relationships as a foundation of interpersonal relatedness in the Rorschach test.

self-concept. People's understanding of who they are in terms of traits and social roles. Considered to be a core feature of the personality, which impacts attachment, self-esteem, and self-efficacy.

self-efficacy. Degree to which people believe they will be successful at a particular task if they put forth sufficient effort; a key construct in social cognitive learning theory.

self-esteem. How people feel about themselves on good versus bad or high versus low dimensions. The evaluative component of self-concept.

self-medicating. One etiological theory of substance use disorders, which posits that individuals come to abuse drugs in an attempt to reduce unwanted psychological symptoms.

semantic dementia. Major neurocognitive disorder in which individuals perform poorly when given tests of vocabulary, general information, and picture naming.

semantic LTM. Relatively permanent recall of factual knowledge acquired through learning.

semantic memory. Refers to general knowledge (i.e., language and information) learned through formal education.

semantics. Principles that pertain to the meaning of words and symbols.

semenarche (or spermarche). In human males, the beginning of sperm development associated with the onset of puberty.

semi-structured clinical interview. Fundamental psychological assessment technique in which a clinician typically employs a flexible strategic inquiry style to gather detailed information in a number of essential content areas of a patient's current and historical functioning. Such areas include a patient's demographic information, presenting symptoms, developmental history, current mental status and behavior, assessment summary, working diagnoses, and treatment recommendations.

sense of reality. As an ego function that regards one's conscious awareness of both self and the world.

sensitivity. Ability of a test to detect the presence of a psychological construct (e.g., ADHD) if it is actually present.

sensorimotor functioning. Motor control that needs neural feedback from the senses for proper coordination, including kinesthetic, tactile, and visual signals.

sensory integration. The "organization of sensation for use" (Ayers, 1979, p. 184).

sensory memory. First stage in the information-processing model wherein an immense amount of raw information from each of our senses is initially registered, although it remains only a few seconds unless retained by means of attention.

sensory over-responsivity disorder. DC:0–5 sensory-processing disorder in which the child experiences exaggerated, intense, or prolonged reactions to incoming sensory stimuli, which causes significant distress or dysfunction. In the PDM–2, this is referred to as hypersensitive disorder that is further linked to differential types of psychopathology.

sensory processing (integration). The organization of sensation for use; a fundamental neurodevelopmental ability that directly impacts people's adaptation to the environments in which they find themselves.

sensory-processing (integration) disorder/s. An impairment in the ability to organize and coordinate sensations from various modalities for purposes of adjustment and adaptation.

Sensory Processing Measure (SPM). Observer-report measure of processing problems in various sensory systems, including vision, hearing, and body awareness, along with several higher-level integrative functions, such as planning and social participation, which is used to facilitate the diagnosis of sensory processing (integration) disorder in children ages 5 years, 0 months through 12 years, 11 months.

Sensory Processing Measure–Preschool (SPM–P). Observer-report measure of processing problems in various sensory systems, including vision, hearing, and body awareness, along with several higher-level integrative functions, which is used to facilitate the diagnosis of sensory-processing (integration) disorder in children ages 2 years, 0 months through 5 years, 11 months.

sensory under-responsivity disorder. DC:0–5 sensory-processing disorder in which the child experiences muted, minimal, neutral, or extremely brief reactions to incoming sensory stimuli, which causes significant distress or dysfunction.

sentence completion test (SCT). Projective technique in which respondents are asked to finish a listing of partial sentences (i.e., stems) such that each communicates a comprehensible idea or thought. Responses are then analyzed for recurring patterns or themes.

sentence completion test–adolescent (SCT–A). Projective technique in which adolescents are asked to finish a listing of partial sentences (i.e., stems) such that each communicates a comprehensible idea or thought. Responses are then analyzed for recurring patterns or themes.

sentence completion test–child (SCT–C). Projective technique in which children are asked to finish a listing of partial sentences (i.e., stems) such that each communicates a comprehensible idea or thought. Responses are then analyzed for recurring patterns or themes.

separation anxiety disorder. Now classified in the *DSM–5* under anxiety disorders, involves excessive fear and distress when separated from specific attachment figures, including intense and constant worry about their safety or one's own safety. Such symptoms must be in excess of that expected for developmental age and manifest for a minimum of four weeks for children and six months for adults.

sequelae. (**sequela**, singular) Common consequences of a prior disorder, disease, or injury.

serifs. Slight projections that finish off strokes of letters, which make it easier for the human eye to glide smoothly across written words and sentences while reading. The Times New Roman font contains such serifs and is one of the most popular typefaces in use today.

severity of symptoms. Feigning strategy in which individuals report most of their symptoms as being unbearable, intolerable, or insufferable.

sexual content (Sx). R–PAS content code that indicates the presence of a sexual concern or preoccupation.

short-term memory. See *short-term working memory (Gwm)*.

short-term working memory (Gwm). Dynamic, transient storage system that permits information, including prior stored knowledge and new sensory inputs, to be held in immediate awareness and manipulated as needed or required.

sign/s. Objectively observed manifestations of a psychological disorder (e.g., loosening of associations).

signal-detection theory. Explanation of how individuals are able to distinguish between a specified target pattern (i.e., the signal) from that of random distractor patterns (i.e., the noise).

simple difference discrepancy analyses. Statistically comparing individuals' measured intellectual competence with their measured achievement by subtracting the selected intelligence test composite score from each obtained achievement standard score.

simple phrases. One-word utterances that are associated with gestures (i.e., holophrases) or two-word utterances that exclude filler words (e.g., "My ball" or "You go").

single ADOS–2 items. Items that are scored based on one observation.

single-score systems. Instrument that includes only a single form of a test.

social anxiety disorder (social phobia). Disproportionate fear response when exposed to the scrutiny of other people, including an excessive concern of being negatively evaluated and/or subject to humiliation. These symptoms must manifest for at least six months.

social cognition. Understanding interpersonal relationships and oneself, including two components; the recognition of emotions and theory of mind.

social desirability. Tendency for examinees to answer items such that they appear to be interpersonally accepted, moral, likeable, and attractive.

social perception. See *social cognition*.

social (pragmatic) communication disorder. New *DSM–5* communication disorder consisting of an inability to use verbal and nonverbal language effectively in social situations. Principally designed to eliminate the need for a pervasive developmental disorders-not otherwise specified (i.e., PDD-NOS) diagnosis by providing an alternative when impaired social communication occurs in the absence of rigid, repetitive, and stereotyped behavior patterns.

Social-Emotional and Adaptive Behavior Questionnaire. Instrument that is part of the Bayley Scales, which is completed by the caregiver and measures social and emotional developmental milestones in individuals ages 1–42 months.

solitary play. Consists of a child playing alone and involved in a task, usually with toys or objects.

spatial delayed-recognition span paradigm. Task in which an examinee is asked to select a change in a target after a specified delay; for example, an examinee is asked to point to a newly added dot to a previous array of dots.

spatial processing. The ability to comprehend the orientation of visual information in two- and three-dimensional space.

specific ability tests. Narrowly defined subtests that measure capabilities at Stratum I of the intelligence construct hierarchy.

specific intelligences. Referred to as *s* factors in Spearman's two-factor theory of intelligence first proposed in 1904, which were purported to contribute to a more complex general intelligence factor or *g* factor.

specific learning disorder/s (SLD). A *DSM–5* neurodevelopmental disorder that now incorporates all previously recognized *DSM–IV–TR* learning disorders (viz., reading disorder, mathematics disorder, and disorder of written expression) as diagnostic specifiers, although with different diagnostic codes. The new empirical standard is that academic performance must be at or below a percentile rank of 78 as measured by a standardized test of achievement.

specific learning disorder, with impairment in mathematics. Disability in one of the skills needed for mathematics, typically consisting of number sense, memorization of arithmetic facts, accurate or fluent calculation, and accurate math reasoning.

specific learning disorder, with impairment in reading. Disability in one of the skills needed for reading, typically consisting of reading accuracy, reading rate or fluency, and reading comprehension.

specificity. Ability of a test to correctly detect a nonclinical, normal, or healthy case.

specifier. Extension to various mental disorders that clarify their onset, course, and/or severity, or which may identify any unique features of prognostic or treatment significance (e.g., childhood onset, severe with psychotic features).

speech sound disorder. A *DSM–5* communication disorder consisting of impairments in pronouncing words when spoken.

speed of lexical analysis (LA). Covariance between the speed at which objects can be accurately named and name-generating facility.

speed of processing. The rate in which the mind manages various kinds of information; in infants, this is measured by how quickly habituation occurs. See also *habituation*.

stability coefficient. Alternate name for a correlation coefficient used within the context of a test–retest reliability study. In addition to addressing test reliability, such a statistic also provides evidence of the amount of consistency possessed by the purported psychological construct over time.

standard battery. In general, refers to an instrument's test or subtests that together measure its basics constructs. As applied to the Woodcock–Johnson achievement test battery, refers to the first 11 tests, which together measure its fundamental clusters (i.e., reading, written expression, and mathematics, along with cross-domain skills [e.g., academic fluency]).

standard deviation (s or *SD*). The average deviation of a sample of scores from the mean in original (raw) test score units. The larger the standard deviation, the greater the dispersion of scores about the mean.

standard error of estimation (SEE). Used with the estimated true score to derive an asymmetrical confidence interval (CI) that accounts for the true score's regression to the mean.

standard error of measurement (SEM). Estimate of how repeated measures of a person on the same test will tend to be distributed around her or his true score.

standard score/s. Uniform score derived by linear transformation on many standardized psychological tests, especially in the domains of neurocognitive and cognitive abilities, with a mean of 100 and standard deviation of 15, with a typical range from 40 to 160, although this varies among the various tests and the constructs they are designed to measure.

standardization sample. See *norm reference sample*.

standards-based education. Approach to teaching within the schools that requires (a) an unequivocal delineation of course content and subjects to be taught and learned at each grade level, (b) a clear definition of the required levels of performance so they can be measured, and (c) a guarantee that all students will be afforded the opportunity to learn the material according to their needs.

Stanford-Binet Intelligence Scale. Immediate successor to the Binet-Simon intelligence scale that was translated into English in 1908 and revised as the first edition of this test in the United States in 1916.

Stanford-Binet Intelligence Scales, Fifth Edition (SB5). Individually administered intelligence test for individuals ranging in age from 2 years, 0 months through 85 years, 11 months, which includes (a) a standardization sample covering the largest age range compared to other intelligence tests, (b) parallel subtests for verbal and nonverbal abilities, (c) the capability of yielding a nonverbal IQ score for examinees with a severe language disorder, and (d) an incorporated abbreviated IQ.

Stanford–Binet Intelligence Scales, Fifth Edition, Abbreviated Battery IQ (SB5–ABIQ). Individually administered intelligence test for individuals ranging in age from 2 years, 0 months through 85 years, 11 months, which can yield a brief estimate of overall intelligence by means of two subtests; can be used to screen for cognitive impairments.

Stanford–Binet Intelligence Scale, Fourth Edition (SB4). Fourth edition of the test that featured a point scale format and deviation IQ, standard scores for factors, and the introduction of routing subtests that determined the starting points for subsequent subtests.

stanines. Short for "standard nine," consists of a 9-point scale, ranging from 1 to 9, with a mean of 5 and standard deviation of 2; easily compares student performance over a normal distribution.

start point/s. As applied to a standardized subtest wherein the items are sequenced from less to more difficult, including a designated item where test administration is to begin, which is usually determined by an examinee's chronological age or grade level, or by performance on a preceding core subtest (also known as a routing subtest). See also *adaptive testing*; *discontinue rule*; *reversal rule*.

statistical approach. In investigating the number and types of human traits that exist, this approach assumes that trait terms that are highly intercorrelated but have little correlation with other items form factors or latent variables that represent broad-based dispositions of human behavior.

statistical method. Deriving diagnoses by means of collecting and interpreting a profile of standardized psychological test scores.

status offenses. Acts that are illegal for minors but are considered legal if engaged in by adults (e.g., curfew; consuming alcohol).

stems. Beginning partial sentences that are to be made into complete and comprehensible statements by a respondent. A list of various stems together comprises a sentence completion test (SCT), which is classified by some as a completion projective technique.

stimulus barrier. The lowest absolute level or difference in environmental stimulation the human senses can detect 50% of the time; a sensory threshold or boundary.

stop point/s. In adaptive standardized testing of cognitive abilities or skills, recommended rules for terminating a test or subtest, which can be based on (a) the examinee's age or grade level, and/or (b) the number of consecutive errors, with the assumption that the ensuing items would be inappropriately difficult.

strange situation. Laboratory procedure in which repeated separations and reunions between toddlers, their caretakers, and strangers are done for the purpose of examining attachment style.

stratum. (**strata**, plural) Label given to the level of generality or specificity of a factor within a hierarchical model of intelligence, with Stratum III at the topmost general level, Stratum II at the mid-level of broad factors, and Stratum I at the lowest and most specific level.

stress and distress variables. R–PAS data that are related to past and current environmental events, which are experienced by examinees as threats and out of one's control, along with various feelings of dysphoria.

stress moderators. A construct used by the Millon Behavioral Medicine Diagnostic (MBMD), which involves intrapsychic and interpersonal variables that influence the relationship between psychological status and treatment outcome.

stressors. Environmental events that are interpreted by people as threatening or challenging and thus require some sort of adaptive response.

structured interview. One-on-one conversation for purposes of psychodiagnosis in which questions are asked in a non-modifiable preset order with little or no discretion afforded to the inquiring individual.

Structured Interview of Reported Symptoms, Second Edition (SIRS–2). Strictly designed question-and-answer format that is intended to detect the feigning of psychiatric symptoms by means of (a) an unlikely detection strategy (i.e., the reporting of bizarre or improbable symptoms) and (b) an amplified detection strategy (i.e., the magnification of reasonable symptoms that are typically reported by genuine patients). See also *unlikely detection strategy*; *amplified detection strategy*.

subitizing. Instantly identifying the number of objects in a set without the aid of counting.

subjective descriptors. Within the context of a mental status examination, observations of a client's appearance and behavior that are determined by personal opinion and upon which people can disagree.

substance-related and addictive disorders. General class of *DSM–5* psychopathology that involves the abuse of psychoactive drugs, which cause enduring changes in brain function, along with problematic changes in the way people think, feel, and behave.

substance-related disorder. See *substance-related and addictive disorders*.

subtle symptoms.   Feigning strategy in which individuals report common problems as representing major issues.

suicidal attempt.   Action taken to kill oneself wherein the person survives.

suicidal gesture.   Actions taken to kill oneself without the intention of actually dying.

suicidal ideation.   Thoughts of killing oneself.

suicidal plans.   The formulation of methods designed to kill oneself.

sulci.   (**sulcus**, singular) Creases or valleys that form part of the convolutions of the cerebral cortex.

summary ADOS–2 items.   Averaging across all manifestations of a pertinent kind of behavior (e.g., rapport with the examiner) observed during the entire test administration in determining a score.

summative scale.   Scale in which the item raw scores are aggregated for a total raw score, which is usually further transformed into a standard score for subsequent interpretation.

superego.   In psychoanalytic theory, the third structure of the personality that includes the conscience and the ego ideal, which develops at the age of about five years with the successful resolution of the Oedipus and Electra complexes for boys and girls, respectively.

support staff.   Employees working within the same practice or agency as the clinician, who typically provide ancillary services, such as scheduling appointments, filing medical records, and answering phones.

supraspan learning.   The ability to memorize new information that initially exceeds the capacity of immediate memory storage by means of repeated exposure.

sustained attention.   Maintaining attention over time.

syllogistic thinking.   Consists of a major premise (e.g., all boys are aggressive), a minor premise (e.g., Joey is a boy), and a conclusion (e.g., therefore, Joey is aggressive).

symbiotic attachment(s).   Constitutes a relationship in which there is no interpersonal boundary between the two individuals; usually denotes the presence of psychopathology.

symbolic play.   Ability to use objects, actions, and ideas to represent something they are not for purposes of enjoyment; for example, a child using a wooden block as a toy car by means of imagination.

sympathetic nervous system.   Branch of the autonomic nervous system that controls the body's response to stress and energy expenditure.

symptom/s.   Subjectively reported problems suggestive of a psychological disorder.

symptom combinations.   Feigning strategy in which individuals report co-occurring symptoms that (a) are common and (b) rarely, if ever, occur contemporaneously.

symptom neurosis.   According to psychodynamic theorizing, a stress-related disorder resulting from a temporary faltering of ego defense mechanisms in managing intrapsychic conflict; considered to be healthier than a character neurosis in which unresolved unconscious conflict manifests in the form of ingrained and rigid patterns of behavior or traits.

symptom validity testing (SVT).   Earlier version of a feigning performance test in which the examinee heard a tone and, after a delay, was asked to discriminate between a target tone and distractor nontarget tone; feigning was indicated by lower-than-chance performance.

syndrome/s.   A statistical clustering or covariance of psychological symptoms that represent a recognized mental health disorder; frequently used with the term "clinical," as in clinical syndrome or disorder.

synonym frequency.   The greater the number of similar words for a personality trait, the greater its importance in describing and predicting human behavior; based on the assumption of a positive relationship between the number of alternative terms for the same trait in language and the importance of that trait in human behavior.

syntax.   Principles that direct how words and phrases are to be arranged within sentences.

synthetic-integrative functions.   Refer to whether an individual's attitudes, beliefs, feelings, values, affects, behaviors, and self-representation are sufficiently congruent and consistent such that identity formation is developing in a coherent manner.

T

target.   On the TOMM, line drawing presented to an examinee for later recognition.

target stimulus.   An object or event to which an examinee is asked to respond in some manner when it appears during test administration, usually to measure such things as reaction time, attention, impulse control, memory, and even feigning.

TAS.   Abbreviation for "Test Administration and Scoring," which includes psychological and neuropsychological test administration and scoring services.

T-data.   Scores about an individual's personality that are derived from a performance-based test (e.g., intelligence test, Rorschach Inkblot Test).

temperament. Fundamental individual differences in reacting to the environment that are apparent from infancy and early childhood (e.g., reaction to novelty, quality of mood, activity level), thought to be highly genetic and an influence on later adult personality.

temperament scale. Early personality inventory based on Rosanoff's theory, which was designed to measure individuals' basic dispositions to determine their likely adjustment within a work environment.

temporal lobe. Bilateral areas of the cortex next to each ear, which principally control auditory processing, including speech reception and language comprehension, although it also registers pain and the recollection of emotion.

teratogens. A broad class of agents that have the potential of causing birth defects in an as yet unborn child. These include radiation, alcohol, nicotine, rubella, and lithium carbonate. Also known as *teratogenic substances.*

test administration and scoring services. Tasks undertaken by the examiner that consist of giving the psychological measures according to standardized instructions, then converting the examinee's responses and behaviors into quantitative scores or codes, again according to standardized rules.

test evaluation services. As defined by the Current Procedural Terminology (CPT) guidelines, refers to data interpretation, integration, decision-making, treatment planning, report generation, and interactive feedback.

test format. The particular design of a psychological instrument. Examples of common test formats include personality inventories, observer and self-report symptom rating scales, and performance personality tests.

Test of Memory Malingering (TOMM). Measure of visual recognition memory, consisting of two learning test sequences and one delayed retention trial, which appears difficult but is deceptively easy and also includes corrective feedback to provide an added opportunity for an examinee to feign if indeed such motive is present.

testing the limits. Permitting an examinee to continue working on a test item in violation of standardized instructions for added diagnostic information (e.g., allowing an examinee to continue working on a puzzle beyond time limits to assess perseverance or motivation).

testlets. On the SB5, items grouped into six, six-item clusters, each representing an increasing level of difficulty, and where the examinee's performance on one level (i.e., testlet) determines whether test administration will reverse to a previous easier level (i.e., testlet), progress to a more difficult level (i.e., testlet), or discontinue the subtest entirely.

test-taking response sets. See *response sets.*

TEV. Abbreviation for "Test Evaluation," which includes professional services such as test data interpretation, diagnostic decision-making, addressing referral issues, devising treatment recommendations, report generation, communication in written form, and interactive feedback if desired.

thalamus. Brain structure through which all senses (except smell or olfaction) are processed and relayed to the proper area of the cortex for more complex analysis; also known as the *central relay station.*

the play years. Refers to a period from ages two to five wherein play becomes a pivotal activity for all modes of development, including sensorimotor, cognitive, and social domains.

thema. As manifested in storytelling projective testing techniques, the interaction between needs and presses, along with the story outcomes in terms of the hero's success or failure.

Thematic Apperception Test (TAT). Projective storytelling test, consisting of 20 stimulus cards, with the majority including human figures in various interpersonal scenes, designed to measure various components of ego (i.e., personality) functioning and primary defense mechanisms in children and adults, although considered to be most effective for individuals older than 10 years of age.

theory of mind (ToM). The ability to understand that people possess internal mental states, including feelings, desires, beliefs, and intentions, which direct, guide, and ultimately explain their behavior. ToM is considered a fundamental social cognitive ability that facilitates interpersonal interaction, the ability to understand one's own thoughts and feelings, and to effectively regulate one's own emotions.

third parties. As applied to psychological assessment and testing, additional entities that come to the attention of the examiner sometime during the testing process, which would benefit from having access to the examinee's final psychological assessment report and the results therein, usually for purposes of continuity of care.

thought. Within the context of a mental status examination, refers to the examinee's ability to think.

thought blocking. Speech that suddenly and involuntarily halts and in which the idea is removed from conscious awareness.

thought content. The substance of what a client communicates during a clinical interview.

thought process. The manner in which a person's statements follow a logical, relevant, and coherent sequence; the "how" of thinking.

three stratum hierarchical model of intelligence. John Carrol's 1993 theory of cognitive ability consisting of three levels called strata, including a general and complex *g* factor at the top (i.e., Stratum III), broad mid-level factors in the middle (i.e., Stratum II), and specific abilities (Stratum I) at the bottom of the three ranked levels; evolved into the contemporary CHC theory of intelligence, which is emulated to varying degrees by a number of current intelligence tests.

thumb drive.   Small, solid-state, external device, named for its thumb-like physical appearance, which can be plugged directly into a computer's USB port and used to store and transfer files.

time-rule.   Current Procedural Terminology (CPT) principle that defines a billable service according to a defined range of minutes.

Times New Roman.   Typeface that was originally used by a British newspaper called *The Times* in 1931 and later developed by Stanley Morison in collaboration with Victor Lardent. This font includes serifs that make it easy to read and one of the most popular typefaces currently used and available on most personal computers.

tort law.   Laws that cover injuries inflicted by one citizen upon another, designed to restore the injured party to the preinjury degree of functioning, usually by means of monetary recovery, that is, to make the injured party whole again.

traditional information-gathering model.   Approach to psychological testing that focuses on differential diagnosis, treatment planning, and overall increased understanding of a client's problems and how they may be resolved.

trait theory.   Proposes that human personality comprises a number of broad dispositions that represent habitual patterns of behavior, thinking, and feeling, which can be identified and measured. Also known as *dispositional theory*.

trait.   As defined by the Woodcock–Johnson tests of cognition, any skill, ability, or area of knowledge.

transduction.   The transformation of physical energy into electrochemical neural signals by the sensory receptors, which are the first line of neurons specialized for reaction to physical energy.

transfer.   Discontinuation of one specific type of mental health service whereas the client continues to receive other services within the same facility.

trauma.   Catastrophic event (or series of events) that involves threat of serious injury or death to oneself and/or significant others. Considered a necessary although not sufficient criterion for a diagnosis of acute stress disorder, post-traumatic stress disorder (PTDS), reactive attachment disorder (RAD), and disinhibited social engagement disorder.

Trauma Symptom Checklist for Children (TSCC).   Self-report rating scale of trauma-related psychopathology and its many sequelae, including varying types of dissociation, anxious arousal, and intrusive ideation, for individuals ranging in age from 8 years, 0 months through 16 years, 11 months.

Trauma Symptom Checklist for Young Children (TSCYC).   Observer-based rating scale of trauma-related psychopathology and its many sequelae, including varying types of dissociation, anxious arousal, and intrusive ideation, for children ranging in age from 3 years, 0 months through 12 years, 11 months.

Trauma Symptom Inventory, Second Edition (TSI–2).   Self-report rating scale of trauma-related psychopathology and its many sequelae, including varying types of dissociation, anxious arousal, intrusive ideation, and emerging or present personality dysfunction, for individuals ranging in age from 18 years, 0 months through 90 years, 11 months.

traumatic brain injury (TBI).   Physical insult to the brain from an external mechanical force, which is not congenital and not degenerative, with potential temporary or permanent impairment in one's state of consciousness, neurocognitive functioning, and personality adjustment.

treatment prognostics.   A construct used by the Millon Behavioral Medicine Diagnostic (MBMD), which involves behavioral and attitudinal aspects of a patient that can complicate or subvert treatment efficacy.

true score.   An examinee's hypothetical perfectly accurate score on a construct, which when added to the error of a test is equivalent to the examinee's observed score, this according to classical test theory (CTT).

true zero.   Number that signifies a complete absence of the variable being measured, which is the prime characteristic of a ration scales of measurement. Also known as absolute zero.

T–**score.**   Standard score with a mean of 50 and standard deviation of 10, which includes a range of plus and minus 5 standard deviations; also known as a *fifty plus or minus ten scale*.

turbulent personality/pattern.   Recent personality pattern proposed by the Millon theory that consists of the following traits: enthusiastic, animated, and idealistic; expending much time, energy, and creativity in feeling happy and fulfilled; possible scattered thought process due to being inundated with thoughts of meeting one's needs and goals; hyperactive interpersonal style; and can be socially intrusive.

twelve-point (12-point) font size.   Font size is equal to 1/6th of an inch in height.

type I error.   In hypothesis testing, an incorrect decision that involves concluding that an effect, difference, or relationship exists in the population when in fact it does not.

V

V codes. Categories of stressors listed on axis IV in the *DSM–IV–TR*.

validity. The degree to which a psychological test measures the construct it asserts for its stated purpose, namely, the accuracy of a test.

variability. Specific measure on a Current Procedural Terminology (CPT) test that quantifies an individual's response speed changeability to differing interstimulus intervals (ISIs) relative to his or her own average.

vegetative symptoms. Impairments in fundamental physiological functions controlled by the autonomic nervous system, including disturbances in sleeping and appetite.

veracity scales. Type of validity scale capable of detecting the degree to which parents or primary caregivers overestimate or underestimate symptoms when rating their child or adolescent.

verbally fluent. Someone who exhibits smooth, flowing, and effortless speech.

vigilance. Sustained attention within the context of neuropsychological testing.

Vineland Adaptive Behavior Scales, Second Edition (Vineland-II). Measure of daily activities that promote independence, which is normed on individuals ranging in age from 1 month to 90 years, 11 months. It principally consists of the following three-domain structure: (a) Communication—Expressive, Receptive, Written; (b) Daily Living Skills—Personal, Domestic, Community; and (c) Socialization—Interpersonal Relationships, Play and Leisure Time, Coping Skills. Immediate predecessor to the Vineland-3.

Vineland Adaptive Behavior Scales, Third Edition (Vineland-3). Measure of an individual's performance of daily activities required for personal sufficiency, typically completed by observer-report (e.g., parent, caregiver, or teacher) via structured interview or rating scales, normed for individuals virtually throughout the life span.

Vineland semistructured interview technique. Scheme in which a set of two to six items are grouped together based on similar content, which is preceded by an open-ended interview question designed to potentially address some or most of these items. The objective is to increase the speed and efficiency of the administration process.

visual perception. The interpretation of sensory input that is transmitted from the eyes, through the thalamus, and lastly, into the occipital lobe's visual cortex.

visual-spatial sketchpad. Component of working memory that retains visual-spatial information, especially for single complex images.

visuoconstruction. (1) Test items requiring eye–hand coordination, such as drawing a figure. (2) The ability to organize and manually manipulate spatial information to produce a design.

visuospatial processing. The capacity to understand the orientation of visual information in two- and three-dimensional space. See also *spatial processing*; *visual perception*; *visuoconstruction*.

vocational rehabilitation services. Adjunctive service that assists individuals with documented functional impairments (including psychological disorders) to reenter and remain productive in the job market.

***v*-scale score.** Standard score for subdomain scales on the Vineland-3, with a mean of 15 and standard deviation of 3, which are designed to have a lower range for greater measurement precision at more impaired levels of functioning (versus a *T*-score that offers a mean of only 10).

vulnerability-stress model. Thesis proposing that all psychopathology results from a diathesis, which is an early propensity or weakness (i.e., genetic or environmental) toward developing a particular disorder (e.g., perinatal anoxia or recessive gene pattern), and an environmental stress trigger, the combination of which activates symptom onset.

Vyvanse (lisdexamfetamine dimesylate). Central nervous system psychostimulant that begins to work after 90 minutes by increasing norepinephrine (i.e., a stimulant) and dopamine (i.e., a natural substance that enhances pleasure and reward), and lasts about 14 hours due to a longer-action, steady-release chemical feature, principally for the treatment of ADHD.

U

U.S. census-matched sample. Standardization sample that is based on general population statistics (usually using census data); typically, the sample contains approximately equal proportions of gender and is thereafter stratified according to U.S. census proportions in race/ethnicity, geographic region, and education or another socioeconomic status indicator.

U.S. standard system (or imperial system). Units of measurement utilized in the United States (e.g., feet, inches, pounds).

unbearable. On the SIRS–2, a symptom that is reported to be both present and intolerable.

under-responsivity. Type of sensory-processing disorder that consists of muted, minimal, neutral, or extremely brief responses to sensory stimuli.

undoing. Reaction formation with an additional step that reverses the undesired behavior.

unidimensional tests. Tests in which all items are interrelated and form one general factor or psychological construct. Also referred to as *homogeneous tests*.

uniform *T*–scores (*UT*–scores). Standard scores with a mean of 50 and standard deviation of 10, although are computed to have the same percentile ranks across all substantive scales despite their having various degrees of positive skewness in their raw score distributions.

unlikely detection strategy. Approach to identifying feigners of psychopathology by giving them an opportunity to endorse grossly bogus and thus improbable symptoms that those with genuine disorders do not endorse.

unoccupied play. Consists of random or stereotyped movements that have no meaning or purpose other than simple stimulation.

unspecified neurocognitive disorder. Diagnosis given when all the criteria for a neurocognitive disorder have been met, although with an as yet undetermined etiology or etiologies.

unusual form quality (*FQu*). In R–PAS coding, a percept that is less frequently reported and is a less accurate fit to the inkblot location but is not grossly contrary with respect to the inkblot contours.

USB drive. See *thumb drive*.

USB stick. See *thumb drive*.

useful field of view (UFOV) paradigm. Task in which examinees' scan a scene to point out anything that is different, new, or missing from a similar previous scene (e.g., sitting behind a steering wheel of a car).

utility. The degree to which a test is efficient and practical. Factors include: (a) time for test administration, scoring, and interpretation; (b) amount and relevance of the data yield; (c) degree of invasiveness; (d) portability of test materials; and (e) cost of test materials and maintenance.

W

***W* ability.** Value assigned to an item that represents the degree of skill an examinee possesses if responded to successfully.

***W* difference (W DIFF).** Discrepancy between the examinee's measured ability (e.g., 40% proficiency) and the selected criterion (e.g., 50% proficiency); here W DIFF $= -10$ (i.e., 40% $-50\% = -10$).

***W* difficulty.** Value assigned to an item that represents the degree of effort or skill needed for successful responding. Also known as *W score*.

***W* score.** See *W difficulty*.

Wechsler Adult Intelligence Scale (WAIS). Immediate successor to the Wechsler-Bellevue Intelligence Scale (WB) that retained all 11 WB subtests, including Information, Comprehension, Arithmetic, Similarities, Digit Span, Vocabulary, Digit Symbol, Picture Completion, Block Design, Picture Arrangement, and Object Assembly, although it deleted and replaced many items and scoring rules to simplify matters.

Wechsler Adult Intelligence Scale, Fourth Edition (WAIS–IV). Individually administered test of intelligence, normed on individuals from ages 16 years, 0 months through 90 years, 11 months, which yields a full-scale IQ score, along with several index scores and subtest scores.

Wechsler Adult Intelligence Scale, Revised Edition (WAIS–R). Immediate successor to the WAIS, which included Information, Comprehension, Arithmetic, Digit Span, Similarities, and Vocabulary as verbal subtests, along with Picture Arrangement, Picture Completion, Block Design, Object Assembly, and Digit Symbol as nonverbal subtests.

Wechsler Adult Intelligence Scale, Third Edition (WAIS–III). Edition that introduced three new subtests to the previous 11 contained in the WAIS–R, including Matrix Reasoning, Letter-Number Sequencing, and Symbol Search.

Wechsler Individual Achievement Test. First edition of the Wechsler achievement test and immediate predecessor to the WIAT–II.

Wechsler Individual Achievement Test, Second Edition (WIAT–II). Immediate predecessor of the WIAT–III.

Wechsler Individual Achievement Test, Third Edition (WIAT–III). Individually administered test of a variety of fundamental academic skills, ranging from pre-kindergarten through 12th grade, which was normed on individuals ranging in age from as young as 4 years, 0 months through 50 years, 11 months.

Wechsler Intelligence Scale for Children (WISC). First edition of the Wechsler intelligence test series for children and early adolescence, which was actually a modification of the Wechsler-Bellevue Intelligence Scale (WB) for adults.

Wechsler Intelligence Scale for Children, Fifth Edition (WISC–V). Individually administered test of intelligence, normed on individuals from ages 6 years, 0 months through 16 years, 11 months, which yields a full-scale IQ score, along with several index scores and subtest scores.

Wechsler Intelligence Scale for Children, Fourth Edition (WISC–IV). Edition of the Wechsler intelligence test for children that dropped the theoretical VIQ-PIQ dichotomy and transferred completely to the empirically based four-factor structure.

Wechsler Intelligence Scale for Children, Revised Edition (WISC–R). Second edition of the childhood intelligence test that updated the norms and added one year on both the upper and lower ends of the age spectrum, hence 6–16 years.

Wechsler Intelligence Scale for Children, Third Edition (WISC–III). Third edition of this childhood intelligence test that (a) updated the norms, (b) added a new subtest that measured processing speed, and (c) introduced the empirically based primary index scores.

Wechsler Memory Scale, Fourth Edition (WMS–IV). Comprehensive test of memory functioning in individuals ranging in age from age 16 years, 0 months through 90 years, 11 months.

Wechsler Memory Scale, Fourth Edition, Brief Cognitive Status Exam (WMS–IV–BCSE). Screening measure designed to indicate whether a neurocognitive disorder may be present in older adolescence and adults and is in need of further testing. Data are performance-based.

Wechsler Memory Scale, Third Edition (WMS–III). Memory test that was significantly modified by its successor, the WMS–IV.

Wechsler Preschool and Primary Scale of Intelligence (WPPSI). In response to the increasing need for the preschool assessment of intelligence during the 1950s through the early 1960s, this first edition was developed for children ranging in age from 4 years, 0 months through 6 years, 6 months.

Wechsler Preschool and Primary Scale of Intelligence, Fourth Edition (WPPSI–IV). Individually administered test of intelligence, normed on children ages 2 years, 6 months through 7 years, 7 months, which yields a full-scale IQ score, along with several empirically based index scores and subtest scores.

Wechsler Preschool and Primary Scale of Intelligence, Revised Edition (WPPSI–R). Second edition of the preschool version of the Wechsler series that added a new popular subtest called Object Assembly, which includes putting together puzzle pieces of increasing difficulty and continues to be a core subtest in the current fifth edition.

Wechsler Preschool and Primary Scale of Intelligence, Third Edition (WPPSI–III). Third edition of this version of the Wechsler series extending the age range down further to 2 years, 6 months and apportioning the scale into two age bands or versions that continues in the current fourth edition.

Wechsler-Bellevue Intelligence Scale (WB). Original intelligence test designed specifically for adults, which initiated the evolution of the subsequent WAIS editions for adults.

weighted raw scores. Quantitative value that statistically adjusts raw scores such that they reflect the base rate or percentile rank of the norm reference sample.

Wernicke's area. Brain region usually in the left hemisphere that controls the comprehension of speech or receptive language.

with behavioral disturbance. Neurocognitive diagnostic specifier that indicates the presence of psychiatric symptoms secondary to brain dysfunction, including psychotic symptoms, mood disturbance, agitation, and apathy.

with or without behavioral disturbance. Neurocognitive diagnostic specifier that indicates whether there exist psychiatric symptoms secondary to brain dysfunction.

within normal limits (WNL). Term used in MMPI interpretation for a profile in which there are no statistical elevations among the clinical scales, which denotes an absence of psychopathology.

WMS–IV Scoring Assistant. Previous unlimited computer scoring software for the WMS–IV, which is no longer available.

Woodcock–Johnson IV Tests of Achievement (WJ IV ACH). Individually administered test of a variety of fundamental academic skills, including those in reading, mathematics, and writing, and comprising both a standard battery and an extended battery, along with three parallel forms of the test A, B, and C, in the event retesting is required. Its standardization sample ranges in age from 2 years, 0 months through adulthood.

Woodcock–Johnson Psycho–Educational Battery (WJ). First edition of a comprehensive battery of cognitive tests that was developed based on a pragmatic decision-making model with no underlying theory.

Woodcock–Johnson Psycho–Educational Battery–Revised (WJ R). Second edition of a comprehensive battery of cognitive tests that was developed based on the CHC theory of intelligence.

Woodcock–Johnson, Third Edition (WJ III). Third edition of a comprehensive battery of cognitive tests that was developed based on the CHC theory of intelligence.

Woodworth Personality Data Sheet.   A 116-item self-report inventory, based on clinical experience and logic, developed to assess the emotional stability of a large number of recruits for military service in World War I.

word association test.   Well known early projective technique first proposed by Carl Jung, in which examinees would respond to a sequence of target words with the first word that came to mind.

word generation.   The ability to produce words quickly and accurately according to themes or categories.

word retrieval.   Skill that underlies the Oral Word Fluency component of the Wechsler achievement test battery, which includes the ability to report as many different words as possible, as rapidly as possible, within specified categories (e.g., animals, colors). It is controlled in part by Broca's area located in the dominant frontal lobe (i.e., left hemisphere in most people).

working diagnoses.   A listing of one or more disorders that may be later modified with the addition of assessment information and data.

working memory.   (1) Executive system upgrade of short-term memory when multiple alternative tasks are simultaneously required. (2) Holding immediate memory traces while executing cognitive tasks; an upgrade of the short-term memory system.

World Health Organization (WHO).   International association whose objective is to direct health-related issues within the United Nation's health care system and to lead partners in global health responses.

X

X paradigm.   Continuous performance test task in which the examinee is to respond to a target stimulus (i.e., X) and not to a nontarget stimulus (i.e., not X).

XA paradigm.   Continuous performance test task in which the examinee is to respond to a target stimulus only if there is a preceding stimulus (i.e., AX) but not in the absence of a preceding stimulus.

Xanax (alprazolam).   Benzodiazepine antianxiety psychotropic medication that works by binding to GABA inhibitory receptors, hence stimulating their production.

Z

Z codes.   In the *DSM–5*, environmental, social, or developmental phase problems that are not considered psychological or mental disorders but that may be the focus of mental health intervention. Such problems may precipitate, maintain, or aggravate diagnosed psychological disorders. Also includes T codes and one E code. Previously known as *V codes*.

zero-substitution.   Prorating a total score on a summative scale in which item omissions are assigned a score of zero, typically which indicates no evidence of symptoms or problems; considered to be a conservative strategy that increases the risk of underestimating the true degree of psychopathology present in a case.

zeta distributions.   See *Zipf distributions*.

Zipf distributions.   Phenomenon in which certain objects are perceived very frequently by people while others are perceived much less frequently, with an enormous gap in frequency counts between the two; applied to frequency distributions of objects of different content perceived by people in the Rorschach inkblot cards. Also known as *Pareto distributions*; *zeta distributions*; *rank size distributions*; *power-law distributions*.

Zoloft.   Selective serotonin reuptake inhibitor (SSRI) that is classified as an antidepressant psychotropic medication, although it is also prescribed for chronic anxiety or depression with mixed anxiety. Generic label is *sertraline*.

z–score.   Standard score with a mean of 0.00 and standard deviation of 1.00; converts a test's raw or original scores into uniform standard deviation units by means of a linear transformation process to facilitate test interpretation and comparison among tests; also known as a *zero plus or minus one scale*.

zygote.   Ovum fertilized by a sperm cell; human fertilized egg.

Subject Index

For Product Safety Concerns and Information please contact our EU
representative GPSR@taylorandfrancis.com
Taylor & Francis Verlag GmbH, Kaufingerstraße 24, 80331 München, Germany

www.ingramcontent.com/pod-product-compliance
Lightning Source LLC
Chambersburg PA
CBHW081211220326
41598CB00037B/6743